W0112599

Mental and Behavioral Dysfunction in Movement Disorders

Mental and Behavioral Dysfunction in Movement Disorders

Edited by

Marc-André Bédard, MSc, PhD

Université du Québec à Montréal, Montréal, Canada

Yves Agid, MD, PhD

Hôpital de la Salpêtrière, Paris, France

Sylvain Chouinard, MD

Université de Montréal, Montréal, Canada

Stanley Fahn, MD

Columbia University, New York, NY

Amos D. Korczyn, MD, MSc

Tel-Aviv University Medical School, Tel-Aviv, Israel

Paul Lespérance, MD, MSc

Université de Montréal, Montréal, Canada

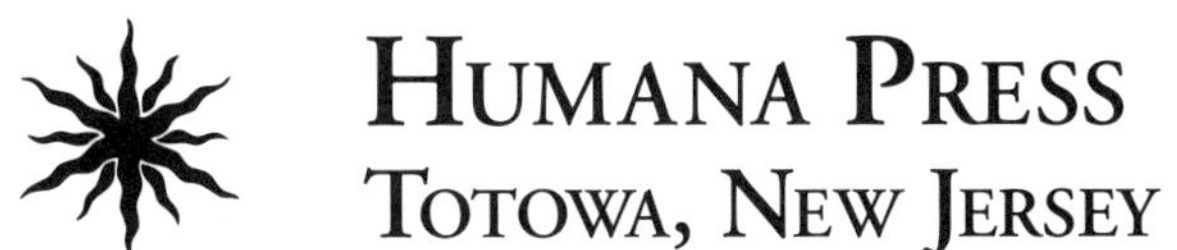

Humana Press
Totowa, New Jersey

999 Riverview Drive, Suite 208
Totowa, New Jersey 07512

www.humanapress.com

Production Editor: Robin B. Weisberg.
Cover Illustration: From Fig. 1 in Chapter 25, "Cortical-Limbic-Striatal Dysfunction in Depression: Converging Findings in Basal Ganglia Diseases and Primary Affective Disorders" by Taresa L. Stefurak and Helen S. Mayberg.
Cover design by Patricia F. Cleary.

For additional copies, pricing for bulk purchases, and/or information about other Humana titles, contact Humana at the above address or at any of the following numbers: Tel.: 973-256-1699; Fax: 973-256-8341; E-mail: humana@humanapr.com or visit our website: humanapress.com

This publication is printed on acid-free paper. ∞
ANSI Z39.48-1984 (American National Standards Institute) Permanence of Paper for Printed Library Materials.

Printed in the United States of America. 10 9 8 7 6 5 4 3 2 1

Library of Congress Cataloging-in-Publication Data

Mental and behavioral dysfunction in movement disorders / edited by Marc-André Bédard ... [et al.].
p. ; cm.
Includes biblographical references and index.
ISBN 1-58829-119-7 (alk. paper); 1-59259-326-7 (e-book)
1. Movement disorders. 2. Cognition disorders. I. Bédard, Marc-André, 1961-.
[DNLM: 1. Movement Disorders—complications. 2. Behavioral Symptoms—complications.
3. Cognition Disorders—complications. WL 390 M549 2003]
RC376.5 .M46 2003
616.7'001'9—dc21

2002027578

Preface

At a time when there is an exponential growth in research related to the neurological and psychological bases of behavior, the mental–motor functional duality of the brain appears progressively unified. This is reflected by the growing commitment of the medical community to better understand and manage mental dysfunctions associated with hypo- and hyperkinetic movement disorders. Fundamental and behavioral sciences also provide the scientific community with plenty of new data that help to conceptualize the basal ganglia and cerebellum as critical structures for many mental processes.

Mental and Behavioral Dysfunction in Movement Disorders is dedicated to both clinicians and scientists working in the fields of the brain and behavioral sciences. The idea of this work grew out of a wish to gather specialists from around the world with wide-ranging research interests and clinical expertise, in order to shed light and establish new standards in the study and the treatment of many cognitive, affective, and behavioral dysfunctions associated with movement disorders.

The aim of *Mental and Behavioral Dysfunction in Movement Disorders* is to provide the reader with an authoritative account of the recent developments in the field set against a background of review material. It will allow scientists and clinicians to better understand and manage mental dysfunctions associated with Parkinson's disease, multiple system atrophy, progressive supranuclear palsy, corticobasal degeneration, Lewy body diseases, Huntington's disease, Tourette syndrome, cerebellar degeneration, and many other related syndromes. The volume gathers some of the world's most renowned scientists and clinicians working on the fundamental and clinical aspects of dementia, depression, psychosis, sleep disorders, and other affective, cognitive, or behavioral conditions associated with movement disorders.

The book is divided into thematic sections containing multiple chapters. Each chapter consists of an in-depth presentation on a specific question. In an introductory chapter (Part I), Parkinson's and Huntington's diseases are depicted from a historical perspective that allows the reader to realize that mental dysfunctions have long been acknowledged, but not adequately emphasized in hypo- and hyperkinetic movement disorders.

Part II discusses the neurobiological evidence showing that cognitive and affective aspects of behavior and mental processes may involve the basal ganglia and the cerebellum.

Parts III and IV are concerned with the cognitive deficits associated with several movement disorders. The topics of attention and intention, memory, as well as language, praxis, and executive functions are all covered in the different chapters. Functional descriptions of the syndromes or models are grouped together in Part III, whereas the physiological, anatomical, and neurochemical aspects form Part IV.

Part V presents the state of the art on neurodegenerative dementia so frequently associated with movement disorders. This section encompasses the diagnosis and treatments, as well as the epidemiology, neuropathology, and genetics of these dementing illnesses.

The chapters in Part VI are devoted to the emerging field of neuropsychiatry in movement disorders. This includes both psychiatric conditions that may be associated with movement disorders and, conversely, abnormal movements that may occur in some specific psychiatric syndromes.

Quality of life in Parkinson's disease is discussed in Part VII. Owing to the high prevalence of this disease and the importance of quality of life in contemporary management of such a neurodegenerative illness, we have dedicated an entire section to this topic. Social and medical determinants as well as sexual dysfunctions and sleep disturbances are presented before concluding the section with a specific chapter on life expectancy in Parkinson's disease.

I hope that this book will succeed in illustrating to the interested scientist and clinician the state of the art on mental and behavioral dysfunctions in movement disorders.

M-A. Bédard, *MSc, PhD*

CONTENTS

VII. Quality of Life in Parkinson's Disease

Contributors

DAG AARSLAND, *School of Medicine, University of Bergen, Section of Geriatric Psychiatry, Rogaland Psychiatric Hospital, Stavanger, Norway*

HERMANN ACKERMANN, *Department of Neurology, University Tübingen and Department of Clinical Neuropsychology, Ruhr-University Bochum, Germany*

YVES AGID, *INSERM U-289 and Hôpital de la Salpêtrière, Paris, France*

MENESKE ALPAY, *Department of Psychiatry, Harvard Medical School, Boston, MA*

KAREN ANDERSON, *Gertrude H. Sergievsky Center, Department of Psychiatry and New York State Psychiatric Institute, Columbia University, New York, NY*

CLIVE G. BALLARD, *Institute for Aging and Health, Wolfson Research Centre, Newcastle General Hospital, Newcastle upon Tyne, UK*

MARC-ANDRÉ BÉDARD, *The André Barbeau Movement Disorder Unit, Centre Hospitalier de l'Universite de Montréal and Cognitive Neuroscience Center, Université du Québec à Montréal, Montréal, Canada*

DEBORAH N. BLACK, *Neuropsychiatric Clinic, Hôpital Louis-H. Lafontaine, Montréal, Canada*

DONALD L. BLIWISE, *Department of Neurology, Emory University, Atlanta, GA*

CHRISTIAN BOCTI, *Clinique de Neuropsychiatrie, Hôpital Louis-H. Lafontaine, Montréal, Canada*

BRADLEY F. BOEVE, *Sleep Disorders Center, Department of Neurology, and Alzheimer's Disease Research Center, Mayo Clinic, Rochester, MN*

GILA BRONNER, *Sex Therapy Clinic, Tel-Aviv Souraski Medical Center and Sackler School of Medicine, Tel-Aviv University, Tel-Aviv, Israel*

EMMANUEL BROUILLET, *CEA CNRS URA 2210 Unit, Service Hospitalier Frédéric Joliot, Orsay, France*

RICHARD G. BROWN, *Department of Psychology, Institute of Psychiatry, London, UK*

DAVID BURN, *Department of Neurology, Royal Victoria Infirmary, Newcastle upon Tyne, UK*

SYLVAIN CHOUINARD, *The André Barbeau Movement Disorder Unit, Centre Hospitalier de l'Universite de Montréal and Department of Neurology, Université de Montréal, Montréal, Canada*

HENRI COHEN, *Cognitive Neuroscience Center and Department of Psychology, Université du Québec à Montréal, Montréal, Canada*

PETER COMO, *Department of Neurology, University of Rochester, Rochester, NY*

FRANÇOISE CONDÉ, *CEA CNRS URA 2210 Unit, Service Hospitalier Frédéric Joliot, Orsay, France*

ROSHAN COOLS, *Department of Experimental Psychology, University of Cambridge, Cambridge, UK*

HARRIET S. CROFTS, *Department of Experimental Psychology, University of Cambridge, Cambridge, UK*

JOSEPH T. DALEY, *Department of Neurology, Emory University, Atlanta, GA*

IRENE DAUM, *Department of Clinical Neuropsychology, Ruhr-University Bochum, Bochum, Germany*

DENNIS W. DICKSON, *Neuropathology Laboratory, Mayo Clinic, Jacksonville, FL and Alzheimer's Disease Research Center, Mayo Foundation, Rochester, MN*

NATAŠA DRAGAŠEVIĆ, *Institute of Neurology CCS, Belgrade, Yugoslavia*

STANLEY FAHN, *College of Physicians and Surgeons, Columbia University, New York, NY*

TIFFANY R. FARCHIONE, *Departments of Psychiatry and Pediatrics, Wayne State University School of Medicine, Detroit, MI*

ANTHONY FEINSTEIN, *Department of Psychiatry, University of Toronto, Ontario, Canada*

TANIS J. FERMAN, *Department of Psychology and Psychiatry, Mayo Clinic, Jacksonville, FL and Alzheimer's Disease Research Center, Mayo Foundation, Rochester, MN*

AMANDA A. FREEMAN, *Department of Neurology, Emory University, Atlanta, GA*

NIR GILADI, *Movement Disorders Unit, Department of Neurology, Sackler School of Medicine, Tel-Aviv University, Tel-Aviv, Israel*

CHRISTOPHER G. GOETZ, *Departments of Neurological Sciences and Pharmacology, Rush University, Chicago, IL*

ALEX D. GOUMENIOUK, *Department of Pharmacology and Therapeutics, University of British Columbia, Canada*

ANN M. GRAYBIEL, *Department of Brain and Cognitive Sciences and the McGovern Institute for Brain Research, Massachusetts Institute of Technology, Cambridge, MA*

MARK GUTTMAN, *Department of Psychiatry and Division of Neurology, University of Toronto, Ontario, Canada*

SUZANNE N. HABER, *Department of Pharmacology and Physiology, University of Rochester School of Medicine and Dentistry, Rochester, NY*

PHILIPPE HANTRAYE, *CEA CNRS URA 2210 Unit and Isotopic, Biochemical and Pharmacological Imaging Unit, Service Hospitalier Frédéric Joliot, Orsay, France*

JOHN HARDY, *Laboratory of Neurogenetics, National Institute of Aging, National Institutes of Health, Bethesda, MD*

KURT A. JELLINGER, *Ludwig Boltzmann Institute of Clinical Neurobiology, Vienna, Austria*

MARY JOHNSON, *Centre for Development in Clinical Brain Aging, Newcastle General Hospital, Newcastle upon Tyne, UK*

ANDREW KERTESZ, *Department of Clinical Neurological Sciences, St. Joseph's Hospital and University of Western Ontario, London, Canada*

AMOS D. KORCZYN, *Department of Neurology, Sackler Faculty of Medicine, Tel-Aviv University Medical School, Tel-Aviv, Israel*

VLADIMIR S. KOSTIĆ, *Institute of Neurology CCS, Belgrade, Yugoslavia*

YASUO KUBOTA, *Department of Brain and Cognitive Sciences and the McGovern Institute for Brain Research, Massachusetts Institute of Technology, Cambridge, MA*

JAIME KULISEVSKY, *Movement Disorders Unit, Department of Neurology, Sant Pau Hospital, Autonomous University, Barcelona, Spain*

ANTHONY E. LANG, *Movement Disorders Clinic, Toronto Western Hospital, and Division of Neurology, Department of Medicine, University of Toronto, Toronto, Ontario, Canada*

JAN PETTER LARSEN, *School of Medicine, University of Bergen and Department of Neurology, Central Hospital, Stavanger, Norway*

EDWARD C. LAUTERBACH, *Department of Psychiatry and Behavioral Sciences, Mercer University School of Medicine, Macon, GA*

JAMES F. LECKMAN, *Child Study Center and the Departments of Pediatrics, Psychiatry and Psychology, Yale University, New Haven, CT*

RAMÓN LEIGUARDA, *Raúl Carrea Institute of Neurological Research, FLENI, Buenos Aires, Argentina*

SIMON LEMAY, *The André Barbeau Movement Disorder Unit, Centre Hospitalier de l'Universite de Montréal and Cognitive Neuroscience Center, Université du Québec à Montréal, Montréal, Canada*

IRA LEROI, *Department of Psychiatry, Johns Hopkins School of Medicine, Baltimore, MD*

PAUL LESPÉRANCE, *The André Barbeau Movement Disorder Unit, Centre Hospitalier de l'Universite de Montréal and Department of Psychiatry, Université de Montréal, Montréal, Canada*

MAXIME LÉVESQUE, *Cognitive Neuroscience Center, Université du Québec à Montréal, Montréal, Canada*

GILBERTO LEVY, *Gertrude H. Sergievsky Center, Columbia University, New York, NY*

IRENE LITVAN, *Movement Disorders Program, Department of Neurology, University of Louisville, Louisville, KY*

JOHN LUCAS, *Department of Psychology and Psychiatry, Mayo Clinic, Jacksonville, FL and Alzheimer's Disease Research Center, Mayo Foundation, Rochester, MN*

SHAUNA N. MACMILLAN, *Departments of Psychiatry and Pediatrics, Wayne State University School of Medicine, Detroit, MI*

KAREN MARDER, *Gertrude H. Sergievsky Center and Department of Neurology, College of Physicians and Surgeons, and the Taub Institute for Research on Alzheimer's Disease and the Aging Brain, Columbia University, New York, NY*

HELEN S. MAYBERG, *Rotman Research Institute and Departments of Neurology and Psychiatry, University of Toronto, Ontario, Canada*

IAN G. MCKEITH, *Wolfson Research Centre, Newcastle General Hospital, Newcastle upon Tyne, UK*

FRANK A. MIDDLETON, *Department of Neurobiology, University of Pittsburgh School of Medicine, Pittsburgh, PA*

MARTHA A. NANCE, *Department of Neurology, University of Minnesota School of Medicine and Hennepin County Medical Center, Rochester, MN*

STÉPHANE PALFI, *CEA CNRS URA 2210 Unit, Service Hospitalier Frédéric Joliot, Orsay cedex, France*

FRANÇOIS PAQUET, *Cognitive Neuroscience Center, Université du Québec à Montréal, Montréal, Canada*

JOSEPH E. PARISI, *Laboratory of Medicine and Pathology, Mayo Clinic and Alzheimer's Disease Research Center, Mayo Foundation, Rochester, MN*

JANE S. PAULSEN, *Departments of Psychiatry and Neurology, University of Iowa, Iowa City, IA*

ELAINE K. PERRY, *Centre for Development in Clinical Brain Aging, Newcastle General Hospital, Newcastle upon Tyne, UK*

ROBERT PERRY, *Centre for Development in Clinical Brain Aging, Newcastle General Hospital, Newcastle upon Tyne, UK*

RONALD C. PETERSEN, *Department of Neurology, Mayo Clinic and Alzheimer's Disease Research Center, Mayo Foundation, Rochester, MN*

MARGARET A. PIGGOTT, *Centre for Development in Clinical Brain Aging, Newcastle General Hospital, Newcastle upon Tyne, UK*

WERNER POEWE, *Department of Neurology, University Hospital Innsbruck, Innsbruck, Austria*

SAŠKA POTREBIĆ, *Institute of Neurology CCS, Belgrade, Yugoslavia*

FRANCOIS RICHER, *The André Barbeau Movement Disorder Unit, Centre Hospitalier de l'Université de Montréal and Cognitive Neuroscience Center, Université du Québec à Montréal, Montréal, Canada*

TREVOR W. ROBBINS, *Department of Experimental Psychology, University of Cambridge, Cambridge, UK*

ANGELA C. ROBERTS, *Department of Anatomy, University of Cambridge, Cambridge, UK*

MARY M. ROBERTSON, *Department of Psychiatry and Behavioural Sciences, University College London and The National Hospital for Neurology and Neurosurgery, Queen Square, London, UK*

DAVID R. ROSENBERG, *Departments of Psychiatry and Pediatrics, Wayne State University School of Medicine, Detroit, MI*

ADAM ROSENBLATT, *Department of Psychiatry, Johns Hopkins School of Medicine, Baltimore, MD*

VLADIMIR ROYTER, *Department of Neurology, Tel-Aviv Souraski Medical Center and Sackler School of Medicine, Tel-Aviv University Medical School, Tel-Aviv, Israel*

ALLEN RUBIN, *Departments of Psychiatry and Neurology, University of Iowa College of Medicine, IA*

DAVID B. RYE, *Department of Neurology, Emory University, Atlanta, GA*

DANIEL S. SA, *Movement Disorders Clinic, Toronto Western Hospital, and Division of Neurology, Department of Medicine, University of Toronto, Toronto, Ontario, Canada*

JEAN A. SAINT-CYR, *Departments of Surgery and Psychology, University of Toronto and University Health Network, Morton and Gloria Shulman Movement Disorders Centre, Toronto Western Hospital, Toronto, Ontario, Canada*

JEREMY D. SCHMAHMANN, *Department of Neurology, Harvard Medical School and Ataxia Unit, Cognitive/Behavioral Neurology Unit, and Geriatric Neurobehavior Clinic, Massachusetts General Hospital, Boston, MA*

JAY S. SCHNEIDER, *Department of Pathology, Anatomy and Cell Biology, Thomas Jefferson University, Philadelphia, PA*

ANETTE SCHRAG, *Sobell Department of Motor Neuroscience and Movement Disorders, Institute of Neurology, London, UK*

CAROLINE SELAI, *Sobell Department of Motor Neuroscience and Movement Disorders, Institute of Neurology, London, UK*

Russ Sethna, *Markham Stoufferille Hospital, Markham, Ontario, Canada*

Michael H. Silber, *Sleep Disorders Center and Department of Neurology, Mayo Clinic, Rochester, MN*

Glenn E. Smith, *Departments of Psychology and Psychiatry, Mayo Clinic and Alzheimer's Disease Research Center, Mayo Foundation, Rochester, MN*

Elka Stefanova, *Institute of Neurology CCS, Belgrade, Yugoslavia*

Taresa L. Stefurak, *Rotman Research Institute and Departments of Neurology and Psychiatry, University of Toronto, Ontario, Canada*

Julie C. Stout, *Department of Psychology, Indiana University, Bloomington, IN*

Alan Thomas, *Institute for Aging and Health, Wolfson Research Centre, Newcastle General Hospital, Newcastle upon Tyne, UK*

John L. Waddington, *Department of Clinical Pharmacology, Royal College of Surgeons in Ireland, Dublin, Ireland*

I
Introduction

1

Historical Issues in the Study of Behavioral Dysfunction in Movement Disorders

Christopher G. Goetz, MD

1. INTRODUCTION

The interface between behavioral and motor function is a characteristic of all movement disorders and has long been appreciated. The historical study of this interface gathers the names and works of several neurological luminaries from the 19th and 20th centuries. This chapter focuses on one hypokinetic disorder, Parkinson's disease (PD), and one hyperkinetic disorder, Huntington's disease (HD). As a historical essay, the chapter presents the background for contemporary topics discussed elsewhere in this volume.

2. PARKINSON'S DISEASE

Mental function received attention even in James Parkinson's original 1817 *Essay on the Shaking Palsy (1)*. His patient series included six patients, some of whom were never examined by him, but he nonetheless concluded; "Senses and intellect are uninjured." This association went unchallenged until the celebrated French neurologist, Jean-Martin Charcot studied PD. In his *Complete Works: Lectures on Diseases of the Nervous System (volume 1)*, he developed a thorough discussion of PD and commented without ambiguity on the depressive affect, dementia, and, rarely, hallucinations that develop among parkinsonian patients *(2)*. Charcot examined many patients with PD during his clinical case presentations (*Tuesday Lessons*) *(3)*, drawn from the extensive inpatient population at the Salpêtrière hospital and from his outpatient clinic. His database, therefore, was far more extensive than Parkinson's. The two views of these seminal figures highlight the dichotomy of historical views on the interface between behavior and motor dysfunction in PD and introduce five relevant questions that remain unanswered in their entirety.

2.1. *Do Mental Aberrations Occur in PD?*

Shortly after his arrival at the Salpêtrière hospital, Charcot joined his colleague, Vulpian, in a systematic examination and categorization of patients with neurological disorders. In a two-part publication (1861–1862), they described PD and detailed the motor, autonomic, and other aspects of the clinical presentation *(4)*. Based on this series, in his concise style, Charcot concluded, "In general, psychic faculties are definitely impaired." He added to this description at a later date, "At a given point, the mind becomes clouded and memory is lost *(2)*." Subsequently, multiple studies from France reiterated Charcot's claim. Ball (1882) reported on seven patients, and Parant, among others, reported individual case histories *(5,6)*. The descriptions suggested that dementia and depression were frequently encountered aspects of PD and that hallucinations could even occur in the context of the untreated illness.

From: *Mental and Behavioral Dysfunction in Movement Disorders*
Edited by: M-A. Bédard et al. © Humana Press Inc., Totowa, NJ

Outside of France, however, most 19th- and early 20th-century researchers agreed more closely with Parkinson's assertion that mental function was unaffected. Wollenberg (1899), Oppenehim (1911), and Konig (1912) concluded that Parkinson's disease was not associated with dementia *(7–9)*. As was typical of the period, scientific attitudes often polarized along geographical lines, partly because of language barriers, partly because of nationalistic temperaments in the wake of the Franco-Prussian war, and partly because of the enormous power and influence that individual professors exerted on their students and communities. In this latter regard, Charcot was a man who radiated a strong and ever-present halo. He was extremely powerful throughout Europe and did not encourage disagreement *(10)*. On the other hand, he based his conclusions on a vast clinical experience drawn from direct patient interview and observation.

After the first decade of the 20th century, a 40-yr hiatus occurred with very few neurobehavioral studies in PD. The advent of systematic neuropsychology tools prompted renewed interest, and in 1949, Mjones reported psychological and neurological evaluations of 194 PD patients using limited but systematic testing batteries *(11)*. After eliminating depressed and delirious patients, he found that dementia (termed "senile psychosis") occurred in 3% of PD subjects. This number was compared to the less than 1% prevalence of dementia in the general Swedish population of the time. A later cross-sectional study of dementia prevalence prior to the introduction of widespread use of levodopa restricted the assessment to PD and not other forms of parkinsonism, finding that dementia occurred in 8% of patients *(12)*. Together, these studies confirm the original statement of Charcot over Parkinson's assessment and document that the study of behavioral aspects of PD is justified.

2.2. *How Should Dementia, Depression, and Psychosis Be Differentiated?*

Charcot and his French colleagues were clear in their enumeration of multiple behavioral aspects of PD *(2,3)*. With a careful reading of Parkinson's *Essay,* allusions to depression can also be found in the words "melancholy" and "dejected," although no further amplification was provided *(1)*. In 1923, Lewy reported on mental alterations in PD, finding 64% of patients affected, although he did not distinguish between dementia and depression *(13)*. In focusing on this distinction, Jackson and colleagues cited five PD patients in a state mental hospital who were markedly depressed but categorically not demented *(14)*. They emphasized that depression could be a prominent and disabling feature of PD, even more disabling than the motor elements. Psychotic behavior and paranoia were elements of depression in some patients, but memory was fully intact.

In terms of etiology, depression has historically been argued to be both an endogenous part of the biochemical lesions of PD as well as a reaction to the loss of autonomy and independence. General assumptions in this paradigm have been that if the depression is reactive, there should be a low prevalence of depression before the onset of PD motor symptoms and that the depression should clear as motor disability is improved with medication. In fact, however, Mayeux and colleagues found that 43% of depressed patients with PD were depressed before the appearance of any motor signs and that there was no relationship between severity of depression and motor disability *(15)*. The question remains a debated one, and ancillary techniques, which include positron emission tomography of frontal lobe function, have been applied to chart the temporal development and interplay between depression and motor dysfunction *(16)*.

In dealing with the complex distinction between depression and dementia, investigators have wrestled with the memory blunting that can occur during depressive episodes *(15,17)*. Conversely, Lieberman and colleagues found that 25% of mildly demented patients with PD also fulfilled diagnostic criteria for depression *(18)*. These studies suggest that the two mental disorders, once confounded, then separated, should be reconsidered as coincident in many patients.

In contrast to the higher prevalence of dementia and depression in PD, psychotic behavior and hallucinations have always been considered rare in nonmedicated patients. Charcot's psychiatric colleague, Ball, described the infrequent occurrence of hallucinations in patients, and it is not clear from these case histories whether the patients had PD or more probably, Lewy Body Dementia *(5)*. In the context of medication treatment, hallucinations, specifically well-formed and stereotypic visual hallucinations, occur in approx 30% of patients *(19)*. The pathophysiology and neuropharmacological basis of these hallucinations remain undetermined, but are a focus of significant research efforts. Whereas hallucinations occur when patients are treated chronically with dopaminergic drugs and decrease or disappear when drugs are stopped, the behavior is not a simple intoxication because high doses of intravenous levodopa in daily hallucinators do not precipitate the behavior *(20)*.

2.3. Is Bradyphrenia an Element of PD?

In 1922, Naville introduced the term "bradyphrenia" to describe the slowing of cognitive processing and impairment of concentration seen in parkinsonian patients, even in the absence of frank dementia *(21)*. Although most of these patients had postencephalitic parkinsonism, some had PD. Bradyphrenia, also known as psychic akinesia, was introduced to parallel the motor slowness of bradykinesia, although most reports posited a psychological basis for the behavior *(22,23)*. Coincident with the development of levodopa, the focus returned to neurological hypotheses, because clinical studies showed a strong correlation between bradykinesia and bradyphrenia *(24)*. Jovoy-Agid and Agid suggested that lesions in the mesocorticolimbic dopaminergic pathways may be important to both behaviors *(25)*. Whereas bradyphrenia can be considered an element of parkinsonism, questions of continued controversy relate to its biochemical and anatomical basis as well as the overlap of bradyphrenia with depression. Neuroimaging techniques using functional magnetic resonance scanning may provide tools to examine these issues.

2.4. Is There a PD Personality?

Current theories of a possible latent period of many years between the induction of dopaminergic cell loss and clinical signs of PD have prompted renewed interest in premorbid signs of the condition. Among the many areas of research, personality traits have historically been a focus and remain an area of investigation. Charcot stressed the interplay among behavior, hereditary illness, and neurological disorders *(2,3,10)*, but the definition of a specific PD personality developed out of psychoanalytic theories in the first half of the 20th century. These studies, reviewed by Todes and Lees, described the prototypic patients as introspective, emotionally rigid, well-controlled, and predisposed to depression *(26)*. Before motor signs appeared, these patients tended to be law-abiding citizens, diligent, trustworthy, but often lacking in adventurous initiative and the willingness to take risks. Studies of twin pairs, one with and one without PD, revealed the affected twin, even as a child, more likely to be self-controlled, conservative, and a follower. These findings have been complemented by studies suggesting that cigaret smoking reduces the risk of PD *(27)*. To the extent that smoking can be considered a risk-taking or extroverted behavior, these findings would support the personality profile suggested by these early studies. These arguments, however, have not been universally accepted, and some researchers have adamantly rebuffed these hypotheses *(28,29)*. In the context of these historical controversies, the need for early detection of subjects at high risk for PD is pivotal to testing putative neuroprotective strategies. Without a clear biological marker of PD, interest in behavioral studies in the premorbid state have rekindled with applications of more sophisticated psychological assessment tools and neuroimaging.

2.5. Is the Prevalence of Mental Changes in PD Increasing?

This question is raised when one compares representative early studies on populational prevalence of dementia in PD and the more recent reports from the levodopa era. In 1949, Mjones *(11)* found the prevalence of dementia to be 3%; in Pollack's and Hornabrook's study from 1966 *(12)*, they documented a prevalence of slightly less than 10%; and Boller's 1980 review of recent reports found 30% prevalence of dementia *(30)*. Multiple explanations can be offered, including higher indices of suspicion, more careful assessments, and drug exposure. Barbeau claimed that after levodopa was introduced, PD patients showed more cognitive impairment than previously observed *(31)*. These studies introduce an important clinical issue on the possible changing phenotype of PD, but also highlight the important issues of methodology implicit to modern epidemiological research alluded to in this volume.

2.6. Future Issues in PD

In addition to introducing the questions just discussed, past investigators have set the stage for studies of other issues related to behavior and PD. Implicit to all research is the development of effective measurement tools, and an important research focus for future study must be the refined definition of rating scales for the overlapping elements of behavioral dysfunction. Likewise, advances in molecular biology offer the possibility of defining subgroups of patients with behavioral complications. Because no behavioral syndrome is universally seen in PD patients, studies of genetic polymorphisms may help to identify those potentially at higher risk for each abnormality. Although the interplay between heredity and environment was suggested in the 19th century *(10)*, it remains to be specifically defined for PD in the 21st century.

3. HUNTINGTON'S DISEASE

As the prototypic hyperkinetic movement disorder, HD presents a variety of behavioral aberrations. Unlike PD, where the very presence of behavioral changes was not originally appreciated, in HD, a wide gamut of cognitive and emotional deficits was documented in even the earliest descriptions by Huntington and others. These reports and a large body of medical research from the 20th century address several questions on the interface between behavior and motor signs in HD, some of which are addressed here from a historical perspective.

3.1. What Is the Character of HD Dementia?

The first recognition of hereditary chorea with dementia predates George Huntington's 1872 description *(32)*. C. O. Waters included a brief account in his 1842 entry for Dunglison's *Practice of Medicine (33)*; "It gradually includes a state of more or less perfect dementia." Lund, writing in 1860, described a Norwegian cohort of patients possibly afflicted with HD and commented that mental decline, termed "fatui," occurred late in the disease's evolution *(34)*. In 1862, Lyon commented on social ostracism of families with hereditary chorea, but did not specifically mention dementia *(35)*. The lack of standardized diagnostic definitions from this era and the variety of mental changes that can affect HD patients make these early reports difficult to interpret with accuracy.

Huntington, likewise, did not specifically allude to the word dementia in his original article, but used the words "a tendency to insanity and suicide" *(32)*. Writing with empathy and clarity, he recounted his observations, showing that he recognized dementia, "The mind becomes more or less impaired, in many, amounting to insanity, while in others, mind and body both gradually fail until death relieves them of their sufferings."

Charcot presented several HD patients in his Tuesday amphitheater conferences at the Salpêtrière hospital *(3)*. He noted "mania, melancholia all ending as dementia…at the terminal stage, choreic movement becomes intense enough to make standing and walking impossible and intellectual function deteriorates to the lowest level so the unfortunate patient is reduced to a bedridden state now prone to every destructive force imaginable" *(3)*. Interestingly, Charcot did not appreciate the diagnostic distinction between HD and Sydenham's chorea, but agreed that in the cases of adult onset, a progressive dementia and chronic, unremitting clinical decline were characteristic *(3)*.

In the early 20th century, the appreciation of cognitive impairment was widespread, prompting Hallock to term HD, "dementia choreica" *(36)*. He did not posit that the dementia had characteristics specific to HD, but only emphasized that he considered dementia as a universal accompaniment of the disease. In the same year, Roasenda published on rare HD cases where cognition was spared, but these exceptional cases served primarily to emphasize the general rule of cognitive involvement *(37)*. The development of standardized neuropsychological testing tools introduced the concept of cortical and subcortical dementia syndromes and allowed distinctions to be drawn between the cognitive decline that typifies HD in contrast to Alzheimer's disease and PD *(38)*. These studies, along with biochemical and neuroimaging studies reported in this volume, address some of these issues.

3.2. What Are the Psychotic and Depressive Manifestations of HD?

Whereas hallucinations are rare in HD patients *(39)*, delusions of grandeur, religious fervor, and persecution are common and are often seen in the early phases of the disease *(40)*. Likened to behaviors seen in schizophrenia by Neff in 1917, these observations built support for hypotheses of schizophrenia as a biochemical illness *(41)*.

Depression occurs more frequently than psychosis and usually forms an important part of the early manifestations of HD, often associated with prominent anxiety and irritability. Huntington himself commented on the "nervous temperament" so characteristic of the HD families *(42)*. Impulsivity and erratic uninhibited behaviors were demonstrated by Charcot in one of his case presentations *(3)*:

> Here is one anecdote among many: while living in Brioude, this patient left his home one day, a sack on his back with no money and walked all the way to Paris. He begged for things along the roadsides and survived on bread crusts. Apparently, his goal was to get to the *Marché du Temple* marketplace where old second-hand clothing was sold. He then returned by foot, having bought a shirt and hat from his native local region. Clearly, this man was not completely stable, having developed intermittent, but quite characteristic, episodes of erratic behavior.

Regarding the same problem of disinhibition and unpredictable patterns of behavior, Huntington recounted on sexual improprieties *(32)*:

> I know of two married men whose wives are living and who are constantly making love to some young lady, not seeming to be aware that there is any impropriety to it. They are men of about 50 years of age, but never let an opportunity to flirt with a girl go past unimproved. The effect is ridiculous in the extreme.

3.3. What Is the Temporal Development of Mental Changes Relative to Motor Changes?

In the historical literature on HD, cases of behavioral changes occurring before, after, and in parallel with motor abnormalities can be found. Meerburg's study from 1923 was historically important, because she identified families who confidently identified those to become afflicted with HD even in early childhood by their distinctive behavior *(43)*. Attempting to match maternal instinct by scientific precision, researchers currently are following genetically identified, but asymptomatic subjects with HD to detect the clinical and neuroimaging changes that occur in the natural progression of illness.

3.4. Future Issues in HD

The identification of a biological marker for HD provides researchers with a tool yet unavailable in PD. Furthermore, because there is no consistently effective therapy for the disease and its symptoms, the natural history of the disorder from the earliest genetic detection can be monitored. The definition of neuropsychological tests, which specifically examine striatal–frontal cortical circuitry, permit increasingly sophisticated clinical tools for the examination of behaviors related to HD. Although neurotherapeutics have advanced much more rapidly for PD than for HD, the development of well-designed assessment tools and the clear definition of the untreated illness provides researchers with background knowledge that is not available for untreated PD at its various states. As therapies are developed, this information will place researchers in an excellent position to assess changes in both motor and behavioral indices of the illness.

4. WILLIAM OSLER AND THE STUDY OF BEHAVIORAL ASPECTS OF PD AND HD

Because the origin of this volume was a congress sponsored by the Movement Disorder Society that took place in Montreal, it is appropriate to review the contributions of the city's native medical luminary, William Osler. Studies of movement disorders received priority in Osler's neurological work. Of particular note, his seminal work on Sydenham's chorea provided a large data set of experience and helped to close the previous controversy on whether Sydenham's chorea and HD were one and the same *(44)*. In this dispute, Osler challenged Charcot and ultimately proved himself correct in separating the two conditions *(45)*.

In regards to PD, Osler identified and accurately described the major clinical features of the illness, although he did not appreciate the distinction between bradykinesia and weakness. Although a skilled pathologist, he did not identify the brainstem lesion of PD, but he felt the lesion was one involving the corticospinal systems and related to premature aging. This stand was important, because Osler nosographically removed PD from its former classification as a névrose or neurosis, a term used to describe neurological illnesses with no presumed or yet-identified anatomical basis. In terms of behavioral involvement, he sided with James Parkinson more than with Charcot, writing in his *The Principles and Practice of Medicine* (1892), "The mental condition rarely shows any change" *(46)*.

Regarding HD, Osler's contributions were more substantial. In addition to his firm stand against coalescing HD with Sydenham's chorea, his *On Chorea and Choreiform Affections* provides elegantly composed descriptions of behavioral problems encountered in HD *(45)*. He commented on suicides risks in the context of depression and impulsivity. He examined autopsy material from patients with HD, but did not identify consistent abnormalities, concluding, "So far, nothing has been found which is peculiar to the disease or is in any way specific" *(45)*.

Perhaps Osler's most important contribution to the understanding of HD was his inclusion of Huntington's complete description of hereditary chorea within the text of *On Chorea and Choreiform Affections*. Because Huntington's original description was published in a minor and only locally circulated journal, Osler's widely read monograph expanded the availability of Huntington's description. Commenting on Huntington's work, Osler stated, "In the history of medicine, there are few instances in which a disease has been more accurately, more graphically, or more briefly described" *(45)*.

REFERENCES

1. Parkinson, J. (1817) *An Essay on the Shaking Palsy*, Sherwood, Neeley and Jones, London.
2. Charcot, J.-M. (1892): Leçon 5. De la paralysie agitante, in *Oeuvres Complètes*, Vol. 1, Bureaux du Progrès Médical, Paris, pp. 155–189. (In English: On paralysis agitans, in *Lectures on Diseases of the Nervous System*, translated by G. Sigerson, 1879, H.C. Lea and Company, Philadelphia, pp. 105–127.
3. Charcot, J.-M. (1887): *Leçons du Mardi à la Salpêtrière. Policliniques 1887-1888*: Notes de Cours de M.M. Blin, Charcot et Colin. Bureaux du Progrès Médical, Paris. (In English: *Charcot the Clinician: The Tuesday Lessons*, translated with commentary by Christopher G. Goetz, 1987, Raven Press, New York.
4. Charcot, J.-M. and Vulpian, A. (1861, 1862) De la paralysie agitante. *Gaz Hebdomadaire Med. Chir.* 1861; **8,** 765–767; 1862; **9,** 54–59.
5. Ball, B. (1882) De l'insanité dans la paralysie agitante. *Encéphale J. Mal. Ment. Nerv.* **2,** 22–32.
6. Parant, V. (1883) La Paralysie agitante examinée comme cause de folie. *Rev. Méd. Toulouse* **17,** 266–280.
7. Wollenberg, R. (1899) Paralysis agitans, in *Specielle Pathologie und Therapie*. (Nothnagel, H., ed.), Vienna, Alfred Holder, pp. 234–254.
8. Oppenheim, H. (1911) *Textbook of Nervous Diseases,* Otto Schulze and Company, Edinburgh.
9. Konig, H. (1912) Zur psychopathologie der paralysis agitans. *Arch. Psychiatr. Nervenkrankheit* **50,** 285–305.
10. Goetz, C.G., Bonduelle, M., and Gelfand, T. (1995) *Charcot: Constructing Neurology.* Oxford University Press, New York.
11. Mjones, H. (1949) Paralysis agitans. *Acta Psychiatr. Neurol.* **54(Suppl. 21),** 1–195.
12. Pollock, M. and Hornabrook, R.W. (1966) The prevalence, natural history and dementia of Parkinson's disease. *Brain* **89,** 429–448.
13. Lewy, F.H. (1923) Die Lehre Von tonus und der bewegung zugleich systematiche Untersuchinger sur Klinik, in *Physiologie, Pathologie und Pathogenese der Paralysis Agitans,* Springer, Berlin, pp. 45–58.

14. Jackson, J.A., Free, G.B.M., and Pike, H.V. (1923) The psychic manifestations in paralysis agitans. *Arch. Neurol.* **10,** 680–684.
15. Mayeux, R., Stern, Y., San, M., et al. (1988) The relationship of serotonin to depression in Parkinson's disease. *Mov. Disord.* **3,** 237–244.
16. Kiyosawa, M., Bosley, T.M., and Kushner, M. (1990) Middle cerebral artery strokes causing homonymous hemianopia: Positron emission tomography. *Ann. Neurol.* **28,** 180–183.
17. Brown, G.L. and Wilson, W.P. (1972) Parkinsonism and depression. *South. Med. J.* **654,** 540–545.
18. Lieberman, A., Dziatlowski, M., and Coppersmith, M. (1979) Dementia in Parkinson's disease. *Ann. Neurol.* **6,** 355–359.
19. Goetz, C.G. (1999) Hallucinations in Parkinson's disease: the clinical syndrome. *Adv. Neurol.* **80,** 419–423.
20. Goetz, C.G., Pappert, E.J., Blasucci, L.M., et al. (1998) Intravenous levodopa in hallucinating Parkinson's disease patients: high-dose challenge does not precipitate hallucinations. *Neurology,* **50,** 515–517.
21. Naville, F. (1922) Les complications et les séquelles mentales de l'encéphalite épidemique. *Encéphale* **17,** 369–375, 423–436.
22. Jelliffe, S.E. (1940) The parkinsonian body posture, some considerations of unconscious hostility. *Review* **27,** 467–479.
23. Booth, G. (1948) Psychodynamics in parkinsonism. *Psychom. Med.* **10,** 1–14.
24. Rogers, D., Lee, A.J., Smith, E., et al. (1987) Bradyphrenia in Parkinson disease and psychomotor retardation in depressive illness. *Brain* **110,** 761–776.
25. Jovoy-Agid, R. and Agid, Y. (1980) Is the mesocortical dopamienrgic system involved in Parkinson's disease? *Neurology* **30,** 1326–1331.
26. Todes, C.J. and Lees, A.J. (1985) The pre-morbid personality of patients with Parkinson's disease. *J. Neurol. Neurosurg. Psychiatry* **48,** 97–100.
27. Checkoway, H., Franklin, G.M., and Costa-Mallen, P. (1998) A genetic polymorphism of MAO-B modifies the association of cigarette smoking and Parkinson's disease. *Neurology* **50,** 1458–1461.
28. Ajuriaguerra, de J. (1971) Etude psychopathologique des Parkionsoniens, in *Monoamines, Noyaux Gris Centraux, et Syndrome de Parkinson* (Ajuriaguerra, de J. and Gauthier, G., eds.), Masson, Paris, pp. 327–351.
29. Riklan, M., Weiner, H., and Diller, L. (1959) Somato-psychologic studies in Parkinson's disease. An investigation into the relationship of certain disease factors to psychological functions. *J. Nerv. Ment. Dis.* **129,** 263–272.
30. Boller, F. (1980) Mental status of patients with Parkinson disease. *J. Clin. Neuropsychol.* **2,** 157–172.
31. Barbeau, A. (1972) *Dopamine and Mental Function. L-Dopa and Behavior.* Raven Press, New York, pp. 9–33.
32. Huntington, G. (1872) On chorea. *Med. Surg. Reporter* **26,** 320–321.
33. Waters, C.O. (1842) Description of chorea, in *Practice of Medicine* (Dunglison, R., ed.), Lea and Blanchard, Philadelphia, pp. 312–313.
34. Lund, J.C. (1860) Chorea sancti Viti I Saetesdalen. *Beretning om sundhedstilstanden og medicinalforholdene i Norge*, Oslo (no publisher).
35. Lyon, R.L.L. (1962) Huntington's chorea in the Moray Firth area. *BMJ* **1,** 1301–1306.
36 Hallock, F.K. (1898) A case of Huntington's chorea with remarks upon the propriety of naming the disease 'dementia choreica'. *J. Nerv. Ment. Dis.* **25,** 851–864.
37. Roasenda, G. (1908) Sui disturbi psichici e sulla patogenesi della corea ereditaria di Huntington. Un caso di corea di Huntington senza alterazioni mentali. *Riv. Neuropatol.* **2,** 41–50.
38. Mayeux, R., Stern, Y., Rosen, J., et al. (1981) Subcortical dementia: a recognizable clinical syndrome. *Ann. Neurol.* **10,** 100–101.
39. Rosenbaum, D. (1941) Psychosis with Huntington's chorea. *Psychiatr. Q.* **15,** 93–99.
40. Hamilton, A.S. (1908) A report of twenty-seven cases of chronic progressive chorea. *Am. J. Insan.* **64,** 403–475.
41. Neff, M.E. (1917) Über Psychosen bei Chorea. *Mschr. Psychiatr. Neurol.* **41,** 65–87.
42. Huntington, G. (1909) Recollections of Huntington's chorea as I saw it in East Hampton, Long Island during my boyhood. *Proc. NY Neurol. Soc.* pp. 97–99. Reprinted in *Adv. Neurol.* 1973, **1**, 37–39.
43. Meerburg, G. (1923) *Huntington's disease: family dimensions.* Thesis. Univer Leiden, Leiden.
44. Goetz, C.G. (2000) William Osler: on Charcot: on chorea. *Ann. Neurol.* **47,** 404–407.
45. Osler, W. (1894) *On Chorea and Choreiform Affections*, Blakiston, Philadelphia.
46. Osler, W. (1892) *The Principles and Practice of Medicine.* Appleton, New York.

II

Mental Processing in the Motor Structures of the Brain

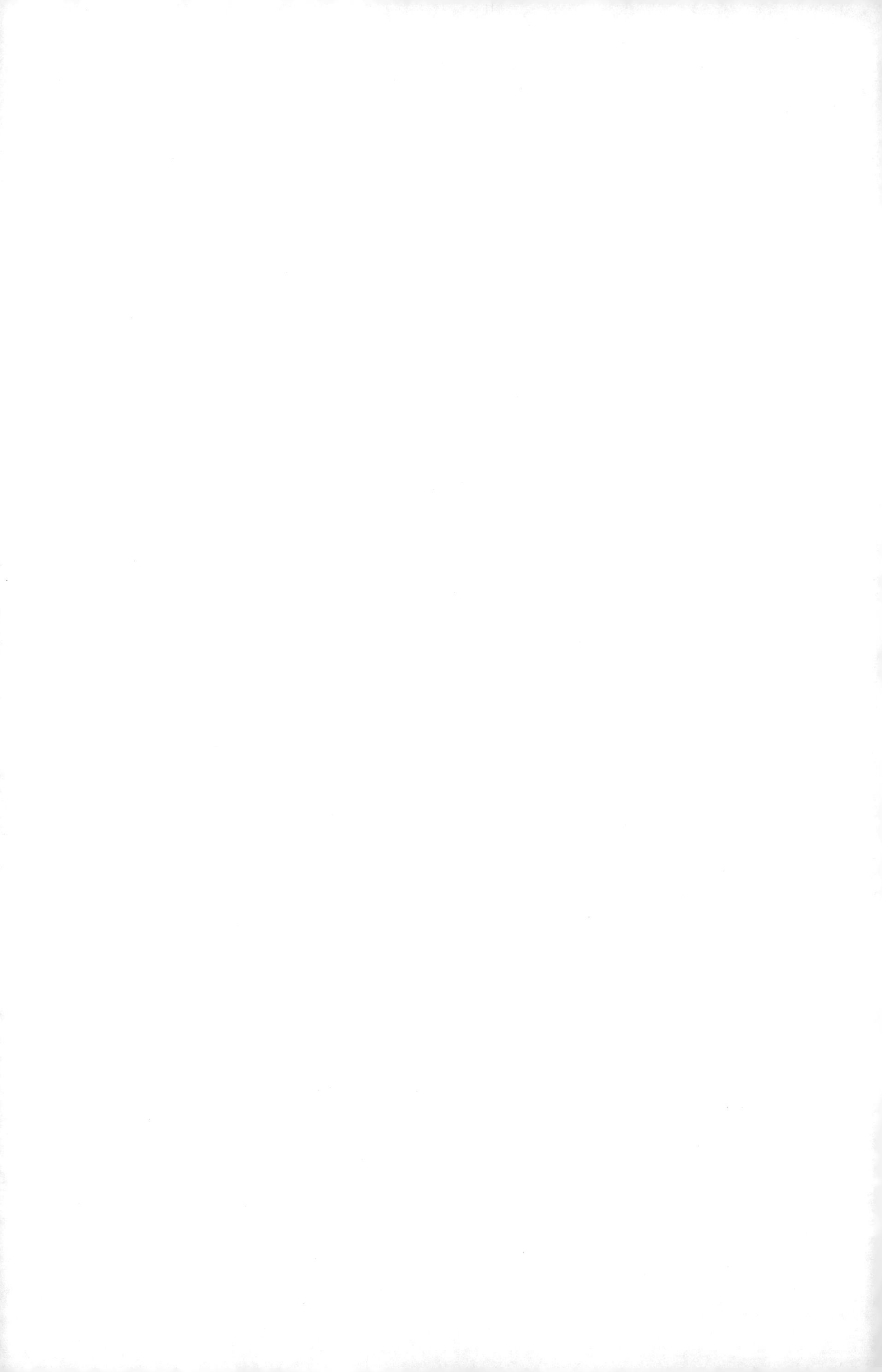

2

Fundamental and Clinical Evidence for Basal Ganglia Influences on Cognition

Frank A. Middleton, PhD

1. INTRODUCTION AND OVERVIEW OF THE BASAL GANGLIA

1.1. Structures and Subdivisions

Over the past century, the term "basal ganglia" has at one time or another been used to indicate a wide variety of brain structures. In its present and most restrictive use, however, the term is generally reserved for three groups of brain structures called the "striatum," "pallidum," and "substantia nigra," and an additional structure termed the "subthalamic nucleus" (STN). Table 1 outlines the basic subdivisions of the basal ganglia. The striatum can be separated into two general components, the dorsal striatum, which consists of the caudate and putamen, and the ventral striatum, which consists of the nucleus accumbens, septum, and olfactory tubercle. The nucleus accumbens, in turn, is subdivided into a lateral core region and medial shell region. In a similar manner, the pallidum can also be divided into multiple divisions, including a lateral or external segment of the globus pallidus (GPe), a medial or internal segment of the globus pallidus (GPi), and a portion that lies ventral and anterior to the anterior commissure, designated the ventral pallidum (VP). The GPi is further divided anatomically by a distinct fiber bundle into a lateral outer portion and a medial inner portion. Finally, the substantia nigra is also composed of more than one component, a cell group rich in neuromelanin called the pars compacta (SNpc), which is responsible for the black appearance of the nucleus in gross specimens, and an unpigmented cell group known as the pars reticulata (SNpr). Further subdivision of the SNpr is also possible, due to the presence of a distinct subpopulation of cells located dorsolaterally in the SNpr, and is referred to as the pars lateralis.

1.2. Connections Between Basal Ganglia Subdivisions

The basic connections between the different components of the basal ganglia are now well described *(1–4)*. According to the simplest classification scheme, the nuclei within the basal ganglia can be subdivided into sets of "input," "output," and "intermediate" structures. Input structures include the caudate, putamen, and nucleus accumbens. Collectively, these input structures receive direct projections from nearly the entire cerebral cortex. These input structures then project to intermediate structures as well as output structures.

Intermediate structures within the basal ganglia include the STN, GPe, and SNpc. An additional structure, the pedunculopontine nucleus (PPN), is also occasionally viewed as an intermediate component of the basal ganglia due to its dense interconnectivity with other basal ganglia structures. In general, intermediate structures project most heavily to other basal ganglia nuclei, including the output structures as well as other intermediate structures.

From: *Mental and Behavioral Dysfunction in Movement Disorders*
Edited by: M-A. Bédard et al. © Humana Press Inc., Totowa, NJ

Table 1
Basal Ganglia Subdivisions

Basal ganglia structure	Primary subdivision	Secondary subdivision	Tertiary subdivision
Striatum	Dorsal striatum	Caudate	
		Putamen	
	Ventral striatum	Nucleus accumbens	Core
			Shell
		Septum	
		Olfactory tubercle	
Globus pallidus	External segment		
	Internal segment	Outer portion	
		Inner portion	
	Ventral pallidum		
Substantia nigra	Pars compacta		
	Pars reticulata	Pars lateralis	
Subthalamic nucleus			

The three principal output structures of the basal ganglia include the GPi, SNpr, and VP. For the most part, these output structures send their efferent projections to different subdivisions of the ventroanterior–ventrolateral (VA/VL), mediodorsal (MD), and intralaminar (IL) groups of thalamic nuclei (particularly the centrum medianum and parafasicularis intralaminar nuclei [CM/PF]) *(1–5)*. The VA/VL and MD nuclei of the thalamus, in turn, project largely back upon the cerebral cortex. Thus, one of the major features of basal ganglia anatomy is their participation in what has become known as cortical-basal ganglia-thalamocortical circuits (hereafter referred to as simply cortical-basal ganglia circuits). Notably, however, some of the neurons in VA/VL and MD, and many of the neurons in CM/PF, send projections to the striatum, and thus form a recurrent thalamic feedback loop with the basal ganglia. Although most early depictions of basal ganglia circuitry have emphasized the unidirectional flow of signals within these loops, as Fig. 1 illustrates, there is an increasing awareness of the importance that recurrent projections from the thalamus, as well as most intermediate and output structures, can play in modulating basal ganglia function.

1.3. Cellular Organization

Superimposed on the macro-organization of cortical-basal ganglia circuits are well-characterized relationships between the various cell types that comprise these circuits. Some of the early and most comprehensive studies of the cellular anatomy of the basal ganglia were made using purely morphological criteria and did not attempt to impose functional distinctions on the cell types. Recent investigations have used a more heuristic approach to describing the cellular components of the basal ganglia, which classifies them initially as either interneurons or projection neurons and differentiates them further within these classes based on morphological, neurochemical, physiological, and hodological features (Table 2) *(2–4,6)*.

1.4. The Basic Cortical-Basal Ganglia Circuit in Action

Many features of the cellular, neurochemical, and physiological organization of the basal ganglia are particularly important in understanding how the basal ganglia process information. Most of the cortical input to the basal ganglia is derived from layer V pyramidal cells that use glutamate (GLU) as a neurotransmitter. These cortical projection neurons can innervate one or more of several types of basal ganglia circuits. Most of the inputs from motor and higher association areas of cortex synapse on medium spiny cells in the striatum that are part of either the direct path or indirect path (see below)

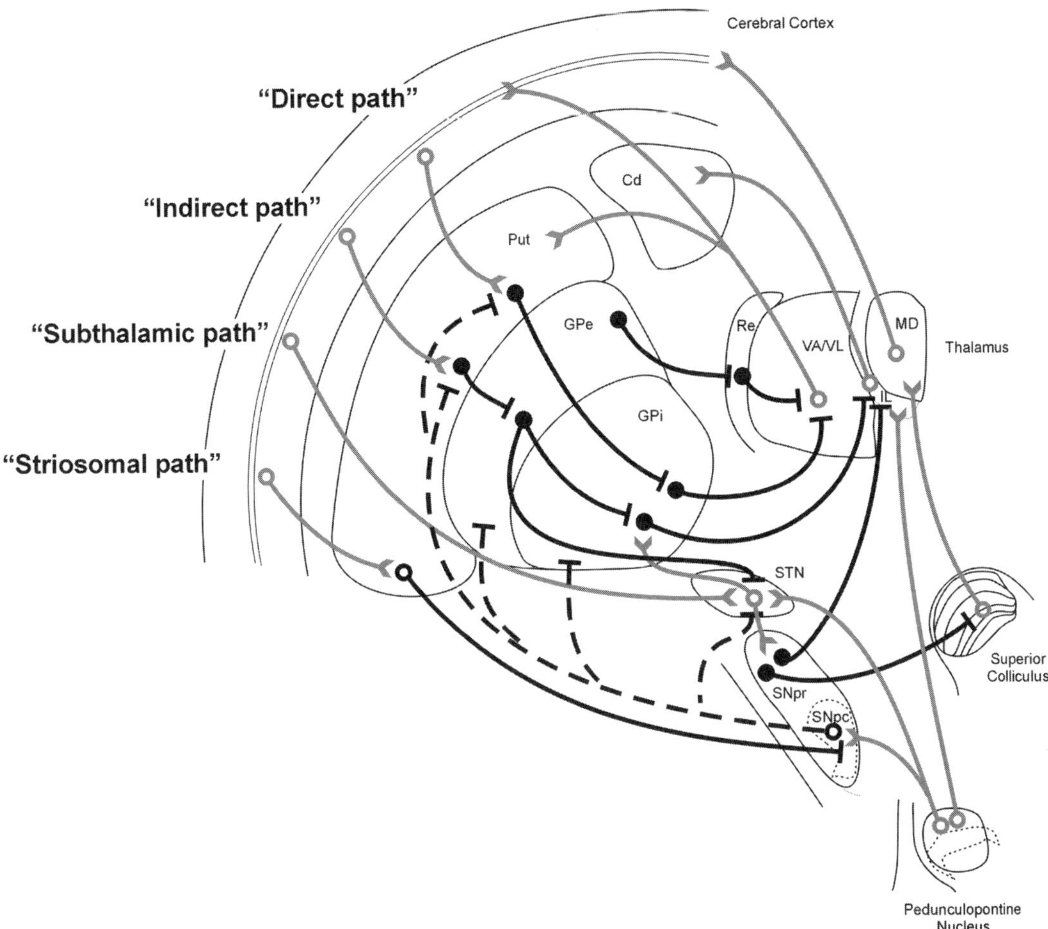

Fig. 1. Basic cortical-basal ganglia circuitry. The organization of connections between different components of the basal ganglia and the cerebral cortex, thalamus, superior colliculus, and pedunculopontine nucleus are shown. Much of the cortical influences on the circuitry of the basal ganglia can be grouped into one or more pathways (direct, indirect, subthalamic, or striosomal). Excitatory connections are shown in gray, and inhibitory connections are shown in black. Note that the influence of dopamine inputs from the SNpc to neurons in the striatum (broken line) can be both excitatory and inhibitory and is fundamentally different in nature from the signals processed in the other components of basal ganglia circuitry. Also note that nearly every component of these circuits has both a principal projection, which follows the direction of information flow within the circuit, as well as a recurrent projection to other basal ganglia components. Abbreviations as in text.

(Fig. 1). Many of these same cortical areas also contain cells that project directly to the STN and, thus, constitute a subthalamic path *(1–4,7)*. Notably, while the striatal inputs from motor and higher association areas in the cerebral cortex target neurons in the striatal matrix, which contain high levels of acetylcholinesterase, the inputs from many orbitofrontal and temporal limbic regions of the cortex target regions of the striatum called patches, or striosomes, which express low levels of acetylcholinesterase *(7,8)*. Neurons in the striosomes do not participate in the same types of circuitry as neurons in the striatal matrix. While medium spiny neurons in the matrix project largely to the γ-amino butyric acid (GABA)-ergic cells of the pallidum and nigra (GPe, GPi, or SNpr), the medium spiny cells in the striosomes project largely to dopamine synthesizing cells in the SNpc *(2–4)*. Thus, at least at the

Table 2
Major Cell Types and Chemical Properties of Basal Ganglia Neurons

Class	Name	Location	Main inputs	Main outputs	Transmitter	Representative markers
Projection	Striatal medium spiny neuron	Striosome	Limbic cortex, SNpc	SNpc	GABA	D1, substance P, GAD NMDA receptor (NR) 1/2B/2A, cannabinoids
		Matrix	Cortex, striatal interneurons, SNpc	GPe	GABA	D2, G(o), G(i), enkephalin, dynorphin, neurotensin, GAD, adenosine A2A receptors, NR1/2B/2A
			Cortex, striatal interneurons, SNpc	GPi, SNpr	GABA	D1, G(s), substance P, GAD, NR1/2B/2A, cannabinoids
	Spindle neurons	GPe	Striatum	Thalamic reticular N, GPi, STN	GABA	GABA subunits (α_{1-4}, β, γ_2, δ), GAD
		GPi	Striatum, GPe, STN	VA/VL	GABA	Cannabinoid receptor, 5HT2C receptor, GABA subunits (α_{1-4}, β, γ_2, δ), GAD
		SNpr	Striatum, Gpi	VA/VL, MD SC, reticular formation	GABA	Cannabinoid receptor, 5HT2C receptor, GABA subunits (α_{1-3}, $\beta_{,2-3}$, γ_2, δ), GAD, CCK
	Excitatory	STN	Cortex, GPe	GPi, SNpr, PPN	GLU	GABA subunits (α_{1-3}, β_{2-3}, γ_2, δ), Glu receptor types
	Pigmented	SNpc	Striatum, SNpr	Striatum, GPi, SNpr, STN	DA	Neuromelanin, Nurr1, Reelin, D1, D2 GABA subunits (α_{3-4}, β_{1-3}, γ_2, δ), torsin A, neurokinin
Interneuron	Large cholinergic	Striatum	Mostly thalamic and striatal projection neurons	Mostly striatal matrix	ACh	Acetylcholinesterase, D1/2, GluR1/4, m1/2/4, GAP-43, NR2C/D
	Medium	Striatum PV positive	Cortex	Adjacent striatal regions	GABA	PV, GAT-1, GAD-67, GluR1/2/3/4
		Striatum CR positive	Other CR positive cells, probably other striatal cells	Other CR positive cells	GABA	CR, GABA, GAD-67
		Striatum SS-NPY-NOS, positive	Cortex	Mostly striatal matrix	NPY, NO	SS, NPY, GAD-67, NOS, acetylcholinesterase, D1, m1/4, NR1/2B/2D, neurokinin, CB

Abbreviations: ACh, acetylcholine; CCK, cholecystokinin; CR, calretinin; CB, calbindin; D1/D2, dopamine receptor subtypes; DA, dopamine; GABA, γ amino-butyric acid; GAD, glutamate decarboxylase; GAP, growth associated protein; GAT-1, GABA transporter; G(i)/G(o)/G(s), G protein subtype; GLU, glutamate; GluR, glutamate receptor subtype; m, muscarinic receptor subtype; NO, nitric oxide; NOS, nitric oxide synthase; NPY, neuropeptide Y; NR, *N*-methyl-D-aspartate (NMDA) receptor subtype; PPN, pedunculopontine nucleus; PV, parvalbumin; SC, superior colliculus; SS, somatostatin, STN, subthalamic nucleus.

input stage of processing, a fourth type of circuit, the corticostriosomal path can be envisioned. The functional properties of these different paths are presented in a later section.

SNpc cells project densely back to widespread regions of the striatum (as well as the STN and pallidum) where they maintain high levels of extracellular and synaptic dopamine pools. The net effect of the dopamine on striatal cells depends largely on the types of receptors present on the target cells. For example, striatal cells in the direct path (that project to the GPi or SNpr) express high levels of D1 receptors, as well as substance P and dynorphin *(2–4)*. Activation of D1 receptors on these cells results in increased cellular activity and responsiveness through G(s)-mediated second messenger systems. In contrast, striatal cells in the indirect path (that project to the GPe) express high levels of D2 receptors as well as enkephalin (ENK) *(2–4)*. Activation of D2 receptors on these cells results in decreased cellular responsiveness and activity through G(i)- and G(o)-mediated second messenger mechanisms.

Despite the differences in the effects of dopamine on the direct and indirect pathways, the medium spiny cells in both of these circuits utilize GABA to inhibit their targets. Because the GPe cells that receive D2-mediated input project largely to the GPi, then the net effect of activation of the direct and indirect pathways in the presence of normal levels of dopamine is the same in terms of information flow; that is, cortical excitation of the basal ganglia input structures leads to less inhibition of the thalamus and increased activity of these circuits *(9–11)*. Importantly, however, cells in the GPe also send inhibitory inputs to the STN, which in turn exert a powerful excitatory influence on the GPi and SNpr. Thus, D2-mediated inhibition of the GPe can promote activity of the STN and allow the basal ganglia to increase inhibition of the thalamus. This effect would be further promoted by the action of direct cortical excitatory inputs to cells in the STN. In summary, the major projection systems within the basal ganglia contain at least two different pathways that lead to increased thalamocortical activation (the direct and indirect paths) and one that can lead to decreased thalamocortical activation (the subthalamic path).

Aside from the projection systems just outlined, however, several of the interneuronal populations of the basal ganglia also exert powerful influences on basal ganglia circuitry *(2,6)*. In the striatum, one important class of interneuron is the large or giant cholinergic interneuron (Table 2). These neurons receive most of their input from thalamic cells in CM/PF and other striatal cell types and a small input from the cortex. In turn, giant cholinergic cells have widespread projections to other striatal cells, largely within the matrix *(6)*. Giant cholinergic cells also express high levels of acetylcholinesterase activity, as well as D1, D2, and selected muscarinic and glutamatergic receptors *(6)*. Within sensorimotor regions of the striatum, these cells are thought to change their basic physiologic properties (tonic irregular firing) as an association is built between a sensory stimulus and an appropriate response *(12)*. Thus, by virtue of their connections with both input level and output level signals, the presence of multiple neurotransmitter phenotypes (including those associated with both direct and indirect pathways), and their widespread axonal collaterals in the striatum, the giant cholinergic cells may represent one of the most important interfaces between basal ganglia circuits that operate in different behavioral modalities.

Although the roles of the other interneuronal cell types in the basal ganglia have been less characterized, most of them appear to exert more local influences on other neurons within the structure they are found. Interneurons in the pallidum and STN, for example, appear to be more similar to the classical concept of a local circuit neuron, which connects adjacent or nearby cells *(2)*. In the striatum, however, at least two other classes of interneurons receive some cortical input (Table 2) *(6)*. It is also interesting to note the recent findings that most interneurons in the striatum and cerebral cortex are derived from a common set of precursor cells in the medial ganglionic eminences during brain development *(13)*. Thus, although basal ganglia interneurons are often overshadowed by projection neurons in terms of their influence on cortical-basal ganglia circuitry, such observations open the possibility that the wiring of basal ganglia circuits with the cerebral cortex could depend in part on cues left behind by these migrating interneurons during development, long before the circuits even become active. In fact, this migration may help define which circuits exist between the cerebral cortex and the basal ganglia altogether.

Table 3
Evolution of Theories of Basal Ganglia Function

Period	Theories	Main influences
Renaissance era—20th century	Basal ganglia influence all aspects of behavior and sensation.	Gross anatomists.
Early 20th century	Basal ganglia primarily influence the control of movement.	Early neuroanatomists and neuropathologists.
Middle 20th century	Basal ganglia solely involved in the control of movement.	Early neurophysiologists.
Late 20th century	Basal ganglia influence motor and nonmotor behavior, including many types of cognitive processing. Basal ganglia involved in goal-directed behavior and simple S-R associations.	Later neurphysiologists and neuroanatomists, neuroimagers, neuropsychologists, neurosurgeons.
Early 21st century	Major influences of basal ganglia on all forms of cognition may be driven by goals and rewards.	Neurophysiologists and neuroimagers.

1.5. Basal Ganglia Circuits with the Cerebral Cortex: How Many, Open, or Closed?

There is general agreement about the properties of the basal ganglia that have been discussed thus far. However, the basic theories regarding the function of the basal ganglia have evolved slowly over the past few centuries and continue to do so today (Table 3). One of the more recent controversies concerned the issue of how many cortical areas participated in basal ganglia circuits, and how the information from different cortical areas was processed within these circuits. Historically, at the input level of processing, the projections from the cerebral cortex to the basal ganglia were recognized as a highly organized and topographic projection system *(1,14,15)*. For example, anterior cortical areas were seen to project to anterior striatal regions, and posterior cortical areas were observed projecting to posterior striatal regions. Likewise, ventromedial regions of cortex projected to ventromedial striatal regions, whereas dorsolateral areas of cortex projected to dorsolateral striatal regions. However, beyond these features, most theories of basal ganglia function held that there was a great deal of convergence both within the striatum and in the projections from the striatum to the intermediate and output levels of processing. In other words, the basal ganglia were thought to have the ability to integrate sensory, limbic, and cognitive information with the commands for movement. In its extreme form, this theoretical concept was even used to argue that the basal ganglia were ultimately only concerned with the control of movement *(14)*.

There were two main reasons for the widespread acceptance of this viewpoint. The first reason was that the symptoms of basal ganglia dysfunction most often include characteristic motor abnormalities. Any cognitive or emotional disturbances also seen in patients with basal ganglia disease were often attributed to other causes and ruled secondary. The second major reason that the basal ganglia were viewed solely as a motor-related structure was the lack of substantive evidence for basal ganglia projections back to nonmotor regions of the cerebral cortex.

In 1986, Alexander, DeLong, and Strick *(1)* reviewed the results of numerous anatomical studies and suggested that rather than serving as a funnel for information from widespread cortical areas, the basal ganglia actually participated in multiple parallel segregated circuits with different regions of the frontal lobe. These regions included cortical areas concerned with skeletomotor and oculomotor control and three regions of the prefrontal cortex involved in cognitive and limbic functions. Recent experimental evidence has supported and expanded on this proposal. In a recent review *(16)*, it was suggested that the original five circuit scheme, proposed by Alexander and colleagues *(1)*, should be broadened to include seven general categories of circuits: skeletomotor, oculomotor, dorsolateral prefrontal, lateral orbitofrontal, medial orbitofrontal, cingulate, and inferotemporal–posterior parietal. Within each of these categories, anatomical evidence supports the existence of multiple (between two and seven) parallel cortical-basal ganglia circuits. This amount of finely tuned parallel anatomical circuitry may not be surprising to neuroanatomists. However, the diversity of functions that these circuits have the potential to influence is impressive. By virtue of their reciprocal connections with posterior cortical areas involved in visual and spatial perception, the basal ganglia would have the potential ability to influence an even broader range of behaviors than those proposed in the model by Alexander and colleagues *(1)*. In that model, the basal ganglia inputs from posterior cortical areas were integrated in basal ganglia circuits and ultimately influenced only regions of the frontal lobe.

Finally, although there is considerable evidence that much of the basal ganglia circuitry comprising the direct, indirect, and subthalamic pathways (Fig. 1) is topographically organized at multiple levels, there is much less evidence to suggest that the striosomal path (see Fig. 1) is similarly organized. Indeed, the recurrent projections from the SNpc to widespread regions of the striatum may represent the means for the basal ganglia to integrate information about primary reward and behavioral state received from limbic and sensory cortical areas with the modality-specific information being processed in the cortical-basal ganglia circuits. As such, these connections clearly represent an open-loop component of basal ganglia circuitry. The implications of this arrangement in terms of basal ganglia influences on cognition are reviewed in a later section.

2. BASAL GANGLIA INFLUENCES ON COGNITION

2.1. *What Cognitive Functions Are Likely to be Influenced by the Basal Ganglia?*

The anatomical substrate exists for the basal ganglia to process large amounts of information related to skeletomotor, oculomotor, cognitive, limbic, and sensory functions. Evidence suggests that at least some component of this processing takes place within multiple parallel circuits with different functionally defined cortical areas. However, these types of anatomical data do not establish the nature of the basal ganglia influence on cognitive function and whether this influence is independent of basal ganglia influences on limbic and motor function. Such issues can only be resolved by examining the behavioral relevance of these circuits. As a first step, it is helpful to define the specific types of cognitive operations that could be processed by such circuits by briefly reviewing the properties of three cortical areas within the prefrontal cortex that are known to participate in both cognitive function as well as basal ganglia circuits.

Areas 9, 46, and 12 are now known to participate in basal ganglia circuits. Areas 9 and 46 project to adjacent regions of the dorsal and lateral caudate, which in turn innervate adjacent regions of the rostral and dorsal GPi and SNpr. These regions of the GPi and SNpr are now known to project back upon areas 9 and 46 via neurons in VA/VL and MD *(16)*, thus completing the parallel circuit with these cortical areas. Area 12, in contrast, projects more ventrally in the caudate and appears to receive its input largely from the SNpr, but not GPi *(16)*. Nonetheless, it is clear that the physiological properties of each of these three prefrontal areas have the potential to drive basal ganglia circuits and, in turn, to be strongly influenced by the output of basal ganglia processing.

2.1.1. Physiological Studies

The physiological properties of the dorsal and lateral prefrontal cortex have been the subject of several in-depth analyses *(17–21)*. These studies have revealed that areas 9, 46, and 12 each appear to be involved in at least four different types of cognitive functions. First, many neurons in these areas display changes in activity related to the performance of delayed-response tasks. These tasks require sensory cues to be stored for a brief period of time and then used to generate a specific response. During such tasks, selective changes in neuronal activity can be seen during the presentation of cues (cue-related activity), the delay period following cue presentation (delay-related activity), and the response preparation and execution periods (response-related activity) *(17–30)*. Depending on the area of the prefrontal cortex in which one records or studies, there are additional task parameters that will determine the relative proportion of neurons involved in the performance of these delayed response tasks. For example, within areas 9 and 46, many neurons have cue- and delay-related activity that is tuned to the spatial position of stimuli (spatially-tuned activity) or the order in which the stimuli are present (sequentially-tuned activity). In contrast, within area 12, neurons appear to be much less involved in spatial and sequential information and more involved in remembering the identity of particular objects (object-tuned activity). Throughout areas 9, 46, and 12, there are also many neurons that appear to be more involved in the learning and remembering of specific rules or associations used in the performance of conditional response (forced choice) tasks (rule-related activity). An example of this type of task is the classic go/no-go task, in which one cue instructs the animal to make a response, while a different cue instructs the animal to withhold that response *(27–31)*. Finally, a relatively small but consistent proportion of neurons in areas 9, 46, and 12 also display changes in activity that coincide with the expectation or anticipation of primary reinforcement or food rewards (reward-related activity) (e.g., ref. *30*).

2.1.2. Lesion Studies

Lesion studies support some of the physiological observations regarding areas 9, 46, and 12. Bilateral damage to area 9 in monkeys produces severe and long-lasting impairments in the performance of tasks that require animals to monitor the order and identity of different objects (but not their spatial position), particularly when the sequence of cues to be remembered is self-ordered *(32)*. These deficits are similar to those found in human patients with dorsal prefrontal lesions *(33)*. In addition, patients with prefrontal lesions have been shown to be deficient in tasks that require the categorization and sorting of different stimuli, including card sorting tasks *(34)*, or the planning and monitoring of script events or sequential actions *(35–37)*. These types of tasks are thought to impose significant demands on planning and short-term (or working) memory for objects or sequential actions. Experimental lesions of area 46 result in an inability of animals to perform spatial delayed-response tasks, spatial delayed-alternation tasks, and go/no-go tasks *(17–21,38)*. These deficits are similar to the problems in attention, planning, working memory, and response inhibition reported in humans with lateral prefrontal lesions *(21,35,37,39,40)*. Finally, lesions of area 12 in monkeys have been shown to produce what has been referred to as an inability of animals to make switches in behavioral set. This deficit leads to perseverative responses on delayed-response tasks, in which the identity of different objects or colors must be remembered (object matching, object reversal, or object alternation tasks), or inappropriate responses in auditory-cued go/no-go tasks *(41–45)*. In addition, there is also evidence that large lesions of area 12 produce deficits in the learning and performance of visual discrimination tasks that do not involve delayed-responses *(46)*.

2.1.3. Functional Imaging Studies

Functional imaging studies in humans support many of the physiological and behavioral findings. Tasks that require difficult planning, the monitoring of sequences of hand movements, or the learning of new movement sequences *(47–55)* produce sites of peak activations in lateral portions of area 9, as do tasks that employ verbal working memory (including word generation tasks) *(56–62)*. Medial portions of area 9 have been shown to be activated by the processing of script events that requires monitoring the categories of events, which took place *(63)*. Kawashima and colleagues *(64)* also reported several foci of activation in area 9 when human subjects performed a go/no-go task, when compared with a simple response selection condition. Similar to area 9, area 46 is particularly active during spatial working memory tasks, difficult planning tasks, go/no-go tasks, some nonspatial object and verbal working memory tasks, and verb generation tasks *(51,65–77)*. Area 46 has also been shown to be active during the generation and monitoring of multiple movement sequences involving the hand or fingers *(47,48,50,53,54,64)*. Many of these studies have concluded that the prefrontal activations in areas 9 and 46 are related to the elaboration or learning of novel sequences, since these activations are most apparent when comparing task performance during the learning phase with that seen after the task is well learned *(53,54,78)*. In contrast to areas 9 and 46, the human equivalent of area 12 (area 47) has been shown to be active during tasks that employ verbal working memory, including word generation tasks *(56,57,71,79,80)*, but not during spatial working memory tasks.

In summary, based on all the evidence presented thus far, one might predict that the influence of the dorsal and lateral prefrontal-basal ganglia circuits on behavior would be strongest for those functions related to spatial and object working memory, rule-based learning, and the monitoring of sequential or serial information used to guide future actions (i.e., planning), while information related to reward may also be present within these circuits, though to a lesser degree.

2.2. *What Is the Evidence for Basal Ganglia Influences on Cognition?*

Having defined a set of functions that are subserved by cognitive regions of the prefrontal cortex, we can now examine the evidence for basal ganglia influences on the same type of cognitive processes. We begin by discussing the results from selected physiological recording studies in awake primates and humans.

2.2.1. *Physiological Studies*

2.2.1.1. Input Stages of Basal Ganglia Processing

There have been hundreds of studies on the physiological properties of striatal cells. Only a small fraction of these, however, have examined the properties of striatal cells that could relate to cognitive processing. With few exceptions, these studies have focused on locating cells with activity related to a type of task and determining under what conditions such task-related activity is enhanced or suppressed.

In a study that examined the effect of task difficulty on caudate nucleus properties in humans, Abdullaev and colleagues *(81)* recorded from human subjects during reading, naming, recognition memory, categorization, and lexical decision making tasks. They found that, during visual processing of words, caudate cells exhibited excitatory responses related to both semantic and phonological-articulatory encoding and that the delay-related firing of cells was increased whenever semantic processing was required. Comparing the properties of striatal cells with those seen in the prefrontal (Broca's) area and in the temporal and parietal lobe areas, the authors found that the caudate cells had properties that were "strikingly similar" to those in Broca's area. Since portions of the prefrontal cortex are often activated during the same types of verbal tasks that activate Broca's area (reviewed in subheading 2.1.3.), it is possible that basal ganglia inputs from these areas also contributed to the findings of this study.

Striatal cell activity during sequential task performance has also been examined. Kermadi and Joseph *(82)* examined the properties of striatal cells during a task that required monkeys to engage in a sequential working memory task. They found that many of the cells with task-related activity had visual-related responses that varied according to the order of a given target, and moreover, that many of the caudate cells seemed to anticipate the fixation of specific targets. Such findings are similar to some of those reported in studies of areas 9 and 46 reviewed above.

Striatal cell activity has also been recorded during conditional task performance. Schultz and Romo *(83)* found many neurons with cue, delay, and response preparatory activity in the caudate and putamen of monkeys trained to perform a go/no-go task. They interpreted their results to indicate that most of these task-related neurons in the striatum were involved in response preparation. A slightly different conclusion was reached by Shuvaev and Shefer *(84)* in another conditional response task in monkeys. They found that the task-related striatal cells they recorded could be separated into two distinct groups.

While one group of cells was clearly tuned to response execution, another group of cells appeared to be more involved in the instructional decision-making process.

In contrast to these experiments that focused solely on formal cognitive operations, Nishino and colleagues *(85)* found that a small proportion of neurons in the head of the caudate nucleus of monkeys responded specifically to the sight of food or food rewards. Furthermore, the results from several recent studies strongly suggest that such reward-related properties can directly affect the cognitive properties of striatal cells. Using a memory-guided saccade task, Kawagoe and colleagues *(86)* demonstrated that the visual and memory responses of caudate cells were so affected by the expectation of reward, that their spatial tuning characteristics often changed specifically toward the rewarded direction, with subsequent responses in this direction becoming earlier and faster. These authors concluded that the caudate contributes to the determination of oculomotor outputs by connecting information about reward with visual signals. In a similar finding, Hassani and colleagues *(87)* observed that during a spatial-delayed response task, in which different picture cues were associated with specific rewards, many neurons in the anterior caudate, putamen, and ventral striatum of monkeys displayed different levels of task-related activity depending on the type of reward being offered and whether it was a preferred or nonpreferred reward of that animal. These authors concluded that their data support the concept that the striatum might help maintain a mental image of the outcome of an action, while the proper behavioral action is performed.

These studies provide clear evidence that striatal cells are involved in many of the same elements of cognitive processing as cells in the prefrontal cortex (including cue, delay, conditional responses, and reward periods of task performance). However, unlike some of the studies that have recorded from the output nuclei of the basal ganglia (see subheading 2.2.1.2.), most studies of striatal physiology have not been conducted with the goal of precisely defining the location or circuit relationship of the neurons involved in specific components of task performance. Thus, it is simply not possible to ascertain whether this involvement reflects the properties of particular basal ganglia circuits.

2.2.1.2. Output Stages of Basal Ganglia Processing

There have also now been numerous single unit recording studies carried out on the output nuclei of the basal ganglia of the human and primate. Results from these studies clearly show that only specific regions of the GPi and SNpr contain neurons whose activity is related to skeletomotor or oculomotor commands *(88–95)*. These regions of the GPi and SNpr largely coincide with the regions that have been shown to project to skeletomotor or oculomotor regions of cortex (reviewed in ref. *96*). In contrast, large portions of the GPi and SNpr contain neurons whose activity is not modulated by simple skeletomotor or oculomotor tasks. Many of these regions fall within the regions that innervate areas of prefrontal cortex involved in cognitive processing *(96)*. Evidence to support the involvement of some of these neurons in cognitive processing is also available. Hikosaka and Wurtz *(89)* and Hikosaka and colleagues *(97)* recorded the activity of neurons in the SNpr of monkeys trained to perform an oculomotor spatial-delayed response task. A considerable number of SNpr neurons were found whose activity was modulated during the delay period of the task. Many of these delay-related cells appeared to be separate from SNpr cells, which were purely saccade-related, but not delay-related, and a number of them were spatially tuned. As reviewed earlier, neuronal properties similar to these have been found in studies of area 46. Thus, nigral outputs to prefrontal cortex could be directly involved in tasks that involve spatial working memory and the planning of eye movements.

Similar conclusions about the presence of delay-related neurons, as well as the existence of sequence-related neurons, were reached by Mushiake and Strick *(98)*, who recorded from the GPi in monkeys trained to remember the spatial sequence (order and position) of three light flashes in a manual delayed-response task. They found that a small but consistent proportion of task-related neurons in the GPi had changes in activity during the instruction period in which the flashes occurred or during the delay period immediately following the instruction. Some of these neurons displayed activity that was specific for the particular sequence of cues the animal had to remember. Moreover, the location of these instruction-related neurons tended to be within dorsomedial portions of the pallidum, a region that both receives input from and projects back upon areas 9 and 46 (via the striatum and thalamus, respectively) *(96,99)*. Thus, spatial and sequential aspects of delayed task performance were found within basal ganglia circuits that subserve prefrontal areas known to be involved in the same type of tasks.

Additional information about the involvement of the basal ganglia output nuclei in conditional response performance and reward processing is also available. In one of the earliest studies of pallidal physiology in awake trained primates, Travis and Sparks *(100)* recorded from the globus pallidus of squirrel monkeys trained to perform a go/no-go task. Surprisingly, only 3 of 89 pallidal neurons in their sample displayed activity related to gross motor movements, suggesting that they were not sampling the skeletomotor circuitry within GPi and may instead have been recording from regions with outputs to prefrontal cortex. Indeed, more than 40% of their task-related cells displayed changes in activity during the instruction period preceding the movement in the go tasks or during the period after the movement prior to the delivery of the reward. DeLong *(101)* pointed out that some of the cells that Travis and Sparks were recording were probably not true pallidal cells, but rather cells that lay in the border region between GPe and GPi. Nevertheless, Travis and Sparks concluded that many pallidal neurons displayed "attention, set, or anticipation activity," as well as activity "related to voluntary sequences of behavior leading to primary reinforcement." Such conclusions are quite similar to those reached decades later by other investigators recording from pallidal neurons. Gdowski and colleagues *(102)* recorded GPi activity during a manual delayed-response task in which monkeys received a reward for correctly executed movements, whereas movements during the return phase of the arm were not rewarded. The authors found that many GPi neurons discharged in a context-dependent manner, being specifically modulated during the cued rewarded movements, but not during the similar self-paced unrewarded movements.

In summary, the physiological properties of many neurons in the striatum and pallidum of humans and nonhuman primates appears to be similar in many respects to those reported in studies of the physiology of the prefrontal cortex. In addition, compared with the prefrontal cortex, there appears to be an increase in the relative proportion of neurons in the basal ganglia whose activity is significantly influenced by the expectation of reward. Thus, although the concept that parallel basal ganglia circuits can subserve different types of tasks appears valid, there clearly appears to be another system operating across circuit boundaries that integrates information about the rewarding value of a behavioral act. Shultz *(103)* proposed that the neural substrate for this reward system is the phasic activity of dopamine synthesizing cells in the SNpc, which conveys information about primary reinforcement and behavioral state to cells in the striatum. Because such influences exist throughout the striatum, it is quite likely that many, if not all, basal ganglia circuits utilize reward-related information to modify the properties of cells within them in order to carry out meaningful behavioral acts.

2.2.2. Functional Imaging Studies

Functional magnetic resonance imaging (fMRI) and positron emission tomography (PET) have been used to examine the activity of the basal ganglia and prefrontal cortex during the performance of tasks involving specific cognitive functions. To date, these studies have not been done on the SNpr. In one of these studies, Jueptner and colleagues *(53,54)* listed significant activations in areas 9 and 46, dorsolateral portions of the caudate, rostrodorsal portions of the globus pallidus, and thalamic sites in VA and paralaminar MD in subjects during the learning of new sequences of eight key presses, compared with activations seen during previously learned sequences. Thus, nearly all of the brain regions that are thought to participate in basal ganglia circuits with the dorsolateral prefrontal cortex were activated during a sequence-learning task in humans.

In another PET study, Owen and colleagues *(104,105)* compared the activity of normal subjects and Parkinson's disease patients during the performance of a difficult planning task (the Tower of London task), a spatial working memory task, and a simple visually guided movement task. Previous studies from this group had strongly implicated areas 9 and 46 in the performance of both the planning and spatial working memory tasks *(51,52)*. These investigators found that Parkinson's disease patients had very little GPi activation during the cognitive tasks, while normal subjects had greatly increased GPi activation during the same tasks. Furthermore, the amount of this differential activation was directly correlated with task difficulty, i.e., the greatest differences occurred in the tasks with the most cognitive demands, whereas there were no differences in GPi activation between normal and parkinsonian subjects in the simple motor task. Because patients with Parkinson's disease had previously been shown to be impaired in the performance of the same cognitive tasks *(106,107)*, the authors concluded that the GPi outputs to the dorsolateral prefrontal cortex (areas 9 and 46) played an important role in these tasks.

Finally, a number of recent studies have examined the functional activation of the basal ganglia and prefrontal cortex during cognitive tasks (mainly card gambling games) that have an artificial reward component *(108,109)*. In one of these studies *(108)*, the investigators obtained strong evidence for the involvement of the striatum, bilateral pallidum, and ventral anterior thalamus in context-dependent responses to increasing levels of rewards. Interestingly, in another study comparing normal and schizophrenic subjects during the performance of a similar task, abnormalities in the activation patterns were found in schizophrenic subjects specifically within the left dorsolateral prefrontal cortex, basal ganglia, and thalamus *(110)*. Moreover, such abnormalities were associated with poorer task performance in the schizophrenic subjects.

Collectively, these studies highlight the convergence of evidence from functional imaging and physiological recording studies on the basal ganglia of humans and nonhuman primates. Such evidence strongly supports a specific role of prefrontal-basal ganglia circuits in maintaining a working knowledge about the location and order of stimuli presented in a task, the rules or arbitrary associations involved in this task, and the planning of sequences of actions that lead to primary reinforcement in these tasks. Moreover, at least some components of the basal ganglia (e.g., neurons within the striatum and pallidum) appear to capable of performing all of these functions concurrently and, thus, may form part of the neuronal substrate for directing goal-oriented behavior.

2.2.3. *Basal Ganglia Pathology*

The results of animal lesion studies and human clinicopathological studies clearly established over a century ago that damage to the basal ganglia results in the production of characteristic motor symptoms and deficits *(111–113)*. The majority of these deficits are now thought to be due to interruption of basal ganglia outputs with motor areas of cortex, although other deficits are clearly due to more direct influences on descending pathways. It is surprising to note, however, that for nearly the same amount of time, basal ganglia lesions were also associated with higher order cognitive and behavioral symptoms (see refs. *1,111,114–116*).

The physiological and functional imaging studies discussed thus far lead to the prediction that a lesion of basal ganglia circuitry involving areas 9 and 46 would lead to disruption of spatial working memory, planning and sequential working memory, and rule-based behavior. It is also possible that such deficits would be particularly manifest in tasks that required reward information to be integrated with a behavioral act. In actual fact, however, it is not likely that lesions of single basal ganglia circuits exist. Most of the clinical and pathological reports of patients with basal ganglia damage indicate that these patients display a number of different symptoms, including both motor and nonmotor ones, and it is quite likely that these symptoms are due to involvement of several subcortical projection systems. Despite these limitations, it is possible to reach some conclusions about the relative involvement of the basal ganglia in cognitive function based on the analysis of fairly localized pathology of the input and output levels of processing.

2.2.3.1. Input Level Pathology

Reversible lesion studies in monkeys have shown that the anterior striatum is particularly important for the learning of new movement sequences, while middle regions of the striatum appear to be more involved in the performance of previously learned movement sequences *(117)*. These findings are consistent with some of the previously discussed observations that portions of the striatum appear to be activated during the learning and the monitoring of sequences of motor acts that must be performed to complete some tasks. Interestingly, some patients with Parkinson's disease and Huntington's disease are also impaired on various tests of sequence learning and sequential task performance *(118–120)*. In view of the evidence, already reviewed, that dorsolateral prefrontal areas may be involved in aspects of sequential task performance, such as the learning and monitoring of sequences or behavioral actions, it is possible that damage to basal ganglia circuits with these areas could disrupt performance of these types of cognitive tasks.

The performance of spatial and nonspatial working memory and rule-based tasks is also affected by striatal pathology. In monkeys, experimental lesions of the dorsal caudate nucleus produce deficits in spatial delayed-response tasks that resemble the deficits seen after lesions of area 46 *(121)*. In contrast, lesions of the ventral caudate produce deficits in nonspatial delayed-response tasks that resemble those seen after area 12 lesions *(121)*. In humans, damage of some of these same striatal regions occurs in Huntington's disease and Parkinson's disease *(122,123)*. Detailed examinations of patients with these disorders have revealed striking deficits in spatial working memory and other cognitive tasks that precede the development of prominent motor symptoms *(124–132)*. Interestingly, recent studies using two of the animal models of Parkinson's disease and Huntington's disease also support these findings. Examination of primates early in the course of chronic low-dose 3-nitropropionic acid (3-NP) or 1-methyl-4-phenyl-1, 2, 3, 6-tetrahydropyridine (MPTP) treatment has revealed the presence of profound cognitive deficits that precede the development of gross motor impairments *(133–136)*. Thus, one conclusion from these studies is that the initial striatal pathology selectively alters prefrontal-basal ganglia circuits to produce these cognitive deficits, while sparing (in most cases) motor circuits.

2.2.3.2. Output Level Pathology

An "isolated" bilateral lesion of the SNpr was reported in one elderly patient diagnosed with peduncular hallucinosis *(114)*. This individual demonstrated deficits in working memory and other cognitive functions, visual hallucinations, and mild neurological symptoms. It is possible that this lesion affected nigral outputs to the prefrontal as well as inferotemporal areas of cortex to produce the complex cognitive and perceptual symptoms that he displayed, while alterations of the outputs to motor areas may have led to his motor difficulties *(137)*.

Parallel findings have been reported in patients with "localized" lesions of the globus pallidus. In addition to varying degrees of motor deficits, the majority of these patients suffered from cognitive deficits such as working memory and card sorting difficulties, compulsive behaviors, and "psychic akinesia," or a lack of a desire to move *(138,139)*. Perhaps the best evidence for the involvement of the globus pallidus in cognitive function, however, has come from the careful evaluation of subjects who have undergone surgical pallidotomy for the treatment of Parkinson's disease. As one recent analysis has shown *(140)*, these subjects often display prominent cognitive impairments on tasks that would normally engage prefrontal-subcortical networks. Moreover, the degree of these impairments is directly related to the anatomical location of the pallidal lesion. Lesions confined to more rostral and dorsomedial regions of GPi produce the greatest cognitive deficits in the patients, consistent with the fact that these GPi regions contain neurons that project to prefrontal areas 9 and 46. In contrast, surgical lesions in more posterior and ventrolateral regions of GPi (which project to skeletomotor areas of cortex) have the greatest effect on motor symptoms. The authors of that study concluded that their results provide further evidence for the segregation of motor and cognitive circuitry within the basal ganglia.

Finally, there is some evidence that abnormalities in basal ganglia circuits may underlie some of the hallmark cognitive deficits seen in certain neuropsychiatric disorders, including schizophrenia, depression, obsessive–compulsive disorder, Tourette's syndrome, autism, and attention deficit disorder. In schizophrenia in particular, there is growing evidence that patients early in the course of the illness have profound deficits in formal tests of planning, working memory, and rule formation *(141–143)* In fact, it appears that these deficits are very often present years before the onset of florid psychosis and may represent one of the best predictors of the course of the illness *(144)*. Obviously, for any serious mental illness, there is always the potential confound of medication on findings, and such concerns should be of paramount importance in the interpretation of findings regarding the basal ganglia. However, Early and colleagues *(145)* demonstrated conclusively that in 10 never-medicated subjects with schizophrenia, there was a consistent abnormality in blood flow within the globus pallidus that was not present in any of 20 control subjects. When this evidence is viewed along with the strong evidence for prefrontal, striatal, and thalamic abnormalities in schizophrenia *(146)*, it is tempting to think that there is a prefrontal-basal ganglia circuit dysfunction in this illness. Although there are now numerous theories describing how this dysfunction could contribute to the pathophysiology of schizophrenia, it is likely that Mettler *(147)* was the first to suggest that schizophrenia was a perceptual disorder caused by primary striatal and pallidal dysfunction, which resulted in secondary cortical dysfunction. Whether such a causal relationship exists remains to be seen.

2.2.4. Molecular Clues to Basal Ganglia Influences on Cognition

With the advent of modern molecular biological approaches to the study of complex disease states, it is now possible to rapidly screen the expression of thousands of genes at a time in different neurological and psychiatric disorders, as well as map the normal expression patterns of these genes through the brain. It is only a matter of time before the anatomical maps of gene expression in the brain rival the resolution of the anatomical maps of human brain activation produced by functional imaging studies. The incorporation and analysis of this vast amount of new information will require a thorough understanding of how all the pieces of the basal ganglia puzzle fit together. Space does not permit a complete or even partial review of the literature that is available on the effects of different agents on cognitive function that could be due to direct influences on prefrontal-basal ganglia circuits. Nonetheless, a few of the molecules, with rather striking patterns of expression in the basal ganglia, do appear to have the potential to be involved in cognitive processing and are briefly mentioned here.

2.2.4.1. Enkephalin

As previously noted, cells in all parts of the striatum that project to the external segment of the globus pallidus (and form part of the indirect pathway) express high levels of enkephalin. In early Huntington's disease, there appears to be a preferential loss of the enkephalin-containing cells in the caudate compared to substance P-containing cells that project to GPi *(148,149)* and, thus, a qualitatively different effect on the indirect versus the direct pathway. Recent reports of monkeys early in the course of MPTP treatment indicates that there is overexpression of preproenkephalin in dorsolateral regions of caudate and putamen, as well as the caudal body of the caudate, which occurs without any motor symptoms *(150)*. Thus, in early Huntington's disease and experimentally induced Parkinson's disease, some of the same neuronal populations could be affected in the same portions of the striatum; namely, those regions that receive input from cognitive areas and visual association areas of the cerebral cortex. This fact is all the more interesting in light of the evidence already presented that patients, early in the course of these disorders, as well as primates being treated with neurotoxins to mimic these disorders, all develop well-described impairments in cognitive and visual functions, often in the absence of gross motor impairments *(129–136)*.

Although it may not immediately be apparent how the preferential dysfunction of enkephalin-containing neurons in nonmotor regions of the striatum could arise, one remote possibility is that such findings may be related to the regional differences in dopamine receptor subtype expression within the striatum. For example, enkephalin-containing cells are known to be D2 positive, and D2 positive cells are most concentrated in the striatal matrix and increase in relative number from rostral to caudal. In contrast, D1 receptor subtypes are expressed most highly in striosomes and increase from caudal to rostral striatal regions. Thus, disruptions of enkephalin-containing cells in early Huntington's and

Parkinson's disease, as well as the animal models of these disorders, may produce more of an affect on cognitive function, because the rostral regions of the striatum would have less reserves of enkephalin and D2 positive cells to draw on to restore normal circuit function. Some indirect support for this possibility was provided in a study of enkephalin knock-out mice by Konig and colleagues *(151)*. Mice homozygous for the mutant gene were viable and fertile and cared for their offspring, but displayed a pattern of distinctive behavioral abnormalities that included hiding under the bedding, "frantic" running or jumping, and prolonged freezing in response to moderate noise. The authors also reported that the mice appeared more anxious and that the males were more aggressive, but none of the mice had gross motor impairments. Such symptoms are consistent with a preferential effect on rostral striatal regions.

2.2.4.2. Cannabinoids

In addition to enkephalin, there is a large body of evidence that cognitive alterations or enhancements can be produced by the selective action of certain receptor subtypes that have localized patterns of expression in the basal ganglia. Some of these include cannabinoids, which

have very well-described effects on motor and cognitive function. Cannabinoid receptors are extremely abundant in the output nuclei of the basal ganglia, in addition to prefrontal regions of the cerebral cortex *(152)*. In fact, cannabinoid binding intensity may be the highest in the SNpr compared to all other brain regions *(152)*. Recent studies that have analyzed formal cognitive processing in cannabis users compared to controls found a significant effect of cannabis abuse on tests of memory, learning, word fluency, speed of processing, and manual dexterity *(153)*. In Huntington's disease, there is an apparent preferential loss of cannabinoid receptors on striatal nerve terminals in the GPe versus GPi in all stages of this illness *(154)*. These observations provide further support for the preferential involvement of the indirect pathway in Huntington's disease, and also suggest that the cognitive effects of cannabinoid use may be strongly mediated through their action on prefrontal-basal ganglia circuits.

2.2.4.3. Adenosine

In contrast to cannabinoids, which impair cognitive processing, caffeine has a clear cognitive enhancing effect, when taken in moderate doses. It is thought that adenosine receptor antagonism by caffeine is the basis for this effect. A recent behavioral study with mice found that selective antagonists of the adenosine A2A receptor produce improvements in learning, but not selective A1 antagonists *(155)*. In the striatum, adenosine A2A receptors are highly expressed in medium spiny neurons in the striatal matrix *(156)*. Interestingly, a recent report found that selective A2A antagonist administration to Parkinson's disease patients had a protective effect, resulting in a slower progression of symptoms *(157)*. The precise mechanism for this effect is not clear, although it is possible that the A2A antagonist administration helped reduce abnormal activity in basal ganglia circuits brought on by loss of dopamine inputs to the striatum because it is known that adenosine and D2 receptors have strong interactions on G(i/o)-mediated second messenger systems in striatal cells.

2.2.4.4. Other Molecules and Directions

Some cholecystokinin receptor subtypes are also highly abundant in regions of the striatum and SNpr that participate in cognitive and limbic processing *(158)*. There is evidence that selective actions of some cholecystokinin receptors can greatly affect cognitive and limbic functions, including recall, anxiety, and satiety in addition to reward-seeking behavior *(158,159)*. Aside from these systems, it is also clear that manipulation of serotonin systems, neuropeptide systems, noradrenergic systems, and cholinergic systems, to name but a few, can produce cognitive impairments or enhancements that may be mediated, in part, by prefrontal-basal ganglia circuits. Such observations should not be viewed as necessarily surprising, but rather simply a reflection of the diverse anatomical and molecular relationships that exist between the prefrontal cortex and basal ganglia. In the near future, it may be possible to exploit new molecular biological technologies to identify circuit-specific genes and proteins and to develop agents that can selectively and therapeutically alter the expression of these molecules to correct a behavioral deficit or restore normal function.

3. SUMMARY AND CONCLUSION

The prefrontal cortex and basal ganglia participate in multiple anatomical circuits. These circuits appear to maintain many of the physiological and behavioral properties of the cortical areas that they subserve. In addition, there appears to be a considerable increase in the relative influence of reward on neurons within prefrontal-basal ganglia circuits compared to neurons in the cortical areas they innervate. Such influences cannot be completely separated from the role that basal ganglia circuits play in cognition, since the ultimate goal of most cognitive acts is the achievement of some predetermined goal or reward. In contrast, the effects of basal ganglia pathology on cognitive processing are clearly distinguishable from effects on motor behavior. However, whether the cognitive deficits that arise from basal ganglia dysfunction are solely a reflection of abnormal cognitive processing or also reflect dissolution of the influence that reward-related signals play on this processing is not clear. Indeed, much additional research is needed to help sort out the precise contributions of the basal ganglia to cognitive behavior.

REFERENCES

1. Alexander, G.E., DeLong, M.R., and Strick, P.L. (1986) Parallel organization of functionally segregated circuits linking basal ganglia and cortex. *Annu. Rev. Neurosci.* **9,** 357–381.
2. Alheid, G.F., Heimer, L., and Switzer, R.C. (1990) Basal ganglia, in *The Human Nervous System*, Academic Press, New York, pp. 483–582.
3. Parent, A. and Hazrati, L.-N. (1995) Functional anatomy of the basal ganglia. I. The cortico-basal ganglia-thalamo-cortical loop. *Brain Res. Rev.* **20,** 91–127.
4. Parent, A. and Hazrati, L.-N. (1995) Functional anatomy of the basal ganglia. II. The place of subthalamic nucleus and external pallidum in basal ganglia circuitry. *Brain Res. Rev.* **20,** 128–154.
5. Percheron, G., Francois, C., Talbi, B., Yelnik, J., and Fenelon, G. (1996) The primate motor thalamus. *Brain Res. Rev.* **22,** 93–181.
6. Kawaguchi, Y., Wilson, C.J., Augood, S.J., and Emson, P.C. (1995) Striatal interneurones: chemical, physiological and morphological characterization. *Trends Neurosci.* **18,** 527–535.
7. Ragsdale, C.W. and Graybiel, A.M. (1981) The fronto-striatal projection in the cat and monkey and its relationship to inhomogeneities established by acetylcholinesterase histochemistry. *Brain Res.* **208,** 259–266.
8. Eblen, F. and Graybiel, A.M. (1995) Highly restricted origin of prefrontal cortical inputs to striosomes in the macaque monkey. *J. Neurosci.* **15,** 5999–6013.
9. DeLong, M.R. (1990) Primate models of movement disorders of basal ganglia origin. *Trends Neurosci.* **13,** 281–285.
10. Carlsson, M. and Carlsson, A. (1990) Interactions between glutamatergic and monoaminergic systems within the basal ganglia—implications for schizophrenia and Parkinson's disease. *Trends Neurosci.* **13,** 272–276.
11. Johnson, A.E., Coirini, H., Kallstrom, L., and Wiesel, F.A. (1994) Characterization of dopamine receptor binding sites in the subthalamic nucleus. *Neuroreport* **5,** 1836–1838.
12. Aosaki, T., Kimura, M., and Graybiel, A.M. (1995) Temporal and spatial characteristics of tonically active neurons of the primate's striatum. *J. Neurophysiol.* **73,** 1234–1252.
13. Marin, O., Anderson, S.A., and Rubenstein, J.L. (2000) Origin and molecular specification of striatal interneurons. *J Neurosci.* **20,** 6063–6076.
14. Kemp, J.M. and Powell, T.P.S. (1971) The connexions of the striatum and globus pallidus: synthesis and speculation. *Phil. Trans. Royal Soc. London B* **262,** 441–457.
15. Asanuma, C., Thach, W.T., and Jones, E.G. (1983) Distribution of cerebellar terminations in the ventral lateral thalamic region of the monkey. *Brain Res. Rev.* **5,** 237–265.
16. Middleton, F.A. and Strick, P.L. (2000) A revised neuroanatomy of frontal subcortical circuits, in *Frontal Subcortical Circuits in Psychiatric and Neurological Disorders* (Lichter, D.G. and Cummings, J.L., eds.), Guilford, New York, pp. 44–58.
17. Rosenkilde, C.E. (1979) Functional heterogeneity of the prefrontal cortex in the monkey: a review. *Behav. Neural. Biol.* **25,** 301–345.
18. Goldman-Rakic, P.S. (1987) Circuitry of primate prefrontal cortex and regulation of behavior by representational memory, in *Handbook of Physiology, Section 1. The Nervous System* (Plum, F., ed.), American Physiological Society, Bethesda, pp. 373–413.
19. Goldman-Rakic, P.S. (1990) Cellular and circuit basis of working memory in prefrontal cortex of nonhuman primates. *Prog. Brain Res.* **85,** 325–336.
20. Passingham, R. (1993) *The Frontal Lobes and Voluntary Action,* Oxford University Press, Oxford.
21. Fuster, J.M. (1997) *The Prefrontal Cortex*, Raven Press, New York.
22. Fuster, J.M., Bauer, R.H., and Jervey, J.P. (1982) Cellular discharge in the dorsolateral prefrontal cortex of the monkey in cognitive tasks. *Exp. Neurol.* **77,** 679–694.

23. Carlson, S., Rama, P., Tanila, H., Linnankoski, I., and Mansikka, H. (1997) Dissociation of mnemonic coding and other functional neuronal processing in the monkey prefrontal cortex. *J. Neurophysiol.* **77,** 761–774.
24. Fuster, J.M. and Alexander, G.E. (1971) Neuron activity related to short-term memory. *Science* **173,** 652–654.
25. Kubota, K. and Niki, H. (1971) Prefrontal cortical unit activity and delayed alternation performance in monkeys. *J. Neurophysiol.* **34,** 337–347.
26. Funahashi, S., Inoue, M., and Kubota, K. (1997) Delay-period activity in the primate prefrontal cortex encoding multiple spatial positions and their order of presentation. *Behav. Brain Res.* **84,** 203–223.
27. Komatsu, H. (1982) Prefrontal unit activity during a color discrimination task with GO and NO-GO responses in the monkey. *Brain Res.* **244,** 269–277.
28. Kubota, K. and Komatsu, H. (1985) Neuron activities of monkey prefrontal cortex during the learning of visual discrimination tasks with GO/NO-GO performances. *Neurosci. Res.* **3,** 106–129.
29. Watanabe, M. (1986) Prefrontal unit activity during delayed conditional Go/No-Go discrimination in the monkey. I. Relation to the stimulus. *Brain Res.* **382,** 1–14.
30. Yamatani, K., Ono, T., Nishijo, H., and Takaku, A. (1990) Activity and distribution of learning-related neurons in monkey (*Macaca fuscata*) prefrontal cortex. *Behav. Neurosci.* **104,** 503–531.
31. Sasaki, K. and Gemba, H. (1986) Electrical activity in the prefrontal cortex specific to no-go reaction of conditioned hand movement with color discrimination in the monkey. *Exp. Brain Res.* **64,** 603–606.
32. Petrides, M. (1995) Impairments on nonspatial self-ordered and externally-ordered working memory tasks after lesions of the mid-dorsal part of the lateral frontal cortex in the monkey. *J. Neurosci.* **15,** 359–375.
33. Petrides, M. and Milner, B. (1982) Deficits on subject-ordered tasks after frontal- and temporal-lobe lesions in man. *Neuropsychologia* **20,** 249–262.
34. Milner, B. (1963) Effects of different brain lesions on card sorting. *Arch. Neurol.* **9,** 90–100.
35. Pascual-Leone, A., Grafman, J., and Hallett, M. (1995) Procedural learning and prefrontal cortex. *Ann. NY Acad. Sci.* **769,** 61–70.
36. Sirigu, A., Zalla, T., Pillon, B., Grafman, J., Dubois, B., and Agid, Y. (1995) Planning and script analysis following prefrontal lobe lesions. *Ann. NY Acad. Sci.* **769,** 277–288.
37. Pascual-Leone, A., Wassermann, E.M., Grafman, J., and Hallett, M. (1996) The role of the dorsolateral prefrontal cortex in implicit procedural learning. *Exp. Brain Res.* **107,** 479–485.
38. Jacobsen, C.F. (1936) Studies of cerebral function in primates: I. The functions of the frontal association areas in monkeys. *Comp. Psychol. Monogr.* **13,** 3–60.
39. Luria, A.R. (1966) *Higher Cortical Functions in Man*, Basic Books, New York.
40. Stuss, D.T. and Benson, D.F. (1986) *The Frontal Lobes*, Raven Press, New York.
41. Butter, C.M. (1969) Perseveration in extinction and in discrimination reversal tasks following selective frontal lobe ablations in *Macaca mulatta*. *Science* **144,** 313–315.
42. Iversen, S.D. and Mishkin, M. (1970) Perseverative interference in monkeys following selective lesions of the inferior prefrontal convexity. *Exp. Brain Res.* **11,** 376–386.
43. Ocsar-Berman, M. (1973) The effects of dorsolateral-frontal and ventrolateral-orbitofrontal lesions on spatial discrimination learning and delayed response in two modalities. *Neuropsychologia* **13,** 237–246.
44. Passingham, R. (1975) Delayed matching after selective prefrontal lesions in monkeys. *Brain Res.* **92,** 89–102.
45. Mishkin, M. and Manning, F.J. (1978) Non-spatial memory after selective prefrontal lesions in monkeys. *Brain Res.* **143,** 313–323.
46. Rushworth, M.F., Nixon, P.D., Eacott, M.J., and Passingham, R.E. (1997) Ventral prefrontal cortex is not essential for working memory. *J. Neurosci.* **17,** 4829–4838.
47. Deiber, M.P., Passingham, R.E., Colebatch, J.G., Friston, K.J., Nixon, P.D., and Frackowiak, R.S. (1991) Cortical areas and the selection of movement: a study with positron emission tomography. *Exp. Brain Res.* **84,** 393–402.
48. Frith, C.D., Friston, K., Liddle, P.F., and Frackowiak, R.S.J. (1991) Willed action and the prefrontal cortex in man: a study with PET. *Proc. R. Soc. London B* **244,** 241–246.
49. Petrides, M., Alivisatos, B., Evans, A.C., and Meyer, E. (1993) Dissociation of human mid-dorsolateral from posterior dorsolateral frontal cortex in memory processing. *Proc. Natl. Acad. Sci. USA* **90,** 873–877.
50. Jenkins, I.H., Brooks, D.J., Nixon, P.D., Frackowiak, R.S., and Passingham, R.E. (1994) Motor sequence learning: a study with positron emission tomography. *J. Neurosci.* **14,** 3775–3790.
51. Owen, A.M., Doyon, J., Petrides, M., and Evans, A.C. (1996) Planning and spatial working memory: a positron emission tomography study in humans. *Eur. J. Neurosci.* **8,** 353–364.
52. Baker, S.C., Rogers, R.D., Owen, A.M., et al. (1996) Neural systems engaged by planning: a PET study of the Tower of London task. *Neuropsychologia* **34,** 515–526.
53. Jueptner, M., Frith, C.D., Brooks, D.J., Frackowiak, R.S., and Passingham, R.E. (1997a) Anatomy of motor learning. II. Subcortical structures and learning by trial and error. *J. Neurophysiol.* **77,** 1325–1337.
54. Jueptner, M., Stephan, K.M., Frith, C.D., Brooks, D.J., Frackowiak, R.S., and Passingham, R.E. (1997b) Anatomy of motor learning. I. Frontal cortex and attention to action. *J. Neurophysiol.* **77,** 1313–1324.
55. Sakai, K., Hikosaka, O., Miyauchi, S., Takino, R., Sasaki, Y., and Putz, B. (1998) Transition of brain activation from frontal to parietal areas in visuomotor sequence learning. *J. Neurosci.* **18,** 1827–1840.
56. Paulesu, E., Frith, C.D., and Frackowiak, R.S.J. (1993) The neural correlates of the verbal component of working memory. *Nature* **362,** 342–345.
57. Petrides, M., Alivisatos, B., Meyer, E., and Evans, A.C. (1993) Functional activation of the human frontal cortex during the performance of verbal working memory tasks. *Proc. Natl. Acad. Sci. USA* **90,** 878–882.

58. Petrides, M., Alivisatos, B., and Evans, A.C. (1995) Functional activation of the human ventrolateral frontal cortex during mnemonic retrieval of verbal information. *Proc. Natl. Acad. Sci. USA* **92,** 5803–5807.
59. Roskies, A.L., Fiez, J.A., Balota, D.A., Raichle, M.E., and Petersen, S.E. (2001) Task-dependent modulation of regions in the left inferior frontal cortex during semantic processing. *J. Cogn. Neurosci.* **13,** 829–843.
60. Buckner, R.L., Petersen, S.E., Ojemann, J.G., Miezin, F.M., Squire, L.R., and Raichle, M.E. (1995) Functional anatomical studies of explicit and implicit memory retrieval tasks. *J. Neurosci.* **15,** 12–29.
61. Grabowski, T.J., Frank, R.J., Brown, C.K., et al. (1996) Reliability of PET activation across statistical methods, subject groups, and sample sizes. *Human Brain Mapping* **4,** 23–46.
62. Herholtz, K., Thiel, A., Wienhard, K., et al. (1996) Individual functional anatomy of verb generation. *Neuroimage* **3,** 185–194.
63. Partiot, A., Grafman, J., Sadato, N., Flitman, S., and Wild, K. (1996) Brain activation during script even processing. *Neuroreport* **7,** 761–766.
64. Kawashima, R., Satoh, K., Itoh, H., et al. (1996) Functional anatomy of GO/NO-GO discrimination and response selection—a PET study in man. *Brain Res.* **728,** 79–89.
65. Petersen, S.E., Fox, P.T., Posner, M.I., Mintun, M., and Raichle, M.E. (1988) Positron emission tomographic studies of the cortical anatomy of single-word processing. *Nature* **331,** 585–589.
66. Grasby, P.M., Frith, C.D., Friston, K.J., Bench, C., Frackowiak, R.S.J., and Dolan, R.J. (1993) Functional mapping of brain areas implicated in auditory-verbal memory function. *Brain* **116,** 1–20.
67. Friedman, H.R. and Goldman-Rakic, P.S. (1994) Coactivation of prefrontal cortex and inferior parietal cortex in working memory tasks revealed by 2DG functional mapping in the rhesus monkey. *J. Neurosci.* **14,** 2775–2788.
68. McCarthy, G., Blamire, A.M., Puce, A., et al. (1994) Functional magnetic resonance imaging of human prefrontal cortex during a spatial working memory task. *Proc. Natl. Acad. Sci. USA* **91,** 8690–8694.
69. Kosslyn, S.M., Alpert, N.M., Thompson, W.L., Chabris, C.F., Rauch, S.L., and Anderson, A.K. (1994) Identifying objects seen from different viewpoints. A PET investigation. *Brain* **117,** 1055–1071.
70. Klein, D., Milner, B., Zatorre, R.J., Meyer, E., and Evans, A.C. (1995) The neural substrates underlying word generation: a bilingual functional-imaging study. *Proc. Natl. Acad. Sci. USA* **92,** 2899–2903.
71. Demb, J.B., Desmond, J.E., Wagner, A.D., Vaidya, C.J., Glover, G.H., and Gabrieli, J.D. (1995) Semantic encoding and retrieval in the left inferior prefrontal cortex: a functional MRI study of task difficulty and process specificity. *J. Neurosci.* **15,** 5870–5878.
72. Schwartz, J.M., Stoessel, P.W., Baxter, L.R. Jr., Martin, K.M., and Phelps, M.E. (1996) Systematic changes in cerebral glucose metabolic rate after successful behavior modification treatment of obsessive-compulsive disorder. *Arch. Gen. Psych.* **53,** 109–113.
73. Smith, E.E., Jonides, J., and Koeppe, R.A. (1996) Dissociating verbal and spatial working memory using PET. *Cereb. Cortex* **6,** 11–20.
74. Haxby, J.V., Ungerleider, L.G., Horwitz, B., Maisog, J.M., Rapoport, S.I., and Grady, C.L. (1996) Face encoding and recognition in the human brain. *Proc. Natl. Acad. Sci. USA* **93,** 922–927.
75. Sweeney, J.A., Mintun, M.A., Kwee, S., et al. (1996) Positron emission tomography study of voluntary saccadic eye movements and spatial working memory. *J. Neurophysiol.* **75,** 454–468.
76. Courtney, S.M., Ungerleider, L.G., Keil, K., and Haxby, J.V. (1997) Transient and sustained activity in a distributed neural system for human working memory. *Nature* **386,** 608–611.
77. Tsujimoto, T., Ogawa, M., Nishikawa, S., Tsukada, H., Kakiuchi, T., and Sasaki, K. (1997) Activation of the prefrontal, occipital and parietal cortices during go/no-go discrimination tasks in the monkey as revealed by positron emission tomography. *Neurosci. Lett.* **224,** 111–114.
78. Raichle, M.E., Fiez, J.A., Videen, T.O., et al. (1994) Practice-related changes in human brain functional anatomy during nonmotor learning. *Cereb. Cortex* **4,** 8–26.
79. Awh, E., Smith, E.E., and Jonides, J. (1995) Human rehearsal processes and the frontal lobes: PET evidence. *Ann. NY Acad. Sci.* **769,** 97–117.
80. Fiez, J.A., Raife, E.A., Balota, D.A., Schwarz, J.P., Raichle, M.E., and Petersen, S.E. (1996) A positron emission tomography study of the short-term maintenance of verbal information. *J. Neurosci.* **16,** 808–822.
81. Abdullaev, Y.G., Bechtereva, N.P., and Melnichuk, K.V. (1998) Neuronal activity of human caudate nucleus and prefrontal cortex in cognitive tasks. *Behav. Brain Res.* **97,** 159–177.
82. Kermadi, I. and Joseph, J.P. (1995) Activity in the caudate nucleus of monkey during spatial sequencing. *J. Neurophysiol.* **74,** 911–933.
83. Schultz, W. and Romo, R. (1992) Role of primate basal ganglia and frontal cortex in the internal generation of movements. I. Preparatory activity in the anterior striatum. *Exp. Brain Res.* **91,** 363–384.
84. Shuvaev, V.T. and Shefer, V.I. (1995) Structure of neuronal activity of the caudate nucleus of monkeys during decision-making and the realization of the motor program in different variants of a delayed spatial choice task. *Neurosci. Behav. Physiol.* **25,** 63–70.
85. Nishino, H., Ono, T., Fukuda, M., Sasaki, K., and Muramoto, K.I. (1981) Single unit activity in monkey caudate nucleus during operant bar pressing feeding behavior. *Neurosci. Lett.* **21,** 105–110.
86. Kawagoe, R., Takikawa, Y., and Hikosaka, O. (1998) Expectation of reward modulates cognitive signals in the basal ganglia. *Nat. Neurosci.* **1,** 411–416.
87. Hassani, O.K., Cromwell, H.C., and Schultz, W. (2001) Influence of expectation of different rewards on behavior-related neuronal activity in the striatum. *J. Neurophysiol.* **85,** 2477–2489.

88. DeLong, M.R. (1971) Activity of pallidal neurons during movement. *J. Neurophysiol.* **34,** 414–427.
89. Hikosaka, O. and Wurtz, R.H. (1983) Visual and oculomotor functions of monkey substantia nigra pars reticulata. I. Relation of visual and auditory responses to saccades. *J. Neurophysiol.* **49,** 1230–1253.
90. DeLong, M.R., Crutcher, M.D., and Georgopoulos, A.P. (1983) Relations between movement and single cell discharge in the substantia nigra of the behaving monkey. *J. Neurosci.* **3,** 1599–1606.
91. Anderson, M.E. and Horak, F.B. (1985) Influence of the globus pallidus on arm movements in monkeys. III. Timing of movement-related information. *J. Neurophysiol.* **54,** 433–448.
92. Schultz, W. (1986) Activity of pars reticulata neurons of monkey substantia nigra in relation to motor, sensory, and complex events. *J. Neurophysiol.* **55,** 660–677.
93. Bakay, R.A., DeLong, M.R., and Vitek, J.L. (1992) Posteroventral pallidotomy for Parkinson's disease. *J. Neurosurg.* **77,** 487–488.
94. Kirschman, D.L., Milligan, B., Wilkinson, S., et al. (2000) Pallidotomy microelectrode targeting: neurophysiology-based target refinement. *Neurosurgery* **46,** 613–622.
95. Baron, M.S., Vitek, J.L., Bakay, R.A., et al. (1996) Treatment of advanced Parkinson's disease by posterior GPi pallidotomy: 1-year results of a pilot study. *Ann. Neurol.* **40,** 355–366.
96. Middleton, F.A. and Strick, P.L. (2000) Basal ganglia output and cognition: evidence from anatomical, behavioral and clinical studies. *Brain Cogn.* **42,** 183–200.
97. Hikosaka, O., Sakamoto, M., and Miyashita, N. (1993) Effects of caudate nucleus stimulation on substantia nigra cell activity in monkey. *Exp. Brain Res.* **95,** 457–472.
98. Mushiake, H. and Strick, P.L. (1995a) Pallidal neuron activity during sequential arm movements. *J. Neurophysiol.* **74,** 2754–2758.
99. Mushiake, H. and Strick, P.L. (1995b) Cerebellar and pallidal activity during instructed delay periods. *Soc. Neurosci. Abstr.* **21,** 411.
100. Travis, R. and Sparks, D.L. (1968) Unitary response and discrimination learning in the squirrel monkey: the globus pallidus. *Physiol. Behav.* **3,** 187–196.
101. DeLong, M.R. (1971) Activity of pallidal neurons during movement. *J. Neurophysiol.* **34,** 414–427.
102. Gdowski, M.J., Miller, L.E., Parrish, T., Nenonene, E.K., and Houk, J.C. (2001) Context dependency in the globus pallidus internal segment during targeted arm movements. *J. Neurophysiol.* **85,** 998–1004.
103. Schultz, W. (1998) Predictive reward signal of dopamine neurons. *J. Neurophysiol.* **80,** 1–27.
104. Owen, A.M., Doyon, J., Dagher, A., Sadikot, A., and Evans, A.C. (1998) Abnormal basal ganglia outflow in Parkinson's disease identified with PET. Implications for higher cortical functions. *Brain.* **121,** 949–965.
105. Owen, A.M. (1997) Cognitive planning in humans: neuropsychological, neuroanatomical and neuropharmacological perspectives. *Prog. Neurobiol.* **53,** 431–450.
106. Owen, A.M., James, M., Leigh, P.N., et al. (1992) Fronto-striatal cognitive deficits at different stages of Parkinson's disease. *Brain* **115,** 1727–1751.
107. Owen, A.M., Beksinska, M., James, M., et al. (1993) Visuospatial memory deficits at different stages of Parkinson's disease. *Neuropsychologia* **31,** 627–644.
108. Delgado, M.R., Nystrom, L.E., Fissell, C., Noll, D.C., and Fiez, J.A. (2000) Tracking the hemodynamic responses to reward and punishment in the striatum. *J. Neurophysiol.* **84,** 3072–3077.
109. Elliott, R., Friston, K.J., and Dolan, R.J. (2000) Dissociable neural responses in human reward systems. *J. Neurosci.* **20,** 6159–6165.
110. Manoach, D.S., Gollub, R.L., Benson, E.S., et al. (2000) Schizophrenic subjects show aberrant fMRI activation of dorsolateral prefrontal cortex and basal ganglia during working memory performance. *Biol. Psychiatry* **48,** 99–109.
111. Wilson, S.A.K. (1912) Progressive lenticular degeneration. *Brain* **34,** 295–509.
112. Lewy, F.H. (1942) Historical introduction, in *The Disease of the Basal Ganglia (*Putnam, T.J., Frantz, A.M., and Ranson, S.W., eds.), William and Wilkins, Baltimore, pp. 1–20.
113. Bhatia, K.P. and Marsden, C.D. (1994) The behavioural and motor consequences of focal lesions of the basal ganglia in man. *Brain* **117,** 859–876.
114. McKee, A.C., Levine, D.N., Kowall, N.W., and Richardson, E.P. (1990) Peduncular hallucinosis associated with isolated infarction of the substantia nigra pars reticulata. *Ann. Neurol.* **27,** 500–504.
115. Rogers, D. (1992) *Motor Disorder in Psychiatry: Towards a Neurological Psychiatry,* Wiley & Sons, Chichester.
116. Partiot, A., Verin, M., Pillon, B., Teixeira-Ferreira, C., Agid, Y., and Dubois, B. (1996) Delayed response tasks in basal ganglia lesions in man: further evidence for a striato-frontal cooperation in behavioural adaptation. *Neuropsychologia* **34,** 709–721.
117. Miyachi, S., Hikosaka, O., Miyashita, K., Karadi, Z., Rand, M.K. (1997) Differential roles of monkey striatum in learning of sequential hand movement. *Exp. Brain Res.* **115,** 1–5.
118. Saint-Cyr, J.A., Taylor, A.E., and Lang, A.E. (1988) Procedural learning and neostriatal dysfunction in man. *Brain* **111,** 941–959.
119. Heindel, W.C., Salmon, D.P., Shults, C.W., Walicke, P.A., and Butters, N. (1989) Neuropsychological evidence for multiple implicit memory systems: a comparison of Alzheimer's, Huntington's, and Parkinson's disease patients. *J. Neurosci.* **9,** 582–587.
120. Pascual-Leone, A., Grafman, J., Clark, K., Stewart, M., Massaquoi, S., Lou, J.S., and Hallett, M. (1993) Procedural learning in Parkinson's disease and cerebellar degeneration. *Ann. Neurol.* **34,** 594–602.
121. Divac, I., Rosvold, H.E., and Swarcbart, M.K. (1967) Behavioral effects of selective ablation of the caudate nucleus. *J. Comp. Physiol. Psychol.* **63,** 184–190.

122. vonSattel, J.P., Myers, R.H., Stevens, T.J., Ferrante, R.J., Bird, E.D., and Richardson, E.P. (1985) Neuropathological classification of Huntington's disease. *J. Neuropathol. Exp. Neurol.* **44,** 559–577.
123. Kish, S.J., Shannak, K., and Hornykiewicz, O. (1988) Uneven pattern of dopamine loss in the striatum of patients with idiopathic Parkinson's disease. Pathophysiologic and clinical implications. *N. Engl. J. Med.* **318,** 876–880.
124. Butters, N., Sax, D., Montgomery, K., and Tarlow, S. (1978) Comparison of the neuropsychological deficits associated with early and advanced Huntington's disease. *Arch. Neurol.* **35,** 585–589.
125. Levin, B.E., Llabre, M.M., and Weiner, W.J. (1989) Cognitive impairments associated with early Parkinson's disease. *Neurology* **39,** 557–561.
126. Taylor, A.E., Saint-Cyr, J.A., and Lang, A.E. (1990) Memory and learning in early Parkinson's disease: evidence for a "frontal lobe syndrome." *Brain Cogn.* **13,** 211–232.
127. Dewick, H.C., Hanley, J.R., Davies, A.D.M., Playfer, J., and Turnbull, C. (1991) Perception and memory for faces in Parkinson's disease. *Neuropsychologia* **29,** 785–802.
128. Farina, E., Cappa, S.F., Polimeni, M., et al. (1994) Frontal dysfunction in early Parkinson's disease. *Acta Neurol. Scand.* **90,** 34–38.
129. Jacobs, D.H., Shuren, J., and Heilman, K.M. (1995) Impaired perception of facial identity and facial affect in Huntington's disease. *Neurology* **45,** 1217–1218.
130. Jacobs, D.H., Shuren, J., and Heilman, K.M. (1995) Emotional facial imagery, perception, and expression in Parkinson's disease. *Neurology* **45,** 1696–1702.
131. Lawrence, A.D., Sahakian, B.J., Hodges, J.R., Rosser, A.E., Lange, K.W., and Robbins, T.W. (1996) Executive and mnemonic functions in early Huntington's disease. *Brain* **119,** 1633–1645.
132. Dubois, B. and Pillon, B. (1997) Cognitive deficits in Parkinson's disease. *J. Neurol.* **244,** 2–8.
133. Schneider, J.S. and Roeltgen, D.P. (1993) Delayed matching-to-sample, object retrieval, and discrimination reversal deficits in chronic low dose MPTP-treated monkeys. *Brain Res.* **615,** 351–354.
134. Roeltgen, D.P. and Schneider, J.S. (1994) Task persistence and learning ability in normal and chronic low dose MPTP-treated monkeys. *Behav. Brain Res.* **60,** 115–124.
135. Schneider, J.S. and Pope-Coleman, A. (1995) Cognitive deficits precede motor deficits in a slowly progressing model of parkinsonism in the monkey. *Neurodegeneration* **4,** 245–255.
136. Palfi, S., Ferrante, R.J., Brouillet, E., et al. (1996) Chronic 3-nitropropionic acid treatment in baboons replicates the cognitive and motor deficits of Huntington's disease. *J. Neurosci.* **16,** 3019–3025.
137. Middleton, F.A. and Strick, P.L. (1996) The temporal lobe is a target of output from the basal ganglia. *Proc. Natl. Acad. Sci. USA* **93,** 8683–8687.
138. Laplane, D., Levasseur, M., Pillon, B., et al. (1989) Obsessive-compulsive and other behavioural changes with bilateral basal ganglia lesions. A neuropsychological, magnetic resonance imaging and positron tomography study. *Brain* **112,** 699–725.
139. Strub, R.L. (1989) Frontal lobe syndrome in a patient with bilateral globus pallidus lesions. *Arch. Neurol.* **46,** 1024–1027.
140. Lombardi, W.J., Gross, R.E., Trepanier, L.L., Lang, A.E., Lozano, A.M., and Saint-Cyr, J.A. (2000) Relationship of lesion location to cognitive outcome following microelectrode-guided pallidotomy for Parkinson's disease: support for the existence of cognitive circuits in the human pallidum. *Brain* **123,** 746–758.
141. Andreasen, N.C., Rezzai, K., Alliger, R., et al. (1992) Hypofrontality in neuroleptic-naive patients and in patients with chronic schizophrenia. *Arch. Gen. Psych.* **49,** 943–958.
142. Berman, K.F., Torrey, E.F., Daniel, D.G., and Weinberger, D.R. (1992) Regional cerebral blood flow in monozygotic twins discordant and concordant for schizophrenia. *Arch. Gen. Psych.* **49,** 927–934.
143. Park, S. and Holzman, P.S. (1992) Schizophrenics show spatial working memory deficits. *Arch. Gen. Psych.* **49,** 975–982.
144. Lewis, D.A. and Lieberman, J.A. (2001) Catching up on schizophrenia: natural history and neurobiology. *Neuron* **28,** 325–334.
145. Early, T.S., Reiman, E.M., Raichle, M.E., and Spitznagel, E.L. (1987) Left globus pallidus abnormality in never-medicated patients with schizophrenia. *Proc. Natl. Acad. Sci. USA* **84,** 561–563.
146. Harrison, P.J. (1999) The neuropathology of schizophrenia. A critical review of the data and their interpretation. *Brain* **122,** 593–624.
147. Mettler, F. (1955) Perceptual capacity, functioning of the corpus striatum and schizophrenia. *Psychiat. Q.* **29,** 89–111.
148. Reiner, A., Albin, R.L., Anderson, K.D., D'Amato, C.J., Penney, J.B., and Young, A.B. (1988) Differential loss of striatal projection neurons in Huntington disease. *Proc. Natl. Acad. Sci. USA* **85,** 5733–5737.
149. Sapp, E., Ge, P., Aizawa, H., et al. (1995) Evidence for a preferential loss of enkephalin immunoreactivity in the external globus pallidus in low grade Huntington's disease using high resolution image analysis. *Neuroscience* **64,** 397–404.
150. Bezard, E., Ravenscroft, P., Gross, C.E., Crossman, A.R., and Brotchie, J.M. (2001) Upregulation of striatal preproenkephalin gene expression occurs before the appearance of parkinsonian signs in 1-methyl-4-phenyl-1,2,3,6-tetrahydropyridine monkeys. *Neurobiol. Dis.* **8,** 343–350.
151. Konig, M., Zimmer, A.M., Steiner, H., et al. (1996) Pain responses, anxiety and aggression in mice deficient in preproenkephalin. *Nature* **383,** 535–538.
152. Glass, M., Dragunow, M., and Faull, R.L. (1997) Cannabinoid receptors in the human brain: a detailed anatomical and quantitative autoradiographic study in the fetal, neonatal and adult human brain. *Neuroscience* **77,** 299–318.

153. Croft, R.J., Mackay, A.J., Mills, A.T., and Gruzelier, J.G. (2001) The relative contributions of ecstasy and cannabis to cognitive impairment. *Psychopharmacology* **153,** 373–379.
154. Richfield, E.K. and Herkenham, M. (1994) Selective vulnerability in Huntington's disease: preferential loss of cannabinoid receptors in lateral globus pallidus. *Ann. Neurol.* **36,** 577–584.
155. Kopf, S.R., Melani, A., Pedata, F., and Pepeu, G. (1999) Adenosine and memory storage: effect of A(1) and A(2) receptor antagonists. *Psychopharmacology* **146,** 214–219.
156. Kull, B., Svenningsson, P., and Fredholm, B.B. (2000) Adenosine A(2A) receptors are colocalized with and activate g(olf) in rat striatum. *Mol. Pharmacol.* **58,** 771–777.
157. Chen, J.F., Xu, K., Petzer, J.P., et al. (2001) Neuroprotection by caffeine and A(2A) adenosine receptor inactivation in a model of Parkinson's disease. *J. Neurosci.* **21,** RC143.
158. Kritzer M.F., Innis, R.B., and Goldman-Rakic, P.S. (1990) Regional distribution of cholecystokinin binding sites in macaque basal ganglia determined by in vitro receptor autoradiography. *Neuroscience* **38,** 81–92.
159. Dauge, V. and Lena, I. (1998) CCK in anxiety and cognitive processes. *Neurosci. Biobehav. Rev.* **22,** 815–825.

3

Integrating Cognition and Motivation into the Basal Ganglia Pathways of Action

Suzanne N. Haber, PhD

1. INTRODUCTION

The involvement of the basal ganglia in motor control is well documented, particularly in its association with the neurological disorders, Parkinson's disease (PD) and Huntington's disease (HD). It is the dorsal basal ganglia that is most affected in these diseases. In contrast, the ventral basal ganglia (the ventral striatum [VS] and ventral pallidum [VP]) are associated with mental health problems including schizophrenia and drug abuse and addiction *(1–5)*. Taken as a whole, the basal ganglia, both dorsal and ventral components, are involved in motor, cognitive, and limbic functions. These functions are thought to be contained in separate, segregated corticobasal ganglia circuits *(6)*. However, although severe motoric dysfunctions are associated with the dorsal striatum, and cognitive, emotional, and motivational problems are associated with the VS diseases effecting these striatal regions often have a mixed set of dysfunctions *(7–15)*. For example, often the earliest detectable symptoms in PD patients occur on cognitive tasks requiring attentional set-shifting and tasks requiring organizational skills and use of working memory. Thus, although different basal ganglia regions are involved in various functions, the basal ganglia as a whole operates in concert with cortex in mediating overall behavioral responses. This involves a complex coordination of motivational, cognitive, and motor elements.

The main driving force of the basal ganglia is cortex, with particular emphasis on frontal cortex. The basic basal ganglia circuit starts with the corticostriatal projection to the striatum. The striatum then projects to the globus pallidus (GP), and substantia nigra, pars reticulata (SNr); the GP/SNr project to the relay nuclei of the thalamus, which project back to the cortex (Fig. 1). Since the identification of the VS/VP as a separate loop of the basal ganglia *(16)*, several additional segregated basal ganglia circuits have been proposed *(17)*. Each circuit begins in a functionally identified region of cortex and projects topographically to each of the basal ganglia nuclei and, via the thalamus, back to the cortical region of origin. These corticobasal ganglia-cortical loops drive the concept of segregated functional circuits, providing few mechanisms by which, for example, limbic circuits might influence cognitive or motor output basal ganglia pathways *(18,19)*. However, several studies also favor mechanisms by which information can flow between corticobasal ganglia circuits *(13,20–23)*. Here, we review aspects of the corticobasal ganglia system that are parallel, but emphasize two mechanisms by which cross-talk between loop systems occurs. Particular focus is on the fundamental role that the dopaminergic neurons play in integrating information across circuits *(22)*. The organization of pathways between the striatum and midbrain allows information from one circuit to influence another circuit in an ordered fashion. In this way, basal ganglia circuits carrying out a cortical command can accommodate to new incoming cortical information. Furthermore, attention is given to the complex relationship between the basal ganglia relay nuclei of the thalamus and frontal cortex *(24)*.

From: *Mental and Behavioral Dysfunction in Movement Disorders*
Edited by: M-A. Bédard et al. © Humana Press Inc., Totowa, NJ

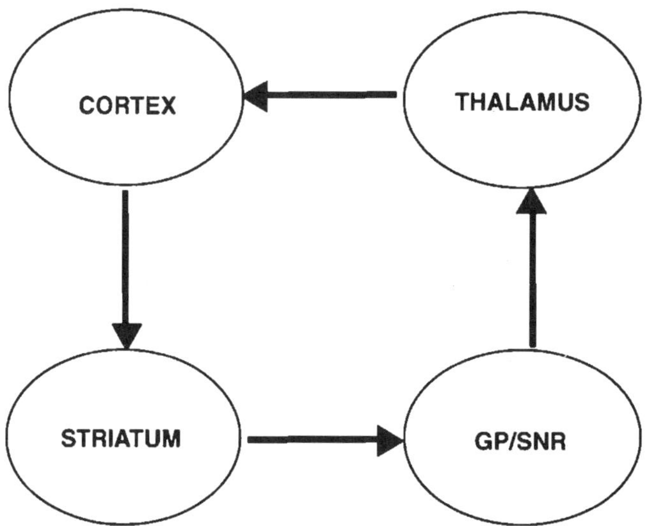

Fig. 1. Illustration of the basic corticobasal ganglia circuit.

2. THE BASIC CORTICOBASAL GANGLIA CIRCUIT IS TOPOGRAPHICALLY ORGANIZED AND RELATES TO CORTICAL FUNCTION

The association of frontal cortex with specific functions is well established. Motor, premotor, supplementary motor cortices, and the cingulate motor area mediate different aspects of motor control *(18, 25–27)*. The dorsolateral prefrontal cortex (DLPFC) is involved in executive functions, such as procedural learning, working memory, strategic planning, and the ability to switch cognitive sets *(28,29)*. This area is often referred to as association cortex. The orbital and medial prefrontal cortex (OMPFC) is involved in linking primary rewards with motivational and emotional features and plays a key role in the development of reward guided behaviors *(30–38)*. We refer to the OMPFC as the area of prefrontal cortex (PFC) related to the limbic system.

The entire frontal cortex is often considered "motor" cortex in the broadest sense, in that it is devoted to action, be it expression of emotion, logical reasoning, or skeletal movement *(39)*. The connectional organization of frontal cortex forms a hierarchy, in which a cascade of pathways from prefrontal regions through premotor regions ultimately terminates in areas that mediate motor expression. In brief, primary motor cortex (M1) is directly and most densely connected to the spinal cord. Caudal premotor areas (PMc) are directly and most densely connected to M1, but also have some connections to the spinal cord. Rostral premotor areas (PMr) are directly and most densely connected to PMc; DLPFC is directly and most densely connected to PMr, and the OMPFC is most densely connected to the DLPFC. This hierarchy of organization is reflected in the cortical projections to the striatum.

Cortical projections to the striatum have a rostral–caudal, medial–lateral, and dorsal–ventral organization *(22,40–47)*. Areas 9 and 10, the most rostral association regions project to the rostral pole of the caudate. As the striatum enlarges, these projections are pushed dorsally, and occupy the central caudate and putamen. At this level, the rostral medial cortical areas 24, 25, and 32 areas project to the rostral, medial, and VS, including the shell of the nucleus accumbens and the ventral medial caudate nucleus. Orbital frontal areas project more laterally in the rostral VS and include the medial putamen. Taken together, the OMPFC projections to the striatum occupy a relatively large ventromedial region just rostral to the anterior commissure (AC). In contrast, the premotor and motor cortical

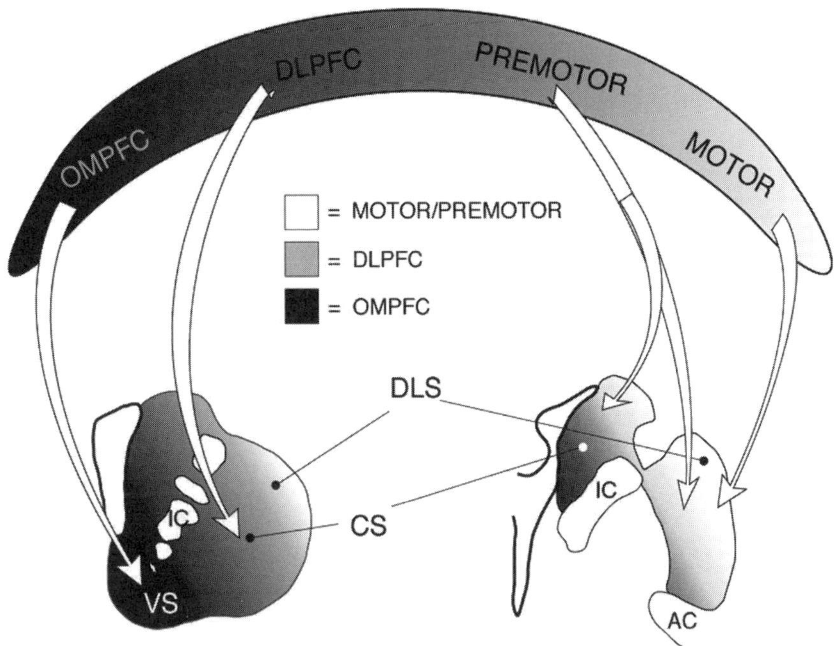

Fig. 2. Schematic illustrating the organization of corticostriatal projections. The shading gradient represents a continuum of inputs from functionally specific regions of frontal cortex, shaded to correspond to the projection. AC, anterior commissure; CS, central striatum; DLPFC, dorsolateral prefrontal cortex; DLS, dorsolateral striatum; IC, internal capsule; OMPFC, orbital and medial prefrontal cortex; VS, ventral striatum.

projections are quite limited here. Posterior to the AC, however, projections from the premotor and motor areas occupy a progressively greater proportion of the striatum. At the level of the two pallidal segments, almost the entire putamen receives input from them. In summary, the OMPFC project to a large region of the rostral striatum, occupying its entire ventral half. The DLPFC projects to the remainder of the rostral striatum, along with a small input from rostral premotor areas. Caudal premotor areas and the motor cortex project to the dorsolateral striatum, including most of the caudal putamen. At this caudal level there are some, albeit few, projections from the OMPFC. Thus, although the basal ganglia is considered as part of the motor system, the motor and premotor cortex projects primarily to the putamen, caudal to the AC, leaving the large rostral striatum connected to the DLPFC and the OMPFC (Fig. 2). We define the VS as the limbic-related region of striatum, in that it receives input from the OMPFC, no input from motor or premotor areas, and little or no input from the DLPFC. This includes the nucleus accumbens and the medial rostral caudate nucleus and putamen. The central striatum (CS), which is defined as the association portion of the striatum, receives input primarily from the DLPFC. The dorsolateral caudate nucleus and caudal putamen (DLS) receives the main input from the motor, premotor, supplementary motor (SMA) cortex, and the cingulate motor area.

The output pathways of the striatum to the GP/SNr, and from the GP/SNr to the thalamus, and then back to the cortex, maintain this topography, thereby creating several functionally discrete circuits (Fig. 3). For example, the output of the striatum to the GP demonstrates a dorsal–ventral medial–lateral topography *(48–55)*. This organization continues in the pallidal projections to the ventral nuclei and the mediodorsal (MD) nucleus of the thalamus, which are the thalamic relay nuclei of the basal ganglia *(19,53,56)*. These thalamic cell groups have specific projections to motor, premotor, cingulate motor, and prefrontal cortical areas *(57–65)*. The organization of these projections back to cortex forms the basis for the parallel and separate basal ganglia loops hypothesis *(18)*.

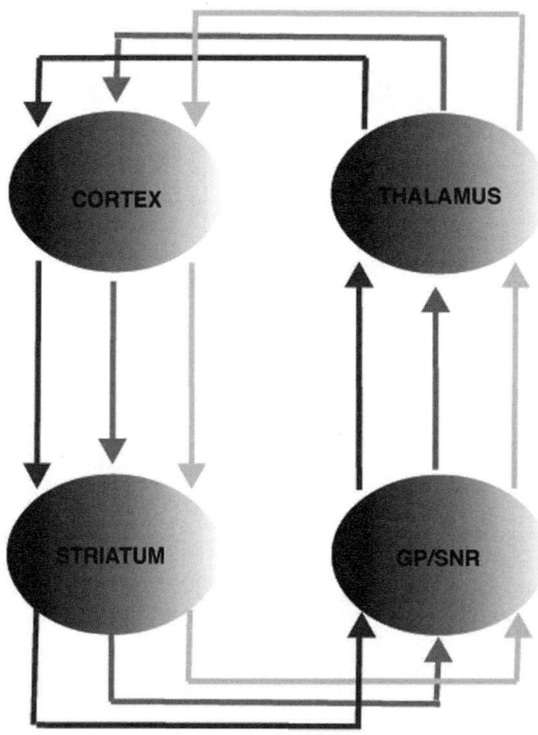

Fig. 3. Diagram of the functional topography of corticobasal gangliathalamocortical circuits. Shading represents different functions. Each functional region of cortex projects to a specific region of the striatum, represented by the same shading. The striatum in turn projects to a specific region of the GP/SNr, also represented by the same shading. The GP/SNr projects to a specific region of thalamus and back to the cortical region of origin. GP, globus pallidus; SNr, substantia nigra, pars reticulata.

3. THE CENTRAL ROLE OF THE DOPAMINE NEURONS IN LINKING ACROSS PARALLEL PATHWAYS

3.1. Dopamine Neurons Are Divided into a Dorsal Tier and a Ventral Tier

The substantia nigra, pars compacta (SNc) is mainly constituted of dopaminergic cell bodies *(66–69)*. The midbrain dopamine (DA) neurons are divided into three groups: (*i*) a dorsal group, also referred to as the pars dorsalis; (*ii*) a main, densocellular region; and (*iii*) the cell columns that extend deep into the pars reticulata (Fig. 1) *(70–72)*. The dorsal group cells are loosely arranged and extend dorsolaterally bordering the ventral and lateral aspects of the superior cerebellar peduncle and the red nucleus. These cells lie just dorsal to the densocellular region, and form a continuous band with the ventral tegmental area (VTA). The dorsal group and the VTA are calbindin-positive and stand out in this respect from the ventrally located densocellular and cells column neurons that are calbindin-negative *(73–75)*. The dendrites of the dorsal group stretch in a mediolateral direction and do not extend into the ventral parts of the pars compacta or into the pars reticulata. In contrast, the dendritic arborizations of the densocellular region and the cell columns are oriented ventrally and occupy the major portion of the pars reticulata in primates. The mRNA expression for dopamine transporter (DAT) mRNA and for the dopamine 2 receptor (D2R) is highest in the densocellular and ventral regions of the primate midbrain DA neurons *(75)* and relatively low in the both the dorsal group and in the VTA. Consistent with this labeling pattern, the dorsal striatum has denser DAT immunocytochemistry than

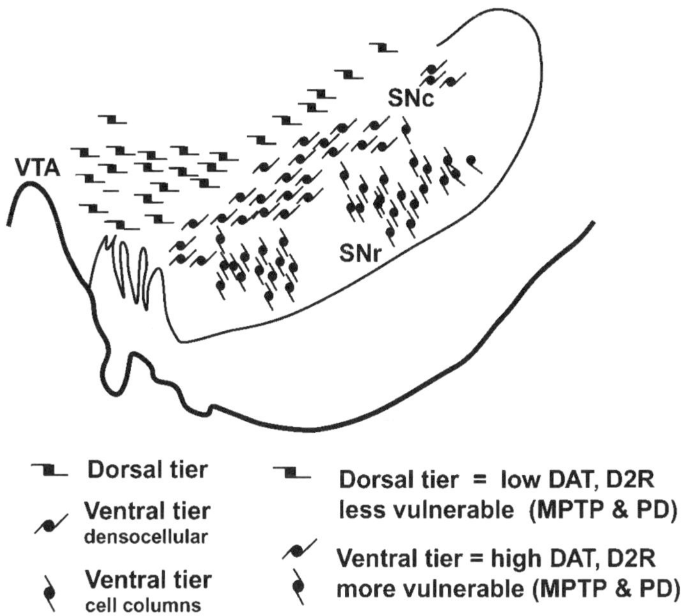

Fig. 4. Schematic illustrating the cell groups of the midbrain dopamine system. DAT, dopamine transporter; D2R, dopamine, 2 receptor; PD, Parkinson's disease; SNc, substantia nigra, pars compacta; SNr, substantia nigra, pars reticulata; VTA, ventral tegmental area.

the VS *(76,77)*. Both the densocellular and cell columns neurons are more vulnerable to toxic insult, including 1-methyl-4-phenyl-1, 2, 3, 6-tetrahydropyridine (MPTP) toxicity, and to degeneration in neurodegenerative diseases, such as PD *(73,78–80)*. The features of these cell groups (cell morphology, calbindin staining, mRNA expression levels, and vulnerability to degeneration) divide the midbrain DA cells into two groups, the dorsal tier cells (the dorsal SNc and the VTA) and the ventral tier group (the densocellular and cell column neurons) (Fig. 4).

3.2. *The Midbrain DA Cells Project to and Receive their Main Input from the Striatum*

The main efferent projection of the DA cells is to the striatum. While emphasis is placed on the SNr as the main recipient of the striatum, the main input to the DA cells is also the striatum. The organization of each of these projections (striatonigral and nigrostriatal) form an inverse dorsal–ventral topography *(71,81–89)*. When considered separately, each limb of the system creates a loose topographic organization, such that the VTA and medial SN are associated with the limbic system, and the lateral and ventral SN are related to the associative and motor striatal regions. However, these two projection systems are typically examined separately, without consideration of their relationship to each other. Here, we focus on this relationship (projections from the striatum to the midbrain and projections from the midbrain to the striatum) from the different functionally defined striatal areas.

3.3. *VS Pathways*

Projections from the VS to the midbrain terminate in the dorsal midbrain, including both the dorsal tier and the dorsal part of the ventral tier extending into the medial and dorsal pars reticulata. These terminal fields are distributed widely throughout the midbrain and concentrated in the medial part rostrally and dorsolaterally at central and caudal levels (Fig. 5A). Terminal labeling from the VS overlaps extensively with the labeled cells that project back to the VS. However, the distribution of midbrain cells that project to the VS are more limited in their distribution and are concentrated primarily in the medial half of the midbrain. In addition, there are cells that project to the VS that lie dorsal to the VS terminal field. There is also a ventrolateral terminal region that does not contain cells that project back to the VS. Thus, there are three components in the striatonigral–nigrostriatal VS projection system: one reciprocal pathway which lies between two nonreciprocal pathways. The reciprocal pathway contains both cells that project to the VS and terminal fibers from the VS. Dorsal to this area is a region that contains only cells that project to the VS, but does not contain terminal fibers. Ventral to the reciprocal component lies a region that contains only a terminal field from the VS, but no cells that project to the VS (Fig. 5A). Both the shell and core striato-nigro-striatal (SNS) projection systems contain the three components in the midbrain: a dorsal group of labeled cells that projects to the shell or core, but does not lie within its reciprocal efferent projection. A central group of cells that lies within its efferent terminal field; and efferent fibers from the shell that terminate cells ventral to it. Cells projecting to the core are located both within the terminal fields of the core and dorsal to it. This dorsal group of cells lies within the ventral terminal field of the shell. In contrast, there is little overlap between efferent fibers originating from the core and labeled cells projecting to the shell. Labeled fibers from the core are also located ventral to the labeled cell population that projects back to the core.

3.4. CS and DLS Pathways

The central SNS field lay primarily within the densocellular region of the midbrain (Fig. 5B). The CS efferent projection is extensive and terminates in the ventral part of the densocellular region and extends into the cell columns and surrounding pars reticulata. Cells that project to the CS are also located throughout the densocellular region, in a wide medial-lateral area. Efferent projections from the dorsal striatum are concentrated in the ventral and lateral half of the SN. Unlike the widespread terminal fields of the VS and CS pathways, the distribution of efferent fibers from the DLS pathway is more restricted. In contrast to its limited efferent projection, the distribution of cells projecting to the DLS is widespread and found in both in the cell columns and in the densocellular area. As seen with the VS, both the CS and DLS SNS projection systems exhibit the three components, one reciprocal and two nonreciprocal components. Cells that project to the CS are found embedded within the CS terminal fields. In addition, cells projecting to the CS are also located dorsal to the main CS terminal projection field, and there are terminals from the CS that lie ventral and not in close approximation to the main population of cells projecting to the CS (Fig. 5B). Likewise, there is a dorsal group of cells that projects to the DLS, but does not lie within its efferent projection field (Fig. 5C); a group of cells projecting to the DLS that does lie within its efferent projection); and a ventral terminal field that does not contain cells that project back to the DLS. The labeled cells in the densocellular region comprise the group that does not lie with the efferent projection from the DLS. This dorsal population of cells is relatively large, compared to those projecting to the VS. Together, the DLS SNS pathway is made up of a widespread cell population that projects to the DLS and a relatively confined DLS efferent terminal field.

3.5. Features of the VS, CS, and DLS Pathways Both Set Them Apart and Unite Them

The VS and DLS have contrasting relationships with the midbrain. They differ in their relative proportional contribution to each limb of the SNS projection. Efferent projections from the VS terminate throughout an extensive region of the dorsal midbrain, while the DLS projection is relatively limited to the ventrolateral SN. The CS pathway occupies an intermediate position between the VS and DLS in the striato-nigral pathway. In contrast, the VS receives a more limited projection from the midbrain, while the DLS receives the largest. These differences in proportions significantly alter their relationship to the midbrain. The VS influences a wide range of DA neurons, but is itself influenced by a relatively limited group of DA cells. On the other hand, the DLS influences a limited midbrain region,

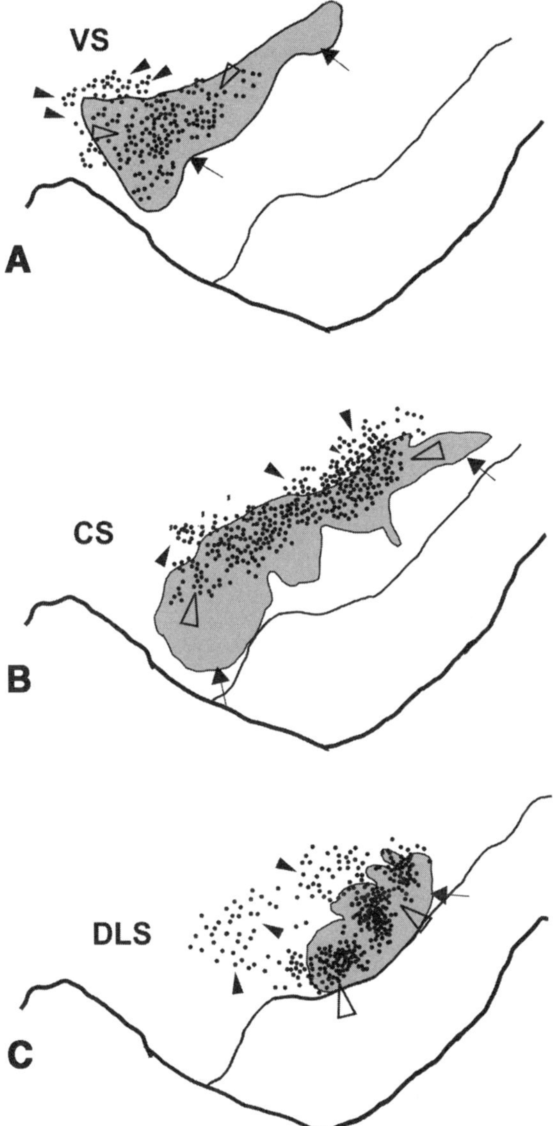

Fig. 5. The VS (**A**), CS (**B**), and the DLS (**C**) SNS projection systems illustrating the three components within the midbrain for each. Each schematic of the midbrain shows the terminal field of axons projecting to the mid-brain from each functional striatal region (shaded area) and the distribution of cells that project to that striatal region (dots). Black arrowheads indicate cells dorsal to terminals, white arrowheads indicate the region of cells within the shell terminal field, and arrows point to terminals ventral or lateral to cells projecting back to the striatal region.

but is affected by a relatively large midbrain region. Of particular importance, is that, for each striatal region, the SNS projection system contains three components in the midbrain: (*i*) a dorsal group of cells that does not lie within its reciprocal terminal field; (*ii*) a group of cells that does lie within its reciprocal terminal field; and (*iii*) a ventral component comprised of the efferent terminals that do not contain a reciprocally connected group of labeled cells. While the overlap between labeled cells and terminals

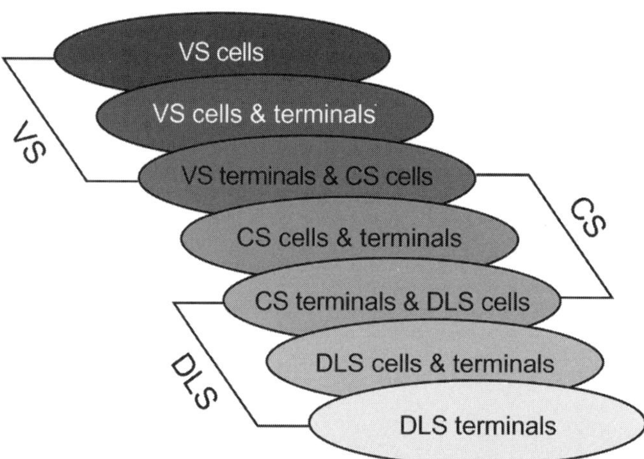

Fig. 6. Diagram of the three SNS components for each striatal region in the midbrain, illustrating an overlapping and interdigitating system. The three midbrain components for each striatal region are represented by three ovals. The top oval in each set corresponds to the region of midbrain cells dorsal to its reciprocal afferent projection. The second oval corresponds to the region of cells within its reciprocal afferent projection. The third oval corresponds to the ventral region of nonreciprocal terminals that overlaps with cells of a more dorsal SNS system. Note that the third midbrain component of a striatal region overlaps the first component of the adjacent dorsal striatal region, resulting in stepwise feedforward projection from ventral to dorsal striatal regions. CS, central striatum; DLS, dorsolateral striatum; VS, ventral striatum.

at the light microscopic level does not demonstrate a direct synaptic connection, it is likely that this close relationship does indicate that the terminals in the region convey information relevant to the cells either directly or indirectly. Likewise, the lack of an overlap between terminal fields and labeled cells in the other two components is not necessarily evidence for a lack of connectivity, which might occur on distal dendrites. However, terminals at the cell bodies and proximal dendrites will be electronically closer to the soma and, therefore, likely to exert a greater influence on spike activity than if they terminate distally *(90,91)*. Thus, the three components of the SNS system represent different levels of interaction. Where cells and terminals overlap, there is likely to be a more direct interface, which we refer to as a reciprocal connection. The dorsal and ventral components, in which the cells and terminals do not overlap, we refer to as nonreciprocal components. These three components for each SNS projection system occupy a different position within the midbrain. The VS system lies dorsomedially, the DLS system lies ventrolaterally, and the CS system is positioned between the two (Fig. 6). This arrangement of overlying regions of cells and terminals within the midbrain, related to different striatal functional areas, mediate interactions between parallel circuits.

3.6 An Ascending Midbrain Spiral Mediates Limbic Input to Motor Outcome

The three midbrain components of the SNS projection system allows information from the limbic system to reach the motor system through a series of connections. The VS receives forebrain input primarily from areas most closely associated with the limbic system and projects to the dorsal tier. However, its efferent projection to the midbrain terminates, not only in the dorsal tier, but also lateral and ventral to the dorsal tier, in the dorsal densocellular region. The area of this terminal projection does not project back to the VS. It projects to the CS. Thus, cortical information that influences the dorsal tier through the VS, also modulates the densocellular region, which projects to the CS (Fig. 7A). The CS is reciprocally connected to the densocellular region, but also projects to the ventral pars reticulata and the cell columns. The cell columns project to the DLS, with a reciprocal connection back

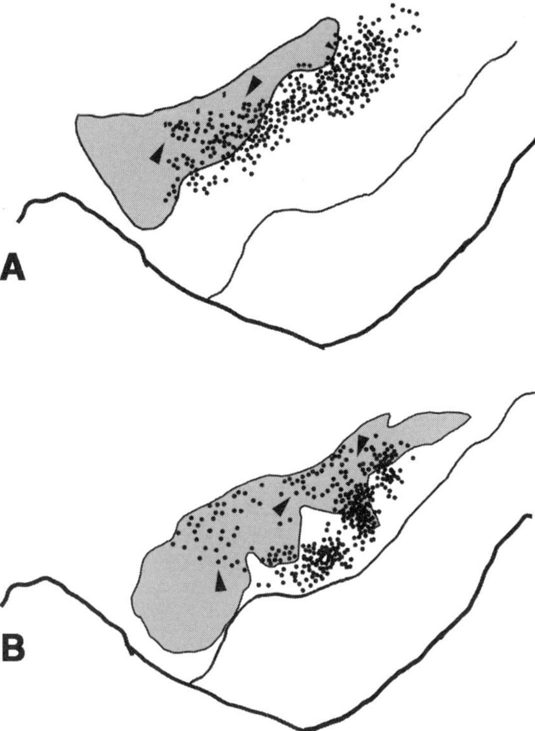

Fig. 7. Schematic demonstrating the cell and terminal overlap in the midbrain between the VS, CS, and DLS. (**A**) Schematic comparing the distribution of the VS terminal field (shaded area) with the distribution of cells (dots) that project to the CS. (**B**) Schematic comparing the distribution of the CS terminal field (shaded area) with the distribution of cells (dots) projecting to the DLS.

to the ventral densocellular region and cell columns. Thus, projections to the DLS are influenced by the terminal fields arising from the CS (Fig. 7B). The confined distribution of efferent DLS fibers limits the influence of the motor striatum to a relatively small region involving the cell columns and the pars reticulata. Taken together, the interface between different striatal regions via the midbrain DA cells is organized in an ascending spiral interconnecting different functional regions of the striatum (Fig. 8).

Dopaminergic neurons play an important role in the acquisition of newly acquired behaviors *(92–95)*. The striatum is a major source afferent control of the DA neurons *(96)* and inhibits neurons in both the pars compacta and the pars reticulata. However, stimulation of the striatum can also increase DA firing through inhibition of γ-amino butyric acid (GABA)ergic interneurons (or pars reticulata cells) that terminate on dopaminergic cells and dendrites. This results in disinhibition of pars compacta cells *(97–99)*. The dual effect of both inhibition and disinhibition may modulate different aspects of the ascending SNS spiral, thus controlling information flow. Likewise, striatal response to DA is complex, and while tonic release of DA attenuates medium spiny neuronal response, phasic release potentiates striatal response *(100)*. DA can both inhibit background corticostriatal input but facilitate (and therefore focus) specific corticostriatal synaptic transmission. Taken together, if the reciprocal component of each limb of the spiral terminated directly on a DA cell, it would result in inhibition of DA burst firing. Conversely, the nonreciprocal feedforward component of the ascending spiral might terminate on GABAergic interneurons and result in disinhibition and an increase of burst firing. Each component of information would send both an inhibitory feedback response, but facilitate transfer of

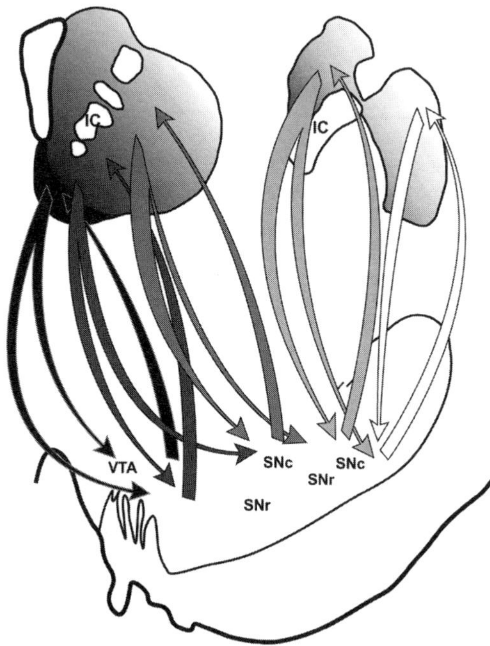

Fig. 8. Diagram of the organization of SNS projections. The shaded gradient in rostral and caudal schematics of the striatum illustrates the organization of functional corticostriatal inputs (see fig. 2). Midbrain projections from the VS target both the VTA and ventromedial SNc (black arrows). Midbrain projections from the VTA to the VS form a "closed," reciprocal SNS loop (black arrow). Projections from the medial SN feedforward to more dorsal areas forming the first part of a spiral (dark gray arrow). The spiral continues through the SNS projections (lighter gray arrows) with pathways originating in the VS and projecting through the CS, and more dorsally, to the DLS (white arrows). In this way, ventral striatal regions influence more dorsal striatal regions via spiraling SNS projections. IC, internal capsule; SNc, substantia nigra pars compacta; SNr, substantia nigra pars reticulata; VTA, ventral tegmental area.

information to the next step in the spiral (via disinhibition). As information about potential reward of a specific behavior from the shell is conveyed to the midbrain, it would inhibit additional information flow from the shell via the reciprocal connection. The nonreciprocal feedforward projection, terminating in proximity to cells projecting to the core, would increase DA burst firing in the core via disinhibition. The reciprocal projection to the core also inhibits its midbrain feedback, but, via the GABAergic interneuron, disinhibits cells projecting to the CS. Thus, information transfer continues from the core to the CS, through the CS to the DLS, and then the final motor outcome (Fig. 8).

Behavioral studies of DA pathways have lead to the association of the mesolimbic pathway and nigrostriatal pathway with reward and motor activity, respectively. But the basal ganglia link between motivation and motor outcomes has focused primarily on pathways of the nucleus accumbens in rodents *(23,101,102)*. Recent primate studies demonstrate that DA's primary function is to direct attention to important stimuli likely to bring about a desired outcome *(103,104)*. This requires processing a complex chain of events beginning with motivation, proceeding through cognitive processing that shapes final motor outcomes. This sequence reflected in the feedforward organization of the SNS connections. The SNS circuit creates a complex feedforward neuronal network through which information from the limbic system can influence cognitive function and cognition can influence motor function *(22)*.

4. THALAMOCORTICAL AND CORTICOTHALAMIC PROJECTIONS CREATE ANOTHER POTENTIAL MECHANISM FOR INFORMATION TO FLOW ACROSS SEPARATE CORTICOBASAL GANGLIA CIRCUITS

The concept of "parallel" processing within basal ganglia pathways relies, in part, on the fact that distinct thalamic relay nuclei, that receive basal ganglia output, project to specific motor, premotor, and prefrontal cortical areas *(6,58,59,63,65,105)*. Thalamic relay nuclei, once thought to simply passively transfer information from afferent systems to cortex, are now known to play an important role in changing the dynamics of cortical processing by setting up different oscillation patterns of frequency and synchrony *(106)*. For example, the resting tremor in PD is thought to be the consequence of changes in thalamic firing frequency due to an increased inhibition of the pallidal input to the ventroanterior (VA)/VL cell groups. This inhibition leads to a hyperpolarization of thalamic cells and changes in its oscillatory firing pattern to cortex *(107)*.

Often ignored in models of basal ganglia function is the large corticothalamic projection. Indeed, this projection is 10 times as great as the thalamocortical projection. This projection controls the oscillatory firing pattern of the thalamus *(108–110)*, through a feedback mechanism that inhibits relay neurons *(111,112)*. Thus, the relationship between the thalamocortical and corticothalamic projection systems of the ventral and MD thalamic nuclei is likely to have an important impact on how information is processed for each basal ganglia circuit. Furthermore, this relationship is likely to have important implications on how information transfer can take place between circuits.

Based on studies in other systems and preliminary results in our laboratory, there are two components to the corticothalamic projection: (*i*) a reciprocal component, in which the cortical area receiving the thalamic input projects back to the same thalamic area; and (*ii*) a nonreciprocal component, in which a given cortical area projects to a region of thalamus that does not receive its input. Thus, corticothalamic terminal fields to a given thalamic region are derived from a wider range of cortical areas than the reciprocal thalamocortical output *(24,106,113–117)*. The nonreciprocal component of the projection arises from large cells in layer V, while the reciprocal component is derived primarily from small cells in layer VI *(118–121)*. The nonreciprocal neurons of layer V are large rapidly conducting cells, which may therefore be responsible for changing the thalamocortical oscillatory patterns. This change in firing pattern would, therefore, effect a different part of cortex providing a mechanism for cortex to synchronize thalamic oscillations in distal cortical regions *(122)*. In this way, specific thalamic relay nuclei modify and facilitate information flow across functional regions of cortex via specific thalamic nuclei, and these thalamic nuclei can modify that information (Fig. 8). Thus, the interactions between cortical and thalamic activity may act in a general way to influence global cortical activity. Alternatively, it may function in a specific feedforward mechanism that facilitates information transfer from one cortical area to another. This has been a proposed mechanism by which primary sensory cortex can influence "higher" cortical association areas *(106,108)*.

Corticothalamic projections to specific VA/VL and MD sites are more widespread than the VA/VL and MD thalamocortical projections. Based on separate experiments that demonstrate the thalamocortical projections and the corticothalamic projections of the basal ganglia thalamic relay nuclei, we can surmize that these nuclei also receive both reciprocal and nonreciprocal corticothalamic inputs *(42,58, 62,63,65,123–126)*. For example, VL has reciprocal connections primarily with caudal motor areas. In addition, it receives a nonreciprocal cortical projection from more rostral motor areas. VA is reciprocally connected with rostral motor areas, and dorsolateral prefrontal areas, but it also receives a nonreciprocal corticothalamic projections from medial areas, as well as lateral orbitofrontal areas. Reciprocal connections with MD are similarly limited, involving primarily dorsolateral prefrontal and lateral orbitofrontal areas. However, nonreciprocal MD inputs also arise from medial, limbic-related, prefrontal areas, such as 24a/b and 32. If the pattern formed by the reciprocal and nonreciprocal limbs of the corticothalamocortical pathway are organized in a similar fashion as the SNS projection system described above, it may create a hierarchy of influence through different cortical regions (Fig. 8) *(24)*.

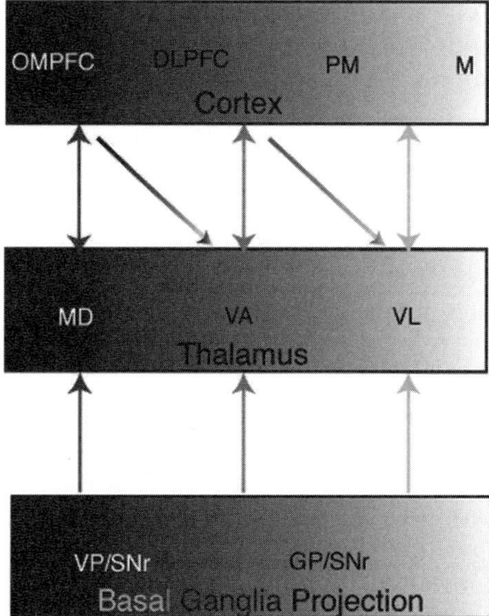

Fig. 9. Illustration of potential information transfer from one area of the cortex to another via a nonreciprocal connection to the thalamic relay nuclei.

Such a hierarchy of information transfer has been described in the visual system *(106)*. Thus, the corticothalamocortical circuit relays information from different basal ganglia loops forming a feed-forward circuit associated with limbic, cognitive, motor planning, to motor execution.

The complexity of the thalamocorticothalamic circuit raises an interesting issue related to the concept of parallel vs nonparallel processing of information through basal ganglia pathways. Information from each thalamic relay nuclei is conveyed back to the cortical region of origin, providing the last link in the parallel and segregated circuits. However, since there is also a nonreciprocal corticothalamic input to each of these thalamic nuclei, the incoming basal ganglia information from each circuit is mixed with cortical inputs from a different circuit (Fig. 9). Since the nonreciprocal input to each thalamic nucleus is derived, at least in part, from more rostral and medial cortical areas, the flow of information from cortex to thalamus is from limbic and cognitive areas into premotor and motor regions of thalamus. Therefore, although the last link to cortex is through the basal ganglia and follows a parallel pathway, the bidirectional connections between cortex and thalamus may have a great influence on how segregated the information is from each loop. The information that the thalamic relay nuclei convey to cortex is, therefore, not only effected by the parallel pathway through the basal ganglia structures, but is also modified by the nonreciprocal corticothalamic pathway, resulting in an integrated feed-forward processing similar to that seen in sensory systems *(126)*.

ACKNOWLEDGMENTS

This work was supported by National Institutes of Health (NIH) grant nos. MH45573 and NS22511.

REFERENCES

1. Koob, G.F. and Nestler, E.J. (1997) The neurobiology of drug addiction. *J. Neuropsychiatry Clin. Neurosci.* **9,** 482–497.
2. Singer, H.S., Butler, I.J., Tune, L.E., Seifert, W.E. Jr., and Coyle, J.T. (1982) Dopaminergic dsyfunction in Tourette syndrome. *Ann. Neurol.* **12,** 361–366.

3. Grace, A.A. (1991) Phasic versus tonic dopmaine release and the modulation of dopamine system responsivity: a hypothesis for the etiology of schizophrenia. *Neuroscience* **41,** 1–24.
4. Swerdlow, N.R. and Koob, G.F. (1987) Dopamine, schizophrenia, mania, and depression: toward a unified hypothesis of cortico-striato-pallido-thalamic function. *Behav. Brain Res.* **10,** 197–245.
5. Cooper, J.A., Sagar, H.J., Doherty, S.M., Jordan, N., Tidswell, P., and Sullivan, E.V. (1992) Different effects of dopaminergic and anticholinergic therapies on cognitive and motor function in Parkinson's disease. A follow-up study of untreated patients. *Brain* **115,** 1701–1725.
6. Alexander, G.E. and Crutcher, M.D. (1990) Functional architecture of basal ganglia circuits: neural substrates of parallel processing. *Trends Neurosci.* **13,** 266–271.
7. Cooper, J.A., Sagar, H.J., Jordan, N., Harvey, N.S., and Sullivan, E.V. (1991) Cognitive impairment in early, untreated Parkinson's disease and its relationship to motor disability. *Brain* **114,** 2095–2122.
8. Owen, A.M., Iddon, J.L., Hodges, J.R., Summers, B.A., and Robbins, T.W. (1997) Spatial and non-spatial working memory at different stages of Parkinson's disease. *Neuropsychologia* **35,** 519–532.
9. Taylor, A.E., Saint-Cyr, J.A., Lang, A.E., and Kenny, F.T. (1986) Parkinson's disease and depression: a critical re-evaluation. *Brain* **109,** 279–292.
10. Taylor, A.E., Saint-Cyr, J.A., and Lang, A.E. (1990) Memory and learning in early Parkinson's disease: evidence for a "frontal lobe syndrome." *Brain Cogn.* **13,** 211–232.
11. Folstein, S.E., Folstein, M.F., and McHugh, P.R. (1979) Psychiatric syndromes in Huntington's disease, in *Advances in Neurology* (Chase, T.N., ed.), Raven Press, New York, pp. 281–280.
12. J, B. (1991) Cognitive impairments in Huntington's disease: insights into the neuropsychology of the striatum, in *Handbook of Neuropsychology* (Boller, F. and Grafman, J., ed.), Elsevier, Amsterdam, pp. 241–264.
13. Kalivas, P.W., Churchill, L., and Klitenick, M.A. (1993) The circuitry mediating the translation of motivational stimuli into adaptive motor responses, in *Limbic Motor Circuits and Neuropsychiatry* (Kalivas, P.W. and Barnes, C.D., eds.), CRC Press, Boca Raton, pp. 237–275.
14. Mogenson, G.J., Wu, M., and Jones, D.L. (1980) Locomotor activity elicited by injections of picrotoxin into the ventral tegmental area is attenuated by injections of GABA into the globus pallidus. *Brain Res.* **191,** 569–571.
15. Mogenson, G.J. and Nielsen, M.A. (1983) Evidence that an accumbens to subpallidal GAGAergic projection contributes to locomotor activity. *Brain Res. Bull.* **11,** 309–314.
16. Heimer, L. and Wilson, R.D. (1975) The subcortical projections of the allocortex: similarities in the neural associations of the hippocampus, the piriform cortex, and the neocortex, in *Golgi Centennial Symposium: Perspectives in Neurobiology* (Santini, M., ed.), Raven Press, New York, pp. 177–193.
17. Alexander, G.E., DeLong, M.R., and Strick, P.L. (1986) Parallel organization of functionally segregated circuits linking basal ganglia and cortex. *Annu. Rev. Neurosci.* **9,** 357–381.
18. Alexander, G.E., Crutcher, M.D., and DeLong, M.R. (1990) Basal ganglia-thalamocortical circuits: parallel substrates for motor, oculomotor, "prefrontal" and "limbic" functions. *Prog. Brain Res.* **85,** 119–110.
19. Middleton, F.A. and Strick, P.L. (1997) New concepts about the organization of basal ganglia output. *Adv. Neurol.* **74,** 57–68.
20. Nauta, W.J.H., Smith, G.P., Faull, R.L.M., and Domesick, V.B. (1978) Efferent connections and nigral afferents of the nucleus accumbens septi in the rat. *Neuroscience* **3,** 385–401.
21. Percheron, G., Yelnik, J., and Francois, C. (1984) The primate striato-pallido-nigral system: an integrative system for cortical information, in *The Basal Ganglia: Structure and Function* (McKenzie, J.S., Kemm, R.E., and Wilcock, L.N., eds.), Plenum Press, London, pp. 87–105.
22. Haber, S.N., Fudge, J.L., and McFarland, N. (2000) Striatonigrostriatal pathways in primates form an ascending spiral from the shell to the dorsolateral striatum. *J. Neurosci.* **20,** 2369–2382.
23. Mogenson, G.J., Jones, D.L., and Yim, C.Y. (1980) From motivation to action: functional interface between the limbic system and the motor system. *Prog. Neurobiol.* **14,** 69–97.
24. Haber, S.N. and McFarland, N.R. (2001) The place of the thalamus in frontal cortical-basal ganglia circuits. *Neuroscientist,* in press.
25. Dum, R.P. and Strick, P.L. (1993) Cingulate motor areas, in *Neurobiology of Cingulate Cortex and Limbic Thalamus: A Comprehensive Treatise* (Vogt, B.A. and Gabriel, M., eds.), Birkhauser, Boston, pp. 415–441.
26. Kurata, K. (1993) Premotor cortex of monkeys: set- and movement-related activity reflecting amplitude and direction of wrist movements. *J. Neurophysiol.* **69,** 187–200.
27. Matsuzaka, Y., Aizawa, H., and Tanji, J. (1992) A motor area rostral to the supplementary motor area (presupplementary motor area) in the monkey: neuronal activity during a learned motor task. *J. Neurophysiol.* **68,** 653–662.
28. Passingham, R.E. (1995) *The Frontal Lobes and Voluntary Action. Oxford Psychology Series,* vol. 21, Oxford University Press, Oxford.
29. Levy, R. and Goldman-Rakic, P.S. (1999) Association of storage and processing functions in the dorsolateral prefrontal cortex of the nonhuman primate. *J. Neurosci.* **19,** 5149–5158.
30. Cummings, J.L. (1995) Anatomic and behavioral aspects of frontal-subcortical circuits. [review]. *Ann. NY Acad Sci.* **769,** 1–13.
31. Filley, C.M. (1995) Frontal lobe syndromes, in *Neurobehavioral Anatomy, 1st ed.* University Press of Colorado, Niwot, pp. 149–162.
32. Schall, J.D. (1997) Visuomotor areas of the frontal lobe, in Ce*rebral Cortex, Vol. 12, Extrastriate Cortex in Primates, 1st ed.* (Rockland, K.S., Kaas, J.H., and Peters, A., eds.), Plenum Press, New York, pp. 527–638.

33. Cummings, J.L. (1993) Frontal-subcortical circuits and human behavior [review]. *Arch. Neurol.* **50,** 873–880.
34. Eslinger, P.J. and Damasio, A.R. (1985) Severe disturbance of higher cognition after bilateral frontal lobe ablation: patient EVR. *Neurology* **35,** 1731–1741.
35. Fuster, J.M. (1989) Lesion studies, in *The Prefrontal Cortex Anatomy, Physiology, and Neuropsychology of the Frontal Lobe, 2nd ed.,* Raven Press, New York, pp. 51–82.
36. Rolls, E.T., Burton, M.J., and Mora, F. (1980) Neurophysiological analysis of brain-stimulation reward in the monkey. *Brain Res.* **194,** 339–357.
37. Carmichael, S.T. and Price, J.L. (1996) Limbic connections of the orbital and medial prefrontal cortex in macaque monkeys. *J. Comp. Neurol.* **363,** 615–641.
38. Butter, C.M. (1969) Perseveration in extinction and in discrimination reversal tasks following selective fronal ablations in macaca mulatta. *Physiol. Behav.* **4,** 163–171.
39. Fuster, J.M. (1989) *The Prefrontal Cortex*, Raven, New York.
40. Künzle, H. (1975) Bilateral projections from precentral motor cortex to the putamen and other parts of the basal ganglia. An autoradiographic study in Macaca fascicularis. *Brain Res.* **88,** 195–209.
41. Künzle, H. (1978) An autoradiographic analysis of the efferent connections from premotor and adjacent prefrontal regions (areas 6 and 9) in macaca fascicularis. *Brain Behav. Evol.* **15,** 185–234.
42. Künzle, H. (1978) An autoradiographic analysis of the efferent connections from premotor and adjacent prefrontal regions (areas 6 and 9) in Macaca fascicularis. *Brain Behav. Evol.* **15,** 185–234.
43. McFarland, N.R. and Haber, S.N. (2000) Convergent inputs from thalamic motor nuclei and frontal cortical areas to the dorsal striatum in the primate. *J. Neurosci.* **20,** 3798–3813.
44. Selemon, L.D. and Goldman-Rakic, P.S. (1988) Common cortical and subcortical targets of the dorsolateral prefronal and posterior parietal cortices in the Rhesus monkey: evidence for a distributed neural network subserving spatially guided behavior. *J. Neurosci.* **8,** 4049–4068.
45. Kunishio, K. and Haber, S.N. (1994) Primate cingulostriatal projection: limbic striatal versus sensorimotor striatal input. *J. Comp. Neurol.* **350,** 337–356.
46. Chikama, M., McFarland, N., Amaral, D.G., and Haber, S.N. (1997) Insular cortical projections to functional regions of the striatum correlate with cortical cytoarchitectonic organization in the primate. *J. Neurosci.* **17,** 9686–9705.
47. Haber, S.N., Kunishio, K., Mizobuchi, M., and Lynd-Balta, E. (1995) The orbital and medial prefrontal circuit through the primate basal ganglia. *J. Neurosci.* **15,** 4851–4867.
48. Wilson, C.J. and Phelan, K.D. (1982) Dual topographic representation of neostriatum in the globus pallidus of rats. *Brain Res.* **243,** 354–359.
49. Shink, E., Sidibé, M., and Smith, Y. (1997) Efferent connections of the internal globus pallidus in the squirrel monkey: II. Topography and synaptic organization of pallidal efferents to the pedunclulopontine nucleus. *J. Comp. Neurol.* **382,** 348–363.
50. Shammah-Lagnado, S.J., Alheid, G.F., and Heimer, L. (1996) Efferent connections of the caudal part of the globus pallidus in the rat. *J. Comp. Neurol.* **376,** 489–507.
51. Kim, R., Nakano, K., Jayaraman, A., and Carpenter, M.B. (1975) Projections of the globus pallidus and adjacent structures: an autoradiographic study in the monkey. *J. Comp. Neurol.* **169,** 263–290.
52. Inase, M. and Tanji, J. (1994) Projections from the globus pallidus to the thalamic areas projecting to the dorsal area 6 of the macaque monkey: a multiple tracing study. *Neurosci. Lett.* **180,** 135–137.
53. Haber, S.N., Groenewegen, H.J., Grove, E.A., and Nauta, W.J.H. (1985) Efferent connections of the ventral pallidum. Evidence of a dual striatopallidofugal pathway. *J. Comp. Neurol.* **235,** 322–335.
54. Maurice, N., Deniau, J.M., Menetrey, A., Glowinski, J., and Thierry, A.M. (1997) Position of the ventral pallidum in the rat prefrontal cortex-basal ganglia circuit. *Neuroscience* **80,** 523–534.
55. Maurice, N., Deniau, J.M., Menetrey, A., Glowinski, J., and Thierry, A.M. (1998) Prefrontal cortex-basal ganglia circuits in the rat: involvement of ventral pallidum and subthalamic nucleus. *Synapse* **29,** 363–370.
56. Parent, A. and De Bellefeuille, L. (1982) Organization of efferent projections from the internal segment of the globus pallidus in the primate as revealed by fluorescence retrograde labeling method. *Brain Res.* **245,** 201–213.
57. Vogt, B.A., Pandya, D.N., and Rosene, D.L. (1987) Cingulate cortex of the Rhesus monkey: I. Cytoarchitecture and thalamic afferents. *J. Comp. Neurol.* **262,** 256–270.
58. Schell, G.R. and Strick, P.L. (1984) The origin of thalamic inputs to the arcuate premotor and supplementary motor areas. *J. Neurosci.* **4,** 539–560.
59. Wiesendanger, R. and Wiesendanger, M. (1985) The thalamic connections with medial area 6 (supplementary motor cortex) in the monkey (macaca fascicularis). *Exp. Brain Res.* **59,** 91–104.
60. Matelli, M., Luppino, G., Fogassi, L., and Rizzolatti, G. (1989) Thalamic input to inferior area 6 and area 4 in the macaque monkey. *J. Comp. Neurol.* **280,** 468–488.
61. Holsapple, J.W., Preston, J.B., and Strick, P.L. (1991) The origin of thalamic inputs to the "hand" representation in the primary motor cortex. *J. Neurosci.* **11,** 2644–2654.
62. Kurata, K. (1994) Site of origin of projections from the thalamus to dorsal versus ventral aspects of the premotor cortex of monkeys. *Neurosci. Res.* **21,** 71–76.
63. Matelli, M. and Luppino, G. (1996) Thalamic input to mesial and superior area 6 in the Macaque monkey. *J. Comp. Neurol.* **372,** 59–87.
64. Nakano, K., Tokushige, A., Kohno, M., Hasegawa, Y., Kayahara, T., and Sasaki, K. (1992) An autoradiographic study of cortical projections from motor thalamic nuclei in the macaque monkey. *Neurosci. Res.* **13,** 119–137.

65. Goldman-Rakic, P.S. and Porrino, L.J. (1985) The primate mediodorsal (MD) nucleus and its projection to the frontal lobe. *J. Comp. Neurol.* **242,** 535–560.
66. Garver, D.L. and Sladek, J.R. (1875) Monoamine distribution in primate brain. I. Catecholamine-containing perikarya in the brain stem of macaca speciosa. *J. Comp. Neurol.* **159,** 289–304.
67. Schofield, S.P.M. and Everitt, B.J. (1981) The organization of catecholamine-containing neurons in the brain of the rhesus monkey (macaca mulatta). *J. Anat.* **132,** 391–418.
68. Pearson, J., Goldstein, M., Markey, K., and Brandeis, L. (1983) Human brainstem catecholamine neuronal anatomy as indicated by immunocytochemistry with antibodies to tyrosine hydroxylase. *Neuroscience* **8,** 3–32.
69. Tanaka, C. (1982) Histochemical mapping of catecholaminergic neurons and their ascending fiber pathways in the rhesus monkey brain. *Brain Res. Bull.* **9,** 255–270.
70. Olszewski, J. and Baxter, D. (1954) *Cytoarchitecture of the Human Brain Stem,* S. Karger, Basil.
71. Lynd-Balta, E. and Haber, S.N. (1994) The organization of midbrain projections to the striatum in the primate: sensorimotor-related striatum versus ventral striatum. *Neuroscience* **59,** 625–640.
72. Poirier, L.J., Giguere, M., and Marchand, R. (1983) Comparative morphology of the substantia nigra and ventral tegmental area in the monkey, cat and rat. *Brain Res. Bull.* **11,** 371–397.
73. Lavoie, B. and Parent, A. (1991) Dopaminergic neurons expressing calbindin in normal and parkinsonian monkeys. *Neuroreport* **2,** 601–604.
74. McRitchie, D.A. and Halliday, G.M. (1995) Calbindin D28K-containing neurons are restricted to the medial substantia nigra in humans. *Neuroscience* **65,** 87–91.
75. Haber, S.N., Ryoo, H., Cox, C., and Lu, W. (1995) Subsets of midbrain dopaminergic neurons in monkeys are distinguished by different levels of mRNA for the dopamine transporter: Comparison with the mRNA for the D2 receptor, tyrosine hydroxylase and calbindin immunoreactivity. *J. Comp. Neurol.* **362,** 400–410.
76. Ciliax, B.J., Heilman, C., Demchyschyn, L.L., et al. (1995) The dopamine transporter: immunochemical characterization and localization in brain. *J. Neurosci.* **15,** 1714–1723.
77. Freed, C., Revay, R., Vaughan, R.A., et al. (1995) Dopamine transporter immunoreactivity in rat brain. *J. Comp. Neurol.* **359,** 340–349.
78. Pifl, C., Schingnitz, G., and Hornykiewicz, O. (1991) Effect of 1-methyl-4-phenyl-1,2,3,6-tetrahydropyridine on the regional distribution of brain monoamines in the rhesus monkey. *Neuroscience* **44,** No. 3, 591–605.
79. Schneider, J.S., Yuwiler, A., and Markham, C.H. (1987) Selective loss of subpopulations of ventral mesencephalic dopaminergic neurons in the monkey following exposure to MPTP. *Brain Res.* **411,** 144–150.
80. Parent, A. and Lavoie, B. (1993) The heterogeneity of the mesostriatal dopaminergic system as revealed in normal and Parkinsonian monkeys. *Adv. Neurol.* **60,** 25–20.
81. Deniau, J.M., Menetrey, A., and Charpier, S. (1996) The lamellar organization of the rat substantia nigra pars reticulata: segretated patterns of striatal afferents and relationship to the topography of corticostriatal projections. *Neuroscience* **73,** 761–781.
82. Szabo, J. (1967) The efferent projections of the putamen in the monkey. *Exp. Neurol.* **19,** 463–476.
83. Szabo, J. (1970) Projections from the body of the caudate nucleus in the rhesus monkey. *Exp. Neurol.* **27,** 1–15.
84. Selemon, L.D. and Goldman-Rakic, P.S. (1990) Topographic intermingling of striatonigral and striatopallidal neurons in the rhesus monkey. *J. Comp. Neurol.* **297,** 359–376.
85. Lynd-Balta, E. and Haber, S.N. (1994) Primate striatonigral projections: a comparison of the sensorimotor-related striatum and the ventral striatum. *J. Comp. Neurol.* **343,** 1–17.
86. Szabo, J. (1980) Organization of the ascending striatal afferents in monkeys. *J. Comp. Neurol.* **189,** 307–321.
87. Parent, A. and Hazrati, L.-N. (1994) Multiple striatal representation in primate substantia nigra. *J. Comp. Neurol.* **344,** 305–320.
88. Carpenter, M.B. and Peter, P. (1971) Nigrostriatal and nigrothalamic fibers in the rhesus monkey. *J. Comp. Neurol.* **144,** 93–116.
89. Parent, A., Mackey, A., and De Bellefeuille, L. (1983) The subcortical afferents to caudate nucleus and putamen in primate: a fluorescence retrograde double labeling study. *Neuroscience* **10,** 1137–1150.
90. Magee, J.C. and Johnston, D. (1997) A synaptically controlled, associative signal for Hebbian plasticity in hippocampal neurons [see comments]. *Science* **275,** 209–213.
91. Spruston, N., Jaffe, D.B., and Johnston, D. (1994) Dendritic attenuation of synaptic potentials and currents: the role of passive membrane properties. *Trends Neurosci.* **17,** 161–166.
92. Schultz, W. (1992) Activity of dopamine neurons in the behaving primate. *Semin. Neurosci.* **4,** 129–138.
93. Schultz, W., Apicella, P., and Ljungberg, T. (1993) Responses of monkey dopamine neurons to reward and conditioned stimuli during successive steps of learning a delayed response task. *J. Neurosci.* **13,** 900–913.
94. Wilson, C., Nomikos, G.G., Collu, M., and Fibiger, H.C. (1995) Dopaminergic correlates of motivated behavior: importance of drive. *J. Neurosci.* **15,** 5169–5178.
95. Richardson, N.R. and Gratton, A. (1996) Behavior-relevant changes in nucleus accumbens dopamine transmission elicited by food reinforcement: an electrochemical study in rat. *J. Neurosci.* **16,** 8160–8169.
96. Smith, I.D. and Grace, A.A. (1992) Role of subthalamic nucleus in the regulation of nigral dopamine neuron activity. *Synapse* **12,** 287–303.
97. Grace, A.A. and Bunney, B.S. (1995) Electrophysiological properties of midbrain dopamine neurons, in *Psychopharmacology: The Fourth Generation of Progress* (Bloom, F.E. and Kupfer, D.J., eds.), Raven Press, New York, pp. 163–177.

98. Francois, C., Percheron, G., Yelnik, J., and Heyner, S. (1979) Demonstration of the existence of small local circuit neurons in the Golgi-stained primate substantia nigra. *Brain Res.* **172,** 160–164.
99. Johnson, S.W. and North, R.A. (1992) Two types of neurone in the rat ventral tegmental area and their synaptic inputs. *J. Physiol.* **450,** 455–468.
100. Cepeda, C. and Levine, M.S. (1998) Dopamine and N-methyl-D-aspartate receptor interactions in the neostriatum. *Dev. Neurosci.* **20,** 1–18.
101. Mogenson, G.J., Brudzynski, S.M., Wu, M., Yang, C.R., and Yim, C.C.Y. (1993) From motiviation to action: a review of dopaminergic regulation of limbic-nucleus accumbens-pedunculopontine nucleus circuitries involved in limbic-motor integration, in *Limbic Motor Circuits and Neuropsychiatry* (Kalivas, P.W. and Barnes, C.D., eds.), CRC Press, Boca Raton, pp. 193-236.
102. Groenewegen, H.J., Wright, C.I., and Beijer, A.V.J. (1996) The nucleus accumbens: gateway for limbic structures to reach the motor system? in *Progress in Brain Research* (Holstege, G., Bandler, R., and Saper, C.P., eds.), Amsterdam, Elsevier Science, pp. 485–511.
103. Schultz, W., Dayan, P., and Montague, P.R. (1997) A neural substrate of prediction and reward [review]. *Science* **275,** 1593–1599.
104. Ljungberg, T., Apicella, P., and Schultz, W. (1992) Responses of monkey dopamine neurons during learning of behavioral reactions. *J. Neurophysiol.* **67,** 145–163.
105. Parent, A. and Hazrati, L.N. (1995) Functional anatomy of the basal ganglia. I. The cortico-basal ganglia-thalamo-cortical loop. *Brain Res. Brain Res. Rev.* **20,** 91–127.
106. Sherman, S.M. and Guillery, R.W. (1996) Functional organization of thalamocortical relays. *J. Neurophysiol.* **76,** 1367–1395.
107. Pare, D., Curro'Dossi, R., and Steriade, M. (1990) Neuronal basis of the parkinsonian resting tremor: a hypothesis and its implications for treatment. *Neuroscience* **35,** 217–226.
108. Jones, E.G. (1998) The thalamus of primates, in *The Primate Nervous System, Part II,* Vol. 14 (Bloom, F. E., Björklund, A., and Hökfelt, T., eds.), Elsevier Science, Amsterdam, pp. 1–298.
109. Contreras, D. and Steriade, M. (1997) Synchronization of low-frequency rhythms in corticothalamic networks. *Neuroscience* **76,** 11–24.
110. Steriade, M. (1999) Coherent oscillations and short-term plasticity in corticothalamic networks. *Trends Neurosci.* **22,** 337–345.
111. Destexhe, A., Contreras, D., and Steriade, M. (1998) Mechanisms underlying the synchronizing action of corticothalamic feedback through inhibition of thalamic relay cells. *J. Neurophysiol.* **79,** 999–1016.
112. Bal, T., Debay, D., and Destexhe, A. (2000) Cortical feedback controls the frequency and synchrony of oscillation in the visual thalamus. *J. Neurosci.* **20,** 7478–7488.
113. Catsman-Berrevoets, C.E. and Kuypers, H.G. (1978) Differential laminar distribution of corticothalamic neurons projecting to the VL and the center median. An HRP study in the cynomolgus monkey. *Brain Res.* **154,** 359–365.
114. Deschenes, M., Veinante, P., and Zhang, Z.W. (1998) The organization of corticothalamic projections: reciprocity versus parity. *Brain Res. Brain Res. Rev.* **28,** 286–308.
115. Murphy, P.C. and Sillito, A.M. (1996) Functional morphology of the feedback pathway from area 17 of the cat visual cortex to the lateral geniculate nucleus. *J. Neurosci.* **16,** 1180–1192.
116. Hoogland, P.V., Welker, E., and Van der Loos, H. (1987) Organization of the projections from barrel cortex to thalamus in mice studied with Phaseolus vulgaris-leucoagglutinin and HRP. *Exp. Brain Res.* **68,** 73–87.
117. Darian-Smith, C., Tan, A., and Edwards, S. (1999) Comparing thalamocortical and corticothalamic microstructure and spatial reciprocity in the macaque ventral posterolateral nucleus (VPLc) and medial pulvinar. *J. Comp. Neurol.* **410,** 211–234.
118. Jones, E.G. and Wise, S.P. (1977) Size, laminar and columnar distribution of efferent cells in the sensory-motor cortex of monkeys. *J. Comp. Neurol.* **175,** 391–438.
119. Giguere, M. and Goldman-Rakic, P.S. (1988) Mediodorsal nucleus: area 1 laminar and tangential distribution of afferents and efferents in the frontal lobe of rhesus monkeys. *J. Comp. Neurol.* **277,** 195–213.
120. Arikuni, T. and Kubota, K. (1986) The organization of prefrontocaudate projections and their laminar origin in the macaque monkey: a retrograde study using HRP-gel. *J. Comp. Neurol.* **244,** 492–510.
121. Chmielowska, J. and Pons, T.P. (1995) Patterns of thalamocortical degeneration after ablation of somatosensory cortex in monkeys. *J. Comp. Neurol.* **360,** 377–392.
122. Destexhe, A., Contreras, D., and Steriade, M. (1999) Cortically-induced coherence of a thalamic-generated oscillation. *Neuroscience* **92,** 427–443.
123. Ray, J.P. and Price, J.L. (1993) The organization of projections from the mediodorsal nucleus of the thalamus to orbital and medial prefrontal cortex in Macaque monkeys. *J. Comp. Neurol.* **337,** 1–31.
124. Russchen, F.T., Amaral, D.G., and Price, J.L. (1987) The afferent input to the magnocellular division of the mediodorsal thalamic nucleus in the monkey, Macaca fascicularis. *J. Comp. Neurol.* **256,** 175–210.
125. Nakajima, S. (1984) Serotonergic mediation of habenular self-stimulation in the rat. *Pharmacol. Biochem. Behav.* **20,** 859–862.
126. McFarland, N.R. and Haber, S.N. (2002) Thalamic relay nuclei of the basal ganglia form both reciprocal and non-reciprocal cortical connections linking multiple frontal cortical areas. *J. Neurosci.* **22,** 8117–8132.

4
Understanding Corticobasal Ganglia Networks as Part of a Habit Formation System

Ann M. Graybiel, PhD and Yasuo Kubota, PhD

1. INTRODUCTION

The basal ganglia are nodal points in corticobasal ganglia circuits that have been implicated in a range of cognitive and motor disorders *(1–4)*. In normal individuals, the basal ganglia may be essential to the development of the kinds of automatic or semiautomatic behaviors that underlie habits in everyday life *(5–9)*. There is no definitive link yet between normal habits and the symptomatology present in the particular clinical disorders attributable to basal ganglia dysfunction. But there is great interest in the possibility that the neural mechanisms that make the habit learning possible are malfunctional in basal ganglia disorders. At the heart of this view is the idea that in order to form a habit, it may be necessary to "chunk" together movements, complex acts or sequences, or cognitive acts by means of developing novel neural firing patterns that represent the entire action sequences or that, at minimum, release the action sequences when triggered by an external or internal stimulus *(10)*. Current electrophysiological evidence suggests that much of the temporal and spatial organization of behavioral sequences is built up in the neocortex, especially in the regions of the frontal and prefrontal cortex, including the supplementary motor areas *(11,12)*. Yet, there is strong experimental evidence that neurons in the basal ganglia also become active preferentially in relation to sequences of movements *(13–18)*. There are massive inputs to the basal ganglia from the frontal cortex, so that much of the neuronal activity in the basal ganglia may depend on the neocortex for its patterning. However, because corticobasal ganglia circuits lead from large parts of the cerebral cortex through basal ganglia nuclei to the frontal cortex, the basal ganglia may actually be important for the development of sequence representation in the frontal cortex.

Imaging studies have already demonstrated coordinate activation of the frontal cortex and the striatum in performance of sequential tasks in normal subjects *(19–25)* and, in the clinical setting, have demonstrated coordinate abnormal activation in the frontal cortex and basal ganglia in disorders ranging from Parkinson's disease to obsessive–compulsive disorder and Tourette syndrome *(2,26,27)*. These studies suggest that neural activity patterns associated with the acquisition and performance of sequences are dynamic. As performance begins, activity is greatest in anterior parts of the frontal cortex and striatum and, with time, activity shifts toward more posterior parts of the frontal cortex and striatum *(28–30)*. This suggests that ensembles of neurons in different regions become coordinately active or inactive during the evolution of complex behaviors. Understanding the dynamics of this process may be critical for understanding the neural mechanisms underlying clinical disorders that, at steady state, have abnormalities in complex motor and cognitive action as major symptomatologies.

From: *Mental and Behavioral Dysfunction in Movement Disorders*
Edited by: M-A. Bédard et al. © Humana Press Inc., Totowa, NJ

2. REORGANIZATION OF NEURONAL ACTIVITY PATTERNS IN THE STRIATUM DURING HABIT LEARNING

To study these issues at a mechanistic level, we have begun to record simultaneously from ensembles of individual neurons in the striatum and the cerebral cortex as animals learn habits. As a first approach, we recorded chronically with multiple electrodes from the striatum of rats as they learned to navigate in simple mazes in order to gain reward at the end of the maze *(31)*. Such a task has the great advantage of involving free unhindered action on the part of the animal. Moreover, the task involves both motor and cognitive operations. The animal must decide when to initiate movement, then learn to carry out the maze run itself, and, in so doing, decide which maze path to follow. In the T-maze task (see Fig. 1) that we have mainly used, we added an auditory conditional cue to instruct the animal about which of the two choice arms to enter in order to reach the reward-bated goal. This allowed us to examine neural activity that might occur with such instruction, as well as anticipation and decision making following the cueing. Altogether, the task involves elements of at least two stages of habit formation: a first stage in which the animal learns to run in the maze, and a second in which its reaction to the instruction cue becomes automatic. We found that the performance of this maze task is dependent on normal operation of the basal ganglia. Excitotoxic lesions in the dorsolateral striatum in rats already trained in the task produced impairment in choice accuracy *(32)*.

During the entire time that the animals learned and performed the maze task, we recorded the activity of striatal neurons with electrodes chronically implanted in the striatum. In the first of these studies, we focused on recording from the projection neurons in the sensorimotor striatum, which receives input from the sensorimotor cortex, so that we could track sensorimotor responses from the time the animals first were exposed to the task until after they had learned the task and then were given extensive overtraining *(31)*. To assess motor performance, we measured the reaction times of the animals to the opening of the start gate that initiated each trial, and we measured the speed of the maze runs. To assess accuracy of the maze performance, we calculated the percent of the time that animals chose the correct choice arm in response to the instruction cue. We then analyzed the neuronal activity patterns in relation to critical points in the task: the start of the maze run, the time that the instruction tone sounded, the times that the animals started and completed the turns into the goal arms, and goal-reaching itself. Altogether, we recorded from about 30 neurons per day from electrodes that moved very little, if at all. As a result, we could compare the activity patterns of local groups of neurons from day to day during the entire experiment.

We found dramatic changes in neuronal activity in the striatum as the animals learned to perform the maze task. Early during the habit learning, over half the task-related neurons responded when the animals executed the selected behavioral response by turning into the goal arm. As the animals learned, however, this kind of task-related activity fell dramatically. By contrast, there were very large increases in the number of task-related neurons that fired at the initiation of the maze run (at the start point) and also large increases in the numbers of task-related neurons that fired as the animals reached the goal. In fact, by the end of the training, large numbers of the striatal neurons responded selectively at the initiation and completion of the maze run, but fired very little during the actual run itself.

We found no selective relation in any of neural changes with any single performance measure that we analyzed. The performance measures did indicate, however, that the learning process might indeed have occurred in two stages, because the motor performance measures (reaction time and run time) tended to change earlier than performance accuracy (percent correct). By the time the animals reached the performance accuracy criterion (72.5% correct), the major changes in the start and turn responses had already occurred. There was a gradual increase in goal-related activity until the end of the experiment.

What could these large-scale changes in activity mean in relation to habit learning? One possibility is that as a habit is acquired, there is a reconfiguration of the neural circuitry involved in producing individual actions that together make up a habit. Early on, each component of the performance is

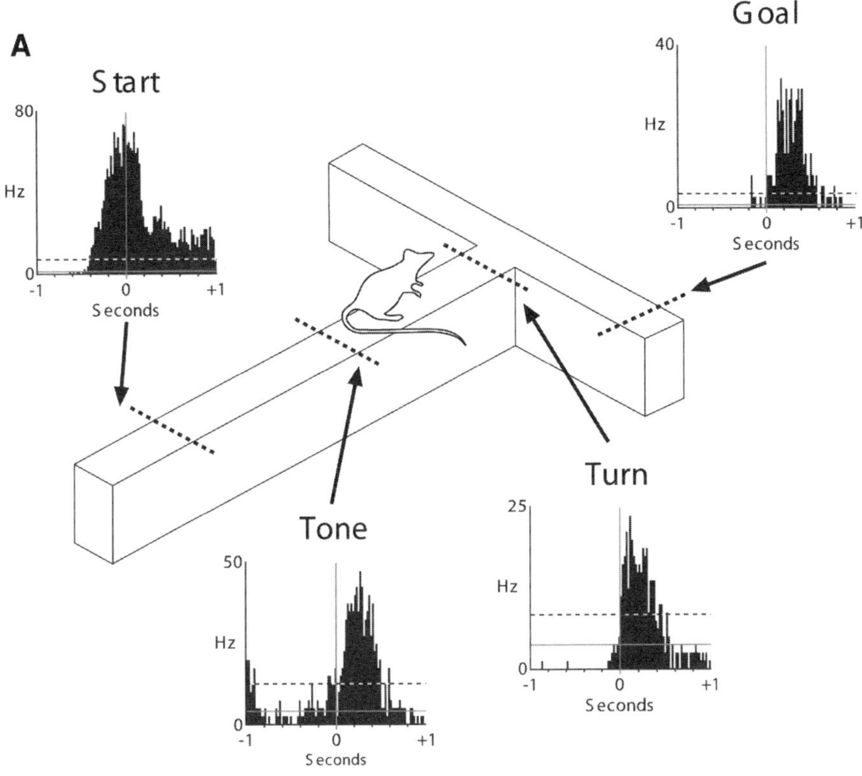

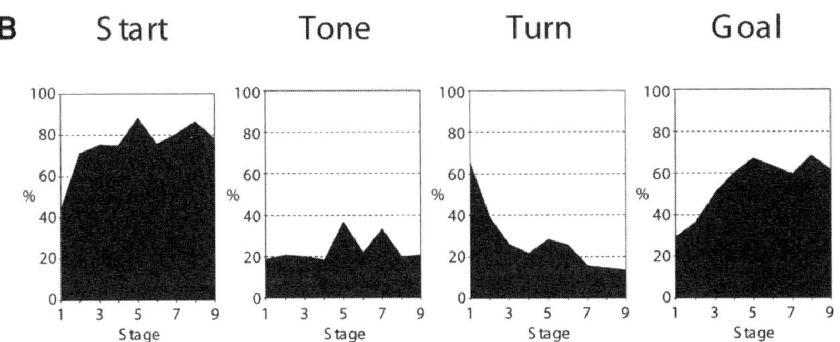

Fig. 1. Ensemble neuronal activity in the dorsolateral striatum in rats during acquisition and performance of a conditional turning task in a T-maze. (**A**) Rats were trained to initiate a maze run when a gate at the start area opened and to turn right or left at the choice point of the elevated T-maze, as instructed by auditory cues (1 or 8 kHz pure tone), in order to obtain a food reward. The tone was turned on when the rat broke a photobeam located along the long maze arm and remained on until the rat reached the goal or made an incorrect turn. Single unit activity of striatal neurons were analyzed in relation to four task events (start of maze run, tone onset, turn onset, and goal reaching). Examples of task-related discharges are shown in peri-event time histograms plotted in 20-ms bins for a 2-s period around each event as labeled. The gray horizontal line in each plot indicates the mean firing rate during the 2-s baseline period before each trial, and a dotted line represents the level of 2 standard deviations above the mean. (**B**) Summary plots showing the percent of all task-related units during acquisition of the T-maze learning task. The numbers on the horizontal axis represent learning stages where 1 and 2 are, respectively, the first and second days of training, and 3 to 9 indicate, respectively, the first to seventh sessions in which the percent correct performance of the rat reached $p < 0.01$ by chi-square test. Note large increase in start responses and goal responses, but dramatic decline in turn-related responses.

salient and represented by the neural activity. With time and repeated performance, some of the neural activity is short-circuited. Instead of having each component represented, a compressed representation occurs. In the case of the maze run, the firing of neurons in relation to the start might be sufficient to set off the habit (the run), and the firing of neurons in relation to goal-reaching might be sufficient to indicate completion of this complex act. In this way, the neural activity would form a chunked representation of the entire behavior sequence—a trigger for action.

If this line of reasoning were correct, then one might expect another remodeling of the circuit to occur if the habit were broken. In on-going experiments, we are testing for this possibility by having animals undergo extinction training, in which a reward is no longer given for correct responses *(33)*. Again, recordings are made in the sensorimotor striatum during acquisition and overtraining, and they are then continued through an extensive extinction period. The data collected so far strongly suggest that remodeling of the response characteristics of striatal neurons occurred as the maze habit is broken. At the end of the extinction training, responses during turning increased, and responses at start and goal reaching decreased, relative to levels acquired by the end of overtraining.

A surprising aspect of these findings is that the habit learning appears to broaden the spectrum of responsivity of neurons in the sensorimotor striatum. Many neurons, after habit learning, fire at the start of the task, even if the animal is not actively moving. This activity could, for example, represent anticipation of the maze run or the eventual reward to be obtained, or represent a general readiness to respond. In either case, these behavioral correlations would suggest cognitive coding by neurons of the sensorimotor striatum. Much the same is true for the firing at goal-reaching, which could have more to do with reward anticipation or marking the end of the task than with deceleration *per se*.

In our initial study of the sensorimotor striatum, we found very few neurons that responded in relation to the presentation of the auditory conditional cues. These cues signaled which goal arm was bated with reward and, thus, were the most salient stimuli for the selection of a behavioral response (turning direction). If the striatum were involved in acquiring new association between salient stimuli and behavioral responses, then striatal neurons should respond to the cue presentations and/or have striatal activity that links the cue information and response selection. The neurons in the sensorimotor striatum, however, do not receive cortical inputs carrying auditory information; neurons in other regions of the striatum, such as medial striatum, which receives inputs from auditory and limbic cortices, should mediate such processes. In fact, in one of the animals, electrodes were placed more medially, and we found more neurons that fired in relation to the cue presentation. Interestingly, the number of neurons with tone-related responses increased during early training stages and decreased with training, so that by the end of the training, most neurons responded only at start and/or at goal-reaching.

3. NEURONAL PLASTICITY EXHIBITED BY INTRINSIC NETWORK NEURONS OF THE STRIATUM DURING REINFORCEMENT-BASED LEARNING

Together, these findings suggest that projection neurons in striatum are highly sensitive to environmental contexts that lead to habit learning, and also suggest that one of the outcomes of such habit learning may be a reconfiguration of neuronal circuit activity within the striatum. The neurons that showed reconfigured ensemble activity were identifiable as projection neurons, which make up more than 90% of all the neurons in the striatum. Changes in patterns of convergent and divergent input to these neurons may have been instrumental in reconfiguring the circuit *(34)*. However, an interesting possibility is that part of the circuit modification resulted from changes in the activity of local circuit neurons, which make up no more than 10% of all neurons in the striatum and which influence these projection neurons *(35)*. There are five classes of striatal interneurons. The best known of these are the tonically active neurons (usually called TANs). These neurons are readily identifiable in the primate striatum by their low irregular firing rates and the by the fact that they do not fire in relation to movement, but instead, fire in response to salient sensory stimuli. TANs are of special interest because they are thought to be the cholinergic interneurons of the striatum and, thus, to have an important role in modulating striatal function in coordination with the actions of dopamine-containing nigrostriatal inputs.

We and our collaborators have carried out experiments in macaque monkeys to test the possibility that these neurons show plasticity in their responsiveness to sensory stimuli as a result of behavioral training *(36)*. The results of these experiments demonstrate that, during sensorimotor conditioning tasks, TANs acquire responses to stimuli that predict the presentation of reward. Remarkably, if the dopamine-containing input to the striatum is then damaged by local infusion of the neurotoxin, 1-methyl-4-phenyl-1,2,3,6-tetrahydoropyridine (MPTP), the acquired responses of the TANs are greatly decreased *(37)*. This result suggests that TANs may have a special role in mediating dopamine-modulated plasticity in the striatum. Most of the cholinergic neuropil of the striatum is in the matrix compartment (the large compartment that receives sensorimotor and association cortical inputs and that gives rise to direct and indirect pathways of the striatum) *(38)*. Interestingly, when we marked the sites at which TANs were identified by physiological recording in monkeys, many of the marked sites turned out to lie at, or very close to, the borders between striosomes and matrix *(39)*. This distribution suggested the notion that TANs may be a part of a mechanism coordinating activity between the sensorimotor matrix and the striosomes, which are thought to be most strongly affiliated with limbic input coming from such sites as the orbitofrontal cortex and medial prefrontal–anterior cingulate cortex *(40)*. If the TANs operate to induce circuit reconfigurations in the striatum, they might be in a good position to do so based on evaluating the significance of the stimuli via limbic input and then exerting effects on the large matrix compartment from which the direct and indirect pathways originate.

Early experiments on TANs suggested that they are primarily part of a reward-based learning circuitry of the striatum, but more recent evidence suggests that they have broader functions *(41–44)*. They respond to neutral stimuli and to aversive stimuli, and they receive inputs not only from reward-sensitive dopaminergic neurons of the substantia nigra, but also from neurons of the intralaminar nuclei, which respond to salient stimuli regardless of reward association *(45)*. Lesions of the intralaminar nuclei in the macaque decreased acquired sensory responses in striatal TANs nearly as much as the lesions of the dopamine-containing substantia nigra *(45)*. These findings suggest that TANs integrate reward-related signals originating in the substantia nigra with signals originating from the intralaminar nuclei, which have been associated with brainstem arousal mechanisms.

Our laboratory recently has found that TANs readily acquire responses to aversive airpuffs directed toward the eye in a macaque monkey performing a classical delayed conditioning task, and that they show equally dramatic loss of such responses as a result of extinction training *(42,43)*. Moreover, the TAN responses increase in proportion to the intensity of sensory stimuli and show systematic habituation with repeated exposure to these stimuli. These results point to the functions of TANs as extending beyond positive reinforcement domain; these striatal interneurons appear to signal the relevance for behavior of ongoing sensory events.

The TANs of the striatum are sparsely distributed, but they are distributed throughout the striatum. Thus, they could influence a large part of the striatum and, consequently, a large part of corticobasal ganglia loop circuitry. This broad distribution suggested the idea that TANs might participate in binding sensorimotor and cognitive processing in the striatum *(34,46)*. There is as yet no full account of how TANs influence other neurons of the striatum, but they are thought to regulate not only cortical and dopaminergic inputs to striatal projection neurons, but also to regulate the activity of other striatal neurons. Given the available evidence in the monkey experiments, they seem likely candidates to contribute neuronal plasticity underlying habit formation.

4. IMPLICATIONS OF STRIATAL PLASTICITY FOR MENTAL AND BEHAVIORAL DYSFUNCTION IN MOVEMENT DISORDERS

A central issue that remains to be resolved is how these activities of neurons in the striatum of normal animals, and their putative relation to habit formation, are affected in basal ganglia disorders.

If the striatum were involved in the chunking of actions and action repertoires to produce habits, and if the plasticity of striatal neurons were involved in this phenomenon, then dysfunctions of striatal circuits could be involved in genesis of symptomatology associated with basal ganglia disorders. There is convincing evidence that patients with Parkinson's disease and Huntington's disease have deficits in learning and performing new behavioral procedures *(8,9,47–52)*. A reduction in the capacity of striatal neurons to form new associations under the modulation of dopaminergic input could underlie this impairment. Particularly striking are symptoms of obsessive–compulsive disorder and Tourette syndrome, in which thoughts and actions, including sometimes complex trains of thought and action, are expressed without intent but with urgency *(1,2)*. If the release of these thoughts and actions were related to striatal dysfunction, they might represent abnormally released, and possibly abnormal chunked, activity patterns of corticobasal ganglia loop function.

ACKNOWLEDGMENTS

This work was supported by the Stanley Foundation, the National Parkinson Foundation, National Institute of Mental Health (NIMH) MH60379, and Javits award National Institute of Neurological Disorders and Stroke (NINDS) NS25529.

REFERENCES

1. Graybiel, A. and Rauch, S. (2000) Toward a neurobiology of obsessive-compulsive disorder. *Neuron* **28,** 343–347.
2. Leckman, J.F. and Riddle, M.A. (2000) Tourette's syndrome: when habit-forming systems form habits of their own? *Neuron* **28,** 349–354.
3. Albin, R.L., Young, A.B., and Penney, J.B. (1989) The functional anatomy of basal ganglia disorders. *Trends Neurosci.* **12,** 366–375.
4. Wichmann, T. and DeLong, M.R. (1996) Functional and pathophysiological models of the basal ganglia. *Curr. Opin. Neurobiol.* **6,** 751–758.
5. Hirsh, R. (1974) The hippocampus and contextual retrieval of information from memory: a theory. *Behav. Biol.* **12,** 421–444.
6. Knowlton, B.J., Mangels, J.A. and Squire, L.R. (1996) A neostriatal habit learning system in humans. *Science* **273,** 1399–1402.
7. Mishkin, M., Malamut, B., and Bachevalier, J. (1984) Memories and habits: two neural systems, in *Neurobiology of Human Learning and Memory* (Lynch, G., McGaugh, J.L., and Weinberger, N.M., eds.), Guilford Press, New York, pp. 65–77.
8. Salmon, D.P. and Butters, N. (1995) Neurobiology of skill and habit learning. *Curr. Opin. Neurobiol.* **5,** 184–190.
9. White, N.M. (1997) Mnemonic functions of the basal ganglia. *Curr. Opin. Neurobiol.* **7,** 164–169.
10. Graybiel, A.M. (1998) The basal ganglia and chunking of action repertoires. *Neurobiol. Learn. Mem.* **70,** 119–136.
11. Tanji, J. and Hoshi, E. (2001) Behavioral planning in the prefrontal cortex. *Curr. Opin. Neurobiol.* **11,** 164–170.
12. Fuster, J.M. (1997) *The Prefrontal Cortex: Anatomy, Physiology, and Neuropsychology of the Frontal Lobe,* Lippincott Williams & Wilkins, Philadelphia.
13. Hikosaka, O., Sakamoto, M., and Usui, S. (1989) Functional properties of monkey caudate neurons I. Activities related to saccadic eye movements. *J. Neurophysiol.* **61,** 780–798.
14. Hikosaka, O., Sakamoto, M., and Usui, S. (1989) Functional properties of monkey caudate neurons. III. Activities related to expectation of target and reward. *J. Neurophysiol.* **61,** 814–832.
15. Hikosaka, O., Sakamoto, M., and Usui, S. (1989) Functional properties of monkey caudate neurons. II. Visual and auditory responses. *J. Neurophysiol.* **61,** 799–813.
16. Kermadi, I. and Joseph, J.P. (1995) Activity in the caudate nucleus of monkey during spatial sequencing. *J. Neurophysiol.* **74,** 911–933.
17. Matsumoto, N., Hanakawa, T., Maki, S., Graybiel, A.M., and Kimura, M. (1999) Role of nigrostriatal dopamine system in learning to perform sequential motor tasks in a predictive manner. *J. Neurophysiol.* **82,** 978–998.
18. Mushiake, H. and Strick, P.L. (1995) Pallidal neuron activity during sequential arm movements. *J. Neurophysiol.* **74,** 2754–2758.
19. Grafton, S.T., Woods, R.P., and Tyszka, M. (1994) Functional imaging of procedural motor learning: relating cerebral blood flow with individual subject performance. *Hum. Brain Mapp.* **1,** 221–234.
20. Jenkins, I.H., Brooks, D.J., Nixon, P.D., Frackowiak, R.S., and Passingham, R.E. (1994) Motor sequence learning: a study with positron emission tomography. *J. Neurosci.* **14,** 3775–3790.
21. Rauch, S.L., Savage, C.R., Brown, H.D., et al. (1995) A PET investigation of implicit and explicit sequence learning. *Hum. Brain Mapp.* **3,** 271–286.
22. Rauch, S.L., Whalen, P.J., Savage, C.R., et al. (1997) Striatal recruitment during an implicit sequence learning task as measured by functional magnetic resonance imaging. *Hum. Brain Mapp.* **5,** 124–132.

23. Seitz, R.J. and Roland, P.E. (1992) Learning of sequential finger movements in man: a combined kinematic and positron emission tomography (PET) study. *Eur. J. Neurosci.* **4,** 154–165.
24. Seitz, R.J., Roland, P.E., Bohm, C., Greitz, T., and Stone-Elander, S. (1990) Motor learning in man: a positron emission tomographic study. *NeuroReport* **1,** 57–60.
25. Shadmehr, R. and Holcomb, H.H. (1997) Neural correlates of motor memory consolidation. *Science* **277,** 821–825.
26. Harrington, D.L. and Haaland, K.Y. (1991) Sequencing in Parkinson's disease: abnormalities in programming and controlling movement. *Brain* **114,** 99–115.
27. Brown, R.G. (1999) The roles of cortico-striatal circuits in learning sequential information, in *Parkinson's Disease* (Advances Neurology, 80) (Stern, G.M., ed.), Lippincott Williams and Wilkins, Philadelphia, pp. 31–39.
28. Sakai, K., Hikosaka, O., Miyauchi, S., Takino, R., Sasaki, Y., and Putz, B. (1998) Transition of brain activation from frontal to parietal areas in visuomotor sequence learning. *J. Neurosci.* **18,** 1827–1840.
29. Jueptner, M., Stephan, K.M., Frith, C.D., Brooks, D.J., Frackowiak, R.S.J., and Passingham, R.E. (1997) Anatomy of motor learning I. Frontal cortex and attention to action. *J. Neurophysiol.* **77,** 1313–1324.
30. Jueptner, M., Frith, C.D., Brooks, D.J., Frackowiak, R.S.J., and Passingham, R.E. (1997) Anatomy of motor learning II. Subcortical structures and learning by trial and error. *J. Neurophysiol.* **77,** 1325–1337.
31. Jog, M., Kubota, Y., Connolly, C.I., Hillegaart, V., and Graybiel, A.M. (1999) Building neural representations of habits. *Science* **286,** 1745–1749.
32. DeCoteau, W., Hu, D., Kubota, Y., and Graybiel, A. (2000) Striatal lesions impair performance of a T-maze procedural learning task in rats. *Soc. Neurosci. Abstr.* **26,** 684.
33. Hu, D., Kubota, K., and Graybiel, A.M. (2001) Successive resculpting of task-related activity patterns in the striatum during action-sequence procedural learning, extinction and relearning. *Soc. Neurosci. Abstr.* **27,** 514.9.
34. Graybiel, A.M., Aosaki, T., Flaherty, A.W., and Kimura, M. (1994) The basal ganglia and adaptive motor control. *Science* **265,** 1826–1831.
35. Kawaguchi, Y., Wilson, C.J., Augood, S.J., and Emson, P.C. (1995) Striatal interneurons: chemical, physiological and morphological characterization. *Trends Neurosci.* **18,** 527–535.
36. Aosaki, T., Tsubokawa, H., Ishida, A., Watanabe, K., Graybiel, A.M., and Kimura, M. (1994) Responses of tonically active neurons in the primate's striatum undergo systematic changes during behavioral sensorimotor conditioning. *J. Neurosci.* **14,** 3969–3984.
37. Aosaki, T., Graybiel, A.M., and Kimura, M. (1994) Effects of the nigrostriatal dopamine system on acquired neural responses in the striatum of behaving monkeys. *Science* **265,** 412–415.
38. Graybiel, A.M., Baughman, R.W., and Eckenstein, F. (1986) Cholinergic neuropil of the striatum observes striosomal boundaries. *Nature* **323,** 625–627.
39. Aosaki, T., Kimura, M., and Graybiel, A.M. (1995) Temporal and spatial characteristics of tonically active neurons of the primate's striatum. *J. Neurophysiol.* **73,** 1234–1252.
40. Eblen, F. and Graybiel, A.M. (1995) Highly restricted origin of prefrontal cortical inputs to striosomes in the macaque monkey. *J. Neurosci.* **15,** 5999–6013.
41. Ravel, S., Legallet, E., and Apicella, P. (1999) Tonically active neurons in the monkey striatum do not preferentially respond to appetitive stimuli. *Exp. Brain Res.* **128,** 531–534.
42. Blazquez, P., Fujii, N., Kojima, J., and Graybiel, A.M. (2000) A network representation of response probability in the striatum. *Neuron* **14,** 973–982.
43. Blazquez, P.M., Fujii, N., DeCoteau, W.E., and Graybiel, A.M. (2001) Tonically active neurons in the primate striatum have responses that correlate with the probability of behavioral respose in reward and aversive Pavlovian conditioning and habituation. *Soc. Neurosci. Abstr.* **27,** 514.8.
44. Shimo, Y., Sato, M., and Hikosaka, O. (2000) Tonically active neurons in monkey caudate nuclei carry spatial, rather than reward, information. *Soc. Neurosci. Abstr.* **26,** 254.10.
45. Matsumoto, N., Minamimoto, T., Graybiel, A.M., and Kimura, M. (2001) Neurons in the thalamic CM-Pf complex supply neurons in the striatum with information about behaviorally significant sensory events. *J. Neurophysiol.* **85,** 960–976.
46. Graybiel, A.M. (1997) The basal ganglia and cognitive pattern generators. *Schizophr. Bull.* **23,** 459–469.
47. Graybiel, A.M. (1995) Building action repertoires: memory and learning functions of the basal ganglia. *Curr. Opin. Neurobiol.* **5,** 733–741.
48. Frith, C.D., Bloxham, C.A., and Carpenter, K.N. (1986) Impairments in the learning and performance of a new manual skill in patients with Parkinson's disease. *J. Neurol. Neurosurg. Psychiatry* **49,** 661–668.
49. Gabrieli, J.D., Stebbins, G.T., Singh, J., Willingham, D.B., and Goetz, C.G. (1997) Intact mirror-tracing and impaired rotary-pursuit skill learning in patients with Huntington's disease: evidence for dissociable memory systems in skill learning. *Neuropsychology* **11,** 272–281.
50. Pascual-Leone, A., Grafman, J., Clark, K., et al. (1993) Procedural learning in Parkinson's disease and cerebellar degeneration. *Ann. Neurol.* **34,** 594–602.
51. Soliveri, P., Brown, R.G., Jahanshahi, M., Caracani, T., and Marsden, C.D. (1997) Learning manual pursuit tracking skills in patients with Parkinson's disease. *Brain* **120,** 963–976.
52. Vriezen, E.R. and Moscovitch, M. (1990) Memory for temporal order and conditional associate-learning in patients with Parkinson's disease. *Neuropsychologia* **28,** 1283–1293.

5

The Role of the Cerebellum in Cognition and Emotion

Jeremy D. Schmahmann, MD

1. INTRODUCTION

The traditional notion regarding cerebellar function has been that it is important for coordinating voluntary motor activity *(1)*. Early studies of patients with degenerative cerebellar diseases or focal cerebellar injuries *(2)* described ataxia (wide-based lurching gait) and dysmetria (inaccuracy and wavering unsteadiness or dysrhythmia of directed extremity movements). These observations led to the conclusion that when cerebellum malfunctions, balance and coordination are impaired, tremor is evident, eye movements are disordered, speech is dysarthric, and handwriting is illegible. Theories of cerebellar function, experiments to test the role of the cerebellum in nervous system, and the interpretation of previously available cerebellar anatomy have been predicated on the hypothesis that cerebellum is a motor control device.

Reconsideration of the clinical and experimental literature, however, revealed that a sizeable body of credible evidence was overlooked in reaching this motor control view, and there were early indications that this did not account for all the observed cerebellar functions *(3–8)*. The understanding of the cerebellum is presently in the midst of a paradigm shift. At the heart of this reevaluation is the recognition that cerebellum may contribute a unique modulating role to a wide array of functions and that loss of cerebellar modulation degrades many different types of behaviors in a unique manner. This change in appreciation of the role of the cerebellum has been facilitated by converging lines of evidence from anatomical, clinical, experimental, and functional neuroimaging data that suggest the motor view was, at best, incomplete (see ref. *9*). This chapter provides an overview of: (*i*) anatomic substrates that may facilitate the cerebellar modulation of mental operations; (*ii*) clinical observations of impairments of intellect and emotion following cerebellar lesions; and (*iii*) a theoretical approach to understanding the fundamental role of the cerebellum in the nervous system. Comprehensive analyses of these topics by this and other authors may be found in Schmahmann *(9–13)*.

2. HISTORICAL CONSIDERATIONS

Clinical reports dating back to the mid-1800s *(3,7)* contain anecdotal descriptions of patients with cerebellar atrophy, degeneration, or agenesis, in whom clinical manifestations included or were characterized predominantly by psychosis, mental retardation, and dementia. The earliest experimental demonstrations of cerebellar influences outside the motor domain were derived from physiological studies of the effects of fastigial nucleus stimulation. This produced changes in the electroencephalographic pattern *(14)* and autonomic phenomena, such as alterations in blood pressure, heart rate, vascular reactivity, and pupil diameter *(15)*. The complex nonstereotyped behaviors of grooming, self-stimulation, sham rage (the "hypothalamic outbursts" of Bard *[16]*), and predatory attack were also elicited

From: *Mental and Behavioral Dysfunction in Movement Disorders*
Edited by: M-A. Bédard et al. © Humana Press Inc., Totowa, NJ

by fastigial nucleus stimulation *(17,18)*. Electrophysiological mapping studies *(19)* indicated topography of motor function within the cerebellum. These "motor" maps, however, were derived from sensory stimulation experiments, and they demonstrated also that there are peripheral and central visual and auditory inputs to vermal lobules VI and VII. Snider, along with others, asserted that cerebellum is involved in nonmotor control and that it has a role to play in the highest levels of human behavior.

The notion that cerebellum is a motor control device was broadened by the demonstration that cerebellum is involved in motor learning *(20,21)*. It was further challenged by evidence that the cerebellum is critical for conditional associative learning in rabbits, ferrets, and in humans (see ref. *22*) and for the procedural learning and memory inherent in spatial navigation in cerebellar mutant mice *(23)* and in rats subject to hemicerebellectomy *(24)*.

3. ANATOMIC ORGANIZATION OF THE CEREBROCEREBELLAR SYSTEM

The cerebellar cortex is characterized by a repeating cytoarchitecture that, with a few exceptions, is essentially constant throughout the structure *(25)*. A repeating sequence is also seen in the chemoarchitectonic divisions within the cerebellar cortex that are identified by alternating bands of neuronal staining induced by monoclonal antibodies *(26)*. In contrast, there is a rich complexity and diversity to the connections between cerebellar hemispheres and cerebellum. The cerebellum has connections with the reticular system that support arousal; the hypothalamus, which is important for autonomic function; the limbic system that subserves the experience and expression of emotion; and the paralimbic and neocortical association areas crucial for cognitive processes and the cognitive dimensions of affect. These anatomic systems provide the necessary substrates to support the notion that there is topographic organization in the cerebellar contribution to both sensorimotor and nonmotor processing and are, therefore, reviewed here in some detail.

3.1. Reticular System

The vermis at the cerebellar midline and the fastigial nucleus are anatomically tightly linked and functionally related *(27)*. Reticular projections to the vermal–fastigial region arise from the pontine raphe and pontine reticular tegmental nucleus, and from the mesencephalic and medullary reticular formation *(28)*. The lateral reticular nucleus sends projections to all the cerebellar nuclei *(29,30)*.

Fastigial nucleus projections to the reticular formation are directed to the medial, lateral, and paramedian reticular nuclei, the vestibular nuclei, nucleus tractus solitarius, nucleus gigantocellularis, and to the nucleus pontis caudalis, the physiological significance of which was underscored by elevation of blood pressure and heart rate following fastigial stimulation *(31)*. The fastigial nucleus also sends efferents to the central mesencephalic reticular formation, the periaqueductal gray and the lateral reticular nucleus *(29)*.

Efferent projections are also directed through the superior cerebellar peduncle to the nonspecific intralaminar thalamic nuclei, notably the central lateral, paracentral, paraventricular, and parafascicular nuclei *(29,30,32–34)* that project widely throughout the cerebral hemispheres and may play a role in arousal as well as in nociception.

Brainstem neurotransmitter systems in the raphe (serotonin), locus ceruleus (norepinephrine), ventral tegmental area (dopamine), and possibly histaminergic structures receive diffuse cerebral cortical input and, in turn, convey their efferents to widespread cerebellar regions *(35–37)*. This may confer a background tone upon which the mossy fiber and climbing fiber systems in the cerebellum exert their more specific and topographically precise influence.

3.2. Autonomic System

Physiological studies have demonstrated the influence of cerebellar stimulation on the autonomic nervous system. Respiratory and vasomotor carotid sinus reflexes are inhibited by stimulation of the anterior vermis *(38)*, and bradycardia, hypotension, mydriasis, altered gastrointestinal motility, length of gestational period, and piloerection are induced by anterior lobe cortex or fastigial nucleus stimulation *(15)*. The cerebellum also influences vasomotor tone *(31,39,40)* and vagally mediated respiratory reflexes *(41)*. Functional imaging studies that reveal cerebellar activation during painful stimulation *(42,43)*, thirst *(44)*, and hunger *(45)* also implicate the cerebellum in these autonomic-limbic behaviors.

Anatomic studies reveal connections between cerebellum and brainstem nuclei that subserve taste (the nucleus tractus solitarius), and nociceptor regions including periaqueductal gray, and the central lateral and paracentral intralaminar thalamic nuclei, previously mentioned. Reciprocal connections link multiple hypothalamic nuclei with all layers of the cerebellar cortex and the deep cerebellar nuclei *(46)*.

3.3. *Limbic System*

Electrical stimulation of the cerebellum influences the physiology of limbic system structures, producing evoked responses in hippocampus and amygdala *(47,48)*, and altered and/or arrested abnormal or epileptiform discharges in the hippocampus *(49,50)*. Heath et al. *(51)* demonstrated facilitation in the septal region, inhibition in the hippocampus, and a mixed pattern of responses in the amygdala in cats and rats following stimulation of the rostral vermis, fastigial nucleus, and intervening midline folia, but not following stimulation of the lateral cerebellar hemispheres and dentate nucleus.

Anatomic studies reveal projections from the fastigial nucleus of cat to the ventral tegmental area (VTA), interpeduncular nucleus, periaqueductal gray, and locus ceruleus, which are themselves interconnected with limbic regions *(52)*. The mesorhombencephalic component of the VTA also has a reciprocal projection back to the cerebellum *(53)*. The medial mammillary bodies are closely linked with the limbic anterior thalamic nuclei through the mammillothalamic tract, and they are also in communication with the cerebellum by way of their projections to the nuclei of the basilar pons *(54)*.

Finally, the cingulate gyrus implicated in depression *(55)* and in obsessive–compulsive disorder *(56)* has direct projections into the feedforward limb of the cerebrocerebellar circuits through the basilar pons *(57,58)*. The rostral cingulate projects to medial pontine nuclei and the caudal cingulate to more lateral regions.

3.4. *Association and Paralimbic Cortices*

The pathways linking the associative and paralimbic regions of the cerebral hemispheres with the cerebellum are critical in the consideration of the anatomic substrates that subserve the cerebellar involvement in cognitive operations. The circuit comprises a two-stage feedforward limb, in which the pontine nuclei serve as the obligatory synaptic step between the corticopontine pathway and the mossy fiber-mediated pontocerebellar pathway, and a two-stage feedback system, in which thalamus is the obligatory synaptic step between the cerebellothalamic and the thalamocortical projections *(59)* (Fig. 1).

3.4.1. Feedforward Limb

The corticopontine projections arise not only from sensorimotor regions *(60–62)*, but from the prefrontal cortex, from multimodal regions of the posterior parietal and temporal lobes, from paralimbic cortices in the cingulate and posterior parahippocampal gyrus, and from the visual association cortices in the parastriate region as well.

3.4.1.1. Prefrontal Cortex

Corticopontine projections from the prefrontal cortices are located in the medial aspects of the rostral half of the basilar pons and are distributed in a topographically precise manner, favoring the median, paramedian, dorsomedial, and medial part of the peripeduncular pontine nuclei *(63,64)* (Fig. 2). The prefrontal projections arise most prominently from the dorsolateral and dorsomedial convexities, from areas concerned with attention as well as with conjugate eye movements (area 8), the spatial attributes of memory and working memory (area 9/46d), planning, foresight, and judgment (area 10), motivational behavior and decision making capabilities (areas 9 and 32), and from areas considered to be homologous to the language area in human (areas 44 and 45) *(63–69)* (Fig. 2).

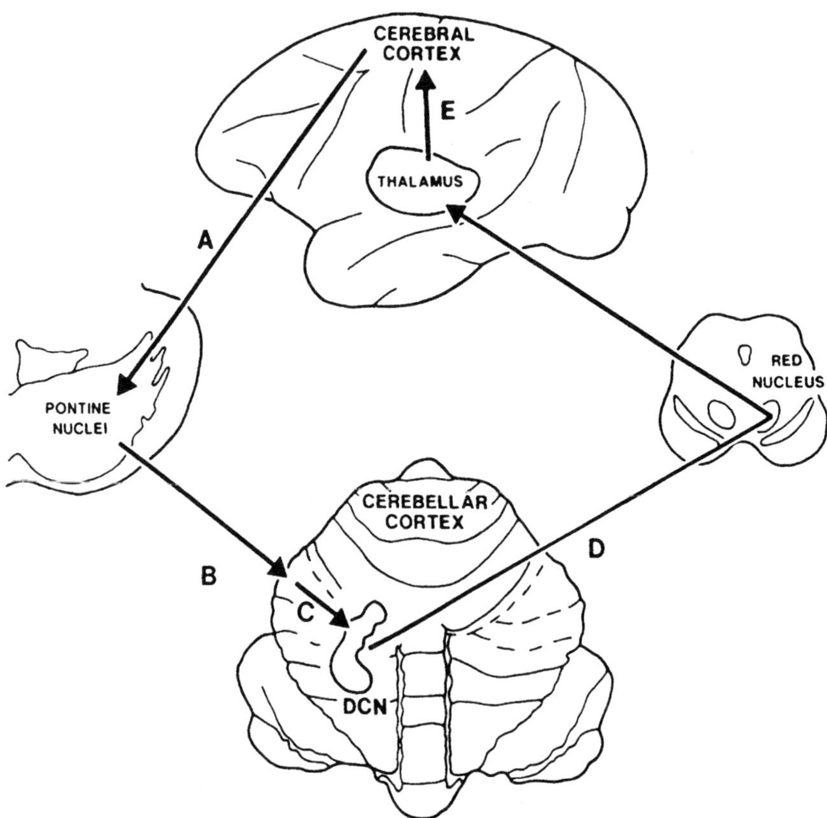

Fig. 1. Diagram of the cerebrocerebellar circuit. Feedforward limb: the corticopontine pathway (**A**) carries associative, paralimbic, sensory, and motor information from the cerebral cortex to the neurons in the ventral pons. The axons of these pontine neurons reach the cerebellar cortex via the pontocerebellar pathway (**B**). Feedback limb: the cerebellar cortex is connected with the deep cerebellar nuclei (DCN) (**C**), which project via the red nucleus to the thalamus (the cerebellothalamic projection) (**D**). The thalamic projection back to cerebral cortex (**E**) completes the feedback circuit. From Schmahmann (1994) ref. *184*.

3.4.1.2. Posterior Parietal Cortex

The superior parietal lobule, concerned with intramodality associative functions (multiple joint position sense, touch, and proprioceptive impulses from similar regions *[70]*) projects throughout the rostrocaudal extent of the pons focusing mostly on the nuclei in the central and lateral region of the basilar pons *(71)* (see Fig. 3). The inferior parietal lobule, important for spatial cognition and strongly implicated in the neglect syndrome *(72,73)*, projects to the rostral half of the pons, with terminations being located more at the lateral and dorsolateral pontine regions *(62,71,74,75)*.

Fig. 2. Diagram showing the distribution within the basilar pons of the rhesus monkey of projections derived from the prefrontal cortices. Injections of anterograde tracers in the medial (**A**) and lateral (**B**) surfaces of the cerebral hemisphere result in terminations (color-coded) in rostrocaudal levels of the pons I–IX. The plane of section through the basilar pons for both Figs. 2 and 3 is at the bottom of the diagram. The prefrontopontine projection is characterized by a complex mosaic of terminations. Each cerebral cortical region has preferential sites of pontine terminations. There is considerable interdigitation of the terminations from some of the different cortical sites, but almost no overlap. From Schmahmann and Pandya (1997) ref. *64*.

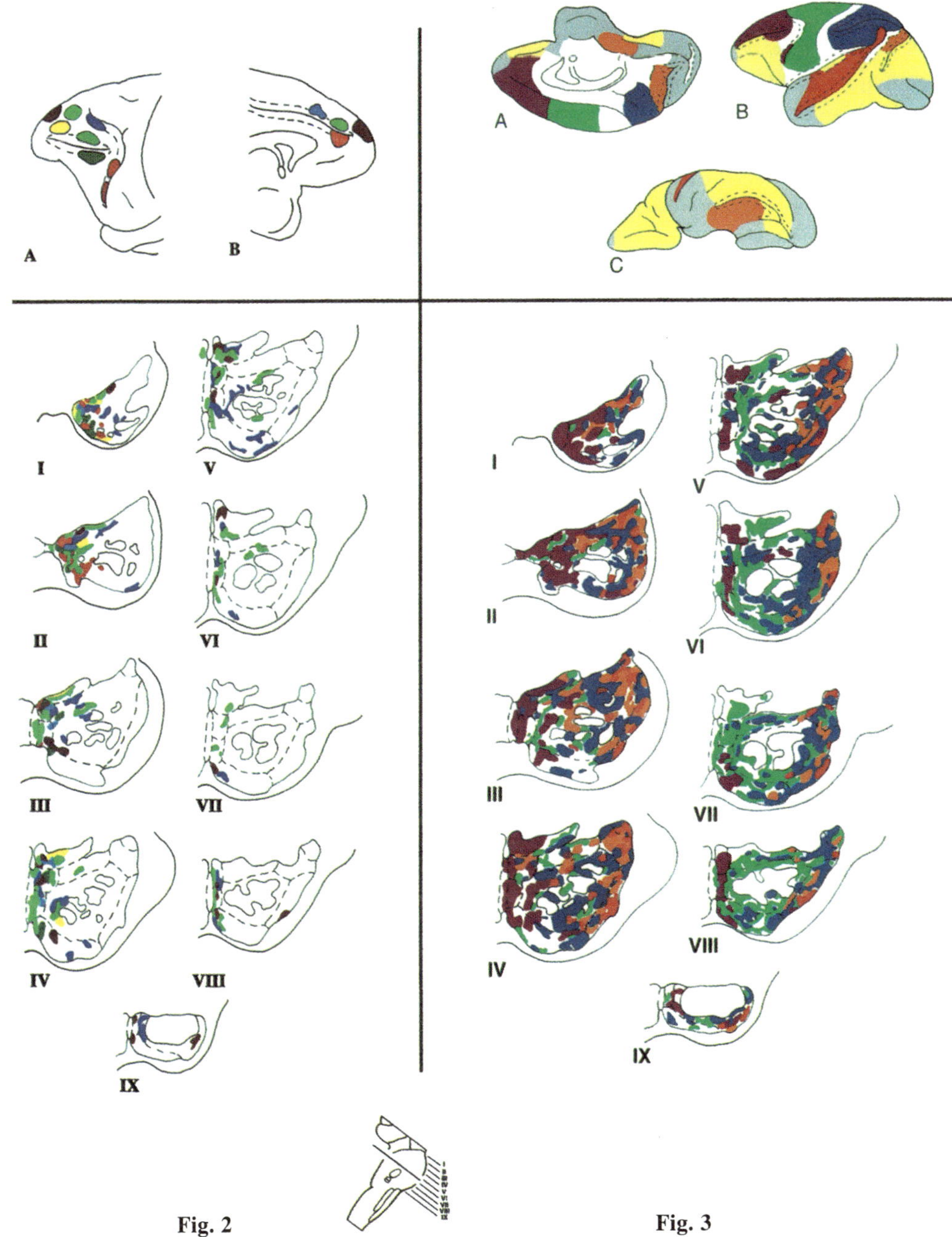

Fig. 3. The figure on the right is a color-coded summary diagram illustrating the distribution within the basilar pons (levels I–IX) of the rhesus monkey of projections derived from association and paralimbic cortices in the prefrontal (purple), posterior parietal (blue), temporal (red), and parastriate and parahippocampal regions (orange), and from motor, premotor and supplementary motor areas (green). The medial (**A**), lateral (**B**), and ventral (**C**) surfaces of the cerebral hemisphere are shown above. Cerebral areas that have been shown to project to the pons by other investigators using either anterograde or retrograde tracers are depicted in white. Areas that have no pontine projections (according to anterograde and retrograde studies) are shown in yellow; those with no pontine projections according to retrograde studies are in gray. Dashed lines on the hemispheres represent sulcal cortices. Dashed lines in the pons represent pontine nuclei, and solid lines demarcate corticospinal fibers. From Schmahmann (1996) ref. *59*.

3.4.1.3. Temporal Lobe

The auditory association areas in the superior temporal gyrus and supratemporal plane are connected with the lateral and dorsolateral pontine nuclei. The upper bank of the superior temporal sulcus is activated during face recognition tasks, influenced by direction of gaze *(76)*, and projects to the lateral, dorsolateral, and extreme dorsolateral pontine nuclei *(77)* (Fig. 3). The areas middle temporal (MT), fundus of the superior temporal (FST), and medial superior temporal (MST), which are responsive to motion and direction of movement, also have pontine connections *(78)*, but the inferotemporal cortex, including the rostral lower bank of the superior temporal sulcus relevant for feature discrimination *(79)*, has no pontine efferents *(62,74,77,80)*.

3.4.1.4. Parastriate Cortices

The medial and dorsal prelunate regions project to the dorsolateral, lateral, and peripeduncular pontine nuclei nuclei, but the ventral prelunate cortices and the inferotemporal regions do not *(74,75,80, 81)*. The medial and dorsal prelunate regions are part of the dorsal visual stream concerned with motion analysis and the visual–spatial attributes of motion, and these connections may facilitate cerebellar involvement in the visual guidance of movement.

3.5.1.5. Paralimbic Cortices

The posterior parahippocampal gyrus is responsive to visual stimuli in the peripheral lower quadrant *(82)* and has been identified as part of the substrate for spatial attributes of memory *(83)*. Pontine connections arising from this region are directed to the lateral, dorsolateral, and lateral aspects of the peripeduncular pontine nuclei *(80)*. The cingulate cortex projections to the pons arise not only from the motor related areas in the depth of the cingulate sulcus *(84)*, but also from regions of the cingulate gyrus thought to be concerned with motivation and drive *(85,86)*. The anterior insular cortex, a cortical component of autonomic and pain modulation systems *(87)*, has been shown in retrograde anatomical studies to have pontine connections *(85)*.

3.4.1.6. Specificity of Connections

The associative and paralimbic projections distributed throughout the basilar pons, but with a rostral predominance, constitute a considerable extent of the pontine nuclear territory and are not overwhelmed by the motor corticopontine projections located mostly in the caudal half of the pons *(59)* (Fig. 3). Further, each cortical area projects to a unique set of terminations within the pons *(64)* (see Fig. 2), and the trajectories of the corticopontine fibers within the cerebral white matter are also discretely organized *(88,89)*. The corticopontine projections are thus distinguishable at each point, from origin, though trajectory, to termination, appear to be organized in parallel, and in this regard resemble the multiple parallel loops that characterize the corticosubcortical interactions with the basal ganglia *(90)*.

3.4.1.7. Climbing Fibers

The interaction between the pontine mossy fiber system input to the cerebellum and the climbing fibers derived exclusively from the inferior olivary nucleus has served as the substrate for hypotheses concerning the cerebellar role in motor learning *(20,21)*. The inferior olive receives little, if any, direct input from the cerebral cortex. Its major source of descending afferents arises from the red nucleus that carries mostly sensorimotor information *(91–93)*. It does, however, also receive some associative cortical input indirectly from brainstem reticular nuclei and from the zona incerta (ZI) *(94)*. The ZI, in turn, receives input from the rostral cingulate, dorsolateral and medial prefrontal, posterior parietal, and medial prestriate cortices *(95)*, thus maintaining the possibility that interaction between the mossy fiber and climbing fiber systems may be relevant for higher function.

3.4.1.8. The Pontocerebellar Pathway

Details of the pontocerebellar system remain unclear, beyond some general organizing principles. Physiological and anatomical studies indicate that both central and peripheral auditory and visual inputs are conveyed to vermal lobules VI and VII and the dorsal paraflocculus via the dorsolateral pontine nucleus and the nucleus reticularis tegmenti pontis *(96,97)*. In addition, the anterior lobe receives afferents from motor, premotor, and rostral parietal cortices; prefrontal cortices are linked with crus I (and to a lesser extent, crus II) of the ansiform lobule, and parietal cortices are linked with crus I, crus II, and lobule VIIB *(62,87,96,98,99)*.

There is a complex pattern of diverging and converging corticopontine and pontocerebellar projections, and this has led to the suggestion that information from one cerebral cortical area is distributed to numerous sites in the cerebellar cortex *(99)*. Preliminary trans-synaptic anterograde tracer experiments in the prefrontal cortex *(100)*, however, reveal that the anterograde projections through the medial pons are directed to focal areas in crus I and crus II and are not widely distributed. This important detail needs further clarification, as it relates directly to the issue of connectional and functional topography in the cerebellum.

3.4.2. Feedback Limb

The cerebellar cortical feedback to the deep cerebellar nuclei is arranged in an orderly manner with medial areas committing efferents mostly to the midline nuclei fastigial nucleus, and lateral cortices projecting to the lateral, or dentate, nucleus *(101–103)*. The dentate nucleus itself has been recognized to be architectonically heterogeneous, and Dow *(104)* elaborated upon this by defining a phylogenetically older dorsomedial part with minimal gyration and large neurons, and a more recently evolved ventrolateral part that is heavily folded and contains small neurons. Leiner, Leiner, and Dow *(6)* later postulated that the newer ventrolateral dentate evolved in concert with the cerebral association areas (prefrontal cortex in particular), to facilitate a cerebellar role in language processing.

The conventional understanding has been that the cerebellar dentate nucleus projects via motor thalamic nuclei back to the motor-related cortices. However, the cerebellar nuclear projections to thalamus arise not only from the dentate nucleus, but from the fastigial and the interpositus nuclei as well *(105)*. Further, the thalamic input is directed not only to the classic cerebellar recipient "motor" thalamic nuclei (subdivisions of ventral lateral, ventral posterolateral nuclei, and nucleus *X* of Olszewski *[106]*), but also to the "nonmotor" thalamic nuclei including the centralis lateralis (CL), paracentralis (Pcn), and centromedian-parafascicular (CM-Pf) complex, and the medial dorsal (MD) nucleus *(107–114)*. The CL nucleus, like other intralaminar nuclei, has widespread cortical connections including the posterior parietal cortex, the multimodal regions of the upper bank of the superior temporal sulcus, the prefrontal cortex, the cingulate gyrus, and the primary motor cortex *(115–120)*, and the Pcn nucleus projections include the parahippocampal gyrus (Blatt, G., Rosene, D.L., Pandya, D.N., 1991, personal communication). The MD thalamic nucleus receives cerebellar afferents mainly in its pars multiformis and pars densocellularis *(110,113)* that have reciprocal connections with the dorsolateral prefrontal cortex *(120–122)*, cingulate gyrus, posterior parietal cortex, and multimodal parts of the superior temporal sulcus *(116–119)*. Moreover, the traditionally motor thalamic nuclei are reciprocally interconnected with the prefrontal periarcuate areas *(66,68,115)*, the multimodal cortex in the upper bank of the superior temporal sulcus *(117)*, and the posterior parietal cortices *(119)*.

The conclusion that cerebellum projects back to the higher order cerebral areas from which the inputs are derived *(7,59)* is supported by direct trans-synaptic retrograde viral tracer studies demonstrating that the cerebellar dentate nucleus sends projections through thalamus to different areas of the frontal lobe in the monkey *(123,124)* (Fig. 4). The dorsomedial dentate sends projections to the motor cortex, whereas the ventrolateral and ventromedial dentate is connected with the prefrontal cortex, including area 9/46. It is likely that this degree of organization in the feedback from the cerebellum to the cerebral hemispheres is reproduced throughout the cerebrocerebellar system, but this remains to be demonstrated.

3.5. Anatomical Synthesis

There is an evolving body of anatomic information that links the cerebellum with systems that subserve every level of behavior, from arousal to autonomic function, motivation, emotion, and the highest forms of cognitive processing. The cerebrocerebellar loops are topographically organized, linking

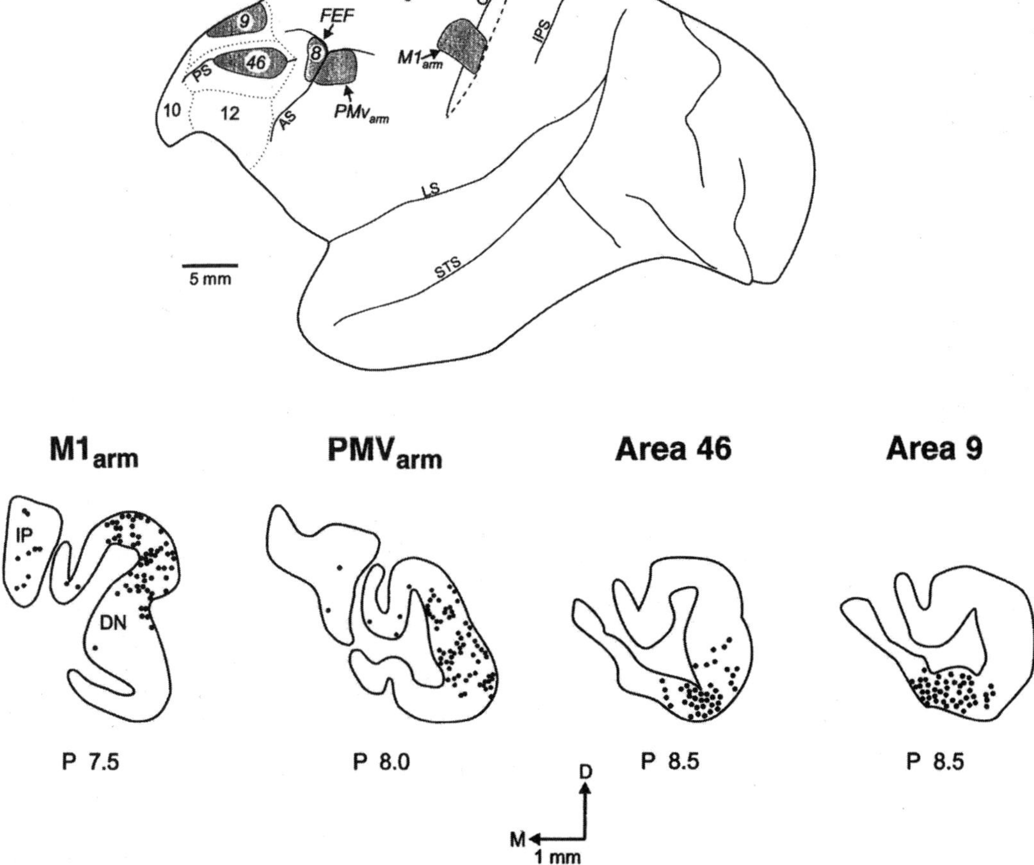

Fig. 4. Lateral view of a cebus monkey brain (top) to show the location of injections of McIntyre-B strain of Herpes simplex virus type-1 in the arm representation of the primary motor cortex ($M1_{arm}$, arm representation of the ventral premotor cortex PMV_{arm}, and areas 9 and 46 of the prefrontal cortex. The resulting retrogradely labeled neurons in the cerebellar dentate and interpositus nuclei (bottom) are indicated by solid dots. Relative antero-posterior locations of the labeled neurons within the dentate nucleus are indicated below each section. Adapted from Middleton and Strick (1997) ref. *124*.

specific cerebral areas with different regions of the cerebellum. The topographic arrangement in the cerebellar connections is superimposed upon an essentially constant pattern of intrinsic cerebellar cortical circuitry. This dichotomy provides support for the dysmetria of thought hypothesis *(7,11)*, predicated on the notion that the cerebellum performs its unique computations in a topographically precise manner on diverse streams of information relating to almost all aspects of behavior including cognition and emotion.

4. PHYSIOLOGICAL CORROBORATION

The reciprocal anatomic connections between the cerebral hemispheres and the cerebellum have been shown to be functionally relevant in recovery from cerebellar injury. When sensory cortex is removed prior to an induced cerebellar lesion, the cerebellar deficits are exaggerated, and recovery is limited *(125)*. When sensory cortex lesions are made subsequent to a cerebellar lesion, and after recovery from the cerebellar deficits, the initially recovered cerebellar deficits reappear. Furthermore, the effects of combined sequential cerebellar and sensory cortical lesions appear worse than expected if the two lesions were merely additive. These results indicate a functional interrelationship dependent upon the cerebrocerebellar system, which facilitates compensation following injury.

The phenomenon of cerebellar diaschisis, functional deactivation at a distance following damage to an interconnected region, has been documented following lesions of the cerebral hemispheres, including language-related cortex in the frontal lobe *(126)*. Conversely, reversed cerebellar diaschisis has also been observed. Lesions of cerebellum are associated with decreased activation in the contralateral cerebral hemisphere, in both sensorimotor, as well as association cortices *(7,127,128)*.

5. COGNITIVE AND PSYCHIATRIC MANIFESTATIONS OF CEREBELLAR PATHOLOGY

The anatomical, physiological, and behavioral investigations of the cerebrocerebellar system have been important in predicting and explaining the nonmotor clinical phenomena observed in some patients with diseases of the cerebellum. Early anecdotal reports of neuropsychiatric presentations in patients with cerebellar anomalies (see ref. *7*) were followed by studies of patients with hereditary ataxia who demonstrated emotional lability, irritability, loss of comprehension, poverty of association, and general intellectual impairment *(129)*, and of patients with olivopontocerebellar degeneration, who displayed deficits in verbal and nonverbal intelligence, memory, and frontal system function including concept formation *(130,131)*. Impaired executive function was demonstrated in patients with cerebellar cortical atrophy, as shown by increased planning times when performing the Tower of Hanoi test *(132)*, and by poor performance on tests of fluency and the initiation–perseveration subtest of the Mattis Dementia Rating Scale *(133)*. Most of the genetically identified spinocerebellar ataxias have now been reported to have cognitive decline as part of the clinical spectrum at some point in the course *(134)*.

Neuropsychological studies in patients with focal cerebellar injuries have revealed visual spatial deficits following focal left hemisphere lesions such as tumor excision *(135)* and left superior cerebellar artery territory infarction *(136)*; and agrammatism *(137)* and impaired error detection and practice-related learning of a verb-for-noun generation task *(138)* following right cerebellar infarction. These accounts did not resolve the question of whether focal lesions of the cerebellum produce cognitive or other behavioral deficits that are clinically relevant. The report of a cerebellar cognitive affective syndrome *(128)* resulting from lesions confined to the cerebellum appears to have added this previously missing important clinical description to the discussion.

5.1. The Cerebellar Cognitive Affective Syndrome

In our original study *(128)*, 20 patients had pathology confined to the cerebellum on clinical and neuroimaging grounds. Thirteen patients suffered stroke, three had postinfectious cerebellitis, three had cerebellar cortical atrophy, and one had a midline cerebellar tumor resected. On bedside mental state testing, all patients were awake, cooperative, and able to give an account of their history, although the level of attention was variable. Eighteen patients demonstrated problems with executive functions. Working memory was poor in 11 (of 16 tested), motor or ideational set-shifting in 16 (of 19), and perseveration of actions or drawings was noted in 16 (of 20). Verbal fluency was impaired in 18 patients, and in some, this was clinically evident as telegraphic speech. In two, speech output was so limited as to resemble mutism. Decreased verbal fluency was unrelated to dysarthria. Some patients with minimal dysarthria in the setting of acute lesions performed more poorly on fluency tests than others with severe dysarthria and disease of greater duration.

Visuospatial disintegration, most marked in attempting to draw or copy a diagram, was found in 19 patients, regardless of lesion acuity or severity of the dysmetria. The sequential approach to the drawing of the diagrams and the conceptualization of the figures was disorganized. Four patients demonstrated simultanagnosia.

Naming was impaired in 13 patients, generally being spared in those with smaller lesions. Six patients had agrammatic speech, most notably in those with bilateral acute disease. Elements of abnormal syntactic structure were noted in others, but less prominently. Prosody was abnormal in eight patients, with tone of voice characterized by a high pitched, whining, childish, and hypophonic quality.

Mental arithmetic was deficient in 14 patients. Verbal learning and recall were mildly abnormal in 11 patients, and visual learning and recall were impaired in 4 (of 13 patients tested). Ideational apraxia was evident in two individuals.

A prominent feature of the bedside mental state examination in 15 patients was the presence of difficulty in modulation of behavior and personality style. The notable exception was those patients whose strokes were either very limited in size or confined to the anterior lobe. Flattening of affect or disinhibition were manifested as overfamiliarity, flamboyant and impulsive actions, and humorous but inappropriate and flippant comments. Behavior was regressive and childlike, particularly following large or bilateral posterior inferior cerebellar artery (PICA) territory infarcts and in the patient with surgical excision of the vermis and paravermian structures. Obsessive–compulsive traits were occasionally observed.

Autonomic changes were a central feature in one patient, whose stroke in a medial branch of the right PICA involved the fastigial nucleus and paravermian cortex region. This manifested as spells of hiccuping and coughing, which precipitated bradycardia and syncope.

The findings on neuropsychological testing were in agreement with the observations from the bedside mental state evaluation with respect to the nature of the deficits detected. The distribution of patients' scores differed significantly from the normal distribution, with the most marked deviation from normal evident in the categories of executive and visual spatial function (see Fig. 5). Attention and orientation and language functions more closely approximated a normal distribution of scores. In addition, performance on the Porteus Mazes Task (a test of visual spatial planning) was very poor, with all subjects scoring at or below a test age of 12 yr. Patients with bilateral lesions and posterior lobe lesions were most impaired, and those with small lesions, or in whom disease was confined to the anterior lobe of the cerebellum, were least affected.

In summary, the Cerebellar Cognitive Affective Syndrome (CCAS), is characterized by:

1. Disturbances of executive function. This includes deficient planning, set-shifting, abstract reasoning, working memory, and decreased verbal fluency.
2. Impaired spatial cognition, including visual–spatial disorganization, and impaired visual–spatial memory.
3. Personality change, characterized by flattening or blunting of affect, and disinhibited or inappropriate behavior.
4. Linguistic difficulties, including dysprosodia, agrammatism, and mild anomia.

The net effect of these disturbances in cognitive functioning is a general lowering of overall intellectual function.

These deficits were clinically relevant, noted by family members and nursing and medical staff, and were associated with detectable abnormalities in the bedside mental state examination. The neurobehavioral presentation in our patients was more pronounced and generalized in patients with large, bilateral, or pancerebellar disorders, and particularly in those with acute-onset cerebellar disease. It was less evident in patients with more insidious disease, in the recovery phase (3 to 4 mo) after acute stroke, and in those with restricted cerebellar pathology. Lesions of the posterior lobe were particularly important in the generation of the disturbed cognitive behaviors, and the vermis was consistently involved in patients with pronounced affective presentations. The anterior lobe seemed to be less prominently involved in the generation of these cognitive and behavioral deficits. The one patient with an autonomic syndrome had a lesion involving the medial posterior lobe, including the fastigial nucleus.

The clinical relevance of the CCAS has been emphasized in subsequent clinical reports. Young adults (ages 18–44) with cerebellar strokes have delayed return to the work force because of cognitive limitations, not motor incapacity *(139)*. The cognitive deficits described in this group of patients was similar to those with the CCAS, proportional to the size of the infarct, and included deficits in

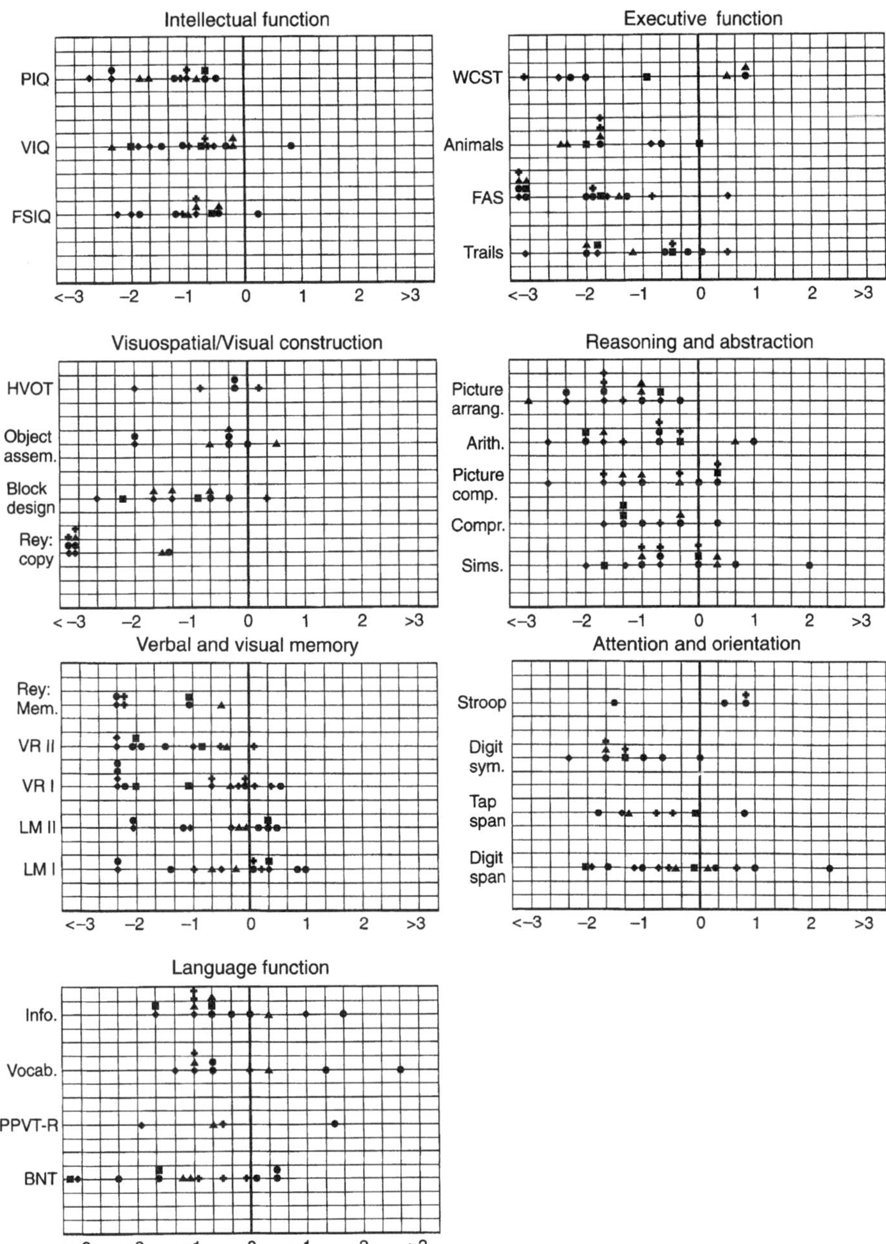

Fig. 5. Distribution graphs of the z-scores for patients (grouped according to disease type and location) showing their performance on neuropsychological tests. Diamonds represent bilateral PICA infarction; circles represent unilateral PICA infarction; squares represent SCA infarction; triangles represent cerebellitis; crosses represent cerebellar cortical atrophy. Abbreviations as follows. Intellectual function: Picture, Verbal, and Full-Scale Intelligence Quotient. Executive function: Wisconsin Card Sorting Test, Animal naming, F-A-S-verbal fluency test, Trails A and B. Visuospatial/Visual construction: Hooper Visual Orientation Test, Object assembly. Reasoning and abstractions: Picture arrangement, Arithmetic, Picture completion, Comprehension, Similarities. Verbal and visual memory: Rey Complex figure memory, Visual Reproduction I and II, Logical Memory I and II. Attention and orientation: Digit symbol. Language function: Information, Vocabulary, Peabody Picture Vocabulary Test-Revised, Boston Naming Test. From Schmahmann and Sherman (1998) ref. *128*.

attention, working memory, the temporary storage of complex information, visuospatial skills, and cognitive flexibility. Performance on the block design task in the early post-stroke period predicted maximal working capacity at 12 mo. Similarly, Neau et al. *(140)* studied 15 patients with cerebellar infarcts (10 PICA, 4 superior cerebellar artery [SCA] and 1 anterior inferior cerebellar artery [AICA]) and reported findings consistent with the CCAS as defined above. Specifically, this included deficits in executive function as revealed by poor performance on phonemic and alternate categorical fluency, naming with and without interference, and a paced auditory serial addition task; and visual spatial deficits with low scores on the Wechster Adult Intelligence Scale-Revised (WAIS-R) Block Design.

Parvizi et al. *(141)* explored the dysequilibrium inherent in the emotional display of some patients with cerebellar lesions, by considering the phenomenon of pathologic laughter and crying (PLC) in a patient in whom the cerebellum was partially deafferented by multiple infarcts in the left lateral cerebral peduncle, midline rostral basilar pons, right middle cerebellar peduncle, and white matter of right cerebellar crus II (inferior semilunar lobule). Cognitive testing also revealed deficits in executive function and visual memory, and relative weakness in abstract reasoning. The authors concluded that PLC arises from lesions of the cerebropontocerebellar pathways. In their view, the normal cerebellum automatically adjusts the execution of laughter or crying to the cognitive and situational context of a potential stimulus. Loss of the cerebellar input requires that the cerebellum operate on the basis of incomplete information about that context, the result of which is inadequate or chaotic behavior.

One study of patients with cerebellar lesions failed to detect neuropsychological deficits *(142)*. The control population had limited education and poor Mini-Mental State Score, however, that may have limited the ability of the investigators to detect significant behavioral impairments in the study group *(143)*. Further, the study included patients with lesions that were more than 6 mo old, and the CCAS from unilateral lesions has been shown to recover with time *(128,140,144)*.

5.2. CCAS in Children

Impairments in intelligence, memory, language, attention, academic skills, and psychosocial function have been reported in children following resection of cerebellar tumors *(145,146)*, but these have been observed in groups that have undergone cerebellar resection as well as cranial radiation and/or chemotherapy. This is problematic, because radiation necrosis is associated with deficits in general intelligence, academic achievement, verbal knowledge and reasoning, and perceptual motor abilities; and methotrexate causes substantial neurological and neurobehavioral impairment *(145,147–149)*.

In order to determine whether the CCAS is observed in children, Levisohn et al. *(150)* performed a retrospective record review of the results of standardized neuropsychological tests in 19 children with cerebellar tumors who received neither methotrexate nor radiation therapy prior to testing. Eleven had medulloblastoma, seven had astrocytoma, one had an ependymoma. The children ranged in age from 3–14 yr at the time of tumor resection. The time between surgery and neuropsychological testing ranged from 1–22 mo (mean 5.1, standard deviation [sd] 6.4). Eight children received chemotherapy prior to neuropsychological testing. Two cases had hydrocephalus that required shunting.

Seven of the 19 patients (37%) met criteria for expressive language deficits. Another four demonstrated word finding difficulties detected in testing (difficulty naming objects in the Picture Completion test) or in spontaneous conversation in the context of otherwise intact language abilities. Seven (37%) had deficits in visual–spatial functions (see Fig. 6). Three (16%) had deficits in both expressive language and visual–spatial functions. In addition to these deficits in expressive language and visual–spatial functions, of 14 children administered the Digit Span test, 8 (57%) performed poorly. Additionally, some with average scores on Digit Span showed perseveration and difficulties establishing set. Five of 15 tested (33%) had verbal memory deficits along with other deficits in visual–spatial and/or language function. Standard measures used to evaluate executive–prefrontal function in this group were limited.

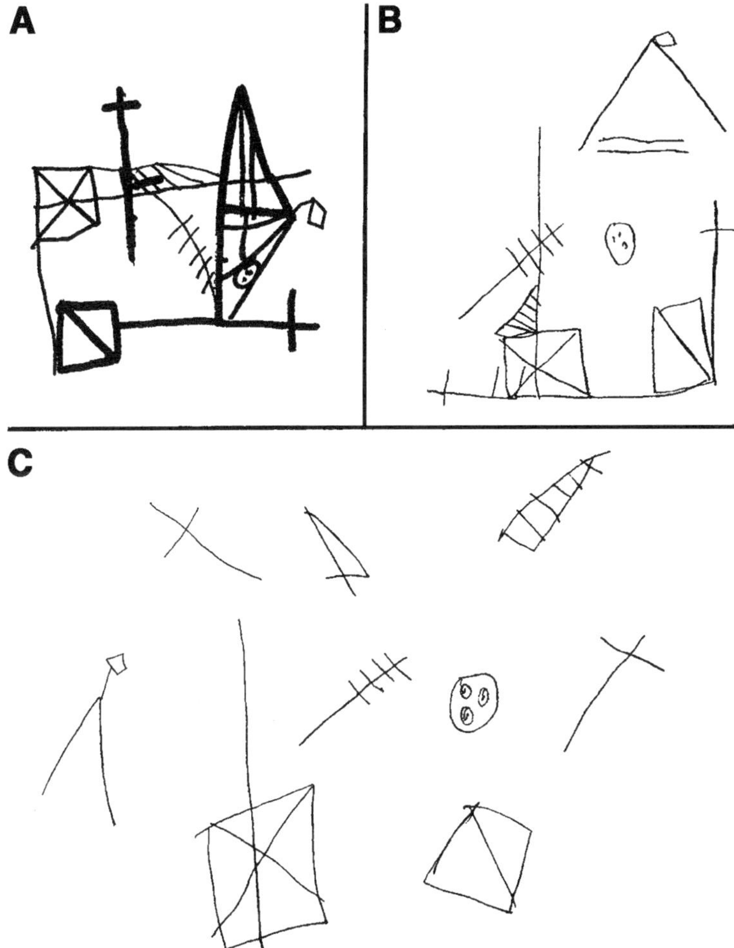

Fig. 6. Drawings of the Rey-Osterrieth figure by a 6-yr-old boy following resection of a left cerebellar astrocytoma. Copy seen in (**A**), immediate recall in (**B**), and 20-min delayed recall in (**C**). From Levisohn et al. (2000) ref. *150*.

Six patients (32%) had deficits in affect regulation, and they all had extensive vermis damage. In contrast, none of the patients without affect problems had extensive vermis damage. Children with extensive vermis damage were more likely to exhibit changes in affect regulation than those with intact vermis or only minimal vermis damage. Five of nine children who sustained extensive vermis damage (56%) exhibited the posterior fossa syndrome postoperatively. Patients who were older at the time of testing were more likely to show neuropsychological deficits. Eight of the 10 patients older than 7 yr had deficits (80%), whereas 3 of the 9 children (33%) younger than 7 yr were impaired. These age effects may have been confounded by tumor type, because medulloblastomas were more common in the older children, and astrocytomas or ependymomas were more common (75%) in the younger children.

Other investigators have replicated the observation that children with cerebellar tumor excision manifest high-level cognitive and emotional deficits. Riva and Giorgi *(151)* evaluated 26 such children and reported that those with right cerebellar hemisphere tumors presented with disturbances of auditory sequential memory and language processing, whereas those with left hemisphere tumors showed deficits on tests of spatial and visual sequential memory. These investigators also found that vermal lesions led to postsurgical mutism, which evolved into speech disorders or language disturbances similar to agrammatism; and behavioral disturbances including irritability, decreased ability to tolerate the company of others, and a general tendency to avoid physical and eye contact. Complex repetitive and rhythmic rocking movements, stereotyped linguistic utterances, and general lack of empathy in one patient met criteria for a diagnosis of autism.

5.3. *The Posterior Fossa Syndrome*

An intriguing neurobehavioral syndrome has been observed in children who undergo resection of midline tumors of the cerebellum *(152–154)*. The phenomenon is marked by the development of mutism within 48 h following surgical approach involving the cerebellar vermis, and in the recovery phase over a period of months it is accompanied by dysarthria and buccal and lingual apraxia. There is no involvement of equilibrium, gait, or appendicular movements, although motor tone is decreased. In addition to the mutism, these children display a behavioral syndrome that includes regressive personality changes, apathy, and poverty of spontaneous movement. Emotional lability is marked, and there is rapid fluctuation of expression of emotion that gravitates between irritability with inconsolable crying and agitation to giggling and easy distractibility. Not all children with the CCAS pass through the stage of the posterior fossa syndrome, as the CCAS develops following unilateral or bilateral damage to the posterior lobes with or without vermal involvement, whereas the posterior fossa syndrome occurs only following midline lesions. Children with the CCAS, whose damage includes the vermis however, have prominent mood dysregulation, and some of these pass initially through the phase of postoperative mutism. Postoperative mutism has been observed in some adults *(155)*. Restriction of verbal fluency, almost to the point of mutism, was present in some patients in the original CCAS series, but was less marked than in the children with posterior fossa syndrome.

5.4. *Developmental Cognitive Abilities*

An interesting series of recent observations suggests a relationship between developmental anomalies of cerebellum and neurobehavioral syndromes. Quantitative morphometry of the cerebellum in attention deficit hyperactivity disorder (ADHD) reveals smaller posterior lobes of the vermis (lobules VIII through X) in both males *(156,157)* and females *(158)*, and early evidence suggests that the size of the vermis is related to the severity of the ADHD.

Allin et al. *(159)* set out to establish whether cognitive and motor impairments in adolescents born very preterm (before 33 wk of gestation) are associated with abnormalities of the cerebellum as revealed by volumetric analysis of brain magnetic resonance imaging (MRI) scans. In their longitudinal study, cognitive and neurological evaluations are performed from ages 1 through 15. The MRI scans of 67 children born very preterm and 50 age-matched, full-term born controls were studied. The preterm-born subjects had significantly reduced cerebellar volume compared with term-born controls ($p < 0.001$). This difference was present after controlling for potential confounders. There was no association between cerebellar volume and motor neurological signs. However, there were significant associations between cerebellar volume and several cognitive test scores. These included impaired executive and visual–spatial functions as revealed by the Similarities, Block Design and Object Assembly subtests of the Wechsler Intelligence Scale for Children-Revised, Riddle interpretation, impaired language skills as revealed by Schonnel reading age, and difficulty decoding and understanding the Kaufman Assessment Battery for Children. The similarity between the major findings of this study and the CCAS in adults and children provides a concordance of information from different spheres of clinical investigation. The impairment of reading is of interest in the light of the finding that individuals with dyslexia demonstrate lower cerebellar activation on positron emission tomography scans compared to controls when performing motor tasks *(160)*. Activation was significantly lower for the dyslexic adults than for the controls in the right cerebellar cortex and the left cingulate gyrus when executing a prelearned sequence of finger movements; and in the right cerebellar cortex when learning a novel sequence. These findings on traditional tests of cerebellar motor coordination in dyslexics suggest a possible cerebellar role in this high level cognitive skill.

Cerebellar agenesis is rare and, until recently, was considered to be asymptomatic. Glickstein *(161)* challenged the accepted notion that cerebellar agenesis is asymptomatic from the perspective of motor control and uncovered historical accounts of children with agenesis showing impairments of coordination, speech, and oro-motor faculties along with delay of motor milestones. Additionally, clinical reports of cerebellar agenesis from the 19th century describe a variety of higher order deficits, including "subnormal intelligence," "mental retardation," and "idiocy" (see ref. *7*). Gardner et al. *(162)* evaluated three patients with near-total absence of the cerebellum in whom only a nubbin of remnant cerebellar tissue is detectable. They reported delayed milestones, mild motor impairments, and intellectual handicap. Chheda et al. *(163)* found that near-complete or partial cerebellar agenesis was accompanied by behavioral and motor deficits in eight patients (six children and two adults), and the location and extent of the agenesis was correlated with the severity and range of the motor, cognitive, and psychiatric impairments. The children presented with gross and fine motor delay, oral motor apraxia, impaired saccades, and vestibulo-ocular reflex cancellation, clumsiness, and mild ataxia. Behavioral features included autistic-like stereotypical performance, obsessive rituals, and difficulty understanding social cues. Tactile defensiveness (avoidance of, and adverse reaction to touch) was a prominent feature in four children. Executive impairments included perseveration, disinhibition, and poor abstract reasoning, working memory and verbal fluency. Spatial cognition was impaired for perceptual organization, visual spatial copying, and recall. Some children presented with expressive language delay as the prin-cipal manifestation, in two instances so severe as to require instruction in sign language. Impaired prosody was evident in all cases, and over-regularization of past tense verbs was noted. In longitudinal follow-up, extensive rehabilitation enhanced motor, linguistic, and cognitive performance. Of the two adults with partial agenesis in this study, one with vermal predominant agenesis suffered from life-long psychotic depression, and the other with subtotal right hemisphere agenesis experienced a psychotic episode in adolescence.

5.5. The Cerebellum and Psychosis

The CCAS includes as part of its spectrum of manifestations the alterations in behavior that extend beyond cognition. Adults and children experience altered regulation of mood and personality, display obsessive–compulsive tendencies, and demonstrate psychotic thinking. The mother of one patient (unpublished) who underwent resection of a midline astrocytoma reported her surprise at witnessing a prominent and persistent behavior change in her son. His personality style had been characterized by impulsiveness and assertiveness to the point of aggression from age 5. The tumor declared itself with nausea, vomiting, vertigo, and ataxia, and at age 12 it was resected. The patient's personality changed from the moment that he recovered from anesthesia. He became passive, immature, and child-like and showed no hint of the previous aggressive behavior. He has remained unchanged for 6 yr. Another patient (Schmahmann, Sherman, Weilburg, unpublished) who underwent resection of a midline tumor at age 6, has slipped in early adulthood into a state of paranoid ideation, bizarre illogical thinking (at times of psychotic proportions), depressed mood, obsessional preoccupation, and personal stereotypical rituals. He has become inaccessible to family and friends, and unable to organize his thoughts and plan his life. Systematic investigations of this putative relationship between acquired cerebellar pathology and psychosis are much needed.

Anecdotal examples from selected patients may be purely coincidental, and a prospective study to evaluate the presence and nature of immediate or delayed postcerebellectomy psychosis has yet to be performed. The disturbances of behavior and emotion that have declared themselves in the series of patients with the CCAS, however, emphasize the relevance of the cerebellum for the psychiatric population, and for clinicians and investigators interested in understanding psychiatric diseases. The descriptions of cognitive and emotional influences in patients with cerebellar diseases are complemented by the investigations of conditions that are defined by their behavioral features, and in which cerebellar anomalies have subsequently been defined. Publications in the 1800s noted deviant and aberrant behaviors in individuals with cerebellar anomalies. These reports were strengthened by later clinical observations of a relationship between the cerebellum and personality, aggression, and emotion, and that linked psychosis, and schizophrenia in particular, with cerebellar structural abnormalities. Heath et al. *(164)* described pathology such as cysts and tumors in the midline cerebellum in patients diagnosed with psychosis. Pollak et al. *(165)* also described seven patients with posterior fossa structural abnormalities who presented with neuropsychiatric symptomatology. Two patients had tumors, two patients had mega-cisterna magna, two patients had Dandy-Walker variants, and in one patient, a fourth ventricle tumor was removed in childhood. Psychiatric diagnoses that met the Diagnostic Statistical Manual of Mental Disorders, fourth edition (DSM-IV) criteria were psychosis (two patients), major depression (one patient), personality disorders (two patients), and somatoform disorders (two patients).

Pathologic anatomical findings have been reported in schizophrenia, including enlargement of the fourth ventricle, smaller cerebellar vermis, and cerebellar atrophy *(166,167)*. More recently, Loeber et al. *(168)* used MRI to measure the volume of individual cerebellar lobules in 19 patients with schizophrenia and 19 healthy comparison subjects. They found that compared to the controls, patients with schizophrenia had a significantly smaller inferior vermis and significantly less cerebellar hemispheric asymmetry. In an MRI study of schizophrenic patients who had no history of using neuroleptic medication, Ichimiya et al. *(169)* found significantly reduced vermis volume in the schizophrenic group, and no significant differences in the volumes of other cerebellar structures or cerebral hemispheres. Furthermore, reduction in the vermal volume correlated with the depression and paranoia subscores of the Brief Psychiatric Rating Scale. Volz et al. *(170)* undertook a morphometric study specifically to explore the dysmetria of thought hypothesis *(7)* as it has been applied to schizophrenia *(171)*. They found reduced volumes in patients with schizophrenia in the left cerebellar hemisphere and the right cerebellar vermis as well as in the frontal lobe, the temporal lobe, and thalamus. Not all studies, however, have demonstrated the smaller cerebellar volumes *(172)*, but this may reflect differences in methodological approach.

Quantitative MRI morphometry *(173,174)* and postmortem analysis of early infantile autism *(175)*, which was once classified as juvenile schizophrenia, have revealed abnormalities in the midline deep cerebellar nuclei, the cortex in the posterior lobes, and the vermis. These contemporary observations lend credence to the notion that midline structures of the cerebellum in patients and monkeys play a role in emotion, aggression, and psychosis *(18,19,51,176–178)*. The activation of midline cerebellar structures on functional imaging studies of panic *(179)* and sadness *(180,181)*, add to the clinical evidence implicating the vermis in the regulation of emotion.

6. THE DYSMETRIA OF THOUGHT HYPOTHESIS

The recognition that there are neurobehavioral syndromes with cognitive and emotional components and psychiatric overtones challenges the notion that the cerebellum is purely a motor control device. The clinical descriptions are consistent with a broader vision of cerebellar function and are encapsulated by the dysmetria of thought hypothesis *(7,11,59)*. This theory proposes that the cerebellar contribution to the nervous system is embodied in a universal cerebellar transform (UCT) applied to multiple domains of neurologic function. The nature of the transform is constant, but the information modulated by the cerebellum is different, determined by the location within cerebellum where the transform is applied, and dependent upon the anatomically precise cerebrocerebellar interconnections with other brain regions. The vermis and midline fastigial nucleus constitute the limbic cerebellum concerned with emotional modulation and autonomic function, whereas the cerebellar hemispheres and more laterally placed dentate nucleus are concerned with high level associative cognitive operations. The cerebellar contribution to these multiple different functions is to act as an oscillation dampener, smoothing out performance around a homeostatic baseline. The cerebellum regulates not only the rate, force, rhythm, and accuracy of movements, but also the speed, capacity, consistency, and appropriateness of mental or cognitive processes.

Following a cerebellar lesion, the hypothesis holds, the UCT that modulates the function subserved by the lesioned region is lost. The universal cerebellar impairment (UCI) that results is dysmetria. The UCI from lesions in the sensorimotor cerebellum manifests as ataxia and dysmetria. The UCI in the behavioral realm is dysmetria of thought, manifesting as the various components of the CCAS *(7,11)*. Dysmetria of movement is matched by an unpredictability and illogic to social and societal interaction. The overshoot and inability in the motor system to check parameters of movement may be equated, in the behavioral realm, with a mismatch between reality and perceived reality and erratic attempts to correct the errors of thought or behavior. Cognitive deficits result from lesions of the cognitive cerebellum in the cerebellar hemispheres, and emotional and psychiatric disturbances follow lesions of the limbic cerebellum in the vermis and fastigial nucleus.

Inherent in the dysmetria of thought hypothesis is the prediction that there is functional topography of cognition and emotion in the cerebellum. Clinical studies support this notion, as do meta-analyses of functional neuroimaging studies *(182,183)*. These results indicate that the anterior lobe is the sensorimotor cerebellum, and the posterior lobe is the cognitive cerebellum. The motor components of articulation activate the anterior lobe vermis, whereas language tasks activate lobule VI and crus I at the vermis and right hemisphere. Verbal working memory tasks activate lobule VI and crus I on the right, in a location slightly rostral to language processing. Attentional modulation is more heavily concentrated in lobule VI on the left; and nonmotor learning is focused particularly in Crus I and Crus II bilaterally. The cerebellar vermis and paravermian regions are activated preferentially in studies of pain, hunger, and thirst.

This dysmetria of thought hypothesis, thus, helps explain the observed clinical phenomena in the CCAS and its different cognitive and psychiatric variants, including psychosis. It has provided a testable model for the evaluation of the anatomic substrates of major psychiatric illnesses, such as schizophrenia, and it helps predict observations and guide experiments directed towards elucidating the anatomic substrates and clinical manifestations of neurobehavioral and psychiatric phenomena. Further neuropsychological and psychiatric observations in patients with known cerebellar lesions, and morphometric and functional imaging studies of cerebellum in psychiatric patients will be important as investigators further evaluate the manifestations of the CCAS, test the dysmetria of thought hypothesis, and extend our understanding of the cerebellar role in the nervous system.

ACKNOWLEDGMENTS

This work was supported in part by the McDonnell Pew Program in Cognitive Neuroscience. Substantial sections of this chapter are derived from Human Brain Mapping 1996;4:174–198[*59*]; Brain 1998;121:561–579[*128*]; Journal of Neurolinguistics 2000;13:189–214[*11*]; International Review of Psychiatry 2001;13:247–260[*12*]; International Review of Psychiatry 2001;13:313–322[*13*].

REFERENCES

1. Adams, R.D. and Victor. M. (2000) *Principles of Neurology*, McGraw Hill, New York.
2. Holmes, G. (1917) The symptoms of acute cerebellar injuries due to gunshot wounds. *Brain* **40,** 461–535.
3. Dow, R.S. and Moruzzi, G. (1958) *The Physiology and Pathology of the Cerebellum,* University of Minnesota Press, Minneapolis.
4. Dow, R.S. (1974) Some novel concepts of cerebellar physiology. *Mt. Sinai. J. Med.* **41,** 103–119.
5. Watson, P.J. (1978) Nonmotor functions of the cerebellum. *Psychol. Bull.* **85,** 944–967.
6. Leiner, H.C., Leiner, A.L., and Dow, R.S. (1986) Does the cerebellum contribute to mental skills? *Behav. Neurosci.* **100,** 443–454.
7. Schmahmann, J.D. (1991) An emerging concept: the cerebellar contribution to higher function. *Arch. Neurol.* **48,** 1178–1187, and (1992) **49,** 1230.
8. Schmahmann, J.D. (1997) Rediscovery of an early concept, in Int. Rev. Neurobiol., volume 41, *The Cerebellum and Cognition* (Schmahmann, J.D., ed.), Academic Press, San Diego, pp. 3–27.

9. Schmahmann, J.D. (Ed.) (1997) Int. Rev. Neurobiol., volume 41, *The Cerebellum and Cognition*, Academic Press, San Diego.
10. Schmahmann, J.D. (1998) Dysmetria of thought. Clinical consequences of cerebellar dysfunction on cognition and affect. *Trends Cogn. Sci.* **2,** 362–370.
11. Schmahmann, J.D. (2000) The role of the cerebellum in affect and psychosis. *J. Neurolinguistics* **13,** 189–214.
12. Schmahmann, J.D. (2001) The cerebrocerebellar system: anatomic substrates of the cerebellar contribution to cognition and emotion. *Int. Rev. Psychiatry* **13,** 247–260.
13. Schmahmann, J.D. (2001) The cerebellar cognitive affective syndrome: clinical correlations of the dysmetria of thought hypothesis. *Int. Rev. Psychiatry* **13,** 313–322.
14. Moruzzi, G. (1947) Sham rage and localized autonomic responses elicited by cerebellar stimulation in the acute thalamic cat. Proc. XVII Internat Congress Physiol Oxford, pp. 114–115.
15. Martner, J. (1975) Cerebellar influences on autonomic mechanisms. *Acta Physiol. Scand.* **425(Suppl.),** 1–42.
16. Bard, P. (1928) A diencephalic mechanism for the expression of rage with special reference to the sympathetic nervous system. *Am. J. Physiol.* **84,** 490–515.
17. Zanchetti, A. and Zoccolini, A. (1954) Autonomic hypothalamic outbursts elicited by cerebellar stimulation. *J. Neurophysiol.* **17,** 475–483.
18. Reis, D.J., Doba, N., and Nathan, M.A. (1973) Predatory attack, grooming and consummatory behaviors evoked by electrical stimulation of cat cerebellar nuclei. *Science* **182,** 845–847.
19. Snider, R.S. (1950) Recent contributions to the anatomy and physiology of the cerebellum. *Arch. Neuro. Psychol.* **64,** 196–219.
20. Marr, D. (1969) A theory of cerebellar cortex. *J. Physiol.* **202,** 437–470.
21. Albus, J.S. (1971) A theory of cerebellar function. *Math Biosc.* **10,** 25–61.
22. Thompson, R.F., Bao, S., Chen, L., et al. (1997) Associative learning, in *The Cerebellum and Cognition* (Schmahmann, J.D., ed.), Academic Press, San Diego, pp. 151–189.
23. Lalonde, R. (1997) Visuospatial abilities, in *The Cerebellum and Cognition* (Schmahmann, J.D., ed.), Academic Press, San Diego, pp. 191–216.
24. Petrosini, L., Molinari, M., and Dell'Anna, M.E. (1996) Cerebellar contribution to spatial event processing: Morris water maze and T-maze. *Eur. J. Neurosci.* **9,** 1896–1996.
25. Voogd, J. and Glickstein, M. (1998) The anatomy of the cerebellum. *Trends Neurosci.* **21,** 370–375.
26. Hawkes, R., Colonnier, M., and Leclerc, N. (1985) Monoclonal antibodies reveal sagittal banding in the rodent cerebellar cortex. *Brain Res.* **6,** 359–365.
27. Haines, D.E. (1981) Zones in the cerebellar cortex. Their organization and potential relevance to cerebellar stimulation. *J. Neurosurg.* **55,** 254–256.
28. Noda, H., Sugita, S., and Ikeda, Y. (1990) Afferent and efferent connections of the oculomotor region of the fastigial nucleus in the macaque monkey. *J. Comp. Neurol.* **302,** 330–348.
29. Qvist, H. (1989) Demonstration of axonal branching of fibres from certain precerebellar nuclei to the cerebellar cortex and nuclei: a retrograde fluorescent double-labelling study in the cat. *Exp. Brain Res.* **75,** 15–27.
30. Gonzalo-Ruiz, A. and Leichnetz, G.R. (1998) Connections of the caudal cerebellar interpositus complex in a new world monkey (Cebus apella). *Brain Res. Bull.* **25,** 919–927.
31. Andrezik, J.A., Dormer, K.J., Foreman, R.D., and Person, R.J. (1984) Fastigial nucleus projections to the brain stem in beagles: pathways for autonomic regulation. *Neuroscience* **11,** 497–507.
32. Miller, R.A. and Strominger, N.L. (1977) An experimental study of the efferent connections of the superior cerebellar peduncle in the rhesus monkey. *Brain Res.* **133,** 237–250.
33. Person, R.J., Andrezik, J.A., Dormer, K.J., and Foreman, R.D. (1986) Fastigial nucleus projections in the midbrain and thalamus in dogs. *Neuroscience* **18,** 105–120.
34. Aumann, T.D. and Horne, M.K. (1996) Ramification and termination of single axons in the cerebellothalamic pathway of the rat. *J. Comp. Neurol.* **376,** 420–430.
35. Snider, R.S. (1975) A cerebellar-ceruleus pathway. *Brain Res.* **88,** 59–63.
36. Dempsey, C.W., Tootle, D.M., Fontana, C.J., Fitzjarrell, A.T., Garey, R.E., and Heath R.G. (1983) Stimulation of the paleocerebellar cortex of the cat: increased rate of synthesis and release of catecholamines at limbic sites. *Biol. Psychiat.* **18,** 127–132.
37. Marcinkiewicz, M., Morcos, R., and Chretien, M. (1989) CNS connections with the median raphe nucleus: retrograde tracing with WGA-apoHRP-gold complex in the rat. *J. Comp. Neurol.* **289,** 11–35.
38. Moruzzi, G. (1940) Paleocerebellar inhibition of vasomotor and respiratory carotid sinus reflexes. *J. Neurophysiol.* **3,** 20–32.
39. Paton, J.F. and Spyer, K.M. (1990) Brain stem regions mediating the cardiovascular responses elicited from the posterior cerebellar cortex in the rabbit. *J. Physiol. (Lond.)* **427,** 533–552.
40. Reis, D.J. and Golanov, E.V. (1997) Autonomic and vasomotor regulation, in *The Cerebellum and Cognition* (Schmahmann, J.D., ed.), Academic Press, San Diego, pp. 121–149.
41. Xu, F. and Frazier, D.T. (1997) Involvement of the fastigial nuclei in vagally mediated respiratory responses. *J. Appl. Physiol.* **82,** 1853–1861.
42. Coghill, R.C., Sang, C.N., Maisog, J.M., and Iadarola, M.J. (1999) Pain intensity processing within the human brain: a bilateral, distributed mechanism. *J. Neurophysiol.* **82,** 1934–1943.
43. Ploghaus, A., Tracey, I., Gati, J.S., et al. (1999) Dissociating pain from its anticipation in the human brain. *Science* **284,** 1979–1981.

44. Parsons, L.M., Egan, G., Liotti, M., et al. (2001) Neuroimaging evidence implicating cerebellum in the experience of hypercapnia and hunger for air. *Proc. Natl. Acad. Sci. USA* **98,** 2041–2046.
45. Tataranni, P.A., Gautier, J.F., Chen, K., et al. (1999) Neuroanatomical correlates of hunger and satiation in humans using positron emission tomography. *Proc. Natl. Acad. Sci. USA* **96,** 4569–4574.
46. Haines, D.E., Dietrichs, E., Mihailoff, G.A., and McDonald, E.F. (1997) The cerebellar-hypothalamic axis: basic circuits and clinical observations, in *The Cerebellum and Cognition* (Schmahmann, J.D., ed.), Academic Press, San Diego, pp. 83–107.
47. Whiteside, D.G. and Snider, R.S. (1953) Relation of cerebellum to upper brain stem. *J. Neurophysiol.* **16,** 397–413.
48. Heath, R.G. and Harper, J.W. (1974) Ascending projections of the cerebellar fastigial nucleus to the hippocampus amygdala and other temporal lobe sites: evoked potential and histological studies in monkeys and cats. *Exp. Neurol.* **45,** 2682–2687.
49. Mutani, R. (1967) Cobalt experimental hippocampal epilepsy in the cat. *Epilepsia* **8,** 223–240.
50. Babb, T.L., Mitchell, A.G. Jr., and Crandall, P.H. (1974) Fastigiobulbar and dentatothalamic influences on hippocampal cobalt epilepsy in the cat. *Electroencephalogr. Clin. Neurophysiol.* **36,** 141–154.
51. Heath, R.G., Dempsey, C.W., Fontana, C.J., and Myers, W.A. (1978) Cerebellar stimulation: effects on septal region, hippocampus, and amygdala of cats and rats. *Biol. Psychiat.* **13,** 501–529.
52. Snider, R.S. and Maiti, A. (1976) Cerebellar contributions to the Papez circuit. *J. Neurosci. Res.* **2,** 133–146.
53. Oades, R.D. and Halliday, G.M. (1987) Ventral tegmental (A10) system: neurobiology. 1. Anatomy and connectivity. *Brain Res.* **434,** 117–165.
54. Aas, J.-E. and Brodal, P. (1988) Demonstration of topographically organized projections from the hypothalamus to the pontine nuclei: an experimental study in the cat. *J. Comp. Neurol.* **268,** 313–328.
55. Ebert, D. and Ebmeier, K.P. (1996) The role of the cingulate gyrus in depression: from functional anatomy to neurochemistry. *Biol. Psychiatry* **39,** 1044–1050.
56. Rauch, S.L., Jenike, M.A., Alpert, N.M., et al. (1994) Regional cerebral blood flow measured during symptom provocation in obsessive-compulsive disorder using oxygen 15-labeled carbon dioxide and positron emission tomography. *Arch. Gen. Psychiatry* **1,** 62–70.
57. Vilensky, J.A. and Van Hoesen, G.W. (1981) Corticopontine projections from the cingulate cortex in the rhesus monkey. *Brain Res.* **205,** 391–395.
58. Brodal, P., Bjaali, J.G., and Aas, J.E. (1991) Organization of cingulo-ponto-cerebellar connections in the cat. *Anat. Embryol. (Berl.)* **184,** 245–254.
59. Schmahmann, J.D. (1996) From movement to thought: anatomic substrates of the cerebellar contribution to cognitive processing. *Hum. Brain Mapping* **4,** 174–198.
60. Sunderland, S. (1940) The projection of the cerebral cortex on the pons and cerebellum in the macaque monkey. *J. Anat.* **74,** 201–226.
61. Nyby, O. and Jansen, J. (1951) An experimental investigation of the corticopontine projection in macaca mulatta. Skrifter utgitt av Det Norske Videnskaps-Akademi: Oslo; 1. *Mat. Naturv. Klasse.* **3,** 1–47.
62. Brodal, P. (1978) The corticopontine projection in the rhesus monkey. Origin and principles of organization. *Brain* **101,** 251–283.
63. Schmahmann, J.D. and Pandya, D.N. (1995) Prefrontal cortex projections to the basilar pons: implications for the cerebellar contribution to higher function. *Neurosci. Lett.* **199,** 175–178.
64. Schmahmann, J.D. and Pandya, D.N. (1997) Anatomic organization of the basilar pontine projections from prefrontal cortices in rhesus monkey. *J. Neurosci.* **17,** 438–458.
65. Astruc, J. (1971) Corticofugal connections of area 8 (frontal eye field) in macaca mulatta. *Brain Res.* **33,** 241–256.
66. Künzle, H. and Akert. K. (1977) Efferent connections of cortical area 8 (frontal eye lid) in Macaca fascicularis. A reinvestigation using the autoradiographic technique. *J. Comp. Neurol.* **173,** 147–164.
67. Fuster, J.M. (1980) *The Prefrontal Cortex: Anatomy, Physiology and Neuropsychology of the Frontal Lobe.* Raven Press, New York.
68. Stanton, G.B., Goldberg, M.E., and Bruce, C.J. (1988) Frontal eye field efferents in the macaque monkey: II. Topography of terminal fields in midbrain and pons. *J. Comp. Neurol.* **271,** 493–506.
69. Petrides, M. and Pandya, D.N. (1994) Comparative architectonic analysis of the human and the macaque frontal cortex, in *Handbook of Neuropsychology,* vol. 9 (Boller, F. and Grafman, J., eds.), Elsevier, New York, pp. 17–57.
70. Hyvarinen, J. (1982) Posterior parietal lobe of the primate brain. *Physiol. Rev.* **62,** 1060–1129.
71. Schmahmann, J.D. and Pandya DN. (1989) Anatomical investigation of projections to the basis pontis from posterior parietal association cortices in rhesus monkey. *J. Comp. Neurol.* **289,** 53–73.
72. Critchley, M. (1953) *The Parietal Lobes.* Hafner Press, New York.
73. Denny-Brown, D. and Chambers, R.A. (1958) The parietal lobe and behavior. *Res. Publ. Assoc. Nerv. Ment Dis.* **36,** 35–117.
74. Glickstein, M., May, J.G., and Mercier, B.E. (1985) Corticopontine projection in the macaque: the distribution of labeled cortical cells after large injections of horseradish peroxidase in the pontine nuclei. *J. Comp. Neurol.* **235,** 343–359.
75. May, J.G. and Andersen, R.A. (1986) Different patterns of corticopontine projections from separate cortical fields within the inferior parietal lobule and dorsal prelunate gyrus of the macaque. *Exp. Brain Res.* **63,** 265–278.
76. Perrett, D.I., Mistlin, A.J., and Chitty, A.J. (1987) Visual neurons responsive to faces. *Trends Neurosci.* **10,** 358–364.
77. Schmahmann, J.D. and Pandya, D.N. (1991) Projections to the basis pontis from the superior temporal sulcus and superior temporal region in the rhesus monkey. *J. Comp. Neurol.* **308,** 224–248.

78. Ungerleider, L.G., Desimone, R., Galkin, T.W., and Mishkin, M. (1984) Subcortical projections of area MT in the macaque. *J. Comp. Neurol.* **223,** 368–386.
79. Desimone, R. and Ungerleider, L.G. (1989) Neural mechanisms of visual processing in monkeys, in *Handbook of Neurophysiology,* vol. 2 (Boller, F. and Grafman, J., eds), Elsevier, Amsterdam, pp. 267–299.
80. Schmahmann, J.D. and Pandya, D.N. (1993) Prelunate, occipitotemporal, and parahippocampal projections to the basis pontis in rhesus monkey. *J. Comp. Neurol.* **337,** 94–112.
81. Fries, W. (1990) Pontine projection from striate and prestriate visual cortex in the macaque monkey: an anterograde study. *Vis. Neurosci.* **4,** 205–216.
82. Boussaoud, D., Desimone, R., and Ungerleider, L.G. (1991) Visual topography of area TEO in the macaque. *J. Comp. Neurol.* **306,** 554–575.
83. Nadel, L. (1991) The hippocampus and space revisited. *Hippocampus* **1,** 221–229.
84. Picard, N. and Strick, P.L. (1996) Motor areas of the medial wall: a review of their location and functional activation. *Cereb. Cortex* **6,** 342–353.
85. Devinsky, O., Morrell, M.J., and Vogt, B.A. (1995) Contributions of anterior cingulate cortex to behaviour. *Brain* **118,** 279–306.
86. Paus, T. (2001) Primate anterior cingulate cortex: where motor control, drive and cognition interface. *Nat. Rev. Neurosci.* **2,** 417–424.
87. Mesulam, M.-M. and Mufson, E.J. (1985) The insula of reil in man and monkey. Architectonics, connectivity, and function, in *Cerebral Cortex,* vol. 4 (Peters, A. and Jones, E.G., eds.), Plenum Press, New York, pp. 179–226.
88. Schmahmann, J.D. and Pandya, D.N. (1992) Fiber pathways to the pons from parasensory association cortices in Rhesus Monkey. *J. Comp. Neurol.* **326,** 159–179.
89. Schmahmann, J.D. and Pandya, D.N. (1997) The cerebrocerebellar system, in *The Cerebellum and Cognition* (Schmahmann, J.D., ed.), Academic Press, San Diego, pp. 31–60.
90. Alexander, G.E., DeLong, M.R., and Strick, P.L. (1986) Parallel organization of functionally segregated circuits linking basal ganglia and cortex. *Annu. Rev. Neurosci.* **9,** 357–381.
91. Kuypers, H.G.J.M. and Lawrence, D.G. (1967) Cortical projections to the red nucleus and the brainstem in the rhesus monkey. *Brain Res.* **4,** 151–188.
92. Humphrey, D.R., Gold, R., and Reed, D.J. (1984) Sizes, laminar and topographic origins of cortical projections to the major divisions of the red nucleus in the monkey. *J. Comp. Neurol.* **225,** 75–94.
93. Kennedy, P.R., Gibson, A.R., and Houk, J.C. (1986) Functional and anatomic differentiation between parvicellular and magnocellular regions of red nucleus in the monkey. *Brain Res.* **364,** 124–136.
94. Saint-Cyr, J.A. and Courville, J. (1980) Projections from the motor cortex, midbrain, and vestibular nuclei to the inferior olive in the cat: anatomical and functional correlates, in *The Inferior Olivary Nucleus: Anatomy and Physiology* (Courville, J., DeMontigny, C., and Lamarre, Y., eds.), Raven Press, New York, pp. 97–124.
95. Shah, V.S., Schmahmann, J.D., Pandya, D.N., and Vaher, P.R. (1997)Associative projections to the zona incerta: possible anatomic substrates for extension of the Marr-Albus hypothesis to non-motor learning. *Soc. Neurosci. Abstr.* **23,** 1829.
96. Allen, G.I., and Tsukahara, N. (1974) Cerebrocerebellar communication systems. *Physiol. Rev.* **54,** 957–1008.
97. Stein, J.R. and Glickstein, M. (1992) Role of the cerebellum in visual guidance of movement. *Physiol. Rev.* **72,** 967–1017.
98. Sasaki, K., Oka, H., Matsuda, Y., Shimono, T., and Mizuno, N. (1975) Electrophysiological studies of the projections from the parietal association area to the cerebellar cortex. *Exp. Brain Res.* **23,** 91–102.
99. Brodal, P. (1979) The pontocerebellar projection in the rhesus monkey: an experimental study with retrograde axonal transport of horseradish peroxidase. *Neuroscience* **4,** 193–208.
100. Strick, P.L. (1999) Symposium: basal ganglia, cerebellum and motor control. *Soc. Neurosci. Abstr.* **25,** 528.
101. Jansen, J. and Brodal, A. (1940) Experimental studies on the intrinsic fibers of the cerebellum. II. The corticonuclear projection. *J. Comp. Neurol.* **73,** 267–321.
102. Chambers, W.W. and Sprague, J.M. (1955) Functional localization in the cerebellum. I. Organization in longitudinal corticonuclear zones and their contribution to the control of posture, both extrapyramidal and pyramidal. *J. Comp. Neurol.* **103,** 105–130.
103. Haines, D.E. (1989) HRP study of cerebellar corticonuclear-nucleocortical topography of the dorsal culminate lobule—lobule V—in a prosimian primate (Galago): with comments on nucleocortical cell types. *J. Comp. Neurol.* **282,** 274–292.
104. Dow, R.S. (1942) The evolution and anatomy of the cerebellum. *Biol. Rev.* **17,** 179–220.
105. Brodal, A. (1981) *Neurological Anatomy in Relation to Clinical Medicine*, Oxford University Press, New York.
106. Olszewski, J. (1952) *The Thalamus of the Macaca Mulatta*, S. Karger, Basel.
107. Strick, P.L. (1976) Anatomical analysis of ventrolateral thalamic input to primate motor cortex. *J. Neurophysiol.* **39,** 1020–1031.
108. Batton, R.R. III, Jayaraman, A., Ruggiero, D., and Carpenter, M.B. (1977) Fastigial efferent projections in the monkey: an autoradiographic study. *J. Comp. Neurol.* **174,** 281–306.
109. Thach, W.T. and Jones, E.G. (1979) The cerebellar dentatothalamic connection: terminal field, lamellae, rods and somatotopy. *Brain Res.* **169,** 168–172.
110. Stanton, G.B. (1980) Topographical organization of ascending cerebellar projections from the dentate and interposed nuclei in Macaca mulatta: an anterograde degeneration study. *J. Comp. Neurol.* **190,** 699–731.

111. Kalil, K. (1981) Projections of the cerebellar and dorsal column nuclei upon the thalamus of the rhesus monkey. *J. Comp. Neurol.* **195,** 25–50.
112. Wiesendanger, R. and Wiesendanger, M. (1985) The thalamic connections with medial area 6 (supplementary motor cortex) in the monkey (*Macaca fascicularis*). *Exp. Brain Res.* **59,** 91–104.
113. Ilinsky, I.A. and Kultas-Ilinsky, K. (1987) Sagittal cytoarchitectonic maps of Macaca mulatta. *J. Comp. Neurol.* **173,** 147–164.
114. Orioli, P.J. and Strick, P.L. (1989) Cerebellar connections with the motor cortex and the arcuate premotor area: an analysis employing retrograde transneuronal transport of WGA-HRP. *J. Comp. Neurol.* **288,** 621–626.
115. Kievet, J. and Kuypers, H.G.J.M. (1977) Organization of the thalamocortical connections to the frontal lobe in the rhesus monkey. *Exp. Brain Res.* **29,** 299–322.
116. Yeterian, E.H. and Pandya, D.N. (1985) Corticothalamic connections of the posterior parietal cortex in the rhesus monkey. *J. Comp. Neurol.* **237,** 408–426.
117. Yeterian, E.H. and Pandya, D.N. (1989) Thalamic connections of the cortex of the superior temporal sulcus in the rhesus monkey. *J. Comp. Neurol.* **282,** 80–97.
118. Vogt, B.A. and Pandya, D.N. (1987) Cingulate cortex of the rhesus monkey: II. Cortical afferents. *J. Comp. Neurol.* **262,** 271–289.
119. Schmahmann, J.D. and Pandya, D.N. (1990) Anatomical investigation of projections from thalamus to the posterior parietal association cortices in rhesus monkey. *J. Comp. Neurol.* **295,** 299–326.
120. Siwek, D.F. and Pandya, D.N. (1991) Prefrontal projections to the mediodorsal nucleus of the thalamus in the rhesus monkey. *J. Comp. Neurol.* **312,** 509–524.
121. Giguere, M. and Goldman Rakic, P.S. (1988) Mediodorsal nucleus: areal, laminar, and tangential distribution of afferents and efferents in the frontal lobe of rhesus monkeys. *J. Comp. Neurol.* **277,** 195–213.
122. Barbas, H., Haswell Henion, T.H., and Cermon, C.R. (1991) Diverse thalamic projections to the prefrontal cortex in the rhesus monkey. *J. Comp. Neurol.* **313,** 65–94.
123. Middleton, F.A. and Strick, P.L. (1994) Anatomical evidence for cerebellar and basal ganglia involvement in higher cognitive function. *Science* **266,** 458–451.
124. Middleton, F.A. and Strick, P.L. (1997) Cerebellar output channels, in *The Cerebellum and Cognition Schmahmann* (Schmahmann, J.D., ed.), Academic Press, San Diego, pp. 61–82.
125. Mackel, R. (1987) The role of the monkey sensory cortex in the recovery from cerebellar injury. *Exp. Brain Res.* **66,** 638–652.
126. Metter, E.J., Kempler, D., Jackson, C.A., et al. (1987) Cerebellar glucose metabolism in chronic aphasia. *Neurology* **37,** 1599–1606.
127. Botez-Marquard, T. and Botez, M.I. (1997) Olivopontocerebellar atrophy and Friedreich's ataxia: neuropsychological consequences of bilateral versus unilateral cerebellar lesions, in *The Cerebellum and Cognition* (Schmahmann, J.D., ed.), Academic Press, San Diego, pp. 387–410.
128. Schmahmann, J.D. and Sherman, J.C. (1998) The cerebellar cognitive affective syndrome. *Brain* **121,** 561–579. (see editorial, *Brain* 1998; **121,** 545–546.)
129. Knoepfel, H.K. and Macken, J. (1947) Le syndrome psycho-organique dans les heredo-ataxies. *J. Belge. Neurol. Psychiat.* **47,** 314–323.
130. Kish, S.J., El-Awar, M., Schut, L., Leach, L., Oscar-Berman, M., and Freedman, M. (1988) Cognitive deficits in olivopontocerebellar atrophy: implications for the cholinergic hypothesis of Alzheimer's dementia. *Ann. Neurol.* **24,** 200–206.
131. Bracke-Tolkmitt, R., Linden, A., Canavan, A.G.M., et al. (1989) The cerebellum contributes to mental skills. *Behav. Neurosci.* **103,** 442–446.
132. Grafman, J., Litvan, I., Massaquoi, S., Stewart, M., Sirigu, A., and Hallett, M. (1992) Cognitive planning deficit in patients with cerebellar atrophy. *Neurology* **42,** 1493–1496.
133. Appollonio, I.M., Grafman, J., Schwartz, V., Massaquoi, S., and Hallett, M. (1993) Memory in patients with cerebellar degeneration. *Neurology* **43,** 1536–1544.
134. Geschwind, D.H. (1999) Focusing attention on cognitive impairment in spinocerebellar ataxia. *Arch Neurol.* **56,** 20–22.
135. Wallesch, C.-W. and Horn, A. (1990) Long-term effects of cerebellar pathology on cognitive functions. *Brain Cogn.* **14,** 19–25.
136. Botez-Maquard, T., Leveille, J., and Botez, M.I. (1994) Neuropsychological functioning in unilateral cerebellar damage. *Can. J. Neurol. Sci.* **21,** 353–357.
137. Silveri, M.C., Leggio, M.G., and Molinari, M. (1994) The cerebellum contributes to linguistic production: a case of agrammatic speech following a right cerebellar lesion. *Neurology* **44,** 2047–2050.
138. Fiez, J.A., Petersen, S.E., Cheney, M.K., and Raichle, M.E. (1992) Impaired non-motor learning and error detection associated with cerebellar damage. A single case study. *Brain* **115,** 155–178.
139. Malm, J., Kristensen, B., Karlsson, T., Carlberg, B., Fagerlund, M., and Olsson, T. (1998) Cognitive impairment in young adults with infratentorial infarcts. *Neurology* **51,** 433–440.
140. Neau, J.P., Arroyo-Anllo, E., Bonnaud, V., Ingrand, P., and Gil, R. (2000) Neuropsychological disturbances in cerebellar infarcts. *Acta Neurol. Scand.* **102,** 363–370.
141. Parvizi, J., Anderson, S.W., Martin, C.O., Damasio, H., and Damasio, A.R. (2001) Pathological laughter and crying: a link to the cerebellum. *Brain* **124,** 1708–1719.

142. Gomez Beldarrain, M., Garcia-Monco, J.C., Quintana, J.M., Llorens, V., and Rodeno, E. (1997) Diaschisis and neuropsychological performance after cerebellar stroke. *Eur. Neurol.* **37,** 82–89.
143. Schmahmann, J.D. and Sherman, J.C. The cerebellar cognitive affective syndrome. (1998) *Brain* **121,** 2203–2205.
144. Botez-Marquard, T., Léveillé, J., and Botez, M.I. (1994) Neuropsychological functioning in unilateral cerebellar damage. *Can. J. Neurol. Sci.* **21,** 353–357.
145. Dennis, M., Spiegler, B.J., Hetherington, C.R., and Greenberg, M.L. (1996) Neuropsychological sequelae of the treatment of children with medulloblastoma. *J. Neurooncol.* **29,** 91–101.
146. Waber, D.P. and Holmes, J.M. (1985) Assessing children's copy production of the Rey-Ostereith complex figure. *J. Clin. Exp. Neuropsychol.* **7,** 264–280.
147. Duffner, P.K., Cohen, M.E., and Thomas, P. (1983) Late effects of treatment on the intelligence of children with posterior fossa tumors. *Cancer* **51,** 233–237.
148. Glauser, T.A. and Packer, R.J. (1991) Cognitive deficits in long-term survivors of childhood brain tumors. *Child's Nerv. Sys.* **7,** 2–12.
149. Radcliffe, J., Packer, R.J., Atkins, T.E., et al. (1992) Three- and four-year cognitive outcome in children with noncortical brain tumors treated with whole-brain radiotherapy. *Ann. Neurol.* **32,** 551–554.
150. Levisohn, L., Cronin-Golomb, A., and Schmahmann, J.D. (2000) Neuropsychological consequences of cerebellar tumour resection in children: cerebellar cognitive affective syndrome in a paediatric population. *Brain* **123,** 1041–1050.
151. Riva, D. and Giorgi, C. (2000) The cerebellum contributes to higher functions during development: evidence from a series of children surgically treated for posterior fossa tumours. *Brain* **123,** 1051–1061.
152. Wisoff, J.H. and Epstein, F.J. (1984) Pseudobulbar palsy after posterior fossa operation in children. *Neurosurgery* **15,** 707–709.
153. Pollack, I.F., Polinko, P., Albright, A.L., Towbin, R., and Fritz, C. (1995) Mutism and pseudobulbar symptoms after resection of posterior fossa tumors in children: incidence and pathophysiology. *Neurosurgery* **37,** 885–893.
154. Catsman-Berrevoets, C.E., Van Dongen, H.R., Mulder, P.G., Pazy Geuze, D., Paquier, P.F., and Lequin, M.H. (1999) Tumour type and size are high risk factors for the syndrome of "cerebellar" mutism and subsequent dysarthria. *J. Neurol. Neurosurg. Psychiatry* **67,** 755–757.
155. Dunwoody, G.W., Alsagoff, Z.S., and Yuan, S.Y. (1997) Cerebellar mutism with subsequent dysarthria in an adult: case report. *Br. J. Neurosurg.* **11,** 161–163.
156. Berquin, P.C., Giedd, J.N., Jacobsen, L.K., et al. (1998) Cerebellum in attention-deficit hyperactivity disorder: a morphometric MRI study. *Neurology* **50,** 1087–1093.
157. Mostofsky, S.H., Mazzacco, M.M., Aakalu, G., Warsofsky, I.S., Denckla, M.B., and Reiss, A.L., et al. (1998) Decreased cerebellar posterior vermis size in fragile X syndrome: correlation with neurocognitive performance. *Neurology* **50,** 121–130.
158. Castellanos, F.X., Giedd, J.N., Berquin, P.C., et al. (2001) Quantitative brain magnetic resonance imaging in girls with attention-deficit/hyperactivity disorder. *Arch. Gen. Psychiatry* **58,** 289–295.
159. Allin, M., Matsumoto, H., Santhouse, A.M., et al. (2001) Cognitive and motor function and the size of the cerebellum in adolescents born very pre-term. *Brain* **124,** 60–66.
160. Nicolson, R.I., Fawcett, A.J., Berry, E.L., Jenkins, I.H., Dean, P., and Brooks, D.J. (1999) Association of abnormal cerebellar activation with motor learning difficulties in dyslexic adults. *Lancet* **353,** 1662–1667.
161. Glickstein, M. (1994) Cerebellar agenesis. *Brain* **117,** 1209–1212.
162. Gardner, R.J., Coleman, L.T., Mitchell, L.A., et al. (2001) Near-total absence of the cerebellum. *Neuropediatrics* **32,** 62–68.
163. Chheda, M.G., Sherman, J.C., and Schmahmann, J.D. (2002) Neurologic, psychiatric and cognitive manifestations in cerebellar agenesis. *Neurology* **58(Suppl. 3),** 356.
164. Heath, R.G., Franklin, D.E., and Shraberg, D. (1979) Gross pathology of the cerebellum in patients diagnosed and treated as functional psychiatric disorders. *J. Nerv. Ment. Dis.* **167,** 585–592.
165. Pollak, L., Klein, C., Rabey, J.M., and Schiffer, J. (1996) Posterior fossa lesions associated with neuropsychiatric symptomatology. *Int. J. Neurosci.* **87,** 119–126.
166. Lippman, S., Manshadi, M., Baldwin, H., Drasin, G., Rice, J., and Alrajech, S. (1981) Cerebellar vermis dimensions on computerized tomographic scans of schizophrenic and bipolar patients. *Am. J. Psychiatry* **139,** 667–668.
167. Moriguchi, I. (1981) A study of schizophrenic brains by computerized tomography scans. *Folia. Psychiatry Neurol. Jpn.* **35,** 55–72.
168. Loeber, R.T., Cintron, C.M., and Yurgelun-Todd, D.A. (2001) Morphometry of individual cerebellar lobules in schizophrenia. *Am. J. Psychiatry* **158,** 952–954.
169. Ichimiya, T., Okubo, Y., Suhara, T., and Sudo, Y. (2001) Reduced volume of the cerebellar vermis in neuroleptic-naive schizophrenia. *Biol. Psychiatry* **49,** 20–27.
170. Volz, H., Gaser, C., and Sauer, H. (2000) Supporting evidence for the model of cognitive dysmetria in schizophrenia —a structural magnetic resonance imaging study using deformation-based morphometry. *Schizophr. Res.* **46,** 45–56.
171. Andreasen, N.C., O'Leary, D.S., Cizadlo, T., et al. (1996) Schizophrenia and cognitive dysmetria: a positron-emission tomography study of dysfunctional prefrontal-thalamic-cerebellar circuitry. *Proc. Natl. Acad. Sci. USA* **93,** 9985–9990.
172. Staal, W.G., Hulshoff Pol, H.E., Schnack, H.G., van Haren, N.E., Seifert, N., and Kahn, R.S. (2001) Structural brain abnormalities in chronic schizophrenia at the extremes of the outcome spectrum. *Am. J. Psychiatry* **158,** 1140–1142.
173. Courchesne, E., Yeung-Courchesne, R., Press, G.A., Hesselink, J.R., and Jernigan, T.L. (1988) Hypoplasia of cerebellar vermal lobules VI and VII in autism. *N. Engl. J. Med.* **318,** 1349–1354.

174. Murakami, J.W., Courchesne, E., Press, G.A., Yeung-Courchesne, R., and Hesselink, J.R. (1989) Reduced cerebellar hemisphere size and its relationship to vermal hypoplasia in autism. *Arch Neurol.* **46,** 689–694.
175. Kemper, T.L. and Bauman, M. (1998) Neuropathology of infantile autism. *J. Neuropathol. Exp. Neurol.* **57,** 645–652.
176. Heath, R.G. (1977) Modulation of emotion with a brain pacemaker. Treatment for intractable psychiatric illness. *J. Nerv. Ment. Dis.* **165,** 300–317.
177. Cooper, I.S., Riklan, M., Amin, I., and Cullinan, T. (1978) A long-term follow-up study of cerebellar stimulation for the control of epilepsy, in *Cerebellar Stimulation in Man* (Cooper, I.S., ed.), Raven Press, New York, pp. 19–38.
178. Berman, A.J., Berman, D., and Prescott, J.W. (1974) The effects of cerebellar lesions on emotional behavior in the rhesus monkey, in *The Cerebellum Epillepsy and Behavior* (Cooper, I.S., Riklan, M., and Snider, R.S., eds.), Plenum Press, New York, pp. 277–284.
179. Reiman, E.M., Raichle, M.E., Robins, E., et al. (1989) Neuroanatomical correlates of a lactate-induced anxiety attack. *Arch. Gen. Psychiatry* **46,** 493–500.
180. Lane, R.D., Reiman, E.M., Ahern, G.L., Schwartz, G.E., and Davidson, R.J. (1997) Neuroanatomical correlates of happiness, sadness, and disgust. *Am. J. Psychiatry* **154,** 926–933.
181. Beauregard, M., Leroux, J.M., Bergman, S., et al. (1998) The functional neuroanatomy of major depression: an fMRI study using an emotional activation paradigm. *Neuroreport* **9,** 3253–3258.
182. Desmond, J.E. and Fiez, J.A. (1998) Neuroimaging studies of the cerebellum: language, learning and memory. *Trends Cog. Sci.* **2,** 355–362.
183. Schmahmann, J.D., Loeber, R.T., Marjani, J., and Hurwitz, A.S. (1998) Topographic organization of cognitive function in the human cerebellum. A meta-analysis of functional imaging studies. *Neuroimage* **7,** S721.
184. Schmahmann, J.D. (1994) The cerebellum in autism: clinical and anatomic perspectives, in *The Neurobiology of Autism* (Bauman, M.L. and Kemper, T.L., eds.), Johns Hopkins University Press, Baltimore, pp. 195–226.

III
Cognition in Movement Disorders

6
Assessing Cognition in Movement Disorders

Julie C. Stout, PhD and Jane S. Paulsen, PhD

1. INTRODUCTION AND OVERVIEW

Movement disorders are associated with a wide range of changes in movement, cognition, and emotion. Changes to the motor system resulting from central nervous system damage or disease are virtually always accompanied by cognitive dysfunction. In fact, the study of movement disorders has fostered a growing debate about the utility of separating motor, cognitive and emotional symptom constructs *(1)*, given their overlapping neural systems, and the convergence of these symptoms within individuals.

This chapter is an overview of neuropsychological assessment for the movement disorders. First, we provide a neurobiological rationale for the co-occurrence of motor and cognitive impairment in the movement disorders. Next, we describe neuropsychological methods for clinical assessment of patients with movement disorders. Finally, we discuss a sample of current issues in the neuropsychological study of movement disorders that symbolize the latest developments and future of this field.

Although cognitive changes are the rule rather than the exception in movement disorders, there is heterogeneity with which cognitive deficits appear. For example, Huntington's disease (HD) is associated with cognitive dysfunction, which occurs early in the course of the disease and eventually develops into dementia. Parkinson's disease (PD) is also associated with cognitive impairment, yet progression of the disease coincides with the development of dementia in only a subset of persons with PD. Cerebellar diseases are rarely associated with dementia, and in many cases, cognitive decline is difficult to substantiate. When a sufficiently sized sample can be constructed for neuropsychological study, and in-depth evaluations of cognition are performed, cognitive differences are usually detected in movement disorder groups as compared to comparison samples. The clinical significance of such findings is not always apparent, however, particularly when the findings are subtle or minimal.

This chapter limits its focus to a subset of movement disorders. HD and PD, both affecting the basal ganglia, receive the greatest attention. For the purpose of comparison, cerebellar disorders are also addressed, however, this volume contains chapters devoted entirely to the neuropsychology of cerebellar disorders, and these should be consulted for a more in depth analysis of this issue (see Chapters 5 and 11 of this book). Complete reviews of the neuropsychological findings associated with individual movement disorders can be found elsewhere *(2)*. The current chapter emphasizes the neurobiological rationale for cognitive deficits and the clinical neuropsychological practices for assessment of individuals with movement disorders. It also highlights new directions that embody the general study of cognition in movement disorders.

From: *Mental and Behavioral Dysfunction in Movement Disorders*
Edited by: M-A. Bédard et al. © Humana Press Inc., Totowa, NJ

2. NEUROBIOLOGICAL EVIDENCE FOR COGNITIVE IMPAIRMENT IN THE MOVEMENT DISORDERS

Historical views have emphasized the importance of cortical rather than subcortical brain regions in cognition. Additionally, the basal ganglia and cerebellum, which are primary sites of neuropathology in most movement disorders, have typically been considered part of the motor system, and were not assumed to play a major role in cognition. Although these views are outdated and incomplete, they continue to influence the studies of cognition in the movement disorders. Nonetheless, there is clear evidence that movement disorders are associated with impairment in cognition.

2.1. *The Basal Ganglia and Cognition*

A direct role of basal ganglia function in cognitive processes is implied by the fact that these structures receive inputs from virtually all levels of the cerebral cortex and have output that modulates the descending motor tracts. The input to output structure of the basal ganglia is described as a many to few arrangement, where actions within the basal ganglia act as filters, amplifying the effects of some inputs and dampening the effects of others. Thus, the basal ganglia aid efficient response selection for those inputs that are relevant.

Some have argued that the basal ganglia have a similar function for cognition, acting to enhance selection of behaviorally relevant cognitive operations. Anatomically this is plausible, because the basal ganglia output nuclei, including the globus pallidus interna and the substantia nigra reticulata project, via the thalamus, toward both motor areas and nonmotor cortical areas. For example, Middleton and Strick *(3)* showed that basal ganglia outputs target the dorsolateral prefrontal cortex, which is associated with executive functions and working memory, as well as the inferotemporal cortex, which is associated with object recognition.

2.2. *The Cerebellum and Cognition*

According to current theories, the cerebellum provides executive neural control of action. A review by Daum and Ackerman *(4)* describes a role for the cerebellum's computational processing in motor learning, timing, and higher cognitive functions. According to this view, the cerebellum receives input from the posterior parietal, superior temporal, motor, premotor, and prefrontal cortex via the pontine nuclei, and provides outputs, via the thalamus, to the dentate nucleus, prefrontal cortex, posterior parietal, and superior temporal cortices, which are all richly connected associations areas. They suggest that the actions of cerebellar computations on cognition are analagous to those on motor tasks. That is, they improve the accuracy of the process (cognitive, motor) by providing feedback and updating that allows modification and improved accuracy of the process. According to this view, ideas and concepts can be targets of cerebellar modulation in a parallel fashion to the modulation of limb activities during movement *(1)*. This cerebellar control assists in cognitive processing by providing automaticity, thus reducing the attention requirement for processing, improving timeliness, and providing scaling operations. Thus, the cerebellum is seen not as a generator of activity, but as a modulator, which can smooth the action of various cerebral processes.

2.3. *Circuitry Models for the Influence of the Basal Ganglia and Cerebellum in Cognition*

2.3.1. *Basal Ganglia Circuitry*

Several authors have contributed to the development of a functional neuroanatomical model of cortical-subcortical brain circuits, which has pervaded the neurological and psychiatric literature for the past 15 years, and about which numerous articles and books have been written *(3,5–9)*. According to these models, there are several circuits that originate in the frontal cortex, project to the basal ganglia and pallidum, which in turn project to the thalamus, and then back to the frontal cortex (see Chapters 2 and 24 of this book for more detailed descriptions of these circuits). Cummings *(6)* articulates this model in the context of neuropsychiatric disorders such as Huntington's and other diseases that affect the basal ganglia and argues that damage at any level of the circuit can produce functional impairment of the circuit and, in turn, cause alterations in the behavioral functions subserved by that circuit. Originally, the nonmotor frontal subcortical circuits were described as three circuits with their frontal origins in the dorsolateral, mesial frontal–anterior cingulate, and orbitofrontal regions. Damage to these circuits was linked to declines in executive functions and working memory (dorsolateral circuit), apathy and akinesia (medial frontal–anterior cingulate circuit), and disinhibition–emotional control (orbitofrontal circuit) *(6,7)*.

Recent evidence has expanded the circuitry model of the basal ganglia to include additional circuits whose cortical targets fall outside of the frontal cortex. For example, Middleton and Strick *(10)* describe at least 11 nonmotor circuits that are linked to frontal, posterior parietal, and temporal cortex. The recent work by Middleton and Strick strongly demonstrates that the basal ganglia are situated to have a pervasive influence on cortical function, thus certainly affecting cognition via this circuitry.

2.3.2. Cerebellar Circuitry

Although less well-characterized thus far, the cerebellum is also known to have projections to nonmotor regions of the cortex. As with the basal ganglia circuits, the cerebellum projections reach the cortex via thalamic "relay" nuclei. For example, the ventral dentate nucleus of the cerebellum projects to prefrontal regions important in planning, working memory, and other high-level executive functions. The outputs from the cerebellum appear to originate from distinct regions of the dentate gyrus and project to distinct regions of the prefrontal cortex *(11)*.

2.4. Widespread Neuropathology in the Movement Disorders

2.4.1. Distribution of Neuropathology in the Cortex in the Movement Disorders

Virtually every movement disorder that has been studied at autopsy has revealed neuropathological findings in the neocortex. For example, in HD, generalized cortical atrophy is frequently observed, with relatively greater effects in posterior than anterior cortical regions *(12)*. In PD, cell death occurs in the pigmented cells of the substantia nigra that innervate the striatum, but also in the ventral tegmental area, which constitutes the mesocortical ascending dopaminergic system. There is also significant cell death in the noradrenergic, serotonergic, and cholinergic cells arising, respectively, from the locus coeruleus, the raphe nuclei, and the basal forebrain, which all constitute major ascending systems to the cortex. In addition, PD is characterized by the presence of Lewy bodies, which affect not only subcortical structures, but also pervade the whole cortex *(13)*. Corticobasal degeneration is associated with cell loss at the frontoparietal junction, the cingulate, and the insula *(14)*. Thus, cognitive dysfunction in the movement disorders is likely caused, at least in part, by the widespread damage to the cortical mantle that appears repeatedly across these diseases (see Chapter 18 of this book for a complete description on the neuropathology of these diseases).

2.5. Neuropsychological Characterization of Movement Disorders

Numerous studies have documented the presence of cognitive deficits in movement disorder patients, and several of the movement disorders have been extensively characterized by neuropsychological methods. We briefly describe neuropsychological findings and related neuroanatomical brain damage in a sample of movement disorders affecting the basal ganglia and cerebellum to illustrate the common patterns of cognitive impairment observed in these diseases.

2.5.1. PD

One of the most well-studied movement disorders is PD, a progressive neurodegenerative disease that is mainly characterized by the presence of a pill-rolling resting tremor, rigidity and bradykinesia (slowed voluntary movements). Neuropsychological studies suggest that the majority of individuals with PD experience subtle cognitive declines *(15)*, which may be recognized under the term subcorticofrontal syndrome (SCFS). The term SCFS is sometimes used to better describe the nature of the intellectual deficiencies frequently observed in patients with basal ganglia dysfunction. The syndrome is nonetheless nonspecific, and it can also be observed in several syndromes accompanied by subcortical pathology *(16)*, such as thalamic lesions, tumors of the third ventricle, normal pressure hydrocephalus, or multiple sclerosis. SCFS in PD is characterized by the executive deficits similar to what is encountered in patients with frontal cortical lesions. In PD, common findings include intellectual inertia or slowing (bradyphrenia), shifting deficits (mental and behavioral inflexibility), planning and sequencing difficulties, and memory deficits *(17,18)*. Memory deficits in SCFS are characteristic and different from those observed in amnesia. Patients may not be able to remember events spontaneously, but may easily recognize them if a choice is offered or if a cue is given. Therefore, contrary to amnestic patients, patients with SCFS do not forget the information *per se*, but rather experience some difficulties in establishing efficient recall strategies to find the preserved memories *(19)*. In general, the SCFS is subtle enough that people with PD function fairly well in their daily activities, despite frequent memory complaints by PD patients and their families *(20)*.

The finding that SCFS is detectable early in the course of PD has been used to argue that these changes are associated at least somewhat with the dopaminergic nigrostriatal changes that occur early in the disease (see Chapter 14 of this book). However, this view has frequently been challenged by clinical and experimental evidence showing that other neurochemical systems, namely the noradrenergic and cholinergic systems could be involved in the SCFS (see Chapters 13 and 15).

In PD, there is also a subset of patients that develop a dementia syndrome, but this issue is not covered in this chapter (see Chapter 20 for a complete review on the epidemiology of dementia in PD).

2.5.2. HD

HD is a genetically transmitted disease of the basal ganglia that is characterized by a triad of clinical symptoms including choreoathetosis, cognitive decline, and psychiatric features. The motor disorder changes over time. Early motor signs often include involuntary movements, a change in saccadic eye movements, balance problems, akathisia, tongue motor impersistence, and impaired rapid alternating movements *(21–24)*. With progression, the severity of chorea tends to level off, and then decline, while rigidity, spasticity, dystonia, and bradykinesia increase *(25,26)*.

Job loss, marital distress, and decline in activities of daily living in HD are associated more strongly with cognitive decline than the movement impairment *(27,28)*. The declines in cognition associated with HD are extensive and get progressively worse, leading eventually to dementia in virtually all individuals with HD. Zakzanis *(29)* conducted an effect-size analysis incorporating meta-analytic principles and summarized neuropsychological performances from 760 HD patients and 943 healthy research participants. The findings indicated that in HD, a SCFS is present with deficits occurring in learning and acquisition of new information, delayed recall, cognitive flexibility, manual dexterity, attention, speed of processing, and verbal skill.

2.5.3. Cognition in Other Parkinsonian and Cerebellar Diseases

Cerebellar disorders are relatively rare, and the opportunities to characterize neuropsychological features in individual subtypes of these conditions have been limited. Multiple system atrophy (MSA) is a group of disorders that includes olivopontocerebellar atrophy (OPCA), Shy-Drager syndrome, and striatonigral degeneration. These individuals exhibit rigidity, bradykinesa, and postural instability, usually in an asymmetric distribution. In addition, autonomic dysfunction is common *(30)*. Dementia syndromes are uncommon in these disorders. Cognitive impairment tends to be relatively mild, and when it appears, resembles the SCFS. Some studies also report visuospatial deficits. One particular example is Fahr's disease, which is a syndrome in the category of bilateral striopallidodentate calcinosis and which is associated with calcium deposits in both the basal ganglia and the cerebellum's dentate nucleus. In Fahr's disease, the neuropsychological picture includes visual spatial misperception, poor learning, and executive dysfunction *(31)*. Similar patterns of cognitive impairment are also observed when cerebellar atrophy appears to be more isolated *(32–34)*. Additionally, more specific cognitive impairments have been identified in studies of persons with cerebellar pathology. For example, relatively isolated cerebellar dysfunction has been associated with impairments in noun–verb and rule-based word *(34)*, timing of two short sequentially presented stimuli *(35)*, reaction times in a task requiring selection of spatial–temporal pattern as a distracter between triggering stimuli *(36)*, and rapid shifts of attention between sensory modalities *(33)*.

3. COGNITIVE ASSESSMENT OF MOVEMENT DISORDERS: THE CLINICAL SETTING

Cognitive assessment relies on the integrity of the motor system for the demonstration of abilities or knowledge. Neuropsychological evaluations require spoken and manual responses, such as writing or gesturing. Therefore, the evaluation of patients with abnormalities in movement requires a special consideration of how test administration procedures and response requirements may interfere with the assessment of cognitive abilities. Test instructions may require modifications, and accommodations may be needed in the speed or precision of movements, thus leading to alternate scoring procedures. These deviations from standard clinical practice limit the utility of normative reference data. Thus, it is essential to understand how adaptations in test procedures can be used for assessment in movement disorders, how such adaptations affect interpretations of data, and how to accurately report results that arise in the course of nonstandardized clinical assessment practices.

Unlike the mental status assessment, more detailed cognitive assessments, such as those performed by clinical neuropsychologists, are not typically used for diagnosis. Cognitive assessments often have a central role in maximizing functioning in persons with impairment by suggesting compensatory techniques and assisting with rehabilitation prescriptions and long-term care or residential plans. Cognitive assessments are also used to evaluate treatment effects of pharmacological and surgical interventions. The following section provides information for clinicians who refer movement disorder patients for neuropsychological assessment.

3.1. Referrals for a Clinical Neuropsychological Evaluation

Historically, cognitive evaluations have not been essential for the diagnosis of movement disorders. Instead, the "gold standard" for diagnosis has been the detection of movement abnormalities in the neurological examination, and the match between the specific abnormal findings and the known symptoms of a particular movement disorder. For example, the diagnosis of HD requires unequivocal presence of choreiform movements, along with a confirmed family history of HD. So, while cognitive and psychiatric findings are nearly always detectable in HD by the time that the chorea can be diagnosed, the description of these changes does not have a role in diagnosis.

Some of the most common referrals for cognitive assessment of movement disordered patients include:

1. Characterization. What cognitive strengths and weaknesses are present, and how can assessment findings be used to maximize functioning? This evaluation would likely encompass measures of attention, language, visuospatial function, learning, memory, psychomotor dexterity, and executive functions.
2. Progression. How has this patient's cognitive function changed across time? Such a question may be posed in response to previous testing results or could be related to an observation by the patient, family, or referring clinician. Although repeat assessments are not always available, neuropsychological evaluation can often determine whether a change in cognitive function has occurred. Ideally, these referral questions are subjected to longitudinal evaluations.
3. Cognitive staging. Has this patient declined in functioning from his or her previous level? Is this patient demented, and, if so, how does he or she function relative to other patients with dementia? What is the pattern of dementia and its likely course? This type of referral question is a request for general information, and instruments to provide an overall qualitative rating (normal, mildly impaired, moderately impaired, and early vs late dementia) may be helpful. There are several instruments that provide a general overview of basic cognitive functions, such as the Mini-Mental Status Examination *(37)* and the Mattis Dementia Rating Scale *(38)* (see Table 1).

Table 1
Neuropsychological Tests and Adaptations for Movement Disorders

Test and description[a]	Motor demands	Possible adaptations
Premorbid Intelligence Quotient (IQ) estimate		
ANART *(52,53)*: Assesses reading ability as a estimate of IQ; difficult for individuals with dysarthria.	Speech output—clear pronunciation is important.	Clarify pronunciations if necessary.
WASI/WAIS-III Vocabulary subtest *(54,55)*: Assesses vocabulary knowledge as estimate of IQ.	Speech output.	Adjusted for diminished speech output.
Barona *(56)*: Uses demographic and education–occupation information to calculate premorbid IQ.	None.	Good alternative if speech output is severely impaired.
Staging–dementia severity		
Mattis Dementia Rating Scale (DRS) *(38,57)*.	Copying drawings, writing, repeating bimanual movements, speech output.	Important to have an awareness of what each item is meant to measure, for example, liberal scoring on visual construction items is allowed (i.e., do not take off points for sloppiness due to chorea).
Mini-Mental Status Exam (MMSE) *(37)*: Less demanding than DRS, but less sensitive.	Copying drawings, writing, speech output.	Important to have an awareness of what each item is meant to measure, score accordingly.
Cognitive screening		
Center to Establish a Registry for Alzheimer's Disease (CERAD; includes MMSE) *(58)*: Assesses basic attention, category fluency, visual and verbal memory.	Copying drawings, writing, speech output.	Important to have an awareness of what each item is meant to measure, score accordingly; liberal scoring on visual construction items is allowed.
Verbal memory and learning		
CVLT-II, CVLT, CVLT-II alternate *(59)*: Two versions and a short form, computerized scoring program.	Speech output.	Ask for repetitions of responses if necessary, extra time for responses if needed; do not assume the patient is finished (always ask).
Logical Memory (WMS-R, WMS-III) *(60,61)*: Assesses ability to recall short stories—immediate and delayed recall scores.	Speech output.	Ask for repetitions of responses if necessary, extra time for responses if needed, do not assume the patient is finished (always ask).
Hopkins Verbal Learning Test-Revised *(62)*: Six versions—good choice for repeat evaluations, somewhat easier than CVLT (shorter list).	Speech output.	Ask for repetitions of responses if necessary, extra time for responses if needed, do not assume the patient is finished (always ask).
Visual memory and learning		
Rey Complex Figure Test *(63)*: Assesses immediate and delayed visual memory, visuo-construction, planning–organizational abilities.	Copy and free recall of a detailed drawing, difficult for people with moderate to severe tremor or chorea.	Disregard the timing aspect and allow breaks if needed, this is often used as a process approach; task—examiner can gain information about strategy, visuoconstruction, and visual memory even if normative data is not applicable.

WMS-III Visual Reproduction *(61)*: Assesses immediate and delayed visual memory, and visuoconstruction.	Drawing of 5 figures, while not as detailed or demanding as Rey-Osterrieth Complex Figure Test (RCFT), but still difficult for those with tremor or chorea.	Liberal scoring, this is a measure of memory, it is not intended to assess drawing ability.
Brief Visuospatial Memory Test *(64–66)*: Assesses memory of both location and form. Three trials adds a learning component; Recognition trial; visual only (no motor component); Simple drawings; not as reliant on visuoconstruction.	Drawing of simple shapes required.	Liberal scoring of responses.
Memory for Faces (from Warrington Recognition Memory Test or WMS-III) *(67)*: No motor demands, visual recognition format only.	None, other than pointing to or stating correct response.	None needed.
Continuous Visual Memory Test *(68,69)*: Assesses visual memory in a recognition format.	None, other than indicating that an item is old or new.	None needed.
Measures of executive functions		
Wisconsin Card Sorting Test *(70,71)*: Assesses set shifting, problem-solving, perseveration. Non-verbal only—good for those with speech output problems.	Moving cards from stack to one of four response locations.	Assist patient with handling of cards: examiner can stack cards in front of patient and then ask patient to point to the stack where the top one should be moved, examiner can move cards for the patient.
Stroop Color Word Interference Test *(72–74)*: Assesses ability to inhibit a dominant response; also used as a measure of processing speed (first two trials).	Speech output, visual tracking.	Place the card on a table so patients do not have to hold it, allow them to point to items in order to mark their place.
Trails B Army Intelligence Test Battery *(75)*: Assesses ability to shift between two sets of stimuli, maintain response set; also relies on visual scanning and speeded motor movement.	Speeded motor movements, visual scanning.	Normative data may not be worthwhile if movement is particularly slow. If the goal is to assess ability to maintain and shift set, then evaluate this in a process oriented manner (i.e., not using the timed norms).
Self-Ordered Pointing Test *(76)*: Assess working memory and strategy abilities; little normative data available	None, other than pointing.	Ask patient to touch the selected item each time, as pointing may be difficult to interpret due to tremor/chorea.
WAIS-III Similarities subtest *(55)*: Assesses verbal abstraction abilities.	Speech output.	Ask patient to repeat if necessary.
Language tests		
Boston Naming Test (BNT) *(77)*: Naming ability.	Speech output.	Clarify responses if necessary.
Verbal Fluency/Controlled Oral Word Association *(78)*: Assesses production of specific word list.	Rapid speech output.	Clarify responses if necessary.
Peabody Picture Vocabulary Test-III *(79)*: Assesses vocabulary and comprehension; good choice when speech is severely impaired.	Pointing.	Ask patient to touch the selected response; pointing may be difficult to interpret due to tremor/chorea.

Table 1 (Continued)

Test and description[a]	Motor demands	Possible adaptations
Language tests *(continued)*		
Token Test *(80,81)*: Assesses comprehension; good choice when speech is severely impaired.	Pointing or touching token.	Ask patient to touch the selected token; pointing may not be accurate due to tremor/chorea. May not be possible to administer the items that require moving and picking up tokens; in this case, use this test in a process approach to assess integrity or impairment of comprehension.
Auditory attention		
Digit Span *(60)*: Assesses verbal working memory.	Speech output.	Clarify responses if necessary.
Brief Test of Attention *(82,83)*: Assesses divided auditory attention.	None.	None required.
Visual attention		
WMS-III Spatial Span *(60,84)*: Assesses visual working memory.	Pointing to a set of blocks in a specified pattern.	Ask patient to touch the blocks; pointing may be difficult to interpret due to tremor/chorea.
Perceptual ability		
Hooper Visual Organization Test *(85)*: Assesses perception and ability to integrate nonverbal material; requires naming—not a good choice if BNT or other tests of word retrieval indicate impairment.	Speech output; single word naming.	For patients with word retrieval/naming problems, examiner can attempt to determine if the perceptual aspect of the task is intact by detecting related words or gestures that indicate the patient accurately recognizes the item.
Test of Visual-Perceptual Skills *(86)*: Designed for children/adolescents, but norms for adults are available; seven subtests assess a variety of visual spatial abilities in the absence of motor demands.	Pointing to responses.	Examiner can select individual tests that are relevant to the evaluation question(s). Ask patient to touch the selected item, as pointing may not be accurate due to tremor/chorea.

[a]Abbreviations for test names: ANART, American National Adult Reading Test; CVLT, California Verbal Learning Test; CERAD, Consortium to Establish a Registry for Alzheimer's Disease; WASI, Wechsler Abbreviated Scale for Intelligence; WAIS-III, Wechsler Adult Intelligence Scale (Third Revision); WMS-R, Wechsler Memory Scale (Revised); WMS-III, Wechsler Memory Scale (Third Revision).

4. Treatment efficacy. Has cognition been affected by treatment? Cognitive changes are known to occur in conjunction with the treatment of psychiatric symptoms (i.e., depression, psychosis, and anxiety) and motor symptoms (chorea and tremor). Cognitive assessment of treatment outcome is an expanding focus of neuropsychological assessment. For such assessments to be sensitive, it has been essential to expand neuropsychological approaches to focus on relatively subtle indices of change, and to consider practice effects that occur with repeated assessment.

In making referrals for neuropsychological assessment, it is essential to provide basic demographic information such as age, sex, and years of education so that appropriate measures can be selected for the evaluation. Knowledge of a patient's age is useful for test selection because normative reference data are not always available for the entire range of ages that one might encounter in the evaluation setting. Education level (i.e., number of years completed successfully) allows the consideration of education in the interpretation of performance. For instance, it is likely that a 40-yr-old with 6 yr of education will perform quite differently than a 40-yr-old with 20 yr of education, irrespective of brain disease. Health status is useful for planning the length of an evaluation, because individuals who are quite ill are usually unable to tolerate extensive testing, while at the other extreme, those who are outpatients and who are able to live independently may often be evaluated more extensively. Finally, knowledge of a patient's physical disabilities, such as impaired use of hands, fingers, or problems with speech production, can help in the process of planning an evaluation. Because several alternative standardized tests tend to be available within a given cognitive domain, it may be possible to select tests that do not rely on motor functions known to be impaired in the patient.

3.2. *Clinical Neuropsychological Assessment of the Movement Disordered Patient*

Neuropsychological assessments generally focus on some combination of the following cognitive domains: attention, language, visuoperceptual functions, complex gestures, learning and memory, psychomotor speed, and executive functions. In addition, measures of emotional function are usually obtained because depressive symptoms can affect cognitive performance and confound the results of an evaluation. Assessment of depression is particularly relevant for the cognitive evaluation of movement disorders. Prevalence of depression in patients with movement disorders has been estimated at two to six times the rate in the general population (see Chapters 24–27 of this book). The effects of depressed mood on cognitive performance can mimic a SCFS with typical slowed speed and inattention.

The attribution of poor test performances to neurological disease can be made only after confounding factors, such as depression or anxiety, are ruled out. General practice guidelines typically suggest the initiation of antidepressant pharmacotherapy for the treatment of depression in movement disorders. Follow-up cognitive assessment following successful improvement in mood can help to disentangle the respective influences of neurological disease and mood or cognition.

Cognitive assessment proceeds in steps, including preparation for the evaluation (i.e., review of history and referral information, preliminary test selection), interview of the patient and a caregiver, standardized cognitive testing, questionnaire completion by patient and caregiver, scoring of tests and questionnaires, data integration, comparison with normative standards, and report writing.

The assessment preparation requires a review of the medical record and referral information in order to develop a test battery adapted to each patient. Following are some examples of situations in which testing accommodations might be made for individuals with movement disorders. Accommodations that are more specific to individual test instruments are described in Table 1.

1. Tremor and bradykinesia in the dominant hand may suggest limited use of manual responses to tests. Multiple choice formats may be more reliable than those based on more extensive response output, such as handwriting or drawing.
2. Hypophonia may require an isolated testing space with the capacity for amplifying speech output.
3. Brief batteries that target only those cognitive domains about which concerns have been expressed are more appropriate for the assessment of some patients than are more broad surveys of cognition. For example, many persons with HD are uncomfortable in novel situations. They sometimes respond to this novelty with akathesia,

which progresses toward agitation. Thus, brief test sessions tend to be more tolerable and, in turn, most likely produce more valuable accurate estimates of cognitive ability.

4. Numerous memory tests exist ranging from the acquisition and recall or recognition of 3–16 words. Advanced information about the severity of a memory problem and its impact on daily life helps the neuropsychologist select memory tests that are challenging but not frustrating for the patient.

The interview is also an important part of the neuropsychological assessment. It provides information about the history and complaints of the patient and allows the clinician to observe the patient's behavior. Regardless of the referral question, a core set of behavioral observations are typically noted: (*i*) the patient's appearance as a reflection of personal hygiene; (*ii*) the quantity, prosody, rate, rhythm articulation, and coherence of the patient's speech output; (*iii*) the degree and consistency of effort put forth to indicate levels of motivation, energy, and fatigue; and (*iv*) the degree and quality of motor activity typically observed at rest, during cognitive performances, and when dual activities are required. Observations specifically important in movement disorders include gait, gross and fine motor coordination, balance, speed of movement, the presence of involuntary or semivoluntary movements, awareness of cognitive and motor changes, awareness of emotion and humor, and facial expressiveness.

Several structured interviews are currently available for standardized assessment of neuropsychiatric symptoms. First, the Huntington Study Group has designed the Unified Huntington's Disease Rating Scale *(39)* for standardized assessment of cognition, motor control, psychiatric symptoms, and functional capacity. Less specific scales are available for any movement disorder. For example, the Neuropsychiatric Inventory *(40)* has been used in a variety of neurological diseases to document psychiatric syndromes, such as mania, depression, obsessiveness, apathy, irritability, and psychoses that are commonly observed in movement disordered patients *(41)*. Thorough assessment of neuropsychiatric symptoms is critical to the interpretation of the cognitive and functional evaluations. For example, apathy is often associated with low motivation, irritability and low frustration tolerance, and mania is associated with impulsivity and working too fast in testing. Litvan has shown that neuropsychiatric symptoms mirror motor symptoms in persons with movement disorders, in that patients with hypokinetic movement disorders (e.g., PD, progressive supranuclear palsy) exhibit greater apathy and akinesia, whereas patients with hyperkinetic movement disorders (e.g., HD and Tourette syndrome) display greater irritability and agitation (see Chapter 26 of this book) *(42)*.

Questionnaires may also be used during the neuropsychological assessment to obtain a description of a patient's symptoms, to identify cognitive complaints, to characterize the level of independence of the patient in activities of daily living, and to measure the degree of mood disturbance. These questionnaires often require patients to report their own behavior and activities. Self-report can be particularly difficult for movement-disordered patients, as they may have reduced awareness or insight *(43)*. With cognitive impairment, they may also have difficulty filling out their forms independently, and if there are specific problems with the hands, written expression may be limited or infeasible. Although the usage of self-report instruments is common in neuropsychological assessment practices, it is important to obtain concomitant cognitive performance data, because self-reports of cognitive impairments are generally found to have only small or moderate relationships with actual cognitive function *(44)*.

Some questionnaires have forms that allow separate completion by the patient and her or his caregiver. Using both a patient's self-report and an "other" report is essential to detect a discrepancy between a patient's and family member's perception of impairments. These data can be useful for identifying poor insight or high levels of caregiver distress. Evidence of reduced insight suggests that formal assessment of potential safety problems is necessary. When unawareness of possible deficits exists, it is important to acquire a comprehensive evaluation of safety-related activities such as driving, cooking, and supervision of children.

The cognitive tests used to assess movement disorders are not specific to these clinical populations, although some authors *(45)* have developed batteries that may be help to distinguish the SCFS of various movement disorders. Factors such as the clinician's training and the availability of time play a role in determining how many and which specific tests are selected. Test selection may also be informed by the need for a repeatable assessment, and by specifics of the movement disorder that will influence the ability to express one's response to the test demands. Table 1 provides a list of some tests commonly used in neuropsychological evaluations for movement disorder and other patients.

Hundreds of neuropsychological tests exist that are designed to evaluate the various areas of cognitive functioning, and most clinicians have a somewhat stable set of preferred tests that they tend to employ across patient groups. Details of many of these tests are described in two volumes *(46,47)* that have catalogued information about the uses of particular tests, summaries of validity and reliability studies, and normative reference tables. In addition, several additional sources of normative tables are available, and updated norms are constantly being published. Several comprehensive sources of normative data are available *(48,49)*.

3.2.1. Adapting Test Procedures for Patients with Movement Disorders

For many patients, adaptations of standardized test procedures may be essential for obtaining valid meaningful test results. Careful use of modified testing procedures should minimize the effects of movement problems on measures of other abilities. Table 1 provides suggestions for modifying some tests for use in movement disorder patients.

Some characteristics, such as fatigue and pain, can contribute to poor test performance and can be unrelated to the specific characteristics of the neurological disease or cognitive test procedures. It is recommended that every effort be made to minimize these effects:

1. Low stamina. Movement disorders are typically associated with reduced physical and mental stamina. Assessment may be conducted across more than 1 day, so that the patient may rest in between sessions. It is also helpful to inquire about the patient's "best time of day," so that the patient can be evaluated during optimal performance. This may be essential in PD patients showing therapeutic fluctuations or dyskinesia. Both movement and anxiety are elevated during these episodes and may certainly affect cognitive performance. Low stamina should also be distinguished from attentional and vigilance fluctuations that may sometimes occur during testing (e.g., such as in dementia with Lewy bodies or depression).
2. Fatigue developing during the evaluation. When fatigue appears to affect test performance, it is necessary to discontinue testing until the patient becomes rested. When testing a participant who is showing signs of fatigue, the addition of this observation to the record is essential, so that when the results are reviewed, the effects of fatigue on particular parts of the assessment can be considered. Performance patterns that suggest fatigue include: (*i*) discrepant results on tests or parts of tests whose scores are usually highly correlated; (*ii*) a consistent decline from the beginning to the end of the evaluation; and (*iii*) poorer performance on longer tasks.
3. Medication effects. Several classes of medications have been associated with cognitive impairments in neuropsychological testing, including lithium, anticholinergics, neuroleptics, tricyclic antidepressants, benzodiazepine, and anticonvulsants *(50)*. Effects of medications have tended to appear in tests of attention, concentration, psychomotor functions, memory, and perception. Although it may be impractical to evaluate patients off of these medications, their possible effects should be considered in the interpretation of data.
4. Bradykinesia. When motor slowing is present, the use of tests that have a speeded motor component will be of limited use. Using a task that requires timed trials will result in very low scores in the bradykinetic patient, which may significantly under represent her/his ability. For this reason, it is useful to select tasks that do not rely on speeded responses to demonstrate ability levels.
5. Speech problems. Movement disorders often affect brain regions that control speech, typically leading to dysarthria or hypophonia (see Chapter 8 of this book). If speech is difficult or very effortful, the examination should be designed to minimize the number of tasks that rely on speech output for correct responses. Also, if it is difficult to comprehend the patient's spoken speech, it may be necessary to make frequent requests for the patient to repeat a response. Although this is often necessary for obtaining accurate data, it can lead to fatigue. Typically, the need for speech repetition does not invalidate test results, although it is important to consider repetition effects on timed tests (verbal fluency) or memory tests, in which repetition may act as an additional rehearsal or learning opportunity for that information.
6. Pain. Patients with movement disorders often experience pain, such as muscle cramping, which may grow worse with physical demands. Rest breaks or opportunities to move freely or stretch can ameliorate these problems and reduce their impact on the evaluation.

3.2.2. Normative Comparisons, Interpretation of Findings, and Reporting the Results of the Cognitive Assessment

Assessment of cognition in patients with movement disorders frequently requires significant modification of standard test administration, and it is essential to question the degree to which test results can be meaningfully compared with available normative data. The lack of population-based norms can complicate the interpretation of test data, but it is essential to bear in mind that some evaluations may rely on alternative references, such as a patient's estimated predisease ability. For example, if evidence gathered indicates a strong likelihood that the patient was functioning at a normal level in an ability area prior to illness, but that patient is now clearly performing below normal, the interpretation that a decline has occurred is relatively straightforward and can be made with confidence.

Similarly, when longitudinal or treatment assessments warrant serial evaluations, normative references are of limited use. As an alternative, raw scores can be plotted over time, and normative data can be helpful for determining the degree to which variability in performance can be used to estimate whether changes over time are of a magnitude sufficient to indicate that the change was greater than simply normal variability would predict. Practice effects must also be considered in repeat testing *(46,47,51)*. Whenever possible, the use of alternate test forms for serial testing can ameliorate the effects of practice. Also, some practice effects come not from the repetition of particular stimuli, but instead from becoming familiar with the test process.

Perhaps the most challenging aspect of evaluating patients with movement disorders is the integration of the data from the record, interview, observation, and cognitive performances. Although the patient's level of effort is a primary consideration in test interpretation, accurate estimates of effort in persons with movement disorders are hindered by the high prevalence of apathy and depression, which can be misinterpreted as poor effort and motivation *(41)*.

Compiling the findings from the various parts of the evaluation into a report requires a judicious combination of art and science, particularly when there are multiple factors that bear on the validity of the assessment. There are several report formats that can be used, and these generally are tailored to the setting from which the referral originated. Many of these are described in several recent books *(23,50)*. Typically, neuropsychological reports include: (*i*) identifying information, presenting complaints, and referral question; (*ii*) medical–neurological–psychiatric exams; (*iii*) interview data and behavioral observations; (*iv*) complete test list with results organized by cognitive domain; (*v*) results of questionnaire–psychiatric symptom testing; (*vi*) summary; (*vii*) interpretations; and (*viii*) recommendations. Some reports also contain a full list of tests administered with corresponding norms, and in the case of nonstandard administration, notes on the alterations from the standard format.

In summary, movement disorders typically require multiple adaptations of the cognitive assessment process. Careful attention to enhancing the validity of cognitive assessments should guide the selection of tests and their adaptations. Interpretations of the data must also be made with the consideration of medical, psychiatric, and pharmacological effects on performance and overall cognitive function. The limitations of the evaluation should be clearly stated. Deviations from standardized evaluation procedures should be acknowledged, and their use should temper one's certainty about the validity of test results.

4. WHAT'S NEW IN COGNITIVE ASSESSMENT OF MOVEMENT DISORDERS?

Cognitive assessment in movement disorders has evolved from a focus on lesion localization to deficit measurement to the detection of subtle declines from premorbid level or alterations in cognitive abilities as a result of treatment. Although the presence of mental disturbances in movement disorders has been recognized for some time, research and clinical practice have only recently embraced cognition. Cognitive assessments have become a central component of early disease detection and a marker of successful treatment and/or negative side effects in experimental treatment paradigms. Cognition is also at the center of the quality of life of these patients (see Chapter 37 of this book).

Early detection of disease has presented challenges for cognitive assessment because of the necessity of detecting very small effects that occur in the context of progression from normal functioning to very mild impairment. The focus on early detection requires the development of new tests, because most existing cognitive tests have been developed to characterize clear impairments following injury and/or disease. Previous validity studies in neuropsychology have relied on findings of significant group differences, while the magnitude of differences in early detection is smaller than could be reliably detected in a cross-sectional group analysis.

Early detection batteries have been implemented for research on Alzheimer's, Parkinson's, Huntington's and schizophrenia. For example, large-scale efforts are underway to detect the earliest cognitive changes in HD in the prodromal phase of illness. For some movement disorders, drug development has pushed beyond the goal of providing palliative interventions to a goal of delaying onset or slowing the progression of disease. In HD, intervention may soon involve medication to delay onset prior to the manifest movement disorder. Detection of early cognitive decline is, therefore, essential in this population to determine when to initiate clinical trials to delay motor onset.

Tests developed in the field of cognitive psychology may provide a source for assessment strategies that are sensitive to subtle variations from baseline levels of function. Rapid developments in cognitive and neural sciences are expanding our understanding of how cognitive processes are implemented in the healthy brain and altered by brain damage. Clinical neuropsychological assessment practices lag behind research discoveries because of the necessity of using standard practices that have widespread acceptance in the clinical community. This lag is, in part, due to the time and financial costs of converting scientific observations into standardized test procedures. Test development for clinical use involves psychometric characterization, collection of adequate normative databases, and validity studies to establish the meaning of differences in test performances for different populations. As in other clinical professions, continuing education, professional meetings, and in recent years, the use of internet-based discussion formats serve as the primary means of disseminating information about new developments for cognitive assessment.

ACKNOWLEDGMENTS

The authors wish to acknowledge Shannon Johnson and Jason Hochman for excellent assistance in the writing of this chapter. The work was supported by RO1 NS40068 and RO3 MH62556.

REFERENCES

1. Bloedel, J.R. and Bracha, V. (1997) Duality of cerebellar motor and cognitive functions. *Int. Rev. Neurobiol.* **41,** 613–634.
2. Paulsen, J.S., Nehl, C., and Guttman, M. (2002) Basal ganglia and movement disorders, in *Principles and Practice of Behavioral Neurology and Neuropsychology* (Rizzo, M. and Eslinger, P., eds.), Harcourt Health Sciences, Philadelphia, in press.
3. Middleton, F.A. and Strick, P.L. (2000) Basal ganglia output and cognition: evidence from anatomical, behavioral, and clinical studies. *Brain Cogn.* **42,** 183–200.
4. Daum, I. and Ackerman, H. (1995) Cerebellar contributions to cognition. *Behav. Brain Res.* **67,** 201–210.
5. Alexander, G.E., DeLong, M.R., and Strick, P.L. (1986) Parallel organization of functionally segregated circuits linking basal ganglia and cortex. *Annu. Rev. Neurosci.* **9,** 357–381.
6. Cummings, J.L. (1993) Frontal subcortical circuits and human behavior. *Arch. Neurol.* **50,** 873–880.
7. Mega, M.S. and Cummings, J.L. (1994) Frontal-subcortical circuits and neuropsychiatric disorders. *J. Neuropsychiatry Clin. Neurosci.* **6,** 358–370.
8. Lichter, D.G. and Cummings, J.L. (2001) *Frontal-Subcortical Circuits in Psychiatric and Neurological Disorders,* Guilford Press, New York.
9. Middleton, F.A. and Strick, P.L. (2000) Basal ganglia and cerebellar loops: motor and cognitive circuits. *Brain Res. Rev.* **31,** 236–250.
10. Middleton, F.A. and Strick, P.L. (2001) Revised neuroanatomy of frontal-subcortical circuits, in *Frontal-Subcortical Circuits in Psychiatric and Neurological Disorders* (Lichter, D.G. and Cummings, J.L., eds.), Guilford Press, New York, pp. 44–58.
11. Middleton, F.A. and Strick, P.L. (2001) Cerebellar projections to the prefrontal cortex of the primate. *J. Neurosci.* **21,** 700–712.
12. Lange, H.W. (1981) Quantitative changes of telencephalon, diencephalon, and mesencephalon in Huntington's chorea, postencephalic, and idiopathic Parkinson's disease. *Verh. Anat. Ges.* **75,** 923–925.

13. Hughes, A.J., Daniel, S.E., Kilford, L., and Lees, A.J. (1992) Accuracy of clinical diagnosis of idiopathic Parkinson's disease: a clinicopathological study of 100 cases. *J. Neurol. Neurosurg. Psychiatry* **55,** 181–184.
14. Watts, R.L., Mirra, S.S., and Richardson, E.P. (1994) Corticobasal ganglionic degeneration, in *Movement Disorders 3* (Marsden, C. and Fahn, S., eds.), Butterworth, London, pp. 282–299.
15. Pirozzolo, F.J., Hansch, E.C., Mortimer, J.A., Webster, D.D., and Kuskowski, M.A. (1982) Dementia in Parkinson's disease: a neuropsychological analysis. *Brain Cogn.* **1,** 71–83.
16. Cummings, J.L. (1990) *Subcortical Dementia*, Oxford University Press, New York.
17. Robbins, T.W., James, M., Owen, A.M., et al. (1994) Cognitive deficits in progressive supranuclear palsy, Parkinson's disease, and multiple system atrophy in tests sensitive to frontal lobe dysfunction. *J. Neurol. Neurosurg. Psychiatry* **57,** 79–88.
18. Taylor, A.E. and Saint-Cyr, J.A. (1995) The neuropsychology of Parkinson's disease. *Brain Cogn.* **28,** 281–296.
19. Pillon, B., Deweer, B., Agid, Y., and Dubois, B. (1993) Explicit memory in Alzheimer's, Huntington's and Parkinson's diseases. *Arch. Neurol.* **50,** 374–379.
20. Dubois, B. and Pillon, B. (1998) Cognitive and behavioral aspects of movement disorders, in *Parkinson's Disease and Movement Disorders* (Jankovic, J. and Tolosa, E., eds.), Williams & Wilkins, Baltimore, pp. 837–858.
21. Harper, P.S., Lim, C., and Craufurd, D. (2000) Ten years of presymptomatic testing for Huntington's disease: the experience of the UK Huntington's Disease Prediction Consortium. *J. Med. Genet.* **37,** 567–571.
22. Siemers, E., Foroud, T., Bill, D.J., et al. (1996) Motor changes in presymptomatic Huntington disease gene carriers. *Arch. Neurol.* **53,** 487–492.
23. Armengol, C.G., Kaplan, E., and Moes, E.J. (2001) The Consumer-Oriented Neuropsychological Report, in *Psychological Assessment Resources,* Lutz, FL.
24. Lasker, A. and Zee, D. (1997) Ocular-motor abnormalities in Huntington's disease. *Vision Res.* **37,** 3639–3645.
25. Penney, J.B. Jr., Young, A.B., Shoulson, I., et al. (1990) Huntington's disease in Venezuela: 7 years of follow-up on symptomatic and asymptomatic individuals. *Mov. Disord.* **5,** 93–99.
26. Koroshetz, W.J., Myers, R.H., and Martin, J.M. (1992) The neurology of Huntington's disease, in *Movement Disorders in Neurology and Neuropsychiatry* (Joseph, A.B. and Young, R.R., eds.), Blackwell Scientific Publications, Boston, pp. 167–185.
27. Marder, K., Zhao, H., Myers, R.H., et al. (2000) Rate of functional decline in Huntington's disease. *Neurology* **54,** 452–458.
28. Rothlind, J.C. and Brandt, J. (1993) A brief assessment of frontal and subcortical functions in dementia. *J. Neuropsychiatry Clin. Neurosci.* **5,** 73–77.
29. Zakzanis, K.K. (1998) The subcortical dementia of Huntington's disease. *J. Clin. Exp. Neuropsychol.* **20,** 565–578.
30. Wenning, G.K., Ben-Shlomo, Y., Magalhaes, M., Daniel, S.E., and Quinn, N.P. (1994) Clinical features and natural history of multiple system atrophy. An analysis of 100 cases. *Brain* **117,** 835–845.
31. Lopez-Villegas, D., Kulisevsky, J., Deus, J., et al. (1996) Neuropsychological alterations in patients with computed tomography-detected basal ganglia calcification. *Arch. Neurol.* **53,** 251–256.
32. Grafman, J., Litvan, I., Massaquoi, S., Stewart, M., Sirigu, A., and Hallet, M. (1992) Cognitive planning deficit in patients with cerebellar atrophy. *Neurology* **42,** 1493–1496.
33. Akshoomoff, N.A., Courchesne, E., Press, G.A., and Iragui, V. (1992) Contribution of the cerebellum to neuropsychological functioning: evidence from a case of cerebellar degenerative disorder. *Neuropsychologia* **30,** 315–328.
34. Fiez, J.A., Petersen, S.E., Cheney, M.K., and Raichle, M.E. (1992) Impaired non-motor learning and error detection associated with cerebellar damage. *Brain* **115,** 155–178.
35. Ivry, R.B., Keele, S.W., and Diener, H.C. (1988) Dissociation of the lateral and medial cerebellum in movement timing and movement execution. *Exp. Brain Res.* **73,** 167–180.
36. Pascuale-Leone, A., Grafman, J., Clark, K., et al. (1993) Procedural learning in Parkinson's disease and cerebellar degeneration. *Ann. Neurol.* **34,** 594–602.
37. Folstein, M.F., Folstein, S.E., and McHugh, P.R. (1975) Mini-mental state. *J. Psychiatr. Res.* **121,** 189–198.
38. Mattis, S. (1988) *Dementia Rating Scale (DRS)*, Psychological Assessment Resources, Odessa, FL.
39. Huntington Study Group. (1996) Unified Huntington's Disease Rating Scale: reliability and consistency. *Mov. Disord.* **11,** 136–142.
40. Cummings, J.L., Mega, M.S., Gray, K., Rosenberg-Thomspson, S., Carusi, D., and Gornbein, J. (1994) The Neuropsychiatric Inventory: comprehensive assessment of psychopathology in dementia. *Neurology* **44,** 2308–2314.
41. Levy, M., Cummings, J.L., Fairbanks, L., et al. (1998) Apathy is not depression. *J. Neuropsychiatry Clin. Neurosci.* **10,** 314–319.
42. Litvan, I., Paulsen, J.S., Mega, M.S., and Cummings, J.L. (1998) Neuropsychiatric assessment of patients with hyperkinetic and hypokinetic movement disorders. *Arch. Neurol.* **55,** 1313–1319.
43. Vitale, C., Pellechia, M.T., Grossi, D., et al. (2001) Unawareness of dyskinesias in Parkinson's and Huntington's diseases. *Neurol. Sci.* **22,** 105–106.
44. Stout, J.C. and Murray, L.L. (2001) Assessment of memory in neurogenic communication disorders. *Semin. Speech Lang.* **22,** 137–145.
45. Dubois, B., Slachevsky, A., Litvan, I., and Pillon, B. (2000) The FAB: a frontal assessment battery at bedside. *Neurology* **55,** 1621–1626.
46. Lezak, M.D. (1995) *Neuropsychological Assessment*, 3rd ed., Oxford University Press, New York.
47. Spreen, O. and Strauss, E. (1998) *A Compendium of Neuropsychological Tests: Administration, Norms, and Commentary*, Oxford University Press, New York.

48. Heaton, R.K., Grant, I., and Matthews, C.G. (1991) *Comprehensive Norms for an Expanded Halstead-Reitan Battery*, Psychological Assessment Resources, Odessa, FL.
49. Mitrushina, M.N., Boone, K.B., and D'Elia, L.F. (1999) *Handbook of Normative Data for Neuropsychological Assessment*, Oxford University Press, New York.
50. Groth-Marnat, G. (2000) *Neuropsychological Assessment in Clinical Practice: a Guide to Test Interpretation and Integration*, John Wiley & Sons, New York.
51. Heaton, R.K., Temkin, N., Dikmen, S., et al. (2001) Detecting change: a comparison of three neuropsychological methods, using normal and clinical samples. *Arch. Clin. Neuropsychol.* **16,** 75–91.
52. Nelson, H.E. and O'Connell, A. (1978) Dementia: the estimation of pre-morbid intelligence levels using the new adult reading test. *Cortex* **14,** 234–244.
53. Nelson, H.E. (1982) *National Adult Reading Test (NART): Test Manual*, NFER Nelson, Windsor, England.
54. Wechsler, D. (1999) *Wechsler Abbreviated Scale of Intelligence (WASI): Professional Manual*, Psychological Assessment and Intervention, San Antonio.
55. Wechsler, D. (1997) *Wechsler Adult Intelligence Scale—Third Edition (WAIS-III)*, Psychological Assessment and Intervention, San Antonio.
56. Barona, A., Reynolds, C.R., and Chastain, R. (1984) A demographically based index of pre-morbid intelligence for the WAIS-R. *J. Consult. Clin. Psychol.* **52,** 885–887.
57. Jurica, P.J., Leitten, C.L., and Mattis, S. (2001) *Dementia Rating Scale-2 (DRS-2)*. Psychological Assessment Resources, Inc., Lutz, IL.
58. Morris, J.C., Heyman, A., Mohs, R.C., et al. (1989) The Consortium to Establish a Registry for Alzheimer's Disease (CERAD). Part I. Clinical and neuropsychological assessment of Alzheimer's disease. *Neurology* **39,** 1159–1165.
59. Delis, D.C., Kramer, J.H., Kaplan, E., and Ober, B.A. (1987) *California Verbal Learning Test: Adult Version*, The Psychological Corporation, San Antonio.
60. Wechsler, D. (1987) *Wechsler Memory Scale-Revised manual*, The Psychological Corporation, San Antonio.
61. Wechsler, D. (1997) *Wechsler Memory Scale—Third Edition (WMS-III)*, Psychological Assessment and Intervention, San Antonio.
62. Brandt, J. and Benedict, R.H.B. (2001) *Hopkins Verbal Learning Test—Revised (HVLT-R): Professional Manual*, Psychological Assessment Resources, Lutz, FL.
63. Osterrieth, P.A. (1944) Le test de copie d'une figure complexe. *Arch. Psychol.* **30,** 206–356.
64. Benedict, R.H.B. and Groninger, L. (1995) Preliminary standardization of a new visuospatial memory test with six alternate forms. *Clin. Neuropsychol.* **9,** 11–16.
65. Benedict, R.H.B., Schretlen, D., Groninger, L., Dobraski, M., and Shpritz, B. (1996) Revision of the Brief Visuospatial Memory Test: studies of normal performance, reliability, and validity. *Psychol. Assess.* **8,** 145–153.
66. Benedict, R.H.B. (1997) *Brief Visuospatial Memory Test-Revised*, Psychological Assessment Resources, Odessa, FL.
67. Warrington, E.K. (1941) *Recognition Memory Test*, NFER-Nelson, Windsor, UK.
68. Hannay, H.J., Levin, H.S., and Grossman, R.G. (1979) Impaired recognition memory after head injury. *Cortex* **15,** 269–283.
69. Hannay, H.J. and Levin, H.S. (no date) *Continuous Recognition Memory Test*, Available from H.J. Hannay, 4046 Grenock, Houston, TX 77025.
70. Grant, D.A. and Berg, E.A. (1948) A behavioral analysis of the degree of reinforcement and ease of shifting to new responses in a Weigl-type card sorting problem. *J. Exp. Psychol.* **38,** 404–411.
71. Berg, E.A. (1948) A simple objective treatment for measuring flexibility in thinking. *J. Gen. Psychol.* **39,** 15–22.
72. Stroop, J.R. (1935) Studies of interference in serial verbal reactions. *J. Exp. Psychol.* **18,** 643–662.
73. Jensen, A.R. and Rohwer, W.D. (1966) The Stroop Color-Word Test: a review, *Acta Psychol.* **25,** 36–93.
74. Golden, C.J. (1978) *Stroop Color and Word Test*, Stoelting, Chicago.
75. Army Individual Testing Battery. (1944) *Manual of Directions and Scoring*, War Department, Adjutant General's Office, Washington, DC.
76. Petrides, M. and Milner, B. (1982) Deficits on subject-ordered tasks after frontal- and temporal-lobe lesions in man. *Neuropsychologia* **20,** 249–262.
77. Kaplan, E.F., Goodglass, H., and Weintraub, S. (1983) *The Boston Naming Test*, 2nd ed., Lea & Febiger, Philadelphia.
78. Benton, A.L. and Hamsher, K. D. (1989) *Multilingual Aphasia Examination*, AJA Associates, Iowa City.
79. Dunn, L.M. and Dunn, L.M. (1981) *Peabody Individual Achievement Test*, American Guidance Service, Circle Pines, MN.
80. Boller, F. and Vignolo, L.A. (1966) Latent sensory aphasia in hemisphere-damaged patients: an experimental study with the Token test. *Brain* **89,** 815–831.
81. De Renzi, E. and Vignolo, L.A. (1962) The Token Test: a sensitive test to detect disturbances in aphasics. *Brain* **85,** 665–678.
82. Schretlen, D., Bobholz, J.H., and Brandt, J. (1996a) Development and psychometric properties of the Brief Test of Attention. *Clin. Neuropsychol.* **10,** 80–89.
83. Schretlen, D., Brandt, J., and Bobholz, J.H. (1996b) Validation of the Brief Test of Attention in patients with Huntington's Disease and amnesia. *Clin. Neuropsychol.* **10,** 90–95.
84. Wechsler, D. (1945) A standardized memory scale for clinical use. *J. Psychol.* **19,** 87–95.
85. Hooper, H.E. (1983) *Hooper Visual Organization Test (VOT)*, Western Psychological Services, Los Angeles.
86. Gardner, M.R. (1982) *TVPT-Test of Visual-Perceptual Skills (non-motor)*, Western Psychological Services, Los Angeles.

7

Disorders of Intention in Parkinsonian Syndromes

Richard G. Brown, PhD

1. INTRODUCTION

In recent years, the symptom of akinesia in parkinsonism has provided a valuable window into the physiological substrate of voluntary movement in man, particularly the role of the basal ganglia and the influence of dopamine. In a similar way, the study of individual nonmotor symptoms in parkinsonism can provide insights into the subsystems underlying discrete aspects of human cognition, emotion, and motivation. Even more importantly perhaps, their study in parkinsonism encourages us to examine the ways in which such diverse functions are integrated and influence broader categories of action and behavior (*see* Chapter 8 in the volume). In doing so, we are led to question whether the term "movement disorder" is the most appropriate term to apply to diseases such as parkinsonism.

This chapter focuses on possible ways in which both the motor and nonmotor functions subserved by the frontostriatal system may interact in the control of intentional behavior. In particular, it focuses on "willed-action" and its impairment in patients with parkinsonism. A model of goal-directed behavior (GDB) is employed as a framework for this discussion. Wherever possible, evidence is presented from the range of parkinsonian syndromes, including progressive supranuclear palsy (PSP) and multiple systems atrophy (MSA). However, in the large majority of published studies, the focus has been exclusively on patients with presumed idiopathic Parkinson's disease (PD).

2. INTENTIONALITY

Although long ignored by empirical science, understanding the nature of intentionality is now one of the major questions being addressed by neuroscience. Before discussing how the study of patients with parkinsonism may contribute to this knowledge, it is helpful to consider the ways in which the term "intentionality" is used.

The Latin root "intentio" refers to the mental equivalent of the pulling a bowstring and contains within it the constructs of mental effort or exertion and of aiming ones attention at a target. Intentionality has long been in the domain of philosophical debate, mainly in relation to mental states, where it has been defined as the energetic directionality of consciousness towards some object *(1)*. Such philosophical definitions focus on the mental state rather than actions themselves, largely because of the belief that definitions based on action need an homunculus. However, it is through action (whether overt of covert) that most people understand and use the concept of intentionality, and it is largely in this sense that it is employed in cognitive science today. In this context, the study of intentionality centers around cognitive processes and representations and their resultant actions concerned with the achievement of some future goal.

From: *Mental and Behavioral Dysfunction in Movement Disorders*
Edited by: M-A. Bédard et al. © Humana Press Inc., Totowa, NJ

In its goal-directedness, intentional behavior is defined as being purposeful, to contrast it with pure perceptual events or random behavior. However not all behavior that serves a purpose would be considered intentional. For example, defensive reflex behaviors (e.g., eye blink) or those that are functional in the early stages of development (e.g., the rooting and grasp reflexes) fail to satisfy the defining characteristics of intentionality in that they are governed by hard-wired neuronal structures and do not derive from a mental state. A more difficult problem for definitions of intentionality is how to view habitual behavior. By definition, such behavior is largely automatic and lacks the characteristic of effort that defines much of intentional behavior. However, such behavior is typically learned, and it is through the process of learning that automaticity grows and the requirement of effort decreases. Thus, the same behavior may require the direction of effort early in learning but not later, or may be performed automatically under some situations but not others. It can, therefore, be argued that the behavior does not change, nor its intentionality, but rather simply the requirements for control according to experience and to the demands of the moment.

This distinction between automatic, skilled, and habitual behavior on one hand and effortful or attention demanding behavior on the other, has been central to psychology and cognitive science since the 19th century. William James *(2)* used the term "ideo-motor" acts to define what we would now call habits and "willed" acts to define those behaviors that depend upon the allocation of the "effort of attention." The same basic distinctions between two broad classes of behavior continues to influence contemporary neuroscience with evidence that they are subserved by distinct, but dynamically related, subsystems (see ref. *3* for a review and Chapter 8 in this volume).

3. IMPAIRMENTS OF INTENTIONAL BEHAVIOR IN PATIENTS WITH PARKINSONISM

This section considers ways in which the behavior observed in parkinsonism can be understood as a disorder of intentionality. In doing so, the primary focus is on behavior (both motor and cognitive) that could be classed "willed," while drawing distinctions with more automatic classes of action. The impact of parkinsonism on willed behavior is illustrated through the use of three main methodological approaches: (*i*) simple reaction time and response preparation; (*ii*) word generation; and (*iii*) learning and memory. First, however, the chapter considers general phenomenon applied to cognitive behavior in parkinsonism and which is directly relevant to the consideration of intentional behavior.

3.1. Bradyphrenia and Cognitive Slowing in Parkinsonism

The term "bradyphrenia" was originally used by Naville *(4)* to refer to a behavioral syndromes of apathy, inertia, and impaired concentration. Although the term is sometimes used in this way today, it more often used to refer to the apparent slowness of cognition within the broader syndrome of subcortical dementia *(5)*. However, the concept of cognitive slowing has also been employed more narrowly to describe a deficit in the actual rate in information processing in patients with parkinsonism, whether demented or not, and irrespective of the class of cognitive operation. The most direct test of this hypothesis come from tasks that look at elemental cognitive processes. Experimental psychology offers a wide range of tasks that permit an estimate to be made on the rate of information processing. These include tasks such as memory scanning, response choice, mental rotation, object naming, and the initiation of sequential motor responses. In these paradigms, increasing the size of the memory set, number of choices, angle of rotation, word frequency, or length of sequence leads to an approximately linear increase in response time, where the slope is taken to indicate the time required to process the particular unit of information involved in the task. Such methods have been widely used in patients with parkinsonism with mixed but largely negative results *(6)* (see refs. *7–12* for examples), with the slopes of the reaction time function (and by inference the rate in information processing) being normal. Such evidence argues strongly against cognitive slowing being a general mechanism in parkinsonism. It is worth noting, however, that the majority of these tasks tap cognitive operations that are largely or fully automatic. In contrast, the behavioral slowness, evidenced clinically or in the types of tasks described below, relates to the time required to exercise a volitional and effort demanding cognitive activity. This suggests that the bradyphrenia observed in patients with PD and particularly those with PSP *(13)* may be most evident in complex behaviors that could be defined as volitional or willed.

3.2. Simple Reaction Time and Response Preparation

In simple reaction time (SRT) tasks, individuals are required to respond as quickly as they can, with a predefined overt motor response, to an external stimulus that is usually constant across the experiment. To make them less predictable, the intervals between stimuli are usually varied. On the surface, such behavior seems a long way from a concept of willed action, particularly as the subject is making a response to an explicit sensory event. However, the invariant nature of the stimulus and response provides the individual with the opportunity to focus their attention on a particular location in space, to prepare their response in advance, and maintain it in a state of readiness to execute it. Such cognitive motor processes are effortful and only occur as a result of a willed intention. The role of the stimulus is simply to trigger the preprogrammed and prepared response. Of course, an individual may be unable, or choose not, to prepare a response, in which case they will carry out all of the cognitive and motor operations to prepare and execute the movement after the stimulus has occurred. While the nature of the response would be the same, there would be a cost in terms of the time taken to execute it. Support for the suggestion that SRT involved effortful and attention demanding processing comes from evidence that when subjects are distracted by another concurrent task their RT increases *(14)*. Because they are no longer able to carry out the effortful willed processes, they are forced into responding reactively to the stimulus with a corresponding increase in response time.

SRT paradigms have been extensively used in studies of patients with PD (although rarely in PSP and MSA). Although it is difficult to generalize across studies, the overall conclusion from such research is that patients are differentially slowed on those tasks on which control subjects are fastest, particularly those such as SRT, which afford the opportunity for willed action (see ref. *15* for a review). In PSP, marked slowing in SRT is also observed, although at least some of this may be due to an inability of the motor cortex to benefit from the tonic excitatory input associated with motor readiness *(16)* rather than a lack of readiness *per se*. Such motor cortical deficits do not seem to contribute to the slowing in PD *(17)*. Instead, their slowness comes in part from a failure to take advantage of the opportunity to prepare a response in advance, operating instead in a more reactive stimulus-driven mode. In support of this, patients with PD show no disadvantage of distraction during the prestimulus period, unlike healthy controls *(14)*, suggesting that they are failing to utilize attention demanding processes during the premovement phase. However, such results do not tell us whether patients with PD are unable to apply the willed processes or choose not to do so, perhaps because of extra effort involved or lack of effectiveness of the result.

These processes have been further investigated using a choice response task (CRT), in which advance information is provided about which one of the stimuli and associated response to expect on that trial. Given time, such precueing allows subjects to reduce their slower CRT response time to the level of SRT. Results suggest that patients with PD are able to make use of such advance information, but require much longer periods of time (>2000 ms) compared to control (400–800 ms) *(18)*. Thus, the preparatory processes may be intact in PD but take longer to carry out. Separate evidence indicates that the largely automatic process of response selection itself is unimpaired in PD *(9)*, indicating that the slowness relates more to the effortful process involved in intentional preparation.

3.3. Word Generation Paradigms

Experimental tasks such as SRT typically constrain individuals in terms of what response they make and when. It may be argued that a more direct test of intentional function would come from tasks that allow individuals more choice about the nature or their response, for example response generation or fluency tasks.

In verbal fluency tasks, individuals are typically given a limited time to generate words belonging to a given class or category of objects (semantic or category fluency) or beginning with a given letter (lexical or letter fluency). The generation of verbs (action fluency) has been less commonly used, as has the production of graphical response (design fluency). In functional imaging studies, verbal fluency has been used as one of the prototypical paradigms for the study of willed action. Evidence points to the involvement of an extensive network of cortical regions, which includes left dorsolateral prefrontal cortex (DLPFC), anterior cingulate cortex (ACC), and superior temporal gyrus. Connectivity analysis *(19)* has supported a model where the DLPFC modulates the associative semantic networks, in which words and their meanings are stored, providing the basic elements of an intentional system of word generation. The same model proposes a more specific attentional role of the ACC in task performance.

Perhaps because verbal fluency tasks are quick and easy to administer, there is an extensive body of data available on their performance in patients with parkinsonism. As with all aspects of cognitive function, the majority of the evidence relates to patients with PD. However, the literature is inconsistent, with some studies finding evidence of impairment in both semantic and lexical fluency task *(20)*, some in semantic only *(21)*, others in lexical only *(22)*, whereas others find impairments in neither *(23)*. Many clinical factors have been examined for sources of this variability. Depression appears not to be a major determinant of impairment *(24)*, although there is some evidence that fluency deficits are more evident in patients with right-side dominant motor symptoms *(25)*, indicating a potential involvement of left fronto-striatal dysfunction. Evidence from positron emission tomography (PET) studies supports a link between striatal dopamine (DA) levels and verbal fluency in PD *(26)*, with performance associated with reduced caudate and prefrontal DA levels, but not levels in the putamen *(27)*. A role of hypodopaminergic stimulation is further supported by evidence of fluency deficits in *de novo* patients with PD, even at the start of the illness *(28)* and a positive impact of levodopa treatment *(29)*. However, the most significant determinant of fluency deficits in PD is the presence of dementia *(30)* with prospective studies suggesting that impairment on fluency tasks is an important predictor of incipient cognitive decline *(31)*. In contrast to the variable pattern of results from studies of PD, studies in patients with PSP, although fewer in number, have consistently reported impairment *(32)*. Evidence of impairment is also found in the few studies of patients with MSA (striatonigral degeneration [SND] type) *(33)*.

Returning to the concept of bradyphrenia, reduced output in fluency tasks could arise from either an overall slowness in word production or the presence of a kind of "mental-freezing," where the patient suddenly stops being able to access the lexicon. "Tip-of-the-tongue" problems have been reported in PD, particularly on confrontation naming tasks *(22)*. However, a study which looked at word generation over a period of several minutes *(20)* demonstrated that the fluency rate in patients paralleled that of control subjects. This suggests a general slowness in accessing lexical semantic long-term store, a conclusion supported by studies using other experimental paradigms *(34)*.

The functional imaging evidence in healthy individuals (see above) points to a critical role for the DLPFC in verbal fluency tasks, a region that is hypofunctional in parkinsonism, even in nondemented patients. This pathophysiological change is presumed to arise from abnormal basal ganglia outflow due to reduced dopamineric input from the substantia nigra *(35)*. However, if the DLPFC's role is in the modulation (and specifically the inhibition) of semantic associative networks, we would expect prefrontal hypofunction to lead to an increase in perseverative or rule breaking responses in fluency tasks, rather than the reduction in overall output observed. Just such an inhibitory failure is observed in the generation of random numbers in PD *(36)*, another form of willed response generation task dependent on the inhibitory function of the DLPFC *(37)*.

Another possible candidate for the impairment in fluency tasks in parkinsonism is pathophysiological change in the ACC, also implicated in fluency tasks by the imaging data. In contrast to the DLPFC, this region forms part of the corticothalamobasal ganglia circuit involving the ventral striatum and receives dopaminergic input from the ventral tegmental area (VTA). VTA degeneration is marked in demented patients with PD and patients with PSP, the groups of patients showing the most clear cut deficits in verbal fluency. As discussed in Subheading 4 and in Chapter 26 in this volume, these same neuronal systems are most closely implicated in the clinical phenomenon of apathy, which may be considered as a global reduction in willed intentional behavior *(38)*.

3.4. Memory

Memory comprises a broad domain of function that involves the common processes of encoding, storage, and retrieval of information. This simple framework, however, masks the diversity of memory function and associated memory systems. It has been recognized for years that some aspects of memory function are relatively automatic, while others depend on the effortful or controlled cognitive processes. The learning and recall of word lists or stories requires a range of active and effort demanding processes. Free recall in particular requires the subject to self-initiate effective retrieval processes from long-term episodic store (just as verbal fluency tasks require such retrieval from semantic memory). This process may be aided by the provision of an explicit retrieval cue, reducing the demands on internally generated retrieval processes, or by using recognition formats where the item to be recalled is presented to the subject, and the judgement becomes one of familiarity, a relatively automatic process.

Within the context of intentionality, we might expect the greatest impairments in parkinsonism on those aspects of memory function that are most dependent on willed or effortful processes (e.g., free recall) and less when external cues and recognition formats are used. This prediction is largely supported by the evidence, at least with regard to episodic memory *(39,40)*. Although free recall deficits are frequently reported in parkinsonism, patients tend to benefit normally from recall cues *(41,42)*, and recognition memory is largely intact *(43)*, although a recent meta-analysis suggests that subtle recognition deficits may occur, particularly in demented patients *(44)*. One reason for impaired free recall may be less efficient encoding of the information at input. It is known, for example, that semantic encoding and other active organizational strategies can facilitate subsequent recall, as retrieval of a single item may cue further information encoded in the same way. Patients with PD have been shown to make less use of semantic clustering strategies *(45)*, with a significant link between the clinical measures of hypokinesia and the use of less effortful but less efficient encoding strategies *(46)*. Thus both effort demanding encoding and retrieval processes are impaired in parkinsonism, whereas relatively automatic and externally cued processes remain relatively intact.

4. APATHY IN PARKINSONIAN SYNDROMES

The evidence considered so far has been based largely on laboratory-based measures, which demonstrate deficits in a range of cognitive and cognitive motor tasks that share the properties of requiring effortful, self-initiated, or self-directed processing. At a clinical level, the deficit in intentional (and specifically willed) behavior is most clearly manifested as the neurobehavioral disorder of apathy. This term has been used at both syndrome *(38)* and symptom level (e.g., as a feature of subcortical dementia). At either, however, apathy is characterized by a general lack of purposeful overt behavior and cognition and diminished emotional responsiveness (see Table 1). Importantly, the diagnosis of apathy requires diminished activity in all of these domains *(47)*.

Although apathy has long been reported anecdotally in patients with parkinsonism, it is only with development of new instruments such as the Apathy Evaluation Scale *(48)* and Neuropsychiatric Inventory *(49)* that we have begun to learn more about the scale and nature of the phenomenon. The population prevalence of apathy in PD has been estimated at 16.5% *(50)*, although clinic-based samples suggest figures of 30–40% *(51)*, while in PSP, the figure is closer to 90% *(51)*. To date, there are no published data on apathy in MSA. Where apathy is observed clinically in parkinsonism, it is closely

Table 1
The Clinical Phenomenology of Apathy

Overt Behavior
- Lack of productivity.
- Lack of effort.
- Lack of time spent on activities of interest.
- Lack of initiative and perseverance.
- Behavioral compliance or dependency on others to structure activities.
- Diminished socialization or recreation.

Cognition
- Lack of interests, lack of interest in learning new things, lack of interest in new experiences.
- Lack of concern about one's personal, health, or functional problems.
- Diminished importance or value attributed to such goal-related domains as socialization, recreation, productivity, initiative, perseverance, and curiosity.

Emotion
- Unchanging affect.
- Lack of emotional responsivity to positive and negative events.
- Euphoric or flat affect.
- Absence of excitement or emotional intensity.

From ref. *38*.

associated with the presence of dementia and, particularly, impairment in executive function. Although sharing some common features with depression, the severity of apathy and depression are unrelated.

Apathy is common in a range of neurological disorders including stroke and Alzheimer's disease and shares many common features with the negative symptoms observed in patients with schizophrenia and depression (see ref. *52* for a review). All of these conditions share the pathological or pathophysiological involvement of prefrontal cortex and their associated subcortical structures, although there is no evidence that disorder within a single structure or circuit is responsible for the symptoms in each condition. However, the main focus of attention at present is the limbic-ventrostratopallidal system or "motive circuit," suggested as the key to the translation of motivation into action *(53)*. Many limbic structures, including the amygdala and hippocampus, send outputs to the ventral striatum and, from there, into the dorsal striatothalamocortical circuits. Direct limbic input into the same circuit is also provided at the level of the thalamus, where it coincides with the indirect amygdalostriatopallidal signal and to the medial orbitofrontal cortex and ACC *(54)*.

As noted above, the VTA provides dopamine-mediated input to the ventral striatum and other limbic structures, as well as to the cortex itself, via the mesolimbic and mesocortical systems. The cortical DA release modulates descending corticostriatal fibers, thus potentially influencing the activity of the various striatothalamocortical circuits. Another such modulatory opportunity is offered by the output from the ventral striatum, influenced by both limbic and descending cortical input, which diffusely and nontopographically innervates the substantia nigra pars compacta *(55)* and from there affects most of the rest of the frontal cortex.

Nondopamine-related pathology, such as the degeneration of the cholinergic tegmenal pedunculopontine nuclei, might contribute to the high levels of apathy in PSP *(56)* and AD. This structure forms another possible center for the integration of the motor information provided by the dorsal striatum with the motivational or limbic information and is implicated in a range of neurological and psychiatric disorders *(57)*. The roles of such structures and circuits in the domains of cognition, emotion, and motivation have been reviewed in detail elsewhere *(58)* and in Chapter 3 in this volume.

5. A MODEL OF GOAL-DIRECTED BEHAVIOR

In attempting to operationalize intentionality and its disorders, including apathy, the most common framework within neuroscience is that of goal-directed behavior (GDB). It avoids the problems of defining intentionality in relation to the direction of effort, attention, or mental energy and, instead, considers a number of parallel routes to action, which subserve GDB and are applied according to current situational demands and constraints, and the experience of the organism.

GDB is construed as a set of related processes by which an internal state (derived from an internal or external event) is translated, through action, into the attainment of a goal. The goal essentially defines the act as distinct from the action and constituent behavior of movement. For example, the desire to greet somebody is the intended act, the greeting itself the action, and the handshake comprises the overt movement by which the goal is achieved. The directedness of GDB is an essential component of formulations of intentionality as described above. Because, by definition, the goal state is something that does not currently exist and will occur only in the future, it follows that GDB must be mediated by a representation of that goal. A further assumption that has to be made is that there is some knowledge within the system (although not necessarily conscious awareness) of the contingency between the action and the desired outcome.

In essence, GDB models serve as a way of formulating intentionality within cognitive neuroscience. They seek to integrate diverse processes served by different neuronal systems to provide a more meaningful description of how the brain controls voluntary action. In particular, they have sought to integrate motivational, emotional, cognitive, and motor processes making them ideal for considering the experimental findings in parkinsonism and the clinical phenomenon of apathy.

There is no one model of GDB, although all have at least some of the elements shown in Fig. 1. This particular model attempts to synthesise the key characteristics and prerequisites of GDB as reflected in contemporary cognitive and neurophilosphical theory.

- In the model, purposeful behavior is driven by an internal process or intention (indicated by [A] in Fig. 1). This may be a conscious wish, desire, or urge, perhaps arising from another cognitive event, or a relatively automatic state-change in response to an environmental stimulus.
- These internal states have motivational properties [B]. These may be either innate (primary reinforcers) or learned through experience. Motivators, by definition, change the probability of a particular behavior being pursued and are typically labeled emotionally [C].
- As noted, it is a prerequisite of GDB that there must be an internal representation of the goal [D] together with knowledge (although not necessarily conscious awareness) of a causal relationship [E] between a particular course of action and its outcome. That knowledge may exist as a conscious expectation or an associative connection.
- To succeed, the individual needs to assemble an appropriate serially ordered action program designed to achieve the goal, perhaps evaluating it against alternatives and selecting the most appropriate [F]. These serially ordered subtasks may each be considered intentional, even if they are not subject to a conscious desire or urge. Such intention to action *(59)* may exist in the absence of primary prior intention when the GDB is directly triggered by an external event or occurs in the context of a repetitive or habitual task [G].
- In some instances, the individual may need to exert conscious control [H], perhaps inhibiting some habitual response tendencies, which might be inappropriate in the present context, or other internal states that may interfere with the current process. These executive processes involve conscious, controlled, and effort-demanding activity in the control of action.
- The action or action sequence must be initiated and executed effectively [I] with the intensity and effort determined, in part, by the associated drive properties of the motivational state associated with the goal [J].
- Control and maintenance of the activity is achieved through on-line evaluation of goal outcome against the goal representation [K]. Output from this comparison process will serve to maintain or stop the ongoing action [L] and may influence the on-line modification of the action as the situation demands [M]. Where the goal is distant, the action may be sustained by motivating properties of the goal representation [N].
- Outcome is associated with a change in the motivational state [O] and associated with the emotional and hedonic response [P]. Goal attainment and reward produces positive responses, maintaining the causal link between the internal state and the action used to achieve the goal, and to further increase the likelihood of

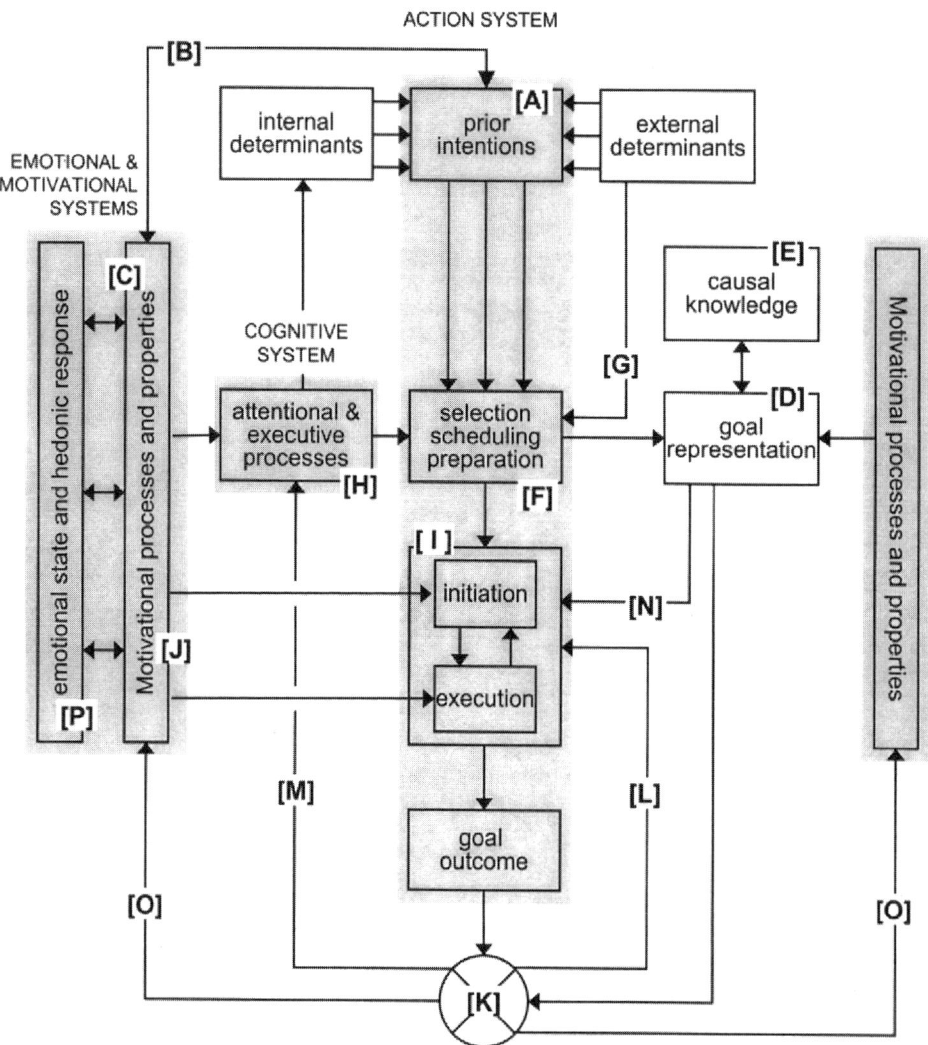

Fig. 1. Schematic model of the representations and processes involved in GDB. The scheme shows the processing flow in the central Action system from initial intention to goal outcome, through processes of selection, scheduling, and performance of the action itself. Control and modulation of these stages is achieved through a combination of factors, including active attentional and executive processes (Cognitive system), and multiple direct and indirect motivational inputs (Emotional and Motivational systems). Affective and motivational processes are in turn influenced by the goal outcome, thus facilitating the adaptation of existing action repertoires and the learning of new associations to guide future behavior. See the main text for further details and for an explanation of the labels [A–P] (adapted from ref. *52* with permission).

the behavior being chosen in the future through a process of incentive learning. Similarly, failure to achieve the goal leads to a negative response, supporting the adoption of alternative action plans, both immediately and in the future.

This model, although descriptive rather than heuristic, serves to point to possible routes by which intentional behavior may be disrupted by neurological disorder. Although complex, the model probably reflects only some of the processes, representations, and their interactions involved in the huge array of behavior that comprises intentional behavior.

6. COGNITIVE, EMOTIONAL, AND MOTIVATIONAL ASPECTS OF INTENTIONALITY IN PARKINSONISM

What evidence do we have that cognitive, emotional, and motivational processes have a direct causal role in intentional impairments? Even in the absence of such evidence, what roles might they play?

Perhaps the clearest and most consistent pattern to emerge is the association between reductions in intentional behavior and indicators of cognitive dysfunction and particularly frontal executive impairment. This would support the importance of the cognitive system [H] in Fig. 1. However, it is still unclear how much the cognitive deficits contribute directly to the lack of intentional action, or whether they are simply co-morbid features of a more general neuronal disorder. Although dysexecutive problems, such as disinhibition and perseveration, are observed in parkinsonism, it is difficult to see how these would directly causes a reduction in willed behavior. More likely is that both the positive (disordered) and negative (apathetic) features are different aspects of the same impairment in self-directed limited capacity cognitive processes. These may make the patient less likely to initiate behavior spontaneously in the absence of external triggers, while at the same time making them more sensitive to irrelevant environmental cues and contexts.

What of the role of motivation and the hedonic processes? These are grey areas in the field of human neuroscience, and we can only speculate on the possible mechanisms by which problems might influence intentional behavior. First, as described earlier, there may be a primary disorder resulting in pathological and pathophysiological changes to the circuits underlying motivation and emotion. These might lead to: (*i*) the failure of internal or external cues to signal future reward, thus disrupting the basic link between the intention and the motivating aspect attached to the goal outcome; or (*ii*) a loss of hedonic response, reducing the reward value of goal achievement and decreasing the probability of the behavior occurring in the future. It is also possible to consider reductions in behavior that occur as a learned response in the absence of a fundamental motivational deficit: (*i*) previous actions may have failed to achieve the intended goal due to cognitive of motor deficits, leading to loss of reinforcement and extinction of the behavior; or (*ii*) the goals may have been achieved only at the expense of uneconomic effort, altering the cost–benefit value of inaction over action.

Whether a primary deficit or a learned response, a loss of motivation could lead to a decreased probability that a willed intention is formed in the first place, a decreased likelihood that the necessary cognitive and physical effort would be expended to ensure the action is performed effectively, and a further reduction in the likelihood that a particular behavior would be repeated in the future.

However, while such processes and mechanisms can be suggested, almost nothing can be said about their validity, as motivational functioning in parkinsonism has barely begun to be studied. This is despite the clinical and experimental indications and the presence of a neurobiological substrate for motivational disturbance. To date, there is limited imaging evidence in PD for absent *(60)* or abnormal *(61)* neuronal response in the circuits normally associated with reward processing. However, the one published behavioral study to date found no abnormality in the impact of financial incentive on a vigilance task with PD *(62)*. It is clear that the detailed study of motivational and emotional processing in parkinsonism is necessary to fully understand the nature of intentional disorder in parkinsonism and its underlying mechanisms.

Such research is important in two main respects. First, through studying of the breakdown of global aspects of behavior, such as intentionality, we can learn more about how distinct domains, such as motor function, cognition, emotion, and motivation, are integrated within the brain. Such an approach is important to move us on from the more narrow reductionist view that treats each domain as a discrete function with its own segregated substrate within the nervous system. Second, at a clinical level, parkinsonism continues to be identified and treated as a disorder of movement, with drugs and surgical treatments targeted at managing the motor symptoms. Yet such treatments are rarely effective at treating the other aspects of disorder that contribute to the overall loss of intentional behavior. At the point that the patient starts to dement and manifests significant apathy, the burden of the disease grows dramatically from that caused by the motor symptoms alone. Patients experience greater handicap, medical management is complicated, and caregivers experience greater strain and burden *(63)*. Despite this, only gradually are treatments emerging that appear to be effective in counteracting these non-motor symptoms in neurodegenerative disease including parkinsonism *(64,65)*. Further development depends on a better understanding of these phenomena at a clinical, cognitive, and neurobiological level.

REFERENCES

1. Brentano, F. (1973) *Psychology from an Empirical Standpoint (1874), (Edited by Kraus, O. and translated from the German by Rancrello, A.C., Terrel, D.B., and McAlister, L.L.)*, Routledge and Kegan Paul, London.
2. James, W. (1890) *The Principles of Psychology,* Holt, New York.
3. Jahanshahi, M. and Frith, C.D. (1998) Willed action and its impairments. *Cognit. Neuropsychol.* **15,** 483–533.
4. Naville, D. (1922) Étude sur les complications et les séquelles mentale de l'encéphalite épidémique. La bradyphrénie. *Encéphale* **17,** 369–436.
5. Cummings, J.L. and Benson, D.F. (1984) Subcortical dementia. Review of an emerging concept. *Arch. Neurol.* **41,** 874–879.
6. Smith, M.C., Goldman, W.P., Janer, K.W., Baty, J.D., and Morris, J.C. (1998) Cognitive speed in nondemented Parkinson's disease. *J. Int. Neuropsychol. Soc.* **4,** 584–592.
7. Russ, M.O. and Seger, L. (1995) The effect of task complexity on reaction times in memory scanning and visual discrimination in Parkinson's disease. *Neuropsychologia* **33,** 561–575.
8. Howard, L.A., Binks, M.G., Moore, A.P., and Playfer, J.R. (1994) How convincing is the evidence for cognitive slowing in Parkinson's disease? *Cortex* **30,** 431–443.
9. Brown, R.G., Jahanshahi, M., and Marsden, C.D. (1993) Response choice in Parkinson's disease. The effects of uncertainty and stimulus—response compatibility. *Brain* **116,** 869–885.
10. Brown, R.G. and Marsden, C.D. (1986) Visuospatial function in Parkinson's disease. *Brain* **109,** 987–1002.
11. Gamsu, C.V. (1986) Confrontation naming in parkinsonian patients: post-operative anomia revisited. *Neuropsychologia* **24,** 727–729.
12. Rafal, R.D., Inhoff, A.W., Friedman, J.H., and Bernstein, E. (1987) Programming and execution of sequential movements in Parkinson's disease. *J. Neurol. Neurosurg. Psychiatry* **50,** 1267–1273.
13. Dubois, B., Pillon, B., Legault, F., Agid, Y., and Lhermitte, F. (1988) Slowing of cognitive processing in progressive supranuclear palsy. A comparison with Parkinson's disease. *Arch. Neurol.* **45,** 1194–1199.
14. Goodrich, S., Henderson, L., and Kennard, C. (1989) On the existence of an attention-demanding process peculiar to simple reaction time: converging evidence from Parkinson's disease. *Cognit. Neuropsychol.* **6,** 309–331.
15. Gauntlett-Gilbert, J. and Brown, V.J. (1998) Reaction time deficits and Parkinson's disease. *Neurosci. Biobehav. Rev.* **22,** 865–881.
16. Molinuevo, J.L., Valls-Sole, J., and Valldeoriola, F. (2000) The effect of transcranial magnetic stimulation on reaction time in progressive supranuclear palsy. *Clin. Neurophysiol.* **111,** 2008–2013.
17. Valldeoriola, F., Valls-Sole, J., Tolosa, E., Ventura, P.J., Nobbe, F.A., and Marti, M.J. (1998) Effects of a startling acoustic stimulus on reaction time in different parkinsonian syndromes. *Neurology* **51,** 1315–1320.
18. Jahanshahi, M., Brown, R.G., and Marsden, C.D. (1992) Simple and choice reaction time and the use of advance information for motor preparation in Parkinson's disease. *Brain* **115,** 539–564.
19. Friston, K.J., Frith, C.D., Liddle, P.F., and Frackowiak, R.S. (1991) Investigating a network model of word generation with positron emission tomography. *Proc. R. Soc. Lond. B Biol. Sci.* **244,** 101–106.
20. Flowers, K.A., Robertson, C., and Sheridan, M.R. (1996) Some characteristics of word fluency in Parkinson's disease. *J. Neurolinguistics* **9,** 33–46.
21. Auriacombe, S., Grossman, M., Carvell, S., Stern, M., and Hurtig, H.I. (1993) Verbal fluency deficits in Parkinson's disease. *Neuropsychology* **7,** 182–192.
22. Matison, R., Mayeux, R., Rosen, J., and Fahn, S. (1982) "Tip-of-the-tongue" phenomenon in Parkinson disease. *Neurology* **32,** 567–570.
23. Troster, A.I., Fields, J.A., Testa, J.A., et al. (1998) Cortical and subcortical influences on clustering and switching in the performance of verbal fluency tasks. *Neuropsychologia* **36,** 295–304.
24. Troster, A.I., Stalp, L.D., Paolo, A.M., Fields, J.A., and Koller, W.C. (1995) Neuropsychological impairment in Parkinson's disease with and without depression. *Arch. Neurol.* **52,** 1164–1169.
25. Rey, G.J., Tomer, R., Levin, B.E., Sanchez, R.J., Bowen, B., and Bruce, J.H. (1995) Psychiatric symptoms, atypical dementia, and left visual field inattention in corticobasal ganglionic degeneration. *Mov. Disord.* **10,** 106–110.
26. Broussolle, E., Dentresangle, C., Landais, P., et al. (1999) The relation of putamen and caudate nucleus 18F-Dopa uptake to motor and cognitive performances in Parkinson's disease. *J. Neurol. Sci.* **166,** 141–151.
27. Rinne, J.O., Portin, R., Ruottinen, H., et al. (2000) Cognitive impairment and the brain dopaminergic system in Parkinson disease: [18F]fluorodopa positron emission tomographic study. *Arch. Neurol.* **57,** 470–475.
28. Cooper, J.A., Sagar, H.J., Jordan, N., Harvey, N.S., and Sullivan, E.V. (1991) Cognitive impairment in early, untreated Parkinson's disease and its relationship to motor disability. *Brain* **114,** 2095–2122.

29. Lange, K.W., Paul, G.M., Naumann, M., and Gsell, W. (1995) Dopaminergic effects on cognitive performance in patients with Parkinson's disease. *J. Neural. Transm. Suppl.* **46,** 423–432.
30. Piatt, A.L., Fields, J.A., Paolo, A.M., Koller, W.C., and Troster, A.I. (1999) Lexical, semantic, and action verbal fluency in Parkinson's disease with and without dementia. *J. Clin. Exp. Neuropsychol.* **21,** 435–443.
31. Mahieux, F., Fenelon, G., Flahault, A., Manifacier, M.J., Michelet, D., and Boller, F. (1998) Neuropsychological prediction of dementia in Parkinson's disease. *J. Neurol. Neurosurg. Psychiatry* **64,** 178–183.
32. Pillon, B., Dubois, B., and Agid, Y. (1991) Severity and specificity of cognitive impairment in Alzheimer's, Huntington's, and Parkinson's diseases and progressive supranuclear palsy. *Ann. NY Acad. Sci.* **640,** 224–227.
33. Pillon, B., Gouider-Khouja, N., Deweer, B., et al. (1995) Neuropsychological pattern of striatonigral degeneration: comparison with Parkinson's disease and progressive supranuclear palsy. *J. Neurol. Neurosurg. Psychiatry* **58,** 174–179.
34. Gurd, J.M. (1996) Word search in patients with Parkinson's disease. *J. Neurolinguistics* **9,** 207–218.
35. Wichmann, T. and DeLong, M.R. (1998) Models of basal ganglia function and pathophysiology of movement disorders. *Neurosurg. Clin. N. Am.* **9,** 223–236.
36. Brown, R.G., Soliveri, P., and Jahanshahi, M. (1998) Executive processes in Parkinson's disease: random number generation and response suppression. *Neuropsychologia* **36,** 1355–1362.
37. Jahanshahi, M., Profice, P., Brown, R.G., Ridding, M.C., Dirnberger, G., and Rothwell, J.C. (1998) The effects of transcranial magnetic stimulation over the dorsolateral prefrontal cortex on random number generation. *Brain* **121,** 1533–1544.
38. Marin, R.S. (1991) Apathy: a neuropsychiatric syndrome. *J. Neuropsychiatry Clin. Neurosci.* **3,** 243–254.
39. Bak, T.H. and Hodges, J.R. (1998) The neuropsychology of progressive supranuclear palsy. *Neurocase* **4,** 89–94.
40. Taylor, A.E. and Saint-Cyr, J.A. (1995) The neuropsychology of Parkinson's disease. *Brain Cogn.* **28,** 281–296.
41. Knoke, D., Taylor, A.E., and Saint-Cyr, J.A. (1998) The differential effects of cueing on recall in Parkinson's disease and normal subjects. *Brain Cogn.* **38,** 261–274.
42. Pillon, B., Blin, J., Vidailhet, M., et al. (1995) The neuropsychological pattern of corticobasal degeneration: comparison with progressive supranuclear palsy and Alzheimer's disease. *Neurology* **45,** 1477–1483.
43. Robbins, T.W., James, M., Owen, A.M., et al. (1994) Cognitive deficits in progressive supranuclear palsy, Parkinson's disease, and multiple system atrophy in tests sensitive to frontal lobe dysfunction. *J. Neurol. Neurosurg. Psychiatry* **57,** 79–88.
44. Whittington, C.J., Podd, J., and Kan, M.M. (2000) Recognition memory impairment in Parkinson's disease: power and meta-analyses. *Neuropsychology* **14,** 233–246.
45. Massman, P.J., Delis, D.C., Butters, N., Levin, B.E., and Salmon, D.P. (1990) Are all subcortical dementias alike? Verbal learning and memory in Parkinson's and Huntington's disease patients. *J. Clin. Exp. Neuropsychol.* **12,** 729–744.
46. Berger, H.J., van Es, N.J., Van Spaendonck, K.P., et al. (1999) Relationship between memory strategies and motor symptoms in Parkinson's disease. *J. Clin. Exp. Neuropsychol.* **21,** 677–684.
47. Marin, R.S. (1990) Differential diagnosis and classification of apathy. *Am. J. Psychiatry* **147,** 22–30.
48. Marin, R.S., Biedrzycki, R.C., and Firinciogullari, S. (1991) Reliability and validity of the Apathy Evaluation Scale. *Psychiatry Res.* **38,** 143–162.
49. Cummings, J.L., Mega, M., Gray, K., Rosenberg Thompson, S., Carusi, D.A., and Gornbein, J. (1994) The Neuropsychiatric Inventory: comprehensive assessment of psychopathology in dementia. *Neurology* **44,** 2308–2314.
50. Aarsland, D., Larsen, J.P., Geok Lim, N., et al. (1999) Range of neuropsychiatric disturbances in patients with Parkinsons's disease. *J. Neurol. Neurosurg. Psychiatry* **67,** 492–496.
51. Levy, M.L., Cummings, J.L., Fairbanks, L.A., et al. (1998) Apathy is not depression. *J. Neuropsychiat. Clin. Neurosci.* **10,** 314–319.
52. Brown, R.G. and Pluck, G. (2000) Negative symptoms: the "pathology" of motivation and goal-direct behaviour. *Trends Neurosci.* **23,** 412–417.
53. Mogenson, G.J., Jones, L.D., and Yim, C.Y. (1980) From motivation to action: functional interface between the limbic system and the motor system. *Prog. Neurobiol.* **14,** 69–97.
54. Price, J.L., Camichael, S.T., and Drevets, W.C. (1996) Networks related to the orbital and medial prefrontal cortex: a substrate for emotional behavior?, in *Progress in Brain Research,* vol. 107 (Holstege, G., Bandler, R., and Saper, C.B., eds.), Elsevier Science BV, Amsterdam, pp. 523–536.
55. Haber, S.N., Kunishio, K., Mizobuchi, M., and Lynd-Balta, E. (1995) The orbital and medial prefrontal circuit through the primate basal ganglia. *J. Neurosci.* **15,** 4851–4867.
56. Jellinger, K. (1988) The pedunculopontine nucleus in Parkinson's disease, progressive supranuclear palsy and Alzheimer's disease. *J. Neurol. Neurosurg. Psychiatry* **51,** 540–543.
57. Erro, E. and Gimenez-Amaya, J.M. (1999) Pedunculopontine tegmental nucleus. Anatomy, functional considerations and physiopathological implications. *An. Sist. Sanit. Navarra* **22,** 189–201.
58. Davidson, R.J. and Irwin, W. (1999) The functional neuroanatomy of emotion and affective style. *Trends Cogn. Sci.* **3,** 11–21.
59. Searle, J.R. (1983) *Intentionality. An Essay on the Philosophy of Mind,* Cambridge University Press, Cambridge.
60. Leenders, K., Kuenig, G., Martin, Ch., and Schultz, W. (1999) Reward processing in the Parkinson's disease brain. *Parkinsonism Rel. Disord.* **5,** S61.
61. Goerendt, I.K., Lawrence, A.D., and Brooks, D.J. (1999) Reward processing in the Parkinsonian brain: an activation study using PET. *Parkinsonism Rel. Disord.* **5,** S58.

62. Hart, R.P., Wade, J.B., Calabrese, V.P., and Colenda, C.C. (1998) Vigilance performance in Parkinson's disease and depression. *J. Clin. Exp. Neuropsychol.* **20,** 111–117.
63. Aarsland, D., Larsen, J.P., Karlsen, K., Lim, N.G., and Tandberg, E. (1999) Mental symptoms in Parkinson's disease are important contributors to caregiver distress. *Int. J. Geriatr. Psychiatry* **14,** 866–874.
64. Galynker, I., Ieronimo, C., Miner, C., Rosenblum, J., Vilkas, N., and Rosenthal, R. (1997) Methylphenidate treatment of negative symptoms in patients with dementia. *J. Neuropsychiat. Clin. Neurosci.* **9,** 231–239.
65. McKeith, I., Del Ser, T., Spano, P., et al. (2000) Efficacy of rivastigmine in dementia with Lewy bodies: a randomised, double-blind, placebo-controlled international study. *Lancet* **356,** 2031–2036.

8
Cognitive Control in Frontostriatal Disorders

Francois Richer, PhD and Sylvain Chouinard, MD, FRCP

1. INTRODUCTION

There is now ample evidence that cognitive symptoms observed in striatal disorders bear strong similarities with those associated with frontal cortex lesions. The most characteristic cognitive deficits in frontostriatal disorders are cognitive control (executive control) deficits. Cognitive control symptoms affect functions such as attention, decisions, action planning, and retrieval from memory *(1–6)*. These symptoms can easily be observed in patients with Huntington's disease (HD) and in a majority of patients with parkinsonian syndromes. They also represent the most ubiquitous cognitive symptoms in psychiatric disorders.

Cognitive control symptoms can be observed in a large variety of tasks. The apparent heterogeneity of these symptoms is linked to the rich diverse connections of the frontostriatal brain systems to sensory, motor, cognitive, and motivational systems. However, this heterogeneity is also due to the fact that frontostriatal systems are involved in general purpose processes, which influence many functions. Cognitive control deficits affect many functions at once, not through a basic functional loss, but through an impaired regulation of processing. Cognitive control deficits affect the control of cognitive processing by goals *(7)*. Goals provide bias signals that modulate processing. Goals are ubiquitous in behavior, and many cognitive processes can be considered goal-directed or voluntary in a general sense. However, only some processing is goal-controlled, i.e., systematically biased in relation to the goal as opposed to automatic processing that runs mainly on the basis of learned associations. Cognitive control processes regulate the speed, progression, and outcome of cognitive processes such as response selection, perceptual selection, and information retrieval. Because of this regulatory function, cognitive control deficits have a high impact on daily activities. They can affect decision points in behavior, information retrieval, communications, calculations, and learning.

2. COGNITIVE CONTROL SYMPTOMS ARE SENSITIVE TO TASK PARAMETERS

Cognitive control symptoms are most apparent in special conditions. A first set of conditions involves novel or ambiguous contexts, which are associated with weak associative cues. For example, their performance difficulties are more apparent in novel combinations of movements (e.g., Luria's serial gestures: palm-edge-fist) than in familiar ones (e.g., palm-fist-palm) and are more apparent in new problems than in practiced problems.

From: *Mental and Behavioral Dysfunction in Movement Disorders*
Edited by: M-A. Bédard et al. © Humana Press Inc., Totowa, NJ

A second set of conditions that can help detect cognitive control deficits involves interference from competing stimuli or responses. This is well illustrated in attention tasks such as the Stroop task, in which color words are written in a color that conflicts with the word (e.g., red written in blue). The competition between the reading response and the color naming response in this task affects patients with cognitive control deficits much more than controls *(8)*. Other conditions that help bring out cognitive control symptoms include processing demands, precision demands, and time limitations. For example, cognitive control deficits will affect response choices, especially if they are rapid and involve a nonautomatic decision rule. In more practiced or less demanding conditions, performance is less dependent on cognitive control mechanisms and can rely more on automatic control processes, in which learned associations provide selection cues. Cognitive control symptoms are often said to be linked to cognitive difficulty (processing demands or effortful processing). Whereas task difficulty or cognitive effort may often be linked to goal-controlled processing, these general terms are insufficient to explain the underlying mechanisms of cognitive control symptoms.

3. COGNITIVE CONTROL EPISODES ARE PART OF MOST TASKS

Consider a task involving the retrieval of the last number in the two following series: (52-53- ?) and (70-62- ?). The stimuli are similar, the response is identical but, for most people, the latter series requires a more prolonged cognitive episode. This cognitive episode involves activating and integrating several types of information such as the main rule (minus 8) and learned information (ex: 12 – 8 = 4). It also involves maintaining the representation of the first digit of the correct response *(5)*, inhibiting interference from competing responses (e.g.,58), and maybe verifying the answer (54 + 8 = 62).

Most tasks probably require multiple alternating episodes of goal-controlled and automatic processing during different phases. Cognitive control episodes are constructed ad hoc to integrate sensory input, memory information, premovement information, and motivational signals linked to a goal. Depending on the task examined, cognitive control episodes are sometimes called intentional sets, attentional engagements, or retrieval episodes. In frontostriatal disorders, these episodes are often disrupted or delayed.

Even when an action is simple or highly practiced, cognitive control processes may still be needed during brief intervals. They may be needed before initiating responses, at critical decision points, or other more demanding intervals when learned habits and associative cues cannot adequately specify the response. Because cognitive control deficits can affect small intervals in prolonged tasks, tasks may vary widely in sensitivity depending on the impact of these critical intervals on performance. For example, choice tasks, which require switching from one conditional rule to another, are more sensitive to cognitive control deficits than ordinary choice tasks *(9)*. Switching tasks generally involve a high degree of cognitive control at switching points. However, learned associations can reduce the impairment in switching *(9)*.

The fact that most tasks involve automatic and goal-controlled episodes can give rise to paradoxical interpretations. For example, patients will often complete a task with more effort and time than controls, suggesting that they make more use of cognitive control processes. How can that be if they have impaired cognitive control processes? Patients appear to make more use of cognitive control processes, because their cognitive control episodes are prolonged and inefficient. They may not solve the task with these processes more often than controls, they may simply spend more time in unsuccessful cognitive control episodes.

4. COGNITIVE CONTROL ERRORS REFLECT COMPETITIVE PROCESSING

Cognitive control deficits often lead to errors from an incorrect selection of an alternative response. The selection of responses is especially impaired when there is competition from other responses or when selection cues are weak as in memory-guided responses *(4,6,10,11)*. The correct response is often replaced by prepotent well-learned responses that lead to capture errors or by recent responses that lead to perseverative errors. Errors can also be responses that would normally follow the correct response, as in sequential inversion errors, which are frequent in rapid motor sequences or in speech. Incorrect answers may also simply share some features with the correct responses (e.g., general location). This suggests that cognitive control influences competition between responses.

5. COGNITIVE CONTROL AS COMPETITIVE CONSOLIDATION EPISODES

Cognitive control symptoms are still poorly understood. They are often described as lists of symptoms or with general functions such as planning or working memory difficulties. One reason for the lack of adequate models of cognitive control symptoms is that they cut across many cognitive domains such as attention, memory, decision, or movement depending on the tasks examined.

Several general hypotheses have been proposed to account for frontostriatal cognitive functions. Some have emphasized the capacity of these circuits to maintain information in short-term memory *(12)*. Other authors have highlighted their supervisory functions, and others have highlighted their associative learning functions *(13)*. However, several portions of the brain have short-term memory capacity, and several are involved in associative learning. Frontostriatal systems are unique in having a dominant contribution to cognitive control functions *(7)*. These functions certainly depend on short-term memory, and they can be useful in many learning situations, but their main role is goal-controlled regulation of processing. Models more specifically adapted to the cognitive control functions of frontostriatal circuits have emphasized processes such as the temporal integration between sensory and motor processes *(6)* or response selection processes *(4,14)*.

Recent evidence suggests that two properties of frontostriatal systems are important to understand cognitive control symptoms: (*i*) bias signals, and (*ii*) slow consolidation.

Frontostriatal systems interact with sensory and other systems to bias processing in relation to goals *(15)*. Sensory systems in posterior cortex show competitive activity when multiple stimuli are present and frontal-posterior networks play a role in biasing this activity toward goals. Biased competition mechanisms can help select perceptions according to templates of target stimuli in attention tasks. Similar mechanisms may also help select responses according to their relevance to task rules. Cognitive control symptoms are probably linked to the dynamics of biased competition in neural networks. A major function of cognitive control could involve the regulation of competition between alternatives in perceptual selection, response selection, and information retrieval.

The second important characteristic of cognitive control episodes is that they involve a progressive consolidation of goal-relevant information. Networks between frontostriatal systems and other brain regions integrate multiple sources of information on the basis of relevance to the goal. This activity circulates through the network and takes time to converge toward a final configuration. Consolidation time can be affected by the rate of accumulation of goal-relevant information and by the interfering effects of competing stimuli or responses.

Frontostriatal systems must use some criterion or control variables to bias the consolidation process towards the intended goal. These control variables are used as a common currency in networks that integrate many types of information. One control variable proposed for motor decisions is reward prediction error, which provides information on the adequacy of alternative responses for the prediction of reward *(16)*. Predicition error can be used as a form of anticipatory feedback on response selection circuits to help bias consolidation in favor of the most correct action for the context. Frontostriatal neurons can code for prediction error. Different variables may be used to consolidate different types of cognitive control episodes, and future work may help identify several other control variables.

Competitive consolidation mechanisms can account for many of the properties of cognitive control symptoms, including their sensitivity to factors such as novelty, interference, task demands, and temporal limitations. In a model involving competitive consolidation episodes, goal-relevant information is consolidated in neural networks during brief intervals. Errors occur because cognitive control states are suceptible to interference during consolidation. Interference could distort the consolidation of cognitive control episodes. Competitive consolidation mechanisms can also be affected by novelty since this factor reduces the amount of automatic processing and learned information that can be used in a task, and performance must then rely more heavily on cognitive control episodes. Task demands also increase the amount of cognitive control necessary to succesfully complete the task. Finally, time limitations put pressure on the termination of cognitive control episodes, which may compromise the quality of consolidation. Thus, time limitations represent a stress test for cognitive control processes and will increase the probability of incorrect consolidation in people with cognitive control deficits.

6. PERFORMANCE SLOWING AND TIMING VARIABILITY REFLECT CONSOLIDATION PROBLEMS

The slowing of performance is one of the major symptoms of frontostriatal disorders, affecting initiation and execution of movements *(17,18)*. More complex tasks exacerbate this slowing, suggesting that it is partly linked to processing complexity. This control-related slowing is probably not the only source of slowing associated with frontostriatal disorders, but it may compound slowing originating from other sources. Cognitive control problems also lead to a high variability in performance speed, with normally fast responses alternating with very slow responses *(19,20)*. This variability suggests that response selection episodes can consolidate properly, but that their control is impaired.

Slowed and variable performance may result from the same control problems that produce performance errors. Cognitive control episodes take more or less time to complete, depending on the difficulty of accessing goal-relevant information and on the level of interference present. These variables can be influenced by the strength and quality of frontostriatal biasing signals, and thus, slowing may partly index the efficiency of cognitive control episodes. Neurophysiological evidence indicates that variations in response speed in rapid choices are linked to the rate of increase in frontal cortex activity *(21)*. Frontostriatal disorders may influence the rate of consolidation of cognitive control episodes during response selection by making them more sensitive to variables like interference, choice complexity, or lack of associative cues.

Cognitive control problems can also affect the timing of responses, either in rhythmic intervals or in individual preparatory intervals *(20,22)*. Initiation timing requires cognitive control to coordinate different preparation processes in different portions of the nervous system from the cortex to the spinal cord. The variability in initiation timing can be reduced by timing cues such as countdowns *(23)*, suggesting that the control of performance by stimuli can compensate the variability in the rate of response consolidation associated with cognitive control deficits.

7. DEFICITS IN SERIAL MOVEMENTS REFLECT INCREASED SUSCEPTIBILITY TO INTERFERENCE

Frontostriatal disorders have long been known to affect serial responses *(4,24,25)*. This has been shown for complex problems or mazes, but also for short sequences of movements *(26–31)*. Response sequences require the retrieval or selection of multiple responses in close temporal contiguity. In these situations, cognitive control processes help complete response selections according to task rules, with minimal interference from response alternatives and within a short interval. They also help coordinate transitions between responses. Neural activity in frontostriatal structures indicates that they have a major role in the preparation and execution of movement sequences *(4,32,33)*. Also, sequential or overlapping tasks often produce net increases in functional brain activation in frontal cortex compared to the activation observed in single tasks *(34–38)*.

Patients with frontostriatal disorders show response selection errors in sequences, particularly when response speed is increased. This suggests that adjacent response selection episodes interfere with each

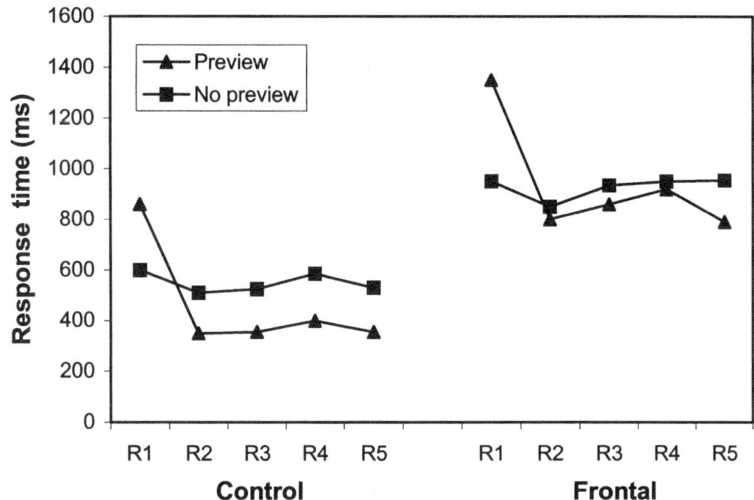

Fig. 1. Serial response times in a task involving typing a sequence of 5 letters presented either one at a time (no preview) or all at once before initiation (sequence preview). Advance information does not accelerate responses in patients as it does in controls.

other more in patients with cognitive control deficits than in controls. Another indication of this is that patients are limited in their use of advance information for serial response selections. Advance information on responses to be executed allows some processing to take place concurrently (e.g., retrieving a response while executing the previous one in a series) in control subjects. Patients may be able to prepare one response in advance in a sequence, but knowing multiple responses in advance does not speed up responses in frontostriatal patients as it does in controls (see Fig. 1) *(19,39–44)*. This suggests that individual decisions are more susceptible to interference by adjacent decisions in frontostriatal disorders.

8. COGNITIVE CONTROL DEFICITS AFFECT PERCEPTUAL CONSOLIDATION

Cognitive control episodes can be investigated in perceptual attention tasks. Perceptual decisions about stimuli are often made in distracting or ambiguous contexts that require cognitive (attentional) control. Frontostriatal circuits interact with sensory cortex and some of these interactions are involved in the attentional biasing of sensory systems according to goals *(15,45–48)*. Frontostriatal activity is involved in selecting target objects among distractors, and it is also involved in selecting a categorical interpretation of stimuli *(48–52)*.

Frontostriatal disorders can produce significant deficits in perceptual attention tasks. They affect the search for target stimuli among distractors in different modalities and in spatial as well as temporal domains *(1,8,53–55)*. They also affect rapid perceptual decisions made under interference. For example, when a specified target–stimulus must be identified in a rapid series of brief stimuli, patients with frontostriatal damage make significantly more errors than controls when a masking distractor follows the target closely (see Fig. 2) *(56,57)*. Identifying a target followed closely by a masking distractor produces a brief perceptual competition, which affects the consolidation of the target and increases the probability of seeing the distractor instead of the target *(58–60)*. This perceptual competition is resolved by a transient attentional response, which biases processing in favor of the target. Attentional responses can last more than half a second, and during this period, they can prevent new perceptual decisions from being completed *(59)*. Frontostriatal disorders increase the consolidation period during which perceptual consolidation episodes are susceptible to perturbation.

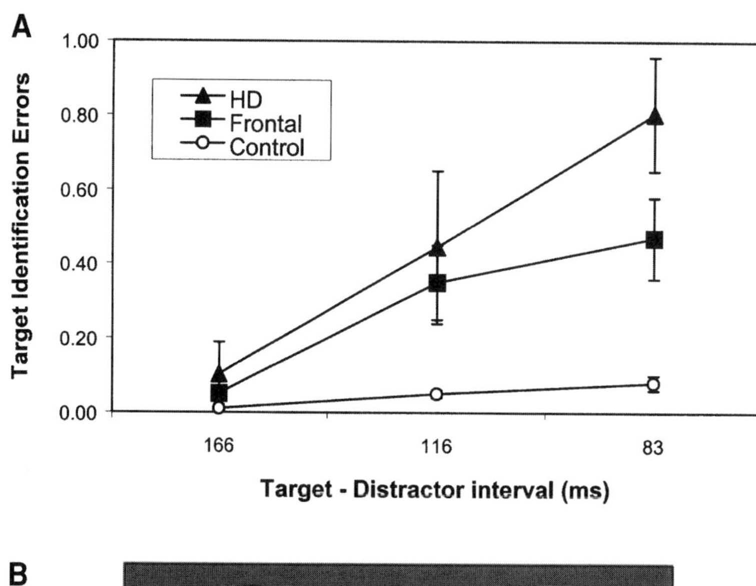

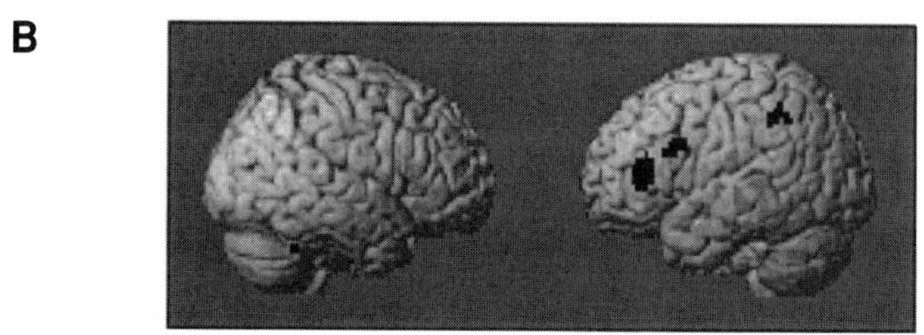

Fig. 2. (**A**) Identification of target letters in rapid series when the target and following distractor were separated by 83, 116, or 166 ms. (**B**) Functional brain activation (fMRI) of frontoparietal circuits associated with the attentional response to a target–stimulus when it is followed by a masking distractor after 83 vs 166 ms.

Functional brain imaging during perceptual decision tasks shows that frontal circuits are involved *(60)*. When trying to identify targets in rapid visual streams, masking interference increases activation in frontal and parietal cortical regions (Fig. 2). Interactions between these regions may underlie cognitive control processes necessary for perceptual decisions under interference.

These data lend support to the hypothesis that frontostriatal systems play an important role in perceptual decisions that require attentional responses. They also suggest that cognitive control episodes involve a brief period of consolidation through regional interactions and that they are susceptible to interference during this period. One of the control variables, which has been proposed for the cognitive control of perceptual decisions, is the likelihood ratio that provides a comparative evaluation of the various alternatives based on available information *(61)*. Likelihood ratios can guide the perceptual consolidation of sensory inputs, and there is evidence that frontostriatal neurons can code for this variable as they code for reward prediction error during response selection.

9. COGNITIVE CONTROL DEFICITS AFFECT LEARNING

Sensorimotor learning involves shifts in the control processes underlying performance. Initially, performance strongly relies on cognitive control for resolving competition between alternative movements with weak associative links and to use error feedback. With practice, appropriate associative links or motor programs develop and the control of movements shifts from frequent episodes of cognitive control to increasing degrees of automatic or predictive control *(62)*. There is evidence from

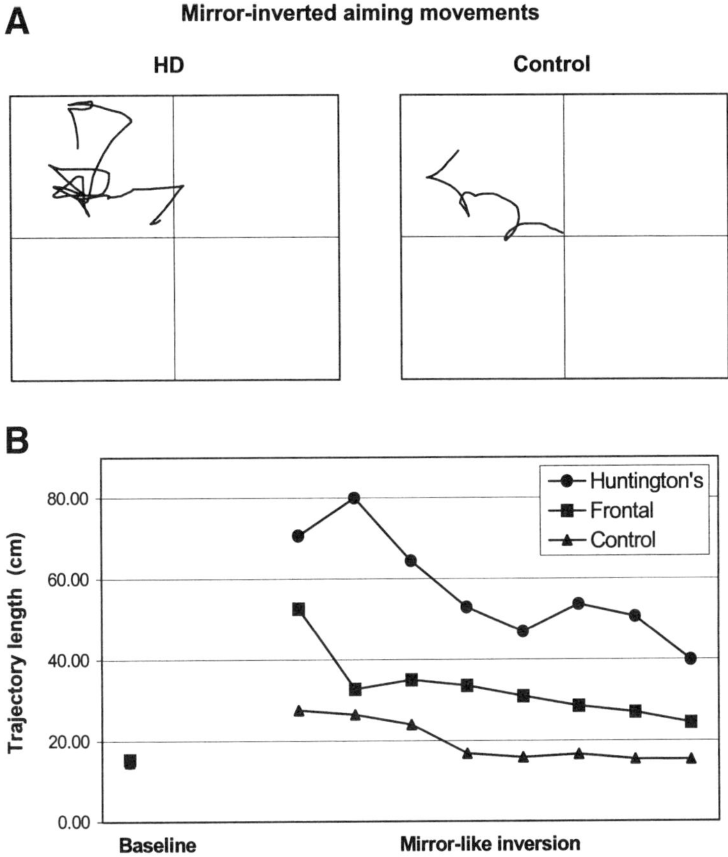

Fig. 3. (**A**) Sample trajectories in the first trials of mirror-inverted aiming movements on a graphics tablet by a patient with early HD and a control subject. Movements were made from the center to a peripheral target. (**B**) Average lengths of trajectories in aiming movements on a graphics tablet in baseline conditions and after a mirror-like inversion of visual feedback.

cellular neurophysiology and functional brain imaging that frontostriatal systems show changes in activity linked to sensorimotor learning *(63,64)*. However, it is still unclear how much of these activity changes reflect changes in the degree of cognitive control involved in the movements during learning as opposed to other aspects of learning.

Cognitive control deficits can affect movements in novel contexts. For example, patients with HD show poor initial performance in sensorimotor learning tasks. In mirror-inverted movements, patients show significant trajectory control problems (see Fig. 3) *(57,65–67)*. In visuomotor tracking tasks, patients require lower speeds to maintain normal precision levels. Thus, frontostriatal disorders affect the cognitive control of novel movements in learning tasks.

In addition to initial performance problems, learning problems have also been reported in HD patients in some tasks (e.g., predictable visuomotor tracking) but not in others (e.g., random motion tracking or mirror-inverted movements) *(68–71)*. Cognitive control deficits may partly account for these task differences in skill acquisition in frontostriatal disorders. For example, it has been reported that acquisition of predictable visuomotor pursuit is more impaired than acquisition of mirror drawing in HD *(68–70)*. However, mirror drawing has a higher learning rate than predictable visuomotor pursuit, which may indicate that automatic motor control takes over portions of the movement more quickly

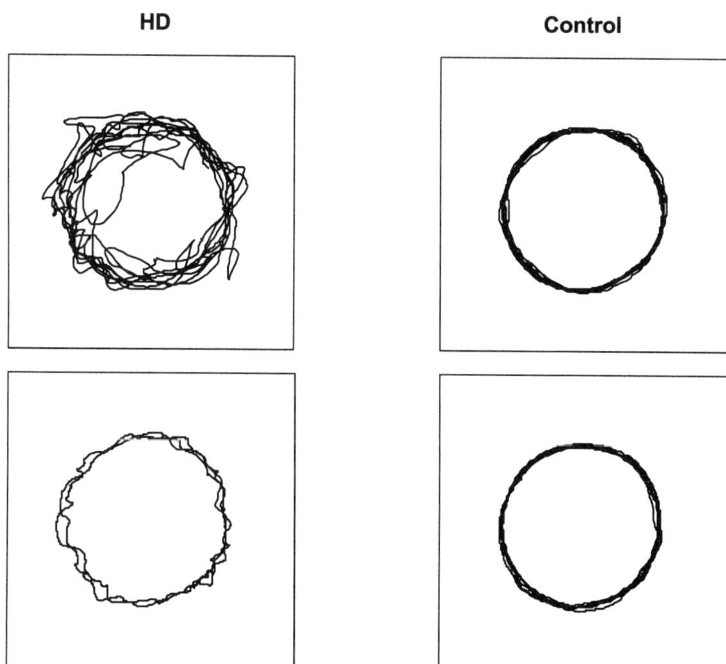

Fig. 4. Sample tracing performance in a circular path with borders separated by 2.5 mm in patients with early HD and controls.

in mirror drawing. The availability of automatic control processes can help patients bypass cognitive control deficits. Thus, the degree to which cognitive control deficits can be bypassed may be an important factor in determining acquisition impairments in different tasks.

The deficits observed in novel visually guided movements also have implications for the interpretation of the effects of visual guidance. Visual guidance can help movements in frontostriatal disorders *(17)*. It has been suggested that frontostriatal disorders produce a deficit in the control of movement based on learned internal representations, which would lead to a greater reliance on the visual control of movement *(17,39)*. However, visually guided tasks are often less demanding than memory-guided tasks *(54)*, so an alternative explanation is that visual guidance may help bypass deficient cognitive control processes. This explanation would better account for the significant impairment observed in patients when movements require precise visual control as is the case in novel contexts *(57)*. Thus, frontostriatal disorders do not dissociate internal from external control, but they do dissociate goal-related control from automatic control.

In addition to the deficits observed in novel movements, patients also show cognitive control deficits in movements made under high precision demands. For example, when HD patients are asked to trace simple paths within borders, reducing the width of the tracing corridor increases the control impairment (Fig. 4) *(72)*. Also, when brief perturbations are applied during a movement, HD patients show significant problems in controlling movement corrections *(73)*. Thus, frontostriatal systems appear to be necessary for the cognitive control of visually guided movements. Cognitive control processes may be recruited during movement because of the lack of learned programs, high precision demands, or when interference, such as movement perturbations, is present.

Several studies have suggested that frontostriatal disorders produce problems in the learning of arbitrary stimulus–response associations or categorization rules *(10,23,69,74–78)*. Because cognitive control problems affect response selection in novel contexts, it is difficult to disentangle learning problems from control problems in these situations. Before a conditional stimulus–response association is well learned, response selection involves resolving competition between correct and incorrect associations, which is a process that requires cognitive control. Thus, the difficulty may lie as much in the retrieval of poorly learned information as in the acquisition of the conditional associations.

The link between cognitive control deficits and acquisition is still unclear. As Wise pointed out, much work needs to be done on the performance control functions of frontostriatal circuits before their role in learning can be adequately understood *(14)*. The effects of frontostriatal disorders on sensorimotor learning tasks should be reexamined to determine how much of the reported learning deficits are due to cognitive control deficits.

10. CONCLUSIONS

Our understanding of cognitive control deficits is still in its infancy. However, recent work suggests that neuroscientific models can be developed for these symptoms. Some basic principles that may help develop these models are already apparent.

1. Frontostriatal systems interact with other systems to bias competitive processing in relation to goals and other top-down influences. The biasing functions of frontostriatal systems may help explain why cognitive control deficits affect general purpose regulatory functions instead of specific skills.
2. Frontostriatal systems regulate transient episodes that are recruited at critical intervals during complex behavior. These episodes integrate sensory, memory, and motivational information relevant to task demands. The consolidation of these episodes is dependent on the relative strength of goal-relevant information and irrelevant interference. This helps explain why cognitive control symptoms are exacerbated by weak associative cues, competitive interference, and task demands.

Future progress on modeling cognitive control processes will require work in a number of directions. Neurophysiology studies will be needed to clarify the contributions of different portions of frontostriatal circuits, including striatal, diencephalic, and brain stem nuclei, to goal-related bias signals and control variables. Other work will need to clarify the network interactions between frontostriatal systems and other brain regions, which underly the consolidation of cognitive control episodes. Finally, future work will need to better specify the neural events underlying the effects of factors such as interference, novelty, and task demands. These studies will help develop more precise models of cognitive control deficits that are needed to predict performance in daily activities.

ACKNOWLEDGMENTS

This work was supported in part by grants from the Canadian Institutes of Health Research and the Fonds de Recherche en Santé du Québec.

REFERENCES

1. Brown, R.G. and Marsden, C.D. (1988a) Subcortical dementia: the neuropsychological evidence. *Neuroscience* **25,** 363–387.
2. Sagar, H.J. and Sullivan, E.V. (1988) Patterns of cognitive impairment in dementia, in *Recent Advances in Clinical Neurology,* vol. 5 (Kennard, C., ed.), Edinburgh, Churchill Livingstone, pp. 47–86.
3. Owen, A.M., James, M., Leigh, P.N., et al. (1992) Fronto-striatal cognitive deficits at different stages of Parkinson's disease. *Brain* **115,** 1727–1751.
4. Passingham, R. (1993) *The Frontal Lobes and Voluntary Action,* Oxford University Press, New York.
5. Lawrence, A.D., Sahakian, B.J., Hodges, J.R., Rosser, A.E., Lange, K.W., and Robbins, T.W. (1996) Executive and mnemonic functions in early Huntington's disease. *Brain* **119,** 1633–1645.
6. Fuster, J.M. (1997) *The Prefrontal Cortex,* Lippincott-Raven, Philadelphia.
7. Shallice, T. (1988) *From Neuropsychology to Mental Structure,* Cambridge University Press, New York.
8. Richer, F. Decary, A., Lapierre, M.F., Rouleau, I., Bouvier, G., and Saint-Hilaire, J.M. (1993) Target detection deficits in frontal lobectomy. *Brain Cogn.* **21,** 203–211.
9. Lawrence, A.D., Sahakian, B.J., Rogers, R.D., Hodges, J.R., and Robbins, T.W. (1999) Discrimination, reversal, and shift learning in Huntington's disease: mechanisms of impaired response selection. *Neuropsychologia* **37,** 1359–1374.

10. Petrides, M. (1985) Deficits on conditional associative-learning tasks after frontal- and temporal-lobe lesions in man. *Neuropsychologia* **23,** 601–614.
11. Decary, A. and Richer, F. (1995) Response selection deficits in frontal excisions. *Neuropsychologia* **33,** 1243–1253.
12. Goldman-Rakic, P.S. (1987) Circuitry of primate prefrontal cortex and regulation of behavior by representational memory, in *Handbook of Physiology—The Nervous System, V* (Plum, F., ed.), American Psychological Society, New York.
13. Graybiel, A. (1998) The basal ganglia and chunking of action repertoires. *Neurobiol. Learn. Mem.* **70,** 119–136.
14. Wise, S.P. (1996) The role of the basal ganglia in procedural memory. *Semin. Neurosc.* **8,** 39–46.
15. Miller, E.K. and Cohen, J.D. (2001) An integrative theory of prefrontal cortex function. *Ann. Rev. Neurosci.* **24,** 167–202.
16. Schultz, W. and Dickinson, A. (2000) Neuronal coding of prediction errors. *Ann. Rev. Neurosci.* **23,** 473–500.
17. Brown, R.G. and Marsden, C.D. (1988) Internal versus external cues and the control of attention in Parkinson's disease. *Brain* **111,** 323–345.
18. Bhatia, K. and Marsden, C.D. (1994) The behavioural and motor conšerquences of focal lesions of the basal ganglia in man. *Brain* **117,** 859–876.
19. Jahanshahi, M., Brown, G., and Marsden, C.D. (1993) A comparative study of simple and choice reaction time in Parkinson's, Huntington's and cerebellar disease. *J. Neurol. Neurosurg. Psychiatry* **56,** 1169–1177.
20. Richer, F. and Boulet, C. (1999) Frontal lesions and fluctuations in response preparation. *Brain Cogn.* **40,** 234–238.
21. Hanes, D.P. and Schall, J.D. (1996) Control of voluntary movement initiation. *Science* **274,** 427–430.
22. Halsband, U., Ito, N., Tanji, J., and Freund, H.J. (1993) The role of premotor cortex and the supplementary motor area in the temporal control of movement in man. *Brain* **116,** 243–166.
23. Maddox, W.T. and Filoteo, J.V. (2001) Striatal contributions to category learning: quantitative modeling of simple linear and complex non-linear rule learning in patients with Parkinson's. *J. Int. Neuropsychological Soc.* **7,** 710–727.
24. Luria, A.R. (1966) *Higher Cortical Functions in Man,* Basic Books, New York.
25. Benecke, R., Rothwell, J.C., Dick, J.P.R., Day, B.L., and Marsden, C.D. (1987) Disturbance of sequential movements in patients with Parkinson's disease. *Brain* **110,** 361–379.
26. Shallice, T. (1982) Specific impairments of planning. *Philos. Trans. R. Soc. Lond. B Biol. Sci.* **288,** 199-209.
27. Canavan, A.G.M., Passingham, R.E., Marsden, C.D., Quinn, N., Wyke, M., and Polkey, C.E. (1989) Sequence ability in parkinsonians, patients with frontal lobe lesions and patients who have undergone unilateral temporal lobectomies. *Neuropsychologia* **27,** 787–798.
28. Owen, A.M., James, M., Leigh, P.N., et al. (1990) Planning and spatial working memory following frontal lobe sessions in man. *Neuropsychologia* **28,** 1021–1034.
29. Glosser, G. and Goodglass, H. (1990) Disorders in executive control functions among aphasic and toher brain-damaged patients. *J. Clin. Exp. Neuropsychol.* **12,** 485–501.
30. Karnath, H.O. and Wallesch, C.W. (1992) Inflexibility of mental planning: a characteristic disorder with prefrontal lesions? *Neuropsychologia* **30,** 1011–1016.
31. Richer, F., Bédard, S., Lepage, M., and Chouinard, M.J. (1998) Frontal lesions produce a dual task deficit in simple rapid choices. *Brain Cogn.* **37,** 173–175.
32. Barone, R. and Joseph, J.P. (1989) Prefrontal cortex and spatial sequencing in macaque monkey. *Exp. Brain Res.* **78,** 447–464.
33. Mushiake, H., Inase, M., and Tanji, J. (1991) Neuronal activity in the primate premotor, supplementary, and precentral motor cortex during visually guided and internally determined sequential movements. *J. Neurophysiol.* **66,** 705–718.
34. D'Esposito, M., Detre, J.A., Alsop, D.C., Shin, R.K., Atlas, S., and Grossman, M. (1995) The neural basis of the central executive system of working memory. *Nature* **378,** 279–281.
35. Bunge, S.A., Klingberg, T., Jacobsen, R.B., and Gabrieli, J.D.E. (2000) A resource model of the neural basis of executive memory. *Proc. Natl. Acad. Sci. USA* **97,** 3573–3578.
36. Adcock, R.A., Constable, R.T., Gore, J.C., and Goldman-Rakic, P.S. (2000) Functional neuroanatomy of executive processes involved in dual-task performance. *Proc. Natl. Acad. Sci. USA* **97,** 3567–3572.
37. Corbetta, M., Miezin, F.M., Dobmeyer, S., Shulman, G.L., and Petersen, S.E. (1991) Selective and divided attention during visual discriminations of shape, color, and speed: functional anatomy by positron emission tomography. *J. Neurosci.* **11,** 2383–2402.
38. Fink, G.R., Dolan, R.J., Halligan, P.W., Marshall, J.C., and Frith, C.D. (1997) Space-based and object-based visual attention: shared and specific neural domains. *Brain* **120,** 2013–2028.
39. Bradshaw, J.L., Phillips, J.G., Dennis, C., et al. (1992) Initiation and execution of movement sequences in those suffering from and at-risk of developing Huntington's disease. *J. Clin. Exp. Neuropsychol.* **14,** 179–192.
40. Lepage, M. and Richer, F. (1996) Inter-response interference contributes to the sequencing deficit in frontal lobe lesions. *Brain* **119,** 1289–1295.
41. Lepage, M. and Richer, F. (2000) Frontal brain lesions affect the use of advance information during response planning. *Behav. Neurosci.* **114,** 1034–1040.
42. Bloxham, C.A., Mindel, T.A., and Frith, C.D. (1984) Initiation and execution of predictable and unpredictable movements in Parkinson's disease. *Brain* **107,** 371–384.
43. Willingham, D.B., Koroshetz, W.J., Treadwell, J.R., and Bennett, J.P. (1995) Comparison of Huntington's and Parkinson's disease patients' use of advance information. *Neuropsychology* **9,** 39–46.
44. Georgiou, N., Bradshaw, J.L., Phillips, J.G., Chiu, E., and Bradshaw, J.A. (1995) Reliance on advance information and movement sequencing in Huntington's disease. *Mov. Disord.* **10,** 472–481.

45. Fuster, J.M., Bauer, R.H., and Jervey, J.P. (1985) Functional interactions between inferotemporal and prefrontal cortex in a cognitive task. *Brain Res.* **25,** 299–307.
46. Colby, C.L. and Goldberg, M.E. (1999) Space and attention in parietal cortex. *Ann. Rev. Neurosci.* **22,** 319–349.
47. Hopfinger, J.B., Buonocore, M.H., and Mangun, G.R. (2000) The neural mechanisms of top-down attentional control. *Nat. Neurosci.* **3,** 284–291.
48. Kastner, S. and Ungerleider, L.G. (2000) Mechanisms of visual attention in the human cortex. *Ann. Rev. Neurosci.* **23,** 315–341.
49. Reynolds, J.H., Chelazzi, L., and Desimone, R. (1999) Competitive mechanisms subserve attention in macaque areas V2 and V4. *J. Neurosci.* **19,** 1736–1753.
50. Rainer, G., Assad, W.F., and Miller, E.K. (1998) Selective representation of relevant information by neurons in the primate prefrontal cortex. *Nature* **393,** 577–579.
51. Kim, J.N. and Shadlen, M.N. (1999) Neural correlates of a decision in the dorsolateral prefrontal cortex of the macaque. *Nat. Neurosci.* **2,** 176–185.
52. Thompson, K.G. and Schall, J.D. (1999) The detection of visual signals by macaque frontal eye field during masking. *Nat. Neurosci.* **2,** 283–288.
53. Brouwers, P., Cox, C., Martin, A., Chase, T., and Fedio, P. (1984) Differential perceptual-spatial impairment in Huntington's and Alzheimer's dementias. *Arch. Neurol.* **41,** 1073–1076.
54. Brown, R.G. and Marsden, C.D. (1991) Dual task performance and processing resources in normal subjects and patients with Parkinson's disease. *Brain* **114,** 215–231.
55. Sharpe, M.H. (1990) Distractibility in early Parkinson's disease. *Cortex* **26,** 239–246.
56. Richer, F. and Lepage, M. (1996) Frontal lesions increase post-target interference in rapid visual streams. *Neuropsychologia* **34,** 509–514.
57. Richer, F., Boulet, C., Chouinard, M.J., Bédard, M.A., and Chouinard, S. Impaired attentional control of unpracticed movements in early Huntington's disease, submitted.
58. Di Lollo, V., Enns, J.T., and Rensick, R.A. (2000) Competition for consciousness among visual events: the psychophysics of reentrant visual processes. *J. Exp. Psychol. Gen.* **129,** 481–507.
59. Raymond, J.E., Shapiro, K.L., and Arnell, K.M. (1992) Temporary suppression of visual processing in an RSVP task: an attentional blink? *J. Exp. Psychol. Hum. Percept. Perform.* **18,** 849–860.
60. Richer, F., Marcantoni, W.S., Lévesque, M., Mansour, B., Beaudoin, G., and Bourguoin, P. Distinct brain systems for masking interference and inter-target interference in visual attention, submitted.
61. Gold, J.I. and Shadlen, M.N. (2001) Neural computations that underlie decisions about sensory stimuli. *Trends Cogn. Sci.* **5,** 10–16.
62. Schmidt, R.A. (1982) Motor control and learning. *Human Kinetics,* Champaign, IL.
63. Shadmehr, R. and Holcomb, H.H. (1997) Neural correlates of motor memory consolidation. *Science* **277,** 821–825.
64. Petersen, S.E., van Mier, H., Fiez, J.A., and Raichle, M.E. (1998) The effects of practice on the functional anatomy of task performance. *Proc. Natl. Acad. Sci. USA* **95,** 853–860.
65. Chouinard, M.J., Rouleau, I., and Richer, F. (1998) Closed-loop sensorimotor control and acquisition after frontal lesions. *Brain Cogn.* **37,** 178–182.
66. Richer, F., Chouinard, M.J., and Rouleau, I. (1999) Frontal lesions impair the attentional control of movements during motor learning. *Neuropsychologia* **37,** 1427–1435.
67. Lemay, S., Lévesque, M., Chouinard, S., Blanchet, P., Richer, F., and Bédard, M.A. (2001) Parkinson's disease affects movements in transformed visual feedback [abstract]. *Mov. Disord.* **16(Suppl. 1),** S28.
68. Gabrieli, J.D.E., Stebbins, G.T., Singh, J., Willingham, D.B., and Goetz, C.G. (1997) Intact mirror-tracing and impaired rotary-poursuit skill learning in patients with Huntington's disease: evidence for dissociable memory systems in skill learning. *Neuropsychology* **11,** 272–281.
69. Willingham, D.B. and Koroshetz, W.J. (1993) Evidence for dissociable motor skills in Huntington's disease patients. *Psychobiol.* **21,** 173–182.
70. Willingham, D.B., Koroshetz, W.J., and Peterson, E.W. (1996) Motor skills have diverse neural bases: spared and impaired skill acquisition in Huntington's disease. *Neuropsychology* **10,** 315–321.
71. Heindel, W.C., Butters, N., and Salmon, D.P. (1988) Impaired learning of a motor skill in patients with Huntington's disease. *Behav. Neurosci.* **10,** 141–147.
72. Boulet, C., Chouinard, S., Lesperance, P., and Richer, F. (2001) Attentional demands affect visuomotor precision in early Huntington's disease [abstract]. *Mov. Disord.* **16(Suppl. 1),** S28–S29.
73. Smith, M.A., Brandt, J., and Shadmehr, R. (2000) Motor disorder in Huntington's disease begins as a dysfunction in error feedback control. *Nature* **403,** 544–549.
74. Knopman, D. and Nissen, M.J. (1987) Procedural learning is impaired in Huntington's disease: evidence from the serial reaction time task. *Neuropsychologia* **29,** 245–254.
75. Saint-Cyr, J.A., Taylor, A.E., and Lang, A.E. (1988) Procedural learning and neostriatal dysfunction in man. *Brain* **111,** 941–959.
76. Pascual-Leone, A., Grafman, J., Clark, K., et al. (1993) Procedural learning in Parkinson's disease and cerebellar degeneration. *Ann. Neurol.* **34,** 594–602.
77. Jackson, G.M., Jackson, S.R., Harrison, J., Henderson, L., and Kennard, C. (1995) Serial reaction time learning and Parkinson's disease: evidence for a procedural learning deficit. *Neuropsychologia* **33,** 577–593.
78. Doyon, J., Gaudrea, D., Laforce, R., et al. (1997) Role of the striatum, cerebellum and frontal lobes in the learning of a visumotor skill. *Brain Cogn.* **34,** 218–245.

9

Disorders of Speech and Language in Parkinson's Disease

Henri Cohen, PhD

> Cases occur in which the muscles duly excited into action by the impulse of the will, do then, with an unbidden agility, and with an impetus not to be repressed, accelerate their motion, and run before the unwilling mind. It is a frequent fault of the muscles belonging to speech, nor yet of these alone... (Gaubius; cited in ref. *1*, p. 24).

> What words he still could utter were monosyllables, and these came out, after much struggle, in a violent expiration, and with such a low voice and indistinct articulation, as hardly to be understood but by those who were constantly with him. (Case A.B.; cited in ref. *1*, p. 40).

1. INTRODUCTION

Parkinson's disease (PD) is the functional model of hypokinetic extrapyramidal disorders. It is characterized by a massive loss of dopaminergic neurons in the substantia nigra (*pars compacta*) as well as by other neurochemical and anatomical changes. Tremor, akinesia, and rigidity, as well as bradykinesia are the cardinal signs of limb and gait disorders in PD. Limb and posture perturbations may also be associated with specific speech motor and linguistic disorders. The physiological processes associated with the various stages in the motor realization of speech are complex, and the planning, initiation, and execution of motor speech acts require the activation of different, hierarchically organized, neural substrates (e.g., see ref. *2* for a detailed presentation). Speech production is a motor activity and requires the integration and coordination of precise movements of articulators, muscles, and mechanisms (diaphragm, abdomen, thoracic cage, larynx, tongue, lips, lower jaw).

2. SPEECH DISORDERS IN PD

Speech disturbances are very common in PD and have a devastating effect on patients' personal relationships. An early epidemiological study by Atarachi and Uchida *(3)* revealed speech disorders in more than two-thirds of individuals afflicted with PD. Today, it is generally agreed that nearly half of all PD patients exhibit some kind of speech disorder.

One of the earliest efforts to define speech disturbances in populations with subcortical damage is by Peacher *(4)*, who attempted to correlate features of dysarthria with lesions of the central and peripheral nervous system. Drawing on previous classifications of dysarthrias, Peacher refers to a number of clinicians who had contributed to a rather wide-ranging neurological classification of this speech disorder. First, Zentay (1937) (cited in ref. *4*) proposed three subdivisions based on neuroanatomical involvement: cortico-bulbar, cortico-striato-pallido-rubro-bulbar-extra-pyramidal, and fronto-ponto-cerebellar.

From: *Mental and Behavioral Dysfunction in Movement Disorders*
Edited by: M-A. Bédard et al. © Humana Press Inc., Totowa, NJ

Later, Foreschel's (1943) (cited in ref. *4*) classification included pyramidal, extrapyramidal, frontopontine, and cerebellar distinctions. Brain's (1948) (cited in ref. *4*) classification encompassed upper motor neurons, corpus striatum, and lower motor neuron lesions, myopathies, and disorders of coordination. Finally, Cobb (1943) (cited in ref. *4*) offered the following classification from a neuropsychiatric perspective: neuromuscular and cranial nerve disturbance (dysarthria), cortico-bulbar and cerebellar dysfunction (dysarthria), symbolic disturbances (agnosia, aphasia, apraxia), and social and personal disturbances (stuttering and reading problems). From his own observations, Peacher *(4)* reported that chewing, swallowing, and articulation are affected in paralysis agitans (PD); he also noted that speech is usually slow and monotonous, with little variation in pitch, and that complete anarthria may occur in advanced cases of PD. Peacher concluded that all dysarthrias share a basic set of impairments, i.e., in articulation, phonation, respiration, rhythm, and resonation, but that certain features are more prominent than others depending on the locus of the lesion. For example, rhythm may be more affected in cerebellar dysfunction, articulation in pyramidal dysfunction, and respiration and phonation in basal ganglia disorders. Peacher cites Rutherford (1939), who observed that "... speech in the basal ganglia type tended to be more irregular, louder, lower pitched, monotonous, and aspirate which was felt to be due to interference with the respiratory apparatus" (ref. *4*, p. 262). Finally, Peacher noted that neurologists have traditionally attributed descriptive terms to several central nervous system (CNS) and peripheral nervous system lesions; the description for paralysis agitans was "weak and expressionless." He concluded that "pure dysarthria" (misarticulation alone) rarely occurs with CNS lesions, but is more frequently encountered after peripheral nervous system lesions. More recent classification schemes have since evolved and effectively replaced these first efforts *(5)*.

Sarno's investigation *(6)* represents the first systematic attempt to characterize the speech behavior of patients with PD and to evaluate the benefits of a rehabilitation program designed specifically for them. Previous observations had revealed several speech problems such as decreased intensity, narrow pitch range, variability in rate, indistinctness or unintelligibility, and performance below the normal range in diadochokinetic and sustained phonation tasks. Sarno noted that the decreased rate of movement of the articulators, common in many patients with PD, significantly impairs speech. She concluded that therapeutic efforts were probably of greatest benefit to the patients' psychological well-being rather than their ability to speak, since no improvement was observed with treatment.

The work of Darley, Aronson, and Brown *(7–9)* is characteristic of the first comprehensive examinations of speech in neurologically impaired populations. The earliest study *(7)* aimed at specifying the dysarthria associated with each of seven neurological impairments, including PD. The groups were evaluated by three judges (the authors) on 38 deviant speech dimensions, grouped into seven categories (pitch characteristics, loudness, vocal quality, respiration, prosody, articulation, and overall/general impression). The dysarthria in the parkinsonian group was characterized by several disorders in the categories of pitch (monopitch, low pitch), loudness (monoloudness), vocal quality (harsh voice, breathy voice), prosody (reduced stress, inappropriate silences, short rushes of speech, variable rate), and articulation (imprecise consonants). Since then, many studies have consistently shown that PD tends to produce hypokinetic dysarthria as characterized by imprecise articulation, prosodic abnormalities, disturbance of speech rate, and low vocal volume *(9–16)*. Also, some patients with PD speak more slowly than controls, and others speak more rapidly *(9,10,17,18)*. Reduced volume is frequently observed in the speech of parkinsonian patients and has been described as a prominent clinical feature of the disease *(19,20)*.

Darley and his colleagues *(8)* also identified "clusters" of deviant speech. One such cluster, prosodic insufficiency (monopitch, monoloudness, reduced stress, short phrases), was found in the PD group and was attributed to a reduced range of movements. Accompanying features of this cluster (short rushes of speech, variable rate, imprecise consonants) were seen only in the parkinsonian group. Other speech dimensions, which did not constitute a cluster by themselves, were also observed in parkinsonian speech: inappropriate silences due to difficulty in initiating articulatory movements; breathy voice,

harsh voice, and low pitch ascribed to rigidity of laryngeal musculature. On the basis of their observations, these authors delineated five types of dysarthria, with one type, hypokinetic dysarthria, proposed to designate the complex speech profile in PD. Darley et al. *(9)* also examined how language changes after thalamotomy and pallidectomy, for the alleviation of parkinsonian symptoms in a large sample of patients (n = 123). Their observations revealed that 23% of the patients showed language changes after one or more surgical procedures. The incidence of language impairment was greater after left than right thalamotomy, greater after multiple than single unilateral thalamotomy, and greater after mixed pallidectomy–thalamotomy than thalamotomy alone. The impairment was manifested predominantly in the higher language functions.

Although there is extensive variation in speech and movement problems, it is generally accepted that motor impairments and fairly consistent articulatory errors are signal features of hypokinetic dysarthria, regardless of context or task *(21)*. Some researchers *(22)* have proposed that speech impairments are consistent across speech tasks, since the found very little difference in articulatory accuracy between automatic and volitional speech. However, there is evidence that speech deficits do not reliably occur in PD and that dysarthric signs can vary across speech tasks. For instance, speaking loudly can improve speech intelligibility and patients are generally more intelligible when reading aloud than when speaking spontaneously *(23)*. Canter and Van Lancker *(24)* examined the speech of a patient with PD who had undergone bilateral thalamic surgery and made the same observation: the patient was more intelligible when reading aloud than when speaking spontaneously. Treatment programs for hypokinetic dysarthria now exist that specifically emphasize the improvement of vocal volume *(25)*.

Earlier studies, which mainly relied on clinical judgment, also sought to evaluate whether antiparkinsonian drugs improved speech intelligibility and labial movement. Nakano, Zubida, and Tyler *(26)*, in a double-blind study with 18 patients (who also served as their own controls), compared the influence of levodopa (L-dopa) with other forms of medication (placebo and procyclidine hydrochloride). They observed a significant increase in speech intelligibility with L-dopa therapy, with the exception of two patients who experienced excessive iatrogenic extrapyramidal signs. Changes in labial movement were measured with labial needle electrodes and were associated with improved speech intelligibility. The study also noted that micrographia was improved with L-dopa. It was concluded that the general improvement in bradykinesia and rigidity may have induced the improved articulation in PD patients. A similar conclusion was reached in a more recent study, in which it was also found that fundamental frequency, a measure of pitch, was significantly increased after medication, whereas measures of noise and speech tremor decreased *(27)*. The improvement was attributed to a decrease in laryngeal hypokinesia and rigidity.

Voice quality and speech production of PD patients before L-dopa treatment were also examined by Séguier et al. *(28)*. In accord with previous observations, their data showed alterations of timbre (harsh voice; 62%), inadequate articulation (43%), voice tremor (32%), decreased intensity (only severe manifestations were noted; 10%), and monotonous voice in one-third of the sample. Correlations between speech deficits and clinical symptoms revealed an association between a mask-like face and rate variability, festination and timbre alteration with pitch variability and rate variability. It is interesting to note that there was no correlation between the clinical sign of tremor and any of the speech deficits.

In an effort to determine the frequency of vocal tract dysfunctions and the specific phonemes affected by the reduction in lingual or labial control in PD, Logemann et al. *(20)* first investigated the sequence of degeneration in vocal-tract control in a large sample (n = 200) of PD patients (idiopathic or postencephalitic). Several parameters were extracted from reading and spontaneous speech tasks and four groups of vocal-tract disturbances were identified: (*i*) laryngeal disorders (89%); (*ii*) articulatory disorders (45%)—the consonants most affected were those requiring greatest constriction of the vocal tract (i.e., obstruents, fricatives, and affricates); (*iii*) speech rate disorders (20%); and (*iv*) hypernasality (10%). A small number of patients (11%) were free of any vocal-tract dysfunction. Co-occurrence of errors in articulation was also analyzed and complex patterns of co-occurring misarticulations were revealed. The authors offer two interpretations of their findings: (*i*) clusters of symptoms are indicative of a progressive dysfunction, beginning with laryngeal changes and increasing to include other areas of neuromuscular control of the vocal tract, such as the lips and tongue; or (*ii*) patterns of coexistence of various vocal-tract dysfunctions may reveal natural subgroups of PD patients. Logemann and Fisher *(29)* carried out a more detailed description of the articulatory errors of this large sample of parkinsonian patients. In the earlier study, 90 patients had produced articulatory errors, mostly with stop consonants and fricatives (see their Table 1 in ref. *29*). In their reexamination of the data, the authors showed that patients were consistent in their errors—when a given patient misarticulated a phoneme, the nature of the misarticulation was maintained in other occurrences of the same phoneme. Moreover, patients showed interindividual consistency in their errors; that is all patients produced the same substitution errors. Finer analysis of the stop consonants misarticulations revealed that patients could not completely close the articulators, resulting in a continuous emission of the air stream. The results of these analyses suggested to the authors that the effects appear to be related entirely to an alteration of neuromuscular control of the articulators, as determined by an incapacity to achieve the requisite degree of vocal tract constriction for particular phonemes. It should be noted that these data are not evidence of reduced strength in the muscles involved in articulation. These results corroborate those of an earlier electromyographic study by Netsell et al. *(14)*, which revealed an "articulatory undershoot" in PD patients, similar in nature to the incomplete contact of the articulators.

The hypothesis that parkinsonian subjects are unable to appreciate perceived or produced prosodic features of speech as well as aspects of facial expression and gesture was tested by Scott, Caird, and Williams *(30)*, who evaluated discrimination of prosodic contrasts, matching of speech and facial expression, discrimination of the affective and grammatical functions of prosody, production of anger, and production of question and declarative forms in both PD subjects and normal elderly controls. Differences were found in the discrimination of prosodic contrasts and production of declarative forms. A specific impairment of the production and perception of prosody in PD was also found by Caekebeke et al. *(31)*, who explored the association between dysprosody and cognitive, affective, and perceptual variables in PD patients and normal controls. They found that patients were less efficient both at mimicking anger and in a storytelling task. Although they concluded that a failure to process emotional information is not a necessary feature of PD, they nevertheless proposed that PD patients with cognitive deterioration displayed receptive and expressive dysprosody based on such a failure. More recently, Pell *(32)* investigated the ability of PD subjects to identify linguistic and emotional attributes of prosodic stimuli and observed a reduction in their ability to comprehend the linguistic and emotional meaning of sentence-level prosody. There was, however, no loss of the ability to discriminate prosodic patterns.

Dementia also appears to exacerbate speech impairments in PD. Cummings et al. *(33)* compared patients with Alzheimer's disease (DAT) with demented and nondemented PD patients on aspects of speech production and language. The speech of all PD patients was found to be more affected than that of DAT patients. Moreover, demented PD patients were more affected on the motor aspects of speech production than nondemented patients. The authors concluded that demented PD patients and DAT patients can be contrasted on the basis of speech and language characteristics.

As we have seen, parkinsonian speech has been the focus of several perceptual and acoustical investigations. Acoustic analyses, however, have generally been concerned with only one aspect of speech or voice in PD. Cohen and Fraïle *(11)* compared the speech perturbations in two basal ganglia movement disorders with contrasting pathophysiology and behavioral manifestations. They investigated the speech production profiles (temporal organization of speech and prosodic abilities) associated with PD, a hypokinetic disorder, and Tardive Dyskinesia (TD), a hyperkinetic disorder, to help understand the functional implication of the basal ganglia in the control of action-oriented behavior. The subjects in their study were administered three speech production tasks: repeated syllables (normal and fast speaking rates), intonation (vowels produced at high and low pitch), and sentence production (imita-

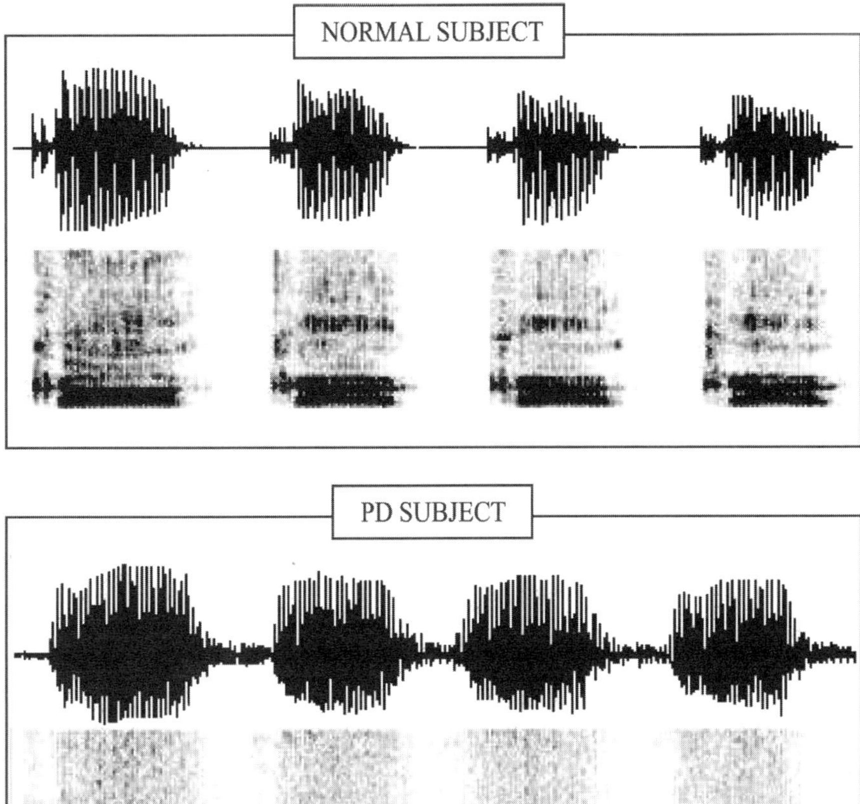

Fig. 1. Production of syllable /ka/, fast speaking rate, by a control subject and PD (light) patient. Note the concentration of resonating energy in the lower frequencies and the imprecise VOT articulation in the speech of the parkinsonian subject.

tion/auditory and free/reading in three linguistic modes). Measures of voice onset time (VOT), voicing duration, pauses, and fundamental frequency were extracted from the digitized speech samples. In PD, the analyses revealed a timing control impairment in the production of both simple and more complex sequences (e.g., fast vs normal speaking rate; see Figs. 1 and 2) and a reduction in the maximal modulation of F0. A dissociation in performance was also found between sentence production conditions, with generally normal intonation when repeating auditorily presented sentences and significantly reduced intonation when reading sentences in the exclamatory or interrogative modes. This suggests that PD patients find it difficult to reach optimal performance in the absence of external cues to guide production. PD patients' dependence on guides or external cues has already been suggested in the context of executing motor and cognitive tasks. In TD, the analyses also revealed anomalies in the temporal organization of speech. Relative to PD, disturbances in phonatory timing control were more generalized in

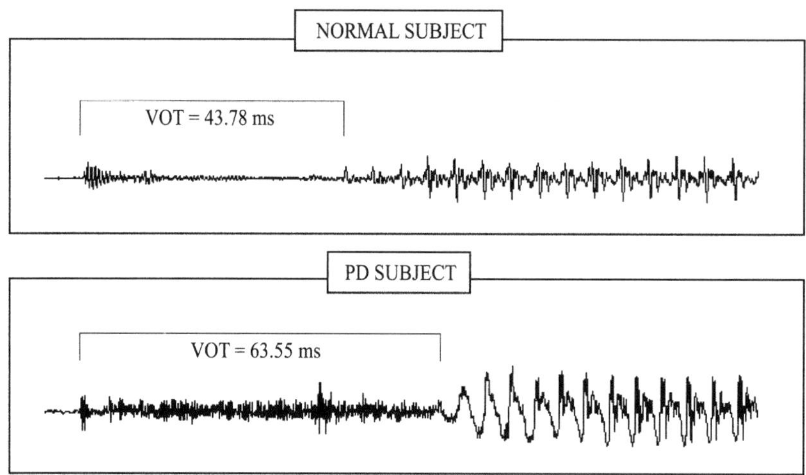

Fig. 2. Production of syllable /ka/, normal speaking rate. VOT measures are fairly stable across speakers of English. The longer VOT duration in PD speech reflects inadequate control of the vocal cords.

TD, and deficiencies were also observed with fast VOT. In contrast to PD, prosodic ability was normal in TD.

These observations indicate that hypokinetic (PD) and hyperkinetic (TD) movement disorders may present with similar difficulties in voluntary motor responses, such as those seen in the temporal organization of sequential movements. The observed dissociation in PD between differing conditions of linguistic intonation production suggests that basal ganglia dysfunction perturbs the dynamic interactions between specific neuronal networks and may lead to more central deficits—the manifestations of which are globally apparent in oriented responses.

It thus appears that speech disorders in PD, and with basal ganglia impairment in general, are associated with abnormal movements. Although the programming aspect of speech articulation is relatively unimpaired, it is the motor programs during articulation that are most affected. Also, strategic processes involved in the production of speech sequences appear weakened in PD, suggesting that the nature of the speech disorder is not only motor but may implicate functional executive-type deficits.

3. LANGUAGE DISORDERS IN PD

In his description of the "shaking palsy," James Parkinson *(1)* did not link intellectual impairment to the disease, which he saw as a strictly motor disorder. Deterioration of intellectual functions in PD was first reported by Trousseau *(34)*; since then, a wide range of cognitive deficits have been identified in PD patients. Indeed, there is a growing consensus that cognitive (and linguistic) impairments are among the complex manifestations of PD. Traditionally, impaired cognitive functioning was ascribed to bradyphrenia (or slow thinking). Several studies now suggest that impairments in procedural memory *(35–38)*, reasoning *(39)*, and attention *(40)* are found in patients with PD.

With respect to language abilities, it was believed, until recently, that they were well preserved and showed only gradual deterioration with the progression of the disease *(41)*. The first investigations of language in PD, using either standard aphasia batteries or Wechsler Adult Intelligence Scale (WAIS) subtests *(42)*, generally concluded that language is relatively intact. However, it is clear that some aspects of language processing are affected in PD (for a review, see refs. *43* and *44*). For instance, there are many studies assessing the comprehension of sentences in PD. Grossman et al. *(45)* found that a majority of their PD patients were compromised in their ability to answer simple questions (e.g., "The eagle chased the hawk that was fast. Which bird was chased?") and that the impairment was more pronounced with sentences of greater syntactic complexity. Grossman et al. *(46)* also noted that most PD subjects show a language-sensitivity deficit in appreciating grammatical information. According to these authors, this difficulty in processing grammatical information is one of the factors implicated in the language deficiencies of PD subjects. For Grossman and colleagues *(45)*, sentence comprehension problems in PD may be affected by frontal lobe-mediated attentional deficits. In a positron emission tomography (PET) study, they found that impaired sentence comprehension in some patients was correlated with reduced mesial frontal lobe glucose metabolism, suggesting an association with frontal lobe attentional mechanisms. In essence, Grossman and colleagues have attributed the comprehension deficiency of PD patients to limited cognitive and attention resources, involving the dysfunction of the striatum as well as of the dorsolateral and medial frontal cortices *(47–49)*. More recently, De Vita et al. *(50)* monitored regional brain activity with functional magnetic resonance imaging (fMRI) in PD and control subjects in tasks where grammatical features and cognitive load were manipulated. These authors suggest a specific neural basis for the sentence comprehension difficulty in PD. There was little caudate recruitment and reduced right posterolateral temporal activation with sentences that create a greater cognitive load (see also ref. *51*). In summary, the results of studies conducted by Grossman and his colleagues on sentence comprehension in PD generally support the view that limited cognitive resources are mainly responsible for the linguistic impairments observed in these patients.

It is, however, possible that the origin of sentence comprehension difficulties in PD, as in the case of complex syntactic forms, does not necessarily result from memory or attentional-cognitive overload. It already appears, from the literature, that individuals with PD are impaired on tasks that rely on procedural memory *(35,38)*, namely those tasks that have been acquired through practice rather than explicit teaching. Consequently, one would expect that patients with PD will show impairments in those aspects of language that rely on procedural memory, namely those that are acquired incidentally, stored implicitly and used automatically without any conscious knowledge of the underlying structure of the forms produced. We refer to those aspects of language that are derived by rule (i.e., generalizations), such as the marking of regular plurals and the past tense of regular verbs, in the context of well-preserved use of irregular verbs and lexical items (nouns, adjectives, adverbs; for a lucid discussion of implicit and explicit linguistic competence, see ref. *52*). Individuals with PD would be expected to show the same form of impairment as individuals with Broca's aphasia and genetic dysphasia *(53)*. They are expected to exhibit a double dissociation from individuals with Alzheimer's disease, who are impaired in tasks that rely on declarative memory and, hence, have difficulty with lexical items rather than inflectional morphology and with irregular rather than with regular verbs *(54)*. This view would help us to understand the pattern of linguistic deficits seen in PD: fairly consistent difficulties in tasks that require processing of sentences with complex syntax, which rely on procedural skills, and highly variable results with lexical decision tasks, which are affected by cognitive or memory load.

Naming is the linguistic production task that has been most frequently investigated in PD. Impairments in picture naming have been reported, but mostly with demented individuals *(33,55)* or with patients apparently not screened for dementia *(56)*. With nondemented PD patients, picture naming performance is equivocal: impairments are reported in some studies *(57)*, while normal performance is reported in others *(58,59)*. A similar performance profile is also observed in generative naming tasks, as measured by verbal fluency, where subjects are asked to retrieve words belonging to specific semantic categories or beginning with a particular letter. The pattern of impairments in generative naming is, here again, equivocal. In some studies, PD patients are more impaired on semantic retrieval tasks *(60)*; in other studies, they are more impaired on letter fluency tasks *(61)*. A possible explanation for these discrepant observations has been suggested by Azuma and colleagues *(62)*, who found that verbal fluency was influenced by the nature of the individual categories used. Their results also indicated that individual fluency tasks are differentially sensitive to the mental status of the PD patients, suggesting that closer attention to the nature of the categories may help clarify the inconsistent effects of PD on verbal fluency.

4. CONCLUSION

Speech and language disorders are frequently observed in individuals with PD. Although the manifestations of speech disturbances have been well studied, it remains to be determined the extent to which these anomalies are exacerbated by the progression of the disease. With respect to the often observed linguistic disorders, in particular the difficulties in appreciating syntax complexity, it is still an open question whether these are part and parcel of the parkinsonian syndrome, or whether they can be explained in terms of deficiencies associated with attention and cognitive load or, alternatively, in terms of an impairment of specific cognitive systems, such as procedural memory.

ACKNOWLEDGMENTS

I thank Michel Paradis for his comments on an earlier version of this chapter.

REFERENCES

1. Parkinson, J. (1817) *Essay on the Shaking Palsy,* Sherwood, Neely, and Jones, London.
2. Crosson, B. (1992) *Subcortical Functions in Language and Memory,* Guilford Press, New York.
3. Atarachi, J. and Uchida, E. (1959) A clinical study of parkinsonism. *Recent Adv. Res. Nervous System* **3,** 871–882.
4. Peacher, W.G. (1950) The etiology and differential diagnosis of dysarthria. *J. Speech Hear. Disord.* **15,** 252–265.
5. Mariotti, C. and Di Donato, S. (2001) Cerebellar/spinocerebellar syndromes. *Neurol. Sci.* **22(Suppl. 2),** S88–S92.
6. Sarno, M.T. (1968) Speech impairment in Parkinson's disease. *Arch. Phys. Med. Rehabil.* **49,** 269–275.
7. Darley, F.L., Aronson, A.E., and Brown, J.R. (1969a) Differential diagnostic patterns of dysarthrias. *J. Speech Hear. Res.* **12,** 246–269.
8. Darley, F.L., Aronson, A.E., and Brown, J.R. (1969b) Clusters of deviant speech dimensions in the dysarthrias. *J. Speech Hear. Res.* **12,** 462–496.
9. Darley, F.L., Aronson, A.E., and Brown, J.R. (1975) *Motor Speech Disorders,* WB Saunders Company, Philadelphia.
10. Canter, G.J. (1965) Speech characteristics of patients with Parkinson's disease: I. Intensity, pitch, and duration. *J. Speech Hear. Disord.* **28,** 221–229.
11. Cohen, H. and Fraïle, V. (2001) Acoustical analysis of speech disorders in basal ganglia dysfunction, 4th International Speech Motor Conference, Nijmegen, NL, June 13–16.
12. Cohen, H., Laframboise, M., and Labelle, A. (1995) Dysprosody in Parkinson's disease. *J. Int. Neuropsychol. Soc.* **4,** 389.
13. Duffy, J. (1995) *Motor Speech Disorders: Substrates, Differential Diagnosis and Management,* Mosby, St. Louis.
14. Netsell, R., Daniel, B., and Celesia, G.G. (1975) Acceleration and weakness in parkinsonian dysarthria. *J. Speech Hear. Disord.* **40,** 170–178.
15. Weismer, G. (1984) Acoustic descriptions of dysarthric speech: perceptual correlates and physiological inferences, in *Current Views of Dysarthria* (Rosenbek, J., ed.), Thieme-Stratton, New York.
16. Weismer, G. (1997) Motor speech disorders, in *Handbook of Phonetic Sciences* (Hardcastle, W. and Laver, J., eds.), Blackwell Publishers, Oxford, pp. 191–219.
17. Caligiuri, M.P. (1989) The influence of speaking rate on articulatory hypokinesia in Parkinsonian dysarthria. *Brain Lang.* **36,** 493–502.
18. Adams, G.G. (1994) Accelerating speech in case of hypokinetic dysarthria, in *Motor Speech Disorders. Advances in Assessment and Treatment* (Till, J., Beukelman, D., and Yorkston, K., eds.), Brookes, Baltimore, pp. 213–228.
19. Darley, F.L. and Sprietersbach, D.C. (1978) *Diagnostic Methods in Speech Pathology,* Harper and Row, New York.
20. Logemann, J.A., Fisher, H.B., Boshes, B., and Blonsky, E.R. (1978) Frequency and cooccurrence of vocal tract dysfunctions in the speech of a large sample of Parkinson patients. *J. Speech Hear. Disord.* **18,** 47–57.
21. Yorkston, K.M., Beukelman, D.R., and Bell, K.R. (1988) *Clinical Management of Dysarthric Speakers,* College Hill Press, Boston.
22. Shames, G.H. and Wiig, E.H. (1990) *Human Communication Disorders,* Merrill Publishing Company, Columbus.
23. Frearson, B. (1985) A comparison of the A.I.D.S. sentence list and spontaneous speech intelligibility scores for dysarthric speech. *Aust. J. Hum. Commun. Disord.* **13,** 5–21.

24. Canter, G.J. and Van Lancker, D. (1985) Disturbances of the temporal organization of speech following bilateral thalamic surgery in a patient with Parkinson's disease. *J. Commun. Disord.* **18,** 329–349.
25. Ramig, L.O., Countryman, S., Thompson, L.L., and Horii, Y. (1995) Comparison of two forms of intensive speech treatment of Parkinson's disease. *J. Speech Hear. Res.* **38,** 1232–1251.
26. Nakano, K.K., Zubick, H., and Tyler, H.R. (1973) Speech deficits of Parkinsonian patients. *Neurology* **23,** 865–870.
27. Sanabria, J., Garcia Ruiz, P., Gutierrez, R., et al. (2001) The effect of levodopa on vocal function in Parkinson's disease. *Clin. Neuropharmacol.* **24,** 99–102.
28. Séguier, N., Spira, A., Dordain, M., Lazar, P., and Chevrie-Muller, C. (1974) Étude des relations entre les troubles de la parole et les autres manifestations cliniques dans la maladie de Parkinson. *Folia Phoniatr (Basel)* **26,** 108–126.
29. Logemann, J. A. and Fisher, H. B. (1981) Vocal tract control in Parkinson's disease: phonetic feature analysis of misarticulations. *J. Speech Hear. Disord.* **46,** 348–352.
30. Scott, S., Caird, F., and Williams, B. (1984) Evidence of an apparent sensory speech disorder in Parkinson's disease. *J. Neurol. Neurosurg. Psychiatry* **47,** 840–843.
31. Caekebeke, J.F.V., Jennekens-Schinkel, A., van der Linden, M.E., Buruma, O.J.S., and Roos, R.A.C. (1991) The interpretation of dysprosody in patients with Parkinson's disease. *J. Neurol. Neurosurg. Psychiatry* **54,** 145–148.
32. Pell, M.D. (1996) Receptive prosody and Parkinson's disease. *Brain Cogn.* **32,** 316–318.
33. Cummings, J.L., Darkins, S., Mendez, M., Hill, M.A., and Benson, D.F. (1988) Alzheimer's disease and Parkinson's disease: comparison of speech and language alterations. *Neurology* **38,** 680–684.
34. Trousseau, A. (1868) Lecture XV: senile trembling and paralysis agitans, in *Lectures on Clinical Medicine Delivered at Hôtel-Dieu, Paris,* Sydenham Society, London.
35. Saint-Cyr, J.A., Taylor, A.E., and Lang, A.E. (1988) Procedural learning and neostriatal dysfunction in man. *Brain* **111,** 949–959.
36. Saint-Cyr, J.A., Taylor, A.E., and Nicholson, K. (1995) Behavior and the basal ganglia. *Adv. Neurol.* **65,** 1–28.
37. Allain, H., Lieury, H., Quemener, V., and Thomas, V. (1995) Procedural memory and Parkinson's disease. *Dementia* **6,** 174–178.
38. Cohen, H., Pourcher, E., and Lussier, J. (2001) Dopaminergic damage on procedural learning in Parkinson's disease. Intact encoding, impaired long-term retrieval. *J. Cogn. Neurosci. Suppl.* 36.
39. Cohen, H., Bouchard, S., Scherzer, B.P., and Whitaker, H.A. (1994) Language and verbal reasoning in Parkinson's disease. *Neuropsychiatry Neuropsychol. Behav. Neurol.* **7,** 166–175.
40. Brown, R.G. and Marsden, D.C. (1988) Internal versus external cues and the control of attention in Parkinson's disease. *Brain* **111,** 323–345.
41. Levin, B.E. and Tomer, R. (1992) A prospective study of language abilities in Parkinson's disease. *J. Clin. Exp. Neuropsychol.* **14,** 34.
42. Bentin, S., Silverberg, R., and Gordon, H.W. (1981) Asymmetrical cognitive deterioration in demented and Parkinson patients. *Cortex* **17,** 533–543.
43. Cohen, H. (1998) Language impairment in Parkinson's disease, in *Handbook of Neurolinguistics* (Stemmer, B. and Whitaker, H.A., eds.), Academic Press, Orlando, pp. 475–483.
44. Lieberman, P., Kako, E., Friedman, J., Tajchman, G., Feldman, L.S., and Jimenez, E.B. (1992) Speech production, syntax comprehension, and cognitive deficits in Parkinson's disease. *Brain Lang.* **43,** 169–189.
45. Grossman, M., Carvell, S., Gollomp, S., Stern, M.B., Vernon, G., and Hurtig, H.I. (1991) Sentence comprehension and praxis deficits in Parkinson's disease. *Neurology* **41,** 1620–1626.
46. Grossman, M., Stern, M.B., Gollomp, S., et al. (1994) Verb learning in Parkinson's disease. *Neuropsychology* **8,** 413–423.
47. Grossman, M., Carvell, S., Stern, M.B., Gollomp, S., and Hurtig, H.I. (1992) Sentence comprehension in Parkinson's disease: the role of attention and memory. *Brain Lang.* **42,** 347–384.
48. Grossman, M., Carvell, S., Gollomp, S., et al. (1993) Cognitive and physiological substrates of impaired sentence processing in Parkinson's disease. *J. Cogn. Neurosci.* **5,** 480–498.
49. Grossman, M. (1999) Sentence processing in Parkinson's disease. *Brain Cogn.* **40,** 387–413.
50. De Vita, C., Cooke, A., Lee, C., et al. (2001) The neural basis for sentence comprehension difficulty in Parkinson's disease. *Brain Lang.* **79,** 11–12.
51. Lee, C., Grossman, M., Zurif, E., et al. (2001) Sentence comprehension and information processing in Parkinson's disease. *Brain Lang.* **71,** 13–14.
52. Paradis, M. (1994) Neurolinguistic aspects of implicit and explicit memory: implications for bilingualism, in *Implicit and Explicit Learning of Second Languages* (Ellis, N., ed.), Academic Press, London, pp. 393–419.
53. Paradis, M. and Gopnik, M. (1997) Compensatory strategies in genetic dysphasia: declarative memory. *J. Neurolinguistics* **10,** 173–185.
54. Ullman, M.T., Corkin, S., Coppola, M., and Hickock, G. (1997) A neural dissociation within language: evidence that the mental dictionary is part of declarative memory, and that grammatical rules are processed by the procedural system. *J. Cogn. Neurosci.* **9,** 266–276.
55. Cooper, J.A., Sagar, H.J., Jordan, N., Harvey, N.S., and Sullivan, E.V. (1991) Cognitive impairment in early untreated Parkinson's disease and its relationship to motor disability. *Brain* **114,** 2095–2122.
56. Matison, R., Mayeux, R., Rosen, J., and Fahn, S. (1982) "Tip of the tongue" phenomenon in Parkinson's disease. *Neurology* **29,** 951–956.

57. Goldman, W.P., Baty, J.D., Buckles, V.D., Sahrmann, S., and Morris, J.C. (1998) Cognitive and motor functioning in Parkinson's disease. *Arch. Neurol.* **55,** 674–680.
58. Gurd, J.M. and Ward, C.D. (1989) Retrieval from semantic and letter-initial categories in patients with Parkinson's disease. *Neuropsychology* **11,** 180–186.
59. Staab, J. (2001) Cognitive and motor contributions to picture naming latencies in Parkinson's disease. M.A. Thesis, Department of Psychology, Université du Québec à Montréal.
60. Auriacombe, S., Grossman, M., Carvell, S., Gollomp, S., Stern, M.B., and Hurtig, H.I. (1993) Verbal fluency deficits in Parkinson's disease. *Neuropsychology* **7,** 182–192.
61. Zec, R.F., Landreth, E.S., Fritz, S., et al. (1999) A comparison of phonemic, semantic, and alternating word fluency in Parkinson's disease. *Arch. Clin. Neuropsychol.* **14,** 255–264.
62. Azuma, T., Bayles, K.A., Cruz, R.F., et al. (1997) Comparing the difficulty of letter, semantic and name fluency tasks for normal elderly and patients with Parkinson's disease. *Neuropsychology* **11,** 488–497.

10

Distinctive Features of Apraxia in Corticobasal Degeneration and Other Neurological Illnesses

Ramón Leiguarda, MD

1. INTRODUCTION

Apraxia is a term used to denote a wide spectrum of higher order motor disorders that result from acquired brain disease affecting the performance of skilled and/or learned movements with or without preservation of the ability to perform the same movement outside the clinical setting in the appropriate situation or environment. The disturbance of purposive movements cannot be termed apraxia, however, if the patient suffers from any elementary motor or sensory deficit (i.e., paresis, dystonia, ataxia), which could fully explain the abnormal motor behavior, or if it results from a language comprehension disorder or from dementia *(1,2)*. Nevertheless, praxic errors are well defined clinically and kinematically and can be superimposed on elementary motor disorders *(3,4)*. Praxic disturbances may affect specific parts of the body (i.e., limb apraxia, buccofacial apraxia, gait apraxia) and may involve both sides of the body (i.e., ideational and ideomotor apraxias), preferentially one side (i.e., limb-kinetic apraxia) or, alternatively, interlimb coordination, as in the case of gait apraxia.

Apraxias are common disorders that can result from a wide variety of focal or diffuse brain damage. Limb apraxia is a hallmark clinical feature and one of the presenting clinical manifestations of corticobasal degeneration (CBD); it is seen in about 80% of patients *(5–11)*. Apraxia is also a salient and frequent neurocognitive deficit in patients with Alzheimer (AD) type of dementia *(12–14)*, as well as in those with primary progressive aphasia (PPA) *(15)*. However, it is only an occasional and late finding in cases of frontotemporal dementia (FTD) *(15)*. Roughly 25 and 70% of patients with Parkinson's disease (PD) and progressive supranuclear palsy (PSP), respectively, may exhibit limb apraxia *(16)*. It also seems to be a relatively frequent motor-behavioral deficit in Huntington's disease (HD) *(17)*.

Contemporary ideas concerning apraxia stem from the classic work of Liepmann, whose initial description and classification of three types of apraxia, ideational (IA), ideomotor (IMA), and limb-kinetic (LKA), has such clarity and influence that it still underlies the most widely used existing schemes of apractic disturbances *(18)*.

A systematic evaluation of limb praxis is critical in order: *(i)* to identify the presence of apraxia; *(ii)* to classify correctly the nature of limb praxis deficit according to the errors committed by the patient; and *(iii)* to gain an insight into the underlying mechanism of the patient's abnormal motor behavior, which may be further defined by kinematic analysis.

Several movement types are used in the evaluation of praxis, and it is not an uncommon finding that praxic patients perform some but not all movements in a particularly abnormal fashion and/or that individual differences appear in some but not all components of a given movement. Therefore, the dissimilar complexity and features of movements should be considered to analyze and interpret praxic

From: *Mental and Behavioral Dysfunction in Movement Disorders*
Edited by: M-A. Bédard et al. © Humana Press Inc., Totowa, NJ

errors accurately. For instance: *(i)* movements may or may not be repetitive in nature (e.g., hammering vs using a bottle opener to remove the cap); *(ii)* an action may consist of sequential movements (e.g., to reach for a glass and take it to the lips in drinking); *(iii)* a movement may primarily reflect proximal limb control (transport) such as transporting the wrist when carving a turkey, proximal and distal limb control such as reaching and grasping a glass of water, or primarily distal control as when the patient is asked to manipulate a pair of scissors; and *(iv)* movements may be performed away from the body in the peripersonal space (e.g., carving a turkey), in body-centered space (e.g., toothbrushing), or require the integration of both, such as the drinking action *(4)*.

Analysis of a patient's performance is based on both accuracy and error patterns (Table 1). Patients with IA or conceptual apraxia (CA) commit content errors, whereas those with IMA show primarily temporal and spatial errors. Three-dimensional (3D) motion analysis of the spatiotemporal features of gestural movements has provided an accurate method to capture objectively the nature of the praxis errors observed at clinical examination. Thus, patients with IMA, due to focal left hemisphere lesions *(19,20)* and diverse asymmetric cortical degenerative syndromes *(15,21)*, have shown slow and hesitant build-up of hand velocity, irregular and nonsinusoidal velocity profiles, abnormal amplitudes, alterations in the plane of motion and the direction and shape of wrist trajectories, decoupling of hand speed and trajectory curvature, and loss of interjoint coordination. All these studies have evaluated gestures, such as carving a turkey or slicing a loaf of bread, which mainly explore the transport or reaching phase of the movement. However, the majority of transitive gestures included in most apraxia batteries are prehension (reaching and grasping) movements reflecting proximal (transport) and distal limb control (grasping), as well as coupling of transport and grasping components. The analysis of prehension movements in apraxic patients has shown disruption in both the transport and grasp phases of the movements, as well as transport-grasping uncoupling *(21,22)*. Furthermore, the analysis of manipulating finger movements has disclosed abnormal workspace and the breakdown in temporal profiles of scanning movements in patients with LKA *(21)*. Thus, exploration into the kinematics of reaching, grasping, and manipulating not only provides information regarding the specific neural subsystems involved in patients with diverse types of limb praxic disorders, but may also help to understand how these systems are integrated with those involved in object representation.

Most of the errors exhibited by IMA cases are equally seen in left or right hemisphere-damaged patients when they pantomime nonrepresentative and representative–intransitive gestures, but are observed predominantly in left hemisphere-damaged patients when they pantomime transitive movements, because it is this action type that is performed outside the natural context *(23)*. The left hemisphere would not only be dominant for the "abstract" performance (i.e., pantomiming to verbal command) of transitive movements, but also for learning and reproducing novel movements, such as meaningless actions and sequences *(24)*. Rushworth et al. proposed that the left hemisphere is also dominant for learning to select a limb movement that is appropriate for the use of an object; one of the difficulties experienced by apraxia patients may involve selecting the appropriate action given the context *(25)*.

2. TYPES OF LIMB APRAXIA

2.1. *Ideational Apraxia*

Liepmann defined IA as an impairment in tasks requiring a sequence of several acts with tools and objects *(18)*. However, other authors use the term to denote a failure to use single tools appropriately *(2)*. To overcome this confusion, Ochipa et al. *(26)* have suggested restricting the term IA to a failure to conceive a series of acts leading to an action goal and introduced the term CA to denote loss of diverse types of tool-action knowledge, as proposed by Roy and Square *(1)*. However, patients with IA not only fail on tests of multiple object use, but also when using single objects *(27)*; thus, a strict difference between IA and CA is not always feasible. Patients with IA or CA exhibit, primarily, content errors in the performance of transitive movements (Table 1), because they are unable to associate tools

Table 1
Types of Praxis Errors

Temporal
S = sequencing: some pantomimes require multiple positionings that are performed in a characteristic sequence. Sequencing errors involve any perturbation of this sequence including addition, deletion, or transposition of movement elements as long as the overall movement structure remains recognizable.
T = timing: this error reflects any alterations from the typical timing or speed of a pantomime and may include abnormally increased, decreased, or irregular rate of production or searching or groping behavior.
O = occurrence: pantomimes may involve either single (i.e., unlocking a door with a key) or repetitive (i.e., screwing in a screw with a screwdriver) movement cycles. This error type reflects any multiplication of single cycles or reduction of a repetitive cycle to a single event.

Spatial
A = amplitude: any amplification, reduction, or irregularity of the characteristic amplitude of a target pantomime.
IC = internal configuration: when pantomiming, the fingers and hand must be in specific spatial relation to one another to reflect recognition and respect for the imagined tool. This error type reflects any abnormality of the required finger and/or hand posture and its relationship to the target tool. For example, when asked to pretend to brush teeth, the subject's hand may close tightly into a fist with no space allowed for the imagined toothbrush handle.
BPO = body-part-as-object: the subject uses his/her finger, hand, or arm as the imagined tool of the pantomime. For example, when asked to smoke a cigarette, the subject might puff on his or her index finger.
ECO = external configuration orientation: when pantomiming, the fingers, hand, and/or arm and the imagined tool must be in a specific relationship to the "object" receiving the action. Errors of this type involve difficulties orienting to the object or in placing the object in space. For example, the subject might pantomime brushing teeth by holding his hand next to his mouth without reflecting the distance necessary to accommodate an imagined toothbrush. Another example would be when asked to hammer a nail, the subject might hammer in differing locations in space reflecting difficulty in placing the imagined nail in a stable orientation or in a proper plane of motion (abnormal planar orientation of the movement).
M = movement: when acting on an object with a tool, a movement characteristic of the action and necessary to accomplish the goal is required. Any disturbance of the characteristic movement reflects a movement error. For example, a subject, when asked to pantomime using a screwdriver, may orient the imagined screwdriver correctly to the imagined screw but instead of stabilizing the shoulder and wrist and twisting at the elbow, the subject stabilizes the elbow and twists at the wrist or shoulder.

Content
P = perseverative: the subject produces a response that includes all or part of a previously produced pantomime.
R = related: the pantomime is an accurately produced pantomime associated in content with the target. For example, the subject might pantomime playing a trombone for a target of a bugle.
N = nonrelated: the pantomime is an accurately produced pantomime not associated in content with the target. For example, the subject might pantomime playing a trombone for a target of shaving.
H = the patient performs the action without benefit of a real or imagined tool. For example, when asked to cut a piece of paper with scissors, he or she pretends to rip the paper.

Other
C = concretization. The patient performs a transitive pantomime not on an imagined object, but instead on a real object not normally used in the task. For example, when asked to pantomime sawing wood, the patient pantomimes sawing on his or her leg.
NR = no response.
UR = unrecognizable response: the response shares no temporal or spatial features of the target.

Adapted from ref. *3* with permission.

and objects with their corresponding action. They may also lose the ability to associate tools with the objects that receive their action; thus, when a partially driven nail is shown, the patient may select a pair of scissors rather than a hammer from an array of tools to perform the action. Not only are patients unable to select the appropriate tool to complete an action, but they may also fail to describe a function of a tool or point to a tool when the function is described by the examiner, even when the patient names the tool properly when shown to him or her *(26)*. These patients may also be impaired in the sequencing of tool and/or object use *(2,18)*. Patients with IA or CA are disabled in everyday life, because they use tools and/or objects improperly, misselect tools and/or objects for an intended activity, or perform a complex sequential activity (e.g., make express coffee) in a mistaken order or entirely fail to complete the task *(3)*.

IA was traditionally allocated to the left parieto-occipital and parietotemporal regions *(2,18)*. However, frontal and frontotemporal lesions may also cause IA *(27)* as well as CA *(28)*.

2.2. *Ideomotor Apraxia*

IMA has been defined as "a disturbance in programming the timing, sequencing, and spatial organization of gestural movements"*(3)*. Patients with IMA mainly exhibit temporal and spatial errors. Movements are incorrectly produced, but the goal of the action can usually be recognized, although on occasion, performance is so severely deranged that the examiner cannot recognize the movement. Transitive movements are more affected than intransitive ones on pantomiming to command. Patients usually improve on imitation when performance is compared to responses to verbal command, and acting with tools and/or objects is usually carried out better than pantomiming their use, but even so, movements are not normal *(2,3)*.

IMA is commonly associated with damage to the parietal association areas, less frequently with lesions of the premotor cortex (PM) and supplementary motor area (SMA), and usually with disruption of the intrahemispheric white matter bundles interconnecting them, as well as with basal ganglion and thalamic damage *(4)*. Although small lesions of the basal ganglia may cause IMA, most patients sustained larger lesions to the basal ganglia and/or thalamus together with the internal capsule and periventricular and peristriatal white matter, interrupting association fibers, in particular those of the superior longitudinal fasciculus and frontostriatal connections *(29)*. Most studies examining possible clinicoanatomical correlation for IMA have found a strong association of apraxia with large cortico-subcortical lesions in the suprasylvian, perirolandic region of the left dominant hemisphere, but no specific lesion site correlating with apraxia. It seems that white matter damage with disruption of cortico-cortical and corticosubcortical connections is crucial for the occurrence of apraxia *(30)*.

2.3. *Limb-Kinetic Apraxia*

This type of apraxia was originally described by Kleist, who called it "innervatory apraxia" to stress the loss of hand and finger dexterity, due to the inability to connect and to isolate individual innervation, and attributed it to damage to the PM cortex *(31,32)*. The deficit is mainly confined to finger and hand movements contralateral to the lesion, regardless of its hemispheric side, with preservation of power and sensation. Manipulatory finger movements are predominantly affected, but in most cases, all movements, whether complex or routine, independent of the evoking modality, are coarse and mutilated. The virtuosity given to movements by practice is lost, and they become clumsy, awkward, and "amorphous." Fruitless attempts usually precede wrong movements, which in turn are often contaminated by extraneous movements. Imitation of finger postures is also abnormal, and some patients use the less affected or normal hand to reproduce the requested posture. The deficit clearly interferes with daily activities *(31,33–36)*.

LKA has been scantily reported with focal lesions *(33)*. There are basically two potential explanations: *(i)* most PM lesions also involve the precentral cortex, so that the contralateral paresis or paralysis precludes expression of the praxic deficit; and *(ii)* bilateral activation of the PM cortex is often observed with unilateral movements. Thus, a unilateral lesion would not be enough for the deficit to become clearly manifested, since bilateral involvement would be most likely necessary. As a matter of fact, all recently pathologically confirmed cases of LKA had undergone a degenerative process, such as corticobasal degeneration and Pick's disease, involving frontal and parietal cortices, or, predominantly, the PM cortex *(4)*.

3. THE NATURE OF APRAXIA IN CORTICOBASAL DEGENERATION

We have studied for the presence of apraxia 16 right-handed patients, aged 56–78 yr, who met accepted clinical criteria for the diagnosis of CBD *(9,21,36)*. Disease duration ranged from 2–6 yr. To minimize confounding effects imposed by the elementary motor disorder, the original 10 patients were assessed in the less affected limb, whereas in the last 6, both limbs were evaluated. Thirteen patients exhibited IMA; spatial and temporal errors were more frequently observed when performing transitive than intransitive movements, either to command, imitation, and even with the use of the real object and/or tool. Spatial errors, such as incorrect positioning of the hand to grasp the tool (internal configuration errors), difficulty in orienting the hand with respect to the body and the tool with respect to the object receiving the tool's action in extrapersonal space (external configuration errors), abnormal movement trajectories, and timing errors were those more frequently found, whereas body-part-as-object and sequencing errors were not so common. All these patients have difficulties when imitating meaningful and meaningless postures and movements, and some exhibited even more errors when imitating rather than pantomiming gestures to command. Patients with the most severe praxic disturbances also exhibit errors (i.e., omissions, misuse, mislocations, intrusions) when performing sequential arm movements, and four patients committed content errors, three of whom also showed deficits on gesture recognition.

The praxis disorders were more frequent in patients who had initial symptoms in the right limb (left hemisphere dysfunction) than in the left limb (right hemisphere dysfunction) in agreement with the fact that most right-handers develop IMA, as well as IA, predominantly with left hemisphere lesions. IMA and IA scores significantly correlated with Mini-Mental State Examination (MMSE) scores. IMA scores also correlated with a task sensitive to frontal lobe dysfunction, and alien limb behavior was only seen in patients with IMA. On the other hand, primitive reflexes were particularly evident in patients with IA.

We found no LKA in our original 10 patients, most likely due to the fact that we only assessed the less affected limb *(9)*, as also happened with Jacobs et al. study *(37)*. Four out of the last six patients we evaluated with the classical clinical picture of CBD presented a clear-cut unilateral limb-kinetic type of praxic deficit in addition to bilateral IMA *(36)*. Patients showed slow, awkward, and mutilated finger and hand movements; on occasion, movements were amorphous and contaminated by extraneous movements. Difficulties were particularly evident with motor skills requiring fractionated or sequential fingers movements. Imitation of finger postures was abnormal, and some patients used the other hand to move the abnormal one to reproduce the requested posture. At times, the fingers and hand remained in an abnormal posture while the patient performed other tasks with the contralateral hand. Perseveration of postures and movements was commonly observed. Patients were aware of the poor performance, but were unable to correct their errors. Kinematic studies in these patients showed severe disruption of manipulative movements with marked interfinger uncoordination *(36)*.

Jacobs et al. *(37)* studied four patients with clinical diagnosis of CBD of brief duration. Testing the less affected upper extremity, they found ideomotor types of praxis errors on gesture to command as well as imitation with relative preservation on gesture discrimination and novel gesture learning *(37)*. Pillon et al. evaluated 15 right-handed patients with probable CBD (mean age ± standard deviation [SD]: 67.8 ± 8 yr) and disease duration less than 10 yr. They found a bilateral though asymmetric praxis disorder, which they identified as IMA *(38)*. Finally, Blondel et al. found, in three right-handed patients with clinical diagnosis of CBD, a severe IMA with "some traits of LKA" *(39)*. Comparing performance on gestures to command with imitation and the use of the real object and/or tool, no consistent pattern emerged, since some patients may have more difficulties when imitating than pantomiming gestures, and occasionally patients performed worse when handling the objects than pantomiming to command or the reverse, showing a dramatic improvement when holding the tool and/or object *(40)*.

The limb-kinetic type of apraxia has also been frequently reported in CBD *(21,34–36,41)*. Okuda et al. described two patients with presumed CBD who had difficulty making fine finger movements, imitating finger patterns, and manipulating objects *(41)*. Three patients in the Pillon et al. study had a unilateral limb type of deficit which "might correspond to LKA" *(38)*. Denes et al. recently reported five patients (three presumed to have CBD) with a type of limb apraxia, whose characteristics perfectly fit the definition of LKA originally proposed by Kleist and Liepmann; three of them also had IMA, and one had oral apraxia *(34)*. Another recent study also stressed the derangement of finger and hand movements characteristic of LKA in patients with CBD *(35)*.

IA has been scarcely reported in patients with CBD. However, Kertesz et al. studied 44 patients with the clinical diagnosis of CBD, 35 prospectively and six by retrospective file review. Eleven cases with autopsy had CBD or other forms of Pick's complex. Fifteen patients presented with movement disorders and 20 with cognitive manifestations, either progressive aphasia or frontotemporal dementia. Limb apraxia, usually ideational and ideomotor, was described in 34 out of 35 patients; however, apraxia was formally tested in only 19 patients, whereas in the remainder, it was obtained by history *(42)*. Orofacial apraxia has not been so frequent in CBD. Pillon et al. found orofacial apraxia in their patients though milder than limb apraxia *(38)*. We only demonstrated orofacial apraxia in 4 out of 16 patients *(9)*, but Jacobs et al. and Blondel et al. failed to mention it in their studies *(37,39)*. However, in a recent study by Ozsancak et al., orofacial apraxia, as evaluated by means of simple and sequential gestures, was found in 9 of 10 patients with a clinical diagnosis of CBD *(43)*.

In summary, patients with CBD usually have severe bilateral, though asymmetric, ideomotor type of apraxia, which, in many cases, coexists with unilateral or, infrequently, bilateral limb-kinetic praxis deficits. An ideational or conceptual defect may also be observed in advanced stages of the disease or in patients who presented with cognitive disorders.

4. APRAXIA IN OTHER NEUROLOGICAL ILLNESSES

4.1. *Basal Ganglion Diseases*

Few studies on apraxia in PD have been published *(16,44–46)*. Sharpe et al. evaluated 14 patients with PD and found that they performed at a lower gestural level on representational tasks (representation of implement usage) and made significantly more spatial errors on the nonrepresentational tasks (imitation of nonrepresentational gestures) than normal controls *(44)*. Goldenberg et al. studied 42 patients with moderate to severe PD; execution of movement sequence and a "total apraxia score" were worse in patients than in controls, and such deficits appeared to correlate with visuospatial disabilities *(45)*. The ability of 22 nondemented patients with PD to execute two gestural tasks was evaluated by Grossman et al. *(46)*. PD patients made significantly more errors than controls, and such errors were not explained convincingly by bradykinesia *(46)*. We studied 45 nondemented PD patients with a standard comprenhensive praxia battery in "on" and "off" states. We found bilateral IMA for transitive movements, which improved on imitation and became almost normal with the use of tool and/or objects in 12 out of 45 PD patients. Spatial errors (i.e., external configuration, internal configuration, and trajectory) were those most frequently found, whereas hesitation, occurrence, and sequence errors were unusual, and content errors were not observed. Patients also had difficulties in imitating hand and finger postures, but comprehension of pantomimes was normal. Dopaminergic therapy failed to modify apraxia. IMA scores correlated with deficits in frontal lobe-related neuropsychological tasks; there was also a clear trend towards significance between deficits on visuospatial cognition and apraxia *(16)*. We further studied by means of 3D motion analysis, 10 patients with PD in the "on" state while performing a bread-loaf slicing action. We demonstrated impairment of spatial precision of movements and the disruption of velocity-curvature relationship and interjoint coordination *(47)*. Since these kinematic abnormalities tended to be more severe in apraxic PD patients, they are likely the expression of some of the praxic errors observed on clinical examination.

Limb apraxia, particularly of the ideomotor type, has been occasionally reported in PSP patients *(48–50)*. We have found bilateral IMA for transitive movements in 8 out of 12 patients with PSP; 5 of whom also had IMA for intransitive movements. Performance improved on imitation and with tactile cues provided by the tool and/or object. Spatial (i.e., external and internal configuration, body-part-as-object, and trajectory) were more prominent than temporal errors (i.e., hesitation, delay), and sequencing errors occurred rarely. In addition to the ideomotor type of praxis errors, five patients also showed an abnormal motor behavior compatible with LKA. IA scores correlated significantly with cognitive deficits as measured with MMSE *(16)*.

Shelton and Knopman found IMA in three out of nine patients with HD. Apraxia correlated significantly with disease duration and postural abnormalities, but not with other individual aspects of elementary motor and cognitive functions *(17)*.

4.2. *Cortical Dementia and Asymmetric Cortical Degenerative Syndromes*

Apraxia has traditionally been considered as one of the salient neurocognitive deficits of AD. However, conflicting results have been obtained regarding both the frequency of apraxia during the progression of the disease and the relationship between apraxia and the ability to perform activities of daily life. IMA has been found in about one-third of cases of mild AD type of dementia and in 70–90% of cases in advanced stages of the disease, whereas IA has been described predominantly in patients with moderate or severe dementia *(12)*. However, Ochipa et al. found that most patients with AD scored lower than controls in conceptual tasks, and a double dissociation on language performance as well as IMA and CA were observed *(26)*. Derousné et al. recently evaluated 22 patients with mild-to-moderate dementia of the Alzheimer type and found conceptual types of praxic deficits throughout and IMA in 17 *(14)*. Impaired ability to perform activities of daily life correlated with CA, although other authors have demonstrated relationships only between activities of daily life and IMA *(12)*.

Apraxia is not a common clinical feature of FTD, and mild-to-moderate IMA may only be found in advanced stages of the disease, most likely disclosing the progression of pathological changes towards the PM cortex and the association with striatal and/or late parietal involvement *(15)*.

Both IMA and orofacial apraxia are frequent findings in patients with nonfluent PPA, whereas those with fluent PPA may show IMA as well as IA. Although in most PPA patients, IMA is mild and slowly progressive, PPA cases with more severe apraxic deficits may later develop the full CBD syndrome. On the other hand, the presence of IA may herald the progression towards an Alzheimer type of dementia *(15)*.

5. THE PATHOPHYSIOLOGY OF LIMB APRAXIAS

Hand use for object grasping and manipulation requires a sequential motor performance starting with the reaching or transport movement component, the assumption of an adequate hand posture during object acquisition, and the grasping and object manipulation *(51)*. These processes seem to be subserved by several parallel parietofrontal circuits performing sensorimotor transformation for posture, reaching, and grasping, as well as for coding peripersonal space for limb movements *(52)*. The movement transport component combines information about spatial location of the object with information about initial arm configuration and position to compute a motor command for the muscles that will move the hand toward the target. This reaching process is subserved by a complex parietofrontal network. The parietal regions, all in the superior parietal lobule (SPL) and upper bank of the intraparietal sulcus (IPS), contain populations of neurons coding retinal and gaze positional information for target localization in the posterior part, neurons tuned to arm position in the intermediate part, and neurons with arm movement-related activity on the rostral part, with functional overlap among regions *(53)*. These parietal regions are reciprocally connected with the PM dorsal cortex and primary motor area (M1) *(52,53)*.

The grasping component requires information concerning intrinsic object properties (such as size and shape) for the determination of a suitable grasping pattern or adequate hand configuration. Thereafter, object exploration and manipulation depend on the ability to generate independent finger movements and on delicate somatotosensory control processes *(54)*.

Studies in monkeys have shown a distal hand movement representation in area F5 (rostral-most part of the ventral PM cortex), which is directly connected with the hand area of the M1 *(55)*. In F5, a variety of neuron populations would encode diverse motor acts (schemas), such as grasping, holding, and tearing, others would indicate how objects are to be grasped, and the effectors (fingers) appropriate for the action. The motor schemas would be action segments and form a basic "vocabulary" from which many skilled movements may be constructed as coordinated control programs *(54)*. Area F5 is reciprocally connected with the anterior intraparietal area (AIP) located within the IPS and receives projections from the second somatosensory area (S_{II}) and from parietal area 7b *(56)*. Some neurons in AIP discharge in response to the presentation of specific 3D objects, while others respond to finger and hand movements. Still other manipulation-related neurons discharge both during active finger movements and in response to 3D stimuli congruent in size and shape with the coded grasping movement *(57)*. A recent functional magnetic resonance imaging (MRI) study has demonstrated that grasping and manipulation of complex objects leads to the activation of the ventral PM cortex and of a region located within the IPS, basically the same areas found in monkeys to be involved in the circuit for visuomotor transformation for grasping *(58)*. In addition, activation was also observed in a sector of the SPL, mostly related to proprioception, as well as in S_{II}, where neurons respond primarily to tactile activation. Thus, S_{II} would provide essential tactile input to ventral PM cortex for accurate control and direct finger movements during object manipulation in the absence of visual guidance *(58)*.

All the motor areas of the cerebral cortex, as well as of the prefrontal cortex, send projections as a part of parallel segregated circuits to diverse regions of the basal ganglia *(59)*. The parietal areas, reciprocally interconnected with such areas of the motor cortex making up the parietofrontal circuits, also send extensive projections to the basal ganglia *(60)*. Thus, it seems likely that the basal ganglia are an integral part of a series of specialized circuits for sensorimotor transformation. As regards reaching, Burnod et al. have recently suggested that the basal ganglia could provide the cortex with gating signals capable of triggering the sequence of movements at the appropriate time and in the appropriate order, when several outputs are possible for a given task and when the decision has to be made between concurrent tasks *(53)*. Thus, in addition to their putative roles in sensorimotor transformation for reaching and grasping, the basal ganglia may participate in praxis in other ways, whether in the selection of the kinematics and direction of arm movements, by encoding peripersonal space for limb movements, by contributing to diverse mechanisms of response selection, or by acting as an integral part of brain systems involved in the representation of action sequences *(30)*.

It has been previously suggested that disruption of the parietofrontal circuits, and their subcortical connections, subserving transformation of sensory information into action, may give rise to most of the praxic errors observed in patients with IMA and LKA *(4)*. Damage to the circuits devoted to sensorimotor transformation for reaching and posture, transformation of body part location into information necessary for the control of body part movement, as well as the circuit subserving the representation of peripersonal space somatotopically, would produce praxic errors, such as inappropriate arm configuration, faulty movement orientation, and movement trajectory abnormalities. Incorrect hand posture may result if the parietal node of the circuit devoted to grasping is also involved. These errors may be similarly observed in the limb contralateral to a left or right hemisphere lesion, if an associated elemental motor or sensory deficit does not preclude their proper interpretation. However, they would be particularly reflective of IMA, and thus also observed in the limb ipsilateral to a left hemisphere lesion, when the patient pantomimes a transitive movement to verbal command and/or reproduces novel movements. Involvement of the circuits subserving sensorimotor transformation for grasping may produce some of the ideomotor type of praxis errors confined to hand movements. However, it seems quite likely that damage to this circuit, particularly when there is bilateral involvement of the ventral PM cortex, would primarily disrupt action segments and the specificity for diverse hand and finger movements and configurations. The "motor vocabulary" necessary for the proper selection of finger and hand movements *(54)* would be impaired, and a limb-kinetic type of praxis deficit would appear in the hand contralateral to the more affected hemisphere, regardless of the pattern of cerebral dominance. Finally, IA would reflect an inability to select and use tool and/or objects due to the disruption of the complex integration processes between systems subserving functional knowledge of actions (i.e., reaching, grasping and manipulating, sequencing) and those devoted to knowledge of objects and tools *(4)*.

The brunt of the pathology in CBD is located in the superior frontal gyrus, which is more often affected than the middle and inferior gyri, the pre- and postcentral regions, the anterior corpus callosum, the caudate, putamen, globus pallidus, thalamus, and substantia nigra with atypical asymmetric distribution *(61)*. Functional brain imaging studies have disclosed a decreased metabolism in the frontoparietal region, particularly in the superior prefrontal cortex, the lateral and mesial premotor areas, in the sensorimotor and parietal association cortices, as well as in the caudate, lenticular, and thalamic regions with striking interhemispheric asymmetries; the hemisphere contralateral to the more affected limb proving more severely involved *(62)*.

The particular distribution of the pathological process in patients with CBD clearly explains the disruption of the cortical and subcortical components of the circuits subserving transformation of sensory information into action and, hence, the severe IMA and LKA observed in these patients. The limb-kinetic type of praxic deficit may be further aggravated by derangement of independent finger movements and by dysfunction of somatosensory control of manipulation *(36)*. Involvement of inhibitory areas in the inferior and superior frontal gyri and damage to subcortical structures may reduce facilitation of inhibitory interneurons, causing defective cortical inhibition, which in turn may also interfere with the selection and control of finger muscle activity. We found reduced cortical inhibition, as reflected by a short silent period, in CBD patients with LKA *(36)*. Finally, an associated sensory defect due to parietal damage may interfere with the kinesthetic and tactile information necessary for somatosensory control of manipulation. However, as a defect in somesthesis may not be present and parietal involvement may be absent in patients with CBD, LKA may, basically, result from bilateral dysfunction of nonprimary cortical motor areas *(36)*.

Limb apraxia is observed in some but not all patients with PSP, PD, and HD *(16,17)*. As described above, apraxia scores in PSP significantly correlated with low MMSE, whereas in PD they correlated with neuropsychological tests reflecting frontal lobe dysfunction and visuospatial cognition deficits *(16)*. Thus, apraxia in these patients most likely results from the combination of basal ganglion and cortical pathology. Cortical degeneration is now recognized to be common in PSP and identified mainly in the cingulate, superior, and medial frontal gyri *(63)*. In PSP patients with limb apraxia, specific pathological changes may be confined to premotor and motor cortices or coexist with AD pathology *(16,50)*.

In PD patients, impairment of neuropsychological tests reflecting frontal lobe function correlated with reduced fluorodopa uptake in the caudate nucleus *(64)*, and proton magnetic resonance spectroscopy (MRS) may detect temporoparietal cortical dysfunction in nondemented patients with PD *(65)*. Therefore, it seems plausible that the subgroups of PD patients developing limb apraxia and more severe kinematic abnormalities in the spatial precision of movements and interjoint coordination *(47)* are those with greater caudate nucleus and frontal lobe involvement with or without temporoparietal cortical dysfunction *(30)*. Thus, basal ganglion pathology *per se* would not cause overt apraxia. However, when combined with dysfunction of the cortical components of the neural circuits devoted to sensorimotor transformation, sequencing, and response selection, various types of praxic deficits would become clinically manifested. As a matter of fact, the most severe examples of limb apraxia are usually seen in patients with CBD, in whom frontoparietal and basal ganglion damage coexists *(30)*.

REFERENCES

1. Roy, E.A. and Square, P.A. (1985) Common considerations in the study of limb, verbal, and oral apraxia, in *Neuropsychological Studies of Apraxia and Related Disorders* (Roy, E.A., ed.), Elsevier Science Publishers B.V., Amsterdam, The Netherlands, pp. 111–161.
2. De Renzi, E. (1989) Apraxia, in *Handbook of Neuropsychology* (Boller, F. and Grafman, J., eds.), Elsevier Science, Amsterdam, pp. 245–263.
3. Rothi, L.J. and Heilman, K.M. (eds.) (1997) *Apraxia: the Neuropsychology of Action,* Psychology Press, East Sussex, UK.
4. Leiguarda, R. and Marsden, C.D. (2000) Limb apraxias: higher-order disorders of sensorimotor integration [review]. *Brain* **123**, 860–879.
5. Rebeiz, J.J., Kolodny, E.H., and Richardson, E.P. (1968) Corticodentatonigral degeneration with neuronal achromasia. *Arch. Neurol.* **18,** 20–33.
6. Riley, D.E., Lang, A.E., Lewis, A., et al. (1990) Corticobasal ganglionic degeneration. *Neurology* **40,** 1203–1212.
7. Gibb, W.R., Luthert, P.J., and Marsden, C.D. (1989) Corticobasal degeneration. *Brain* **112,** 1171–1192.
8. Rinne, J., Lee, M., Thompson, P., and Marsden, C.D. (1994) Corticobasal degeneration: a clinical study of 36 cases. *Brain* **117,** 1183–1196.
9. Leiguarda, R., Lees, A.J., Merello, M., Starkstein, S., and Marsden, C.D. (1994) The nature of apraxia in corticobasal degeneration. *J. Neurol. Neurosurg. Psychiatry* **57,** 455–459.
10. Kampoliti, K., Goetz, C.G., Boeve, B.F., et al. (1998) Clinical presentation and pharmacological therapy in corticobasal degeneration. *Arch. Neurol.* **55,** 957–961.
11. Litvan, I., Agid, Y., Goetz, C., et al. (1997) Accuracy of the clinical diagnosis of corticobasal degeneration: a clinicopathologic study. *Neurology* **48,** 119–125.
12. Edwards, D.F., Denel, R.K., Baum, C.M., and Morris, J.C. (1991) A quantitative analysis of apraxia in senile dementia of Alzheimer type: a stage-related differences in prevalence and type. *Dementia* **2,** 142–149.
13. Luchelli, F., Lopez, O., Faglioni, P., and Boller, F. (1993) Ideomotor and ideational apraxias in Alzheimer's disease. *Int. J. Ger. Psych.* **8,** 413–417.
14. Derousné, C., Lagha-Pierucci, S., Thibault, S., Bandouin-Madec, V., and Lacomblez, S. (2000) Apraxic disturbances in patients with mild to moderate Alzheimer's disease. *Neuropsychologia* **38,** 1760–1769.
15. Leiguarda, R. and Starkstein, S. (1998) Apraxia in the syndromes of Pick Complex, in *Pick's Disease and Pick Complex* (Kertesz, A. and Muñoz, D.G., eds.), Wiley-Liss, New York, pp. 129–143.
16. Leiguarda, R., Pramstaller, P., Merello, M., Starkstein, S., Lees, A.J., and Marsden, C.D. (1997) Apraxia in Parkinson's disease, progressive supranuclear palsy, multiple system atrophy, and neuroleptic induced parkinsonism. *Brain* **120,** 75–90.
17. Shelton, P.A. and Knopman, D.S. (1991) Ideomotor apraxia in Huntington's disease. *Arch. Neurol.* **48,** 35–41.
18. Liepmann, H. (1920) Apraxia. *Ergeb Gesamten Medizin* **1,** 516–543.
19. Clark, M.A., Merians, A.S., Kothari, A., et al. (1994) Spatial planning deficits in limb apraxia. *Brain* **117,** 1093–1106.
20. Poizner, H., Clark, M.A., Merians, A.S., Macauley, B., Gonzalez Rothi, L.J., and Heilman, K.M. (1995) Joint coordination deficits in limb apraxia. *Brain* **118,** 227–242.
21. Leiguarda, R., Merello, M., and Balej, J. (2000) Apraxia in corticobasal degeneration, in *Corticobasal Degeneration and Related Disorders. Advances in Neurology,* vol. 82 (Litvan, I., Goetz, C.G., and Lang, A., eds.), Lippincott, Williams &Wilkins, Philadelphia, pp. 103–121.
22. Caselli, R.J., Stelmach, G.E., Caviness, J.V., et al. (1999) A kinematic study of progressive apraxia with and without dementia. *Mov. Disord.* **14,** 276–287.
23. Haaland, K.Y. and Flaherty, D. (1984) The different types of limb apraxia errors made by patients with left vs. right hemisphere damage. *Brain Cogn.* **3,** 370–384.
24. Rapcsak, S.Z., Ochipa, C., Beeson, P.M., and Rubens, A. (1993) Apraxia and the right hemisphere. *Brain Cogn.* **23,** 181–202.
25. Rushworth, M.F.S., Nixon, P.D., Wade, D.T., Renowden, S., and Passingham, R.E. (1998) The left hemisphere and the selection of learned actions. *Neuropsychologia* **36,** 11–24.
26. Ochipa, C., Rothi, L.J.G., and Heilman, K.M. (1992) Conceptual apraxia in Alzheimer's Disease. *Brain* **115,** 1061–1071.
27. De Renzi, E. and Lucchelli, F. (1988) Ideational apraxia. *Brain* **113**, 1173–1188.
28. Heilman, K.M., Maher, L.H., Greenwald, L., and Rothi, L.J. (1997) Conceptual apraxia from lateralized lesions. *Neurology* **49,** 457–464.
29. Pramstaller, P.P. and Marsden, C.D. (1996) The basal ganglia and apraxia [review]. *Brain* **119,** 319–340.
30. Leiguarda, R. (2001) Limb-apraxia: cortical or subcortical. *Neuroimage* **14,** 5137–5141.
31. Kleist, K. (1907) Kortikate (innervatorische) Apraxie. *J. Psychiatr. Neurol.* **25,** 46–112.
32. Kleist, K. (1931) Gehirnpathologische und lokalisatorische Ergebnisse: das Stirnhirn im engeren Sinne und seine Störungen. *Z. ges Neurol. und Psychiat.* **131,** 442–448.
33. Faglioni, P. and Basso, A. (1985) Historical perspectives on neuroanatomical correlates of limb apraxia, in *Neuropsychological Studies of Apraxia and Relates Disorders* (Roy, E.A., ed.), Elsevier Science Publishers B.V., Amsterdam, The Netherlands, pp. 3–44.
34. Denes, G., Mantovan, M.C., Gallana, A., and Cappelletti, J.V. (1998) Limb-kinetic apraxia. *Mov. Disord.* **13,** 468–476.
35. Blasi, V., Labruna, L., Soricelli, A., and Carlomagno, S. (1999) Limb-kinetic apraxia: a neuropsychological description. *Neurocase* **5,** 201–211.

36. Leiguarda, R., Merello, M., Nouzeilles, M.I., Balej, J., Rivero, A., and Nogués, M. (2001) Limb-kinetic apraxia: clinical and kinematic features. *Mol. Disord.,* in press.
37. Jacobs, D.H., Adair, J.C., Macauley, B.L., Gold, M., Gonzalez Rothi, L.J., and Heilman, K.M. (1999) Apraxia in corticobasal degeneration. *Brain Cogn.* **40,** 336–354.
38. Pillon, B., Blin, J., Vadailhet, M., et al. (1995) The neuropsychological pattern of corticobasal degeneration: comparison with supranuclear palsy and Alzheimer's disease. *Neurology* **45,** 1477–1483.
39. Blondel, A., Eustache, F., Schaeffer, S., Maire, R., Lechvalier B., and Sayette, V. (1997) Etudie clinique et cognitive de l'apraxie dans l'atrophie cortico-basale. *Rev. Neurol.* (Paris) **153,** 737–747.
40. Graham, N.L., Zenan, A., Young, A.W., Patterson, K., and Hodges, J.R. (1999) Dyspraxia in a patient with corticobasal degeneration: the role of visual and tactile inputs to action. *J. Neurol. Neurosurg. Psychiatry* **67,** 334–344.
41. Okuda, B., Tachibana, H., Kawabata, K., Takeda, M., and Sugita, M. (1992) Slowly progressive limb-kinetic apraxia with a decrease in unilateral cerebral blood flow. *Acta Neurol. Scand.* **86,** 76–81.
42. Kertesz, A., Martínez-Lange, P., Davidson, W., and Muñoz, D.G. (2000) The corticobasal degeneration síndrome overlaps progressive aphasia and frontotemporal dementia. *Neurology* **14,** 1368–1375.
43. Ozsancak, C., Auzou, P., and Hannequin, D. (2000) Dysarthria and orofacial apraxia in corticobasal degeneration. *Mov. Disord.* **15,** 905–910.
44. Sharpe, M.H., Cermak, S.A., and Sax, D.S. (1983) Motor planning in Parkinson patients. *Neuropsychologia* **21,** 455–462.
45. Goldenberg, G., Wimmer, A., Auff, E., and Schnaberth, G. (1986) Impairment of motor planning in patients with Parkinson's disease: evidence for ideomotor apraxia texting. *J. Neurol. Neurosurg. Psychiatry* **49,** 1266–1272.
46. Grossman, M., Carbell, S., Gollomp, S., Stern, M.B., Bernon, G., and Hurtig, H.I. (1991) Sentence comprehension and praxis deficits in Parkinson's disease. *Neurology* **41,** 1620–1626.
47. Leiguarda, R., Merello, M., Balej, J., Starkstein, S., Nogués, M., and Marsden, C.D. (2000) Disruption of spatial organization and interjoint coordination in Parkinson's disease, progressive supranuclear palsy and multiple system atrophy. *Mov. Disord.* **15,** 627–640.
48. Cambier, J., Masson, M., Viader, F., Limodin, J., and Strube, A. (1985) Le syndrome frontal de la paralysie supranucléaire progressive. *Rev. Neurol.* (Paris) **141,** 528–536.
49. Collins S.J., Ahlskog, J.E., Parisi, J.E., and Maraganore, D.M. (1995) Progressive supranuclear palsy: neuropathologically based diagnostic clinical criteria. *J. Neurol. Neurosurg. Psychiatry* **58,** 167–173.
50. Bergeron, C., Pollamen, M.S., Weyer, L., and Lang, A.E. (1997) Cortical degeneration in progressive supranuclear palsy. A comparison with cortical-basal ganglionic degeneration. *J. Neuropathol. Exp. Neurol.* **56,** 726–734.
51. Jeannerod, M. (1966) Cortical coding of visual object attributes during object-oriented behaviour, in *Vision and Movements Mechanisms in the Cerebral Cortex* (Caminitti, R., Hoffmann, K.P., Lacquanti, F., and Altman, J., eds.), Human Frontier Science Program, Strasbourg, pp. 15–23.
52. Rizzolatti, G., Luppino, G., and Matelli, M. (1998) The organization of the cortical motor system: new concepts [review]. *Electroencephalogr. Clin. Neurophysiol.* **106,** 283–296.
53. Burnod, Y., Baraduc, P., Battaglia, A., et al. (1999) Parieto-frontal coding of reaching: an integrated framework. *Exp. Brain Res.* **129,** 325–346.
54. Jeannerod, M., Arbid, M.A., Rizzolatti, G., and Sakata, H. (1995) Grasping objects: the cortical mechanisms of visuomotor transformation. *Trends Neurosci.* **18,** 314–320.
55. Rizzolatti, G., Camarda, R., Fogassi, M., Gentilucci, M., Luppino, G., and Matelli, M. (1988) Functional organization of inferior area 6 in the macaque monkey: II Area F5 and the control of distal movements. *Exp. Brain Res.* **71,** 491–507.
56. Pandya, D. and Kuypers, H.G. (1969) Cortico-cortical connections in the rhesus monkeys. *Brain Res.* **13,** 13–36.
57. Sakata, H., Taira, M., Mine, S., and Murata, A. (1992) Hand-movements related neurons of the posterior parietal cortex of the monkey: their role in visual guidance of hand movements, in *Control of Arm Movements in Space: Neurophysiological and Computational Approaches* (Caminiti, R., Johnson, P.B., and Burnod, Y., eds.), Springer, Berlin, pp. 185–198.
58. Binkofski, F., Buccino, G., Posse, S., Seitz, R.J., Rizzolatti, G., and Freund, H.J. (1999) A fronto-parietal circuit for object manipulation in man: evidence from an fMRI study. *Eur. J. Neurosci.* **11,** 3276–3286.
59. Alexander, G.E., DeLong, M.R., and Strick, P.L. (1986) Parallel organization of functionally segregated circuits linking basal ganglia and cortex. *Ann. Rev. Neurosci.* **9,** 357–381.
60. Yeterian, E.H. and Pandya, D.N. (1993) Striatal connections of the parietal association cortices in rhesus monkeys. *J. Comp. Neurol.* **332,** 175–197.
61. Dickson, D.W., Liu, W.K., Reding, H.K., and Yen, S.H. (2000) Neuropathologic and molecular considerations, in *Corticobasal Degeneration and Related Disorders. Advances in Neurology,* vol. 82 (Litvan, I., Goetz, C.G., and Lang, A.E., eds.), Lippincott, Williams & Wilkins, Philadelphia, pp. 9–28.
62. Brooks, D.J. (2000) Functional imaging studies in corticobasal degeneration, in *Corticobasal Degeneration and Related Disorders. Advances in Neurology,* vol. 82 (Litvan, I., Goetz, C.G., and Lang, A.E., eds.), Lippincott, Williams & Wilkins, Philadelphia, pp. 209–216.
63. Daniel, S.E., de Bruin, V., and Lees, A.J. (1995) The clinical and pathological spectrum of Steele-Richardson-Olszewski syndrome (progressive supranuclear palsy): a reappraises [review]. *Brain* **118,** 759–770.
64. Rinne, J., Portin, R., Ruottinen, H., et al. (2000) Cognitive impairment and the brain dopaminergic system in Parkinson disease. *Arch. Neurol.* **57,** 470–475.
65. Hu, M.T.M., Taylor-Robinson, S.D., Ray Chaudhuri, K., et al. (1999). Evidence for cortical dysfunction in clinically non-demented patients with Parkinson's disease: a proton MR spectroscopy study. *J. Neurol. Neurosurg. Psychiatry* **67,** 20–26.

11
Neuropsychological Deficits in Cerebellar Syndromes

Hermann Ackermann, MD, MA and Irene Daum, PhD

1. INTRODUCTION

Based on ablation experiments in a variety of subhuman species, Rolando (1809) proposed cerebellar lesions to compromise motor functions but to spare the sensory and intellectual domains (for a review, see refs. *1,2*). The seminal work of Gordon Holmes on the clinical sequels of posterior fossa pathology in humans during the first two decades of the 20th century corroborated this concept. Sporadic case reports pointing to a possible contribution of cerebellar dysfunctions to the development of dementia went rather unnoticed or were considered to reflect concomitant supratentorial disorders. Snider (1950) first called for a broader concept emphasizing modulation of the limbic and autonomic system by the cerebellum. This notion has received some empirical support by clinical observations of affective abnormalities in patients with cerebellar disorders. During the past decade, considerable interest in eventual contributions of the cerebellum to cognition, beyond the realm of vegetative functions and emotional behavior, emerged. First, the extensive reciprocal cerebellar connections with various areas of supratentorial association cortex provide the anatomical prerequisites for any modulatory influences on cognitive functions *(3)*. Second, Ivry and Keele *(4)* were able to document a distinct perceptual deficit in cerebellar patients. Third, the seminal positron emission tomography (PET) studies of Petersen and coworkers *(5)* revealed right hemisphere hemodynamic responses to lexical operations at the level of the cerebellum.

The following paragraphs aim at a critical evaluation of the empirical evidence indicating a distinct contribution of the cerebellum in nonmotor functions. Classical conditioning of eyelid reactions or motor skill acquisition will not be considered, since participation of cerebellar structures in these activities is well-established *(6)*. Emotional and affective abnormalities associated with cerebellar lesions are not covered either (see Chapter 5 of this book and ref. *7* for detailed reviews on these topics).

2. MENTAL RETARDATION AND BEHAVIORAL ABNORMALITIES IN CEREBELLAR MALFORMATIONS

Because of a rather long course of maturation, developmental abnormalities of the cerebellum are not uncommon. Assuming cerebellar participation in nonmotor functions, an impaired intellectual status of subjects with partial (vermis, either hemisphere) or complete aplasia of that organ must be expected. Indeed, most cases presented with signs of intellectual retardation. Nevertheless, cerebellar aplasia not necessarily yields cognitive deficits compromising activities of daily life: sometimes these conditions incidentally were detected at postmortem examination in patients who had achieved normal age in the absence of a history of disordered motor coordination or mental disruption (for a

From: *Mental and Behavioral Dysfunction in Movement Disorders*
Edited by: M-A. Bédard et al. © Humana Press Inc., Totowa, NJ

review, see refs. *2,8*). Thus, even the most severe variants of a cerebellar malformation characterized by small amounts of undifferentiated tissue within the posterior fossa may fail to cause intellectual retardation or behavioral abnormalities.

Children with cerebellar hypoplasia in terms of a reduced volume of more or less the entire organ often present with mental disorders. However, structural anomalies of the brainstem and/or supratentorial structures have been documented in several variants of this constellation, e.g., pontoneocerebellar hypoplasia or Gillespie-syndrome. If at all, primary degeneration of the granular layer represents a malformation fairly restricted to the cerebellum. Apart from congenital ataxia, these subjects, as a rule, have been reported to exhibit intellectual deficits. Nevertheless, the available data fail to establish a firm causal relationship between mental retardation and cerebellar hypoplasia. For example, even in cases with unaltered supratentorial structures at macroscopic examination, histoanatomic abnormalities of the cerebral cortex comparable to those in oligophrenia have been observed.

3. INTELLECTUAL DETERIORATION IN CEREBELLAR LESIONS AND DISEASES WITH CLINICAL MANIFESTATION IN ADULTHOOD

Hereditary as well as idiopathic degenerative cerebellar ataxias have been reported eventually to give rise to dementia. In most of these cases, however, the disease process extended beyond the cerebellum. The majority of patients with damage restricted to cerebellar structures as confirmed at postmortem examination, furthermore, had no history of intellectual decline. Finally, progressive mental deterioration in more advanced age, many years after onset of ataxia, could be attributed to generalized cerebrovascular disease (for a review, see ref. *2*). Ischemia restricted to the cerebellum does not seem to result in dementia. Similarly, there is little evidence that cerebellar tumors, which do not affect adjacent structures, lead to global cognitive impairment. Indeed, a large clinical study reported "psychological changes" in about one-third of the patients with cerebellar tumors. Given the nature of the problems (confusional states or psychomotor slowing), these deficits reflect raised intracranial pressure rather than selective cerebellar dysfunction.

4. MORPHOLOGICAL ABNORMALITIES OF THE CEREBELLUM IN PSYCHOPATHOLOGICAL AND BEHAVIORAL DISORDERS

Electrical stimulation of cerebellar structures modulates the activity of neurons in various regions of the forebrain, such as the septal nuclei. Therefore, this procedure had been considered a therapeutical option for the alleviation of behavioral abnormalities in otherwise intractable patients. During implantation of cerebellar pacemakers, Heath and coworkers *(9)* first noted gross pathological changes of the vermis in subjects with functional psychosis such as schizophrenia. Whereas several computerized tomography (CT) studies reported atrophy of cerebellar midline structures in at least a subgroup of the schizophrenic patients, unrelated to alcohol intake or neuroleptic medication, other CT and magnetic resonance imaging (MRI) investigations, however, failed to corroborate these findings or observed significantly reduced volume in male subjects only. Even an enlarged size of the vermis in schizophrenic patients as compared to control subjects has been reported *(10)*. Besides CT and MRI data, the available neuropathological postmortem investigations also yielded inconsistent findings. Apart from its questionable pathophysiological significance, a higher prevalence of vermal atrophy in schizophrenia has not yet been established so far. Furthermore, patients with cerebellar ataxia apparently do not show an increased incidence of psychotic syndromes, and the sporadic ataxic subjects with concomitant psychiatric disorders published in the literature also exhibited signs of extracerebellar dysfunctions (see ref. *2*).

The syndrome of early infantile autism, among others, is characterized by atypical social interactions, disordered cognitive skills, and an obsessive insistence on sameness. Among others, a cerebellar contribution to the development of this syndrome has been discussed. A neuropathological single-case study by Bauman and Kemper (1985) (for a review, see Bauman et al. *[11]*) first documented histoanatomic abnormalities both at the level of the limbic system and the cerebellum. Subsequent microscopic investigations of a series of brains obtained from autistic subjects revealed a reduced number of Purkinje cells, either throughout the cerebellum or restricted to the two hemispheres. Absence of any significant glial hyperplasia and missing retrograde loss of inferior olivary neurons indicates that the observed cerebellar abnormalities in autism must have emerged early in development, i.e., prior to wk 30 of gestation. However, structural abnormalities also could be documented at the level of the forebrain. Any inferences, therefore, on a causal relationship between cerebellar pathology, on the one hand, and behavioral abnormalities, as well as cognitive deficits, on the other, are still premature. So far, in vivo morphometric analyses of the cerebellum in autistic subjects using MRI technology yielded inconsistent data. Courchesne and coworkers *(12)* first reported hypoplasia of vermal lobules VI and VII (taxonomy of Larsell). Several following investigations of a similar design failed, however, to detect any significant volume reduction of these structures (for a review, see Bauman et al. *[11]*). Only a subgroup of autistic patients showed any evidence of vermian atrophy, which, when present, did not correlate with the severity of autistic symptoms. Beyond that and most importantly, the MRI findings of vermal hypoplasia in autism are at variance with the available microanatomic findings. Furthermore, a recent structural MRI study documented grey matter alterations in a variety of supratentorial parts of the brain *(13)*. Thus, the various cognitive and behavioral abnormalities cannot unambiguously be assigned to morphological alterations of the cerebellum.

Neuropsychological investigations suggest compromised executive functions, in terms of a failure to inhibit or delay behavioral responses, to be the core pathomechanism of attention-deficit hyperactivity disorder (ADHD). Assuming cerebellar participation in these cognitive domains, structural and/or biochemical alterations of infratentorial structures must be expected. Morphometric MRI studies found a significantly decreased volume of the inferior posterior vermis (lobules VIII to X) in male patients *(14)*. Fragile X syndrome, a constellation resembling mutism in some aspects, also seems to be characterized by a reduced size of this area, more so in male than in female subjects *(15)*. However, these components of the cerebellum are predominantly interconnected with the spinal cord and the vestibular system rather than the forebrain *(16)*. Thus, the relevance of structural alterations at the level of the posterior inferior vermis with respect to any cognitive deficits needs further clarification. In addition to language-related difficulties, dyslexic subjects may exhibit cerebellar-like motor disorders and time estimation deficits. In line with these suggestions, MR spectroscopy provided some evidence for biochemical cerebellar asymmetries in male patients *(17)*. Morphometric alterations in dyslexia at the level of the cerebellum have not yet been reported.

5. FORMAL NEUROPSYCHOLOGICAL TESTING OF PATIENTS WITH DEGENERATIVE DISEASES OR ISCHEMIC LESIONS OF THE CEREBELLUM

5.1. *Introduction*

The following review focuses on degenerative diseases and ischemic lesions of the cerebellum. In case of careful patient selection, these constellations provide a feasible clinical model of cerebellar dysfunctions. Whereas investigations from the early 1990s often included subjects with extracerebellar signs and symptoms (see below), more recent studies are based on subjects with pathology restricted to that organ, as determined by clinical and neuroradiologcal data. Friedreich's ataxia was excluded from the following analyses, since this entity compromises the cerebellar cortex only in later stages of the disease. Recent molecular genetic techniques established a classification of spinocerebellar ataxias based on the chromosomal position of the relevant mutation(s). As a rule, the available neuropsychological studies in degenerative cerebellar disorders do not refer to these criteria. Therefore, molecular genetic classification of spinocerebellar ataxias will not be further considered.

5.2. General Intellectual Abilities and Declarative Memory Functions

As degenerative cerebellar diseases have occasionally been reported to give rise to dementia, the investigation of intellectual capacities in these patients by means of standardized neuropsychological tests is of considerable interest. Although some studies reported reduced scores of either the verbal or both the verbal and performance subtests of the Wechsler Adult Intelligence Scale-Revised *(18–20)*, other investigations found scores in the normal or even the superior range *(21–23)*. Since the former investigations also included patients with signs of extracerebellar pathology, the observed deficits of general intellectual functions might be, in a similar vein as clinical observations of dementia in congenital and acquired ataxic syndromes, contingent upon the presence of extracerebellar dysfunctions. A more recent study in subjects with cerebellar infarctions corroborates these suggestions: as a group, these patients were unimpaired with respect to verbal and nonverbal intelligence *(24)*.

Declarative memory functions, e.g., word list recall, were largely found intact in several studies on patients with cerebellar degeneration or infarct *(19,21–24)*. At some variance with these data, a recent investigation of paired associates learning found subjects suffering from isolated cerebellar degeneration significantly impaired *(25)*.

5.3. Time Estimation in Auditory, Visual, and Somatosensory Modalities

For the first time, Ivry and Keele *(4)* observed disrupted time perception in patients with cerebellar pathology; these subjects performed worse as compared to healthy and clinical controls when asked to compare two successive intervals bound by clicks each, the second stimulus being either shorter or longer than the first one. Subsequent studies corroborated these findings and documented, in addition, impaired representation of temporal information within the somatosensory and visual domains *(26)*. Since at least some cerebellar motor deficits, e.g., enlarged variability of finger tapping in response to external stimuli, might be due to disordered central timing mechanisms, the cerebellum was considered an "internal clock" ("generalized timing hypothesis" *[26]*) subserving precise representations of temporal information across motor and sensory functions (see Subheading 6.1.).

5.4. Visuospatial Abilities

The reciprocal connections between the cerebellum and the parietal cortex provide the theoretical basis for the suggestion of a cerebellar participation in visuospatial capabilities. So far, only a few empirical studies addressing these issues are available. Both deficient visuospatial recall and impaired visuospatial manipulations have been documented in patients with cerebellar pathology. Furthermore, children who had undergone resection of a left hemisphere cerebellar tumor were found impaired in visual sequential memory as compared both to controls and peers with contralateral pathology *(27)*. Other investigatiors, however, did not observe visuospatial processing deficits in adult patient samples. In this regard, investigations based on more comprehensive test batteries including all the relevant various subcomponents of higher order visual functons are needed (for a review, see ref. *8*).

5.5. Working Memory and Anticipatory Planning

Since cerebellar projections target the frontal lobes and vice versa, the idea of a "frontal-like" impairment of executive functions in posterior fossa pathology has received considerable interest. Furthermore, a multitude of neuroimaging studies has, thus far, documented a functional relationship between these areas of the brain. Anticipatory planning, as assessed by the Tower of Hanoi test, was found to be impaired in cerebellar atrophy patients *(28)*; these subjects solved fewer problems and needed more time to plan their moves. Cerebellar patients did not show perseverative tendencies or other deficits on the Wisconsin card sorting test, a traditional probe of frontal lobe function *(19,21,23)*.

The severe problems of cerebellar subjects in shifting attention between modalities, however, would be consistent with impaired cerebellofrontal interactions giving rise, e.g., to deficient implementation of the "frontal" plan to change attentional behavior *(20)*.

Several studies found cerebellar patients by and large unimpaired with respect to short-term memory functions in terms of word and digit spans (for a review, see ref. *8*). A recent investigation of subjects suffering from infratentorial infarction corroborated these findings *(24)*. However, more complex task conditions, i.e., repetition of words while subjects simultaneously tried to analyze sentences ("listening span task"), significantly compromised performance. Obviously, therefore, short-term or working memory functions in cerebellar disorders depend on load effects.

5.6. Implicit (Procedural) Learning

Patients with degenerative cerebellar disease were found impaired at acquiring visuomotor associations in a serial reaction time task *(29)*. Furthermore, subjects who had suffered predominantly unilateral focal damage to the cerebellum exhibited slowed procedural learning of a motor sequence within the context of a similar paradigm *(30)*. Since the changes in reaction time measurements were not separately analyzed for movement initiation and execution components, it is difficult to rule out an eventual contribution of motor performance deficits (e.g., differential fatigue effects). Some theoretical accounts have suggested that the cerebellar participation in skill acquisition may not be limited to motor learning, but may extend into the domain of nonmotor learning paradigms. However, a controlled group study found normal performance of cerebellar patients on standard perceptual and cognitive skill learning tasks (mirror reading, tower of Hanoi test) *(23)*.

5.7. Verbal Fluency Tasks and Verbal Response Selection

Verbal fluency tasks require subjects to name as many items of a certain category (semantic rule) or words starting with a certain letter (orthographic–phonological rule) under time constraints. Two early patient studies reported compromised performance in both domains *(20,22)*. However, a subsequent investigation did not corroborate these findings (see ref. *26*). So far, Molinari and coworkers *(30)* conducted the most comprehensive study in this regard utilizing three distinct cerebellar patient groups (atrophy of mainly vermal and paravermal regions and focal lesions restricted to lateral parts of either hemisphere). As a group, the cerebellar subjects scored at a lower level than their matched controls, the orthographic–phonological task being more severely compromised. Furthermore, patients suffering from predominant atrophy of midline structures were found less impaired than those with more lateralized lesions in spite of more severe ataxia. Finally, the right-focal group performed worse than patients with left-sided cerebellar damage. These findings provide first evidence for a differential role of midline and lateral structures of the cerebellum in verbal fluency tasks and indicate phonological processing predominantly to be related to the right hemisphere.

A PET study by Petersen and coworkers *(5)* first documented a contribution of the cerebellum to lexical operations. Among others, these authors asked their subjects to (*i*) overtly repeat a visually presented noun and (*ii*) generate a semantically associated verb in response to the same lexical items and to utter this verb aloud. Subtracting the hemodynamic responses to the first task from the activation pattern bound to the second one should allow, within some limits, the identification of the areas subserving verbal response generation or response selection. Under these conditions, a hemodynamic response of the lateral aspects of the right cerebellum, concomitant with left frontal structures adjacent to Broca's area, could be noted. A subsequent single-case study corroborated the suggestion of cerebellar participation in word generation and/or selection *(21)*. Despite high-level conversational skills and normal performance on standard language tests, such as various components of the Boston Diagnostic Aphasia Exam, the patient with right hemisphere cerebellar infarction was found impaired in a semantic word generation task and did not show any clear evidence of learning with increasing practice.

6. SPEECH–LANGUAGE PATHOLOGY IN CEREBELLAR DISORDERS

6.1. Speech Perception

Within some limits, distinct features of the acoustic signal characterize the various classes of speech sounds (phonemes) of any language system. Among others, durational parameters contribute to phoneme specification. For example, syllables with initial voiced and unvoiced stop consonant, such as /da/ and /ta/, differ in voice onset time (VOT), i.e., the time interval between initial burst and vowel onset (see Subheading 5.3.). The generalized timing hypothesis predicts impaired discrimination or identification of verbal utterances in cerebellar subjects given that phonological processing depends upon precise representation of temporal information. Phoneme-boundary effects should provide a feasible test of this hypothesis. As a rule, a series of syllables or words varying in a distinct durational parameter are perceived in a categorical manner. Thus, English-speaking adults asked to label monosyllabic stimuli ranging in VOT from –150 ms, yielding the percept /da/, to +150 ms, recognized as /ta/, show a rather abrupt shift between these two responses at a value of about +35 ms. Assuming impaired representation of temporal information, cerebellar pathology must be expected to compromise the phoneme-boundary effect in speech perception. At variance with this suggestion, similar identification curves across a continuum of verbal utterances varying in VOT of the initial stop consonant have been observed in cerebellar subjects and their controls *(31)*. However, the encoding of durational parameters of the acoustic speech signal does not necessarily require an explicit time representation. It is well established that listeners may utilize all available acoustic cues during phonological encoding. Besides VOT, the sound energy of the aspiration phase, i.e., the loudness of this noise segment, contributes to the perceived voicing contrast of stop consonants (see ref. *31* for additional references). Thus, categorical voicing distinction just might reflect backword masking; aspiration noise must exceed a given intensity threshold in order to be detected.

The English word rapid is characterized by a short period of silence (occlusion time [OT]) signaling the intraword stop consonant /p/. Variation of OT from 20–130 ms gives rise to a phoneme-boundary effect; long intraword pauses yield the percept rapid, whereas short OTs lead to the recognition of rabbit, with a rather abrupt transition from one response type to the other in-between. Under these conditions, listeners cannot make use of sound intensity parameters. It must be expected, therefore, that word recognition solely depends upon encoding of a durational acoustic cue, i.e., OT concomitant with the intraword stop consonants /p/ and /b/. Using a German analogue of the *r*abbit/rapid paradigm (Boten, /boddn/ (= long OT), "messengers" versus Boden, /bodn/ (= short OT), "floor"), patients with diffuse cerebellar atrophy, indeed, failed to exhibit any significant phoneme-boundary effect *(31)*. In accordance with the general timing hypothesis, cerebellar dysfunctions, thus, seem selectively to compromise temporal aspects of speech perception *(32)*.

Functional compartmentalization represents a widely established principle of cerebellar organization. In order to further delineate the subsystem participating in speech perception, functional MRI (fMRI) measurements were performed using again the Boten/Boden series as test material *(32a)*. In order to exclude any interferences with other cognitive functions, a carefully selected control situation was added that just differed in the temporal structure of the stimuli, everything else being equalized. Functional imaging data point at a possible contribution of the cerebellum to distinct lexical operations *(33)*. Furthermore, this organ has been suggested to participate in the regulation of attentional resources as well as executive functions *(20)*. Hierarchical subtraction designs comparing phonetic discrimination with passive listening to acoustic stimuli or encoding of nonspeech auditory materials as a control condition may, thus, be confounded by interactions with other processes *(26)*. The control condition takes advantage of the fact that a given sound category may often be cued by more than a single acoustic feature (trading relations). Apart from OT, the difference in sound structure between the lexical items Boten and Boden soley can be signaled by the VOT of the wordmedial stop consonants /t/ and /d/ (/Bo:t^{h}en/ versus /Bo:den/, the /t/-sound of /Bo:t^{h}en/ being characterized by a short aspiration noise). Therefore, a second series of verbal utterances with constant OT, but systematically varying in wordmedial VOT, was generated. Thus, subjects had to discriminate the same lexical items, i.e., Boten versus Boden, either by analysis of a durational parameter (experimental condition) or a noise segment (control condition). As expected, subtraction of the hemodynamic responses to the VOT series from the activation pattern obtained during application of the OT series yielded a circumscript activation focus within the lateral parts of the right cerebellar hemisphere. There is, thus, convergent evidence from a clinical group study and a functional imaging investigation for a specific contribution of the cerebellum to word recognition in terms of the encoding of temporal speech features.

6.2. *Agrammatic Speech Production*

Silveri et al. *(34)* reported for the first time signs of agrammatic speech, concomitant with slightly reduced verbal fluency, subsequent to a large ischemic lesion within the right cerebellar hemisphere. Repeated CT and MRI failed to detect any relevant supratentorial structural abnormalities accounting for the observed linguistic deficits. The patient's speech utterances were characterized by omissions of free-standing grammatic morphemes and use of infinitive in place of inflected forms. Apart from the deficient morphologic component of spontaneous speech, language examination otherwise was entirely unremarkable. A similar case study of rather exclusive agrammatism, in terms of short telegraphic sentences during spontaneous speech characterized by frequent omissions of function words and grammatical morphemes in the presence of unimpaired auditory comprehension and written language, has been published by Zettin and coworkers *(35)*.

More recent models of syntax processing assume that the production of grammatically correct sentences requires orderly integration of a variety of separate linguistic functions bound to different neural circuits. Based on these suggestions, Molinari et al. *(30)* considered the cerebellum an "interarea functional coordinator" subserving precisely timed sequential organization of verbal utterances. Cerebellar agrammatism, thus, might reflect temporal dissociation, due to compromised articulatory planning processes, between the application of syntactic rules and the availability of grammatical morphemes temporarily stored in working memory *(35)*. As an alternative explanation, "crossed cerebral diaschisis," i.e., a decrease of blood flow, supposedly reflecting functional suppression, within the contralateral cerebral cortex subsequent to a cerebellar lesion, must be taken into account. Whereas structural neuroimaging failed to detect any evidence for supratentorial lesions in the two case studies referred to, single-photon emission computerized tomography (SPECT) revealed, however, marked hypoperfusion of the entire dominant hemisphere. During further follow-up, improvement of language deficits was paralleled by an increase of left hemisphere cerebral perfusion.

6.3. *Aphasic Disorders Subsequent to Right Hemisphere Cerebellar Dysfunctions*

Apart from rather exclusive agrammatism *(34,35)* or deficient word generation *(21)*, patients with right hemisphere cerebellar infarction may show a profile of speech–language pathology resembling transcortical motor or amnesic aphasia *(36–39)*. Hassid *(36)* first provided evidence that crossed cerebral diaschisis also might account for these more extensive constellations of disrupted verbal communication. Besides signs of ataxia, the 17-yr-old left-handed man showed moderate anomia, mildly impaired speech comprehension and reading performance, as well as severe difficulties in writing and mathematics subsequent to a wedge-shaped right-sided infarct of the cerebellum. Structural imaging (CT and MRI) failed to disclose any relevant supratentorial lesions. In contrast, SPECT revealed, in addition to the contralateral cerebellar hemisphere, relative hypoperfusion at the level of frontal, temporal, and parietal regions of the dominant cortex. These observations were corroborated by a follow-up study of Marien and coworkers *(37,38)* documenting a rather parallel development of speech–language pathology, on the one hand, and perfusion patterns, on the other, in a 73-yr-old right-handed patient with ischemic infarction in the vascular territory of the right superior cerebellar artery. A striking dissociation between severe diminution of spontaneous speech and rather well-preserved "imposed" language during naming and repetition tasks concomitant with unimpaired comprehension of daily language, a constellation resembling transcortical motor aphasia, evolved during a period of 2 d after onset of clinical signs of posterior fossa dysfunction. The sparse self-generated verbal utterances were characterized by considerable word-finding difficulties as well as expressive and receptive agrammatism. Again, structural imaging studies (CT and MRI) did not reveal any relevant supratentorial lesions, whereas, however, SPECT investigations documented marked hypoperfusion within the right cerebellar hemisphere and at the level of the contralateral cerebral cortex encroaching on middle and inferior frontal gyri as well as pre- and postcentral areas. Parallel to the improvement of speech–language pathology, left frontoparietal perfusion patterns had significantly increased at follow-up investigations 6 mo and 5 yr after infarction.

6.4. Transient Cerebellar Mutism

The "fossa posterior syndrome" or "transient cerebellar mutism with subsequent dysarthria" predominantly occurs in children subsequent to resection of a hindbrain tumor, especially at the level of the cerebellar vermis (incidence up to 15%). Sporadically, this constellation also may be observed in adults (for a review, see ref. *40*). Apart from surgery, transient cerebellar mutism could be documented in association with traumatic injuries as well as viral cerebellitis. Disrupted speech production, frequently associated with a variety of further behavioral abnormalities, typically develops within a time interval of one to several days after surgical intervention. Initial speechlessness may evolve either into a syndrome of predominant dysarthria or a constellation of agrammatism concomitant with diminished speech initiation and prosodic abnormalities (flattened intonation), auditory speech comprehension, as well as repetition capabilities being well-preserved under both conditions *(27)*.

Bilateral lesions of the anterior mesiofrontal cortex may give rise to the syndrome of akinetic mutism. Furthermore, damage to left hemisphere supplementary motor area and/or the respective projections to the anterior perisylvian "language zone" may yield impaired spontaneous speech production resembling the syndrome of transcortical motor aphasia *(41)*. Therefore, the connections of the mesiofrontal cortex to the anteror perisylvian language zone have been assumed to subserve motivational aspects of verbal communication and/or speech initiation mechanisms. Dependent upon lesion site, i.e., closeness to Broca's area, further linguistic deficits have been observed. Based on these considerations, transient cerebellar mutism might reflect a diaschisis effect at the level of dorsolateral prefrontal and/or mesiofrontal cortex. Accordingly, a follow-up study by Marien and coworkers *(40)* in several children who underwent resection of a fossa posterior tumor revealed a close correlation between frontal-like neurobehavioral dysfunctions and location, as well as the degree of crossed cerebral diaschisis. For instance, SPECT disclosed severe bifrontal hypoperfusion in a 10-yr-old right-handed boy during a 3-wk period of akinetic mutism after resection of a astrocytoma. Subsequent to initial speechlessness, he displayed dynamic aphasia, agrammatism, and slight behavioral alterations. Repeated SPECT still documented bilateral frontal perfusion deficits, being now, however, significantly more pronounced at the left side.

7. CONCLUSIONS

Even the most severe variants of a cerebellar malformation may fail to cause mental retardation, compromising activities of daily life. Furthermore, diseases or lesions of the cerebellum with a clinical manifestation in adulthood do not necessarily give rise to overt cognitive decline. In line with these clinical data, formal neuropsychological testing in patients with pathology restricted to the cerebellum did not provide conclusive evidence for significant deterioration of global intellectual abilities.

As concerns speech–language pathology, it is well-established that cerebellar disorders may give rise to ataxic dysarthria characterized by compromised articulatory and phonatory functions *(42)*. Sporadically, linguistic deficits beyond the domain of speech motor control, e.g., agrammatism, word finding difficulties, dysgraphia, or transcortical motor aphasia, arise subsequent to lesions restricted to the cerebellum. Transient mutism following resection of posterior fossa tumors may evolve into similar language disorders. Preliminary perfusion studies provide first evidence for "crossed cerebral diaschisis" as a possible mechanism of impaired linguistic capabilities subsequent to cerebellar disorders *(40)*. The observed deficits, thus, seem to reflect suppression of the frontal "language zones" rather than disruption of inherent cerebellar functions.

So far, formal neuropsychological studies addressing learning and memory functions or executive capacities yielded, even in patient groups with well-documented pathology restricted to the cerebellum, controversial findings, e.g., with respect to paired associates learning or problem solving. Conceivably, severity of cerebellar pathology accounts for the observed discepancies. Differences in task demands or experimental constraints must be considered an alternative explanation (e.g., a recent investigation found short-term memory dysfunctions in cerebellar patients to depend upon load effects). The specific role of the cerebellum in these complex nonmotor tasks remains to be established *(26)*.

Several well-controlled group studies indicate participation of the cerebellum in perceptual tasks requiring precise representation of temporal information. Among others, encoding of durational parameters of verbal utterances has been found to hinge upon cerebellar structures. Thus, under these conditions, the auditory cortex might join up with cerebellar structures in order to facilitate processing of spoken language. In line with these suggestions, functional imaging revealed activation of the right cerebellar hemisphere in association with the encoding of temporal speech information during word recognition tasks.

Speech sound categories (phonemes) are considered the building blocks of the word forms of the mental lexicon. These entities are not specified in terms of distinct VOT or OT values, but rather abstract phonetic features, such as "+/– voicing." However, inner speech (auditory imagery) or working memory rehearsal mechanisms might require, within some limits, the encoding of the temporal structures of word and sentence forms. Durational parameters represent a basic and ubiquitous element of verbal utterances. Assuming higher proficiency of the cerebellum as compared to the auditory cortex, in precise representation of these features, infratentorial disorders, consequently, might compromise any cognitive functions depending upon verbal working memory or auditory speech imagery, such as lexical search processes or problem solving *(43)*. Since, besides temporal structure, other parameters of the acoustic speech signal, e.g., spectral features, also contribute to the specification of phonetic/phonological information, the engagement of cerebellar structures during cognitive functions and/or the severity of neuropsychological deficits subsequent to cerebellar damage might depend upon task demands such as temporal constraints of behavioral performance or increased load of working memory.

REFERENCES

1. Schmahmann, J.D. (1991) An emerging concept: the cerebellar contribution to higher function. *Arch. Neurol.* **48,** 1178–1187.
2. Ackermann, H. and Daum, I. (1995) Cerebellum and cognition: the neuropsychological and neuroradiological evidence. *Fortschr. Neurol. Psychiat.* **63,** 30–37.
3. Leiner, H.C., Leiner, A.L., and Dow, R.S. (1993) Cognitive and language functions of the human cerebellum. *Trends Neeurosci.* **16,** 444–447.
4. Ivry, R.B. and Keele, S.W. (1989) Timing functions of the cerebellum. *J. Cogn. Neurosci.* **1,** 136–152.
5. Petersen, S.E., Fox, P.T., Posner, M.I., Mintun, M., and Raichle, M.E. (1988) Positron emission tomographic studies of the cortical anatomy of single-word processing. *Nature* **331,** 585–589.
6. Daum, I. and Ackermann, H. (1995) Cerebellar contributions to cognition. *Behav. Brain Res.* **67,** 201–210.
7. Schmahmann, J.D. and Sherman, J.C. (1998) The cerebellar cognitive affective syndrome. *Brain* **121,** 561–579.
8. Daum, I. and Ackermann, H. (1997) Neuropsychological abnormalities in cerebellar syndromes: fact or fiction? *Int. Rev. Neurobiol.* **41,** 455–471.
9. Heath, R.G., Franklin, D.E., and Shraberg, D. (1979) Gross pathology of the cerebellum in patients diagnosed and treated as functional psychiatric disorders. *J. Nerv. Ment. Dis.* **167,** 585–592.
10. Levitt, J.J., Mc Carley, R.W., Nestor, P.G., et al. (1999) Quantitative volumetric MRI study of the cerebellum and vermis in schizophrenia: clinical and cognitive correlates. *Am. J. Psychiatry* **156,** 1105–1107.
11. Bauman, M.L., Filipek, P.A., and Kemper, T.L. (1997) Early infantile autism. *Int. Rev. Neurobiol.* **41,** 367–386.

12. Courchesne, E., Yeung-Courchesne, R., Press, G.A., Hesselink, J.R., and Jernigan, T.L. (1988) Hypoplasia of cerebellar vermal lobules VI and VII in autism. *N. Engl. J. Med.* **318,** 1349–1354.
13. Abell, F., Krams, M., Ashburner, J., et al. (1999) The neuroanatomy of autism: a voxel-based whole brain analysis of structural scans. *Neuroreport* **10,** 1647–1651.
14. Berquin, P.C., Giedd, J.N., Jacobsen, L.K., et al. (1998) Cerebellum in attention-deficit hyperactivity disorder: a morphometric MRI study. *Neurology* **50,** 1087–1093.
15. Mostofsky, S.H., Mazzocco, M.M.M., Aakalu, G., Warsofsky, I.S., Denckla, M.B., and Reiss, A.L. (1998) Decreased cerebellar posterior vermis size in fragile X syndrome: correlation with neurocognitive performance. *Neurology* **50,** 121–130.
16. Dichgans, J. (1984) Clinical symptoms of cerebellar dysfunction and their topodiagnostical significance. *Hum. Neurobiol.* **2,** 269–279.
17. Rae, C., Lee, M.A., Dixon, R.M., et al. (1998) Metabolic abnormalities in developmental dyslexia detected by 1H magnetic resonance spectroscopy. *Lancet* **351,** 1849–1852.
18. Kish, S.J., El-Awar, M., Schut, L., Leach, L., Oscar-Berman, M., and Freedman, M. (1988) Cognitive deficits in olivopontocerebellar atrophy: implications for the cholinergic hypothesis of Alzheimer's dementia. *Ann. Neurol.* **24,** 200–206.
19. Bracke-Tolkmitt, R., Linden, A., Canavan, A.G.M., et al. (1989) The cerebellum contributes to mental skills. *Behav. Neurosci.* **103,** 442–446.
20. Akshoomoff, N.A., Courchesne, E., Press, G.A., and Iragui, V. (1992) Contribution of the cerebellum to neuropsychological functioning: evidence from a case of cerebellar degenerative disorder. *Neuropsychologia* **30,** 315–328.
21. Fiez, J.A., Petersen, S.E., Cheney, M.K., and Raichle, M.E. (1992) Impaired non-motor learning and error detection associated with cerebellar damge. *Brain* **115,** 155–178.
22. Appollonio, I.M., Grafman, J., Schwartz, V., Massaquoi, S., and Hallett, M. (1993) Memory in patients with cerebellar degeneration. *Neurology* **43,** 1536–1544.
23. Daum, I., Ackermann, H., Schugens, M.M., Reimold, C., Dichgans, J., and Birbaumer, N. (1993) The cerebellum and cognitive functions in humans. *Behav. Neurosci.* **107,** 411–419.
24. Malm, J., Kristensen, B., Karlsson, T., Carlberg, B., Fagerlund, M., and Olsson, T. (1998) Cognitive impairment in young adults with infratentorial infarct. *Neurology* **51,** 433–440.
25. Drepper, J., Timmann, D., Kolb, F.P., and Diener, H.C. (1999) Non-motor associative learning in patients with isolated degenerative cerebellar disease. *Brain* **122,** 87–97.
26. Ivry, R.B. and Fiez, J.A. (2000) Cerebellar contributions to cognition and imagery, in *The New Cognitive Neurosciences, 2nd ed.* (Gazzaniga, M.S., ed.), MIT Press, Cambridge, MA, pp. 999–1011.
27. Riva, D. and Giorgi, C. (2000) The cerebellum contributes to higher functions during development: evidence from a series of children surgically treated for posterior fossa tumours. *Brain* **123,** 1051–1061.
28. Grafman, J., Litvan, I., Massaquoi, S., Stewart, M., Sirigu, A., and Hallett, M. (1992) Cognitive planning deficite in patients with cerebellar atrophy. *Neurology* **42,** 1493–1496.
29. Pascual-Leone, A., Grafman, J., Clark, K., et al. (1993) Procedural learning in Parkinson's disease and cerebellar degeneration. *Ann. Neurol.* **34,** 594–602.
30. Molinari, M., Leggio, M.G., and Silveri, M.C. (1997) Verbal fluency and agrammatism. *Int. Rev. Neurobiol.* **41,** 325–339.
31. Ackermann, H., Gräber, S., Hertrich, I., and Daum, I. (1997) Categorical speech perception in cerebellar disorders. *Brain Lang.* **60,** 323–331.
32. Ackermann, H., Gräber, S., Hertrich, I., and Daum, I. (1999) Cerebellar contributions to the perception of temporal cues within the speech and nonspeech domain. *Brain Lang.* **67,** 228–241.
32a. Mathiak, K., Hertrich, I., Grodd, W., and Ackermann, H. (2002) Cerebellum and speech perception: a functional magnetic resonance imaging study. *J. Cogn. Neurosci.* **14,** 902–912.
33. Fiez, J.A. and Raichle, M.E. (1997) Linguistic processing. *Int. Rev. Neurobiol.* **41,** 233–254.
34. Silveri, M.C., Leggio, M.G., and Molinari, M. (1994) The cerebellum contributes to linguistic production: a case of agrammatic speech following a right cerebellar lesion. *Neurology* **44,** 2047–2050.
35. Zettin, M., Cappa, S.F., D'Amico, A., et al. (1997) Agrammatic speech production after a right cerebellar haemorrhage. *Neurocase* **3,** 375–380.
36. Hassid, E.I. (1995) A case of language dysfunction associated with cerebellar infarction. *J. Neuro. Rehab.* **9,** 157–160.
37. Marien, P., Saerens, J., Nanhoe, R., et al. (1996) Cerebellar induced aphasia: case report of cerebellar induced prefrontal aphasic language phenomena supported by SPECT findings. *J. Neurol. Sci.* **144,** 34–43.
38. Marien, P., Engelborghs, S., Pickut, B.A., and De Deyn, P.P. (2000) Aphasia following cerebellar damage: fact or fallacy? *J. Neuroling.* **13,** 145–171.
39. Gasparini, M., Di Piero, V., Ciccarelli, O., Cacioppo, M.M., Pantano, P., and Lenzi, G.L. (1999) Linguistic impairment after right cerebellar stroke: a case report. *Eur. J. Neurol.* **6,** 353–356.
40. Marien, P., Engelborghs, S., Fabbro, F., and De Deyn, P.P. (2001) The lateralized linguistic cerebellum: a review and a new hypothesis. *Brain Lang.* **79,** 580–600.
41. Ackermann, H., Hertrich, I., Ziegler, W., Bitzer, M., and Bien, S. (1996) Acquired dysfluencies following infarction of the left mesiofrontal cortex. *Aphasiology* **10,** 409–417.
42. Ackermann, H. and Hertrich, I. (2000) The contribution of the cerebellum to speech processing. *J. Neuroling.* **13,** 28–40.
43. Ackermann, H., Wildgruber, D., Daum, I., and Grodd, W. (1998) Does the cerebellum contribute to cognitive aspects of speech production? A functional magnetic resonance imaging (fMRI) study in humans. *Neurosci. Lett.* **247,** 187–190.

IV

Neurophysiology of Cognition in Movement Disorders

12

Induction and Reversal of Cognitive Deficits in a Primate Model of Huntington's Disease

Stéphane Palfi, MD, PhD, **Emmanuel Brouillet,** PhD, **Françoise Condé,** PhD, **and Philippe Hantraye,** PhD

1. INTRODUCTION

Huntington's disease (HD) is an inherited, autosomal dominant, neurodegenerative disorder characterized by involuntary choreiform movements, progressive cognitive decline, psychiatric manifestations, and a neuronal degeneration primarily affecting the striatum. Neuropathological examination indicates that striatal γ-amino butyric acid (GABA)ergic projecting neurons are preferentially affected, whereas striatal interneurons are relatively spared *(1)*. The gene responsible for the disease (IT15) has been cloned, and the molecular abnormality has been identified as an expanded polyglutamine tract in the N-terminal region of a protein of unknown function, named huntingtin *(2)*. Recent studies showed that huntingtin interacts with a number of proteins; some of them with well identified functions. Thus, it has been suggested that alterations in glycolysis, vesicle trafficking, or apoptosis may play a role in the physiopathology of HD *(3–6)*. Other data derived from positron emission tomography, magnetic resonance spectroscopy, and postmortem biochemistry, showing evidences for a defect in succinate oxidation, have suggested the potential implication of a primary impairment of mitochondrial energy metabolism *(6)*. Based on this mitochondrial hypothesis, phenotypic animal models of HD have been elaborated both in rodents and nonhuman primates, employing a chronic blockade of succinate oxidation by systemic administration of the mitochondrial toxin, 3-nitropropionic acid (3-NP) *(7–11)*. Historically, initial experimental studies in nonhuman primates used unilateral striatal injections of glutamatergic agonists, such as quinolinic and ibotenic acid, to induce abnormal movements. More recently, experimental studies used a systemic injection of 3-NP in nonhuman primates to induce both choreiform and dystonic movements associated with bilateral selective striatal lesions ressembling those observed in HD *(12)*. Further, to elaborate a complete behavioral model of HD, including both motor and a subcortical frontal-type cognitive deficit reminiscent of HD, a prolonged 3-NP intoxication has been developed in nonhuman primates.

Early neurological manifestations in the common form of HD often include a frontal-type subcortical dementia, long before abnormal movements are detected *(1)*. The concept of frontal subcortical dementia was indeed suggested for the first time in the 1970s by McHugh and Folstein *(13,14)*. Although still controversial, this neuropsychological concept seems to be currently accepted by an increasing number of clinicians. Cognitive deficits observed in Parkinson disease *(15)*, Wilson's disease *(16)*, supranuclear palsy *(14)*, and HD *(13)* can be clinically differentiated from those involved in other neurodegenerative diseases affecting in priority the cerebral cortex, such as Alzheimer's disease, Creutzfeldt-Jakob, or

From: *Mental and Behavioral Dysfunction in Movement Disorders*
Edited by: M-A. Bédard et al. © Humana Press Inc., Totowa, NJ

Pick's disease. If subcortical dementia remains essentially a clinical concept, HD cognitive symptoms do not include the classical triad of aphasia-apraxia-agnosia triad observed in cortical dementia diseases, but rather a more diffuse syndrome marked by the association of memory losses, frontal-type deficits, as well as signs of motor abnormalities. Additionally, qualitative cognitive performance analysis in diseases associated with subcortical dementia have suggested that alterations in cognitive programming may not take place, but rather a series of disruptions in initiation, planning, and use of these cognitive programs. Thus, cortical and subcortical dementia differ from each other by the disruption of these functions used to regulate cognitive behavior and by a relative preservation of instrumental "activities," including, for example, memory and language *(17–19)*.

It is no surprise to observe, in HD patients, a prevalent frontal type cognitive deficit, since the majority of the head of the caudate nucleus receives fibers arising from the dorsolateral prefrontal cortex and from the orbitofrontal cortex *(16,20,21)*. Indeed, cardinal features of HD dementia include difficulties in retrieving memories, slowed information processing, cognitive inflexibility, preservative behavior, as well as a severe impairment in the ability to elaborate set-shifting strategies *(16,22)*. In parallel, the cognitive deficits observed in patients displaying lesions limited to the dorsolateral prefrontal cortex affect verbal fluency *(17)*, intellectual flexibility, and the ability to operate mental changes *(23)*, which are also symptoms often detected in HD patients. Thus, patient performances in the Wisconsin card sorting test are often disrupted early in HD *(23)*, as well as the "attentional set-shifting test" (an analogous of Wisconsin card sorting test) in nonhuman primates bearing prefrontal cortex lesions *(24)*. Additionally, the hypothesis that a primary striatal lesion could be associated with a frontal-type syndrome has been further reinforced by observations in patients presenting uni- or bilateral stroke lesions in the caudate nucleus and who exhibit cognitive alterations very similar to those observed in HD *(25)*. All these observations, therefore, suggest that the dementia observed in HD is of a frontal type, associated with subcortical damage, and very similar to that observed in patients with lesion of a dorsolateral prefrontal cortex *(16,26)*.

2. INDUCTION OF A COGNITIVE DEFICIT IN A PRIMATE MODEL OF HD

2.1. *Chronic 3-NP Treatment in Primates as a Model of HD*

3-NP neurotoxicity was studied in adult macaques (*Macaca fascicularis*) and baboons (*Papio papio, P. anubis*). 3-NP was daily injected intramuscularly in two half doses, 5 d/wk. Behavioral deficit was studied first using motor qualitative testing, time-sampled neurological observations (under spontaneous conditions or following intramuscular administration of 0.5–1 mg/kg apomorphine), and rated using a dyskinesia rating scale *(27)*. Furthermore, a quantitative analysis employing a video movement analysis and tracking system (VMA) of the animal's displacements spontaneously and during the apomorphine test was used to confirm clinical observations *(12,27)*. Finally, cognitive performances of the animals were assessed with the object retrieval detour task (ORDT), a sensitive test for detecting frontal-type cognitive deficits in nonhuman primates *(28)*.

2.2. *General Features of the Chronic 3-NP Lesion Model in Nonhuman Primates*

To develop a primate model of progressive striatal degeneration, a prolonged treatment of daily doses of 3-NP was initiated in baboons for 20 wk (Fig. 1). Baboons were treated with 3-NP at an initial dose of 10 mg/kg/d, which was progressively increased to 28 mg/kg/d (1 mg/kg increment at weekly intervals). During the first 6 wk of the protocol, no spontaneous or even apomorphine-induced abnormal movements could be observed (nonsymptomatic phase). As soon as 8–10 wk of 3-NP treatment, apomorphine administration resulted in the appearance of choreiform movements, frontal-type cognitive deficits, indicating that at this stage animals had entered into a "presymptomatic" phase *(27)*. Moreover, severity of motor abnormalities after apomorphine administration increased as the 3-NP intoxication progressed. Starting after 12 wk of intoxication, all 3-NP-animals displayed spontaneous foot dyskinesias, entering into a "symptomatic phase." At the end of the neurotoxic treatment, both

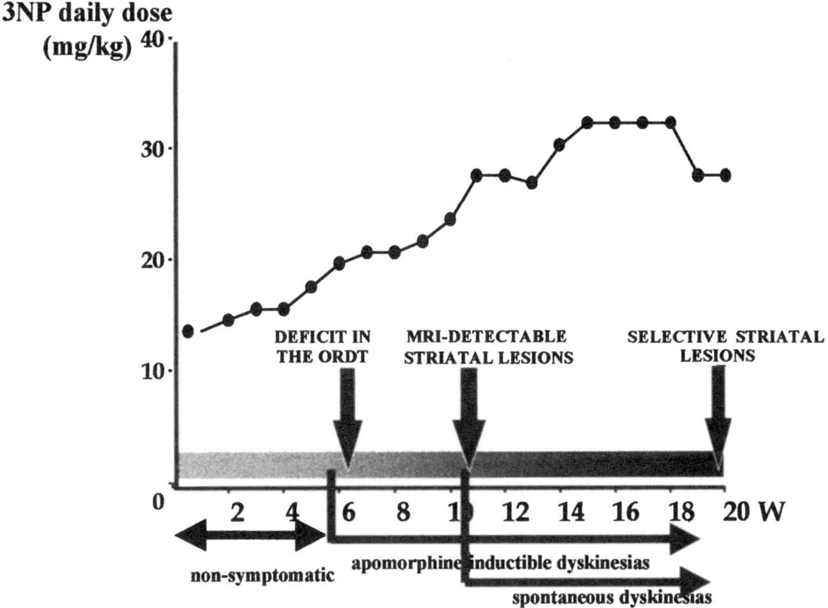

Fig. 1. Schematic representation of the 3-NP intoxication regimen used in nonhuman primates (baboons) to induce progressive striatal degeneration. Starting from 10 mg/kg/d, the daily dose of 3-NP is progressively increased to 29 mg/kg/d. The doses of 3-NP is incremented at weekly intervals to induce progressive succinate dehydrogenase (SDH) inhibition. A first dose increment (2 mg/kg/d) from wk 1 to wk 6 is followed by a dose increment of 0.5 mg/kg/d from wk 6 to wk 25. Such a dose regimen is associated with a progressive body weight loss and the progressive appearance of motor and cognitive deficits.

magnetic resonance imaging (MRI) examination performed prior to the sacrifice and anatomopathological examination confirmed the presence of the bilateral striatal lesions without any detectable extra-striatal lesions (Fig. 2).

2.3. *Cognitive Evaluation*

As described in the introduction section, frontal type cognitive deficit is a typical feature of HD dementia. Replicating such a frontal-type cognitive deficit in a primate model of HD appears essential to evaluate new therapeutic strategies in a preclinical phase. Thus, as the frontal-type cognitive deficit is known to appear early in the disease course, cognitive performances of 3-NP-treated baboons were assessed in the early (nonsymptomatic) phase of the 3-NP intoxication protocol using the ORDT *(29,30)*, a task especially designed to detect frontal-type deficits in human and nonhuman primates *(28)*. This cognitive task was selected because it requires complex sequential motor planning and is particularly sensitive to frontal cortex lesions or striatal dysfunction *(28,31–35)*. Indeed, the ORDT is capable of assessing the ability of the animals to retrieve an object (in the present case, a piece of fruit) from inside a transparent box only open on one side (Fig. 3A). The level of difficulty can be modified by the experimenter by varying the location of the box, the location of the reward in the box, and finally the orientation of the open side of the box in relation to the subject (Fig. 3A). As shown by previous studies in human and nonhuman primates, the ORDT involves cerebral circuits implicated in cognition as well as in motor skills. However, in the majority of the trials in which the opening of the box is not facing the animal, primates must inhibit their natural tendency to reach straight for what they want and must make a detour around the transparent side of the box to the open side of the box

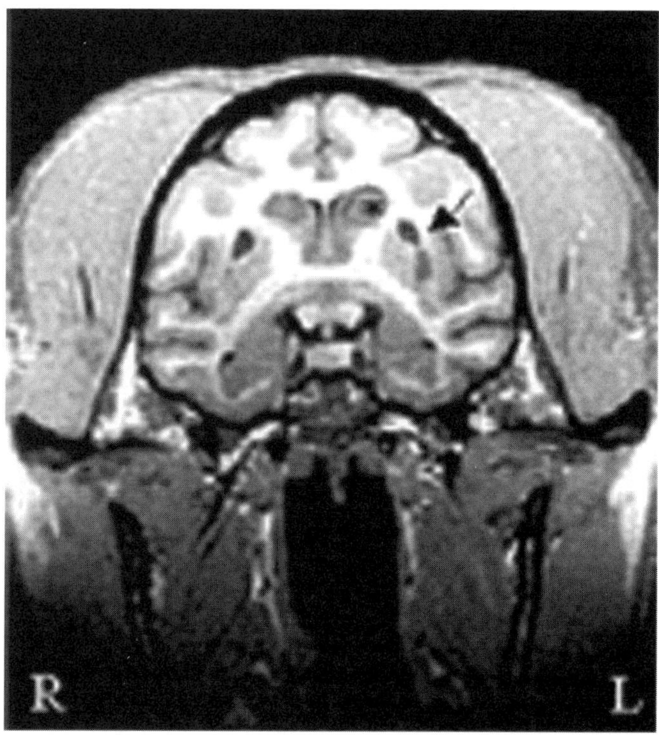

Fig. 2. Coronal T1-weighted MRI (1.5 T General Electric magnet) in a 3-NP-treated primate at an advanced stage of the neurotoxic treatment at the anterior commissural level. Bilateral lesions detected as hyposignals (black), are restricted to the dorsal aspect of the caudate nucleus and putamen (arrow). No other damage was identified in any other brain area.

(Fig. 3B). It has been shown that the inhibition of this natural tendency specifically requires the functional integrity of the frontostriatal system *(28)* and is not affected by lesions in other brain regions such as the hippocampal formation or the parietal cortex *(32)*. Each ORDT test session consisted of 15 trials corresponding to different configurations related to either the position of the reward in the box or the position of the box on the tray facing the animals (Fig. 3A). The reward was only visible for the animal after raising an opaque screen placed between him and the box. Subjects were then allowed a 60-s time period to retrieve the reward, after which the screen was put back in place and the box set up for the next trial. The animals' responses were video recorded and measures of performance included: the number of "success" responses (retrieval of the reward on the first attempt of the trial), the number of "correct" responses (retrieval of the reward within the 60-s time period, whatever the strategy used by the animal to retrieve the piece of fruit). This correct response represents the ability for the baboon to perform the task. Finally, "barrier hits" responses (hitting the closed transparent side of the box instead of making a detour) and "motor problems" responses (reaching the open side of the box but failing to retrieve the reward) were quantified.

Starting after 4 wk of 3-NP treatment, 4 consecutive ORDT test sessions were performed in a weekly basis in 3 baboons intoxicated with 3-NP, and their performances were compared to those of 10 control animals. Compared to intact animals, 3-NP-treated animals were significantly less successful in obtaining the reward on the first reach and were making more barrier hits, indicating that they were impaired in their ability to respond using the appropriate strategy. In contrast, 3-NP-intoxicated animals were not impaired in motor problems or correct responses, indicating that they were as able as the controls to get the rewards (Fig. 4).

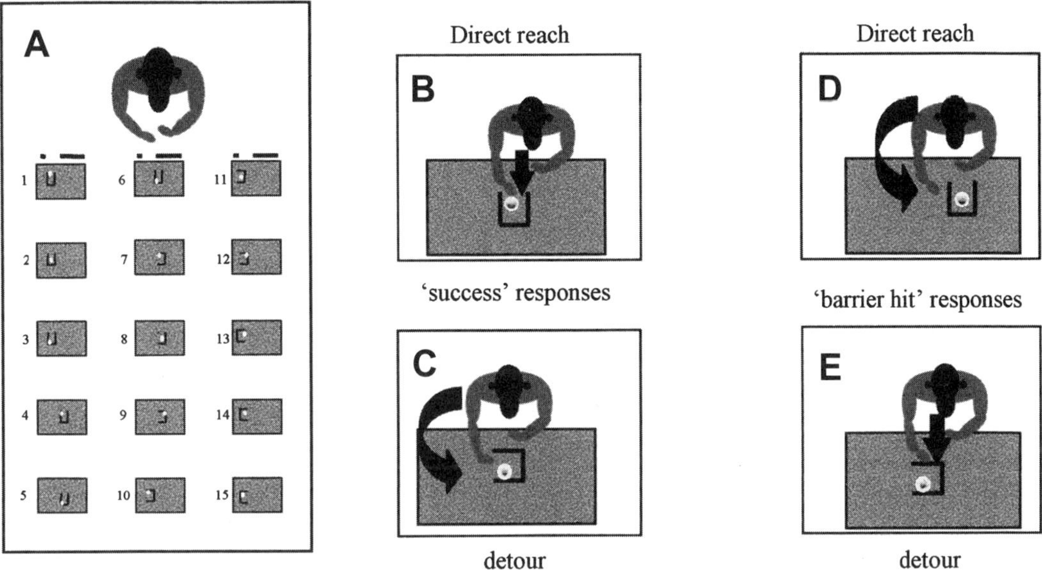

Fig. 3. The ORDT: experimental set-up and principles. In the ORDT, the ability of monkeys to retrieve an object from inside a transparent box only open on one side can be assessed. (**A**) A total of 15 different configurations are randomly presented to the animals. Measures of performance include: (**B,C**) number of success responses (retrieval of the reward on the first reach of the trial); (**D,E**) barrier hit responses (hitting the closed transparent side of the box instead of making a detour). Examples of easy trials (direct reach possible; B and D) and difficult trials (i.e., when a detour around the transparent side of the box is required; C and E) are illustrated.

The frontal syndrome observed in HD patients is primarily characterized by deficits in executive function, motor programming, and organizational strategies for learning tasks. Careful analysis of the time-course of the success, barrier hits, and correct responses indicated that 3-NP-treated baboons showed no significant improvement in their performances from the first to the fourth test day, whereas controls significantly improved their performances from one test session to the other. The deficit noted in 3-NP-treated baboons suggests an impairment in organizational strategy, which resembles the cognitive alterations typically associated with HD. Further studies employing other cognitive tasks specifically designed to assess frontal-type deficits, memory disturbances, and organizational strategies are still required to further characterize the extent of the cognitive alterations associated with chronic 3-NP treatment.

2.4. Neuropathological Findings

Postmortem neuropathological examination of animals presenting spontaneous symptoms at 20 wk of 3-NP treatment invariably detected two types of histological abnormalities restricted to the striatum *(12,27,30)*. The first type of lesion was seen in animals submitted to the 15- to 20-wk experimental protocol. The lesion always began in the most lateral part of the putamen (as shown on MRI; Fig. 2), later encompassing the dorsolateral aspect of the body of the caudate nucleus *(12,29)*. In the core of the lesion, the loss of neurons and processes was almost complete. Surrounding the core of the lesion, a transition area was observed, in which nicotinamide-adenine dinucleotide phosphate, reduced form (NADPH)-diaphorase and cholinergic positive interneurons were found to be relatively preserved, whereas the number of calbindin positive neurons was greatly reduced. In the rostral part of the caudate anterior to the lesion core, a gradient of calbindin immunoreactivity was found, the dorsal part being more affected than the ventral part. The second type of 3-NP lesion was found in animals submitted to a

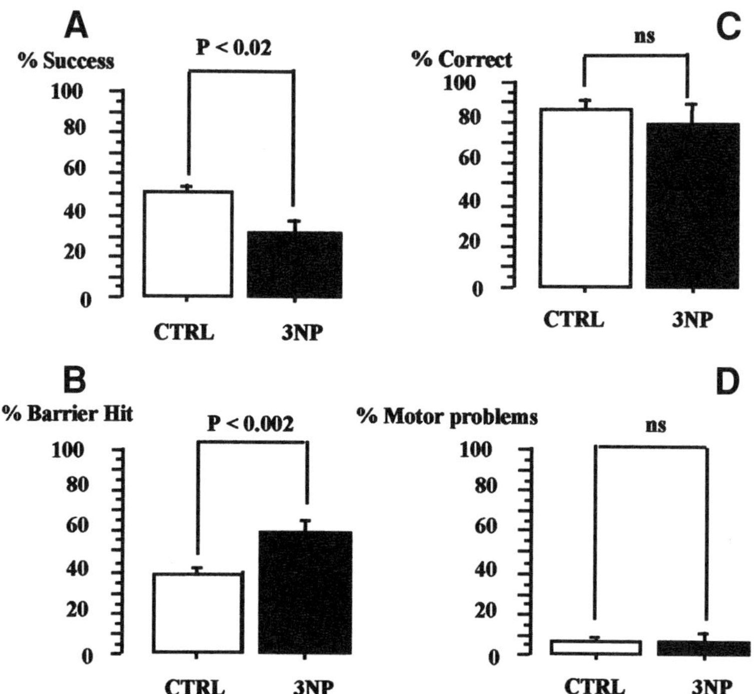

Fig. 4. Frontal-type cognitive deficits in 3-NP-treated baboons compared to age-matched control animals. The percentage of (**A**) success, (**B**) barrier hits, (**C**) correct, and (**D**) motor problems responses are represented as a mean of four consecutive test sessions performed at weekly intervals. Open bars represent control animals (n = 10), and solid black bars represent 3-NP-treated animals (n = 3). Values are mean ± standard error of the mean (SEM). Note that performances of the two groups differ in success and barrier hits responses, but not in correct responses (which represent the ability of each animal to finally reach the reward) nor in motor problems. Consequently, neither alterations in motor control nor a disinterest of the animals in the task could explain the differences observed between the two experimental groups.

longer intoxication protocol (25–35 wk) (Figs. 5 and 8) and was characterized by the absence of detectable changes in MRI signal, even in presence of persistent abnormal movements (leg dystonia). Nevertheless, using image analysis systems on calbindin or DARPP32-immunostained sections, a clear dorsal to ventral loss of immunoreactive cells could be observed, corresponding to a loss of projection neurons (Fig. 7). Markers of the other striatal neuronal populations (choline-acetyl-transferase [ChAT], NADPH-diaphorase) were unchanged (data not shown). This suggests that a selective dysfunction of the striatal projection neurons (as examplified by the loss of calbindin immunoreactivity) may be sufficient to result in clinically overt motor and cognitive deficits. These findings are of great relevance for the design of new therapeutic strategies for HD, especially for neuroprotective clinical trials, in which the treatment should be introduced before a massive loss of striatal neurons has taken place.

3. RESTORING COGNITIVE DEFICITS IN NONHUMAN PRIMATES

3.1. Effect of Fetal Striatal Allografts

In contrast to Parkinson disease, in which the main objective of neural grafting is the release of dopamine in a localized part of the brain, the goal of neural transplantation in HD is to reconstruct a damaged neuronal circuitry. Thus, intracerebral transplantation in HD can only be envisaged if one can compensate for a loss of a well-defined neuronal population, in the present case the GABAergic

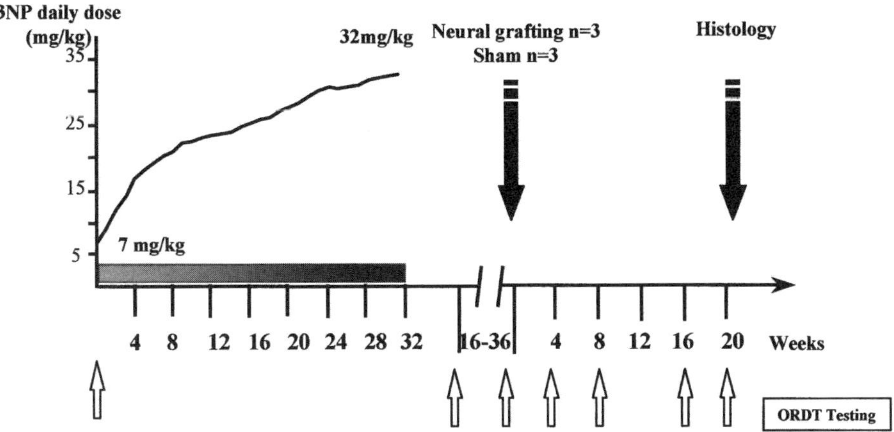

Fig. 5. Schematic representation of the 3-NP treatment and experimental protocol used in striatal allografting experiments. The six macaques (*M. fascicularis*) were intoxicated on a chronic basis with 3-NP and regularly tested on motor and cognitive (ORDT) tasks before and after surgery (open arrows). Animals were sacrificed immediately after the last behavioral testing.

neurons, into a precise site of the brain (the striatum). However, degeneration of GABAergic striatal neurons in HD not only results in severe losses of striatal GABAergic concentrations, but also interrupts a chain of informations originating upstream of the striatum and traveling towards downstream target zones. To reconnect this interrupted circuitry, the chain must be entirely reconstructed, and new grafted striatal neurons must direct themselves to the exact anatomic place in which the host neurons have degenerated. As shown extensively in previous rat studies, specific graft-to-host reinnervation and host-to-graft axonal regeneration must occur, to expect any clinical benefit for the patient.

The only source of tissue currently available for neural grafting in HD is the embryonic striatal primordial tissue derived from the ganglionic eminences dissected from human embryos (gestational age 7 wk). Before any therapeutic trials in HD patients could be initiated, both structural and functional primate studies had to be carried out to evaluate whether fetal striatal grafts could survive, develop, and create synaptic connections with the host tissue. Over the past 20 yr, a number of rat and nonhuman primate studies had already demonstrated that fetal striatal-grafted neurons could survive and mature within the adult host brain (for review, see ref. *36*). Thus, the anatomic maturation of the grafted neurons into the host tissue obtained in various animal models was shown to result in an effective reconstruction of the entire corticostriatopallidal circuitry. In addition, at a functional level, this reconstruction of circuitry regarding the functional effect of striatal grafting and the abilities to obtain a functional compensation in motor behavior has been first studied in rat and nonhuman primate models of HD using xenografting (human tissue to rat, rat tissue to nonhuman primate) and later using allografting procedures *(36–38)*. In nonhuman primates previously receiving a unilateral excitotoxin injection, intrastriatal xenografting of striatal neuroblasts significantly reduced both the apomorphine-induced turning behavior and the choreiform movements typically observed in this model *(37)*. Following cyclosporine A withdrawal, which resulted in graft rejection in this xenograting paradigm, the progressive reappearance of the motor deficits attested that motor improvement was specifically derived from functional implants. Similarly, striatal allografts carried out in a similar excitotoxic lesion model in marmosets, demonstrated good survival, differentiation, and integration of striatal allografts within the host striatum, which was further associated with significant recovery in a test of skilled motor performance *(38)*.

The recent development of the chronic 3-NP lesion model gave us the unique opportunity to assess whether a striatal allograft could also reverse a frontal-type cognitive deficit in nonhuman primates.

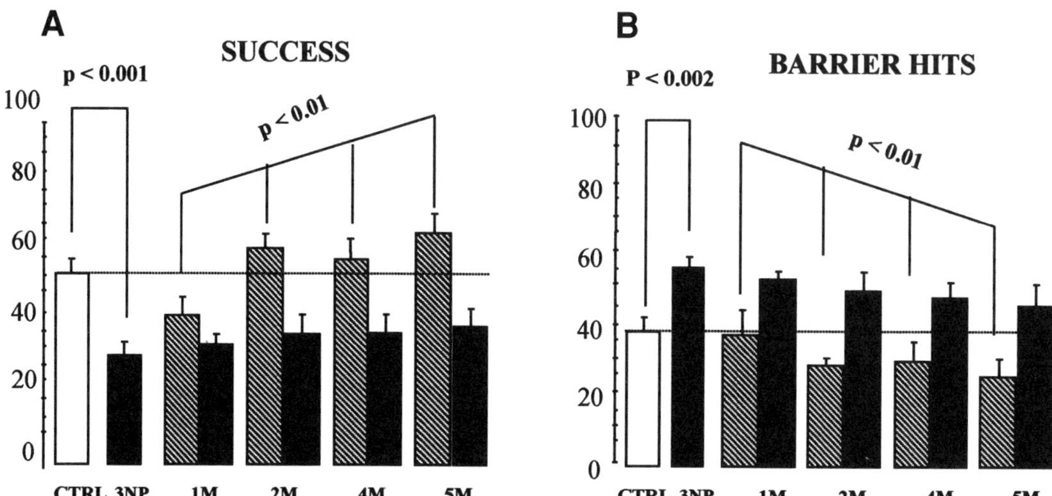

Fig. 6. ORDT results for success (**A**) and barrier hit responses (**B**) before and after chronic 3-NP lesion and fetal striatal allografting. Before striatal allografting, all *M. fascicularis* monkeys treated with 3-NP were significantly less successful compared to controls in reaching the reward at their first attempt (success responses; A) and made significantly more reaching errors (barrier hit responses; B). As early as 2 mo postgrafting, a significant increase in success responses (A) was observed in grafted macaques compared to sham-operated animals. Similarly, starting 2 mo postimplantation, a significant decrease in the number of reaching errors was observed in grafted macaques compared to sham-operated macaques (B). All data are expressed as mean ± SEM.

In this experiment, six macaques received a prolonged systemic 3-NP treatment for 35 wk according to the dose regimen described in Fig. 5. The neurotoxic treatment was adapted to yield a linear increase in dosage until the onset of persistent dystonic abnormal movements in all animals. Nine age-matched control animals were used in parallel for behavioral or histological studies.

Daily clinical examination of the animals revealed intermittent dystonic abnormal movements located in the hindlimbs as early as 3 mo after the initiation of the 3-NP treatment. Dyskinesia subsequently extended to the forelimbs and the face at the end of the 3-NP treatment. No spontaneous reversal of the dystonia was observed thereafter in lesioned control animals.

Two weeks after completion of the 3-NP treatment, the severity of the striatal lesion was assessed on cognitive and motor parameters using the ORDT and the apomorphine test, respectively. ORDT showed that the 3-NP-treated animals were significantly less successful in obtaining the reward on the first reach during testing and made significantly more barrier hits when performing the task, as compared to controls (Fig. 6). These differences could not be attributed to a physical disability of the 3-NP-treated subjects, as motor problems did not differ significantly between the two groups ($p > 0.4$). In the motor test, apomorphine administration elicited a significant increase in abnormal movements in all 3-NP-treated animals compared to control.

After a delay allowing stabilization of degenerative phenomena (4–9 mo), the six 3-NP-treated macaques were distributed into two equivalent groups according to motor and cognitive impairments. The graft group ($n = 3$) received, bilaterally into the striatum, a cell suspension derived from the lateral ganglionic eminence of E51–E55 macaque embryos. The sham operated group ($n = 3$) received saline injections instead. Four injection needle tracks were performed on each side, two into the rostral caudate and two into the rostral-lateral putamen. In order to achieve maximal functional recovery on motor and frontal-type cognitive deficits, the grafts were aimed at caudate territories innervated by the prefrontal cortex *(39)*, whereas they were aimed at the rostral part of the lateral putamen, which receives sensory-motor afferents *(40)* and is implicated in experimental dystonia.

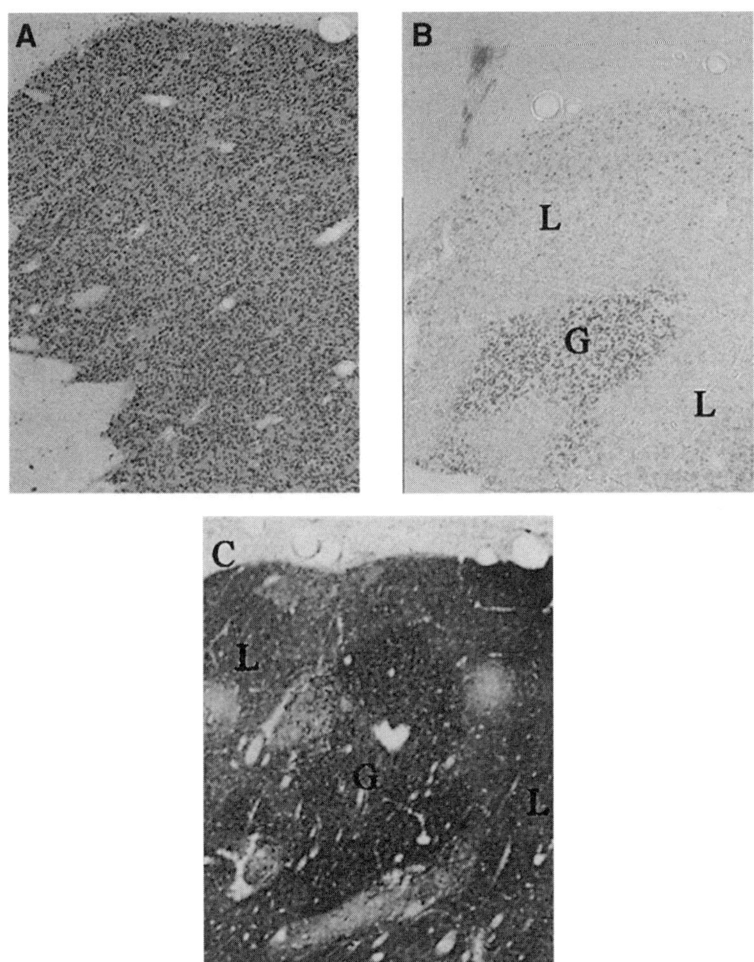

Fig. 7. Fetal striatal allografts in primates immunostained for Neu-N and calbindin-DK28. Neu-N is a neuronal specific marker; calbindin-DK28 a specific marker of a subpopulation of GABAergic neurons located in the striatum. (**A**) Photomicrograph of Neu-N-ir structures in the left precommissural caudate nucleus of a control normal monkey. (**B**) Photomicrograph of Neu-N-ir and (**C**) calbindin-DK28-ir structures in the left precommissural caudate nucleus of one macaque grafted with fetal striatal neuroblasts. Note the central area containing high density of grafted (G) Neu-N-ir or calbindin-ir cells surrounded by a lesioned area devoid of any immunoreactivity (L).

Clinical observations of spontaneous and apomorphine-induced behavior and ORDT were carried out on a monthly basis. The sham-operated animals did not show any significant improvement either in motor or cognitive (Fig. 6) functions. In sharp contrast, the three grafted macaques displayed a progressive improvement in cognitive functions in the ORDT, which led to a complete recovery as early as 2 mo post-grafting, and persisted for the remaining 3 mo before sacrifice (Fig. 6). Dystonia gradually improved in parallel, with significant recovery observed at 4 and 5 mo postgrafting.

As compared to controls, in the sham-operated animals, an overall decrease of 50% in the number of calbindin immunoreactive neurons was observed (Fig. 7), both in caudate and putamen nuclei. In contrast, striatal interneurons were spared.

In the grafted animals, fetal allografts were identified both in caudate and putamen nuclei. These grafts appeared as areas of high cell density expressing calbindin and surrounded by lesioned areas of low calbindin-D28k immunoreactivity (Fig. 7). Within the grafts, calbindin immunoreactive neurons had a stellate-shaped body with strongly immunoreactive processes, whereas in the host striatum, calbindin immunoreactivity was concentrated in the cell body of the few remaining calbindin-D28k immunoreactive cells, as in the control striatum.

These results have provided evidence for recovery in cognitive functions after intrastriatal neural transplantation in the adult primate brain. They bring the anatomofunctional capacity of intracerebral transplantation one step further by establishing that neurons implicated in higher brain functions can also be replaced to correct cognitive deficits in the nonhuman primate. They also confirm previous demonstrations that neural grafts can provide modulatory inputs that are beneficial for cognitive performances in models of learning and memory impairments related to cholinergic denervation of the hippocampus (for a review, see ref. *36*). These series of studies showed that not only modulatory systems, but also pathways requiring a specific neuronal circuitry for the correct processing and integration of informations, can be reconstructed after injury. As mentioned above, this requires a complete anatomofunctional reconstruction of the neuronal relay including graft-to-host and host-to-graft connections, whereas graft-to-host interactions are only required for modulatory systems. Pioneering works suggested that complete rewiring of a cognitive relay system is possible, leading to functional recovery of cognitive functions in rat HD models *(41)*. However, these implications were limited by considerations related to the volume and complexity of brain structures and the more complex nature of the behavioral repertoire of primates. The cognitive recovery observed in the primate model of HD after fetal striatal allografting provided a rationale for the clinical grafting trials in HD patients *(36, 42)*. Interestingly, we could demonstrate in a recent pilot clinical trial, a significant improvement in motor and cognitive function, as well as indices of increased striatal metabolic activity in three patients out of five grafted patients with HD *(42)*, suggesting that behavioral observations in grafted 3-NP-treated primates can be predictive of clinical efficacy.

3.2. *Effects of Ciliary Neurotrophic Factor*

Ciliary neurotrophic factor (CNTF) is a protein belonging to the interleukin 6 cytokine family with proven neuroprotective efficacy in the unilateral excitotoxic rat and primate HD models *(43,44)*. In order to prepare a potential clinical neuroprotective trial in HD patients, we initiated a functional experimental study of both motor and cognitive behavior in 3-NP-treated primates *(45)*. CNTF delivery to the striatum was achieved by implantation into the striatum of encapsulated cells, which were genetically engineered to produce CNTF in situ.

To this aim, six fascicularis monkeys were treated for 25 wk with 3-NP, as described in Fig. 8. Following 10 wk of neurotoxic treatment, performances in motor and cognitive tests (apomorphine tests and ORDT) were assessed, and animals were then distributed into two experimental groups, matched for their respective motor and cognitive deficits. One animal group [CNTF(+), $n = 3$] received CNTF-producing fibroblasts (baby hamster kidney [BHK]-CNTF cells) in a capsule of perm-selective biopolymer bilaterally implanted into the post-commissural putamen and into the lateral cerebral ventricle. The second group of animals [CNTF(-), $n = 3$] were submitted to the same surgical procedure, except that the encapsulated cells were native BHK cells. For all animals, the neurotoxic treatment was then continued for the remainder of the experiment, i.e., for an additional 15-wk time period. During this postimplantation period, the clinical status as well as the motor (Fig. 8) and cognitive (Fig. 8) performances of both groups of animals were assessed on a monthly basis.

Following 10 wk of 3-NP treatment and before capsule implantation, all 3-NP-treated animals displayed significant hyperkinesia compared to controls. At the same time point, all animals displayed severe functional impairment of the frontostriatal pathway as evidenced by a significant decrease in the success score and a significant increase in the barrier hit score at the ORDT (Fig. 9).

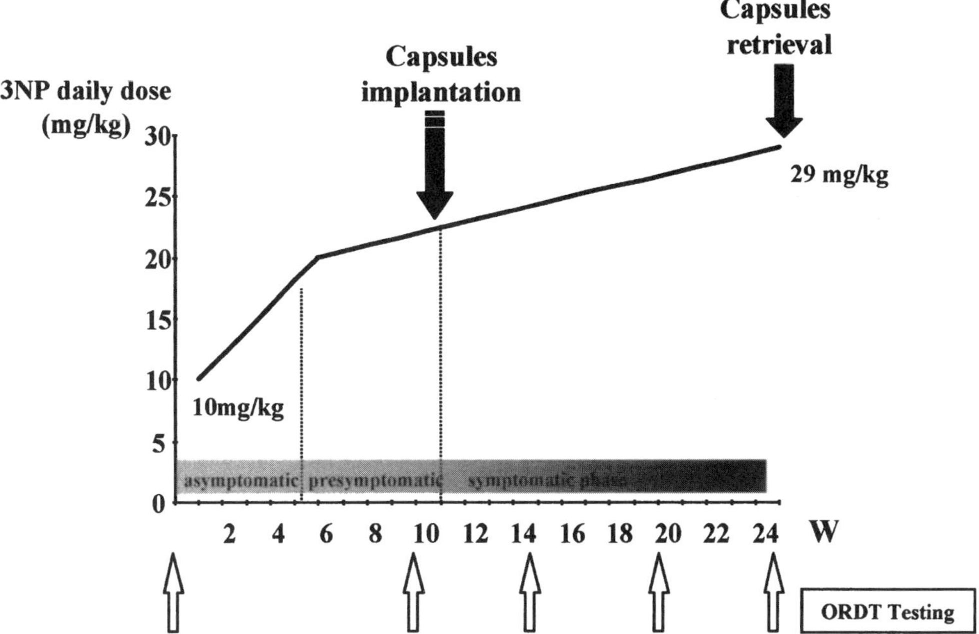

Fig. 8. Schematic representation of the experimental protocol used in the CNTF experiments. Six macaque monkeys were treated daily (5 d/wk) with 3-NP and regularly tested on motor and cognitive tasks (ORDT), i.e., before neurotoxic treatment, immediately before capsule implantation and on a monthly basis after capsule implantation (open arrows). Note that 3-NP treatment was continued following surgery. Animals were sacrificed immediately after the last behavioral testing and retrieval of capsules (i.e., 3 mo postsurgery).

Following implantation of the capsules, behavioral evaluation of these animals showed that, whereas the motor and cognitive deficits of the CNTF(-) animals increased continuously, a progressive significant recovery in both motor and cognitive deficits was observed in the CNTF(+) group of animals, in spite of continuing 3-NP treatment. The motor analysis indicated that, whereas all sham-operated animals displayed persistent dystonia in the lower limbs leading to a significant decrease in locomotor activity at 3 mo postimplantation, no such aggravation in motor symptoms was observed in the CNTF(+) animals, in which normal motor performances were restored as early as 2 mo postimplantation (Fig. 9).

Similarly, starting 1 mo postimplantation, CNTF(+) animals showed a significant improvement in their performances in the ORDT (increase in success score and decrease in barrier hits score), whereas the CNTF(-) animals did not show any significant improvement. This difference between groups was maintained throughout the remainder of the experiment, CNTF(+) animals performing significantly better than CNTF(-) animals at 3 mo postimplantation (Fig. 9).

Postmortem histological analysis confirmed the presence of a severe depletion of calbindin-D28k positive neurons in both caudate nucleus and putamen of the CNTF(-) animals compared to controls. In contrast, CNTF(+) animals displayed a significant neuroprotective effect of the cytokine on 3 out of the 5 anatomical levels compared to CNTF(-) animals.

These results show that CNTF, a cytokine displaying neuroprotective effects on striatal neurons in various lesion models *(43,44,46)*, can also exert restorative and neuroprotective effects in vivo in a primate model of ongoing striatal degeneration. As such, these data demonstrate the strong potential of CNTF as an efficient neuroprotectant for HD.

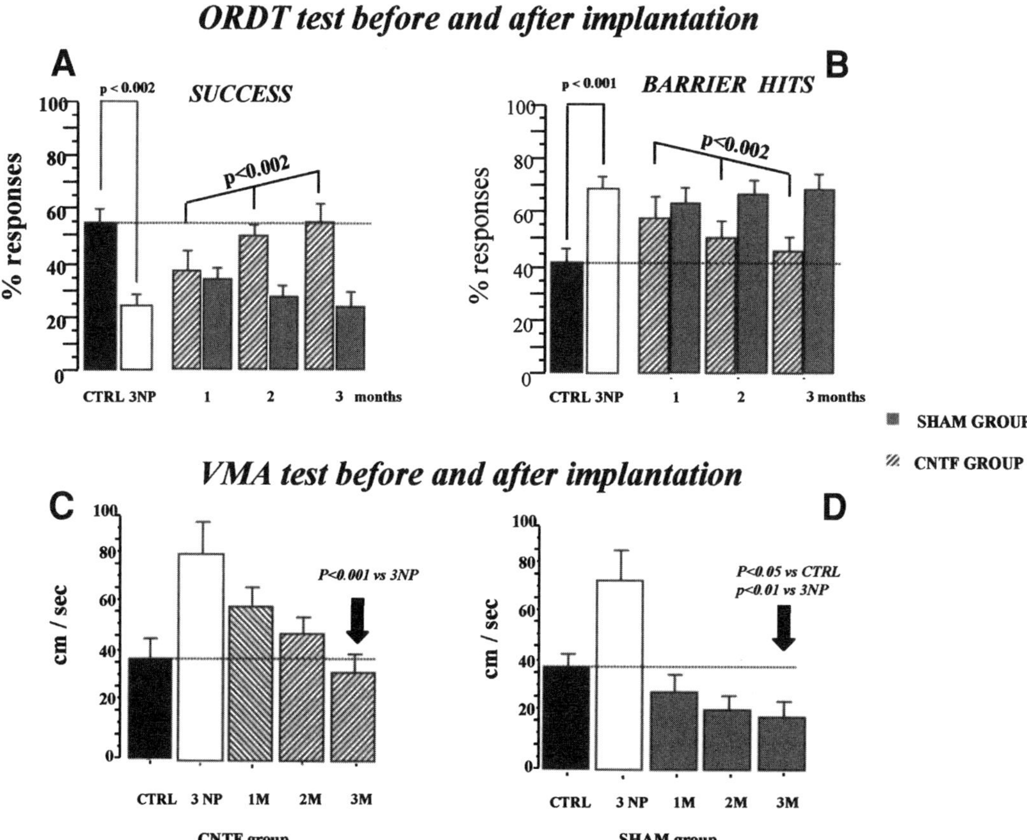

Fig. 9. (**A,B**) ORDT of cognitive performances in CNTF-treated animals (cross-hatched bars) and animals implanted with native BHK cells (grey bars). CNTF-treated and sham-operated animals were tested before (control [Ctrl]), following 10 wk of 3-NP treatment (i.e., just before surgical implantation: 3-NP), and every month following surgery (1, 2, and 3 mo). Before capsule implantation, a severe decrease in the success score (**A**) and a significant increase in the barrier hit score (**B**) evidenced a frontal-type cognitive deficit in all 3-NP-treated animals. For both cognitive indices, the performances of the CNTF-treated animals progressively improved after surgery until they reached control values, whereas those of the sham-operated animals remained severely impaired. VMA test of motor performances in CNTF-treated animals (**C**) and animals implanted with native BHK cells (**D**). The mean peak tangential velocity (PTV) was measured in cm/s in the two experimental groups before (Ctrl), after 10 wk of 3-NP treatment, i.e., just before surgical implantation of capsules (3-NP), and every month following implantation of the encapsulated cells (1, 2, and 3 mo). Following 10 wk of 3-NP administration, PTV significantly increased in both groups, but after implantation, animals from the CNTF-treated group recovered a normal PTV value, whereas animals from the sham-operated group became significantly bradykinetic (decrease in PTV below normal value) due to the occurence of severe dystonia.

4. CONCLUDING REMARKS

The present chapter points to the similarities between the neurodegenerative phenotype associated with prolonged 3-NP neurotoxicity in primates and the motor and cognitive deficits observed in Huntington's patients. Specifically, the development of a primate model that could replicate many of the main phenotypical features of HD, including a subcortical frontal-type cognitive deficit, provided an unique opportunity to evaluate new therapeutic strategies in carefully planned preclinical studies. This is particularly important when considering the potential use of new approaches, such as cellular or gene therapies, for which efficacy and safety should be determined before any trials are initiated in patients.

ACKNOWLEDGMENTS

The authors wish to acknowledge the following persons who have been involved in the studies described above: P. Aebischer, C. Dautry, M. Peschanski, and A. Zurn. We thank Dr. M. Mazière and Prof. A. Syrota for their continuing support and C. Genty, C. Jouy, D. Marchand, and F. Sergent for their help and their oustanding care of the primate colony. This work was supported by grants from Association Francaise contre les Myopathies, Association France-Huntington, Association France Parkinson, Commissariat a l'Energie Atomique (CEA), and Centre National de la Recherche Scientifique (CNRS) (France).

REFERENCES

1. Harper, P.S. (1991) *Huntington's Disease* (Harper, P.S., ed.), WB Saunders Company Ltd, London.
2. The Huntington's Disease Collaborative Group (1993) A novel gene containing a trinucleotide repeat that is expanded and unstable on Huntington's disease chromosomes. *Cell* **72,** 971–983.
3. Wellington, C.L., Brinkman, R.R., O'Kursky, J.R., and Hayden, M.R. (1997) Toward understanding the molecular pathology of Huntington's disease. *Brain Pathol.* **7,** 979–1002.
4. Li, X.J., Sharp, A.H., Li, S.H., Dawson, T.M., Snyder, S.H., and Ross, C.A. (1996) Huntingtin-associated protein (HAP1): discrete neuronal localization resemble those of neuronal nitric oxide synthase. *Proc. Natl. Acad. Sci. USA* **93,** 4839–4844.
5. Burke, J.R., Enghild, J.J., Martin, M.E., et al. (1996) Huntingtin and DRPLA proteins selectively interact with the enzyme GAPDH. *Nat. Med.* **2,** 347–350.
6. Brouillet, E., Condé, F., Beal, M.F., and Hantraye, P. (1999) Replicating Huntington's disease phenotype in experimental animals. *Prog. Neurobiol.* **59,** 427–468.
7. Beal, M.F. (1992) Does impairment of energy metabolism result in excitotoxic neuronal death in neurodegenerative illnesses? *Ann. Neurol.* **31,** 119–130.
8. Beal, M.F., Brouillet, E., Jenkins, B., et al. (1993) Neurochemical and histological characterization of the striatal excitotoxic lesions produced by the mitochondrial toxins 3-nitropropionic acid. *J. Neurosci.* **13,** 1481–1492.
9. Brouillet, E., Jenkins, B., Hyman, B., et al. (1993) Age-dependent vulnerability of the striatum to the mitochondrial toxin 3-nitropropionic acid. *J. Neurochem.* **60,** 356–359.
10. Guyot, M.-C., Hantraye, P., Dolan, R., Palfi, S., Mazière, M., and Brouillet, E. (1997) Quantifiable bradykinesia, gait abnormalities and Huntington's disease-like striatal lesions in rats chronically treated with 3-nitropropionic acid. *Neuroscience* **79,** 45–56.
11. Ouary, S., Bizat, N., Alterac, S., et al. (2000) Major strain differences in response to chronic systemic administration of the mitochondrial toxin 3-nitropropionic acid in rats: implications for neuroprotection studies. *Neuroscience* **97,** 521–530.
12. Brouillet, E., Hantraye, P., Ferrante, R.J., et al. (1995) Chronic mitochondrial energy impairment produces selective striatal degeneration and abnormal choreiform movements in primates. *Proc. Natl. Acad. Sci. USA* **92,** 7105–7109.
13. McHugh, P.R. and Folstein, M.F. (1975) Psychiatric syndromes of Huntington's chorea: a clinical and phenomenologic study, in *Psychiatric Aspects of Neurologic Diseases* (Benson, D.F. and Blumer, D., eds.), Grune & Stratton, New York, pp. 267–285.
14. Albert, M.L. (1978) Subcortical dementia, in *Alzheimer's Disease: Senile Dementia and Related Disorders* (Katzman, R., Terry, R.D., and Bick, K.L., eds.), Raven Press, New York, pp. 173–180.
15. Albert, M.L., Feldman, R.G., and Willis, A.L. (1974) The "subcortical dementia" of progressive supranuclear palsy. *J. Neurol. Neurosurg. Psychiatry* **37,** 121–130.
16. Cummings, J.L. (1993) Frontal-subcortical circuits and human behavior. *Arch. Neurol.* **50,** 873–880.
17. Butters, N., Sax, D., Montgomery, K., and Tarlow, S. (1978) Comparison of the neuropsychological deficits associated with early and advanced Huntington's disease. *Arch. Neurol.* **35,** 585–589.
18. Brandt, J., Folstein, S.E., and Folstein, M.F. (1988) Differential cognitive impairment in Alzheimer's disease and Huntington's disease. *Ann. Neurol.* **23,** 555–561.
19. Pillon, B., Dubois, B., Ploska, A., and Agid, Y. (1991) Severity and specificity of cognitive impairment in Alzheimer's, Huntington's, and Parkinson's diseases and progressive supranuclear palsy. *Neurology* **41,** 634–643.
20. Alexander, G.M., De Long, M.R., and Strick, P.L. (1986) Parallel organization of functionnally segregated circuits linking basal ganglia and cortex. *Ann. Rev. Neurosci.* **9,** 357–381.
21. Parent, A. (1990) Extrinsic connections of the basal ganglia. *Trends Neurosci.* **13,** 254–258.
22. Lawrence, A.D., Sahakian, B.J., Hodges, J.R., Rosser, A.E., Lange, K.W., and Robbins, T.W. (1996) Executive and mnemonic functions in early Huntington's disease. *Brain* **191,** 633–1645.
23. Josiassen, R.C., Curry, L.M., and Mancall, E.L. (1983) Development of neuropsychological deficits in Huntington's disease. *Arch. Neurol.* **40,** 791–796.

24. Roberts, A.C., De Salvia, M.A., Wilkinson, L.S., et al. (1994) 6-hydroxydopamine lesions of the prefrontal cortex in monkeys enhance performance on an analog of the Wisconsin Card Sort Test: possible interactions with subcortical dopamine. *J. Neurosci.* **14,** 2531–2544.
25. Mendez, M.F., Astorna, N.E., and Skoog-Lewandowski, K. (1989) Neurobehavioral changes associated with caudate lesions. *Neurology* **39,** 349–355.
26. Weinberger, D.R., Berman, K.F., Iadarola, M., Driesen, N., and Zec, R.F. (1988) Prefrontal cortical blood flow and cognitive function in Huntington's disease. *J. Neurol. Neurosurg. Psychiatry* **51,** 94–104.
27. Hantraye, P., Riche, D., Mazière, M., and Isacson, O. (1990) An experimental primate model of Huntington's disease: anatomical and behavioural studies of unilateral excitotoxic lesions of the caudate-putamen in the baboon. *Exp. Neurol.* **108,** 91–104.
28. Diamond, A. (1990) Developmental time course in human infants and infant monkeys, and the neural bases of inhibitory control in reaching. *Ann. NY Acad. Sci.* **608,** 637–669.
29. Palfi, S., Ferrante, R.J., Brouillet, E., et al. (1996) Chronic 3-nitropropionic acid treatment in baboons replicates the cognitive and motor deficits of Huntington's disease. *J. Neurosci.* **16,** 3019–3025.
30. Palfi, S., Condé, F., Riche, D., et al. (1998) Fetal striatal allografts reverse cognitive deficits in a primate model of Huntington disease. *Nat. Med.* **4,** 963–966.
31. Diamond, A. and Goldman-Rakic, P.S. (1985) Evidence for involvement of prefrontal cortex in cognitive changes during the first year of life: comparison of performances of human infant and rhesus monkeys on a detour task with transparent barrier. *Soc. Neurosci. Abstr.* **11,** 832.
32. Diamond, A., Zola-Morgan, S., and Squire, L.R. (1989) Successful performance by monkeys with lesions of the hippocampal formation on AB- and object retrieval, two tasks that mark developmental changes in human infants. *Behav. Neurosci.* **103,** 526–537.
33. Taylor, J.R., Elsworth, J.D., Roth, R.H., Sladek, J.R. Jr., and Redmond, D.E. Jr. (1990a) Improvements in MPTP-induced object retrieval deficits and behavioral deficits after fetal nigral grafting in monkeys. *Prog. Brain Res.* **82,** 543–559.
34. Taylor, J.R., Elsworth, J.D., Roth, R.H., Sladek, J.R. Jr., and Redmond, D.E. Jr. (1990b) Cognitive and motor deficits in the acquisition of an object retrieval/detour task in MPTP-treated monkeys. *Brain* **113,** 617–637.
35. Schneider, J.S. (1992) Behavioral and neuropathological consequences of chronic exposure to low doses of the dopaminergic neurotoxin MPTP, in *The Vulnerable Brain and Environmental Risks* (Isaacson, R.L. and Jensen, K.F., eds.), Plenum Press, New York, pp. 293–308.
36. Peschanski, M., Césaro, P., and Hantraye, P. (1995) Rationale for intrastriatal grafting of striatal neuroblasts in patients with Huntington's disease. *Neuroscience* **68,** 273–285.
37. Hantraye, P., Riche, D., Mazière, M., and Isacson, O. (1992) Intrastriatal transplantation of cross-species fetal striatal cells reduces abnormal movements in a primate model of Huntington's disease. *Proc. Natl. Acad. Sci. USA* **89,** 4187–4191.
38. Kendall, L.A., Rayment, F.D., Torres, E.M., Baker, H.F., Ridley, R.M., and Dunnett, S.B. (1998) Functional integration of striatal allografts in a primate model of Huntington's disease. *Nat. Med.* **4,** 727–729.
39. Selemon, L.D. and Goldman-Rakic, P.S. (1985) Longitudinal topography and interdigitation of corticostriatal projections in the Rhesus monkey. *J. Neurosci.* **5,** 776–794.
40. Künzle, H. (1975) Bilateral projections from precentral motor cortex to the putamen and other parts of the basal ganglia. An autoradiographic study in Macaca fascicularis. *Brain Res.* **88,** 195–209.
41. Dunnett, S.B. and Iversen, S.D. (1981) Learning impairments following selective kainic acid induced lesions within the neostriatum of rats. *Behav. Brain Res.* **2,** 189–209.
42. Bachoud-Levi, A.C., Rémy, P., Nguyen, J.P., et al. (2000) Motor and cognitive improvements in patients with Huntington's disease after neural transplantation. *Lancet* **356,** 1975–1979.
43. Emerich, D.F., Lindner, M.D., Winn, S.R., Chen, E.Y., Frydel, B.R., and Kordower, J.H. (1996) Implants of encapsulated CNTF-producing fibroblasts prevent biological deficits and striatal degeneration in a rodent model of Huntington's disease. *J. Neurosci.* **16,** 5168–5181.
44. Emerich, D.F., Winn, R.S., Hantraye, P.M., et al. (1997) Protective effect of encapsulated cells producing neurotrophic factor CNTF in a monkey model of Huntington's disease. *Nature* **386,** 395–399.
45. Mittoux, V., Joseph, J.M., Condé, F., et al. (2000). Restoration of cognitive and motor functions with ciliary neurotrophic factor in a primate model of Huntington's disease. *Hum. Gene Ther.* **11,** 1177–1187.
46. Anderson, K.D., Panayotatos, N., Cordoran, T.L., Lindsay, R.M., and Wiegan, S.J. (1996) Ciliary neurotrophic factor protects striatal output neurons in an animal model of Huntington's disease. *Proc. Natl. Acad. Sci. USA* **93,** 7346–7351.

13

Induction and Reversal of Cognitive Deficits in a Primate Model of Parkinson's Disease

Jay S. Schneider, PhD

1. INTRODUCTION

Parkinson's disease (PD) is typically characterized by the presence of at least two of the four cardinal motor signs typically associated with the disorder: bradykinesia (inability to execute movements with appropriate speed), rigidity, postural instability, and tremor. PD patients also suffer from other motor abnormalities, such as akinesia (inability to initiate movement in a timely manner) and hypokinesia (inability to produce movements of appropriate amplitude once begun). Historically, PD has been considered to be distinctly a disorder of motor function. However, it is now well accepted that cognitive impairment (without dementia) is a common feature of PD, in the early (and perhaps preclinical stages) as well as in the later stages of the disease *(1–4)*. Although PD patients may develop neuropsychological deficits across a range of cognitive functions *(5–8)*, many of these impairments resemble those associated with frontal lobe dysfunction. These deficits include executive function deficits and specifically involve difficulty in attention set shifting and set formation *(9,10)*, temporal ordering, sequencing, and planning *(3)*, impaired nonverbal and verbal short-term recall, impaired spatial short-term memory *(11)*, and impairments in focused attention *(12,13)*. Several lines of evidence suggest that at least some of the cognitive difficulties experienced by early as well as more progressed PD patients may be related to impaired attention mechanisms *(10,12,13)* or a disturbance in the frontal regulation of attention processes *(14)*. Parkinson's disease patients have difficulty in shifting and sustaining attention and have increased distractibility *(10,12,15)*, suggesting an attention deficit involving the selection of relevant from irrelevant stimuli for further information processing *(12,13)*.

2. MODELING THE COGNITIVE DEFICITS OF PD IN NONHUMAN PRIMATES

One advantage of modeling the cognitive deficits associated with PD in nonhuman primates is that it allows for the study of these deficits and their response to various pharmacological agents without the confound of age, chronic treatment effects, and possible co-existing pathologies that accompany the study of cognition in PD patients. In the mid-1980s, we initiated studies to develop the chronic low dose (CLD) 1-methyl-4-phenyl-1,2,3,6-tetrahydropyridine (MPTP) model of parkinsonism in monkeys to enable us to explore issues concerning the evolution of motor and nonmotor aspects of parkinsonism and to allow development of new therapeutic strategies aimed at these deficits *(16,17)*. The neurotoxin MPTP is commonly administered to macaque monkeys in relatively high doses over a short period

From: *Mental and Behavioral Dysfunction in Movement Disorders*
Edited by: M-A. Bédard et al. © Humana Press Inc., Totowa, NJ

of time (typically a over a few days to a few weeks) to produce animals with severe parkinsonian symptoms of akinesia, rigidity, bradykinesia, and stooped posture *(18–20)*. Such animals have proved to be a valuable model of PD, however, the presence of severe motor disability that evolves over a short time period precludes the study of cognitive disability, can be inconsistent with long-term survival, and does not model the progressive nature of human PD. By carefully titrating the dose of MPTP administered, it is possible to produce animals with little or no motor impairment, as well as animals with primarily early appearing cognitive impairment that, with continued exposure to MPTP, progress to have a classic parkinsonian motor deficit *(21)*. Although the time frame in which this syndrome develops is much compressed compared to human PD, these animals nonetheless mimic a progression of cognitive and motor symptoms that reflect the progression of symptoms in PD patients *(22,23)*. The use of these animals as a model for the evolution of parkinsonian symptoms is supported by the finding that MPTP-exposed humans that are asymptomatic for a parkinsonian motor disorder have cognitive deficits similar to those observed in idiopathic PD patients, as well as reduced striatal dopamine (DA)ergic function *(24)*.

A number of cognitive deficits have now been described in monkeys following chronic administration of low doses of the DAergic neurotoxin MPTP *(16,17,25)*. In particular, deficits were observed in performance of spatial delayed response (both with fixed and variable delays), delayed alternation, delayed matching-to-sample, visual discrimination reversal, and object retrieval tasks. In the variable delayed response task, monkeys perform a spatial delayed response task with different delay lengths randomly distributed over the trials that make up a daily test session. These delay conditions yield approximately chance performance at the longest delay, and normal monkeys perform this task showing a delay-dependent increase in errors commensurate with the limits of their short-term spatial memory. Chronic low dose MPTP-treated monkeys are significantly impaired on this task performance and show a delay-independent pattern of responding on this task. That is, they are just as likely to perform poorly on short delay trials as on long delay trials, suggesting attentional as well as short-term spatial memory deficits. Consistent with an attentional deficit, we have also reported that chronic low dose MPTP-treated monkeys, with clinical features that mimic "early" parkinsonism, have increased restlessness and distractibility and a problem with response maintenance *(26)*. Correct performance of all of the above-mentioned tasks is believed to be dependent upon the integrity of frontostriatal circuits *(27–29)*. The monkeys used in our studies had virtually normal motor functioning and retained the ability to perform a visual pattern discrimination task, the performance of which is most likely dependent upon the integrity of the inferotemporal cortex *(27)*.

Other laboratories have also described cognitive deficits in MPTP-treated monkeys. Taylor et al. *(30,31)* described deficits in acquisition and performance of an object retrieval task that can vary in the cognitive and motor difficulty of individual trials. The object retrieval task is a detour reaching task that has been used to assess cognitive development and problem solving in humans and nonhuman primates *(32)*. In this task, monkeys have to retrieve food from a transparent box with one open side. The open side of the box can face toward or away from the monkey, and the position of the food in the box can be such that the reach is motorically easy or difficult. A cognitive error occurs when the monkey reaches to a closed side of the box rather than making a detour reach to the open side. In one study *(31)*, monkeys were administered MPTP and either became severely symptomatic or showed no gross motor impairment, despite major depletions in striatal DA levels. When these animals were tested on an object retrieval task 8–12 mo later, they made a significant number of cognitive errors as well as displayed awkward motor behavior during task performance. Thus, cognitive and motor deficits in the acquisition of this task were observed 8–12 mo after toxin exposure, even in animals that never showed parkinsonian motor deficits. Both cognitive and motor impairments on this task performance remained stable for at least 3 to 4 mo *(30)*.

Fernandez-Ruiz et al. *(33)* administered MPTP to rhesus monkeys and reported that these animals had impaired performance of a spatial delayed response task with both fixed and random delays when tested 10 yr after MPTP exposure. These results show persistent spatial deficits in MPTP-treated monkeys. In addition to work with monkeys, other researchers have also described spatial working memory impairments in mice following MPTP exposure *(34)*.

Slovin et al. *(35)* showed that low dose MPTP treatments in rhesus monkeys produced frontal cognitive deficits (assessed as deficits in performance of a spatial delayed response task with frequent alternations between go and no-go behavioral modes) that were not associated with parkinsonian motor dysfunction. However, self-initiated saccadic eye movements were impaired in these animals, suggesting that frontal-type cognitive impairment and saccadic deficits may be the first signs of MPTP-induced parkinsonism.

Cognitive deficits have also been described in monkeys with MPTP-induced hemiparkinsonism. Animals with unilateral striatal dopamine depletion have been shown to have neglect of contralateral visual stimuli, suggesting perhaps a deficit in selective attention *(36,37)*. More detailed studies of hemiparkinsonian monkeys showed that the hemi-inattention or hemineglect in monkeys with unilateral nigrostriatal lesions were neither purely the result of a primary motor impairment nor a primary sensory impairment, but most likely the result of an impairment in the delivery of appropriate sensory information to the striatum, the faulty processing of sensory information within the striatum or a disturbed sensory-to-motor linkup resulting in abnormal responsiveness to inputs *(38)*.

3. NEUROCHEMICAL DEFECTS IN COGNITIVELY IMPAIRED MPTP-TREATED MONKEYS

PD and MPTP-induced parkinsonism are characterized primarily by loss of substantia nigra DAergic neurons and striatal DA depletion. It is evident though that DAergic defects alone cannot explain all of the various cognitive symptoms of PD or MPTP-induced parkinsonism in monkeys. Although DA replacement therapies have proven useful in relieving the motor disturbances seen in PD, the effect of these therapies on cognitive deficits associated with the disorder are less obvious. Some studies have shown a deleterious effect of levodopa on cognition at doses having a beneficial effect on motor symptoms *(39)*. In a study assessing short-term memory and temporal ordering in early PD, a greater deficit was found in patients treated with DA replacement therapy as compared to *de novo*, untreated patients. In another study, levodopa had no positive effect on cognitive slowing in a visual perception task *(40)*. Nevertheless, some studies have reported beneficial effects of levodopa on at least some cognitive functions, including working memory and attention *(15,41)*. Our own studies of PD patients have shown that some cognitive tasks (i.e., conditional associative learning, attention set shifting) are not performed as well under the levodopa-medicated condition, while other tasks (visuospatial memory) are performed better while medicated (unpublished observations).

Up to this point, neurochemical and neuropathological studies performed on CLD MPTP monkeys have been relatively limited, since most animals have been studied for long periods of time, and post-mortem material has been scarce. However, in CLD MPTP-treated monkeys with cognitive but no gross motor deficits, cortical DA levels were not significantly decreased in any of the cortical regions sampled, and norepinephrine (NE) levels were decreased in the frontal pole and the orbital cortex. Levels of serotonin (5-HT) and its major metabolite 5-hydroxyindoleacetic acid (5-HIAA) were elevated in dorsolateral prefrontal cortex, dihydroxy phenylacetic acid DA (DOPAC), and homovanillio acid (HVA) levels were decreased in all striatal regions, with the dorsolateral caudate most affected, and nucleus accumbens least affected *(42)*. Putamen DA levels were also depleted, but to a lesser extent than in the caudate. An ongoing clinical study in our laboratory examining the relationships between cognitive functioning and DA transporter levels (visualized by SPECT imaging) in early mild PD patients, suggests that those patients with discrete frontostriatal cognitive deficits may have lower DA transporter levels (i.e., possibly reflecting lower DA innervation) in the caudate rather than in the putamen (unpublished observation). These findings are supported by a recent report describing the relationship between cognitive impairment in PD and caudate and putamen DAergic function, using fluorodopa positron emission tomography (PET) scanning *(43)*. Thus, it is possible that lower DAergic innervation of the caudate compared to the putamen may be more associated with impaired cognitive functioning in PD and perhaps in cognitively impaired MPTP-treated monkeys.

In cognitively impaired motor asymptomatic monkeys, postmortem NE levels were also significantly decreased in the caudate nucleus, while 5-HT levels were significantly increased in all striatal regions. While this is in contrast to the reductions in 5-HT levels typically reported in postmortem studies of the human PD brain, it must be remembered that these animals represent a very early stage of parkinsonism, which is rarely observed in human postmortem material. It is quite possible that this increase in 5-HT seen in these animals is a possible compensatory response that contributes to the maintenance of motor function in these animals. Continued study of these early parkinsonian animals, as well as longitudinal study of those that progress through this phase to develop full-blown parkinsonism, might confirm this possibility as well as suggest the existence of other possible compensatory mechanisms. Indeed, preliminary data from our laboratory now shows that animals that were chronically parkinsonian and developed parkinsonian motor symptoms slowly have significantly lower 5-HT levels in cortex and striatum (similar to those observed in acutely symptomatic parkinsonian monkeys) compared to cognitively impaired motor asymptomatic monkeys. Such findings are consistent with a previous report by Pifl et al. *(44)* that also showed significantly higher 5-HT and NE levels in numerous brain regions in MPTP-exposed asymptomatic monkeys vs acutely symptomatic animals, although no behavioral assays were employed in that study.

4. DRUG EFFECTS ON MPTP-INDUCED COGNITIVE DEFICITS IN MONKEYS

4.1. *DAergic Therapies*

We have undertaken numerous studies designed to assess the effects of various pharmacological agents on the cognitive deficits in low dose MPTP-treated monkeys in an effort to obtain a more complete understanding of the neurochemical defect that might underlie these deficits. In view of the DAergic dysfunction known to exist in CLD MPTP-treated monkeys, we have investigated the effects of various DAergic agents on the cognitive deficits in these animals. Levodopa has been found to be generally ineffective in reversing deficits in delayed response or delayed matching-to-sample performance in low dose MPTP-treated monkeys *(45)*. Furthermore, in monkeys with both cognitive and motor deficits associated with long-term MPTP exposure, levodopa was found to significantly improve motor components of object retrieval task performance, but had no effects on the cognitive deficits associated with this task. At low doses, the stimulant methylphenidate and the DA D2 receptor agonist quinpirole decreased the number of omission errors made by CLD MPTP-treated monkeys on delayed response tasks, but had no effects on the number of commission errors these animals made on the same tasks *(46)*. Similarly, Slovin et al. *(35)* showed that combined DAergic therapy (i.e., levodopa and bromocritpine) decreased omission errors, but did not improve commission errors in low dose MPTP-treated monkeys with frontal cognitive deficits. The partial DA D1 receptor agonist SKF-38393 had no effects on omission or commision errors made during delayed response performance *(47)*. However, dihydrexidine, a full DA D1 receptor agonist, significantly decreased both omission and commission errors and significantly improved overall task performance *(47)*. While these results may suggest different influences of D1 and D2 receptors on the behavioral deficits measured in these studies, this interpretation is complicated by the pharmacology of dihydrexidine, which has been shown to not only be a full efficacy DA D1 receptor agonist, but to be a potent releaser of acetylcholine in both the striatum and cortex *(48)*. Thus, the cognition-enhancing activity of this drug may have as much to do with its acetylcholine-releasing properties as its D1 agonist properties. This is particularly significant in view of the known beneficial effects of neuronal acetylcholine receptor agonists on the cognitive dysfunctions in MPTP-treated monkeys (see discussion in Subheading 4.2.).

4.2. *Effects of Nicotinic Acetylcholine Receptor Agonists*

In light of the general lack of effect of direct acting DAergic agents on the cognitive deficits associated with MPTP exposure in monkeys, we undertook a series of studies designed to assess the effects of other pharmacological agents on the behavioral problems of these animals. The nicotinic system was of particular interest, since nicotine had been shown to improve a variety of cognitive problems in animals and improved attention in adults with attention deficit–hyperactivity disorder *(49)* and improved perceptual and visual attentional deficits in Alzheimer's disease patients *(50)*. Because of dose-limiting side effects of nicotine on the gastrointestinal and cardiovascular systems, we chose to study subtype selective nicotinic receptor agonists. Compounds that selectively activate central nicotinic acetylcholine receptor (nAChR) subtypes stimulate the release of DA, acetylcholine, and NE from presynaptic terminals. Our thought was that compounds with such pharmacological profiles might be more effective therapeutic agents for correcting cognitive dysfunction in MPTP-treated monkeys.

The nAChR agonist (S)-(-)-5-ethynyl-3-(1-methyl-2-pyrrolidinyl)pyridine (SIB-1508Y) improved performance of the shortest delay trials in a variable delayed response task, suggesting that SIB-1508Y may enhance attentional abilities *(45)*. It is uncertain as to the extent to which SIB-1508Y may enhance short-term working memory, since SIB-1508Y did not improve performance on long delay trials (that were performed poorly even when the animals were normal), but did improve performance on intermediate length delay trials. The beneficial effect of SIB-1508Y was not paradigm-specific, as marked improvement was also observed in performance of 0- and 3-s delay trials on a delayed matching-to-sample (DMS) task *(45)*. The use of these relatively short duration delays in the DMS task puts little demand on short-term memory, and correct task performance more likely depends on intact attentional processes.

In another study, SIB-1508Y alone did not significantly improve either the cognitive or motor aspects of object retrieval task performance in monkeys with symptomatic parkinsonism *(21)*. Levodopa treatment significantly improved motor aspects of performance, but not cognitive performance deficits. However, the combination of SIB-1508Y and levodopa caused significant improvements in both cognitive and motor aspects of task performance and did so at one-third to one-sixth the levodopa dose necessary to improve motor function alone. Low doses of levodopa alone may provide a necessary but insufficient drive to frontostriatal circuits involved in cognition, and SIB-1508Y may provide a necessary but insufficient requirement for improved cognitive performance in these motor symptomatic animals. However, in combination, these 2 drugs may provide sufficient DAergic and other neurochemical drive to improve cognition in motor-symptomatic monkeys. The combination of these drugs may address the DA deficiency of the parkinsonism while also addressing noradrenergic and possibly cholinergic dysfunctions as well.

In contrast to effects of SIB-1508Y on cognition in low dose MPTP-treated monkeys, another nAChR agonist, SIB-1553A, improved performance on both short and long delay trials on a variable delayed response task, suggesting effects on both attention and short-term spatial memory *(51)*. The differences in effects on task performance between these compounds may be explained by their nAChR subtype selectivity. While SIB-1508Y has prominent selectivity at $\alpha4\beta2$ receptors, SIB-1553A has prominent effects at $\alpha2\beta4$ receptors *(52)*. Additionally, SIB-1553A is very effective in stimulating hippocampal acetylcholine release, whereas SIB-1508Y is much less effective. Both compounds stimulated striatal DA release and stimulate significant NE release from frontal cortex *(52)*. The slightly different profiles of these drugs on neurotransmitter release may underlie their different abilities to improve cognitive functioning in MPTP-treated monkeys.

4.3. *Effects of Other Neuropharmacologic Agents*

We have recently investigated other novel approaches to the amelioration of cognitive performance deficits in low dose MPTP-treated monkeys. Although it is still unclear as to the therapeutic usefulness of N-methyl-D-aspartic acid (NMDA) antagonists in treating the motor dysfunctions of

PD, there may be a role for stimulation of the NMDA receptor in treating some of the nonmotor or cognitive sequelae of PD. Several reports have suggested that positive modulation of the NMDA receptor might be useful for the treatment of various learning and memory impairments. Activation of the NMDA receptor leads to long-term potentiation (a mechanism of synaptic modification related to memory formation and learning) *(53)*, and antagonism of NMDA receptors results in disruption of learning and memory preocesses *(54,55)*. Use of a partial agonist at the glycine modulatory site of the NMDA receptor might circumvent the problem of excitotoxicty associated with NMDA receptor stimulation, while allowing functional NMDA receptor activation. The glycine-B site on the NMDA receptor is a modulatory site wherein glycine, in the presence of glutamate, acts synergistically with glutamate to promote channel opening and excitatory neurotransmision. One such partial glycine agonist is the antibiotic D-cycloserine. As a partial agonist, D-cycloserine, at low concentrations, acts as an agonist mimicking glycine's effects and stimulating NMDA receptors *(56,57)*. At high concentrations, it can antagonize the effects of endogenous glycine, blocking excess stimulation.

Single administration of D-cycloserine significantly improved performance on a variable delayed response task in low dose MPTP-treated monkeys *(58)*. Since D-cycloserine improved performance at both short (2-s) and long (20-s) duration delays, there is the possibility that this drug may have effects on both attention as well as memory components of task performance. The effects of D-cycloserine on cognition in chronic MPTP-treated monkeys may be related to stimulation of neurotransmitter release and enhanced function in a variety of interrelated cortical and subcortical systems. D-cycloserine may act in part to increase cortical and striatal DA activity, since activation of NMDA receptors releases DA and increases DA neuronal firing, particularly in prefrontal cortex *(59)*. Previous studies have also shown NMDA-induced release of acetylcholine in striatum *(59)* and medial septum *(60)* and cholinergic-glutamatergic interactions in cognitive function *(61,62)*. Thus, as observed with nAChR agonists, effects of D-cycloserine on cognitive dysfunction in chronic MPTP-treated monkeys may be related to release of various neurotransmitters at several cortical and subcortical sites, as well as nonspecific effects of directly enhancing glutamatergic neurotransmission.

In addition to deficits in levels of various neurotransmitters in PD and in animal models of PD, decreased levels of various neuropeptides may also contribute to parkinsonian symptomatology *(63)*. Several neuropeptides, particularly substance P, have been implicated in learning and memory *(64)* and are present endogenously in cortex and striatum. Since proline-containing neuropeptides, such as substance P, vasopressin, and thyrotropin-releasing hormone, have all been implicated as potential cognition enhancers *(65)*, a possible therapeutic approach to the cognitive deficits associated with parkinsonism might be enhancement of endogenous neuropeptide levels. This could be accomplished through protection of neuropeptides from degradation with peptidase inhibitors. Proline endopeptidase is a serine endo-oligopeptidase involved in the degradation of various neuropeptides in vitro and in vivo *(66)*. S 17092 is a highly potent orally active cell permeant inhibitor of proline endopeptidase in brain *(67,68)*. S 17092 can at least partially reverse scopolamine-induced amnesia and age-associated spatial delayed alternation deficits in mice, as well as increase striatal substance P immunoreactivity *(69)*.

Seven-day oral administration of S 17092, followed by single dose administration of the same dose on the day of testing, significantly improved overall performance on variable delayed response and DMS tasks. S 17092 did not significantly improve performance on long duration delay trials (≥20 s) in the variable delayed response task, but did improve performance at short and intermediate (≤10 s) length delays *(70)*. Thus, S 17092 appeared to improve memory within its normal limits in these animals and may also have enhanced attentional abilities (evidenced by improved performance at short duration delays).

Chronic oral pretreatment with S 17092 for 7 d prior to administration of the test dose of drug and cognitive testing was necessary in order to observe cognition-enhancing effects. During the first 3 d of the 7 d pretreatment period, S 17092 did not improve any of the cognitive functions measured, which was consistent with other reports that showed chronic oral administration of S 17092 to be more effective than acute administration in inhibiting brain postproline cleaving enzyme activity, thus improving learning and memory performances in both young scopolamine-treated and aged mice *(69)*.

5. CONCLUSIONS

The cognitive deficits in CLD MPTP-treated monkeys and in PD patients most likely arise from dysfunction of several cortical and subcortical neurotransmitter systems and functional circuits, such that DAergic treatments alone cannot sufficiently normalize behavior. The superior effects of nAChR agonists, D-cycloserine, and proline–endopeptidase inhibitors may be due to the ability of these drugs to modulate release of DA and other neurotransmitters, including NE and acetylcholine from various cortical and subcortical sites.

REFERENCES

1. Levin, B.E., Llabre, M.M., and Weiner, W.J. (1989) Cognitive impairments associated with early Parkinson's disease. *Neurology* **39,** 557–561.
2. Heitanen, M. and Teravainen, H. (1986) Cognitive performance in early Parkinson's disease. *Acta Neurol. Scand.* **73,** 151–159.
3. Cooper, J.A., Sagar, H.J., Jordan, N., Harvey, N.S., and Sullivan, E. (1991) Cognitive impairment in early, untreated Parkinson's disease and its relationship to motor disability. *Brain* **114,** 2095–2122.
4. Owen, A.M., James, M., Leigh, P.N., et al. (1992) Fronto-striatal cognitive deficits at different stages of Parkinson's disease. *Brain* **115,** 1727–1751.
5. Lees, A.J. and Smith, E. (1983) Cognitive deficits in the early stages of Parkinson's disease. *Brain* **106,** 257–270.
6. Taylor, A.E., Saint-Cyr, J.A., and Lang, A.E. (1986) Frontal lobe dysfunction in Parkinson's disease. *Brain* **109,** 845–883.
7. Brown, R.G. and Marsden, C.D. (1988) 'Subcortical dementia': the neuropsychological evidence. *Neuroscience* **25,** 363–387.
8. Boller, F., Passafiume, D., Keefe, N.C., et al. (1984) Visuospatial impairments in Parkinson's disease: role of perceptual and motor factors. *Arch. Neurol.* **41,** 485–490.
9. Flowers, K.A. and Robertson, C. (1985) The effect of Parkinson's disease on the ability to maintain a mental set. *J. Neurol. Neurosurg. Psychiatry* **48,** 517–529.
10. Downes, J.J., Roberts, A.C., Sahakian, B.J., Evenden, J.L., Morris, R.G., and Robbins, T.W. (1989) Impaired extradimensional shift performance in medicated and unmedicated Parkinson's disease: evidence for a specific attentional dysfunction. *Neuropsychologia* **27,** 1329–1343.
11. Freedman, M. and Oscar-Berman, M. (1986) Selective delayed response deficits in Parkinson's and Alzheimer's disease. *Arch. Neurol.* **43,** 886–890.
12. Sharpe, M.H. (1990) Distractability in early Parkinson's disease. *Cortex* **26,** 239–246.
13. Sharpe, M.H. (1992) Auditory attention in early Parkinson's disease: an impairment in focused attention. *Neuropsychologia* **30,** 101–106.
14. Stam, C.J., Visser, S.L., Op de Coul, A.A.W., et al. (1993) Disturbed frontal regulation of attention in Parkinson's disease. *Brain* **116,** 1139–1158.
15. Lange, K.W., Robbins, T.W., Marsden, C.D., James, M., Owen, A.M., and Paul, G.M. (1992) L-dopa withdrawal in Parkinson's disease selectively impairs cognitive performance in tests sensitive to frontal lobe dysfunction. *Psychopharmacology* **107,** 394–404.
16. Schneider, J.S., Unguez, G., Yuwiler, A., Berg, S.C., and Markham, C.H. (1988) Deficits in operant behavior in monkeys treated with MPTP. *Brain* **111,** 1265–1285.
17. Schneider, J.S. and Kovelowski, C.J. (1990) Chronic exposure to low doses of MPTP. I. Cognitive deficits in motor asymptomatic monkeys. *Brain Res.* **519,** 122–128.
18. Burns, R.S., Chiueh, C.C., Markey, S.P., Jacobowitz, D.M., and Kopin, I.J. (1983) A primate model of parkinsonism: selective destruction of dopaminergic neurons in the pars compacta of the substantia nigra by N-methyl-4-phenyl-1,2,3,6-tetrahydropyridine. *Proc. Natl. Acad. Sci. USA* **80,** 4546–4550.
19. Schultz, W., Studer, A., Romo, R., Sundstrom, E., Jonsson, G., and Scarnati, E. (1989) Deficits in reaction times and movement times as correlates of hypokinesia in monkeys with MPTP-induced striatal dopamine depletion. *J. Neurophysiol.* **61,** 651–668.
20. Schneider, J.S., Yuwiler, A., and Markham, C.H. (1987) Selective loss of subpopulations of ventral mesencephalic dopaminergic neurons in the monkey following exposure to MPTP. *Brain Res.* **411,** 144–150.
21. Schneider, J.S., Van Velson, M., Menzaghi, F., and Lloyd, G.K. (1998) Effects of the nicotinic acetylcholine receptor agonist SIB-1508Y on object retrieval performance in MPTP-treated monkeys: comparison with levodopa treatment. *Ann. Neurol.* **43,** 311–317.
22. Schneider, J.S. and Pope-Coleman, A. (1995) Cognitive deficits precede motor deficits in a slowly progressing model of Parkinsonism in the monkey. *Neurodegeneration* **4,** 245–255.

23. Pope-Coleman, A., Tinker, J., and Schneider, J.S. (1998) Effects of chronic GM1 ganglioside treatment on cognitive and motor deficits in a slowly progressing model of Parkinsonism in non-human primates. *Restorative Neurol. Neurosci.* **12,** 255–266.
24. Stern, Y., Tetrud, J.W., Martin, W.R.W., Kutner, S.J., and Langston, J.W. (1990) Cognitive change following MPTP exposure. *Neurology* **40,** 261–264.
25. Schneider, J.S. and Roeltgen, D.P. (1993) Delayed matching-to-sample, object retrieval, and discrimination reversal deficits in chronic low dose MPTP-treated monkeys. *Brain Res.* **615,** 351–354.
26. Roeltgen, D.P. and Schneider, J.S. (1994) Task persistence and learning ability in normal and chronic low dose MPTP-treated monkeys. *Behav. Brain Res.* **60,** 115–124.
27. Divac, I., Rosvold, H.E., and Schwarcbart, M.K. (1967) Behavioral effects of selective ablation of the caudate nucleus. *J. Comp. Physiol. Psychol.* **63,** 184–190.
28. Battig, K., Rosvold, H.E., and Mishkin, M. (1960) Comparison of the effects of frontal and caudate lesions on delayed response and alternation in monkeys. *J. Comp. Psychol.* **53,** 400–404.
29. Brozoski, T.J., Brown, R.M., Rosvold, H.E., and Goldman, P.S. (1979) Cognitive deficit caused by regional depletion of dopamine in prefrontal cortex of rhesus monkey. *Science* **205,** 929–932.
30. Taylor, J.R., Elsworth, J.D., Roth, R.H., Sladek, J.R., and Redmond, D.E. (1990) Cognitive and motor deficits in the acquisition of an object retrieval/detour reaching task in MPTP-treated monkeys. *Brain* **113,** 617–637.
31. Taylor, J.R., Roth, R.H., Sladek, J.R., and Redmond, D.E. (1990) Cognitive and motor deficits in the performance of an object retrieval task with a barrier-detour in monkeys (*Cercopithecus aethiops sabeus*) treated with MPTP: long-term performance and effect of transparency of the barrier. *Behav. Neurosci.* **104,** 564–576.
32. Diamond, A. (1990) Developmental time course in human infants and infant monkeys, and the neural basis of inhibitory control in reaching. *Ann. NY Acad. Sci.* **608,** 637–669.
33. Fernandez-Ruiz, J., Doudet, D.J., and Aigner, T.G. (1995) Long-term cognitive impairment in MPTP-treated rhesus monkeys. *Neuroreport* **7,** 102–104.
34. Tanila, H., Bjorlund, M., and Riekkinen, P. Jr. (1998) Cognitive changes in mice following moderate MPTP exposure. *Brain Res. Bull.* **45,** 577–582.
35. Slovin, H., Abeles, M., Vaadia, E., Haalman, I., Prut, Y., and Bergman, H. (1999) Frontal cognitive impairments and saccadic deficits in low-dose MPTP-treated monkeys. *J. Neurophysiol.* **81,** 858–874.
36. Apicella, P., Legallet, E., Nieoullon, A., and Trouche, E. (1991) Neglect of contralateral visual stimuli in monkeys with unilateral striatal dopamine depletion. *Behav. Brain Res.* **46,** 187–195.
37. Bankiewicz, K.S., Oldfield, E.H., Plunkett, R.J., et al. (1991) Apparent unilateral visual neglect in MPTP-hemiparkinsonian monkeys is due to delayed initiation of motion. *Brain Res.* **541,** 98–102.
38. Schneider, J.S., McLaughlin, W.W., and Roeltgen, D.P. (1992) Motor and non-motor behavioral deficits in monkeys made hemi-parkinsonian by intracarotid MPTP infusion. *Neurology* **42,** 1565–1573.
39. Gotham, A.M., Brown, R.G., and Marsden, C.D. (1988) 'Frontal' cognitive function in patients with Parkinson's disease 'on' and 'off' levodopa. *Brain* **111,** 299–321.
40. Pillon, B., Dubois, B., Bonnet, A.M., et al. (1989) Cognitive slowing in Parkinson's disease fails to respond to levodopa treatment: the 15-objects test. *Neurology* **39,** 762–768.
41. Cooper, J.A., Sagar, H.J., Doherty, S.M., Jordan, N., Tidswell, P., and Sullivan, E.V. (1992) Different effects of dopaminergic and anticholinergic therapies on cognitive and motor function in Parkinson's disease. *Brain* **115,** 1701–1725.
42. Schneider, J.S. (1990) Chronic exposure to low doses of MPTP. II. Neurochemical and pathological consequences in cognitively-impaired, motor asymptomatic monkeys. *Brain Res.* **534,** 25–36.
43. Rinne, J.O., Portin, R., Ruottinen, H., Nurmi, E., Bergman, J., Haaparanta, M. (2000) Cognitive impairment and the brain dopaminergic system in Parkinson's disease. *Arch. Neurol.* **57,** 470–475.
44. Pifl, C., Bertel, O., Schingnitz, G., and Hornykiewicz, O. (1990) Extrastriatal dopamine in symptomatic and asymptomatic rhesus monkeys treated with MPTP. *Neurochem. Int.* **17,** 263–270.
45. Schneider, J.S., Tinker, J.P., Van Velson, M., Menzaghi, F., and Lloyd, G.K. (1999) Nicotinic acetylcholine receptor agonist SIB-1508Y improves cognitive functioning in chronic low dose MPTP-treated monkeys. *J. Pharmacol. Exp. Ther.* **290,** 731–739.
46. Schneider, J.S., Sun, Z.-Q., and Roeltgen, D.P. (1994) Effects of dopamine agonists on delayed response performance in chronic low dose MPTP-treated monkeys. *Pharmacol. Biochem. Behav.* **48,** 235–240.
47. Schneider, J.S., Sun, Z.-Q., and Roeltgen, D.P. (1994) Effects of dihydrexidine, a full dopamine D-1 receptor agonist, on delayed response performance in chronic low dose MPTP-treated monkeys. *Brain Res.* **663,** 140–144.
48. Steele, T.D., Hodges, D.B. Jr., Levesque, T.R., and Locke, K.W. (1997) D1 agonist dihydrexidine releases acetylcholine and improves cognition in rats. *Pharmacol. Biochem. Behav.* **58,** 477–483.
49. Levin, E.D., Conners, C.K., Sparrow, E., et al. (1995) Nicotine effects on adults with attention-deficit/hyperactivity disorder. *Psychopharmacology* **123,** 55–63.
50. Jones, G.M.M., Sahakian, B.J., Levy, R., Warburton, D.M., and Gray, J.A. (1992) Effects of nicotine on attention, information processing and short-term memory in Alzheimer's disease. *Psychopharmacology* **108,** 485–494.
51. Tinker, J., Van Velson, M., Menzaghi, F., Lloyd, G.K., and Schneider, J.S. (1998) Effects of SIB-1553A, a novel subtype selective nAChR agonist, on cognition in chronic MPTP-treated monkeys. *Soc. Neurosci. Abstr.* **24,** 333.
52. Lloyd, G.K., Menzaghi, F., Bontempi, B., et al. (1998) The potential of subtype-selective neuronal nicotinic acetylcholine receptor agonists as therapeutic agents. *Life Sciences* **62,** 1601–1606.

53. Collingridge, G.L. and Bliss, T.V.P. (1987) NMDA receptors-their role in long-term potentiation. *Trends Neurosci.* **10,** 288–293.
54. Bischoff, C. and Tiedtke, P.I. (1992) Competitive and non-competitive NMDA receptor antagonists in spatial learning tasks. *Eur. J. Pharmacol.* **213,** 269–273.
55. Ogura, H. and Aigner, T.G. (1993) MK 801 impairs recognition memory in rhesus monkeys: comparison with cholinergic drugs. *J. Pharmacol. Exp. Ther.* **266,** 60–64.
56. Lanthorn, T.H. (1994) D-Cycloserine: agonist turned antagonist. *Amino Acids* **6,** 247–260.
57. Watson, G.B., Bolanowski, M.A., Baganoff, M.P., Deppeler, C.L., and Lanthorn, T.H. (1990) D-cycloserine acts as a partial agonist at the glycine modulatory site of the NMDA receptor expressed Xenopus oocytes. *Brain Res.* **510,** 158–160.
58. Schneider, J.S., Tinker, J.P., Van Velson, M., and Giardiniere, M. (2000) Effects of the partial glycine agonist D-cycloserine on cognitive functioning in chronic low dose MPTP-treated monkeys. *Brain Res.* **860,** 190–194.
59. Ransom, R.W. and Deschenes, N.L. (1989) Glycine modulation of NMDA-evoked release of [3H] acetylcholine and [3H] dopamine from rat striatal slices. *Neurosci. Lett.* **96,** 323–328.
60. Nishimura, L.M. and Boegman, R.J. (1990) N-methyl-D-aspartate-evoked release of acetylcholine form the medial septum/diagonal band of rat brain. *Neurosci. Lett.* **115,** 259–264.
61. Aigner, T.G. (1995) Pharmacology of memory: cholinergic-glutamatergic interactions. *Curr. Opin. Neurobiol.* **5,** 155–160.
62. Matsuoka, N. and Aigner, T.G. (1996) The glycine/NMDA receptor antagonist HA-966 impairs visual recognition memory in rhesus monkeys. *Brain Res.* **731,** 72–78.
63. Mauborgne, A., Javoy-Agid, F., Legrand, J.C., Agid, Y., and Cesselin, F (1983) Decrease in substance P-like immunoreactivity in the substantia nigra and pallidum in Parkinsonian brains. *Brain Res.* **268,** 167–170.
64. Huston, J.P. and Hasenohrl, R.U. (1995) The role of neuropeptides in learning: focus on the neurokinin substance P. *Behav. Brain Res.* **66,** 117–127.
65. Toide, K., Iwamoto, Y., Fujiwara, T., and Abe, H. (1995) JTP-4819: a novel prolyl endopeptidase inhibitor with potential as a cognitive enhancer. *J. Pharmacol. Exp. Ther.* **274,** 1370–1378.
66. Checler, F. (1993) Neuropeptide-degrading peptidase, in *Methods in Neurotransmitters and Neuropeptides Research, Part 2,* vol. 11 (Nagatsu, et al., eds.), Elsevier, Amsterdam, pp. 375–418.
67. Barelli, H., Petit, A., Hirsch, E., et al. (1999) S 17092, a highly potent, specific and cell permeant inhibitor of human proline endopeptidase. *Biochem. Biophys. Res. Commun.* **257,** 657–661.
68. Lepagnol, J., Lebrun, C., Morain, P., De Nateuil, G., and Heidet, V. (1996) Cognition enhancing effects of S 17092, a potent inhibitor of post-proline cleaving enzyme (PPCE). *Soc. Neurosci. Abstr.* **22,** 142.
69. Lestage, P., Lebrun, C., Iop, F., et al. (1998) S 17092, a new post-proline cleaving enzyme inhibitor: memory enhancing effects and substance P neuromodulatory activity. *Adv. Behav. Biol.* **49,** 653–660.
70. Schneider, J.S., Giardiniere, M., and Morain, P. (2002) Effects of the prolyl endopeptidase inhibitor S 17092 on cognitive deficits in chronic low dose MPTP-treated monkeys. *Neuropsychopharmacology* **26,** 176–182.

14

Catecholamines and Cognition

Bridging the Gap Between Animal Studies and Clinical Syndromes

Trevor W. Robbins, PhD, Harriet S. Crofts, PhD, Roshan Cools, PhD, and Angela C. Roberts, PhD

1. INTRODUCTION

There is little doubt that Parkinson's disease (PD) is associated with a cognitive deficit syndrome, although there is variability in the extent to which it is expressed with the motor symptoms. From the earliest descriptions of "subcortical dementia," it is evident that parkinsonian syndromes have distinct patterns of cognitive impairment, and there is still considerable debate about their exact nature, as well as their relationship to the dementia that can occur later in the course of the disease in a significant proportion of PD patients. Much of what we understand about the cognitive syndrome in PD has been stimulated, or even elucidated, by research in experimental animals, as this chapter seeks to establish.

As schematized in Fig. 1, the multivariate pathology of PD *(1,2)* makes it very difficult to attribute the cognitive deficits to a particular source of pathology, in the way that has been possible for the motor symptoms. Thus, are the cognitive problems due to the loss of dopamine (DA) subcortically, specifically in the striatum, or, alternatively do they arise from cortical losses, especially in the prefrontal cortex (PFC)? The deficits may even arise as effects of the medication used to treat the motor symptoms, whether based on dopaminergic remediation or (sometimes) anticholinergic therapy. PD is also associated with significant nondopaminergic pathology, including changes in several of the other chemically identified ascending neurotransmitter systems of the isodendritic core, for example, the noradrenergic locus coeruleus, the serotoninergic mesencephalic raphe nuclei, or the cholinergic basal forebrain (nucleus basalis of Meynert) *(1)*. Any single one or any combination of these could potentially affect cognitive function, for example, via neuromodulatory influences exerted on neocortical function. This chapter will make it clear that, potentially, all of these various candidate mechanisms, both cortical and subcortical, and dopaminergic as well as nondopaminergic, may contribute to the cognitive picture in PD.

The two main psychological hypotheses of the characteristics of parkinsonian cognitive deficit syndrome are: (*i*) that it includes executive impairments frequently associated with frontal lobe damage, such as working memory, cognitive flexibility, and planning *(3,4)*; and (*ii*) that it includes impairments in procedural memory and habit learning as distinct from the deficits seen in declarative memory commonly associated with medial temporal lobe amnesia *(5)*. The relationships between these "clusters" of impairment are unclear, both from neural and psychological perspectives. The possibility that different parts of the cognitive syndrome in PD actually depend on damage to separate neural systems is

From: *Mental and Behavioral Dysfunction in Movement Disorders*
Edited by: M-A. Bédard et al. © Humana Press Inc., Totowa, NJ

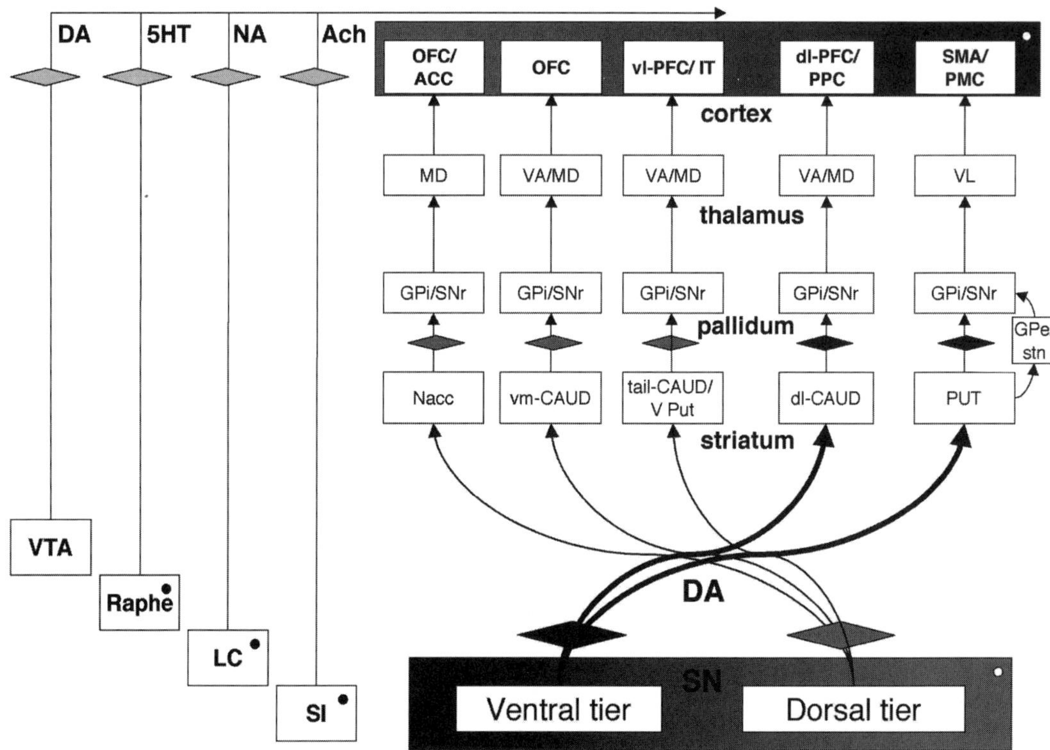

Fig. 1. Schematic to show the chemical neuropathology of PD, as distributed across several corticostriatal loops. See refs. *1* and *2* for further commentary and refs. *63* and *67* on the basic neuroanatomical organization of the corticostriatal circuitry. The darkness of shading in the cortex or in the "lozenges" indicates the degree of DA loss from the corticostriatal loops; the partly hatched lozenges indicate mild degrees of loss (for the chemical neuromodulatory systems projecting to the cortex and also for DA loss in the different striatal segements). The black or white dots indicate the presence of Lewy bodies, which are most common in the substantia nigra (SN), locus coeruleus (LC), substantia innominata (SI), dorsal and medial raphe nucleus, and within certain classes of neurons in the cortex *(2)*. Abbreviations: OFC, orbitofrontal cortex; ACC, anterior cingulate cortex; vl-PFC, ventrolateral prefrontal cortex; IT, inferotemporal cortex; dl-PFC, dorso-lateral prefrontal cortex; PPC, posterior parietal cortex; SMA, supplementary motor area; PMC, premotor cortex; MD, dorsomedial nucleus of thalamus; VA, ventral anterior thalamus; VL, ventrolateral thalamus; GPi, globus pallidus, internal segment; SNr, substantia nigra, pars reticulata; Nacc, nucleus accumbens (ventral striatum); vm-caud, ventromedial caudate; tail caud, tail of the caudate nucleus; V Put, ventral putamen; dl-CAUD, dorsolateral caudate; PUT, putamen; VTA, ventral tegmental area.

entirely plausible. Moreover, different cognitive deficits could also be modulated differentially by pathology in different ascending neurotransmitter pathways.

2. AN INFLUENTIAL EARLY MODEL: SPATIAL WORKING MEMORY

2.1. *Evidence from Animal Studies*

An important development in the working memory hypothesis of prefrontal function in humans derives from the spatial delayed response task used to demonstrate deficits in monkeys with lesions of the sulcus principalis. Following this classic work, Brozoski, Goldman-Rakic, and their colleagues demonstrated the importance of the mesocortical DA projection in mediating this behavior by a landmark study *(6)* using a delayed response type procedure to show that 6-hydroxydopamine (6-OHDA)-induced depletion of DA in the vicinity of the principal sulcus of the dorsolateral PFC in macaques produced an impairment every bit as profound as ablation of the region itself. Depletion of either noradrenaline or serotonin (5-HT) in the PFC had little effect. Further evidence for a specific role of DA came from additional findings that the deficits could be remediated by systemic treatment with drugs such as apomorphine and levodopa (L-dopa). It is these observations in particular that have held great significance for understanding cognitive deficits in PD, as it is apparent that dopaminergic medication can remediate cognitive functions, which may well be impaired in PD as a consequence of prefrontal DA depletion. These striking discoveries have lent hope to the possibility of defining causal mechanisms underlying PD cognitive deficits by using animal models. Further work by the Goldman-Rakic group has been able to identify specific contributions of the D1 receptor to spatial working memory and also to highlight the (intriguing, but somewhat controversial) possibility of different mechanisms in the control of spatial and nonspatial (e.g., faces) working memory within distinct portions of the prefrontal cortex *(7)*. As the anatomical relationships between the cortex and striatum are topographically organized to some extent, and because of the known spatiotemporal course of DA depletion from the striatum *(8)*, quite selective resultant patterns of cognitive deficit in PD are plausible.

2.2. *Relevance to Human PD*

Although the spatial delayed response task is an effective way of assessing cognitive functions of the PFC in humans, it has until recently been less clearly related to human deficits *(9)*. Our own research strategy *(10,11)* has been to devise cognitive tests that effectively bridge the gap between animal and human studies, either by constructing paradigms based on effective animal tests, such as spatial delayed response, or by deconstructing complex tests of human cognition such as the Wisconsin Card Sorting Test (WCST). The latter classical test has been shown to be sensitive to deficits, not only in patients with frontal lobe lesions *(12)*, but also in patients with PD *(13)*. Such decompositions enable them to be employed in tests, for example, using monkeys. The cognitive tests we have used from the so-called Cambridge Neuropsychological Test Automated Battery (CANTAB) *(11)* (Fig. 2), which seem most sensitive to frontal lobe dysfunction, include a suite of programs for testing different aspects of spatial working memory, with tests of spatial planning, using a computerized form of the Tower of London task, and a suite of tests that decomposes the WCST into its constituent elements *(14)*. As will be seen below, this suite has been employed, not only for monkeys, but also to probe more selectively for the nature of WCST deficits in humans.

The spatial working memory and planning battery from CANTAB includes several distinct, but interrelated tests (Fig. 2). For example, it includes a test of spatial span based on the Corsi "Blocks" task, in which subjects have to remember a spatial sequence of a gradually increasing number of stimuli (boxes in distinct locations) immediately after presentation, (similar to "digit span") by responding in the correct spatiotemporal sequence to an array of stimuli presented on a video monitor equipped with a touch-sensitive screen. Subjects are also required to recognize in which spatial locations stimuli (open boxes) have been presented by selecting the familiar versus the novel location in a two choice test. This test, thus, requires not only that the subjects hold stimuli in a spatial memory "buffer" and simply reproduce them, but also to carry out some further transformation or manipulation of these contents of the short term spatial memory store, analogous to "backwards digit span." The third test requires yet further processing, as the subjects themselves must select stimuli from a spatial array in whichever sequence they choose (a self-ordered task), based on, but distinct from, the types of test used by Petrides and Milner *(15)* to assess frontal lobe functioning in humans and monkeys (see Fig. 2). In fact, this test is inspired by the forms of optimal foraging tests of spatial memory employed in rats *(16)* and monkeys *(17)*. The humans, just like the animals, must search through an array of spatial locations and select those most likely to contain food (for the experimental animals) or reward tokens (for humans). Thus, a key principle is that subjects should not return to locations that have previously

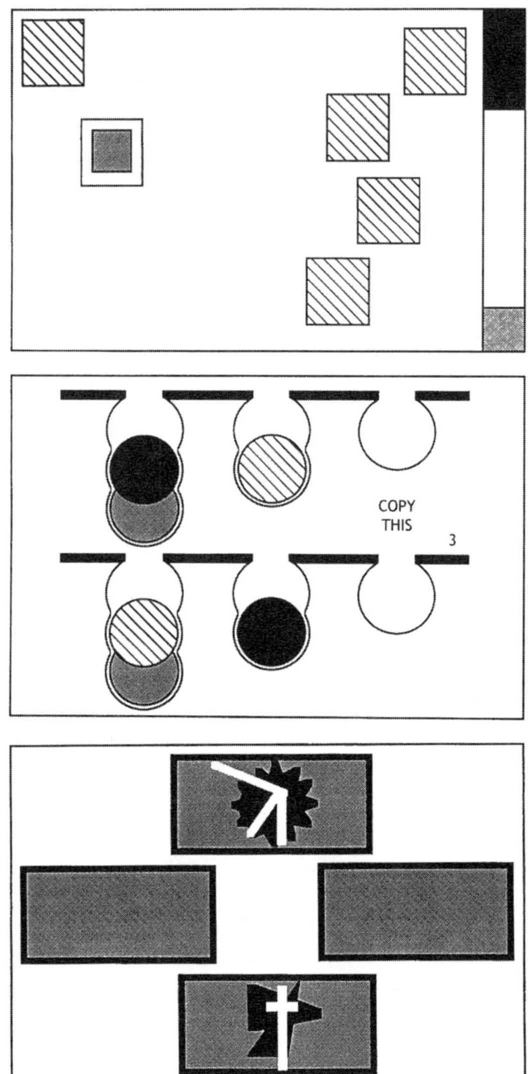

Fig. 2. Tests from the CANTAB. Computerized tests using a touch-sensitive screen from the CANTAB shown to be sensitive to frontal lobe dysfunction and also PD *(4,11)*. (Top panel) Self-ordered spatial working memory task. In this task, subjects are required to search in the array of red boxes for blue tokens to be placed in the vertical column on the right hand side of the array. The number of blue tokens involved matches the number of boxes in the array (which gradually increase on separate trials from 2, 3, 4, 6, to 8.) The subject learns the rule early on that they will not find a blue token in a box that has previously contained a blue token on that trial. However, blue tokens are only available probabilistically from opening a red box. Subjects, thus, have to remember not to return to locations where they have previously found a blue token. (Middle panel) Tower of London Planning task (the Stockings of Cambridge). In this version of the Tower of London test of planning, subjects are required to move the colored balls in the bottom array (by simply touching them and their intended location) to positions that match the positions shown in the top goal arrangement. They are told the required minimum number of moves for perfect solutions, and latencies to move the balls, as well as errors, are noted by the computer. The problems can be of 2, 3, 4, or 5 moves levels of difficulty. A yoked control test plays back the moves actually used by the subjects in the top array and requires the subject to match these responses, thus providing control scores for sensorimotor aspects of moving the balls that can be subtracted from overall latencies to provide estimates of thinking time.

hidden rewards, optimal performance depending to some extent on the construction of a strategic search plan which alleviates some of the burden on working memory processes. Thus, this self-ordered spatial working memory task can index not only short-term spatial memory capacity, but also aspects of strategy use *(18)*. A final component of the battery is a test of spatial planning based on the Tower of London *(19)*. In this task, subjects have to move colored balls around a screen to reach a specified goal position in a minimum number of moves (Fig. 2). There are controls for the sensorimotor aspects of this task, which can be employed to provide estimates of thinking time as well as accuracy in solving the problems.

These tasks have also been employed in functional neuroimaging studies in normal volunteers using positron emission tomography (PET) with $H_2{}^{15}O$ to index changes in regional cerebral blood flow (rCBF) *(20–22)*. For example, the self-ordered spatial working memory task produces activations in both the ventrolateral and dorsolateral PFC *(21)*. This pattern is consistent with Petrides' *(23)* two-stage model, which proposes that the function of holding memories "on-line" depends on the ventrolateral PFC, whereas the task of monitoring choices (for example, the strategy by which they are sequenced and their association with reinforcement) may recruit additional dorsolateral PFC activation. The pattern of activation is quite similar for the Tower of London test of planning, which also, however, shows considerable parieto-occipital activation. However, this similarity is consistent with evidence of psychometric associations between the two tasks *(24)*. The Tower of London task has also been shown to activate the caudate nucleus *(25)*, thus also targeting a structure known to be heavily depleted of DA in PD.

2.2.1. CANTAB in the Evaluation of Cognitive Performances in PD

The CANTAB has been shown to be sensitive to cognitive deficits in PD across the entire course of the disease, from the newly diagnosed nonmedicated stage, through its initial mild course and medication, to its later generally more severe stages, in which cognitive impairment is often more evident in terms of activities of everyday living. The main findings have been reviewed previously *(26,27)* and will be summarized here. Deficits in self-ordered spatial working memory are often more evident than in parallel tasks, tapping nonspatial (e.g. visual and verbal) memory *(28,29)* (see Fig. 3). There is a progressive deficit in performance on the self-ordered spatial working memory task, in terms of "between-search" errors (i.e., returning incorrectly to previously correct locations) The overall pattern of deficit, however, is somewhat different from that seen in patients with frontal damage. Specifically, PD patients exhibit less evidence of strategic deficits than do frontal patients, and they also make fewer "within-search" errors (which entail repeating the just-performed response) than frontals *(4,18)*.

As might be expected, PD patients are also impaired in performance on the Tower of London test, being slower initially to think about the problems before initiating their solutions, but later exhibiting a more frontal pattern of less efficient solutions in terms of errors made *(4,30,31)*. It is of considerable significance that many of these deficits in spatial planning and working memory are sensitive to dopaminergic therapy. This is evident not simply from cross-sectional comparison of medicated and never medicated PD, but also from a study in which L-dopa was withdrawn to demonstrate selective impairments in several tests sensitive to frontal lobe dysfunction *(31,32)* (see Fig. 4). This DA-dependent set of deficits prominently included the tests of spatial memory function, including spatial span,

---

Fig. 2. (Continued). (Bottom panel) ID/ED set-shifting paradigm, which is a computerized analogue of the WCST. This screen shows the types of compound stimuli subjects are required to discriminate on the basis of trial-and-error feedback in different stages of a suite of discrimination tests, which include simple discrimination learning, simple reversal learning, compound discrimination learning and reversal, ID set-shifting and reversal, and finally, ED set-shifting and reversal. The pairs of stimuli are presented at any two of the four locations (to render spatial location irrelevant) and comprise line and shape dimensions with elements that can occur in any combination to form compound shape-line stimuli. Different sets of exemplars are used at the ID set-shift and ED set-shift stages. See refs. *11* and *14* for further explanation.

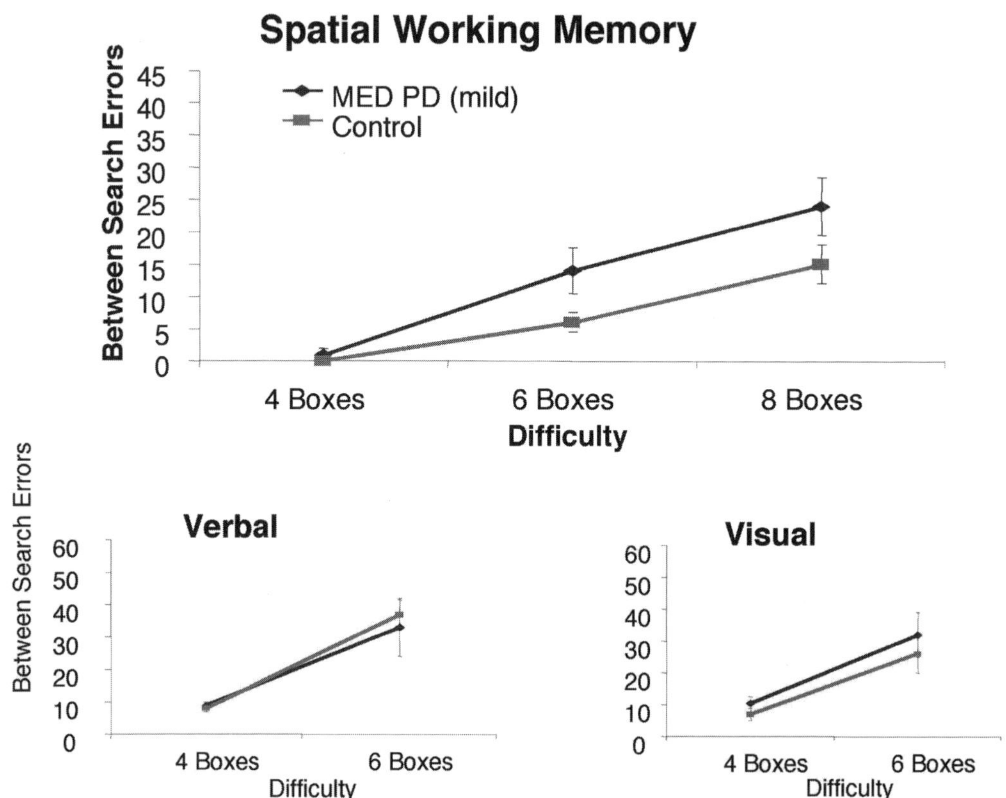

Fig. 3. Deficits in self-ordered spatial working memory versus self-ordered visual or verbal memory in early PD *(28)*.

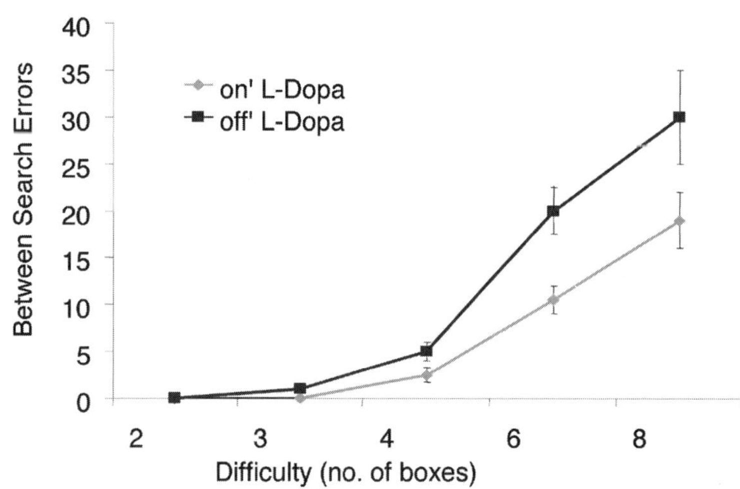

Fig. 4. Detrimental effects of L-dopa withdrawal on self-ordered spatial working memory performance in PD *(32)*.

self-ordered spatial working memory, and spatial planning. Significantly, however, on certain other tests of nonspatial recognition memory and visual learning, there was no significant demonstrable amelioration of existing deficits by L-dopa, suggesting that some of the PD cognitive impairments, at least later in the course of the disease, are nondopaminergic in nature.

While the impairments in spatial working memory were quite prominent in PD, the most discriminating CANTAB test we used for evaluating PD patients was the extradimensional (ED) shifting analogue of the WCST (see Fig. 2), which was sensitive to deficits in some patients, even prior to medication, at the earliest stages of the disease *(14)*. However, it has proved more problematic to establish a dopaminergic contribution to cognitive shifting performance, e.g., in the L-dopa withdrawal study described above *(32)*, the basic discrimination learning capacity of the PD patients was profoundly impaired by L-dopa withdrawal, rendering an assessment of its effects on cognitive shifting difficult to measure.

This brief summary makes it clear that, from an heuristic perspective, the use of paradigms derived from animal neuropsychology has been proven useful for analyzing further the nature of the cognitive deficit in PD. Subsequent developments in these animal models and their application are described below.

2.3. Further Development of the Spatial Working Memory Model

In view of the possible behavioral interpretation that the striking effects of frontal DA loss on spatial delayed response performance might reflect some possible action of dopaminergic manipulations on the performance of mediating responses which obviate the necessity to hold specific information on-line, Goldman-Rakic and Sawaguchi employed an oculomotor delayed saccade procedure, in which monkeys have to hold fixation of a central spot before shifting and making an eye movement to the location of a brief visual stimulus, which was presented a few seconds previously. Selective disruptions in the accuracy of the memory saccades were produced by iontophoretic application to the PFC of doses of DA D1, but not D2, receptor antagonists *(33)*. These findings have been supported by our own experiments with a delayed response procedure in marmosets, which removed the possibility of mediating responses by distracting the animal to the back of the testing chamber during the delay period *(34)*. Once again, DA depletion from the PFC was found to impair the acquisition of a spatial delayed response task, though not to quite the same extent as an excitotoxic lesion of most parts of the PFC itself (Fig. 5) *(34)*.

A key finding from this study *(34)* was the sparing of the capacity to self-order responses without perseveration following mesocortical DA depletion (but which was greatly impaired following excitotoxic lesions of the PFC in marmosets, as might have been expected following effects of frontal lesions in humans on within-search errors on the self-ordered spatial working memory task (ref. *18* and see above). Thus, in conjunction with the findings of deficits on the more conventional spatial delayed response task (Fig. 5), it appeared from the results of this study that DA normally modulates mnemonic functions associated with the working memory task rather than the executive operations of producing the optimal response sequence. This is consistent with the clinical findings, reviewed above, which indicate that the nature of the deficit on the self-ordered spatial working memory task may be more closely related to the spatial memory component rather than the executive processes engaged by the task, as indexed by the strategy measure and the lack of significant within-search errors *(4)*, compared to patients with frontal lobe damage with otherwise comparable degrees of impairment *(18)*.

Although these data support the hypothesis that PFC D1 receptor mechanisms contribute to efficient spatial working memory performance, there have been recent indications that the situation, at least for the intact brain, is more complex. For example, there is evidence, from electrophysiological findings in monkeys *(35)* and pharmacological evidence using tests of spatial working memory in rats *(36)*, that overstimulation of D1 receptors may lead to memory deficits. Thus far, there has been no clear evidence of deficits produced by L-dopa in PD patients, although the possibility of impairments

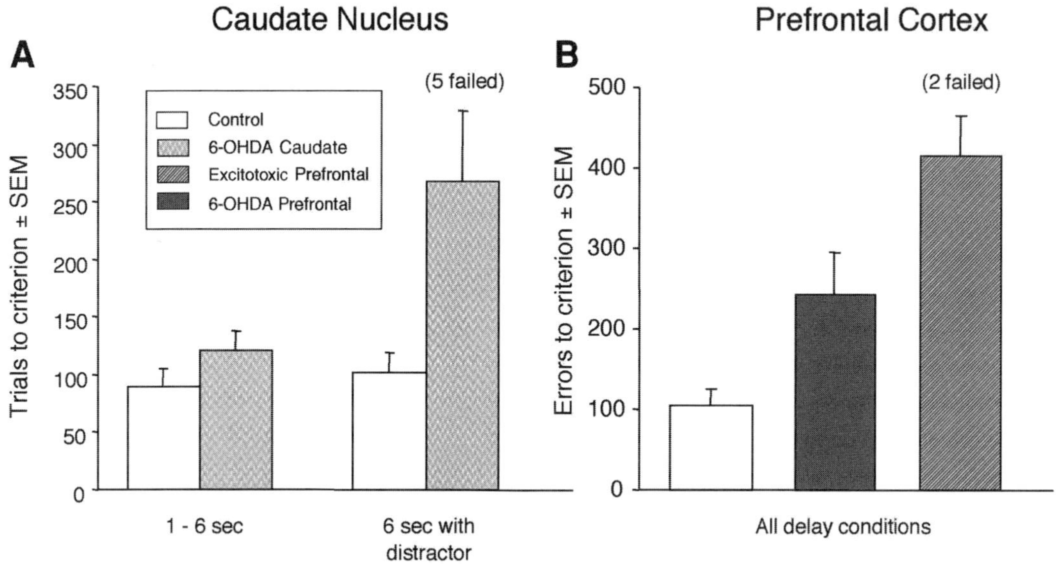

Fig. 5. Summary of effects of lesions of the PFC or striatum on spatial delayed response performance in the marmoset. Comparison of the effects of dopaminergic lesions of the caudate nucleus (**A**) *(45)* and dopaminergic and excitotoxic lesions of the PFC (**B**) *(34)* of marmosets on the ability to acquire the spatial delayed response task.

on certain tests will be reconsidered below *(37,38)*. Presumably, the DA depletion in PD makes it more likely on balance that dopaminergic therapy ameliorates, rather than impairs, cognitive function.

The evidence reviewed so far is consistent with the hypothesis that some of the cognitive deficit in PD is produced by PFC DA loss. Direct tests of this hypothesis, however, have been lacking, until a recent study using PET with $H_2{}^{15}O$ has been used in order to quantify changes in rCBF during performance of spatial working memory and planning tasks in PD patients tested both on and off L-dopa *(39)*. As shown previously *(21)*, these tasks activated a discrete network, including the PFC and parietal cortex, and the striking finding that the relative reduction of rCBF in this network is a consequence of L-dopa medication. This finding is consistent with other evidence we have accumulated, that drugs, such as methylphenidate, which facilitate catecholaminergic neurotransmission in healthy volunteers, may reduce rCBF in critical circuits activated by spatial working memory tasks while actually enhancing performance on those tasks *(40)*. Precise interpretation of these intriguing results is beyond the scope of this chapter, although they may suggest that these drugs in some way enhance the efficiency of processing in cortical networks. The findings clearly provide evidence in favor of a PFC locus of action of effect of dopaminergic therapy on cognitive function in PD. However, it should be noted that these findings do not exclude a possible role for striatal DA in the modulation of spatial working memory, e.g., at the D2 receptor. We have recently found that sulpiride, a selective D2 receptor antagonist, reproduces to some extent the profile of cognitive deficits in normal volunteers, which is seen in PD *(41)*. As D2 receptors are much less densely found in the PFC than D1 receptors and are much more evident in the striatum, this is consistent with a striatal locus of action.

Investigators have hitherto been rather slow to test the hypothesis of possible striatal involvement in working memory function using delayed response performance in monkeys, although the recent study by Levy et al. *(42)*, indicating differential metabolic activation of the caudate nucleus in macaques by spatial and nonspatial working memory tasks, is consistent with the known patterns of projection from the cortex to the striatum (see Fig. 1) and is of particular relevance to the similar pattern for working memory performance we and others have identified for PD (see Fig. 3). Arnsten et al. *(43)* showed beneficial effects of DA D2 receptor agonists in aged macaques, suggesting a possible striatal role in view of the much greater density of D2-like receptors in this region as compared with the PFC. Schneider and colleagues *(44)* have tested spatial delayed response performance in monkeys following treatment with the neurotoxin 1-methyl-4-phenyl-1,2,3,6-tetrahydropyridine (MPTP), which is a notable model of PD, and found significant deficits. However, MPTP produces DA lesions that are not restricted to the striatum nor, indeed, to DA itself. Following from our earlier work describing effects of DA loss in the marmoset, Collins et al. *(45)* have recently produced selective lesions of the caudate DA system, using infusions of 6-OHDA in the terminal fields, and also found evidence for a spatial delayed response deficit, but again only when the possibility of mediating responses is diminished by a distracting stimulus (food), which orients the marmoset away from the response panel (Fig. 5). Taken together, these data indicate that either striatal or PFC DA loss can impair spatial working memory performance in monkeys, possibly via D1 or D2-like receptors. These deficits could both arise because of actions at distinct loci within a common corticostriatal system mediating spatial working memory, and presumably, both deficits may contribute to the impairment in PD itself.

3. DISCRIMINATION AND REVERSAL LEARNING AND ATTENTIONAL SET-SHIFTING

As mentioned above, the deficits in attentional set-shifting and some aspects of discrimination learning were present at the earliest stages of PD, even prior to medication *(4,14)*. These deficits are of particular interest for animal modeling, because the so-called intradimensional, extradimensional (ID/ED) set-shifting paradigm was developed expressly, not only to decompose the WCST, but also to present its major components in a format that can be used with infrahuman primates *(46)*. Indeed, the paradigm has been employed to demonstrate distinct frontal substrates for the different forms of shifting and reversal learning incorporated in the paradigm. Thus, excitotoxic lesions of the marmoset lateral frontal cortex (possibly homologous with human Brodmann areas 9/46) were shown specifically to impair ED shifting, but not ID shifting or reversal learning *(47)*. By contrast, lesions to the marmoset orbitofrontal cortex selectively impaired reversal learning, but not ID set-shifting or ED shifting *(47)*. Various control experiments suggested that these deficits could not be explained easily in terms of impaired working memory functions *(48)*. Moreover, a similar separation of different types of shifting function according to lateral versus orbitofrontal lesions was observed in a very different functional context, based on the rather more naturalistic object-retrieval test *(49)*, further suggesting the fundamental significance of the dissociation.

The significance to PD has emerged from studies that have sought to determine the effects of prefrontal versus striatal DA depletion, using 6-OHDA *(50)*. The first of these studies provided rather provocative findings shown in Fig. 6, by demonstrating the apparent enhancement of ED shifting performance following PFC DA loss, which averaged about 80% (although cortical noradrenaline [NA] was also compromised by over 60%). Additional data led to two possible accounts of these findings: (*i*) observations made using in vivo dialysis of apparent up-regulation of dopaminergic function in the striatum, consequent upon prefrontal DA loss, pointed to a possible overactivity of striatal DA function, which promoted attentional set-shifting opposite to the direction expected from striatal DA loss and, hence, PD; or (*ii*) a possible attentional lability in the prefrontal DA-depleted monkeys, which was undetected in animals that had received extensive preoperative training, but may have led to a tendency to shift more readily to a previously irrelevant dimension and may, thus, have been advantageous in the context of an ED shift. The two accounts are also, of course, not incompatible. A third hypothesis, that the lesion was somehow overcompensated in functional terms, producing the opposite effect to that expected of PFC DA loss, seems less likely in the face of the deficits shown by the same monkeys on the spatial delayed response task (see above). In fact, it is worth noting that the attentional lability hypothesis may also account for this delayed response impairment, especially as the monkeys are required to orient away from the location of the hidden reward before making their choice.

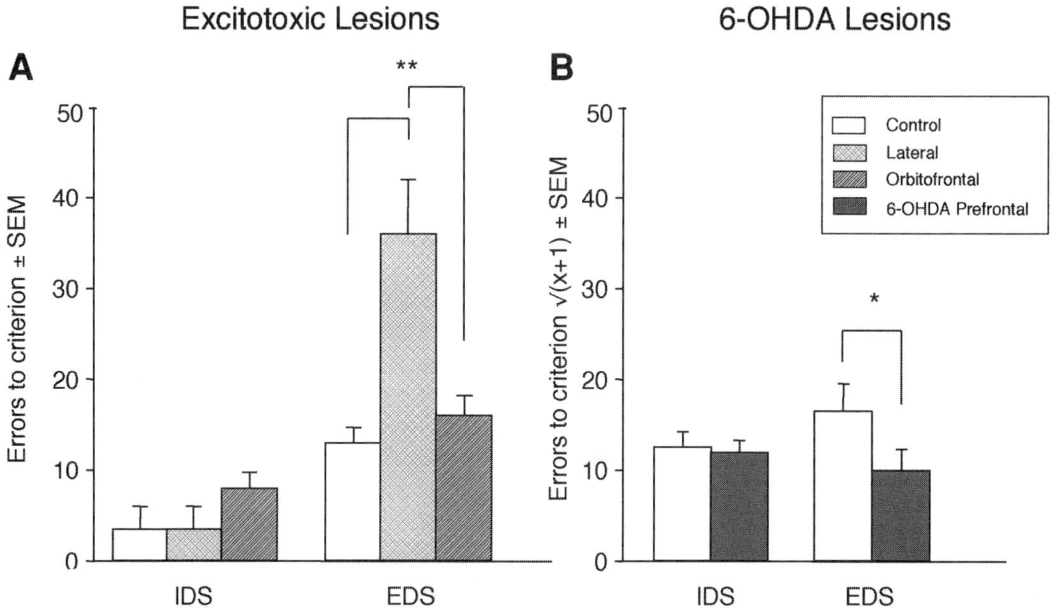

Fig. 6. Contrasting effects of excitotoxic *(47)* and dopaminergic *(50)* lesions of the PFC of the marmoset on the ability to shift an attentional set. $*p < 0.05$. $**p < 0.01$.

Recent evidence has been provided for the attentional lability notion from a follow-up study in which marmosets received minimal preoperative training on the discrimination tasks, thus making them more susceptible to exhibiting attentional lability on other stages of the test *(51)*. In fact, marmosets with lesions with depletions of both DA and NA (to a slightly greater extent for NA than previously) were impaired in the way hypothesized, showing significant deficits in: (*i*) ID shifting, in which the animal is required to generalize a previously acquired discrimination to different exemplars within the same perceptual dimension, thereby demonstrating the formation of attentional "set," and (*ii*) distraction, which disruptions of discrimination performance in a probe test in which the stimuli in the irrelevant dimension are varied, thus measuring the degree to which the animal has selectively attended to the target dimension *(51)* (Fig. 7). Moreover, the DA-depleted monkeys were again quicker to make the ED shift, in terms of errors made, at least for some conditions. More specifically, the lesioned monkeys were superior at ED shifts in which they had to shift from the less-preferred dimension (in fact "lines," the dimension with which they had the most difficulty initially in discriminating) to the more preferred one. Crofts et al. *(51)* interpet this finding in terms of a specific impairment in "top-down," as opposed to "bottom-up," attentional function.

This extensive set of findings for effects of prefrontal catecholamine (probably mainly DA) loss is not, however, what is generally seen in patients with PD performing ostensibly similar tests. Enhanced attentional lability is not, for example, what is observed in PD in the ID/ED test, although some patients are impaired when an irrelevant dimension is initially introduced at the compound discrimination *(4, 14)*. On the other hand, for entirely different paradigms for selective attention or Posner's covert spatial orienting paradigm, there are some indications that PD patients exhibit losses of selective attention *(52)*, or a tendency to disengage too readily, in the covert orienting procedure *(53)*, respectively. Thus, the main deficits of PD patients on the ID/ED tests are not simulated by prefrontal DA loss, suggesting that they are not at the root of the parkinsonian impairment. This is a significant conclusion, consistent with growing clinical evidence that the parkinsonian cognitive deficit in patients is often correlated with an up-regulation of frontal DA function, as indexed using indirect measures with PET *(54)*.

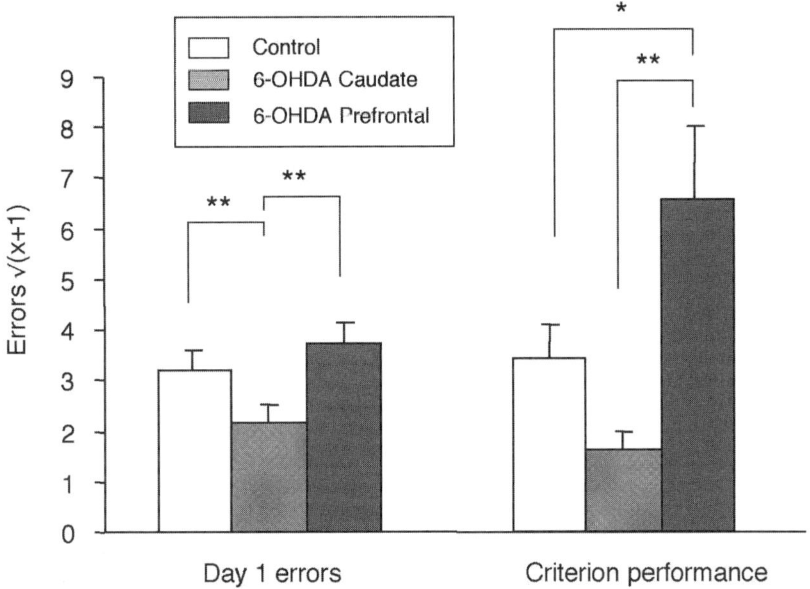

Fig. 7. Results for a probe distraction test administered while performing a visual discrimination task (similar to that shown in Fig. 2, bottom panel) in marmosets with DA depletion from the caudate nucleus or PFC *(51)*. Day 1 errors refers to the initial disruption, which was significantly smaller in the case of the marmosets with caudate DA depletion. The monkeys with PFC DA depletions were significantly slower than the other two groups to reattain criterion levels of performance. $^{*}p < 0.05$. $^{**}p < 0.01$.

The alternative hypothesis entertained above was that it is the changes in striatal DA that are primary. This hypothesis was assessed directly by examining the effects of striatal DA lesions, also affected by 6-OHDA and leading to the depletion of caudate DA to about 20% of control values, i.e., to levels commonly found in the brains of PD patients postmortem. Some limited evidence was found to support this viewpoint *(45,51)*. In the latter study, the enhanced distractibility of monkeys with prefrontal catecholamine loss was complemented by reduced distractibility in marmosets with caudate DA depletion, as seen on the probe test described above (Fig. 7). This does point to a possible change that is compatible with the ED shift impairment in PD. When the ED shift itself was tested in another study *(45)*, however, there was no impairment produced by caudate DA loss at that stage of the test; in fact, at none of the initial stages of the ID/ED paradigm were any deficits revealed. Again, the possibility of functional compensation seems unlikely in the face of a standard deficit in spatial delayed response. One further variant of the ED shift task did separate the lesioned and sham-operated marmosets, in which the monkeys were required to make an additional ED shift back to the previously relevant dimension. Sham-operated controls accomplished this shift more effectively than did caudate DA-depleted animals. Thus, an ED shift impairment was eventually revealed, though not in the standard form of the task.

The "ED shift back" deficit has not been systematically tested in large groups of PD patients in order to provide exact parallels, but there may be an analogue of this impairment in what at first appears to be a somewhat different form of paradigm, namely task set switching.

3.1. Task Set-Shifting Impairments in PD

One problem of interpretation posed by the ID/ED shift paradigm is its possible confounding of learning with shifting performance factors. This is evident in the trivial sense, such that it is in the nature of the paradigm that PD patients may not perform the discrimination learning tasks sufficiently well even to qualify for the ED shift. There is also considerable evidence that interpreting ED shift deficits may be complicated by the learning requirements of these tasks, the fact that PD patients may have such learning problems *(5)*, possibly ameliorated by L-dopa therapy *(32)*, and consistent with a mooted role for striatal DA in reinforcement learning *(54a)*. One way of avoiding such possible confounds of learning is to investigate shifting between two previously well-established response sets, and this is the basis of the task-set shifting paradigm *(55)*. Specifically, subjects are pretrained to switch between two response rules, e.g., naming digits and letters, for digit and letter stimuli presented in compound. Previously, Rogers et al. *(56)* were able to show that patients with left frontal lesions were particularly prone to deficits on this task, even though either right or left frontal lesions impaired the initial acquisition of these conditional response rules. The Rogers et al. study included a comparison group of medicated PD patients, but found no specific impairments that resembled the left frontal switching impairment *(56)*. However, a subsequent study employing a modified procedure to minimize the effect of possible fatigue has reported a specific deficit in task set switching in PD, in a condition in which possible interference between the tasks is enhanced by conditions encouraging "cross-talk" between the two *(57)*. The possible parallel between the ED shift back deficit observed following caudate DA loss in marmosets and the task set switching impairment can clearly be drawn. Thus, in the ED shift back task, the requirement is to switch between two response sets that have previously been established (as habits) by training, as in the case of the task set switching procedure. The results certainly have relevance for understanding the functions of the striatum *(45)*.

However, we are left with the puzzle of the ED shift impairment in PD itself, for which it is difficult to find evidence for either prefrontal mediation (at least via prefrontal DA) or striatal mediation. Nevertheless, other evidence is certainly compatible with the relative noninvolvement of striatal DA in ED shift performance: e.g., (*i*) a functional imaging paradigm using PET has shown a frontal but not a striatal locus for the ED shift in humans *(58)*; and (*ii*) a recent ON-OFF study of effects of L-dopa in PD has shown no evidence of a DA-dependent impairment in ED shifting, although the group of patients did show an overall deficit in this capacity *(38)* (Fig. 8). One must be careful of concluding too much from this group of PD patients with mild disability. However, their impairment on other cognitive tests was L-dopa-dependent *(38)*. One distinct possibility, however, is that the ED impairment in PD is more dependent on other aspects of its pathology. Evidence from both monkey and human studies suggests that the cortical noradrenergic system may be most relevant to ED shift performance. For example, a recent human psychopharmacological study showed specific modulation by noradrenergic agents of ED shifting, though in a manner that remains to be elucidated *(59)*. By contrast, there has been relatively little evidence for mediation by serotoninergic manipulations *(60)* or by cholinergic depletion from the PFC *(61)*. As there is certainly some evidence of enhancement of basic attentional performance in PD by a noradrenergic agonist *(62)*, this remains an intriguing hypothesis.

4. EVIDENCE FOR DA-DEPENDENT NEURAL DISSOCIATIONS IN COGNITIVE PERFORMANCE IN PD

The discussion above highlights the possibility considered in previous studies that the neural basis of the cognitive deficits in PD is potentially quite complex. Our early studies of effects of L-dopa withdrawal are also consistent with that theme, as different deficits in PD appeared to be differentially susceptible to L-dopa withdrawal. That study *(32)* for example, raised the possibility that some of the impairments, e.g., in visual memory commonly associated with temporal lobe damage, were dependent on acetylcholine, rather than being DA-dependent. The concept that L-dopa differentially affects symptoms (including cognitive impairments) in a manner that plausibly relates to the degree of DA loss in the corticostriatal neural pathways differentially implicated in distinct motor and cognitive functions has previously been suggested *(37)*. The previous theorizing emphasised the difference in DA loss between the caudate and putamen based on the classical postmortem work of Kish and colleagues

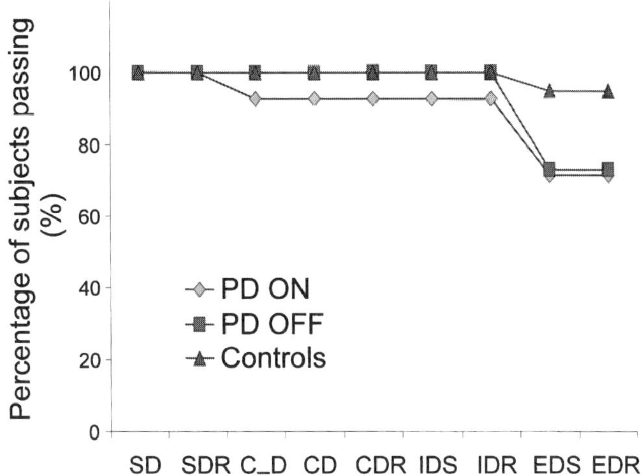

Fig. 8. Failure to exacerbate ED shift deficits in PD following L-dopa withdrawal in PD *(38)*.

(8), in which the putamen is far more affected by PD than the caudate nucleus (see Fig. 1). This pattern is consistent with the hypothesis that reversing the putamen-dependent motor functions by L-dopa therapy may lead to a relative overdose of the drug in caudate and other circuits less depleted by the disease, which may have a greater role in cognition (see Fig. 9). This overdosing in turn may actually lead to impairment rather than correction of function, as proposed in recent theoretical analyses of the functions of cortical DA *(36)*.

We have recently applied this analysis to cognitive tasks mediated by different corticostriatal loops, including those involving the ventral striatum (including the nucleus accumbens) *(63)* (see Fig. 1), which are also relatively spared of DA depletion in PD, to a greater extent than for either the caudate or putamen because of the differential involvement of the dorsal and ventral tier DA neurons *(8)* (Figs. 1 and 9). The improvements commonly seen on the spatial working memory tasks following L-dopa therapy might have been predicated on the basis of the considerable loss of caudate DA in PD, as well as the fact that the dorsolateral PFC projects to the caudate, and is consistent with the known role of the caudate in spatial delayed performance *(34,42)*. Similar predictions can be made about the effects of L-dopa on task set switching, on the basis of studies of patients with frontal lesions or PD, and also of functional imaging studies in normal healthy volunteers *(64)*. In fact, such predictions have recently been confirmed for the detrimental effects of L-dopa withdrawal on the switch-cost associated with task set switching (Fig. 10). However, we might expect deficits on tasks depending on brain regions less depleted by DA loss, including the tail of the caudate nucleus and the mesolimbic DA projections to the ventral striatum *(8)* (Fig. 1).

What might such tasks involve? Some clues may be gained from some of our previous work with marmosets. Recall that reversal learning was impaired by a distinct neural substrate than for ED shifting, implicating the orbitofrontal, rather than the lateral frontal circuitry *(47,48)*. The PET imaging study by Rogers et al. *(58)*, in fact, found no firm evidence for an orbitofrontal substrate. However, there was significant evidence of activations by reversal learning in the ventral striatum, which is connected to the orbitofrontal cortex in a common neural system *(58)*. The failure to observe orbitofrontal activation could conceivably have been a product of the slow temporal resolution of the technique, but a further possible reason for the lack of orbitofrontal activation with reversal could have arisen from the relatively easy nature of the reversal task itself. For this reason, we have designed another task for humans called probabilistic learning and reversal, in which the subjects initially learn a 80:20

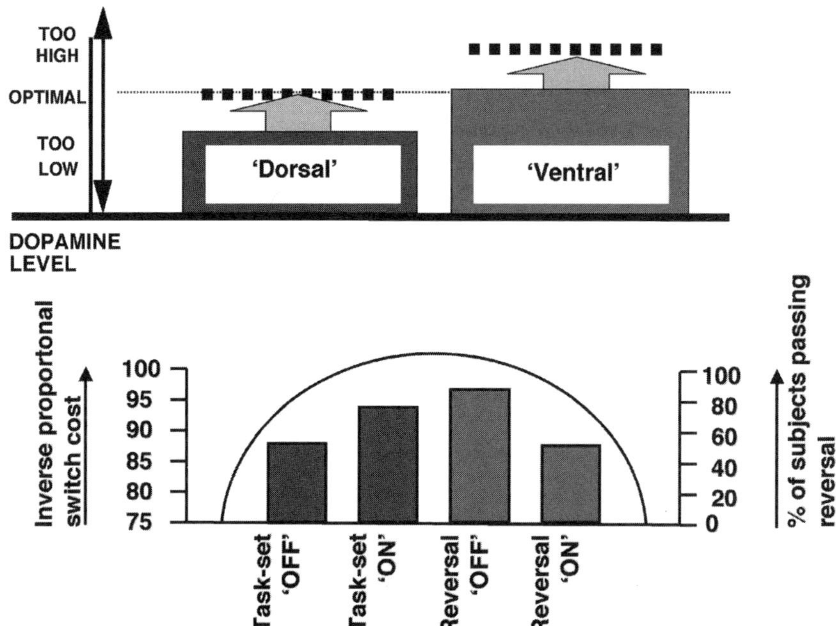

Fig. 9. Schematic showing possible inverted U relationship between dopaminergic activity and cognitive function (bottom panel), as hypothesised by ref. *36*, and how the present data for PD fit the hypothesis (see ref. *38* for more details). (Top panel) How the effects of L-dopa medication may be explained by its interactions with the pattern of DA loss from the dorsal and ventral tiers, projecting to the caudate and putamen, and nucleus accumbens (ventral striatum), respectively.

two-choice discrimination, in which they have to consistently respond to the more densely reinforced visual discriminandum (i.e., the stimulus that is rewarded 80% of the time) *(65)*. Having learned this discrimination, it is then reversed according to a 20:80 rule. Obviously, it is much harder to detect the reversal contingency in this case. PD patients are typically impaired on the reversal phase (and sometimes the initial discrimination, too) *(65)*. However, that study showed that it was the patients on dopaminergic medication who were doing relatively worse, even though the drug was evidently benefiting some aspects of their cognitive performance (spatial memory), as well as their motor symptoms. It was just possible that the superior performance of the unmedicated patients arose from their being in a slightly less advanced phase of the disease (and so had been relatively slow to receive medication). However, an ON-OFF study found essentially the same result: PD patients tested off L-dopa performed significantly better than the same patients tested on drug (*38*, Fig. 11). What was perhaps more striking was that these were the same PD patients who had benefited from L-dopa for task set switching and had been unaffected for attentional set-shifting. Thus, remarkably, for three different aspects of cognitive shifting (ED shifting, task set switching, and reversal learning) and with different cortico-striatal substrates (respectively and hypothetically, PFC, dorsolateral PFC-caudate, and orbitofrontal-ventral striatal), PD patients exhibit differential responses to dopaminergic therapy; no effect, improvement, and impairment, respectively. These findings clearly have major implications for understanding the nature of executive functioning itself and how it may be modulated by DA loss or drugs (see Fig. 9).

While not all of these findings can be ascribed specifically to prior behavioral experimentation with monkeys, most of them can. Indeed, it can be argued that a rich interchange between the human and animal work has been of enormous heuristic value to these lines of research. Given the classical findings that visual discrimination learning implicates projections from the inferotemporal cortex to

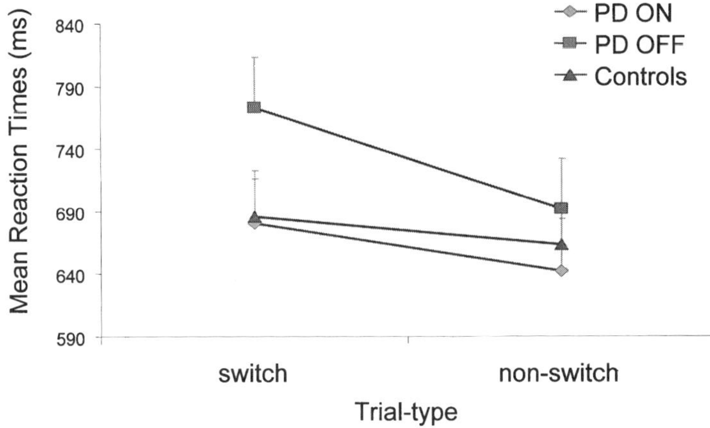

Fig. 10. Detrimental effects of L-dopa withdrawal on task set switching performance in PD *(38)*.

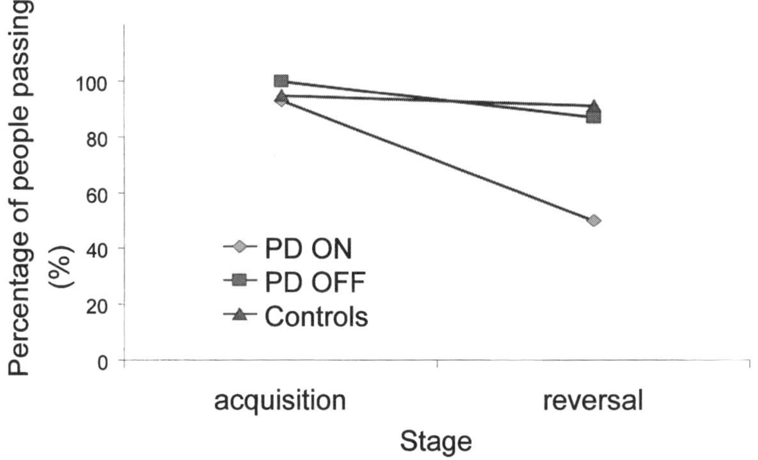

Fig. 11. Beneficial effects of L-dopa withdrawal on probability reversal performance in PD *(38)*.

the tail of the caudate *(66)* and other portions of the striatum *(67)*, similar paradoxical effects of dopaminergic therapy might have been expected for discrimination learning *per se* (if sufficiently difficult). For the present, we need to confirm, through functional neuroimaging studies, that the probabilistic reversal task does implicate an orbitofrontal-ventral striatal circuitry, as presumed, and that it may be modulated by dopaminergic drugs possibly leading to impairment in PD. The cognitive paradigm we have employed for both humans and animals, in conjunction with functional imaging methodology and psychopharmacological investigations, will be invaluable for assessing the newer forms of therapy for PD with dopaminergic drugs or novel neurosurgical procedures. What can be confirmed with confidence from these analyses at present is the heterogeneous nature of cognitive deficits in PD and their likely dependence on different aspects of the chemical neuropathology of this disease.

ACKNOWLEDGMENTS

This work was supported by a Wellcome Trust Programme Grant to T.W. Robbins, B.J. Everitt, A.C. Roberts, and B.J. Sahakian, and completed within the MRC Cooperative Group in Brain, Behaviour, and Neuropsychiatry. R. Cools holds the C.D. Marsden Parkinson's Disease Society Studentship. We are grateful to all of our colleagues for their collaborative assistance, particularly Dr. R. Barker.

REFERENCES

1. Agid, Y., Ruberg, M., Dubois, B., and Pillon, B. (1987) Anatomoclinical and biochemical concepts of subcortical dementia, in *Cognitive Neurochemistry* (Stahl, S.M., Iversen, S.D., and Goodman, E.C., eds.), Oxford University Press, Oxford, pp. 248–271.
2. Cornford, M.E., Chang, L., and Miller, B.L. (1995) The neuropathology of Parkinson's disease: an overview. *Brain Cogn.* **28,** 321–341.
3. Taylor, A.E., Saint-Cyr, J.A., and Lang, A.E. (1986) Frontal lobe dysfunction in Parkinson's disease. *Brain* **109,** 845–883.
4. Owen, A.M., James, M., Leigh, P.H., et al. (1992) Fronto-striatal cognitive deficits at different stages of Parkinson's disease. *Brain* **115,** 1727–1751.
5. Knowlton, B.J, Mangels, J.A., and Squire, L.R. (1996) A neostriatal habit learning-system in humans. *Science* **273,** 1399–1402.
6. Brozoski, T.J., Brown, R., Rosvold, H.E., and Goldman, P.S. (1979) Cognitive deficit caused by regional depletion of dopamine in the prefrontal cortex of rhesus monkeys. *Science* **205,** 929–931.
7. Goldman-Rakic, P.S. (1998) The cortical dopamine system: role in memory and cognition. *Adv. Pharmacol.* **42,** 707–711.
8. Kish, S., Shannak, K., and Hornykiewicz, O. (1988) Uneven patterns of dopamine loss in the striatum of patients with idiopathic Parkinson's disease. *N. Engl. J. Med.* **318,** 876–880.
9. Partiot, A., Verin, M., Pillon, B., Teixeira-Ferreira, C., Agid, Y., and Dubois, B. (1996) Delayed response tasks in basal ganglia lesions in man: further evidence for a striato-frontal co-operation in behavioural adaptation. *Neuropsychologia* **34,** 709–721.
10. Robbins, T.W. (1998) Homology in behavioural pharmacology: an approach to animal models of human cognition. *Behav. Pharmacol.* **9,** 509–520.
11. Robbins, T.W., James, M., Owen, A.M., et al. (1998) A study of performance on tests from the CANTAB battery sensitive to frontal lobe dysfunction in a large sample of normal volunteers: implications for theories of executive functioning and cognitive aging. *J. Int. Neuropsychol. Soc.* **4,** 474–490.
12. Milner, B. (1963) Effects of different lesions on card sorting. *Arch. Neurol.* **9,** 100–110.
13. Bowen, F.P., Kamienny, M.A., Burns, M.M., and Yahr, M.D. (1975) Parkinsonism: effects of levodopa treatment on concept formation. *Neurology* **25,** 701–704.
14. Downes, J.J., Roberts, A.C., Sahakian, B.J., Evenden, J.L., Morris, R.G., and Robbins, T.W. (1989) Impaired extra-dimensional shift performance in medicated and unmedicated Parkinson's disease: evidence for a specific attentional dysfunction. *Neuropsychologia* **27,** 1329–1343.
15. Petrides, M.P. and Milner, B. (1982) Deficits on subject-ordered tasks after frontal and temporal-lobe lesions in man. *Neuropsychologia* **20,** 249–262.
16. Olton, D.S., Becker, J.T., and Handelmans, G.E. (1979) Hippocampus, space and memory. *Behav. Brain Sci.* **2,** 315–365.
17. Passingham, R.E. (1985) Memory of monkeys after lesions in prefrontal cortex. *Behav. Neurosci.* **99,** 3–21.
18. Owen, A., Downes, J.J., Sahakian, B.J., Polkey, C.E., and Robbins, T.W. (1990) Planning and spatial working memory following frontal lobe lesions in man. *Neuropsychologia* **28,** 1021–1034.
19. Shallice, T. (1982) Specific impairments of planning. *Phil. Trans. R. Soc. Lond. B* **298,** 199–209.
20. Baker, S.C., Rogers R.D., Owen A.M., et al. (1996) Neural systems engaged by planning: a PET study of the Tower of London task. *Neuropsychologia* **34,** 515–526.
21. Owen, A.M., Evans, A.C., and Petrides, M. (1996) Evidence for a two stage model of spatial working memory processing within the lateral frontal cortex: a positron emission tomography study. *Cerebral Cortex* **6,** 31–38.
22. Owen, A.M., Doyon, J., Dagher, A., Sadikot, A., and Evans, A.C. (1998) Abnormal basal ganglia outflow in Parkinson's disease identified with PET: implications for higher cortical functions. *Brain* **121,** 949–965.
23. Petrides, M. (1996) Specialized systems for the processing of mnemonic information within the primate frontal cortex. *Philos. Tran. R. Soc. Lond. B Biol. Sci.* **351,** 1455–1461.
24. Robbins, T.W. (1996) Dissociating executive functions of the prefrontal cortex. *Philos. Trans. R. Soc. Lond. B.* **351,** 1463–1471.
25. Elliott, R., Baker, S.C., Rogers, R.D., et al. (1997) Prefrontal dysfunction in depressed patients performing a planning task: a study using positron emission tomography. *Psychol. Med.* **27,** 931–942.
26. Robbins, T.W., Owen, A.M., and Sahakian, B.J. (1998) The neuropsychology of basal ganglia disorders: an integrated cognitive and comparative approach, in *Disorders of Mind and Brain* (Ron, M. and David, A., eds.), Cambridge University Press, New York, pp. 57–83.
27. Cools, R., Swainson, R., Owen, A.M., and Robbins, T.W. (1999) Cognitive dysfunction in non-demented Parkinson's disease, in *Mental Dysfunction in Parkinson's Disease 2* (Wolters, E. Ch., Scheltens, P.H., and Berendse, H.W., eds.), Academic Pharmaceuticals, Utrecht, pp. 142–164.
28. Owen, A.M., Iddon, J.L., Hodges, J.R., Summers, B.A., and Robbins, T.W. (1997). Spatial and non-spatial working memory at different stages of Parkinson's disease. *Neuropsychologia* **35,** 519–532.
29. Postle, B.R., Corkin, S., Jonides, J., Smith, E.E., and Growdon, J.H. (1997) Spatial, but not object, delayed response is impaired in early Parkinson's disease. *Neuropsychology* **11,** 171–179.
30. Owen, A.M., Beksinska, M., James, M., et al. (1993) Visuo-spatial memory deficits at different stages of Parkinson's disease. *Neuropsychologia* **31,** 627–644.

31. Owen, A.M., Sahakian, B.J., Hodges, J.R., Summers, B.A., Polkey, C.E., and Robbins, T.W. (1995) Dopamine-dependent frontostriatal planning deficits in early Parkinson's disease. *Neuropsychology* **9,** 126–140.
32. Lange, K.W., Robbins, T.W., Marsden, C.D., James, M., Owen, A.M., and Paul, G.M. (1992) L Dopa withdrawal in Parkinson's disease selectively impairs cognitive performance in tests sensitive to frontal lobe dysfunction. *Psychopharmacology* **107,** 394–404.
33. Sawaguchi, T. and Goldman-Rakic, P.S. (1991) D1 dopamine receptors in prefrontal cortex: involvement in working memory. *Science* **251,** 947–950.
34. Collins, P., Roberts, A.C., Dias, R., Everitt, B.J., and Robbins, T.W. (1998) Perseveration and strategy in a novel spatial self-ordered sequencing task for nonhuman primates: effects of excitotoxic lesions and dopamine depletions of the prefrontal cortex. *J. Cogn. Neurosci.* **10,** 332–354.
35. Williams, G.V. and Goldman-Rakic, P.S. (1995) Modulation of memory fields by dopamine D1 receptors in prefrontal cortex. *Nature* **376,** 572–575.
36. Zahrt, J., Taylor, J.R., Mathew, R.G., and Arnsten, A.F.T. (1997) Supranormal stimulation of D1 dopamine receptors in the rodent prefrontal cortex impairs spatial working memory performance. *J. Neurosci.* **17,** 8528–8535.
37. Gotham, A.-M., Brown, R.G., and Marsden, C.D. (1988) 'Frontal' cognitive function in patients with Parkinson's disease 'on' and 'off' levodopa. *Brain* **111,** 299–321.
38. Cools, R., Barker, R.A., Sahakian, B.J., and Robbins, T.W. (2001) Enhanced or impaired cognitive function in Parkinson's disease as a function of dopaminergic medication and task demands. *Cerebral Cortex* **11,** 1136–1143.
39. Cools, R., Stefanova, E., Barker, R.A., Robbins, T.W., and Owen, A.M. (2001) Dopaminergic modulation of high-level cognition in Parkinson's disease: the role of prefrontal cortex revealed by PET. *Brain* **125,** 584–594.
40. Mehta, M., Owen, A.M., Sahakian, B.J., Mavaddat, N., Pickard, J.D., and Robbins, T.W. (2000) Methylphenidate enhances working memory by modulating discrete frontal and parietal lobe regions in the human brain. *J. Neurosci.* **20,** RC65, 1–6.
41. Mehta, M.A., Sahakian, B.J., McKenna, P.J., and Robbins, T.W. (1999) Systematic sulpiride in young adult volunteers simulates the profile of cognitive deficits in Parkinson's disease. *Psychopharmacology* **146,** 162–174.
42. Levy, R., Friedman, H.R., Davchi L., and Goldman-Rakic, P.S. (1997) Differential activation of the caudate nucleus in primates performing spatial and non-spatial working memory tasks. *J. Neurosci,* **17,** 3870–3882.
43. Arnsten, A.F.T., Cai, J.X., Murphy, B.L., and Goldman-Rakic, P.S. (1994) Dopamine D-1 receptor mechanisms in the cognitive performance of young adult and aged monkeys. *Psychopharmacology* **116,** 143–151.
44. Schneider, J.S. and Kovelowski, C.J. (1990) Chronic exposure to low doses of MPTP. I. Cognitive deficits in motor asymptomatic monkeys. *Brain Res.* **519,** 122–128.
45. Collins, P., Wilkinson, L.S., Everitt, B.J., Robbins, T.W., and Roberts, A.C. (2000) The effect of dopamine depletion from the caudate nucleus of the common marmoset (*Callithrix jacchus*) on tests of prefrontal cognitive function. *Behav. Neurosci.* **114,** 3–17.
46. Dias, R., Roberts, A.C., and Robbins, T.W (1996) Primate analogue of the Wisconsin Card Sort Test: effects of excitotoxic lesions of the prefrontal cortex in the Marmoset. *Behav. Neurosci.* **110,** 870–884.
47. Dias, R., Robbins, T.W., and Roberts, A.C. (1996) Dissociation in prefrontal cortex of affective and attentional shifts. *Nature* **380,** 69–72.
48. Dias, R., Robbins, T.W., and Roberts, A.C. (1997) Dissociable forms of inhibitory control within prefrontal cortex with an analogue of the Wisconsin card sort test: restriction to novel situations and independence from 'on-line' processing. *J. Neurosci.* **17,** 9285–9297.
49. Wallis, J.D., Dias, R., Robbins, T.W., and Roberts, A.C. (2001) Dissociable contributions of the orbitofrontal and lateral prefrontal cortex to performance on a detour reaching task. *Eur. J. Neurosci.* **13,** 1797–1808.
50. Roberts, A.C., De Salvia, M.A., Wilkinson, L.S., et al. (1994) 6-Hydroxydopamine lesions of the prefrontal cortex in monkeys enhance performance on an analogue of the Wisconsin Card Sorting test: possible interactions with subcortical dopamine. *J. Neurosci.* **14,** 2531–2544.
51. Crofts, H.S., Dalley, J.W., Collins, P., Van Denderen, J.C.M., Everitt, B.J., and Robbins, T.W. (2001) Differential effects of 6-OHDA lesions of the prefrontal cortex and caudate nucleus on the ability to acquire an attentional set. *Cerebral Cortex* **11,** 1015–1026.
52. Maddox, W.T., Filoteo, J.V., Delis, D.C., and Salmon, D.P. (1996) Visual selective attention deficits in patients with Parkinson's disease: a quantitative model-based approach. *Neuropsychology* **10,** 197–218.
53. Wright, M.J., Burns, R.J., Geffen, G.M., and Geffen, L.B. (1990) Covert orientation of visual attention in Parkinson's disease: an impairment in the maintenance of attention. *Neuropsychologia* **28,** 151–159.
54. Leenders, K.L. (1993) Mental dysfunction in patients with Parkinson's disease: PET investigations, in *Mental Dysfunction in Parkinson's Disease* (Wolters, E.C. and Scheltens, P., eds.), Amsterdam, Vrije Universitat, pp. 133–140.
54a. Hollerman, J.R. and Schultz, W. (1998) Dopamine neurons report an error in the temporal prediction of reward during learning. *Nat. Neurosci.* **1,** 304–309.
55. Rogers, R.D. and Monsell, S. (1995) Costs of a predictable switch between simple cognitive tasks. *J. Exp. Psychol.* **124,** 207–231.
56. Rogers, R.D., Sahakian, B.J., Hodges, J.R., Polkey, C.E., Kennard, C., and Robbins, T.W. (1998) Dissociating executive mechanisms of task control following frontal lobe damage and Parkinson's disease. *Brain* **121,** 815–842.
57. Cools, R., Barker, R.A., Sahakian, B.J., and Robbins, T.W. (2001) Mechanisms of cognitive set flexibility in Parkinson's disease. *Brain* **124,** 2503–2512.
58. Rogers, R.D., Andrews, T.C., Grasby, P.M., Brooks, D., and Robbins, T.W. (2000) Contrasting cortical and subcortical PET activations produced by reversal learning and attentional-set shifting in humans. *J. Cogn. Neurosci.* **12,** 142–162.

59. Middleton, H.C., Sharma, A., Agouzoul, D., Sahakian, B.J., and Robbins, T.W. (1999) Idazoxan potentiates rather than antagonizes some of the cognitive effects of clonidine. *Psychopharmacology* **145,** 401–411.
60. Rogers, R.D., Blackshaw, A.J., Middleton, H.C., et al. (1999a) Tryptophan depletion impairs stimulus-reward learning while methylphenidate disrupts attentional control in healthy young adults: implications for the monoaminergic basis of impulsive behavior. *Psychopharmacology* **146,** 482–491.
61. Roberts, A.C., Robbins T.W., Everitt, B.J., and Muir, J.L. (1992) A specific form of cognitive rigidity following excitotoxic lesions of the basal forebrain in monkeys. *Neuroscience* **47,** 251–264.
62. Bedard, M.-A., El Massioui, F., Malapani, C., et al. (1998) Attentional deficits in Parkinson's disease: partial reversibility with napthtoxazine (SDZ NV1-085), a selective noradrenergic alpha-1 agonist. *Clin. Neuropharmacol.* **21,** 108–117.
63. Alexander, G.E. and Crutcher, M.D. (1990) Functional architecture of basal ganglia circuits: neural substrates of parallel processing. *Trends Neurosci.* **13,** 266–271.
64. Sohn, M., Ursu, S., Anderson, J.R., Stenger, V.A., and Carter, C.S. (2000) The role of prefrontal cortex and posterior parietal cortex in task switching. *Proc. Natl. Acad. Sci. USA* **97,** 13,448–13,453.
65. Swainson, R, Rogers, R.D., Sahakian, B.J., Summers, B.A., Polkey, C.E., and Robbins, T.W. (2000) Probabilistic learning and reversal deficits in patients with Parkinson's disease or frontal or temporal lobe lesions: possible adverse effects of dopaminergic medication. *Neuropsychologia* **38,** 596–612.
66. Divac, I., Rosvold, H.E., and Szwarcbart, M.K. (1967) Behavioral effects of selective ablation of the caudate nucleus. *J. Comp. Physiol. Psychol.* **63,** 184–190.
67. Middleton, F.A. and Strick, P.L. (1996) The temporal lobe is a target of output from the basal ganglia. *Proc. Natl. Acad. Sci. USA* **93,** 8683–8687.

15

Nondopaminergic Influences on Cognition in Parkinson's Disease

Marc-André Bédard, PhD, Maxime Lévesque, BSc, Simon Lemay, MPs, and François Paquet, MSc

1. INTRODUCTION

Parkinson's disease (PD) is often associated with a set of neuropsychological dysfunctions referred to as subcorticofrontal syndrome (SCFS), in reference to the subcortical locus of lesions in this disease and to the nature of the cognitive deficits, which mimic those encountered further in patients with frontal cortical lesions *(1,2)* (see also Chapter 6 of this volume). SCFS must be distinguished from other conditions associated with PD that may affect cognitive functions, such as dementia of the Alzheimer type (DAT), or dementia with Lewy body (DLB), which show high prevalence in PD and which are associated with lesions directly located in the cortex (see Chapters 17, 18, and 20 of this volume). Depression must also be clearly identified in PD, given its high prevalence and its worsening effect on SCFS (see Chapter 27 of this volume).

SCFS is nonspecific and can be observed following many subcortical pathologies *(3)*, as well as more systemic illnesses, such as acquired immune deficiency syndrome, chronic obstructive pulmonary disease, or endogenous depression. Clinically, SCFS is characterized by executive dysfunctions *(3–8)*, which may be seen as difficulties in establishing cognitive strategies or in organizing information. For instance, it seems that patients fail *(6)* or succeed *(7)* at performing left/right discrimination or mental-rotation tasks depending on whether they must provide an answer on their own or simply choose the correct answer from among several alternatives. Thus, it is generally accepted *(1,2)* that cognitive deficits related to PD-associated SCFS mainly affects tasks requiring active control over cognitive processes (willed action or processing) (see Chapter 7 of this volume). Conversely, tasks that require only automatic processing or are guided by external cues (i.e., those that do not require "intentional" or voluntarily controlled processes) are usually performed correctly. Some authors *(8)* use the terms "effortful" and "effortless," respectively, to describe these two types of cognitive processing.

Difficulty with tasks requiring effort or intention may result from low cognitive alertness, which is a reduced quantity of the "energetic" resources necessary to process nonautomated mental operations. Although this concept does make sense, the reference to ambiguous functions, such as "energetic resources" or "cognitive alertness," remains nonoperational and, thus, is difficult to study experimentally. Alternatively, a hypothesis drawn from cognitive psychology suggests instead that these energetic resources are poorly distributed among the various mental operations that must be activated in the course of nonautomated reasoning or unusual behavior *(9,10)*. In other words, deficits in willed processing would be related not to a reduction in energetic resources, but rather to the incorrect allocation

From: *Mental and Behavioral Dysfunction in Movement Disorders*
Edited by: M-A. Bédard et al. © Humana Press Inc., Totowa, NJ

of these resources (poor attentional management) to the various cognitive components that must be activated for a given behavior or processing. For instance, despite having preserved memories, PD patients may rely on information or a fragment of information from other sources, thereby inducing memory intrusions. Poor distribution of these resources may also create difficulties with dual tasks *(11,12)*. For instance, a patient may find it hard to maintain a conversation while at the same time pursuing an activity such as cooking or driving.

The misallocation of energetic resources in PD has been measured both by the simultaneous execution of two perceptual cognitive tasks *(11)* and by working memory tasks requiring the retention of one type of information while performing a second task *(12)*. Human and animal studies using this type of dual-task paradigm show that lesions in the frontal lobes or the mesocortical and nigrostriatal dopaminergic systems may induce deficiencies that recall those found in PD *(13)*. Dopamine (DA) depletion in PD could, therefore, be an important factor in SCFS.

2. NEUROCHEMISTRY OF THE COGNITIVE DYSFUNCTION IN PD

2.1. *Dopamine*

Current knowledge of the physiological basis of SCFS in PD remains unclear. The possibility that the characteristic loss of DA-containing neurons of the substantia nigra plays a role has been extensively investigated (see Chapter 14 of this volume). These studies were mainly based on the assumption that PD-associated SCFS results from a reduced dopaminergic modulation of the striatum, which disrupts the flow of information within the circuits that link the striatum and the frontal cortex *(14)*. The mesocortical dopaminergic degeneration observed in PD has also been suggested as a possible pathogenic factor underlying SCFS *(15)*. However, no dopaminergic hypothesis can explain why treatment of PD with dopaminergic substances does not reverse SCFS in these patients. In point of fact, the more severe the SCFS of parkinsonian patients, the poorer their response to dopaminergic treatments *(16,17)*. The slight improvement in performance with levodopa reported in some initial studies *(18,19)* applied only to general intellectual scales and has been mainly attributed to a DA awakening effect (increased vigilance) or a change in affective state. Comparisons of neuropsychological performance "ON" and "OFF" levodopa have also generally been inconclusive *(20–22)*. Indeed, the very few changes observed by some authors were generally task-specific in that, during "ON" phases, performance on some tasks improved, concurrently with a worsening or lack of change in all others. This phenomenon has been observed in many studies, showing that, even though SCFS does not respond well to DA treatment overall, some specific components of the syndrome may improve. For instance, DA treatment of PD has been found to be associated with improved performance on dual tasks such as working memory tasks *(12)* or visuo-auditory concurrent perceptual tasks *(11)*. It has been suggested that DA depletion in PD may induce a difficulty in sharing attention between two or more concurrent tasks *(11,23)*. This hypothesis is in agreement with results obtained from animals with frontal lobe lesions or selective DA depletion (see Chapter 14 of this book). It is not clear, however, whether the mesocortical or the nigrostriatal system is more specifically involved, although some evidence obtained by our team *(23)* and others *(24)* suggests that the involvement of the latter is critical. In spite of these interesting findings on the relationship between DA and certain specific cognitive functions in patients with SCFS, it is clear that DA dysfunction alone cannot account for the entire syndrome in PD patients.

2.2. *Noradrenaline and Serotonin*

Among the nondopaminergic neurochemical lesions in PD, the noradrenergic and serotonergic pathways have been suggested as possible contributing factors to SCFS, but very little evidence supports such a view. The noradrenergic reduction that affects the cortex and the limbic structures in PD is mainly found in patients with severe dementia *(25)*. This depletion is accompanied by an increase in the number of (postsynaptic) β-1 receptors and a reduction in (pre- and postsynaptic) α-2 receptors,

Table 1
The Effect of Naphtoxazine on Tests of Attention in PD

Tests		Naphtoxazine	Placebo	*p*
CPT	(ms)	460.4 (81.9)	459.8 (68.5)	ns
	(% Error)	1.7 (1.9)	2.9 (3.2)	ns
Trail making (B)	(sec)	169.9 (69.1)	167.4 (80.8)	ns
Stroop (3)	(sec)	134.6 (52.4)	217.1(107.7)	*
OMO	(Errors)	6.1 (2.7)	10.5 (4.4)	*
Verbal fluency	(No. of words)	20.7 (6.5)	18.2 (7.6)	ns
15 objects	(No. of pictures)	14.1 (1.7)	13.3 (2.9)	ns
	(sec)	108.1 (51.6)	124.0 (60.2)	ns

CPT, Continuous Performance Test of attention; OMO, Odd Man Out test of Card Classification; ns, not significant.

The drug was found to significantly improve some specific tests of attention (*), but was not effective in reversing the SCFS as a whole. (Taken from ref. *27*).

located mainly in the frontal cortex. However, the role of these noradrenergic abnormalities is not known. Some evidence suggests that these lesions may play a role in the attentional deficiencies associated with PD. In fact, measurement of the cerebrospinal fluid in PD shows that levels of the extracellular metabolite of noradrenaline, 3-methoxy-4-hydroxyphenethyleneglycol (MHPG), are positively correlated with performance on the Continuous Performance Task *(26)*, which is a test of selective attention. Moreover, we have recently shown in PD that the administration of naphtoxazine, an α-1 agonist, can improve performance on some cognitive tests involving selective attention *(27)* (see Table 1). Therefore, it seems that some of the cognitive deficits PD patients experience can be related to the lesion of the ascending noradrenergic systems. However, the evidence is limited, and more studies are needed to support this view.

The same analysis may also apply to lesions of the ascending serotonergic system arising from the raphe nuclei. These neurons have been found to be lesioned in PD. In the cerebral cortex, reduced serotonin concentrations were found in PD patients *(28)*, and this reduction was more specific to the frontal cortex and the cerebral hippocampus. However, no difference was detected between PD patients with or without dementia. The number of serotonergic 5-HT1_A receptors was also found to be upregulated in the striatum in monkeys who developed a parkinsonian syndrome following chronic exposure to 1-methyl-4-phenyl-1,2,3,6-tetrahydropyridine (MPTP) *(29)*. This up-regulation was observed only in the limbic area of the striatum, suggesting an involvement in the affective rather than the cognitive dysfunctions of the disease. This is reinforced by the correlations that have been observed between the low concentrations of the serotonin metabolite 5-hydroxy-indole-acetic acid (5-HIAA) in the cerebrospinal fluid and the severity of depression *(30–32)* in PD.

2.3. *Acetylcholine*

Postmortem studies have shown a massive loss of cholinergic cells in PD patients' brains *(33–37)*. There is a reduced concentration of choline acetyltransferase (CAT) and muscarinic, as well as nicotinic receptors in many areas of the cortex and hippocampus *(38)*. It has, therefore, been suggested that this depletion may contribute to the cognitive deficiencies found in these patients. Unfortunately, these studies have often used the coexistence of dementia as a criterion for cognitive deterioration. The level of degeneration of the innominatocortical and septohippocampal fibers is about 70–80% in PD patients with dementia, while it is around 20% in those patients who do not have an associated dementia *(34)*. But it is difficult to see how cholinergic lesions that affect the cortex as a whole could be involved in the SCFS, which is mainly characterized by specific frontal lobe function deficits.

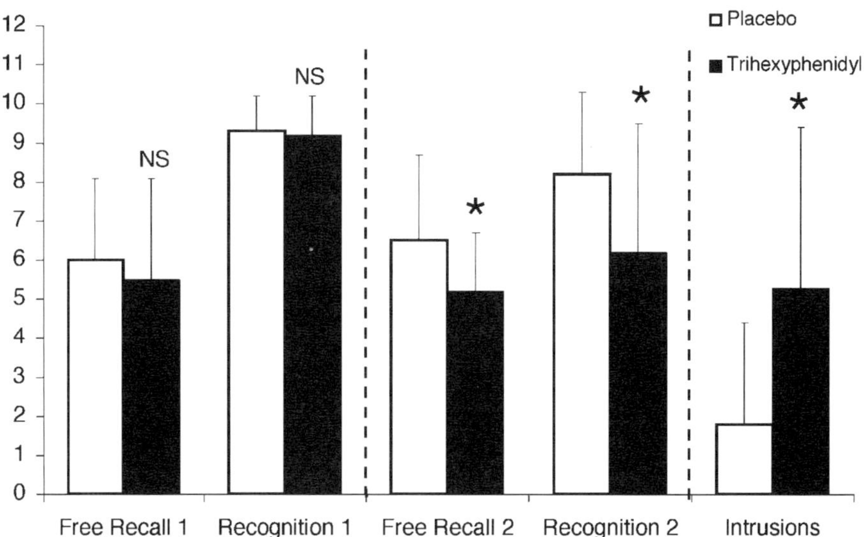

Fig. 1. Selective Reminding Test in PD patients treated with Trihexyphenidyl and placebo. The first free recall was similar between the two groups, so was the recognition of words presented among distracters. However, following this presentation of distracters, a second free recall and recognition revealed lower performances and abnormally high number of intrusions in PD patients. Such a sensitivity to intrusions without forgetting the words is characteristic to a SCFS. (Adapted from ref. *42*.)

Some studies show that PD patients with no cognitive deficiency to whom an anticholinergic treatment is administered may develop a characteristic SCFS in the course of the treatment *(39–42)*. The selectivity of the cognitive deficiency and the low doses used in these studies allow us to eliminate the hypothesis that a confusional syndrome or an Alzheimer-type cognitive decline, sometimes observed with high doses of an anticholinergic *(43)*, has been induced (see Fig. 1). In addition, acute administration of scopolamine at a subclinical dose, which is a dose that has no detectable effect on healthy subjects, produces SCFS in PD patients for the duration of the drug's action *(41–42)* (see Figs. 2–4). The deleterious effects of anticholinergic drugs administered in larger doses to healthy subjects have already been well documented *(43)*. These effects consist of a general cognitive deterioration similar to that observed in Alzheimer-type dementia, suggesting that the effect of anticholinergic drugs on healthy subjects' cognitive functions may be linked to an inhibition of the innominatocortical and septohippocampal cholinergic systems. However, the fact that SCFS, but not Alzheimer-type cognitive deficits, can be induced in PD by using subclinical doses of scopolamine suggests a different mechanism. It is possible that subclinical doses affect only the most damaged cholinergic systems in PD patients and that healthy subjects' better preserved systems may not be affected by such small doses because compensatory processes would take place *(42)*. Such a phenomenon has been demonstrated within the nigrostriatal dopaminergic system in which cell death must be of 70 to 80% before the first motor symptoms can be detected. Cholinergic systems would, therefore, require critical level of degeneration before an SCFS may occur. In PD patients, who do not have this critical level of cholinergic depletion, subclinical doses of scopolamine may precipitate a SCFS by decompensating the residual mechanisms.

Among the cholinergic systems that are most affected in PD, the pedunculopontine (PPTN) and laterodorsal tegmental nuclei (LDTN) may be more specifically involved in SCFS. A significant cell loss has been reported in these nuclei, and this cholinergic loss is correlated with the dopaminergic loss observed in the substantia nigra *(35,36)*. The PPTN and the LDTN are known for their mainly subcortical projections, especially to the mediodorsal nuclei of the thalamus. This thalamic nucleus has a high contingent of projections to the prefrontal cortex and is directly involved in the cognitive and

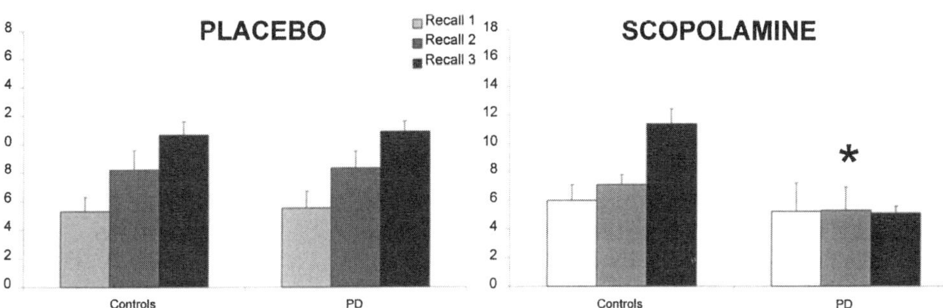

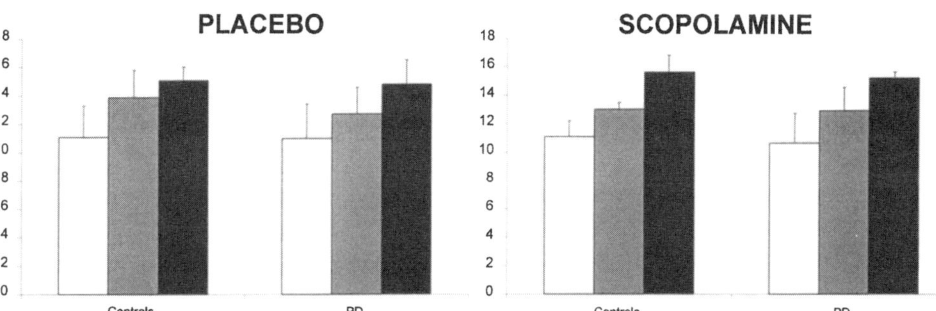

Fig. 2. Grober & Buschke Verbal Memory Test in normal controls and PD patients, both receiving a subclinical dose of scopolamine. The drug did not affect the performance of normal subjects at any time. In PD patients, however, there was no learning effect across the three trials of the Free Recall when they were under the effect of scopolamine. Total Recall (free + Cued recalls) revealed that presenting a cue allows PD patients to retrieve the words that were not recollected during the free recall. This is characteristic to a SCFS. (Adapted from ref. *42*.)

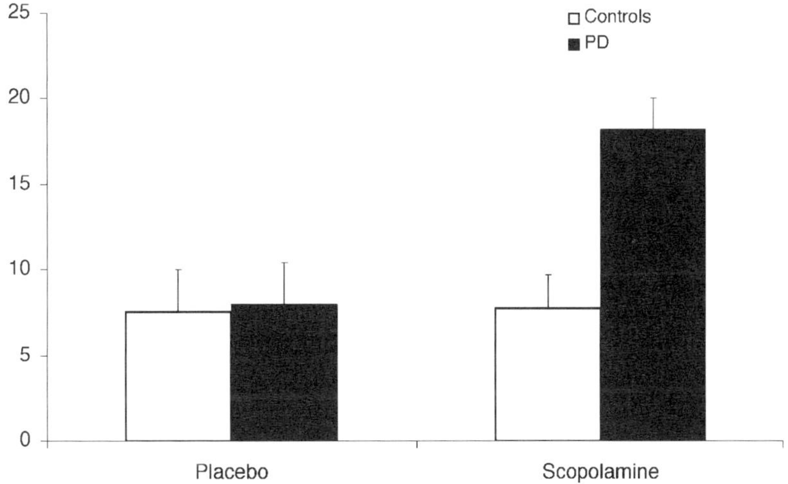

Fig. 3. Self-Ordered Pointing Task in normal controls and PD patients both receiving a subclinical dose of scopolamine. Increased intrusion errors are associated with the drug administration in PD but not in normal controls. (Adapted from ref. *42*.)

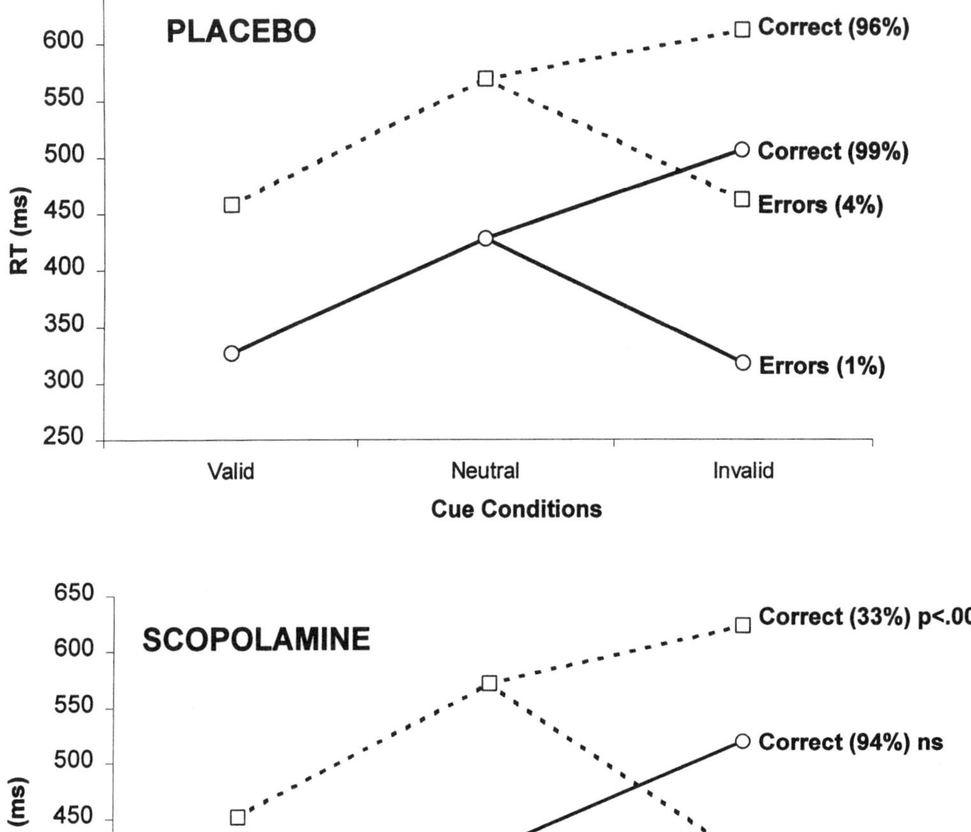

Fig. 4. Shifting Reaction Time Task in normal controls and PD patients, both receiving a subclinical dose of scopolamine. In this task, a target tone is presented to the right or to the left ear, and subject must press the button on the side of the tone. Before the tone, a visual cue is presented to indicate the side to which the tone will be delivered. This allows the subjects to preprogram their responses. There are Valid cues (arrows pointing to the good side); Neutral cues (arrows pointing to the two sides); and Invalid Cues (arrows pointing to the wrong side). Invalid cue condition requires the subjects to inhibit their preprogrammed response (at the moment of the tone) to shift from the wrong to the good side of the tone. Increased number of shifting errors is associated with the drug administration in PD but not in normal controls. (Adapted from ref. *42*.)

limbic portion of the anatomical corticostriatopallidothalamofrontal loop. It is, therefore, possible that this cholinergic demodulation, on its own or in association with the nigrostriatal dopaminergic demodulation, may contribute to the appearance of SCFS in PD. One of the arguments in favor of this hypothesis is that in illnesses such as progressive supranuclear palsy (PSP), multiple system atrophy (MSA), and DLB, in which SCFS is even more severe than in PD, the PPTN and the LDTN are more severely affected than in PD (see Chapter 22 of this volume). In PSP, the PPTN/LDTN are actually the only cholinergic structures affected *(35,37)*. Given that these cholinergic fibers are part of the afferent reticular formation system, one may suggest that a lesion there would have a detrimental impact on cortical alertness, therefore affecting the most effortful or "willed" processes, as is found in SCFS.

The cholinergic hypothesis of SCFS remains to be confirmed. Current research indicates that cholinergic agonists are effective in improving the cognitive performance of some patients with PSP *(44)*, but have no effect on others *(45)*. In animals, the role of PPTN/LDTN could be more specifically demonstrated if lesions restricted to these nuclei were shown to produce behavioral deficiencies that are analogous to those observed following a prefrontal cortical lesion. If these frontal deficiencies are reversed following administration of cholinergic agonists, we could endorse with more certainty the primary role of these cholinergic systems. Positron emission to tomography (PET) studies with ligands of the vesicular acetylcholine transporter *(46)* would also help to establish a relationship between PPTN/LDTN lesions in PD and the clinical symptomatology, including SCFS. Other clinical manifestations of the disease, such as gait disturbances, sleepiness, or rapid eye movement (REM) sleep behavior disorder, could also be related to damage to these nuclei, given that these functions are known to involve the integrity of these cholinergic systems *(47,48)* (see also Chapters 29 and 39 of this volume).

2.4. *Nicotine*

The cerebral areas on which the PPTN/LDTN project are rich in cholinergic nicotinic receptors *(49)*. Nicotinic receptors are generally located on the presynaptic terminals of various neurons, including noncholinergic neurons, and are excitatory, in that they facilitate exocytosis of neurotransmitters (heterosynaptic facilitation) *(50,51)*. For example, studies conducted in vitro have shown that stimulation of the nicotinic receptors located on the ends of nigrostriatal fibers increased the quantity of DA released by these fibers *(50)*. The same phenomenon has also been described for the corticostriatal glutamatergic cells *(51)*. In addition to its action on synaptic transmission, nicotine seems to protect against neurodegeneration. Epidemiological data show that there is a negative correlation between the incidence of PD and smoking frequency *(52,53)*. This protective effect has also been shown in vitro and in animal models of PD *(54–56)*.

Several studies have already administered nicotine to animals or humans to improve cognitive performance. In healthy volunteers *(57)*, nicotine has been found to improve performance on various attentional tasks. Some clinical studies using nicotine have shown an improvement of motor symptoms in PD *(58,59)*, and this effect is thought to result from the stimulating action of the drug on nigrostriatal dopaminergic fibers *(50)*. However, these positive results remain controversial *(60)*. Our own experience with transdermal nicotine patches *(61)* is that more than half of PD patients cannot tolerate the adverse gastrointestinal effects and that even in those who can, there was no improvement in the motor or cognitive symptoms (see Table 2). This has also been observed by others *(62)*. These results may be related to the unspecific action of nicotine; they might have been different with specific nicotinic agonists that do not affect the peripheral autonomous system.

Some pharmaceutical companies have developed their own nicotinic compounds, of which the best known are ABT-418, SIB-1553A, and SIB-1508Y. The effects of these substances on SCFS in PD patients are still unknown, but in the MPTP animal model of PD, SIB-1508Y and SIB-1553A appeared to be effective against akinetic-rigid syndrome *(63)* and to improve cognitive functions *(64)* (see Chapter 13 of this volume).

2.5. *Cholinesterase Inhibitors*

The treatment of dementia in PD is almost the same as for Alzheimer-type dementia. Cholinesterase inhibitors (AhE-I) remain the first choice, although they should be administered with caution, in progressive titrated doses. The aim of such a treatment in dementia is obviously to increase acetylcholine concentration at the synapses, where cholinergic terminals have been found to be reduced.

Table 2
The Effect of Chronic Transdermal Nicotine on Cognitive and Motor Tests in PD

Scores		Mean (standard deviation)		Statistical significance	
		High dose	Baseline	Group	Treatment
Cognitive tasks					
RAVLT					
Total words recalled	PD	42.11 (9.78)	40.78 (11.16)	*	NS
	Ctl	54.00 (7.54)	52.20 (7.98)		
Stroop: (3)					
Completion time (s)	PD	57.54 (13.32)	54.23 (13.58)	*	NS
	Ctl	43.41 (14.06)	39.10 (12.24)		
Alternate fluency					
Total words generated	PD	45.75 (11.61)	48.63 (10.00)	*	NS
	Ctl	56.30 (12.32)	58.30 (9.32)		
Letter-number sequences					
Wechsler Adult Intelligence Scale (WAIS-III) raw score	PD	9.22 (3.80)	9.89 (2.76)	*	NS
	Ctl	12.30 (2.31)	12.70 (2.95)		
Motor tasks					
Diadochokinesimeter					
Velocity (°/s)	PD	41.29 (14.24)	46.21 (21.58)	*	NS
	Ctl	61.98 (18.76)	64.21 (20.54)		
EKM					
Speed accuracy tradeoff	PD	0.184 (0.035)	0.176 (0.030)	*	NS
	Ctl	0.156 (0.028)	0.148 (0.026)		

RAVLT, RET Auditory Verbal Learning Test; EKM, Eurithmokinesi meter; PD, Parkinson's disease; Ctl, control subjects.

For EKM, the lower the score, the better the performance.

Although the tests were generally sensitive enough to distinguish PD patients from healthy subjects (group effect), there was no improvement of performances attributable to nicotine (treatment effect). *, $p < 0.5$; NS, nonsignificant.

Recent studies have showed that AchE-I are effective at improving the cognitive performance of PD patients with dementia *(65–67)*. However, their effect on the SCFS in PD has not yet been assessed, probably because SCFS is not currently considered to be a clinical problem given that its severity does not meet the criteria for dementia. In our opinion, this point of view is questionable given that we have recently demonstrated that SCFS may explain behavioral disorganization during daily functioning better than PD motor impairments *(68)*. Another explanation for the lack of assessment of AchE-I in nondemented PD patients is that these substances increase acetylcholine in the striatum, where it may potentially exacerbate the motor impairments by activating the striatal muscarinic receptors. Recent studies, however, have shown that donepezil *(65)* and rivastigmine *(66)*, the two most prescribed AchE-I, do not worsen the motor symptoms in PD patients with dementia (see Chapter 23 of this volume). It could, therefore, be interesting to verify whether AchE-I would improve SCFS in PD. This might be of some help in improving the quality of life for these patients, which is highly related to their cognitive status (see Chapter 37 of this book). In addition, this would reinforce the hypothesis that Ach depletion in PD may play a primary role in the SCSF.

REFERENCES

1. Brown, R.G. and Marsden, C.D. (1990) Cognitive function in Parkinson's disease: from description to theory. *Trends Neurosci.* **13,** 21–29.
2. Taylor, A.E. (1995) The neuropsychology of Parkinson's disease. *Brain Cogn.* **28,** 281–296.
3. Cummings, J.L. (ed.) (1990) *Subcortical Dementia,* Oxford University Press, Oxford.

4. Pillon, B., Dubois, B., Ploska, A., and Agid, Y. (1991) Severity and specificity of cognitive impairment in Alzheimer's, Huntington's, Parkinson's disease and Progressive Supranuclear Palsy. *Neurology* **41,** 634–643.
5. Pillon, B., Deweer, B., Agid, Y., and Dubois, B. (1993) Explicit memory in Alzheimer's, Huntington's, and Parkinson's diseases. *Arch. Neurol.* **50,** 374–379.
6. Boller, F., Passafiume, D., Keefe, N.C., Rogers, K., Morrow, L., and Kim Y. (1984) Visuospatial impairments in Parkinson's disease. *Arch. Neurol.* **41,** 485–490.
7. Brown, R.G. and Marsden C.D. (1986) Visuospatial function in Parkinson's disease. *Brain* **109,** 987–1002.
8. Weingartner, H., Burns, S., Diebel, R., and Lewitt, P.A. (1984) Cognitive impairment in Parkinson's disease: distinguishing between effort demanding and autonomic cognitive processes. *Psychiatry Res.* **11,** 223–235.
9. Norman, D.A. and Shallice, T. (1980) Attention to action: willed and automatic control of behavior, in *CHIP Report 99*, University of California, San Diego.
10. Baddeley, A. (1986) *Working Memory,* Oxford University Press, Oxford.
11. Malapanis, C., Pillon, B., Dubois, B., and Agid, Y. (1994) Impaired simultaneous cognitive task performance in Parkinson's disease: a dopamine-related function. *Neurology* **44,** 319–326.
12. Dalrymple-Alford, J.C., Kalders, A.S., Jones, R.D., and Watson, R.W. (1994) A central executive deficit in patients with Parkinson's disease. *J. Neurol. Neurosurg. Psychiatry* **57,** 360–367.
13. Goldman-Rakic, P.S. (1995) Cellular basis of working memory. *Neuron* **14,** 477–485.
14. Alexander, G.E., DeLong, M.T., and Strick P.L. (1986) Parallel organization of functionally segregated circuits linking basal ganglia and cortex. *Annu. Rev. Neurosci.* **9,** 357–381.
15. Agid, Y., Ruberg, M., Raisman, R., Hirsch, E., and Javoy-Agid, F. (1990) The biochemistry of Parkinson's disease, in *Parkinson's Disease* (Stern, G., ed.), Chapman & Hall Ltd., London, pp. 99–125.
16. Taylor, A.E., Saint-Cyr, J.A., and Lang, A.E. (1987) Parkinson's disease. Cognitive changes in relation to treatment response. *Brain* **110,** 35–51.
17. Pillon, B., Dubois, B., Cusimano, G., Bonnet, A.M., Lhermitte, F., and Agid, Y. (1989) Does cognitive impairment in Parkinson's disease result from non-dopaminergic lesions? *J. Neurol. Neurosurg. Psychiatry* **52,** 201–206.
18. Beardsley, J. and Puletti, F. (1971) Personality (MMPI) and cognitive (WAIS) changes after levodopa treatment. *Arch. Neurol.* **25,** 145–150.
19. Loranger, A.W., Goodell, H., Le, J.E., and McDowell, F. (1972) Levodopa treatment of Parkinson's syndrome improve intellectual functioning. *Arch. Gen. Psychiatry* **26,** 163–168.
20. Girotti, F., Carella, F., Grassi, M., Soliveri, P., Marano, R., and Caraceni, T. (1986) Motor and cognitive performances of parkinsonian patients in the "ON" and "OFF" phases of the disease. *J. Neurol. Neurosurg. Psychiatry* **49,** 657–660.
21. Gotham, A.M., Brown, R.G., and Marsden, C.D. (1988) Frontal cognitive function in patients with Parkinson's disease "ON" and "OFF" levodopa. *Brain* **111,** 299–321.
22. Lange, K.W., Paul, G.M., Naumann, M., and Gsell, W. (1995) Dopaminergic effects on cognitive performance in patients with Parkinson's disease. *J. Neural. Transm. Suppl.* **46,** 423–432.
23. Duchesne, N., Soucy, J.-P., Masson, H., Chouinard, S., and Bédard, M.-A. (2002) Cognitive deficits and striatal dopaminergic denervation in Parkinson's disease: a SPECT study using Iodine123-beta-CIT in patients ON and OFF levodopa. *Clin. Neuropharmacol.* **25,** 216–224.
24. Muller, U., Wachter, T., Barthel, H., Reuter, M., and von Cramon, D.Y. (2000) Striatal (123I) beta-CIT SPECT and prefrontal cognitive functions in Parkinson's disease. *J. Neural. Transm.* **107,** 303–319.
25. Zweig, R.M., Cardillo, J.E., Cohen, M., Giere, S., and Hedreen, J.C. (1993) The locus ceruleus and dementia in Parkinson's disease. *Neurology* **43,** 986–991.
26. Stern, Y., Mayeux, R., and Coté, L. (1984) Reaction time and vigilance in Parkinson's disease: possible role of norepinephrine metabolism. *Arch. Neurol.* **41,** 1086–1089.
27. Bédard, M.-A., Malapanis, C., El Massioui, F., et al. (1998) Attentional deficits in Parkinson's disease: partial reversibility with naphtoxazine (SDZ NVI 085), a selective noradrenergic alpha 1 agonist. *Clin. Neuropharmacol.* **21,** 108–117.
28. D'Amato, R.J., Zweig, R.M., Whitehouse, P.J., et al. (1987) Aminergic systems in Alzheimer's disease and Parkinson's disease. *Ann. Neurol.* **22,** 229–236.
29. Frechilla, D., Cobreros, A., Saldise, L., et al. (2001) Serotonin 5-HT(1A) receptor expression is selectively enhanced in the striosomal compartment of chronic parkinsonian monkeys. *Synapse* **15,** 288–296.
30. Mayeux, R., Stern, Y., Sano, M., Williams, J.B., and Cote, L.J. (1988) The relationship of serotonin to depression in Parkinson's disease. *Mov. Disord.* **3,** 237–244.
31. Mayeux, R. (1990) Depression in the patient with Parkinson's disease. *J. Clin. Psychiatry* **51(Suppl 20–23),** 24–25.
32. Cummings, J.L. (1992) Depression and Parkinson's disease: a review. *Am. J. Psychiatry* **149,** 443–454.
33. Chang Chui, H. and Perlmutter, L.S. (1992) Pathological correlates of dementia in Parkinson's disease, in *Parkinson's Disease: Neurobehavioral Aspects* (Huber, S.J. and Cummings, J.L., eds.), Oxford University Press, Oxford, pp. 164–177.
34. Perry, E.K., Curtis, M., Dick, D.J., et al. (1985) Cholinergic correlates of cognitive impairment in Parkinson's disease: comparisons with Alzheimer disease. *J. Neurol. Neurosurg. Psychiatry* **48,** 413–421.
35. Hirsch, E., Graybiel, A.M., Duyckaerts, C., and Javoy-Agid, F. (1987) Neuronal loss in the pedunculopontine tegmental nucleus in Parkinson's disease and in Progressive Supranuclear Palsy. *Proc. Natl. Acad. Sci. USA* **84,** 5976–5980.
36. Zweig, R.M., Jankel, W.R., Hedreen, J.C., Mayeux, R., and Price D.L. (1989) The pedunculopontine nucleus in Parkinson's disease. *Ann. Neurol.* **26,** 41–46.

37. Malessa, S., Hirsch, E., Cervera, P., et al. (1991) Progressive Supranuclear Palsy: loss of choline-acetyltransferase-like immunoreactive neurons in the pontine reticular formation. *Neurology* **41,** 1593–1597.
38. Aubert, I., Araujo, D.M., Cecyre, D., Robitaille, Y., Gauthier, S., and Quirion, R. (1992) Comparative alterations of nicotinic and muscarinic binding sites in Alzheimer's and Parkinson's diseases. *J. Neurochem.* **52,** 529–541.
39. VanSpaendonck, K.P.M., Berger, H.J.C., Horstink, M.W.I., Buytenhuijs, E.L., and Cools, A.R. (1993) Impaired cognitive shifting in Parkinsonian patients on anticholinergic therapy. *Neuropsychologia* **31,** 407–411.
40. Dubois, B., Pillon, B., Lhermitte, F., and Agid, Y. (1990) Cholinergic deficiency and frontal dysfunction in Parkinson's disease. *Ann. Neurol.* **28,** 117–121.
41. Dubois, B., Danzé, F., Pillon, B., Cusimano, G., Lhermitte, F., and Agid, Y. (1987) Cholinergic-dependent cognitive deficits in Parkinson's disease. *Ann. Neurol.* **22,** 26–30.
42. Bédard, M.-A., Pillon, B., Dubois, B., Duchesne, N., Masson, H., and Agid, Y. (1999) Acute and long-term administration of anticholinergics in Parkinson's disease: Specific effects on the subcortico-frontal syndrome. *Brain Cogn.* **40,** 289–313.
43. Drachman, D.A. and Leavitt, J. (1974) Human memory and the cholinergic system. *Arch. Neurol.* **30,** 113–121.
44. Litvan, I., Gomez, C., Atack, J., et al. (1989) Physostigmine treatment of Progressive Supranuclear Palsy. *Ann. Neurol.* **26,** 404–407.
45. Kertzman, C., Robinson, D.L., and Litvan, I. (1990) Effects of physostigmine on spatial attention in patients with Progressive Supranuclear Palsy. *Arch. Neurol.* **47,** 1346–1350.
46. Kuhl, D.E., Koeppe, R.A., Fessler, J.A., et al. (1994) In vivo mapping of cholinergic neurons in the human using SPECT and IBVM. *J. Nucl. Med.* **35,** 405–410.
47. Lee, M.S., Rinne, J.O., and Marsden, C.D. (2000) The pedunculopontine nucleus: its role in the genesis of movement disorders. *Yonsei Med. J.* **41,** 167–184.
48. Pahapill, P.A. and Lazano, A.M. (2000) The pedunculopontine nucleus in Parkinson's disease. *Brain* **123,** 1761–1783.
49. Clarke, P.B.S. (1993) Nicotinic receptors in mammalian brain: localization and relation to cholinergic innervation, in *Cholinergic Function and Dysfunction* (Cuello, A.C., ed.), Elsevier, New York, pp. 77–84.
50. Lichtensteiger, W., Hefti, F., Felix, D., Huwyler, T., Mealmed, E., and Schlumpf, M. (1982) Stimulation of nigrostriatal dopamine neurone by nicotine. *Neuropharmacology* **21,** 963–968.
51. Matsubayashi, H., Amano, T., Amano, H., and Sasa, M. (2001) Excitation of rat striatal large neurons by dopamine and/or glutamate released from nerve terminals via presynaptic nicotinic receptor (A4beta2 type) stimulation. *Jpn. J. Pharmacol.* **8,** 429–436.
52. Baron, J.A. (1986) Cigarette smoking and Parkinson's disease. *Neurology,* **36,** 1490–1496.
53. Gorell, J.M., Rybicki, B.A., Johnson, C.C., and Peterson, E.L. (1999) Smoking and Parkinson's disease: a dose-response relationship. *Neurology* **52,** 115–119.
54. Gao, Z.G., Cui, W.Y, Zhang, H.T., and Liu, C.G. (1998) Effects of nicotine on 1-methyl-4-phenyl-1,2,5,6-tetrahydropyridine-induced depression of striatal dopamine content and spontaneous locomotor activity in C57 black mice. *Pharmacol. Res.* **38,** 101–106.
55. Maggio, R., Riva, M., Vaglini, F., Formai, F., Racagni, G., and Corsini, G.U. (1997) Striatal increase of neurotrophic factors as a mechanism of nicotine protection in experimental parkinsonism. *J. Neural. Transm.* **104,** 1113–1123.
56. Jonnala, R.R. and Buccafusco, J.J. (2001). Relationship between the increased cell surface alpha7 nicotinic receptor expression and neuroprotection induced by several nicotinic receptor agonists. *J. Neurosci. Res.* **66,** 565–572.
57. Warburton, D.M. (1992) Nicotine as a cognitive enhancer. *Prog. Neuropsychopharmacol. Biol. Psychiatry* **16,** 181–191.
58. Fagerstrom, K.O., Pomerleau, O., Giordani, B., and Stelson, F. (1994) Nicotine may relieve symptoms of Parkinson's disease. *Psychopharmacology* **116,** 117–119.
59. Ishikawa, A. and Miyatake, T. (1993) Effects of smoking in patients with early-onset Parkinson's disease. *J. Neurol. Sci.* **117,** 28–32.
60. Clemens, P., Baron, J.A., Coffey, D., and Reeves, A. (1995) The short-term effect of nicotine chewing gum in patients with Parkinson's disease. *Psychopharmacology.,* **117,** 253–256.
61. Lemay, S., Blanchet, P., Chouinard, S., et al. (2001) Tolerability and efficacy of a four weeks transdermal nicotine treatment in Parkinson's disease. *Mov. Disord.* **16(Suppl.),** 35.
62. Vieregge, A., Sieberer, M., Jacobs, H., Hagenah, J.M., and Vieregge, P. (2001) Transdermal nicotine in PD: a randomized, double-blind, placebo-controlled study. *Neurology* **25,** 1032–1035.
63. Schneider, J.S., Pope, Coleman, A., Van Velson, M., Menzaghi, F., and Zloyd, G.K. (1998) Effects of SIB 1508Y, a novel neuronal nicotinic acetylcholine receptor agonist, on motor behavior in parkinsonian monkeys. *Mov. Disord.* **13,** 637–642.
64. Schneider, J.S., Van Velson, M., Menzaghi, F., and Lloyd, G.K. (1998) Effects of the nicotinic acetylcholine receptor agonist SIB-1508Y on object retrieval performance in MPTP-treated monkeys: comparison with levodopa treatment. *Ann. Neurol.* **43,** 311–317.
65. Aarsland, D., Laake, K., Larsen, J.P., and Janvin, C. (2002) Donepezil for cognitive impairment in Parkinson's disease: a randomized controlled study. *J. Neurol. Neurosurg. Psychiatry* **72,** 708–712.
66. Korczyn, A.D. (2001) Dementia in Parkinson's disease. *J. Neurol.* **248(Suppl. 3),** III1–III4.
67. Werber, E.A. and Rabey, J.M. (2001) The beneficial effect of cholinesterase inhibitors on patients suffering from Parkinson's disease and dementia. *J. Neural. Transm.* **108,** 1319–1325.
68. Paquet, F., Chouinard, S., Blanchet, P., Masson, H., and Bédard, M.-A. (2001) Impact of the frontal behavioral disturbances in Parkinson's Disease during a daily activity: the meal preparation scale. *Mov. Disord.* **16(Suppl. 1),** 19.

16

Cognitive Consequences of Neurosurgery for Parkinson's Disease

Jean A. Saint-Cyr, PhD, CPsych

1. INTRODUCTION

Despite advances in the pharmacological treatment of Parkinson's disease (PD), there comes a time when symptoms can no longer be adequately controlled, alternating between freezing and dyskinesia, seemingly refractory to the entire panoply of the pharmacopeia at the disposal of neurologists. This has prompted a renewed interest in neurosurgical approaches to treatment, targets for lesions, or deep brain stimulation (DBS) having been identified on the basis of our current understanding of the functional organization of basal ganglia circuits in normal and 1-methyl-4-phenyl-1,2,3,6-tetrahydropyridine (MPTP)-treated subhuman primates *(1,2)*. As confirmed by neurophysiological recording in PD patients during surgery, the disease leads to excessive neuronal discharge in the internal division of the globus pallidus (GPi) and substantia nigra, pars reticulata (SNr), as well as in the subthalamic nucleus (STN). Accordingly, the neurosurgeon aims his intervention at either the GPi or STN. The goal is to reduce or eliminate the pathologically high levels of neuronal drive, which ultimately are responsible for excessive thalamic inhibition. The general clinical outcome is consistent with these models. Both posteroventral pallidotomy (PVP) (usually unilateral) and bilateral or unilateral DBS in the GPi are effective in reducing or eliminating drug-induced dyskinesias. The alternate strategy, STN-DBS, improves the symptoms of tremor and rigidity, permitting a reduction of about 50% of medication, and sometimes more in younger patients who are more responsive to levadopa (L-dopa). Rarely, bilateral lesions of the STN have also been effective, but there remains a danger of inducing ballismus, albeit usually transiently. Systematic clinical evaluation of patient symptoms is usually done with the Unified Parkinson's Disease Rating Scale (UPDRS), following the Core Assessment Program for Surgical Interventional Therapies (CAPSIT) protocol (see refs. *3–7* for comprehensive reviews).

The evaluation of the behavioral consequences of central nervous system (CNS) lesions in animals has a long history in experimental neuropsychology (previously known as physiological or biological psychology and then behavioral neuroscience). It is common wisdom that it is not the function of the area destroyed, which is revealed, but rather the capacity of the remaining brain to manage behavior in its absence. Although obviously incorrect, it is still common to see the impaired processes attributed to the tissue removed. The situation is even more complex in the case at hand, since we have a partially functioning brain due to the pathology to which we add a lesion. This line of critical analysis has been applied to the lesion treatment model of PD as expounded in a seminal paper *(8)*. Succinctly put, this is the Marsden and Obeso paradox: how can loss of tissue lead to improved function? If the basal ganglia play a critical role in motor control and we disable the circuit, how can motor control improve? Indeed, when the circuit malfunctions, we have symptoms such as tremor and rigidity. A

From: *Mental and Behavioral Dysfunction in Movement Disorders*
Edited by: M-A. Bédard et al. © Humana Press Inc., Totowa, NJ

lesion could interrupt the circuit that generates abnormal behavior such as tremor, thus facilitating normalization of overall control due to the action of backup or parallel motor control circuits. In this case, we can draw on motor cortical areas, the cerebellum, rubrospinal, reticulospinal, and vestibulospinal pathways to alter their balance of control. However, intact tissue may also be removed, leading to new symptoms or worsening of those functions for which compensation is inadequate. Thus, we can encounter deterioration of speech (usually hypophonia) and of fine motor control (as in handwriting).

Functional imaging studies have shown that GPi-DBS results in activation of motor cortical areas, previously underactivated in PD *(9)*. Other studies have shown that only clinically effective stimulation of the STN can normalize blood flow to the supplementary and motor association areas, whereas effective stimulation of the GPi has a less specific action *(10)*. These effects were only demonstrable using motor activation paradigms. In a similar paradigm, STN-DBS increased activation (blood flow) of the motor cortical association areas but decreased primary motor cortical activation *(11)*. These studies provide compelling evidence that the DBS effect is related to the recruitment of cerebellar compensatory mechanisms acting through thalamomotor cortical pathways. Again, we are reminded of the position adopted by Mardsen and Obseo *(8)* with regard to the reprogramming of motor control circuits.

Applying the same logic to behavioral and cognitive functions may be conceptually more difficult, since we are still in the process of defining those brain regions and circuits that are responsible for complex mental operations (for reviews, see refs. *12* and *13*). Current functional anatomical models of the basal ganglia emphasize compartmentalization of function with the putamen being the major node for motor control, the caudate for cognitive and the ventral striatum–accumbens for emotional domains *(14)*. Neurosurgeons make every effort to target the purely motor sectors of their targets, using both imaging and neurophysiological guidance to achieve their ends *(15–18)*. However, the anatomical proximity of functionally separate families of fiber pathways makes it difficult, if not impossible to avoid iatrogenic damage to intact circuits *(15–18)*. Consequently, patients may experience behavioral and cognitive costs while also benefiting from a clinical neurological perspective. The systematic study of these cases provides an unique opportunity to study the motor, cognitive, and behavioral consequences of focal lesions or DBS in frontal-subcortical circuits.

The present chapter will briefly review the outcome of neurosurgical interventions in the basal ganglia for the treatment of PD from a neuropsychological perspective.

2. THE BASIC BASAL GANGLIA MODEL

The functional anatomical organization of the basal ganglia has been extensively reviewed *(19,20)*. Briefly, glutamatergic excitatory projections from motor and somatosensory cortical areas terminate in the putamen, forming the first leg of the motor circuit. Inhibitory γ-amino butyric acid (GABA)ergic (i.e., utilizing the neurotransmitter GABA) projections from the putamen project both directly to the GPi/SNr (so-called direct pathway) and also to the external division of the GP (GPe)(so-called indirect pathway). The GPe, in turn also sends inhibitory GABAergic projections to the STN, which then drives the GPi/SNr and all other levels of the basal ganglia through excitatory glutamatergic projections. Superimposed on all of this is the dopaminergic innervation arising largely from the pars compacta of the SN (SNc). Some dopamine (DA) contributions to the ventral striatum also originate in the ventral tegmental area (VTA) and the retrorubral cell groups *(24)*. In order for the model to account for the pathophysiology of PD, a dual action of DA at the putamenal level is proposed, such that the direct pathway is facilitated through D1 receptors while the indirect pathway is inhibited through D2 receptors *(25)*. Thus, loss of the SNc neurons results in decreased inhibition of the GPi/SNr via the direct pathway and, ultimately the excessive drive of the GPi/SNr via the STN. This functionally reduces thalamocortical drive, via relay nuclei ventralis anterior and ventralis lateralis. Thus, motor cortical excitability is reduced, and poverty of movement ensues. Mismatched timing between agonist and antagonist muscles leads to rigidity and cogwheeling, while tremor is generated via oscillating circuits, at least partly within the basal ganglia, but perhaps also influenced by the cerebellum *(26)*. The model is actually much more complex at both the anatomical and transmitter–receptor levels *(3,4,14,27,28)*, but the basic prediction of overly active GPi/SNr and STN nuclei has been confirmed *(2,13,15,16,29, 31)*, thus justifying the neurosurgical approaches.

Parallel circuits subserving nonmotor functions such as cognitive (or protocognitive, see refs. *32* and *33*) processing focus on cortical association areas projecting topographically onto the caudate and caudal-ventral putamen (reviewed in ref. *21*). Similarly, orbitofrontal and anterior cingulate, as well as amygdala inputs to the ventral striatum, tail of the caudate and nucleus accumbens are involved in the processing of emotional information (see recent reviews in refs. *14, 34,* and *35*).

Neuropathological studies have indicated that loss of SNc neurons proceeds along a dorsolateral to ventromedial gradient, which translates into initial denervation of the putamen, followed by the dorsomedial head of the caudate *(36–38)*. In addition, cell loss also occurs in other brain stem nuclei, such as the VTA (DA), locus coeruleus (norepinephrine [NE]), and in the forebrain (nucleus basalis of Meynert, acetylcholine), inter alia. Thus, one would expect motor symptoms to be the most prominent, and cognitive dysfunction to initially target those processes dependent on the integrity of the dorsolateral prefrontal cortex *(39)*. Initial emotional symptoms in PD are typically described as lability *(40)*, although there is often reactive depression *(41)*.

The current model of cognitive dysfunction in PD implies frontostriatal circuit malfunction. We infer that those circuits have not been entirely abandoned, but are still involved in information processing, albeit poorly. One way to conceptualize this is to imagine that the prefrontal cortical areas are in receipt of incomplete or corrupted information from the basal ganglia. This makes decisional choices ambiguous, and the environmental feedback about the consequences of action does not reliably alter reward valence or response probabilities. Thus, the normal feedback essential for trial and error learning (basis for implicit learning, procedural learning, stimulus–response learning, motor skill acquisition, and the automatization of rule and task constraints) fails to alter behavioral shaping. It is on this background that the impact of surgeries must be overlaid (see ref. *42* for a review of basal ganglia nonmotor function).

Specific neuropsychological deficits commonly observed in PD include impaired processes of: working memory, attentional allocation and focus, strategic planning, novel problem solving, sequential organization and information retrieval, initial encoding of information, and initial procedural learning. Thus, the cognitive and behavioral profile expected in PD, based on the neuropathology, has been confirmed in numerous studies (see reviews in refs. *33, 43,* and *44*).

DA replacement therapy should reverse the effects of pathology, and indeed, many motor symptoms are overcome in this way for many years. However, this can only reestablish a tonic DA level in the basal ganglia, with the phasic action of DA in the learning described above remaining uncorrected *(45)*. This may explain why cognitive dysfunction has often remained unchanged by pharmacotherapy (in some cases worse, and selected measures mildly improved) *(46–52)*. Therefore, since at best, STN-DBS results in motor improvement only as good as the best DA action *(53)*, one might suspect that there would be little improvement in cognition other than the indirect effect of alleviating motor control problems and thereby liberating attentional resources to be allocated back to cognitive or behavioral processing *(54)*.

On the other hand, if lesions or stimulation encroach on still functionally intact pathways or cells, then one might expect deterioration of function and perhaps the induction of cognitive or behavioral disorders uncommon in idiopathic PD. Given the anatomical organization, the possibility of behavioral disorders, mood disorders, or impaired cognitive states usually associated with frontal lobe pathology could occur. In addition, the recognition of the presence of such problems could take some time for several reasons. First, the initial recovery period postoperatively may be characterized by confusion and the nonspecific effects of rebalancing medication and DBS programming. Secondly, clinical benefit is usually so dramatic that patients are preoccupied with regaining motor competence and resumption of many activities once abandoned. Thirdly, as patients attempt to fully reengage in activities, they might find that they have become older and deconditioned, falling short of their expectations. Lastly, we have observed both denial and lack of insight, which influence the validity of patients' complaints.

Thus, neuropsychological screening prior to surgery must reflect the expected cognitive profile, despite poor response to pharmacotherapy *(55)*, otherwise a superimposed disease state or misdiagnosis must be suspected *(56)*. Atypical presentation cognitively, a significant psychiatric history, or lack of L-dopa response all are pronostically poor for the outcome of surgery.

3. PVP AND (GPi-DBS)

It is now well established that PVP ameliorates the dyskinesias experienced as adverse effects of DA replacement therapy, although there are no changes in medication or in underlying symptoms *(57,58)*. This is also the case for GPi-DBS *(59,60)*.

It has not been fully explained how these changes come about at the circuit level nor even at the neurobiological level *(1,61,62)*. One might speculate that blocking abnormally functioning circuits provides the simple answer, but, as pointed out by Marsden and Obeso *(8)*, how can elimination of motor circuits lead to better motor control? Careful examination of patients reveals that PVP does lead to faster movement and may eliminate tremor, but fine motor control, such as handwriting and speech articulation may suffer. Thus, the behavior observed must be considered due to the implementation of motor control strategies and circuits other than at least some of the basal ganglia outflow pathways. Speculation focuses on the cerebellum and its outflow pathways as one of the structures principally involved in motor reprogramming.

The question arises about the fate of nonmotor circuits in the basal ganglia, such as those contributing to cognition, self-monitoring, and emotion, to name a few critical functions. Initially, cognitive functions were said to remain intact or even to improve following PVP (see reviews in refs. *63* and *64*) however, subsequent studies with larger groups and more extensive testing indicated hemisphere-specific impairment and executive dysfunction after PVP *(65–67)*. As pointed out by Scott *(68)*, failure to find deficits may be due to failure to ask the right questions or to explore sufficient cognitive domains, perhaps falling prey to poor test sensitivity (e.g., relying on an Mini Mental Status Examination). Trépanier et al. *(65)* adopted a hypothesis-testing approach, targeting cognitive functions known to be at risk in PD.

To the extent that the basal ganglia in these patients are still participating in processing information in cognitive operations, one might expect performance to suffer postoperatively. This was in fact observed by Trépanier et al. *(65)* as well as by Stebbins et al. *(67)*. Thus, both hemisphere-specific effects (recently reviewed in ref. *66*), as well as executive functions *(67)*, were affected. Specific deficits after left PVP, included deterioration in verbal serial list learning, decreased controlled oral word fluency (semantic and phonemic), and impaired working memory *(65,67)*. The deleterious effects of right PVP proved to be more difficult to demonstrate. Trépanier et al. *(65)* found transient impairment of visual constructional abilities and mild reduction of semantic controlled verbal fluency.

Some centers have reported only mild, if any, cognitive changes after surgery *(67,69–71)*, but factors such as the long-term effectiveness, adequacy of neuropsychological assessment, and location of lesion within the pallidum may be critical in this regard. The location of lesions made within the GPi has been shown to be critical, not only with regard to motor outcome *(72)*, but also in terms of impact on cognition *(73)*. These observations suggest that it is possible to demonstrate a functional segregation within the pallidal circuits. In cases of simultaneous or staged bilateral pallidal lesions, all too often, the outcome is characterized by catastrophic declines cognitively and also in behavioral control, with a full-blown frontal syndrome being induced *(64,65,74,75)*.

As is often the case with regard to basal ganglia strokes, bilateral lesions are more likely to result in severe behavioral change than unilateral lesions *(14,32,76)*. In two of three cases of bilateral PVP in our own series and several cases in another report, a catastrophic behavioral syndrome of the frontal type ensued *(64,65)*. Thus, some patients may develop environmental dependence, imitative, and utilization behaviors very much as described by Lhermitte *(77–79)*. In one such case requiring prolonged hospitalization, the patient was able to articulate that he was not depressed or upset by his actions (despite having created public embarrassment to his family). This lack of insight and judgement was quite characteristic, as it was for some cases of unilateral PVP. However, it must be pointed out that this outcome is not obligatory. In one of our cases and in other series, no major behavioral disruption was noted *(64,65,71,75)*, possibly because of location or size of lesion.

The issue of lesion size is controversial, since some studies reported no correlations between size and outcome *(72)*, while Kishore et al. *(80)* have found a relationship. There is little doubt that location is the most important factor, with variability of both clinical motor and cognitive outcome being predicted by region coagulated within the GPi. Specifically, rostrodorsal location within the GPi results in maximal reduction in dyskinesia, while posteroventral lesions optimally reduce akinesia and tremor. The overall optimal location is at the intended posteroventral location *(72)*. Correlations with neuropsychological variables indicated that the rostral lesions were the most toxic, leading to reduced verbal fluency, and, on the left, with impaired verbal encoding *(73)*. That same study also showed that the most caudal lesions led to a modest improvement in attentional capacity. Recently, another study has demonstrated that lesion volume, if segregated into dorsal and ventral compartments within the GPi, is associated with clinical outcome. Specifically, the volume of the posterior component was predictive of reduction of drug-induced dyskinesia *(80)*. The discrepancy with the data from the Gross et al. *(72)* study may be explained by the interruption of pallidofugal fibers originating in the more rostral regions of the GPi and coursing caudally through the larger posterior lesion site of Kishore. GPi-DBS outcome has also been shown to be dependent on the site stimulated within the GPi *(81)*.

Despite insistence by patients that they felt fine, both emotionally (in fact slight postoperative euphoria was often noted) and behaviorally, spouses and caregivers painted a different picture. There were cases of poor judgement, disinhibition, reckless behavior, socially inappropriate behavior, to such an extent that a systematic assessment of personality change was undertaken. It quickly became clear that many of the roughly 25% of patients with such problems had little or no insight into their altered behavior. When noted by the patients, odd or altered behaviors tended to be rationalized and the consequent disruption minimized. The group of patients assessed developed behavioral or personality changes ranging from apathy and abulia to disinhibition and mania *(65)*. Mercifully for the caregivers and medical support staff, the problems often spontaneously resolved within a few months, sometimes responding quite well to a combination of medical therapy and behavioral management interventions. It proved critical to educate the family and caregivers about the organic basis for the behavior and how best to structure the environment and interaction. Patients were also given feedback about their actions and encouraged to trust the advice and guidance of caregivers. Rarely, behavioral alterations persisted beyond 12 mo, requiring ongoing monitoring and treatment. In trying to identify factors that might predispose patients to such reactions, instances of prior psychiatric history were revealed. These may have been considered too remote to be pertinent, may have been considered well-controlled, and rarely, may have been hidden or minimized by patients and family in order to be accepted for surgery. It is now advised that decompensation may be expected, and the treatment team should be ready to deal with such events. For example, if depression was previously a significant factor, then the resumption of treatment with standard antidepressants may prove quite effective in postoperative management.

GPi-DBS may be less cognitively toxic than PVP, possibly because of differential effects on neurons and fibers of passage and the titration of stimulation parameters. This permits bilateral interventions *(75,82)*. As was the case for lesions, location of stimulation within the pallidum (may include portions of GPe) produces differential effects on parkinsonian symptoms in the on and off drug states *(81)*. A comparison of the effects of stimulation at different sites within the pallidum on cognitive function has not been done.

4. STN-DBS

STN-DBS has proven to be most effective to treat PD in that basic symptoms, such as tremor, bradykinesia, and rigidity are significantly reduced or eliminated, thus permitting drastic reductions in medication. Clinically, older patients do not benefit as much as younger ones. In addition, it has been recognized that the most benefit to be expected is equivalent to the best response to medical therapy. However, this benefit is better maintained with reduced periods and severity of disabling freezing and dyskinesia.

In a large series of carefully selected PD patients, GPi- or STN-DBS caused little change in cognitive functions, on a group basis *(82)*. Furthermore, neither presence nor absence of stimulation appeared to alter global cognitive function *(83)*, save for selected executive functions which largely improved. Further studies on these patients, focusing on the executive functions, have shown an improvement with STN-DBS and a decline with GPi-DBS *(84)*.

However, in older PD patients, STN-DBS was shown to reduce cognitive resources *(75,85)*. Behavioral changes of a frontal nature were also observed *(75,85)*. It has become clear that the outcome of DBS is, therefore, predicted by age at surgery, extent of response to DA replacement therapy, and rigorous neuropsychological screening *(75,82)*. The cognitive impact of DBS within the basal ganglia has been interpreted as evidence both for the facilitation of cortically based functions and the interruption of striatally based processing.

Bilateral STN-DBS is currently considered to be the treatment of choice for PD since this fundamentally ameliorates symptoms and permits drastic reductions in medication *(86,87)*. It is thought that DBS blocks the action of the STN, thus reducing its widespread excitatory influence (glutamatergic) throughout the striatal circuitry (and perhaps also directly into the thalamus). In younger patients, cognitive costs are essentially negligible *(82)*. There is evidence for a statistically mild improvement in some executive functions, but this may be without clinical importance *(84)*. It is intriguing that cessation of stimulation does not lead to a loss of this so-called improvement *(83)*, suggesting that other circuits, outside of the sphere of influence of the basal ganglia may permanently take over functions. Alternately, a nonspecific improvement in the allocation of attentional resources may be responsible, and this could take some time to decompensate after the stimulation is interrupted. In contrast, STN-DBS in older patients not only has a clinical motor benefit that is less dramatic, but significant cognitive impairment also ensues *(85)*. The full gamut of cognitive impairment is seen, with those functions dependent on executive mechanisms being at greatest risk. Idiosyncratic behavioral and personality problems also developed, sometimes requiring psychiatric management. It is common to observe transient states of confusion lasting days to months in all patients, even the younger patients.

It is understandable that patients should be delighted with their clinical improvement, and this is typically accompanied by improved mood. STN-DBS has also been reported to induce instantaneous or insidious alterations of mood experienced as euphoria–hilarity or depression–apathy (abulia) *(64,75,88–90)*.

5. REMAINING QUESTIONS

Given the dramatic clinical improvement in PD symptoms after STN-DBS, can these patients be considered to have returned to an earlier stage of their disease, requiring less medication for management? To a certain extent, this may be so, but they are not functionally younger or cognitively improved, nor has their disease process been reversed. In addition, patients are now challenged to engage in activities that have lain fallow for several years. This leads to behavioral complications, including family dynamic issues and conflicts with caregivers. Patients may want to resume driving, managing finances, and rekindle romantic drive, all without the benefit of full judgement or insight. Furthermore, caregivers may no longer treat patients as disabled, requiring special consideration and indulgence, and may start making their own needs felt for the first time in years. This role reversal may be seen as a withdrawal of caring. Often, family counseling may be required to keep the couple together and to reestablish a harmonious relationship.

Another factor, which is significant, is attributable to the impact of altered medical management postoperatively. Patients with the benefit of STN-DBS may decrease L-dopa equivalent dosage from 1500–2000 mg/d to 300–500 mg or less, and this may occur over a relatively short time span. It has been noted that motorically competent patients may become abulic, listless, and unmotivated. It is important to identify this state as opposed to depression or emotional withdrawal, because of the psychosocial issues described above. One also wonders what impact such medical changes could have on cognitive processing, especially in older patients.

6. CONCLUSIONS

As they say in real estate, put your money on location, location, and location. Both with regard to lesions and DBS, misplacement either leads to treatment failure (or limitation) or to iatrogenic problems. The fact that adjacent and partially overlapping circuits within the GPi are difficult to selectively interrupt, accurate positioning is crucial. In the STN, we imagine the presence of areas dedicated to the processing of sensory motor, cognitive, and emotional information. It is clear that all three can be affected by DBS and that both cognitive cost, as well as emotional disturbance, can occur as a result of DBS. What is currently puzzling is that cessation of stimulation leads to fairly rapid return of motor symptoms, while cognitive changes appear to persist. It may be that the instantiation of compensatory cortical processing after stabilization of the effects of DBS, leads to a permanent switch to those processing modes. That is, the basal ganglia truly are eliminated from any further role in the control of those cognitive activities. However, the motor and emotional changes appear to be reversible. That being said, the several cases of suicide reported may or may not be due to the direct action of DBS. Changes in family dynamics, behavioral reactivity to social situations, and medications may all have changed significantly in a relatively short space of time for these patients and their limited capacity to adapt due to age and PD may limit their tolerance.

REFERENCES

1. Benazzouz, A. and Hallett, M. (2000) Mechanism of action of deep brain stimulation. *Neurology* **55(12 Suppl. 6),** S13–S16.
2. Wichmann, T. and DeLong, M.R. (1996) Functional and pathophysiological models of the basal ganglia. *Curr. Opin. Neurobiol.* **6,** 751–758.
3. Lang, A.E. and Lozano, A.M. (1998a) Parkinson's disease—first of two parts. *N. Engl. J. Med.* **339,** 1044–1053.
4. Lang, A.E. and Lozano, A.M. (1998b). Parkinson's disease—second of two parts. *N. Engl. J. Med.* **339,** 1130–1143.
5. Benabid, A.L., Krack, P.P., Benazzouz, A., Limousin, P., Koudsie, A. and Pollak, P. (2000) Deep brain stimulation of the subthalamic nucleus for Parkinson's disease: methodologic aspects and clinical criteria. *Neurology* **55(12 Suppl. 6),** S40–S44.
6. Kumar, R., Lang, A.E., Rodriguez-Oroz, M.C., et al. (2000) Deep brain stimulation of the globus pallidus pars interna in advanced Parkinson's disease. *Neurology* **55(12 Suppl. 6),** S34–S39.
7. Lozano, A.M. (2001) Deep brain stimulation for Parkinson's disease. *Park. Relat. Disord.* **7,** 199–203.
8. Marsden, C.D. and Obeso, J.A. (1994) The functions of the basal ganglia and the paradox of stereotaxic surgery in Parkinson's disease. *Brain* **117,** 877–897.
9. Davis, K.D., Taub, E., Houser, D., et al. (1997) Globus pallidus stimulation activates the cortical motor system during alleviation of parkinsonian symptoms. *Nat. Med.* **3,** 671–674.
10. Limousin, P., Greene, J., Pollak, P., Rothwell, J., Benabid, A.L., and Frackowiak, R. (1997) Changes in cerebral activity pattern due to subthalamic nucleus or internal pallidum stimulation in Parkinson's disease. *Ann. Neurol.* **42,** 283–291.
11. Ceballos-Baumann, A., Boecker, H., Bartenstein, P., et al. (1999). A positron emission tomography study of subthalamic nucleus stimulation in Parkinson's disease: enhanced movement-related activity of motor-association cortex and decreased motor cortex resting activity. *Arch. Neurol.* **56,** 997–1003.
12. Owen, A.M. and Doyon, J. (1999) The cognitive neuropsychology of Parkinson's disease: a functional neuroimaging perspective, in *Parkinson's Disease: Advances in Neurology,* vol. 80 (Stern, C.M., ed.), Lippincott, Williams & Wilkins, Philadelphia, pp. 49–56.
13. Brooks, D.J. (2000) Imaging basal ganglia function. *J. Anat.* **196,** 543–554.
14. Saint-Cyr, J.A., Bronstein, Y.L., and Cummings, J.L. (2002) Neurobehavioral consequences of neurosurgical treatments and focal lesions of frontal-subcortical circuits, in *Principles of Frontal Lobe Function* (Stuss, D. and Knight, R., eds.), Oxford University Press, Oxford, pp. 408–427.
15. Hutchison, W.D., Lozano, A.M., Davis, K.D., Saint-Cyr, J.A., Lang, A.E., and Dostrovsky, J.O. (1994) Differential neuronal activity in segments of globus pallidus in Parkinson's disease patients. *Neuroreport* **5,** 1533–1537.
16. Hutchison, W.D., Allan, R.J., Opitz, H., et al. (1998) Neurophysiological identification of the subthalamic nucleus in surgery for Parkinson's disease. *Ann. Neurol.* **44,** 622–628.

17. Starr, P.A., Vitek, J.L., and Bakay, R.A.E. (1998a) Deep brain stimulation for movement disorders. *Neurosurg. Clin. N. Am.* **9,** 381–402.
18. Starr, P.A., Vitek, J.L., and Bakay, R.A. (1998b) Ablative surgery and deep brain stimulation for Parkinson's disease. *Neurosurgery* **43,** 989–1015.
19. Percheron, G. and Filion, M. (1991) Parallel processing in the basal ganglia: up to a point [letter]. *Trends Neurosci.* **14,** 55–56.
20. Filion, M., Tremblay, L., Matsumura, M., and Richard, H. (1994) Focalisation dynamique de la convergence informationnelle dans les noyaux gris centraux. *Rev. Neurol. (Paris)* **150,** 627–633.
21. Parent, A. and Hazrati, L.N. (1995a) Functional anatomy of the basal ganglia. I. The cortico-basal ganglia-thalamo-cortical loop. *Brain Res. Rev.* **20,** 91–127.
22. Parent, A. and Hazrati, L.N. (1995b) Functional anatomy of the basal ganglia. II. The place of subthalamic nucleus and external pallidum in basal ganglia circuitry. *Brain Res. Rev.* **20,** 128–154.
23. Alexander, G.E. and Crutcher, M.D. (1990) Functional architecture of basal ganglia circuits: neural substrates or parallel processing. *Trends Neurosci.* **13,** 266–271.
24. Prensa, L., Cossette, M., and Parent, A. (2000) Dopaminergic innervation of human basal ganglia. *J. Chem. Neuroanat.* **20,** 207–213.
25. Albin, R.L., Young, A.B., and Penney, J.B. (1989) The functional anatomy of basal ganglia disorders. *Trends Neurosci.* **12,** 366–375.
26. Deuschl, G., Raethjen, J., Baron, R., Lindemann, M., Wilms, H., and Krack, P. (2000) The pathophysiology of parkinsonian tremor: a review. *J. Neurol.* **247(Suppl. 5),** V33–V48.
27. Graybiel, A.M. (1990) Neurotransmitters and neuromodulators in the basal ganglia. *Trends Neurosci.* **13,** 244–254.
28. Parent, A., Lévesque, M., and Parent, A. (2001) A re-evaluation of the current model of the basal ganglia. *Park. Relat. Disord.* **7,** 193–198.
29. Eidelberg, D., Moeller, J.R., Dhawan, V., et al. (1994) The metabolic topography of Parkinsonism. *J. Cereb. Blood Flow Metab.* **14,** 783–801.
30. Eidelberg, D. (1998) Functional brain networks in movement disorders [editorial]. *Curr. Opin. Neurol.* **11,** 319–326.
31. Wichmann, T., Bergman, H., and DeLong, M.R. (1994) The primate subthalamic nucleus. I. Functional properties in intact animals. *J. Neurophysiol.* **72,** 494–506.
32. Saint-Cyr, J.A. and Taylor, A.E. (1992) The mobilization of procedural learning. The „key signature" of the basal ganglia, in *Neuropsychology of Memory*, 2nd ed. (Butters, B. and Squire, L.R., eds.), Guilford Press, New York, pp. 188–202.
33. Saint-Cyr, J.A., Taylor, A.E., and Nicholson, K. (1995) Behavior and the basal ganglia. *Adv. Neurol.* **65,** 1–28.
34. Haber, S.N. and McFarland, N.R. (1999) The concept of the ventral striatum in nonhuman primates. *Ann. NY Acad. Sci.* **877,** 33–48.
35. Nakano, K., Kayahara, T., Tsutsumi, T., and Ushiro, H. (2000) Neural circuits and functional organization of the striatum. *J. Neurol.* **247(Suppl. 5),** V1–V15.
36. Kish, S.J., Shannak, K., and Hornykiewicz, O. (1988) Uneven pattern of dopamine loss in the striatum of patients with idiopathic Parkinson's disease. *N. Engl. J. Med.* **318,** 876–880.
37. Agid, Y. (1991) Parkinson's disease: pathophysiology. *Lancet* **337**, 1321–1324.
38. Braak, H., Braak, E., Yilmazer, D., Schultz, C., De Vos, R.A.I., and Jansen, E.N.H. (1995) Nigral and extranigral pathology in Parkinson's disease. *J. Neural. Transm. Park. Dis. Dement. Sect.* **46(Suppl),** 15–31.
39. Taylor, A.E., Saint-Cyr, J.A., and Lang, A.E. (1986) Frontal lobe dysfunction in Parkinson's disease: the cortical focus of neostriatal outflow. *Brain* **109,** 845–883.
40. Taylor, A.E. and Saint-Cyr, J.A. (1990) Depression in Parkinson's disease: reconciling physiological and psychological perspectives. *J. Neuropsychiatr. Clin. Neurosci.* **2,** 92–98.
41. Brown, R.G. and MacCarthy, B. (1990) Psychiatric morbidity in patients with Parkinson's disease. *Psychol. Med.* **20,** 77–87.
42. Wise, S.P., Murray, E.A., and Gerfen, C.R. (1996) The frontal cortex-basal ganglia system in primates. *Crit. Rev. Neurobiol.* **10,** 317–356.
43. Brown, R.G. and Marsden, C.D. (1990) Cognitive function in Parkinson's disease: from description to theory. *Trends Neurosci.* **13,** 21–29.
44. Dubois, B., Boller, F., Pillon, B., and Agid, Y. (1991). Cognitive deficits in Parkinson's disease, in *Handbook of Neuropsychology,* vol. 5 (Corkin, S., Boller, F., and Grafman, J., eds.), Elsevier Science Publishers B.V., Amsterdam, pp. 195–240.
45. Schultz, W. (1998) Predictive reward signal of dopamine neurons. *J. Neurophysiol.* **80,** 1–27.
46. Gotham, A.M., Brown, R.G., and Marsden, C.D. (1988) 'Frontal' cognitive function in patients with Parkinson's disease 'on' and 'off' levodopa. *Brain* **111,** 299–321.
47. Pullman, S.L., Watts, R.L., Juncos, J.L., Chase, T.N., and Sanes, J.N. (1988) Dopaminergic effects on simple and choice reaction time performance in Parkinson's disease. *Neurology* **38,** 249–254.
48. Lange, K.W., Robbins, T.W., Marsden, C.D., James, M., Owen, A.M., and Paul, G.M. (1992) L-dopa withdrawal in Parkinson's disease selectively impairs cognitive performance in tests sensitive to frontal lobe dysfunction. *Psychopharmacology* **107,** 394–404.
49. Malapani, C., Pillon, B., Dubois, B., and Agid, Y. (1994) Impaired simultaneous cognitive task performance in Parkinson's disease: a dopamine-related dysfunction. *Neurology* **44,** 319–326.

50. Owen, A., Sahakian, B., Hodges, J., Summers, B., Polkey, C., and Robbins, T. (1995) Dopamine-dependent frontostriatal planning deficits in early Parkinson's disease. *Neuropsychology* **9,** 126–140.
51. Kulisevsky, J., Avila, A., Barbanoj, M., Antonijoan, R., Berthier, M.L., and Gironell, A. (1996) Acute effects of levodopa on neuropsychological performance in stable and fluctuating Parkinson's disease patients at different levodopa plasma levels. *Brain* **119,** 2121–2132.
52. Malapani, C., Rakitin, B., Levy, R., et al. (1998) Coupled temporal memories in Parkinson's disease: a dopamine-related dysfunction. *J. Cognit. Neurosci.* **10,** 316–331.
53. Krack, P., Pollak, P., Limousin, P., Benazzouz, A., Deuschl, G., and Benabid, A.L. (1999) From off-period dystonia to peak-dose chorea. The clinical spectrum of varying subthalamic nucleus activity. *Brain* **122,** 1133–1146.
54. Brown, R.G., Dowsey, P.L., Brown, P., et al. (1999) Impact of deep brain stimulation on upper limb akinesia in Parkinson's disease. *Ann. Neurol.* **45,** 473–488.
55. Taylor, A.E., Saint-Cyr, J.A., and Lang, A.E. (1987) Parkinson's disease. Cognitive changes in relation to treatment response. *Brain* **110,** 35–51.
56. Saint-Cyr, J.A. and Trépanier, L.L. (2000) Neuropsychologic assessment of patients for movement disorder surgery. *Mov. Disord.* **15,** 771–83.
57. Lozano, A.M., Lang, A.E., Galvez-Jimenez, N., et al. (1995) Effect of GPi pallidotomy on motor function in Parkinson's disease. *Lancet* **346,** 1383–1387.
58. Lang, A.E., Lozano, A.M., Montgomery, E., Duff, J., Tasker, R., and Hutchinson, W. (1997) Posteroventral medial pallidotomy in advanced Parkinson's disease. *N. Engl. J. Med.* **337,** 1036–1042.
59. Krack, P., Pollak, P., Limousin, P., et al. (1998) Subthalamic nucleus or internal pallidal stimulation in young onset Parkinson's disease. *Brain* **121,** 451–457.
60. Limousin-Dowsey, P., Pollak, P., Van Blercom, N., Krack, P., Benazzouz, A., and Benabid, A. (1999) Thalamic, subthalamic nucleus and internal pallidum stimulation in Parkinson's disease. *J. Neurol.* **246(Suppl. 2),** II42–II45.
61. Ashby, P. and Rothwell, J.C. (2000) Neurophysiologic aspects of deep brain stimulation. *Neurology* **55(12 Suppl. 6),** S17–S20.
62. Beurrier, C., Bioulac, B., Audin, J., and Hammond, C. (2001) High-frequency stimulation produces a transient blockade of voltage-gated currents in subthalamic neurons *J. Neurophysiol.* **85,** 1351–1356.
63. York, M.K., Levin, H.S., Grossman, R.G., and Hamilton, W.J. (1999) Neuropsychological outcome following unilateral pallidotomy *Brain* **122,** 2209–2220.
64. Scott, R., Gregory, R., Hines, N., et al. (1998) Neuropsychological, neurological and functional outcome following pallidotomy for Parkinson's disease. A consecutive series of eight simultaneous bilateral and twelve unilateral procedures. *Brain* **121,** 659–675.
65. Trépanier, L.L., Saint-Cyr, J.A., Lozano, A.M., and Lang, A.E. (1998) Neuropsychological consequences of posteroventral pallidotomy for the treatment of Parkinson's disease. *Neurology* **51,** 207–215.
66. Green, J. and Barnhart, H. (2000) The impact of lesion laterality on neuropsychological change following posterior pallidotomy: a review of current findings. *Brain Cogn.* **42,** 379–398.
67. Stebbins, G.T., Gabrieli, J.D.E., Shannon, K.M., Penn, R.D., and Goetz, C.G. (2000) Impaired fronto-striatal cognitive functioning following posteroventral pallidotomy in advanced Parkinson's disease. *Brain Cogn.* **42,** 348–363.
68. Scott, R.B. (1998) Cognitive function and pallidotomy. *J. Neurol. Neurosurg. Psychiatry* **65,** 148.
69. Ghika, J., Villemure, J.G., Fankhauser, H., Favre, J., Assal, G., and Ghika-Schmid, F. (1998) Efficiency and safety of bilateral contemporaneous pallidal stimulation (deep brain stimulation) in levodopa-responsive patients with Parkinson's disease with severe motor fluctuations: a 2-year follow-up review. *J. Neurosurg.* **89,** 713–718.
70. Ghika, J., Ghika-Schmid, F., Fankhauser, H., et al. (1999) Bilateral contemporaneous posteroventral pallidotomy for the treatment of Parkinson's disease: neuropsychological and neurological side effects. Report of four cases and review of the literature. *J. Neurosurg.* **91,** 313–321.
71. Soukup, V.M., Ingram, F., Schiess, M.C., Bonnen, J.G., Nauta, H.J., and Calverley, J.R. (1997) Cognitive sequelae of unilateral posteroventral pallidotomy. *Arch. Neurol.* **54,** 947–950.
72. Gross, R.E., Lombardi, W.J., Lang, A.E., et al. (1999) Relationship of lesion location to clinical outcome following microelectrode-guided pallidotomy for Parkinson's disease. *Brain* **122,** 405–416.
73. Lombardi, W.J., Gross, R.E., Trépanier, L.L., Lang, A.E., Lozano, A.M., and Saint-Cyr, J.A. (2000) Relationship of lesion location to cognitive outcome following microelectrode-guided pallidotomy for Parkinson's disease: support for the existence of cognitive circuits in the human pallidum. *Brain* **123,** 746–758.
74. Galvez-Jiménez, N., Lozano, A.M., Duff, J., Trépanier, L., Saint-Cyr, J.A., and Lang, A.E. (1996) Bilateral pallidotomy: pronounced amelioration of incapacitating levodopa-induced dyskinesias but accompanying cognitive decline. *Mov. Disord.* **11(Suppl. 1),** 242.
75. Trépanier, L., Kumar, R., Lozano, A., Lang, A., and Saint-Cyr, J.A. (2000) Neuropsychological outcome of neurosurgical therapies in Parkinson's disease: a comparison of GPi pallidotomy and deep brain stimulation of GPi or STN. *Brain Cogn.* **42,** 324–347.
76. Dubois, B., Defontaines, B., Deweer, B., Malapani, C., and Pillon, B. (1995) Cognitive and behavioral changes in patients with focal lesions of the basal ganglia. *Adv. Neurol.* **65,** 29–42.
77. Lhermitte, F. (1986) Human autonomy and the frontal lobes. Part II: patient behavior in complex and social situations: the "environmental dependency syndrome". *Ann. Neurol.* **19,** 335–343.
78. Lhermitte, F., Pillon, B., and Serdaru, M. (1986) Human autonomy and the frontal lobes. Part I: imitation and utilization behavior: a neuropsychological study of 75 patients. *Ann. Neurol.* **19,** 326–334.

79. Lhermitte, F. (1983) 'Utilization behaviour' and its relation to lesions of the frontal lobes. *Brain* **106,** 237–255.
80. Kishore, A., Panikar, D., Balakrishnan, S., Joseph, S., and Sarma, S. (2000) Evidence of functional somatotopy in GPi from results of pallidotomy. *Brain* **123,** 2491–2500.
81. Bejjani, B., Damier, P., Arnulf, I., et al. (1997) Pallidal stimulation for Parkinson's disease. Two targets? *Neurology* **49,** 1564–1569.
82. Ardouin, C., Pillon, B., Peiffer, E., et al. (1999) Bilateral subthalamic or pallidal stimulation for Parkinson's disease affects neither memory nor executive functions: a consecutive series of 62 patients. *Ann. Neurol.* **46,** 217–223.
83. Pillon, B., Ardouin, C., Damier, P., et al. (2000) Neuropsychological changes between "off" and "on" STN and GPi stimulation in Parkinson's disease. *Neurology* **55,** 411–418.
84. Jahanshahi, M., Ardouin, C.M.A., Brown, R.G., et al. (2000) The impact of deep brain stimulation on executive function in Parkinson's disease. *Brain* **123,** 1142–1154.
85. Saint-Cyr, J.A., Trépanier, L.L., Kumar, R., Lozano, A.M., and Lang, A.E. (2000) Neuropsychological consequences of chronic bilateral stimulation of the subthalamic nucleus in Parkinson's disease. *Brain* **123,** 101–118.
86. Krack, P., Limousin, P., Benabid, A.L., and Pollack, P. (1997) Chronic stimulation of sub-thalamic nucleus improves levodopa-induced dyskinesias in Parkinson's disease. *Lancet* **350,** 1676–1680.
87. Kumar, R., Lozano, A.M., Kim, Y.J., et al. (1998a) Double-blind evaluation of the effects of subthalamic nucleus deep brain stimulation in advanced Parkinson's disease. *Neurology* **51,** 850–855.
88. Bejjani, B.P., Damier, P., Arnulf, I., et al. (1999) Transient acute depression induced by high frequency deep-brain stimulation. *N. Engl. J. Med.* **340,** 1476–1480.
89. Krack, P., Kumar, R., Ardouin, C., et al. (2001) Mirthful laughter induced by subthalamic nucleus stimulation. *Mov. Disord.* **16,** 867–875.
90. Stefurak, T.L., Mikulis, D., Mayberg, H., et al. (2001) Deep brain stimulation associated dysphoria and cortico-limbic changes detected by fMRI. *Mov. Disord.* **16(Suppl. 1),** S54–S55.

V

Dementia in Movement Disorders

17

The Clinical Spectrum of Dementia in Movement Disorders

An Overview

Andrew Kertesz, MD

1. INTRODUCTION

It is estimated that in the next decade, dementia and movement disorders will become the second ranking cause of death after cardiovascular disease *(1)*. Dementias and movement disorders are clinically and biologically overlapping manifestations of neurodegenerative disorders. Important areas of overlap are: *(i)* the spectrum of Alzheimer's disease (AD), Parkinson's disease (PD), dementia with Lewy bodies (DLB) (see Table 1); *(ii)* the spectrum of Pick's disease (PiD), frontotemporal dementia (FTD), corticobasal degeneration (CBD), progressive supranuclear palsy (PSP), amyotrophic lateral sclerosis (ALS) (see Table 2); *(iii)* distinct etiologies including Huntington's chorea (HD), Creutzfeldt-Jakob disease (CJD) and vascular dementia (see Table 3).

Differences and overlaps may be observed, namely at a biochemical level. For instance, AD and DLB are generally considered cholinergic, PD dopaminergic, FTD serotoninergic, and HD γ-amino butyric acid (GABA)-ergic deficiency syndromes. Such a single neurotransmitter-based conception of these diseases have significantly influenced the development of their pharmacological treatments. However, it is now well established that these diseases share many neurochemical abnormalities.

Histologically, the degenerative dementias and movement disorders are classified as the tauopathies and synucleinopathies, but these designations also share multiple similarities, and do not correspond to clinical boundaries (see Chapters 18 and 19 of this volume for a complete discussion on the neuropathology and genetics of these diseases). A number of other conditions, such as Wilson's disease or hepatolenticular degeneration, dystonia, and cerebellar degenerations could be included with the movement disorders, but they are rare or infrequently associated with dementia or affect different age groups and have little, if any, overlap with the others. Vascular dementia, on the other hand, has a major clinical overlap with the degenerative diseases associated with dementia and, to a lesser extent, with movement disorders, therefore, it will be included in this overview.

2. PARKINSON'S DISEASE

James Parkinson wrote, that "shaking palsy" does not affect the mind *(2)*. Later day clinicians felt that dementia is relatively common in PD, especially in later stages. The variation concerning the incidence of cognitive impairment in PD is related to the variability in defining both. Most definitions of dementia include intellectual and behavioral decline sufficient to disturb activities of daily living.

There have been extensive reviews on the prevalence of dementia in PD *(3–6)* (see Chapter 20 of this volume for a complete description on this issue). The first study *(3)* found it 32% with an odds

From: *Mental and Behavioral Dysfunction in Movement Disorders*
Edited by: M-A. Bédard et al. © Humana Press Inc., Totowa, NJ

Table 1
Areas of Overlap: The Spectrum of AD, PD, and DLB

	AD plus PD	DLB	Parkinsonism and dementia of Guam and ALS
Presentation	Memory	Fluctuating dementia	Dementia
Major symptom	Parkinsonism	Parkinsonism	Parkinsonism
Distinguishing	Tremor	Visual hallucinations	In Guam
Overlapping	With DLB	With AD + Parkinson's	ALS and FTD
Imaging	Diffuse atrophy	Diffuse atrophy	Diffuse or FTA
Pathology	Plaques, tangles; subcortical Lewy body	Cortical Lewly body; plaques	Tangles only

Table 2
Areas of Overlap: The Spectrum of PiD, FTD, CBD, PSP, and ALS

	FTD	PPA	CBD	PSP
Presentatiaon	Behavior	Aphasia	Akinetic and apractic	Axial rigidity
Major symptom	Aphasia	Behavior	Aphasia or FTD	Dysphagia
Distinguishing	Presenile	Presenile	Alien hand	Vertical gaze
Overlapping	CBD and ALS	CBD and ALS	PSP, FTD, and PPA	CBD, FTD, and PPA
Imaging	Focal atrophy	Focal atrophy	Focal atrophy	Iron in basal ganglia
Pathology	Spongiosis, Pick bodies	ITSNU, Pick cells	Astrocytic plaques	Tufted astrocytes

ITSNU: inclusions tau and synuclein negative, ubiquitinated.

Table 3
Areas of Overlap: CJD, HD, and Vascular Dementia

	CJD	HD	Vascular dementia
Presentation	Dementia	Chorea	Subcortical dementia
Major symptom	Myoclonus	Irritable, aggressive	Parkinsonism
Distinguishing	Rapidity	Family history	Strokes
Differential diagnosis	FTD and ALS, encephalitis	Senile chorea, tardive dyskinesia	FTD and DLB
Laboratory	CSF pro 14-3-3 EEG	Genetic CAG > 40	Leukoaraiosis
Pathology	Spongiform prion	Caudate atrophy	Ischemic

ratio of 10 over controls. A more recent population based study showed 25% of Parkinson patients developed dementia 4 yr after baseline assessment, representing an odds ratio of six compared to age-matched controls *(7)*. Most patients with idiopathic PD are not demented, however, when strict criteria, such as the Diagnosis and Statistical Manual of Mental Disorders, fourth edition (DSM-IV), are used.

In nondemented PD patients, minor cognitive impairments are usually present and characterized by slight frontal lobe syndrome (executive dysfunctions), often called subcortical dementia, in order to distinguish it from the cortical dementias, such as AD and DLB. The neuropsychological evidence for the commonalities and differences between PD and AD or other neurodegenerative diseases has been reviewed extensively elsewhere *(8,9)*. The term subcortical dementia was introduced to describe the cognitive deficit and bradyphrenia of HD *(10)* and PSP *(11)*, and later extended to PD *(9)*. However, while in HD and PSP, the frontal lobe syndrome is usually severe enough to reach the DSM-IV criteria of dementia, this is certainly not the case for most PD patients. It is, therefore, preferable to use the term subcorticofrontal syndrome (SCFS) to describe the minor cognitive changes of the PD patients. This allows the presence of cognitive-executive dysfunctions without necessarily forcing a diagnosis of dementia. If the DSM-IV criteria for dementia are reached, then the term subcortical dementia could be used *(12,13)*.

Subcortical dementia may be difficult to distinguished from AD and DLB, in which executive dysfunctions are also frequent. A certain percentage of AD patients develop extrapyramidal signs. In a study *(14)* (before the identification of Lewy body disease), this was found to be 10%. A smaller subgroup in this study developed myoclonus. More recently, the development of extrapyramidal signs in AD has been considered to be related to the development of DLB *(15–17)*. Late development of extrapyramidal symptoms in degenerative dementia is common across the spectrum and is considered to be a less specific feature, than an early coincidence.

There is a considerable overlap in the clinical, biochemical, and pathological manifestation of dementia in PD and AD. The exact nature of dementia in PD remains unsettled. The following hypotheses have been offered to explain the overlap: *(i)* a subcortical dementia (assumes no cortical degeneration); *(ii)* a coincidence of PD and AD; and *(iii)* cortical and subcortical Lewy body disease.

Although the extent of cortical vs subcortical distribution of Lewy bodies have been proposed as a unitary hypothesis, this has not been accepted by everyone. There may be more than one mechanism to account for different kinds of overlap with more or less resemblance to each other.

3. DEMENTIA WITH LEWY BODIES

Lewy bodies are synuclein and ubiquitin positive intraneuronal inclusions found in the basal ganglia in PD. Their significance in the cortex as a marker of dementia has been recently recognized *(15–17)*. The nosology of DLB is controversial. "Pure" or diffuse Lewy body disease without AD is estimated to be relatively uncommon (less than 5%). "Not so pure" DLB (allowing some neuritic plaques and neurofibrillary tangles) may be 11% *(18)* Mixed DLB and AD or "Lewy body variant" of AD or senile dementia of the Lewy body type (SDLT) is estimated to be about 15–25% of degenerative dementias *(17,19)*. The core symptoms are fluctuation in cognition and attention, visual hallucinations, and parkinsonism *(17)*. Often unexplained falls and hypersensitivity to neuroleptics is observed. False positive diagnosis is uncommon, but some patients with Lewy bodies pathology do not have the typical clinical features and cannot be distinguished from AD (false negatives) *(17)*.

Recent consensus criteria allows two of the three major components of the disease for diagnosis, expanding the clinical prevalence, but also increasing the overlap with AD, which also has hallucinations, extrapyramidal symptoms, and delusions. However, well-formed complex visual hallucinations are more specific in contrast to the reduplication and misidentification delusion common in AD. Fluctuation in cognition is difficult to define and can be subjective, but in DLB, it appears a cardinal feature at times amounting to episodic delirium or even loss of consciousness. They are explained by altered subcortical alerting mechanisms. Lewy body disease, therefore, appears in the differential diagnoses of fluctuating confusional states. Executive and visuospatial dysfunction may precede memory problems *(17)*. The clinical syndrome tends to be seen by geriatricians and geriatric psychiatrists, because of the prevalence in the older age group and the visual hallucinations.

4. PARKINSONISM-DEMENTIA OF GUAM

Parkinsonism-Dementia of Guam, which is clustered in well-defined regions, is behaviorally characterized by a progressive memory disorder resembling AD, and the subsequent development of the extrapyramidal syndrome in a substantially younger age group compared to AD and PD. Neurofibrillary tangles, but few, if any, senile plaques characterize the pathology. It overlaps with endemic ALS clusters in the region. The influence of genetic vs environmental factors continues to be debated. The geographic concentration of these cases led to the suggestion of both genetic and environmental factors. That Chamorros, who were removed from Guam, continue to develop the disease, suggest a genetic etiology, but the environmental camp claimed the cause is damage in utero or in infancy by calcium and aluminum *(20)*. Consumption of the cycad plant has also been implicated. The disease seems to be disappearing.

5. PICK'S DISEASE AND THE PICK COMPLEX: FTD-PPA-CBD-PSP

PiD has been known to have extrapyramidal features *(21)*, but this extrapyramidal variety has been largely forgotten until recent descriptions of CBD were recognized to be equivalent *(22)*. FTD is a recent terminology for PiD without Pick bodies, and it is also used to describe the personality and behavior change characterized by disinhibition and apathy *(23)*. Primary progressive aphasia (PPA) is also a component of PiD/FTD *(24)* and CBD *(25,26)*. CBD has similar pathology to PiD, and lately, it is recognized that it is not only a movement disorder, but many cases have FTD and PPA *(26)*. A great deal of clinical and pathological overlap is recognized between FTD/PPA and CBD, and the term Pick Complex was used to indicate their relationship *(22,24)*. This overlap is estimated to be 20–25% of degenerative dementias. An alternative is to return to the simple clinical term, PiD, but the argument against this is that PiD should be used to designate dementia with Pick bodies. Another claim for specificity is the finding of the different bands, namely the three repeat tau isoforms on Western blots in Pick body dementia, in contrast to the predominance of four repeat tau in CBD and PSP *(22,27)*.

Chromosome 17 localization of familial FTD and parkinsonism (FTDP-17) and the various mutations in the tau gene further confirm the cohesion of this entity. Although there is phenotypic heterogeneity in these families, a frontotemporal disinhibition–apathy dementia, progressive aphasia, and parkinsonism occur in various combinations. Sometimes the same mutation produces different phenotypes even in the same families, and on the other hand, different mutations seemed to be associated with the same phenotypes. Altogether, these variations, rather than reflecting undue heterogeneity, suggest significant overlap of the syndromes. Recently, tau and synuclein negative, and some ubiquitin positive inclusions were found in a substantial number of FTD and PPA cases. These are typical in ALS, but they can be cortical only, without ALS. Some of the tau negative cases may be tau-deficient tauopathies *(28)*. A small portion of Pick complex patients has clear-cut clinical ALS, some with PPA, and some with FTD, and a larger number of ALS patients, have dementia of the FTD type and some even have CBD syndrome *(29)*.

6. CORTICOBASAL DEGENERATION

When corticodentatonigral degeneration was first described *(30)*, the authors considered it a new entity clinically characterized by unilateral rigidity, cortical sensory loss, and apraxia, but recognized the resemblance of the pathological features to PiD. Later, the disease was renamed CBD *(31)*. The extrapyramidal-apraxic syndrome, unresponsive to levodopa, was subsequently described mainly in movement disorder clinics. However, well-documented behavioral, cognitive, and language disturbances, suggestive of frontal and temporal lobe involvement, seem to be frequent features during the course of the disease *(30–33)*. Parietal and frontotemporal cortical atrophy are recognized components of the entity. The view that cognitive presentation is atypical, seems to hamper recognition of the disease *(34,35)*. In some neuropathologically diagnosed CBD series, all patients developed cognitive deficits *(36)*.

Our experience with CBD syndrome showed significant overlap between CBD and the syndromes of FTD/Pick complex *(26)*. All 35 patients with clinical CBD syndrome either had a language disorder or a behavioral and personality change characteristic of FTD. Often the movement disorder and the progressive aphasia or behavioral disorder developed simultaneously, but in the majority of the cases the cognitive disorder came first. Similarly, in all the primary movement presentations, aphasic or behavioral change has developed indicating that CBD should be considered part of the Pick complex. In 11 of our 35 cases with autopsy, 6 cases had CBD pathology, 3 cases had PiD, one had ALS-type inclusions, and one had superficial spongiosis, gliosis, and neuronal loss, also called dementia-lacking-distinctive-histology (DLDH).

7. PROGRESSIVE SUPRANUCLEAR PALSY

Patients with axial dystonia, bradykinesia, falls, dysphagia, and vertical gaze palsy are considered typical of PSP, but lately, the overlap with CBD has been increasingly recognized. Many CBD patients also have vertical gaze palsy and symmetrical extrapyramidal syndrome. Two of our CBD series patients, for instance, received the clinical diagnosis of PSP one time or another. Some studies comparing the SCFS (executive dysfunctions) of PSP and CBD found no significant difference between them *(37)*, although it is generally assumed that SCFS is more severe in PSP *(13)*, while apraxia or other parietal signs (e.g., alien hand) better characterize CBD *(37)*. The pathological features are also considered to be overlapping to a great extent *(38)*. Biochemical and genetic evidence also supports the relationship *(27)*. There is continuing controversy to what extent PSP and CBD can be differentiated, but most experts in the field consider the extent of the overlap significant.

8. HUNTINGTON'S DISEASE

In HD, the psychiatric and memory problems can be prominent even before the movement disorder, but they often follow the chorea *(39)*. Initially, mild failure of attention and memory, especially retrieval and executive dysfunction occur, but subsequently behavioral disorder, irritability, aggression, alcoholism, and psychosis are frequent. The clinical overlap with other conditions is infrequent because of the characteristics of the choreiform movements and the autosomal dominant inheritance of high penetrance. However, there are rigid forms of HD resembling parkinsonism, and an overlap exists with senile chorea in coexistence with AD. Chorea in the elderly is not infrequent and may be related to vascular disease, often due to infarcts in the subthalamic nucleus. The movements may be "ballistic" and in vascular etiology usually unilateral. The differential diagnosis of choreiform tardive dyskinesia, secondary to neuroleptic use, is an important one, especially since neuroleptics are used in psychiatric and dementing conditions.

9. CREUTZFELDT-JAKOB DISEASE

This is a rapidly progressive illness with an average duration of 9 mo overlapping only with other degenerative dementias at the early stages of the illness. The initial cortical type of dementia with memory loss, visual agnosia, and aphasia, changes into an apathetic confusional state with decreasing level of alertness and akinetic mute state, or coma with myoclonic jerks. The characteristic periodic complexes on electroencephalography (EEG) and the recently developed 14-3-3 protein assay in the Cerebrospinal fluid (CSF), are helpful in the differential diagnosis. Biopsies are less frequently done because of the highly infectious nature of the prion proteins. The previously reported overlap with ALS is probably related to faulty pathological diagnosis mistaking the cortical spongiosis of Pick complex for the diffuse spongiform change in CJD before the staining techniques for prion proteins were developed. Antibodies to protease-resistant prion proteins on pathology or the isoforms on Western blot techniques or at times the mutation is needed for definite diagnosis. It is the rapid subacute course of the illness, rather than the specificity of the mental changes, plus the associated laboratory features and the development of the stimulus-sensitive myoclonus that is most helpful in the classical differential diagnosis. Slower progressing, longer duration, ataxic, cerebellar variants may be more difficult to diagnose (Gerstman-Sträussler-Scheinker syndrome). The new variant CJD, relating to bovine spongiform encephalopathy (BSE), affects younger individuals who lived in Europe or had contact with infected cattle or beef products.

10. VASCULAR DEMENTIA

Vascular dementia is poorly defined, controversial, and variable in clinical manifestations. The initiator of the concept of multi-infarct dementia has recently declared it obsolete. Nevertheless, the subcortical variety is often associated with both a frontal type of cognitive deficit and a movement disorder, characterized by gait apraxia, shuffling, bradykinesia, and gegenhalten. Features of vascular dementia, such as impaired executive function, relatively preserved recognition memory, and bradyphrenia are similar to the subcortical dementia and relate to frontal-subcortical disconnection by lacunes and ischemic white matter changes.

Strategically placed infarct, such as in the anterior cerebral aneurysm occlusion syndrome (ACAO) may result in persisting dementia. Thalamic lesions can cause a pure amnestic syndrome with variable recovery. Left thalamic lesions tend to produce loss of language and verbal memory, and right-sided lesions tend to produce neglect, constructional deficit, and visuospatial memory. The limbic system has major thalamic connections, and this accounts for the emotional and motivational aspects of thalamic lesions. Thalamic dementia with bilateral lesions is characterized by deficits of attention, memory, and diminished movements, and responsiveness at times severe enough to approach akinetic mutism.

11. SUMMARY

This overview represents a clinical approach to the overlap between neurodegenerative dementias and movement disorders. The scope of this overview is limited to the clinical aspects somewhat artificially. The clinical nosology and the relationship of the syndromes are often influenced by the underlying pathology, biochemistry, and genetics. Changing concepts and new technologies provide discoveries leading to new approaches and new classifications. However, undue reliance on any single scientific discipline, such as genetics or histochemistry to solve the nosological issues in clinical medicine, is fraught with hazards. As new technologies develop, even "gold standards," such as pathology, change. The same mutation can be associated with divergent clinical phenotypes. None of the current levels of description is able to provide all the questions, let alone the answers to neurodegenerative disease. Therefore, integration of all levels of description becomes crucial, and the clinical approach is only one of the frameworks on which this has to be based.

REFERENCES

1. Lilienfeld, D.E. and Perl, D.P. (1994) Projected neurodegenerative disease mortality among minorities in the United States. *Neuroepidemiology* **13,** 179–186.
2. Parkinson, J. (1897) *An essay on the Shaking Palsy,* Sherwood, London.
3. Lieberman, A., Dziatolowski, M., Kupersmith, M., et al. (1979) Dementia in Parkinson's disease. *Ann. Neurol.* **6,** 355–359.
4. Brown, R.G. and Marsden, C.D. (1984) How common is dementia in Parkinson's disease? *Lancet* **1,** 1262–1265.
5. Mayeux, R., Stern, Y., Rosenstein, R., et al. (1988) An estimate of the prevalence of dementia in idiopathic Parkinson's disease. *Arch. Neurol.* **45,** 260–262.
6. Marder, K., Ming-Xin, T., Cote, L., Stern, Y., and Mayeux, R. (1995) The frequency and associated risk factors for dementia in patients with Parkinson's disease. *Arch. Neurol.* **52,** 695–701.
7. Aarsland, D., Andersen, K., Larsen, J.P., et al. (2001) Risk of dementia in Parkinson's disease: a community-based, prospective study. *Neurology* **56,** 730–736.
8. Appell, J., Kertesz, A., and Fisman, M. (1982) A study of language functioning in Alzheimer patients. *Brain Lang.* **17,** 73–91.
9. Brown, R.G. and Marsden, C.D. (1988) 'Subcortical dementia': the neuropsychological evidence. *Neuroscience* **25,** 363–387.
10. McHugh, P.R. and Folstein, M.F. (eds.) (1975) Psychiatric syndromes of Huntington's chorea: a clinical and phenomenological study, in *Psychiatric Aspects of Neurological Disease* (Benson, D.F. and Blumer, D., eds.), Grune & Stratton, New York, pp. 267–285.
11. Albert, M.L., Feldman, R.G., and Willis, A.L. (1974) The 'subcortical dementia' of progressive supranuclear palsy. *J. Neurol. Neurosurg. Psychiatry* **37,** 121–130.
12. Albert, M. (1978) Subcortical dementia, in *Alzheimer's Disease: Senile Dementia and Related Disorders* (Katzman, R., Terry, R.D., and Bick, K.L., eds.), Raven Press, New York, pp. 173–180.

13. Dubois, B., Pillon, B., Legault, F., Agid, Y., and Lhermitte, F. (1988) Slowing of cognitive processing in progressive supranuclear palsy. *Arch. Neurol.* **45,** 1194–1199.
14. Mayeux, R., Stern, Y., and Spanton, S. (1985) Heterogeneity in dementia of the Alzheimer type: evidence of sub groups. *Neurology* **35,** 453–461.
15. Kosaka, K., Yoshimura, M., Ikeda, K., and Budka, H. (1984) Diffuse type of Lewy body disease: progressive dementia with abundant cortical Lewy bodies and senile changes of varying degree—a new disease? *Clin. Neuropathol.* **3,** 185–192.
16. Gibb, W.R.G., Esiri, M.M., and Lees, A.J. (1985) Clinical and pathological features of diffuse cortical Lewy body disease (Lewy body dementia). *Brain* **110,** 1131–1153.
17. McKeith, I.G., Galasko, D., Kosaka, K., et al. (1996) Consensus guidelines for the clinical and pathologic diagnosis of dementia with Lewy bodies (DLB): report of the consortium on DLB international workshop. *Neurology* **47,** 1113–1124.
18. del Ser, T., Hachinski, V., Merskey, H., and Munoz, D.G. (2001) Clinical and pathologic features of two groups of patients with dementia with Lewy bodies: effect of coexisting Alzheimer-type lesion load. *Alzheimer Dis. Assoc. Disord.* **15,** 31–44.
19. Holmes, C., Cairns, N., Lantos, P., and Mann, A. (1999) Validity of current clinical criteria for Alzheimer's disease, vascular dementia and dementia with Lewy bodies. *Br. J. Psychiatry* **174,** 45–50.
20. Garruto, R.M., Fukatsu, R., Yanagihara, R., et al. (1984) Imaging of calcium and aluminum in neurofibrillary tangle-bearing neurons in parkinsonism-dementia of Guam. *Proc. Natl. Acad. Sci. USA* **81,** 1875–1879.
21. Akelaitis, A.J. (1944) Atrophy of basal ganglia in Pick's disease. A clinicopathologic study. *Arch. Neurol. Psychiatr* **51,** 27–34.
22. Kertesz, A. and Munoz, D.G. (1998) *Pick's Disease and Pick Complex,* Wiley-Liss, New York.
23. The Lund and Manchester Groups (1994) Clinical and neuropathological criteria for frontotemporal dementia. *J. Neurol. Neurosurg. Psychiatry* **57,** 416–418.
24. Kertesz, A., Hudson, L., Mackenzie, I.R.A., and Munoz, D.G. (1994) The pathology and nosology of primary progressive aphasia. *Neurology* **44,** 2065–2072.
25. Frattali, C.M., Grafman, J., Patronas, N., Makhlouf, F., and Litvan, I. (2000) Language disturbances in corticobasal degeneration. *Neurology* **54,** 990–992.
26. Kertesz, A., Martinez-Lage, P., Davidson, W., and Munoz, D.G. (2000) The corticobasal degeneration syndrome overlaps progressive aphasia and frontotemporal dementia. *Neurology* **55,** 1368–1375.
27. Houlden, H., Baker, M., Morris, H.R., et al. (2001) Corticobasal degeneration and progressive supranuclear palsy share a common tau haplotype. *Neurology* **56,** 1702–1706.
28. Zhukareva, V., Vogelsberg-Ragaglia, V., Van Deerlin, V., et al. (2001) Loss of brain tau defines novel sporadic and familial tauopathies with frontotemporal dementia. *Ann. Neurol.* **49,** 165–175.
29. Grimes, D.A., Bergeron, C.B., and Lang, A.E. (1999) Motor neuron disease-inclusion dementia presenting as cortical-basal ganglionic degeneration. *Mov. Disord.* **14,** 674–680.
30. Rebeiz, J.J., Kolodny, E.H., and Richardson, E.P. Jr. (1968) Corticodentatonigral degeneration with neuronal achromasia. *Arch. Neurol.* **18,** 20–33.
31. Gibb, W.R.G., Luthert, P.J., and Marsden, C.D. (1989) Corticobasal degeneration. *Brain* **112,** 1171–1192.
32. Riley, D.E., Lang, A.E., Lewis, M.B., et al. (1990) Cortical-basal ganglionic degeneration. *Neurology* **40,** 1203–1212.
33. Rinne, J.O., Lee, M.S., Thompson, P.D., and Marsden, C.D. (1994) Corticobasal degeneration. *Brain* **117,** 1183–1196.
34. Litvan, I., Agid, Y., Jankovic, J., et al. (1997) Accuracy of clinical criteria for the diagnosis of progressive supranuclear palsy (Steele-Richardson-Olszewski syndrome). *Neurology* **46,** 1–9.
35. Bergeron, C., Davis, A., and Lang, A.E. (1998) Corticobasal ganglionic degeneration and progressive supranuclear palsy presenting with cognitive decline. *Brain Pathol.* **8,** 355–365.
36. Schneider, J.A., Watts, R.L., Gearing, M., Brewer, R.P., and Mirra, S.S. (1997) Corticobasal degeneration: neuropathologic and clinical heterogeneity. *Neurology* **48,** 959–969.
37. Pillon, B., Blin, J., Vidailhet, M., et al. (1995) The neuropsychological pattern of corticobasal degeneration: comparison with progressive supranuclear palsy and Alzheimer's disease. *Neurology* **45,** 1477–1483.
38. Feany, M.B., Mattiace, L.A., and Dickson, D.W. (1996) Neuropathologic overlap of progressive supranuclear palsy, Pick's disease and corticobasal degeneration. *J. Neuropathol. Exp. Neurol.* **55,** 53–67.
39. Butters, N., Tarlow, S., and Cermak, L.S. (1976) A comparison of the information processing deficits of patients with Huntington's chorea and Korsakoff's syndrome. *Cortex* **12,** 134–144.

18

Neuropathological Distinctions and Similarities in Movement Disorders with Dementia

Kurt A. Jellinger, MD

1. INTRODUCTION

Mental and behavioral dysfunctions including dementia in movement disorders have considerable consequences for patients, including increased mortality and risk for nursing home placement *(1,2)*. Their incidence rates in different types of movement disorders are highly variable, but reliable figures are rare. In Parkinson's disease (PD), the reported incidence rates vary between 42.5 *(3)* and 95.3 *(4)* per 1000 person-yr, suggesting that the lifetime risk of developing dementia in patients with PD is two- to almost sixfold increased compared with the normal population *(4,5)*. For many other movement disorders, there are similar deviating data on the incidence rates and variable cognitive profiles of dementia *(6–15)*. The etiology of dementia in movement disorders is a matter of controversy. It may be caused by a variety of neuropathological conditions featured by progressive neuron and synapse loss often associated with cytopathological changes involving specific subcortical and cortical systems and circuits. These neuronal and glial inclusions or neuritic alterations composed of aggregations of insoluble cytoskeletal protein filaments show characteristic immunoreactions, ultra-structure, and biochemistry indicating cytoskeletal mismetabolism. They are important diagnostic signposts that, in addition to the distribution pattern of neurodegeneration, indicate specific vulnerability of neuronal–glial populations, while in some movement disorders with dementia, still no such cyto-pathological hallmarks have been detected. Table 1 presents a (preliminary) classification of movement disorders variably associated with dementia based on morphology and biochemistry of available disease markers. This chapter will present a brief overview of the neuropathological distinctions and similarities of some of the major types of movement disorders associated with mental dysfunctions.

2. SYNUCLEINOPATHIES

This diverse group of neurodegenerative disorders shares a common pathologic lesion composed of aggregates of insoluble α-synuclein (α-S) protein in selectively vulnerable populations of neurons and glia. α-S is a 140-amino acid highly soluble neuron-specific protein of unknown function that is expressed in synaptic terminals *(16)*. Two different pathogenic mutations in the α-S gene on chromosome 4q21.3-q22 have been described in rare kindreds with familial PD *(17,18)*. Abnormal aggregates of α-S are present in Lewy bodies (LB) and Lewy-related neuritic pathology in PD and dementia with Lewy bodies (DLB), but also in glial and neuronal inclusions in multiple system atrophy (MSA) as well as in other neurodegenerative disorders, including familial Alzheimer's disease (AD), Down's syndrome, neurodegeneration with brain iron accumulation (NBIA), thereby expanding the concept of

From: *Mental and Behavioral Dysfunction in Movement Disorders*
Edited by: M-A. Bédard et al. © Humana Press Inc., Totowa, NJ

Table 1
Morphologic and Biochemical Classification of Movement Disorders Associated with Dementia

α-Synucleopathies
- PD (brainstem type of LBD)
- DLB
- DDLB
- LBV-AD (+ neuritic AD pathology)
- MSA
- Neurodegeneration with brain iron accumulation, type I/Hallervorden-Spatz disease

Tauopathies
- PSP (4-repeat tau doublet plus exon 10)
- CBD (similar)
- AGD (similar)
- PDC (3 plus 4-repeat tau triplet)
- PEP (3 plus 4-repeat tau triplet)
- FTDP-17 (tau doublet)
- PPND (4-repeat tau)
- Multiple system tauopathy with presenile dementia (MSTD) (plus 3 intronic mutation)
- PiD (3-repeat tau doublet without exon 10)
- PSG (Neumann-Cohn disease) (4-repeat tau triplet)
- Hallervorden-Spatz disease (with tangles)

Polyglutamine repeat (CAG) disorders
- Huntington's disease
- Choreoacanthocytosis (neuroacanthocytosis)
- Machado-Joseph disease (SCA 3)
- Dentatorubropallidoluysian atrophy (DRLPA)

Other heredodegenerative disorders
- (Non)hereditary striatal degeneration
- Pallidal degeneration and related variants
- Hallervorden-Spatz disease (without α-synucleopathy)
- Wilson's disease
- Inherited dystonias

neurodegenerative synucleinopathies (see ref. *19*). Dementia in synucleinopathies is seen in both PD and DLB and, much less, in MSA *(20)*, which, therefore, are not considered here.

2.1. Parkinson Disease

2.1.1. Basic Neuropathology Findings in PD with Dementia

In PD, both behavioral and cognitive deficits are associated with a wide variety of brain lesions. In a consecutive autopsy series of 210 cases with the clinical diagnosis of parkinsonism, the total prevalence of moderate to severe dementia was 39%. Because 38 cases, or 18%, displayed other pathological syndromes, only 172 cases were confirmed as primary LB disease, including 45 cases of DLB. The prevalence of dementia in this group was 33.7%. Although only 1.3% of PD cases with cognitive impairment showed "pure" PD without concurrent brain lesions, the majority revealed additional brain pathologies, in particular AD or AD-type lesions. Additional cerebrovascular lesions (lacunar state, old infarcts) did not contribute to dementia in PD except for subcortical arteriosclerotic encephalopathy (SAE) or hippocampal sclerosis. DLB in this cohort was associated with dementia in 80%. The incidence of cognitive impairment was much higher in the group of secondary non-LB-related parkinsonian disorders (60.6%), with highest incidence in AD patients presenting with extrapyramidal motor

Table 2
Pathology of PD (1989–2000)

Neuropathology	Total	With dementia n	With dementia %
PD (LB-type)	74	1	1.3
PD plus lacunar state (old infarcts)	23(6)	0	0
PD plus AD (Braak stages V, IV)	5	5	100.0
PD plus limbic AD (Braak stages III, IV)	15	10	66.6
PD plus MIE/SAE[b] (hippocampal sclerosis)[a]	6(2[b], 2[a])	3(2[a])	50.0
PD plus MIX (AD plus MIE)	1	1	100.0
LBV-AD	15	15	100.0
DDLB	30	21	70.0
PD plus other pathology	3	2	66.0
Primary LBD	172	58	33.7
Alzheimer disease (AD)[a]	17(6[a])	17(6[a])	100.0
SAE (MIE)	5(1)	1	40.0
PSP[b]	6(1[b])	1[b]	17.0
MSA[b]	6(2[b])	1[b]	30.0
CBD, PiD	2	2	100.0
Nigral lesion unclassified	2	0	0.0
Secondary Parkinsonian Syndromes	38	23	60.6
TOTAL	210	82	39.0

[a]With nigral lesion.
[b]With AD.
MIE, multi-infarct encephalopathy; SAE, subcortical arteriosclerotic encephalopathy; CBD, corticobasal degeneration; MIX, mixed type dementia; DDLB, diffuse DLB.

Table 3
Pathology of PDD (1989–2000)

Neuropathology	n	%
PD	1	1.7
PD plus lacunar state/infarcts	0	0
PD plus AD/AT pathology	15	25.8
PD plus MIE/SAE	3	5.2
PD plus MIX (AD/MIE)	1	1.7
LBV-AD	15	25.8
DDLB	21	36.2
PD plus other pathology	2	3.5
TOTAL	58	100.0

MIE, multi-infarct encephalopathy; AT, Alzheimer type.

symptoms and, in rare cases, of corticobasal degeneration (CBD), progressive supranuclear palsy (PSP), and MSA associated with AD. The brains of confirmed AD with parkinsonian features showed mild nigral cell loss in 6 out of 17 cases (35.3%), and three of them had additional subcortical LBs in substantia nigra (SN) and/or locus ceruleus (LC) suggesting concurrent PD (Table 2). The inconsistent relationship between clinical parkinsonism and nigral degeneration with LBs in AD was emphasized recently by Ala et al. *(21)*. AD pathology was present in more than 53% of all demented patients with LB-type PD, whereas only 1.7% showed no additional brain lesions, and 7% had concurrent cerebrovascular lesions, mainly MIE/SAE (Table 3).

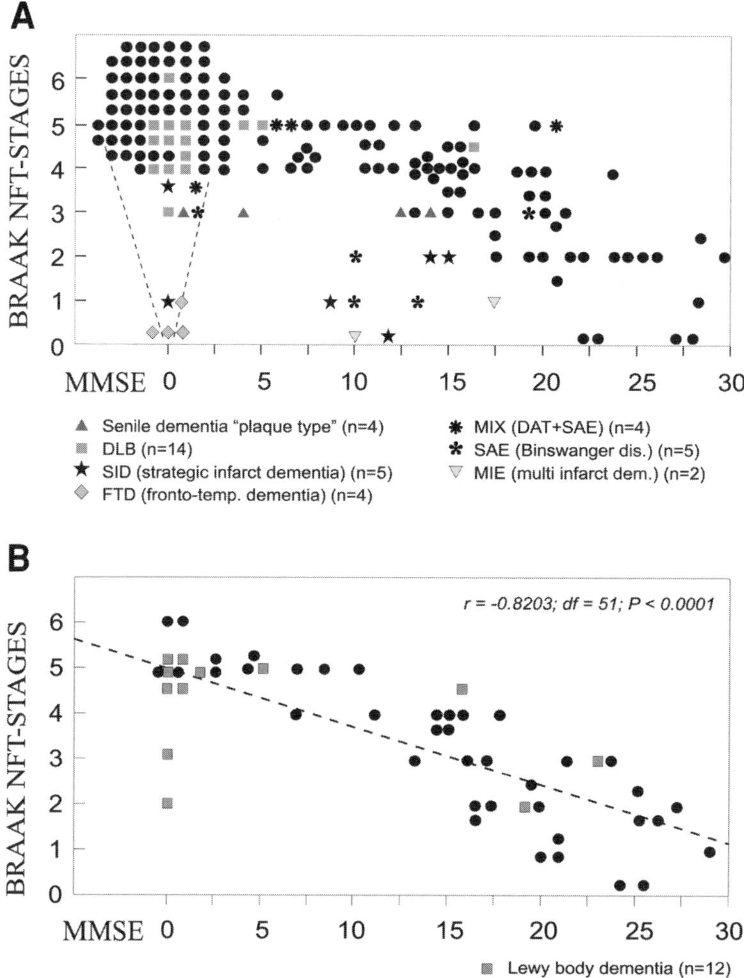

Fig. 1. Relationship between psychostatus assessed by MMSE and Braak stages in 167 consecutive elderly subjects without parkinsonian features—mean age 82.0 yr (**A**), and 51 consecutive autopsy cases of PD—mean age 78.6 yr (**B**).

Neuritic AD pathology is, in general, greater in PD with dementia (PDD) than in nondemented PD subjects. It shows a similar pattern and hierarchic spreading from allocortex to isocortical association areas with early involvement of the (trans)entorhinal regions as in AD *(20,22)*. This has been confirmed by immunochemical detection of abnormally phosphorylated tau protein, the major component of AD neurofibrillary tangles (NFTs) *(23)*: in nondemented PD brain it is restricted to the hippocampus, while PDD subjects show higher amounts of NFT-tau in (pre)frontal, temporal, and entorhinal areas with presevation of cingulate and occipital cortex, suggesting that frontal lobe dysfunction may contribute to cognitive changes. Although this pattern differs slightly from that in AD, with prominent involvement of primary sensory association areas, these data suggest that neuritic AD pathology is a major cause of dementia in PD. Comparative studies of neuritic AD stages and mental status assessed by Mini-Mental State Examination (MMSE) in two prospective autopsy series, 51 patients with PD (mean age 78.6 yr) and 167 aged subjects without parkinsonism (mean age 82.0 ± 8.6 yr), showed highly significant negative correlation between both parameters (Fig. 1). However, contrary to severely demented "pure" AD cases with clustering of Braak stages 5 and 6, PDD patients showed less often isocortical AD stages, while cognitively intact to mild or moderately demented subjects in both groups presented a wide range of AD lesions. Other rare types of dementia, e.g., frontotemporal dementia (FTD) and vascular-type dementias, revealed no correlation between cognitive impairment and severity of AD lesions.

2.1.2. Superimposed AD Pathology as Prognostic Factor

From clinical experience, dementia in PD patients is associated with a poor outcome and a higher risk of mortality compared with nondemented PD subjects *(24–28)*. This has been confirmed in a recent study of 200 consecutive autopsy cases of PD or brainstem type of Lewy body disease (LBD) (male: female ratio 1:1.1; age at death 58–98, mean 77.0 ± 9.5 yr), where major initial clinical symptoms (tremor, akinesia, rigidity), moderate and/or severe dementia documented in 33% of the sample, and duration of illness were assessed retrospectively and correlated with associated AD pathology using Consortium to Establish a Registry for Alzheimer's Disease (CERAD) *(29)*, Braak and Braak *(22)*, and National Insititute on Aging (NIA)-Reagan Institute criteria *(30)*. Although gender had no influence on the clinical motor symptoms and outcome/mortality, tremor dominant type ($n = 56$) had a significantly better outcome than akinetic-rigid forms (n = 144), even after adjustment with age at onset and associated AD pathology ($p = 0.022$). Of those patients classified as having PD without dementia, 97% had a pathologic diagnosis of PD with no signs of additional AD, whereas only 3% of patients with a confirmed LB-type of PD without superimposed neuritic AD lesions were considered during life as demented. In contrast, 94% of patients with clinical signs of moderate to severe dementia had additional cortical AD pathology, whereas only 6% did not ($p < 0.001$) *(31)*. Patients with later onset showed significantly shorter duration of illness irrespective of dementia (mean 5.6 vs 9.85 yr; $p < 0.001$) confirming previous studies on PD *(26,32,33)*. Moderate to severe dementia was significantly correlated with neuritic AD pathology (all three autopsy criteria, i.e., CERAD, Braak, and NIA-Reagan criteria) and showed significantly negative correlation with survival: between CERAD 0-A vs B and C (probable, definite AD), there was a significant difference of odd ratios ($p < 0.001$) (Fig. 2) as was between Braak stages 0–2 (negative and entorhinal), 3–4 (limbic), and 5 (isocortical), but not between Braak stages 3–4 and 5 (Fig. 3). Mean survival in PD cases with co-existent neuritic AD pathology was 4.46 years (95% confidence interval [CI] of mean 3.55–5.37) compared to 10.1 yr (95% CI of mean 9.31–10.9) in the cases without AD. These data confirm the results of previous studies reporting a higher risk of mortality in demented versus nondemented subjects both with PD and the general population *(25–27,34)*. The strong association of dementia with underlying AD pathology suggests that among PD patients, dementia may be a marker of an additional pathological process reducing survival compared to persons with PD alone *(31)*.

2.1.3. Other Pathologies Related to Dementia

In addition to co-existent neuritic AD pathology associated with variable losses of cortical neurons and synapses, the following brain lesions may contribute to cognitive impairment in PD *(20)*: (*i*) Involvement of the cholinergic forebrain system with 50–70% loss of cholinergic neurons in the magnocellular part of nucleus basalis of Meynert (NBM) in PDD cases compared to 30–40% in nondemented ones *(20,26)* and decrease in cholinergic innervation of cortex and hippocampus that may or may not correlate with the severity of NMB cell loss and mental status *(35)*. The loss of cholinergic neurons in the basal forebrain and the pedunculopontine tegmental nucleus (PPN) in the brainstem accounting for 35–40% in PD *(36,37)* may affect hippocampal and prefrontal structures via direct and frontostriatal connections due to dysfunction of the caudate nucleus *(38,39)* and may thus contribute to subcortico-frontal cognitive impairment and behavioral changes in PD *(5,40,41)*. (*ii*) Dysfunctions of other subcorticocortical networks are probably of minor importance for the development of cognitive disorders in PD (see ref. *20*): (a) dopaminergic systems with degeneration of the nigrostriatal loop causing deafferentation of striatoprefrontal circuits and the mesocorticolimbic system (medial SN, ventral tegmentum); (b) noradrenergic deficiency due to neuronal loss and cell shrinkage in the LC, which is the main source of noradrenergic innervation of widespread areas of the CNS and is less severe in nondemented PD subjects than in those with dementia and/or depression, where it approaches the values seen in AD

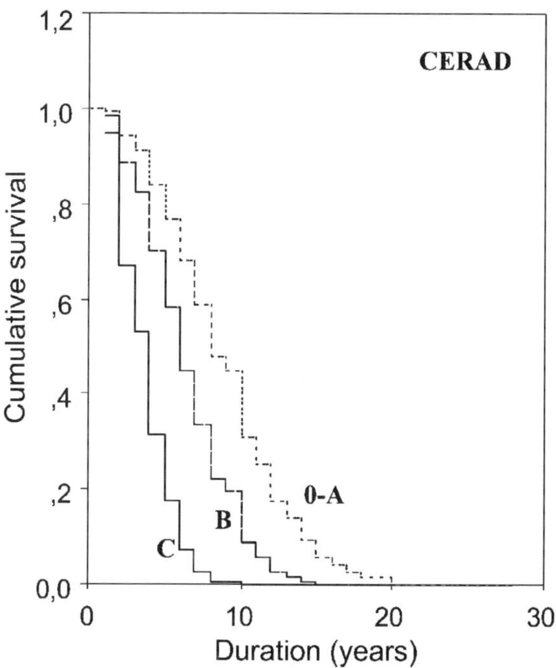

Fig. 2. Kaplan-Mayer curves of survival for PD patients with different CERAD scores of AD pathology.

(42,43); (c) serotonergic deficiency due to loss of serotonin-synthesizing neurons in the dorsal raphe nuclei, which, however, may show no relationship to the extent of cognitive decline *(20,26,44,45)*; (d) involvement of specific nuclei and limbic system appear to have variable effects on cognitive impairment in PD; it is correlated with both the density of dystrophic Lewy neurites in the cornu ammonis (CA) 2–3 subfields of hippocampus, and the periamygdaloid cortex (PAC) *(45)*, suggesting that disruption of the "limbic loop" contributes to dementia *(46)*. On the other hand, involvement of the amygdaloid nucleus in both PD and DLB, being most frequent in the central and accessory nuclei *(47,48)* that receive dense dopaminergic fibers from the SN, has been found to be unrelated to mental impairment, but could be responsible for psychiatric symptoms in patients with PD and DLB *(48)*. This is in contrast to AD, where neuronal loss mainly involves the magnocellular and deep cortical nuclei, which project to frontal and temporal neocortex *(49)*. Destruction of these nuclei may cause "disconnection" of the amygdala from key regions in a similar manner as described for the hippocampus in AD *(50)* (*iii*) The relevance of cortical LB pathology, demonstrable by α-S immunohistochemistry in up to 100% of PD brains *(51,52)*, is still a matter of discussion, and the relationship between LBs and the dementing process has not been well characterized. Recent studies have demonstrated variable correlations between cognitive impairment and the number of cortical LBs *(52,53)* and of Lewy neurites in hippocampus *(46,47)*, while others did not find such an association *(54)*. In contrast, both the density of hippocampal LBs and of neuritic plaques usually correlate well with dementia severity, suggesting an additive process with both LB and neuritic pathology independently contributing to dementia *(20,54)*.

2.2. DLB

2.2.1. Clinical Problems and Prognostic Features

DLB is distinguished from PD or LBD of pure brainstem type by both clinical and morphological features *(55,57)*. This sporadic neurodegenerative disorder comprises a rapidly progressive cognitive

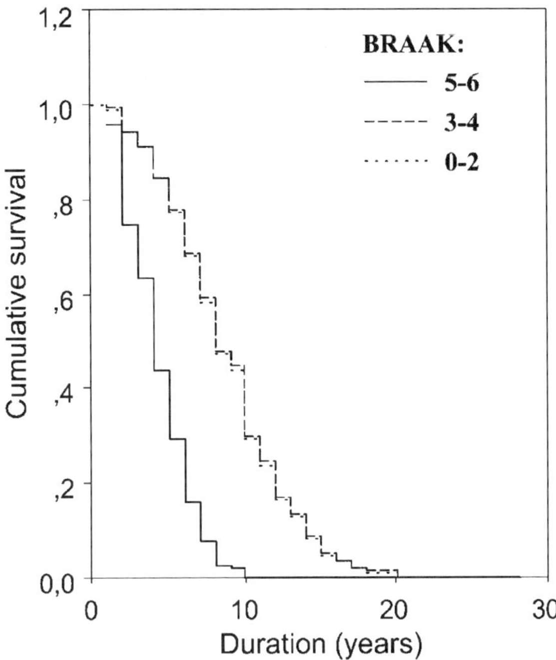

Fig. 3. Kaplan-Mayer curves of survival for PD patients with different Braak stages of neuritic AD pathology.

decline with fluctuating attention, affection of frontal-subcortical skills, visuospatial ability, optic hallucinations, neuroleptic intolerance, and spontaneous parkinsonism. A similar clinicopathological picture may be seen in patients initially presenting with motor deficits of parkinsonism and later development of cognitive impairment and psychosis. Cognitive dysfunction in DLB has specific characteristics that aid in discrimination from AD *(6,58)*. DLB is considered as the second most frequent cause of dementia in the elderly, accounting from 7–30% (mean 15–20%) in several autopsy series *(55,57)*, and was 21% in our recent autopsy cohort of LB-type parkinsonism (Table 2). A community case register study in Camberwell, UK, found 15% of elderly demented subjects to have DLB at autopsy *(59)*. The sensitivity of clinical consensus criteria for probable DLB ranges from 40–83%, the specificity from 22–83%, with a diagnostic validity around 50% *(15,28,59–62)*. In a retrospective study of 62 postmortem-confirmed DLB cases from seven brain banks, the sensitivity of the Consortium on dementia with Lewy bodies (CDLB) criteria at first and last visit for possible DLB was 0.46 and 0.82, respectively, and for probable DLB, 0.26 and 0.69%, respectively. The age at symptom onset was 69.4 ± 10.0 yr, and the average disease duration was 7.5 ± 6.6 yr. Clinical features at first visit included memory impairment (69%), bradykinesia (59%), gait disturbances and frontal lobe behavior (57% each), paranoid delusions (48%), fluctuating attention (37%), and visual hallucinations (36%), with later development of dysarthria (78%), urinary incontinence (71%), and dysphagia (65%) *(61)*. In a recent retrospective clinicopathologic study of 31 cases of DLB, 48 with AD, and 20 PDD, sensitivity of the CDLB criteria for the first visit was low (0.22) with nearly perfect specificity (0.97); for last visit, sensitivity for probable DLB increased (0.60) with decreased specificity (0.85). Specificity in distinguishing DLB from PD and AD at the first visit was 1.0 and 0.96, respectively, and at the last visit was 0.95 and 0.80, respectively. CDLB criteria distinguished DLB from PD with a higher positive predictive value (PPV), first visit 1.00, last visit 0.94, than from AD (first visit 0.71, last visit 0.63), thus suggesting that CDLB criteria for probable DLB may be helpful in the differential diagnosis of DLB *(63)*. Similar results were obtained in another clinicopathologic study on the effect of co-existing AD pathology in DLB *(15)*.

A metaanalysis of 236 postmortem-confirmed DLB cases revealed that dementia, hallucinations, and fluctuating attention at disease-onset were frequently associated with cortical AD pathology and predicted shorter survival (mean 5.7 ± 0.4 yr) than parkinsonism with absence of the above symptoms (mean 8.2 ± 0.6 yr) ($p < 0.0001$), whereas gender, paranoid delusions, and falls were unrelated to prognosis *(64)*.

Temporal evaluation of symptoms in another autopsy series of DLB with concomitant AD showed that most subjects developed either extrapyramidal symptoms or psychosis and hallucinations about 4 yr after onset of cognitive decline, suggesting that clinical diagnostic accuracy of DLB in subjects with concomitant AD is time-dependent *(65)*.

2.2.2. Neuropathologic Comparison with PD and AD

Pathology of DLB, in addition to diffuse brain atrophy, reveals numerous cortical LBs particularly in entorhinal, cingulate cortex, hippocampus, inferior and middle temporal gyri, insula, and amygdala, less often in other isocortical areas, involving small and middle sized neurons in deep cortical laminae *(66)*. LB are demonstrable by immunohistochemistry with α-S antibodies that distinguish them from early NFTs. They are associated with spongy changes in superior cortex, severe loss of neurons in SN and LC associated with subcortical LBs, often indistinghishable in severity and distribution pattern from those in PD, while a minority of cases shows only mild SN damage similar to that in AD *(55,67,68)*. Dystrophic Lewy neurites in the CA 2–3 region of hippocampus are often similar to those in PD, while neuronal loss in the cholinergic magnocellular part of NBM with neocortical cholinergic deficits and up-regulation of cortical muscarinic receptors is more severe than in AD and correlates with dementia *(68–72)*. Recommended criteria for morphologic diagnosis of DLB are a standardized semiquantitative scoring system of cortical LBs (>5 per region *[55,56]*), later simplified *(67)*. These scores may distinguish three pathological categories: brainstem predominant LBD or PD (0–2 cortical LBs), limbic or transitional type (3–6 LBs), and neocortical type (7–10 LBs), but there is no correlation between paralimbic or neocortical and nigral LBs *(66)*.

Pathologic features of AD are also frequently present in DLB, with preponderance of diffuse plaques and different proportion of plaques between DLB (less Aβ-40 than Aβ-42 deposits) and AD *(73)*, the relative absence of neocortical neuritic AD pathology *(57,74)*, or their frequent restriction to the limbic system, corresponding to Braak stages 0–4 or CERAD classes 0–A *(20,57,68)*. By contrast, many PDD patients often show more severe neuritic AD lesions (CERAD B or C; Braak stage 5), with an intermediate likelihood of dementia caused by AD according to the NIA-Reagan Institute criteria *(30)*. Most of the DLB brains have an excess of AD-typical hyperphosphorylated tau protein in the hippocampus when compared with age-matched controls and nondemented PD patients *(69)*. Most, but not all, DLB brains occupy higher Braak stages of neuritic AD pathology than age-matched controls, but lower stages than brains with pure AD *(20,68,69,75–77)* (Fig. 4). The results of a personal comparative study of 57 DLB cases (24 neocortical, 33 limbic), 10 cases each of nondemented PD and PDD, and 30 AD cases are summarized in Table 4. Using the San Diego criteria, 26 of the DLB cases (45.5%) were Lewy body variant (LBV) of AD with mean MMSE of 2.6, CERAD B and C (11 and 15 cases, respectively) and Braak stages 4–5 (mean 4.76). Thirty-one cases (54.5%) were diffuse DLB (DDLB) with mean MMSE of 15.1, CERAD 0 ($n = 17$), A ($n = 9$), and B ($n = 5$), and Braak stages 2–4 (mean 2.6). PDD cases with only few cortical LBs and a mean MMSE of 4.9 showed similar Braak stages as LBV-AD (mean 4.3) and differed from AD with a mean MMSE of 0.5 and a mean Braak stage of 5.5. Correlation between CERAD classes and Braak stages showed considerable differences between DDLB and LBV-AD (Fig. 5A,B). These data are in accordance with those in other DLB cohorts, showing no significant differences in neocortical synapse density and synapse protein (synaptophysin) immunoreactivity versus controls, but severe synapse protein loss comparable to AD in DLB cases with neuritic AD pathology, i.e., LBV-AD *(69,78)*. However, early and more widespread cholinergic losses differentiate DLB from AD *(69,79)*. Since both PD and DLB may be associated with a wide range of AD

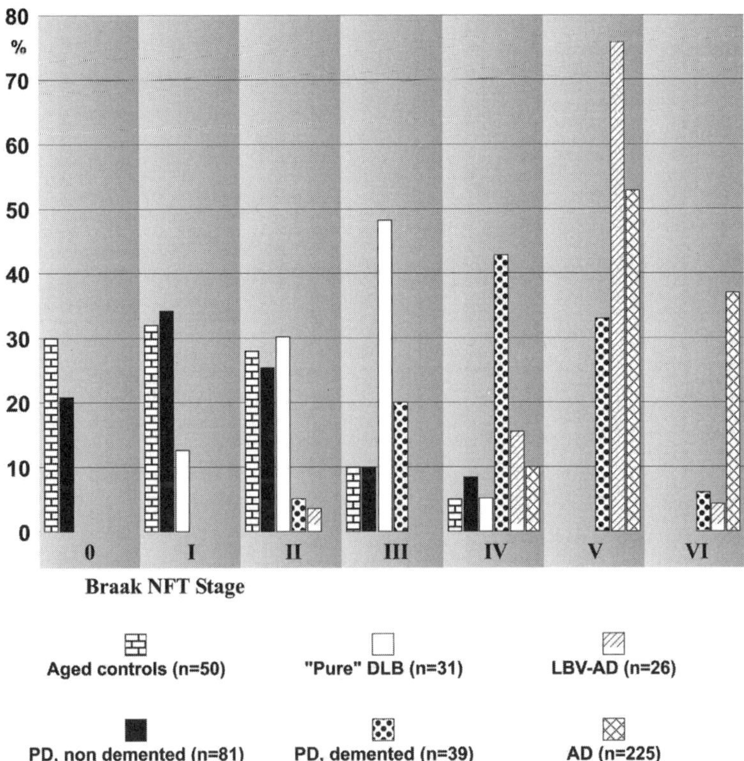

Fig. 4. Extent of neuritic Alzheimer changes using Braak stages in six diagnostic groups. Incidence is expressed as percentage of cases in each diagnostic category.

Table 4
Major Clinical and Alzheimer-Related Changes in LB-Related Disorders, AD Cases, and Age-Matched Controls

	LBV (*n* = 26) x ± (SD)	DDLB (*n* = 31) x ± (SD)	PDD (+AD) (*n* = 10) x ± (SD)	AD (*n* = 30) x ± (SD)	PD nondemented (*n* = 10) x ± (SD)	Controls (*n* = 7) x ± (SD)
Age (yr)	79.8 ± 4.9	76.0 ± 6.1	80.5 ± 5.1	79.0 ± 5.3	77.7 ± 3.2	
Sex (M/F)	8/18	9/22	7/3	25/5	3/7	5/2
Duration (yr)	5.9 ± 2.3	7.4 ± 2.5	7.3 ± 3.2	6.8 ± 3.1	9.5 ± 4.2	—
MMSE (*n* = 12/8)	2.0 ± 1.0	15.1 ± 5.2	4.9 ± 3.2	0.5 ± 0	24.7 ± 1.0	27.0 ± 0.5
Brain weight (g)	1582 ± 112	1206 ± 92	1188 ± 86	1081 ± 48	1246 ± 51	1337 ± 118
DLB limbic/neocortical	16/9	17/14	—	—	—	—
CERAD 0	0	19	2	0	8	7
A	0	9	1	0	1	0
B	11	5	3	1	1	0
C	15	0	4	29	0	0
Braak Stage	4.76 ± 0.2	2.61 ± 0.3	4.3 ± 0.5	5.5 ± 0.2	2.2 ± 0.3	1.3 ± 0.2

SD, standard deviation.

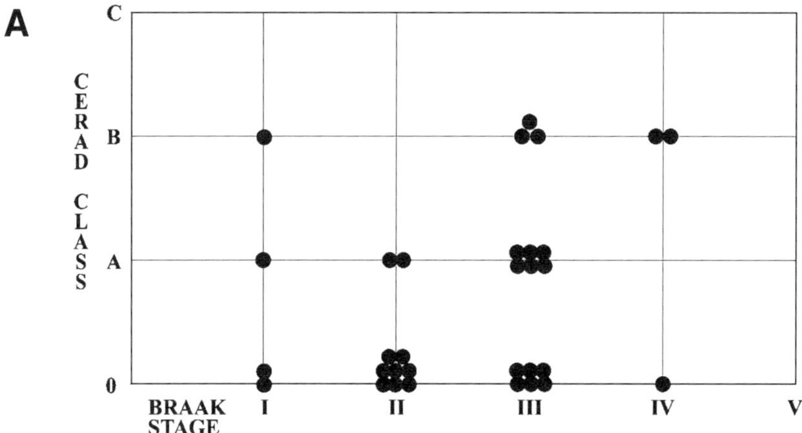

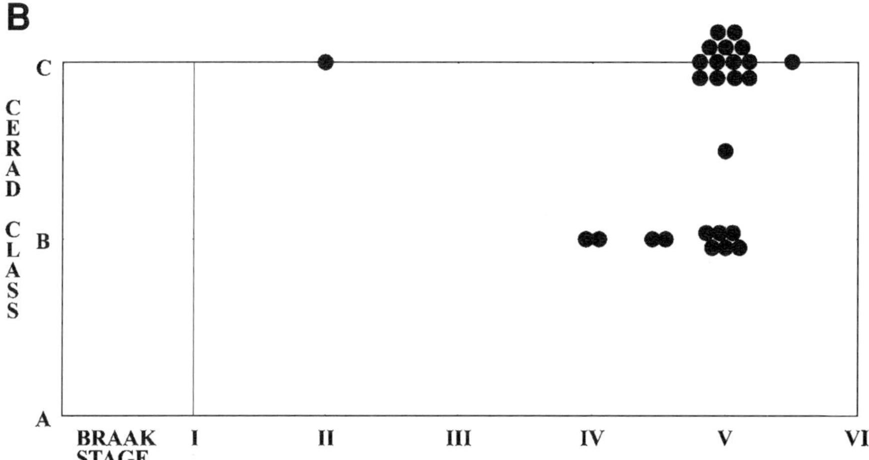

Fig. 5. Correlation between CERAD category and Braak stages in 31 cases of DLBD (**A**) and 26 cases of LBV-AD (**B**).

lesions, the application of the new NIA-Reagan Institute criteria for the postmortem diagnosis of AD *(30)* will provide varying results in these disorders (Table 5).

2.3.3. Distinction Between DLB, PD, and AD

Traditionally, brainstem LBs are pathognomonic for PD, but also occur in all cases of DLB and, occasionally, in AD *(19,83)*, while LBs in the amygdala are common in DLB, familial and sporadic AD, but are rare in other neurodegenerative disorders, e.g., MSA, Pick disease (PiD) or amyotrophic lateral sclerosis (ALS) (84). In many instances, the neuropathology of both nondemented PD and PDD patients is indistinguishable from that in cases with brainstem and limbic DLB *(55,56,66,68)*, and patients with brainstem predominant limbic or neocortical DLB may or may not have dementia. Only a few studies analyzed both demented and nondemented cases with LBs to address the basic issue important for underlying disease mechanisms *(53,54,85)*.

There is neither correlation between LB density in any brain area among DLB patients with cognitive changes or parkinsonism nor between LB density and Braak stages or frequency of neuritic plaques nor between LBs in cortex and SN *(60,66)*. Whereas LB densities, in general, cannot separate DLB from PDD, temporal lobe LBs are usually rare in nondemented PD cases compared with PDD and DLB sub-

Table 5
Likelihood of Dementia (%) Due to AD (NIA-Reagan Institute Criteria)

	CERAD/BRAAK			
Disorder (reference)	Low A/0–II	Intermediate B/III–IV	High C/V–VI	Mean age (yr)
Newell et al. *(80)*				
AD (*n* = 10)	0	20	80	83
DLB (*n* = 9)	44	56	0	81
PSP (*n* = 11)	91	9	0	68
Controls (*n* = 10)	0	0	0	81
Newell et al. *(81)*				
AD (*n* = 33)	0	3	97	83
DLB (*n* = 15)	48	26	26	81
PSP (*n* = 12)	75	17	8	69
Other dementias (*n* = 3)	66	0	34	?
Controls (*n* = 17)	81	19	0	77
Harding et al. *(82)*				
AD (*n* = 31/22-no LB) (CDR 1–3)	26/13	20/27	54/60	77
DLB, neocortical (*n* = 11)	73	18	9	76
PD (*n* = 7) (CDR 0–0.5)	83	17	0	79
Controls (*n* = 18) (CDR 0–0.5)	83	17	0	79
Personal series				
AD (*n* = 90) (MMSE 0–17)	0	22	78	85
DLB (*n* = 57) (MMSE 0–20)	46	15	39	77
PSP (*n* = 10)	70	20	10	72
PD, demented (*n* = 66) (MMSE 0–20)	6	33	61	81
PD, nondemented (*n* = 140) (MMSE >20)	96	4	0	83
Controls (*n* = 20) (MMSE 28–30)	100	0	0	81

CDR, clincial dementia ratio.

jects *(54,68,86)*. The severity and duration of dementia appears to be related to both increasing parahippocampal LB densities and neuritic AD plaque grade. Using a simple screening algorithm for the determination of dementia in PD and DLB, recent studies by Harding and Halliday *(54)* have shown that semiquantitative LB density thresholds in the parahippocampus can distinguish demented from nondemented DLB cases independent of other pathologies (Table 6). However, these studies need further validation.

Despite deposition of nonsoluble α-S in both LBs and Lewy neurites in DLB, no missense mutations of the α-S gene on chromosome 4q observed in familial PD *(87,88)* were reported in DLB. Furthermore, there are differences in the proportion of Aβ-40 and Aβ-42 deposits *(73)*, significantly increased expression of α-S mRNA in DLB than in AD *(89)*, and of tau and cholinergic biochemistry. On the other hand, there are genetic similarities in ApoE ε4 and ε2 allele frequencies *(77,90,91)*, overexpression of ApoEx/genotype in both AD and DLB *(92)*, but lack of association in DLB with the AA genotype of the α-1-antichymotrypsin gene *(93)*, and absence in AD of the CP 206 gene polymorphism observed in PD and DLB *(94,95)*. Additional factors that may also contribute to the development of LBs could be an as yet unidentified gene mapped to the centromeric region of chromosome 12 showing association with DLB independent of ApoEε4 *(96)*. Despite frequent overlap between DLB with both PD and AD, these data support the view that DLB represents an independent nosological entity and not just a special form of either PD or AD.

Table 6
Screening Algorithm for Determination of PDD and DLB

Brainstem Lewy bodies present?

⇓ ⇓

YES — PD or DLB | NO — Neither PD nor DLB

⇓

Did the patient have dementia?

⇓ ⇓

YES — PDD or DLB | NO — PD

⇓

Maximum density of LBs in parahippocampal cortex (2–6 or 7+ LB per 200x field)

⇓ ⇓

(2–6) DLB or PDD | (7+) DLB

Continue to screen for other neurodegenerative disorders.

3. TAUOPATHIES

3.1. Tau Biochemistry and Ultrastructure

A heterogenous group of neurodegenerative disorders is featured by widespread deposition of the hyperphosphorylated microtubule-associated tau protein, previously known to be the key component of AD-NFTs. Tau pathology, which involves both neurons and glia (astroglia and oligodendroglia), varies considerably in both biochemistry and ultrastructure among the different disorders *(97,98)*. Alternative splicing of RNA transcripts generates 6 tau isoforms that can be identified in immunoblots of normal brain tissue; splicing of exon 10 generates tau with either 3- or 4-repeat regions in the microtubule-binding domain, which alters the biophysical properties of tau with respect to interaction with microtubules. While in AD, postencephalitic parkinsonism (PEP), Parkinson-dementia complex of Guam (PDC), and subacute sclerosing panencephalitis (SSPE), all 6 tau isoforms with 3 and 4 microtubule-binding domains are detectable with 3 bands in immunoblots (55, 64, and 69 kDa) forming paired helical and, rarely, straight filaments. PSP, CBD, and argyrophilic grain disease (AGD) reveal 4-R tau isoforms with 2 major bands (55 and 64 kDa) aggregated in coiled filaments or twisted ribbons that are wider (24 nm) and have a longer periodicity (160 nm) than AD paired helical filaments (PHF) (22 nm and 80 nm). PiD, rarely associated with extrapyramidal symptoms, appears different with two isoforms (55 and 64 kDa) of 3-R tau aggregated into twisted ribbons and straight filaments. Frontotemporal dementia with Parkinsonism linked to chromosome 17 (FTDP-17) shows biochemical profiles similar to the tau triplet in AD, but a minor variant at 74 kDa is also found in FTDP-17, PEP, and PDC, while FTDP-17 cases with E-10 mutations, progressive subcortical gliosis (PSG), and pallido-ponto-nigral degeneration (PPND) show a 4-R tau triplet (64, 68, and 72 kDa). The disease-specific types of glial and neuronal tau pathology are summarized in Table 7. The tauopathies exhibit specific patterns of CNS lesions, but may also share both clinical and histopathologic features often causing considerable difficulties in their differential diagnosis *(99)*. Only PiD is associated with distinct neuronal inclusions, Pick bodies, while tau-immunoreactive astrocytis lesions are common in PSP, FTDP-17, CBD, PSG, and PPND, but also in PiD. Astrocytic plaques are characteristic for CBD, other astrocytic lesions are found mostly in neocortex in CBD, FTDP-17, PSG, and PiD and in basal ganglia

Table 7
Disease Specifity of Each Type of Glial and Neuronal Tau Pathology

	Astrocytic			Oligodendroglial				
Disease	Tufted astrocytes	Thorn-shaped astrocytes	Astrocytic plaques	Coiled bodies	Thread-like processes	Neuronal NFTs, neuropil threads	Biochemical composition	Ultrastructure
AD	–	±	–		±	–		+ 3
PEP	±	+	–	–	–	+ 3	PHF-tau 55+64+69(+72+74) kDA;	22 nm PHF
SSPE with NFTs	±	±	–	+	–	+ 2	3+4-R tau triplet	(15–18 nm SF)
PDC	–	±	–	±	–	+		
AGD	–	–	–		+	–	64+69 kDA, 4-R tau	9–18 nm SF + 25 nm TR
PSP	+ 3	±	–	+ 3	+	+	64+69 kDA, 4-R tau doublet, Exon 10	15–18 nm SF + 10–24 nm PHF
CBD	+ 2	±	+ 3	+ 2	+ 3	±	same (no Exon 3)	15–18 nm SF + 24 nm TR
Pick-type FTD	±	±	–	±	±	(+)	55+64 kDA, 3-R tau doublet (no Exon 10)	15–18 nm SF + 15–24 nm TR
FTDP-17	–	–	–	–	+	+ 2 +	variable: (*i*) mutations E-9, -12, -13, all 6 isoforms 55+64+69 (+74) kDA tau triplet; (*ii*) mutations E-10, 64+68+(72) kDA 4-R tau	10–22 nm TR + 15–18 nm SF
PSG	+	±	+	+	–	+	64+68+72 kDA 4-R tau triplet	23 nm TR
PPND	+	(+)	–	+	+	(+)	same	6–22 nm TR
MSTD							same	22–23 nm TR

–, absent; ±, rare; +, mild; +2, moderate; +3, abundant; (+) PHF, paired helical filaments; NFT, neurofibrillary tangles; SF, straight filaments; TR, twisted ribbons; SSPE, subacute sclerosing panencephalitis; FTD, frontotemporal dementia; MSTD, familial multiple system tauopathy with presenile dementia; FTDP-17, FTD and parkinsonism related to chromosome 17; R, repeat.

in PSP, whereas oligodendroglial tau inclusions mainly involving the white matter are similar in all these disorders. Predominant neocortical involvement is seen in CBD, while both neocortex and limbic system are affected in PiD and FTDP-17. The neocortex, except for primary motor areas, is comparatively spared in PSP, while basal ganglia and brainstem pathology is characteristic of PSP, CBD, FTDP-17, and PDC and is also common in PiD. Neurofilament-, αB-cystalline-, and tau-positive ballooned neurons are numerous in the neocortex of CBD and PiD and are also found in FTDP-17, but are rare in PSP. Taken together, the morphology and distribution of neuronal and glial lesions help delineate these disorders, but atypical and overlapping cases challenge inflexible definitions, and molecular and genetic advances may provide further insight into the nosology of these tauopathies *(113)*.

3.2. Comparative Pathology of PSP, CBD, and PD

All three tauopathies share some of their clinical features and also reveal common pathological changes, but also display unique morphological alterations and patterns that allow their recognition as distinct conditions.

3.2.1. PSP

PSP, the most common degenerative akinetic-rigid syndrome after PD, accounting for 3–6% of patients with parkinsonism, is a sporadic, rarely familial, late-onset disorder featured by rigidity, akinesia, postural instability, supranuclear vertical gaze palsy, and frontal lobe dysfunction with relatively spared recognition memory *(13,100)*. Macroscopic changes include atrophy of midbrain and pontine tegmentum with pigment loss from SN and LC and variable frontal lobe atrophy. Histologic features are multisystem neuronal loss and gliosis with widespread globose, non-flame-shaped tangles and neuropil threads composed of 10-24 nm (mean 15 nm) straight tubules with period constrictions at 80–120 nm, which differ from PHF in AD and from twisted ribbons in CBD, with additional 15–18 nm straight filaments in neurons and tau immunodeposits in "tufted" or thorn-shaped astrocytes and oligodendroglia ("coiled bodies," gliofibrillary bundles or thread-like processes), all ocurring throughout the neuraxis *(98,99)*. The brunt of the process is in the brain stem, subcortical nuclei, and cerebellar dentate nucleus with variable cortical involvement, which differs from that in AD. The highest density of tau pathology is seen in prefrontal and angular gyri, with decreasing intensity from frontal, cingulate, hippocampal to temporal and occipital cortex, and principal involvement of the deeper cortical layers contrasting from the bimodal distribution in AD, while entorhinal damage is similar *(101)*. Nigrostriatal dysfunction is a key feature in PSP, with 80–90% loss of dopamine, tyrosine hydroxylase (TH), and postsynaptic D2 receptors in the striatum, while the mesocorticolimbic system is relatively spared. Severe damage to internal and external globus pallidus, SN pars reticulata, and subthalamic nucleus cause considerable dysfunction of the striatal efflux to the motor thalamus *(102)*. Loss of cholinergic neurons in striatum, NBM, and brainstem nuclei with loss of cholinergic innervation of the thalamus may play a role in motor, equilibrium, and cognitive dysfunction *(103)*, while mental decline is ascribed to: (*i*) subcortical pathology with dysfunction of striatoprefrontal circuits due to degeneration of basal ganglia and brainstem tegmental nuclei *(104,105)*; and (*ii*) neuroglial tau pathology in prefrontal areas *(7,12)*. However, no differences in subcortical tau pathology have been observed in PSP cases with and without cognitive impairment, and cortical changes in some PSP patients bear no clear relationship to the degree of cognitive involvement *(106)*. Postmortem diagnosis of PSP is based on consensus criteria *(107)*, the validity of which has been reviewed recently *(13,108)*. Recent studies of the genetics of PSP suggest mutations at intron 6 of the tau gene *(99,109)*.

3.2.2. CBD

CBD, a rare, usually sporadic late-onset disorder with rigid-akinetic syndrome, asymmetric limb apraxia, dystonia, action tremor and myoclonus, pseudobulbar palsy, gaze palsy, and cognitive disturbance may clinically resemble PD or PSP, but also shows clinical differences to PSP *(9,109,110)*. Morphologic features are lobar frontal or parietal atrophy, severe neuronal loss and gliosis in cortex and basal ganglia with microvacuolation of superficial cortical layers and tau-positive ballooned neurons, NFT-like skein inclusions, widespread neuropil threads, and tau-positive astrocytic plaques in the white matter *(98,99)*. Basal ganglia and SN show severe degeneration, and NFT-like neuronal tau deposits are similar to those in PSP, but different from AD-NFTs and Pick bodies *(98,99,110)*. However, recent studies detecting tau isoforms, with sequence endoded by but not without exon 10, suggest that only 4-R tau isoforms aggregate into filaments in both CBD and PSP *(111)*. Cortical inclusions in CBD with the highest density in prefrontal cortex, basal ganglia, thalamus, and brainstem tegmentum point to similarities with PSP, while large numbers of thread-like processes and absence of astrocytic plaques in white matter distinguish PSP from CBD. CBD may be difficult to be distinguished from PiD, with variable overlap between both disorders *(110,112)*, although there are several morphological differences, e.g., Pick-like bodies in CBD are usually absent in the dentate fascia of hippocampus and astrocytic plaques are absent in PiD. Revised consensus criteria for the morphologic diagnosis of CBD are in print *(113)*, and their validation is in progress. Mental decline with a major dysexecutive syndrome are related to degeneration of basal ganglia and frontal cortex, while asymmetric apraxia may be due to tau-related degeneration of prefrontal and parietal cortices. While in PSP several mutations at intron 6 of the tau gene have been reported *(13,109,114)*, no such changes are currently known for CBD, but rare familial forms recently have been classified as FTDP-17 *(99,115)*.

3.2.3. PiD

PiD, or Pick-type of FTD, a rare sporadic or familial dementing disorder, developing extrapyramidal signs in late stages, is macroscopically featured by sharply circumscribed severe frontotemporal lobar atrophy with relative sparing of the sensorimotor area and posterior portion of the superior temporal cortex. There is severe neuronal loss in frontal and limbic areas, with spongy vacuolation and gliosis, and abundant swollen neurons (Pick cells) with argyrophilic tau-positive cytoplamic inclusions (Pick bodies) composed of 3-R tau forming 15–24 nm straight or twisted tubules *(97,116)*. Recent ultrastructural analysis of PiD-derived tau filaments identified three morphologically distinct populations which, however, were indistinguishable from AD-PHFs in mass/nm length and density of the intertwisted filaments *(117)*. They particularly involve the allocortex (granule cell layer of dentate gyrus, CA 1 sector of hippocampus, and entorhinal cortex) and layers 2 and 4 of frontal and temporal cortex. This pattern differs from both AD and non-Pick FTD (Fig. 6), while neuritic AD pathology frequently occurs in PiD *(118)*. Neuronal loss and gliosis with or without Pick bodies are seen in amygdaloid and caudate nuclei and less, in the striopallidonigral system, hypothalamus, brainstem and cerebellum *(116)*. While severe SN damage with parkinsonism is rare and manly occurs in advanced stages of disease *(119)*, single cases with brainstem LBs and FTD with Pick bodies *(120,121)* and of PD with late PiD have been reported *(122)*. The majority of PiD cases does not show mutations of the tau gene, but single cases with mutations at codon 257 or 389 with predominance of either 3- or 4-R domains of the tau gene without aminoterminal inserts have been described recently *(123–125)*. Further studies will be necessary to explain the possibility whether CBD, PSP, PiD, and other frontotemporal degenerations repre-sent distinctive entities or phenotypes of the same disease as a result of modifying gene or gene polymorphism *(126,127)*.

3.3. Distinction Between PSP, Postencephalitic Parkinsonism, and Guam-PD Complex

According to recent immunohistochemical studies, both PEP and PDC are considered to be tauopathies *(128,129)*, although α-S inclusions in amygdala have been reported in brains of PDC patients *(130)*.

3.3.1. PEP

PEP, the late sequela of encephalitis lethargica von Economo and other viral encephalitis, is, at present, rarely seen, but sporadic cases have been reported recently *(128,131–134)*. The clinical features are rather characteristic to enable diagnosis during life *(134)*. Despite epidemiological evidence of an

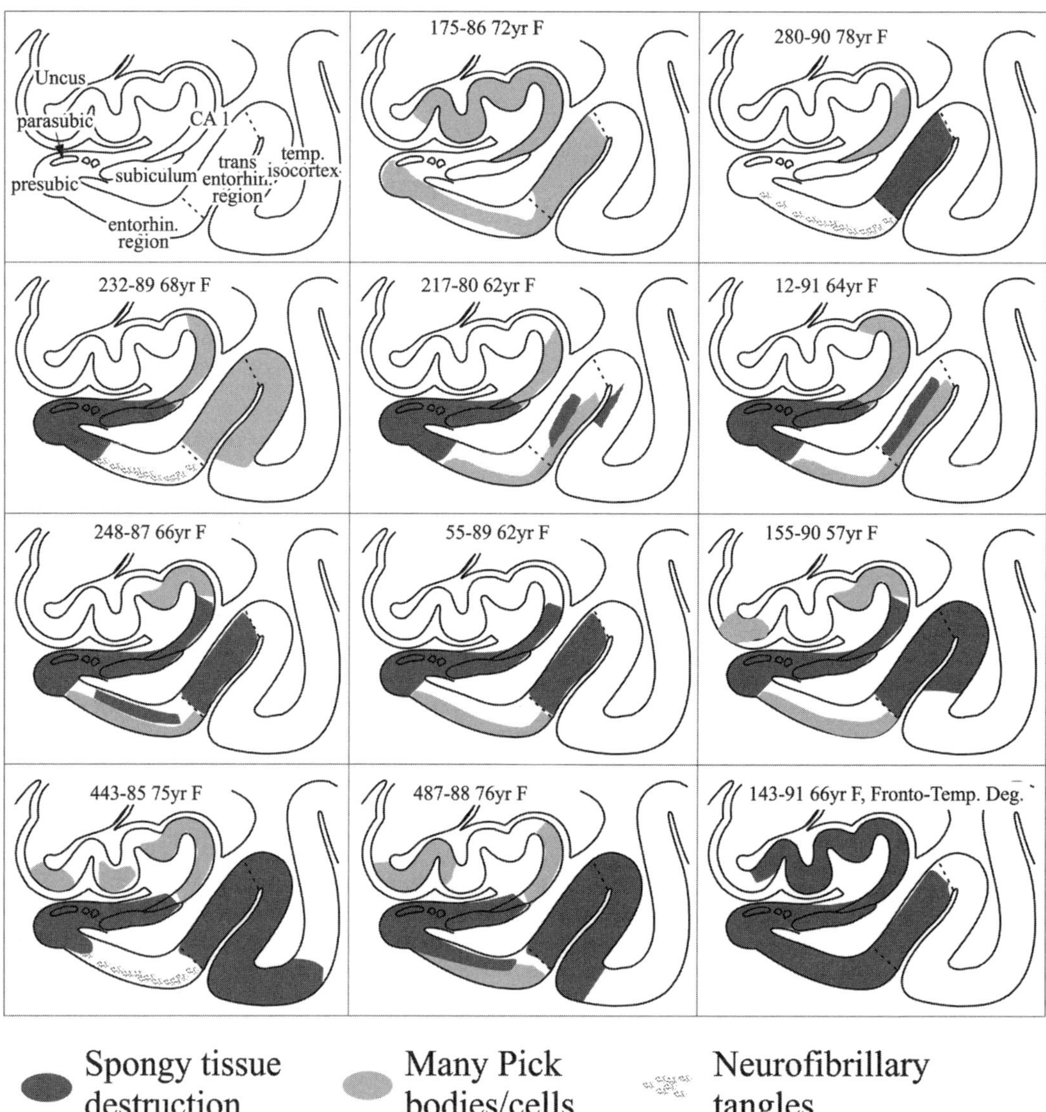

Fig. 6. Distribution of lesions in the hippocampal and parahippocampal formation in PD and one case of frontotemporal degeneration.

influenza virus infection, even with modern molecular methods, this has never been proven definitely *(135)*. The brain may show some mild generalized atrophy with depigmentation of SN and LC. Histology reveals severe, almost complete, and diffuse neuronal loss in SN pars compacta and other parts of the rostral brainstem, e.g., midbrain raphe and pontine tegmentum, with diffuse gliosis and widespread occurrence of tau-positive NFTs and neuropil threads with morphological features identical to those in AD. In addition, they show ubiquitin immunoreactivity, thus differing from NFTs in PSP and CBD (Table 7). Tau-positive astroglia is also seen in affected areas, whereas "tufted astrocytes" and ballooned cells, Pick bodies, and α-S immunoreactive LBs or glial inclusions are absent *(128)*. In contrast to PSP and CBD, there is very little tau pathology in the white matter. The distribution of subcortical tau-positive neuronal and glial inclusions differs from that of other tauopathies including

PSP, e.g., by sparing or only mild involvement of several nuclei usually affected in PSP: striopallidum, thalamus, oculomotor complex, trochlear, vestibular nuclei, pontine basis, inferior olives, and dentate nucleus. However, cholinergic supranuclear centers of gaze movement in some cases of PEP show similar lesions as in PSP, causing gaze palsy and lid apraxia *(133)*. Cortical pathology is common, with tangles mainly in hippocampus, entorhinal, temporal, frontal, and insular areas and preservation of precentral, cingulate, and parietal regions; prominent involvement of layers 2 and 3 differs from that in AD *(136)*.

3.3.1. PDC

PDC, the endemic combination of parkinsonism with dementia in the Chamorro population of Guam, on the Kii peninsula, and in West Guinea, is morphologically featured by frontal and temporal lobe and basal ganglia atrophy, rarely mimicking that in Huntington's disease, and prominent depigmentation of SN and LC. Widespread neuronal loss and gliosis in hippocampus, amygdala, NBM, striopallidum, thalamus, hypothalamus, SN, brainstem tegmentum, and dentate nucleus, are accompanied by abundant NFTs, in hippocampus by granulovacuolar degeneration and Hirano bodies *(137)*. The ultrastructure and biochemistry of NFTs exhibiting twisted tubular structures composed of a 60-, 64-, 68-kDa tau triplet is identical to those in AD; the tau gene shows no mutation *(129)*. In addition, a small number of α-S-positive inclusions reminiscent of cortical LBs have been observed in hippocampus, temporal cortex, and amygdala, often intermingled with pretangles or NFTs *(130)*, which is not seen in CBD, and also showing many pretangles in SN *(138)*. In comparison to PSP and CBD, only a few threads are present in PDC, where many SN neurons degenerate and may disappear via NFTs *(139)*. The distribution pattern of tau pathology, with involvement of hippocampus, frontal and temporal association cortices, brainstem tegmentum, and base, in PDC differs from those in PSP, CBD, and AD, and the loss of large neurons in neostriatum and nucleus accumbens is more severe than in PSP. The latter may be linked to marked degeneration of limbic areas *(138)* and, together with additional subcortical pathology, could be the cause of rapidly progressing cognitive decline in PDC *(140)*. The spinal cord in PDC showing degeneration of the lateral columns and neuronal loss and NFTs in motorneurons is the basis of ALS, which may present as ALS/PDC, a phenotypic variant of a tauopathy caused by genetic abnormalities *(129)*. Despite some morphological similarities, PDC is distinctly different from PSP and CBD, while some similarities between the latter two diseases indicate some common pathomechanisms *(139)*.

3.4. Variable Pathology of FTDP-17

The discovery of more than 20 mutations in the gene encoding the microtubule-associated tau protein in FTDP-17 has shown that dysfunction of the tau protein causes neurodegeneration and dementia *(141,142)*. The disorders caused by mutation of the tau gene in exon 10 (N279K, K280, L284L, P301L, and S305N) are characterized by considerable clinical and morphological heterogeneity. Common clinical manifestations include behavioral and cognitive disturbances, extrapyramidal disorders with parkinsonism (bradykinesia, rigidity, postural instability, with often poor response to levadopa [L-dopa] therapy) appearing early or late in the course, dystonia, oculomotor, and other disorders. Neuropathology shows atrophy of frontal and temporal lobes with neuronal loss and gliosis in basal ganglia, SN, ballooned neurons, and tau deposits in neurons and glia *(141–148)*. In one family with a P301S mutation, there were two different phenotypes, FTD and CBD *(148)*, whereas mutation in codon 305 (S305S) produced a clinical picture with early postural instability and vertical gaze palsy, mild frontotemporal atrophy, and abundant tau pathology with straight and twisted filaments in the basal ganglia, thalamus, and midbrain, reminiscent of PSP *(114)*. Another sporadic multiple system tauopathy with no mutations in either exons 9–13 was morphologically associated with severe temporal lobe atrophy, numerous globular neuronal and glial tau-positive inclusions composed of straight filaments and a 64- and 68-kDa tau doublet in the cortex, nigra, globus pallidus, subthalamic nucleus, and cerebellar dentate nucleus, which is a distribution similar to PSP, but without accompanying neuronal

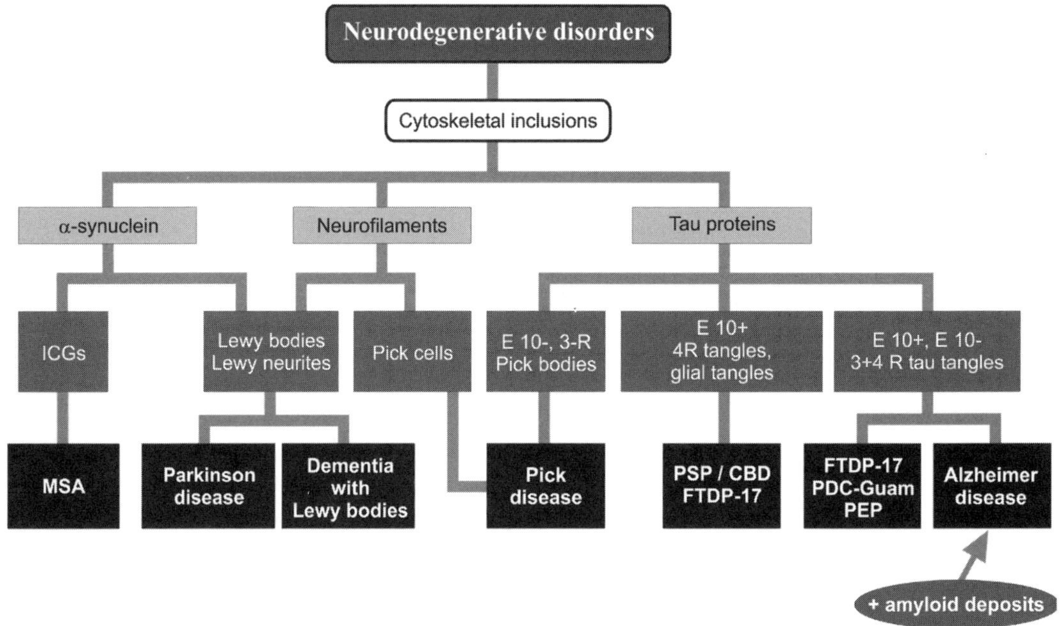

Fig. 7. Schematic distribution of neurodegenerative disorders with α-Synuclein and tau deposition according to major cytoskeletal depositions.

loss or gliosis *(127)*. These and other data underscore the variability in clinical and pathological expression resulting from a given mutation in tau *(149)*. In conclusion, tau mutations, so far, have been shown to give rise to FTD, AD, PD, PSP, CBD, PiD, and progressive subcortical gliosis *(141,148)*. The factors determining these different clinicopathologic phenotypes remain to be discovered.

4. CONCLUSIONS

Dementia in movement disorders is caused by a variety of genetic and neuropathological conditions featured by progressive neuron and synapse loss often associated with cytopathological changes involving specific cortical and subcortical systems (Fig. 7). These neuronal and glial inclusions show characteristic biochemistry, immunoreactions, and ultrastructure indicating cytoskeletal mismetabolism. They are important diagnostic signposts that, in addition to the distribution pattern of neurodegeneration and cytoskeletal pathology, indicate specific vulnerability of neuronal–glial populations, the genetic backgrounds for only some of them have been elucidated so far.

According to the major components of cytoskeletal changes, one can distinguish two major types of movement disorders:

1. Synucleinopathies showing intracytoplasmic inclusions of α-S in Lewy bodies and neurites, the subcellular hallmarks of LB disorders, e.g., PD and DLB, often associated with dementia. In both PD and DLB, the distinction of which despite recent consensus criteria is still debatable, neurodegeneration of subcorticocortical networks (dopamine, noradrenaline, serotonin, and, in particular, cholinergic forebrain systems), together with limbic and/or cortical LB and neuritic AD-type pathologies contribute to cognitive decline, the combination of both indicating a more severe dementia. In both PD and DLB, superimposed neuritic AD pathology is an important prognostic factor reducing survival. DLB, according to the severity of AD lesions, can be separated into diffuse forms and LBV of AD, both showing considerable clinical and morphological differences, but the nosological position of DLB and its pathogenic relationship to both PD and AD is still under discussion.

2. Tauopathies are a heterogenous group of neurodegenerative disorders showing deposition of different isoforms of the hyperphosphorylated microtubule-associated tau protein. They include PSP, CBD, PiD, PEP, DPC, and FTDP-17. All these disorders show multisystem degeneration with tau deposits in neurons, neurites, astroglia, and oligodendroglia of 4-R and, rarely, 3-R tau. In many of these disorders, extensive subcortical tau pathology with involvement of the basal ganglia, striatofrontal, and limbiccortical loops are important factors of mental decline, but may be variably associated with cortical neuron and synapse loss or superimposed AD pathology. The similarities and distinctions of neuropathology in the different types of tauopathies, often associated with different mutations of the tau gene, are critically reviewed.

There are many overlaps and relationships between neurodegenerative movement disorders variably associated with dementia causing considerable differential diagnostic problems that may be clarified by future molecular and genetic studies, and the evolving entities will widely replace currently used clinicopathological classifications.

REFERENCES

1. Louis, E.D., Marder, K., Cote, L., Tang, M., and Mayeux, R. (1997) Mortality from Parkinson disease. *Arch. Neurol.* **54,** 260–264.
2. Aarsland, D., Larsen, J.P., Tandberg, E., and Laake, K. (2000) Predictors of nursing home placement in Parkinson's disease: a population-based, prospective study. *J. Am. Geriatr. Soc.* **48,** 938–942.
3. Hughes, T.A., Ross, H.F., Musa, S., et al. (2000) A 10-year study of the incidence of and factors predicting dementia in Parkinson's disease. *Neurology* **54,** 1596–1602.
4. Aarsland, D., Andersen, K., Larsen, J.P., Lolk, A., Nielsen, H., and Kragh-Sorensen, P. (2001) Risk of dementia in Parkinson's disease: a community-based, prospective study. *Neurology* **56,** 730–736.
5. Dubois, B. and Pillon, B. (2000) Dementia in Parkinson's disease, in *Mental Dysfunctions in Parkinson's Disease II* (Wolters, E.C., Scheltens, P., and Berendse, H.W., eds.), Academic Pharmaceutical Productions, Utrecht, pp. 165–176.
6. Connor, D.J., Salmon, D.P., Sandy, T.J., Galasko, D., Hansen, L.A., and Thal, L.J. (1998) Cognitive profiles of autopsy-confirmed Lewy body variant vs pure Alzheimer disease. *Arch. Neurol.* **55,** 994–1000.
7. Bergeron, C., Davis, A., and Lang, A.E. (1998) Corticobasal ganglionic degeneration and progressive supranuclear palsy presenting with cognitive decline. *Brain Pathol.* **8,** 355–365.
8. Kompoliti, K., Goetz, C.G., Boeve, B.F., et al. (1998) Clinical presentation and pharmacological therapy in corticobasal degeneration. *Arch. Neurol.* **55,** 957–961.
9. Grimes, D.A., Lang, A.E., and Bergeron, C.B. (1999) Dementia as the most common presentation of cortical-basal ganglionic degeneration. *Neurology* **53,** 1969–1974.
10. Gomez-Tortosa, E., del Barrio, A., Garcia Ruiz, P.J., et al. (1998) Severity of cognitive impairment in juvenile and late-onset Huntington disease. *Arch. Neurol.* **55,** 835–843.
11. Soliveri, P., Monza, D., Paridi, D., et al. (1999) Cognitive and magnetic resonance imaging aspects of corticobasal degeneration and progressive supranuclear palsy. *Neurology* **53,** 502–507.
12. Bigio, E.H., Brown, D.F., and White, C. L. III (1999) Progressive supranuclear palsy with dementia: cortical pathology. *J. Neuropathol. Exp. Neurol.* **58,** 359–364.
13. Litvan, I., Dickson, D.W., Buttner-Ennever, J.A., et al. (2000) Research goals in progressive supranuclear palsy. First International Brainstorming Conference on PSP. *Mov. Disord.* **15,** 446–458.
14. Lopez, O.L., Hamilton, R.L., Becker, J.T., Wisniewski, S., Kaufer, D.I., and DeKosky, S.T. (2000) Severity of cognitive impairment and the clinical diagnosis of AD with Lewy bodies. *Neurology* **54,** 1780–1787.
15. Del Ser, T., Hachinski, V., Merskey, H., and Munoz, D.G. (2001) Clinical and pathologic features of two groups of patients with dementia with Lewy bodies: effect of coexisting Alzheimer-type lesion load. *Alzheimer Dis. Assoc. Disord.* **15,** 31–44.
16. Duda, J.E., Lee, V.M.Y., and Trojanowski, J.Q. (2000) Neuropathology of synuclein aggregates. New insights into mechanism of neurodegenerative diseases. *J. Neurosci. Res.* **61,** 121–127.
17. Polymeropoulos, M.H., Lavedan, C., Leroy, E., et al. (1997) Mutation in the α-synuclein gene identified in families with Parkinson's disease. *Science* **276,** 2045–2047.
18. Kruger, R., Kuhn, W., Muller, T., et al. (1998) Ala30Pro mutation in the gene encoding alpha-synuclein in Parkinson's disease. *Nat. Genet.* **18,** 106–108.
19. Galvin, J.E., Lee, V.M., and Trojanowski, J.Q. (2001) Synucleinopathies: clinical and pathological implications. *Arch. Neurol.* **58,** 186–190.
20. Jellinger, K.A. (2000) Morphological substrates of mental dysfunction in Lewy body disease: an update. *J. Neural Transm.* **59(Suppl.),** 185–212.
21. Ala, T.A., Yang, K.H., Sung, J.H., and Frey, W.H. II (2000) Inconsistency between severe substantia nigra degeneration with Lewy bodies and clinical parkinsonism in dementia patients: a cliniconeuropathological study. *Acta Neuropathol.* **99,** 511–516.
22. Braak, H. and Braak, E. (1991) Neuropathological stage of Alzheimer-related changes. *Acta Neuropathol.* **82,** 239–259.

23. Delacourte, A., David, J.P., Sergeant, N., et al. (1999) The biochemical pathway of neurofibrillary degeneration in aging and Alzheimer's disease. *Neurology* **52,** 1158–1165.
24. Mindham, R.H.S., Ahmed, S.W.A., and Clough, C.G. (1982) A controlled study of dementia in Parkinson's disease. *J. Neurol. Neurosurg. Psychiatry* **45,** 969–974.
25. Jellinger, K. (1987) Neuropathological substrates of Alzheimer's disease and Parkinson's disease. *J. Neural Transm.* **24(Suppl.),** 109–129.
26. Piccirilli, M., D'Alessandro, P., Finali, G., and Piccinin, G.L. (1994) Neuropsychological follow-up of parkinsonian patients with and without cognitive impairment. *Dementia* **5,** 17–22.
27. Mindham, R.H. (1999) The place of dementia in Parkinson's disease: a methodologic saga. *Adv. Neurol.* **80,** 403–408.
28. Louis, E.D., Klatka, L.A., Lui, Y., and Fahn, S. (1997) Comparison of extrapyramidal features in 31 pathologically confirmed cases of diffuse Lewy body disease and 34 pathologically confirmed cases of Parkinson's disease. *Neurology* **48,** 376–380.
29. Mirra, S.S., Heyman, A., McKeel, D., et al. (1991) The consortium to establish a registry for Alzheimer's disease (CERAD). Part II. Standardization of the neuropathologic assessment of Alzheimer's disease. *Neurology* **41,** 479–486.
30. Hyman, B.T. and Trojanowski, J.G. (1997) Editorial on Consensus recommendations for the postmortem diagnosis of Alzheimer disease from the National Institute on Aging and the Reagan Institute Working Group on diagnostic criteria for the neuropathological assessment of Alzheimer's disease. *J. Neuropathol. Exp. Neurol.* **56,** 1095–1097.
31. Jellinger, K.A., Seppi, K., Wenning, G.K., and Poewe, W. (2002) Impact of coexistent Alzheimer pathology on the natural history of Parkinson's disease. *J. Neural Transm.* **109,** 329–339.
32. Diamond, S.G., Markham, C.H., Hoehn, M.M., McDowell, F.H., and Muenter, M.D. (1989) Effect of age at onset on progression and mortality in Parkinson's disease. *Neurology* **39,** 1187–1190.
33. Uitti, R.J., Ahlskog, J.E., Maraganore, D.M., et al. (1993) Levodopa therapy and survival in idiopathic Parkinson's disease: Olmsted County project. *Neurology* **43,** 1918–1926.
34. Østbye, T., Hill, G., and Steenhuis, R. (1999) Mortality in elderly Canadians with and without dementia. A 5-year follow-up. *Neurology* **53,** 521–526.
35. Perry, E., Court, J., Goodchild, R., et al. (1998) Clinical neurochemistry: developments in dementia research based on brain bank material. *J. Neural Transm.* **105,** 915–933.
36. Jellinger, K. (1988) The pedunculopontine nucleus in Parkinson's disease, progressive supranuclear palsy, and Alzheimer's disease. *J. Neurol. Neurosurg. Psychiatry* **51,** 540–543.
37. Zweig, R.M., Jankel, W.R., Hedreen, J.C., Mayeux, R., and Price, D.L. (1989) The pedunculopontine nucleus in Parkinson's disease. *Ann. Neurol.* **26,** 41–46.
38. Winn, P., Brown, V.J., and Inglis, W.L. (1997) On the relationships between the striatum and the pedunculopontine tegmental nucleus. *Crit. Rev. Neurobiol.* **11,** 241–261.
39. Sawamoto, N., Honda, M., Hankawa, T., et al. (2001) Pathophysiology of cognitive slowing in Parkinson's disease: a PET study. *Neurology* **56(Suppl. 3),** A269.
40. Litvan, I., Paulsen, J.S., Mega, M.S., and Cummings, J.L. (1998) Neuropsychiatric assessment of patients with hyperkinetic and hypokinetic movement disorders. *Arch. Neurol.* **55,** 1313–1319.
41. Wolters, E.C. and Rrancot, C.M.J.E. (1999) The concept of mental dysfunction in Parkinson's disease, in *Mental Dysfunctions in Parkinson's Disease II* (Wolters, E.C., Scheltens, P., and Berendse, H.W., eds.), Academic Pharmaceutical Productions, Utrecht, pp. 35–48.
42. Zweig, R.M., Cardillo, J.E., Cohen, M., Giere, S., and Hedreen, J.C. (1993) The locus ceruleus and dementia in Parkinson's disease. *Neurology* **43,** 986–991.
43. Hoogendijk, W.J., Pool, C.W., Troost, D., van Zwieten, E., and Swaab, D.F. (1995) Image analyser-assisted morphometry of the locus coeruleus in Alzheimer's disease, Parkinson's disease and amyotrophic lateral sclerosis. *Brain* **118,** 131–143.
44. Chen, C.P., Eastwood, S.L., Hope, T., McDonald, B., Francis, P.T., and Esiri, M.M. (2000) Immunocytochemical study of the dorsal and median raphe nuclei in patients with Alzheimer's disease prospectively assessed for behavioural changes. *Neuropathol. Appl. Neurobiol.* **26,** 347–355.
45. Mattila, P.M., Rinne, J.O., Helenius, H., Dickson, D., and Röyttä, M. (1999) Neuritic degeneration in the hippocampus and amygdala in Parkinson's disease in relation to Alzheimer pathology. *Acta Neuropathol.* **98,** 157–164.
46. Churchyard, A. and Lees, A.J. (1997) The relationship between dementia and direct involvement of the hippocampus and amygdala in Parkinson's disease. *Neurology* **49,** 1570–1576.
47. Braak, H., Braak, E., Yilmazer, D., et al. (1994) Amygdala pathology in Parkinson's disease. *Acta Neuropathol.* **88,** 493–500.
48. Iseki, E., Kato, M., Marui, W., Ueda, K., and Kosaka, K. (2001) A neuropathological study of the disturbance of the nigro-amygdaloid connections in brains from patients with dementia with Lewy bodies. *J. Neurol. Sci.* **185,** 129–134.
49. Vereecken, T.H., Vogels, O.J., and Nieuwenhuys, R. (1994) Neuron loss and shrinkage in the amygdala in Alzheimer's disease. *Neurobiol. Aging* **15,** 45–54.
50. Braak, H., Braak, E., Yilmazer, D., de Vos, R.A., Jansen, E.N., and Bohl, J. (1996) Pattern of brain destruction in Parkinson's and Alzheimer's diseases. *J. Neural. Transm.* **103,** 455–490.
51. Irizarry, M.C., Growdon, W., Gomez-Isla, T., et al. (1998) Nigral and cortical Lewy bodies and dystrophic nigral neurites in Parkinson's disease and cortical Lewy body disease contain α-synuclein immunoreactivity. *J. Neuropathol. Exp. Neurol.* **57,** 334–337.

52. Mattila, P.M., Rinne, J.O., Helenius, H., Dickson, D.W., and Roytta, M. (2000) α-Synuclein-immunoreactive cortical Lewy bodies are associated with cognitive impairment in Parkinson's disease. *Acta Neuropathol.* **100,** 285–290.
53. Hurtig, H.I., Trojanowski, J.Q., Galvin, J., et al. (2000) α-Synuclein cortical Lewy bodies correlate with dementia in Parkinson's disease. *Neurology* **54,** 1916–1921.
54. Harding, A.J. and Halliday, G.M. (2001) Cortical Ley body pathology in the diagnosis of dementia. *Acta Neuropathol.* **102,** 355–372.
55. McKeith, I.G., Galasko, D., Kosaka, K., et al. (1996) Consensus guidelines for the clinical and pathological diagnosis of dementia with Lewy bodies (DLB), report of the consortium on DLB International Workshop. *Neurology* **47,** 1113–1124.
56. McKeith, I.G., Perry, E.K., Perry, R.H., and the Consortium on Dementia with Lewy bodies (1999) Report of the Second Dementia with Lewy body International Workshop (1999) diagnosis and treatment. *Neurology* **53,** 902–905.
57. Ince, P.G., Perry, E.K., and Morris, C.M. (1998) Dementia with Lewy bodies. A distinct non-Alzheimer dementia syndrome? *Brain Pathol.* **8,** 299–324.
58. Calderon, J., Perry, R.J., Erzinclioglu, S.W., Berrios, G.E., Dening, T.R., and Hodges, J.R. (2001) Perception, attention, and working memory are disproportionately impaired in dementia with Lewy bodies compared with Alzheimer's disease. *J. Neurol. Neurosurg. Psychiatry* **70,** 157–164.
59. Holmes, C., Cairns, N., Lantos, P., and Mann, A. (1999) Validity of current clinical criteria for Alzheimer's disease, vascular dementia and dementia with Lewy bodies. *Br. J. Psychiatry* **174,** 45–50.
60. Gomez-Isla, T., Growdon, W.B., McNamara, M., et al. (1999) Clinicopathologic correlates in temporal cortex in dementia with Lewy bodies. *Neurology* **53,** 2003–2009.
61. Seppi, K., Wenning, G.K., Jellinger, K., et al. (2000) Disease progression of dementia with Lewy bodies: a clinicopathological study. *Neurology* **54(Suppl. 3),** A391.
62. Hohl, U., Tiraboschi, P., Hansen, L.A., Thal, L.J., and Corey-Bloom, J. (2000) Diagnostic accuracy of dementia with Lewy bodies. *Arch. Neurol.* **57,** 347–351.
63. Seppi, K., Jellinger, K., Litvan, I., et al. (2000) Accuracy of the clinical criteria of the Consortium on dementia with Lewy Bodies: a clinicopathological study. *Neurology* **54(Suppl. 3),** A127.
64. Wenning, G.K., Seppi, K., Jellinger, K., et al. (2000) Survival of patients with dementia with Lewy bodies: a meta-analysis of 236 postmortem confirmed cases. *Neurology* **54(Suppl. 3),** A391.
65. Chow, T.M., Kaufer, D.L., Lopez, O.L., Hamilton, R.L., Becker, J.T., and DeKosky, S.T. (2000) Temporal evolution of Lewy body phenotype in autopsy-confirmed cases of Alzheimer's disease and dementia with Lewy bodies. *Neurology* **54(Suppl. 3),** A300–A301.
66. Gomez-Tortosa, E., Newell, K., Irizarry, M.C., Albert, M., Growdon, J.H., and Hyman, B.T. (1999) Clinical and quantitative pathologic correlates of dementia with Lewy bodies. *Neurology* **53,** 1284–1291.
67. Harding, A.J. and Halliday, G.M. (1998) Simplified neuropathological diagnosis of dementia with Lewy bodies. *Neuropathol. Appl. Neurobiol.* **24,** 195–201.
68. Jellinger, K.A. and Bancher, C. (1996) Dementia with Lewy bodies: relationship to Parkinson's and Alzheimer's diseases, in *Dementia with Lewy Bodies. Clinical, Pathological, and Treatment Issues* (Perry, R.H., McKeith, I.G., and Perry, E. K., eds.), Cambridge, University Press, New York, pp. 268–286.
69. Samuel, W., Alford, M., Hofstetter, C.R., and Hansen, L. (1997) Dementia with Lewy bodies versus pure Alzheimer's disease: differences in cognition, neuropathology, cholinergic dysfunction, and synaptic density. *J. Neuropathol. Exp. Neurol.* **56,** 499–508.
70. Perry, E., Court, J., and Goodchild, R. (1998) Clinical neurochemistry: developments in dementia research based on brain bank material. *J. Neural Transm.* **105,** 915–934.
71. Lippa, C.F., Smith, T.W., and Perry, E. (1999) Dementia with Lewy bodies: choline acetyltransferase parallels nucleus basalis pathology. *J. Neural Transm.* **106,** 525–535.
72. Shiozaki, K., Iseki, E., Uchiyama, H., et al. (1999) Alterations of muscarinic acetylcholine receptor subtypes in diffuse lewy body disease: relation to Alzheimer's disease. *J. Neurol. Neurosurg. Psychiatry* **67,** 209–213.
73. Lippa, C.F., Ozawa, K., Mann, D.M.A., et al. (1999) Deposition of β-amyloid subtypes 40 and 42 differentiates dementia with Lewy bodies from Alzheimer disease. *Arch. Neurol.* **56,** 1111–1118.
74. Hansen, L.A., Masliah, E., Galasko, D., and Terry, R.D. (1993) Plaque-only Alzheimer disease is usually the Lewy body variant and vice versa. *J. Neuropathol. Exp. Neurol.* **52,** 648–654.
75. Gearing, M. and Mirra, S. (1997) Alzheimer's disease with concomitant Parkinson's disease changes: two subgroups defined by neurofibrillary pathology. *J. Neuropathol. Exp. Neurol.* **56,** 616.
76. Brown, D.F., Dababo, M.A., Bigio, E.H., et al. (1998) Neuropathologic evidence that the Lewy body variant of Alzheimer disease represents coexistence of Alzheimer disease and idiopathic Parkinson disease. *J. Neuropathol. Exp. Neurol.* **57,** 39–46.
77. Rosenberg, C.K., Cummings, T.J., Saunders, A.M., Widico, C., McIntyre, L.M., and Hulette, C.M. (2001) Dementia with Lewy bodies and Alzheimer's disease. *Acta Neuropathol.* **102,** 621–626.
78. Hansen, L.A., Daniel, S.E., Wilcock, G.K., and Love, S. (1998) Frontal cortical synaptophysin in Lewy body diseases: relation to Alzheimer's disease and dementia. *J. Neurol. Neurosurg. Psychiatry* **64,** 653–656.
79. Tiraboschi, P., Hansen, L.A., Alford, M., et al. (2001) Early and widespread cholinergic losses differentiate dementia with Lewy bodies from Alzheimer's disease. *Neurology* **56(Suppl. 3),** A300.
80. Newell, K., Hyman, B., Growdon, J., and Hedley-Whyte, E.T. (1997) Evaluation of the NIA-Reagan Institute criteria for the neuropathological diagnosis of Alzheimer disease. *J. Neuropathol. Exp. Neurol.* **56,** 593.

81. Newell, K.L., Hyman, B.T., Growdon, J.H., and Hedley-Whyte, E.T. (1999) Application of the National Institute on Aging (NIA)-Reagan Institute criteria for the neuropathological diagnosis of Alzheimer disease. *J. Neuropathol. Exp. Neurol.* **58,** 1147–1155.
82. Harding, A.J., Kril, J.J., and Halliday, G.M. (1999) Practical measures to simplyfy the Braak tangle staging method for routine pathological screening. *Acta Neuropathol.* **99,** 199–208.
83. Hamilton, R.L. (2000) Lewy bodies in Alzheimer's disease: a neuropathological review of 145 cases using α-synuclein immunohistochemistry. *Brain Pathol.* **10,** 378–384.
84. Popescu, A. and Lippa, C.F. (2001) Lewy bodies in the amygdala: α-synuclein expression is increased in specific neurodegenerative diseases. *Neurology* **56(Suppl. 3),** 177–178.
85. Haroutunian, V., Serby, M., Purohit, D.P., et al. (2000) Contribution of Lewy body inclusions to dementia in patients with and without Alzheimer disease neuropathological conditions. *Arch. Neurol.* **57,** 1145–1150.
86. Mattila, P.M., Roytta, M., Torikka, H., Dickson, D.W., and Rinne, J.O. (1998) Cortical Lewy bodies and Alzheimer-type changes in patients with Parkinson's disease. *Acta Neuropathol.* **95,** 576–582.
87. Krüger, R., Vieira-Saecker, A.M., Kuhn, W., et al. (1999) Increased susceptibility to sporadic Parkinson's disease by a certain combined α-synuclein/apolipoprotein E genotype. *Ann. Neurol.* **45,** 611–617.
88. Mizuno, Y., Hattori, N., Kitada, T., et al. (1999) Genetic aspects in Parkinson's disease, in *Mental Dysfunction in Parkinson's Disease II* (Wolters, E.C., Scheltens, P., and Berendse, H.W., eds.), Academic Pharmaceutical Productions, Utrecht, pp. 49–61.
89. Honig, L.S. and Chambliss, D.D. (2001) Dementia with Lewy bodies (DLB) symptoms may relate to diffusely increased α-synuclein expression rather than Lewy inclusions. *Neurology* **56(Suppl. 3),** A176–A177.
90. Harrington, C.R., Louwagie, J., Rossau, R., et al. (1994) Influence of apolipoprotein E genotype on senile dementia of the Alzheimer and Lewy body types. Significance for etiological theories of Alzheimer's disease. *Am. J. Pathol.* **145,** 1472–1484.
91. Galasko, D., Saitoh, T., Xia Y., et al. (1994) The apolipoprotein E allele ε4 is overrepresented in patients with the Lewy body variant of Alzheimer's disease. *Neurology* **44,** 1950–1951.
92. Chinnery, P.F., Taylor, G.A., Howell, N., et al. (2000) Mitochondrial DNA haplogroups and susceptibility to AD and dementia with Lewy bodies. *Neurology* **25,** 302–304.
93. Lamb, H., Christie, J., Singleton, A.B., et al. (1998) Apolipoprotein E and α-1 antichymotrypsin polymorphism genotyping in Alzheimer's disease and in dementia with Lewy bodies. Distinctions between diseases. *Neurology* **50,** 388–391.
94. Tanaka, S., Chen, X., Xia, Y., et al. (1998) Association of CYP2D microsatellite polymorphism with Lewy body variant of Alzheimer's disease. *Neurology* **50,** 1556–1562.
95. Cervilla, J.A., Russ, C., Holmes, C., Aitchison, K., et al. (1999) CYP2D6 polymorphisms in Alzheimer's disease, with and without extrapyramidal signs, showing no apolipoprotein E epsilon 4 effect modification. *Biol. Psychiatry* **45,** 426–429.
96. Scott, W.K., Grubber, J.M., Conneally, P.M., et al. (2000) Fine mapping of the chromosome 12 late-onset Alzheimer disease locus: potential genetic and phenotypic heterogeneity. *Am. J. Hum. Genet.* **66,** 922–932.
97. Buée, L. and Delacourte, A. (1999) Comparative biochemistry of tau in progressive supranuclear palsy, corticobasal degeneration, FTD-17 and Pick's disease. *Brain Pathol.* **9,** 681–693.
98. Komori, T. (1999) Tau-positive glial inclusions in progressive supranuclear palsy, corticobasal degeneration and Pick's disease. *Brain Pathol.* **9,** 663–679.
99. Dickson, D.W. (2001) Progressive supranuclear palsy and corticobasal degeneration, in *Functional Neurobiology of Aging* (Hof, R.R. and Mobbs, L.C.K., eds.), Academic Press, New York, pp. 155–171.
100. Geschwind, M.D., Rosen, H.J., Kramer, J., Mychack, P., and Miller, B.L. (2001) Dementia in PSP: subcortical or frontal? *Neurology* **56(Suppl. 3),** A172.
101. Verny, M., Duyckaerts, C., Agid, Y., and Hauw, J. (1996) The significance of cortical pathology in progressive supranuclear palsy. Clinico-pathological data in 10 cases. *Brain* **119,** 1123–1136.
102. Hardman, C.D., Halliday, G.M., McRitchie, D.A., Cartwright, H.R., and Morris, J.G. (1997) Progressive supranuclear palsy affects both the substantia nigra pars compacta and reticulata. *Exp. Neurol.* **144,** 183–192.
103. Shinotoh, H., Namba, H., Yamaguchi, M., et al. (1999) Positron emission tomographic measurement of acetylcholinesterase activity reveals differential loss of ascending cholinergic systems in Parkinson's disease and progressive supranuclear palsy. *Ann. Neurol.* **46,** 62–69.
104. Litvan, I., Paulsen, J.S., Mega, M.S., and Cummings, J.L. (1998) Neuropsychiatric assessment of patients eith hyperkinetic and hypokinetic movement disorders. *Arch. Neurol.* **55,** 1313–1319.
105. Pillon, B., Gouider-Khouja, N., Deweer, B., et al. (1995) Neuropsychological pattern of striatonigral degeneration: comparison with Parkinson's disease and progressive supranuclear palsy. *J. Neurol. Neurosurg. Psychiatry* **58,** 174–179.
106. Daniel, S.E., de Bruin, V.M., and Lees, A.J. (1995) The clinical and pathological spectrum of Steele-Richardson-Olszewski syndrome (progressive supranuclear palsy): a reappraisal. *Brain* **118,** 759–770.
107. Hauw, J.-J., Daniel, S.E., Dickson, D., et al. (1994) Preliminary NINDS neuropathologic criteria for Steele-Richardson-Olszewski syndrome (progressive supranuclear palsy). *Neurology* **44,** 2015–2019.
108. Litvan, I., Grimes, D.A., Lang, A. E., et al. (1999) Clinical features differentiating patients with postmortem confirmed progressive supranuclear palsy and corticobasal degeneration. *J. Neurol.* **246(Suppl. 2),** II1–II5.
109. Morris, H.R., Lees, A.J., and Wood, N.W. (1999) Neurofibrillary tangle parkinsonian disorders—tau pathology and tau genetics. *Mov. Disord.* **14,** 731–736.

110. Litvan, I., Goetz, C.G., and Lang, A.E. (2000) Corticobasal degeneration and related disorders. *Adv. Neurol.* **82.**
111. Sergeant, N., Wattez, A., and Delacourte, A. (1999) Neurofibrillary degeneration in progressive supranucelar palsy and corticobasal degeneration: tau pathologies with exclusively "exon 10" isoforms. *J. Neurochem.* **72,** 1243–1249.
112. Kertesz, A., Martinez-Lage, P., Davidson, W., and Munoz, D.G. (2000) The corticobasal degeneration syndrome overlaps progressive aphasia and frontotemporal dementia. *Neurology* **55,** 1368–1375.
113. Dickson, D.W., Bergeron, C., Chin, S.S., et al. (2002) Office of Rare Diseases neuropathologic criteria for corticobasal degeneration. *J. Neuropathol. Exp. Neurol.* **61,** 935–946.
114. Stanford, P.M., Halliday, G.M., Brooks, W.S., et al. (2000) Progressive supranuclear palsy pathology caused by a novel silent mutation in exon 10 of the tau gene: expansion of the disease phenotype caused by tau gene mutations. *Brain* **123,** 880–893.
115. Brown, J., Lantos, P.L., Roques, P., Fidani, L., and Rossor, M.N. (1996) Familial dementia with swollen achromatic neurons and corticobasal inclusion bodies: a clinical and pathological study. *J. Neurol. Sci.* **135,** 21–30.
116. Dickson, D.W. (1998) Pick's disease: a modern approach. *Brain Pathol.* **8,** 339–354.
117. King, M.E., Ghoshal, N., Wall, J.S., Binder, L.I., and Ksiezak-Reding, H. (2001) Structural analysis of Pick's disease-derived and in vitro-assembled tau filaments. *Am. J. Pathol.* **158,** 1481–1490.
118. Jellinger, K.A. (1996) Structural basis of dementia in neurodegenerative disorders. *J. Neural Transm.* **47(Suppl.),** 1–29.
119. Lang, A.E., Bergeron, C., Pollanen, M.S., and Ashby, P. (1994) Parietal Pick's disease mimicking cortical-basal ganglionic degeneration. *Neurology* **44,** 1436–1440.
120. Kosaka, K., Ikeda, K., Kobayashi, K., and Mehraein, P. (1991) Striatopallidonigral degeneration in Pick's disease: a clinicopathological study of 41 cases. *J. Neurol.* **238,** 151–160.
121. Takauchi, S., Yamauchi, S., Morimura, Y., et al. (1995) Coexistence of Pick bodies and atypical Lewy bodies in the locus ceruleus neurons of Pick's disease. *Acta Neuropathol.* **90,** 93–100.
122. Henderson, J.M., Gai, W.P., Hely, M.A., Reid, W.G., Walker, G.L., and Halliday, G.M. (2001) Parkinson's disease with late Pick's dementia. *Mov. Disord.* **16,** 311–319.
123. Pickering-Brown, S., Baker, M., Yen, S.H., et al. (2000) Pick's disease is associated with mutations in the tau gene. *Ann. Neurol.* **48,** 859–867.
124. Rizzini, C., Goedert, M., Hodges, J.R., et al. (2000) Tau gene mutation K257T causes a tauopathy similar to Pick's disease. *J. Neuropathol. Exp. Neurol.* **59,** 990–1001.
125. Russ, C., Lovestone, S., Baker, M., et al. (2001) The extended haplotype of the microtubule associated protein tau gene is not associated with Pick's disease. *Neurosci. Lett.* **299,** 156–158.
126. Arnold, S.E., Han, L.Y., Clark, C.M., Grossman, M., and Trojanowski, J.Q. (2000) Quantitative neurohistological features of frontotemporal degeneration. *Neurobiol. Aging* **21,** 913–919.
127. Bigio, E.H., Lipton, A.M., Yen, S.H., et al. (2001) Frontal lobe dementia with novel tauopathy: sporadic multiple system tauopathy with dementia. *J. Neuropathol. Exp. Neurol.* **60,** 328–341.
128. Josephs, K.A., Parisi, J.E., and Dickson, D.W. (2002) Alpha-synuclein studies are negative in postencephalic parkinsonism of Von Economo. *Neurology* **59,** 645.
129. Kuzuhara, S., Kokubo, Y., Sasaki, R., et al. (2001) Familial amyotrophic lateral sclerosis and parkinsonism-dementia complex of Kii peninsula of Japan: clinical and neuropathological study and tau analysis. *Ann. Neurol.* **49,** 501–511.
130. Yamazaki, M., Arai, Y., Baba, M., et al. (2000) Alpha-synuclein inclusions in amygdala in the brains of patients with the parkinsonism-dementia complex of Guam. *J. Neuropathol. Exp. Neurol.* **59,** 85–91.
131. Matsumoto, S., Udaka, F., Kameyama, M., Kusaka, H., Ito, H., and Imai, T. (1996) Subcortical neurofibrillary tangles, neuropil threads, and argentophilic glial inclusions in corticobasal degeneration. *Clin. Neuropathol.* **15,** 209–214.
132. Geddes, J.F., Hughes, A.J., Lees, A.J., and Daniel, S.E. (1993) Pathological overlap in cases of parkinsonism associated with neurofibrillary tangles. A study of recent cases of postencephalitic parkinsonism and comparison with progressive supranuclear palsy and Guamanian parkinson-dementia complex. *Brain* **116,** 281–302.
133. Wenning, G.K., Jellinger, K., and Litvan, I. (1997) Supranuclear gaze palsy and eye lid apraxia in postencephalitic parkinsonism. *J. Neural Transm.* **104,** 845–865.
134. Litvan, I., Jankovic, J., Goetz, C.G., et al. (1998) Accuracy of the clinical diagnosis of postencephalitic parkinsonism: a clinicopathologic study. *Eur. J. Neurol.* **5,** 451–457.
135. McCall, S., Henry, J.M., Reid, A.H., and Taubenberger, J.K. (2001) Influenza RNA not detected in archival brain tissue from acute encephalitic lethargica cases of postencephalitic parkinsonism. *J. Neuropathol. Exp. Neurol.* **60,** 606–704.
136. Hof, P.R., Perl, D.P., Loerzel, A.J., Steele, J.C., and Morrison, J.H. (1994) Amyotrophic lateral sclerosis and parkinsonism-dementia from Guam: differences in neurofibrillary tangle distribution and density in the hippocampal formation and neocortex. *Brain Res.* **650,** 107–116.
137. Perl, D.P. (1997) Amyotrophic lateral sclerosis/parkinsonism-dementia complex of Guam, in *The Neuropathology of Dementia* (Esiri, M.M. and Morris, J.H., eds.), Cambridge University Press, Cambridge, pp. 184–203.
138. Oyanagi, K. and Wada, M. (1999) Neuropathology of parkinsonism-dementia complex and amyotrophic lateral sclerosis of Guam: an update. *J. Neurol.* **246(Suppl. 2),** II19–II27.
139. Oyanagi, K., Tsuchiya, K., Yamazaki, M., and Ikeda, K. (2001) Substantia nigra in progressive supranuclear palsy, corticobasal degeneration, and parkinsonism-dementia complex of Guam: specific pathological features. *J. Neuropathol. Exp. Neurol.* **60,** 393–402.

140. Salmon, D.P., Galasko, D., and Craig, U.-K. (2001) Rate of cognitive decline in Parkinson-dementia complex and Marianas dementia in the Chamorro people of Guam. *Neurology* **56(Suppl. 3),** A173.
141. Spillantini, M.C., Van Swieten, J.C., and Goedert, M. (2000) Tau gene mutations in frontotemporal dementia and parkinsonism linked to chromosome 17 (FTDP-17). *Neurogenetics* **2,** 193–205.
142. Tolnay, M. (2001) Probst A. Frontotemporal lobar degeneration—an update on clinical, pathological and genetic findings. *Gerontology* **47,** 1–8.
143. Bird, T.D., Nochlin, D., Poorkaj, P., et al. (1999) A clinical pathological comparison of three families with frontotemporal dementia and identical mutations in the tau gene (P302L). *Brain* **122,** 741–756.
144. Mirra, S.S., Murrel, J.R., Gearing, M., et al. (1999) Tau pathology in a familiy with dementia and P301L mutation in tau. *J. Neuropathol. Exp. Neurol.* **58,** 335–345.
145. Nasreddine, Z.S., Loginov, M., Clark, L.N., et al. (1999) From genotype to phenotype: a clinical, pathological, and biochemical investigation of frontotemporal dementia and parkinsonism (FTDP-17) caused by the P301 L tau mutation. *Ann. Neurol.* **45,** 704–715.
146. Hulette, C.M., Pericak-Vance, M.A., Roses, A.D., et al. (1999) Neuropathological features of frontotemporal dementia and parkinsonism linked to chromosome 17q21-22 (FTDP-17): Duke family 1684. *J. Neuropathol. Exp. Neurol.* **58,** 859–866.
147. Bugiani, O., Murrell, J.R., Giaccone, G., et al. (1999) Frontotemporal dementia and corticobasal degeneration in a family with a P301S mutation in tau. *J. Neuropathol. Exp. Neurol.* **58,** 667–677.
148. Arima, K., Kowalska, A., Hasegawa, M., et al. (2000) Two brothers with frontotemporal dementia and parkinsonism with an N279K mutation of the tau gene. *Neurology* **54,** 1787–1795.
149. Goedert, M., Spillantini, M.G., Crowther, R.A., et al. (1999) Tau gene mutation in familial progressive subcortical gliosis. *Nat. Med.* **5,** 454–457.

19

Homologies Between the Genetic Etiology and Pathogenesis of the Synucleinopathies and Tauopathies

John Hardy, PhD

1. INTRODUCTION

Two major classes of neurodegenerative disease are those in which tangles occur and those in which Lewy bodies occur. Tangles are made up largely of the protein tau *(1)* and Lewy bodies are made up largely of the protein α-synuclein *(2)*. Recent genetic and pathological data show many relationships and similarities between these two classes of disease. Parkinson's disease (PD), lewy body dementia (LBD), progressive supranuclear palsy (PSP), and corticobasal degeneration (CBD) are diseases in which there is intracellular inclusions of synuclein containing Lewy bodies (PD and LBD) or tangles containing tau protein (PSP and CBD). These same lesions can occur in Alzheimer's disease (AD) and prion disease (PrD) when they are secondary to the initiating lesions (amyloïd β [Aβ] in AD and prion protein^{Sc} in PrD).

2. MUTATIONS IN THE COGNATE PROTEIN LEAD TO THEIR DEPOSITION IN AUTOSOMAL DOMINANT VERSIONS OF DISEASE

Mutations in the tau gene lead to the syndrome known as frontal temporal dementia with parkinsonism linked to chromosome 17 (FTDP-17) *(3,4)*. This syndrome is clinically characterized by a variable phenotype and by the variable deposition of tau as tangles, Pick bodies or as wispy tau filaments. The clinical phenotype is also variable *(5)*, and although some of this variability is clearly dependent on the precise mutation, it is not yet clear why a minority of individuals present with a predominantly movement disorder phenotype, while the majority present with a dementia phenotype. Thus, tau-encoded disease leads predominantly to a dementia phenotype, but can lead to a movement disorders phenotype.

Mutations in the α-synuclein gene lead to PD *(6,7)*. In this regard, while it is often stated that the Contursi kindred (in which the first α-synuclein mutation was discovered) has PD, some individuals present with a dementia phenotype (Langston, personal communication). This variability in phenotype is also present in other hereditary "PD" families *(8,9)*; thus, while clearly synuclein-encoded disease predominantly leads to a movement disorder phenotype, it can also lead to a dementia phenotype.

3. GENETIC VARIABILITY IN EXPRESSION OF THE COGNATE GENE PREDISPOSES TO SPORADIC DISEASE

PSP and CBD are the most well characterized sporadic tangle diseases *(10)*; in both cases, tau, mainly the '4-repeat' isoform is deposited as tangles *(11)*. In both variants of disease, the movement disorder

From: *Mental and Behavioral Dysfunction in Movement Disorders*
Edited by: M-A. Bédard et al. © Humana Press Inc., Totowa, NJ

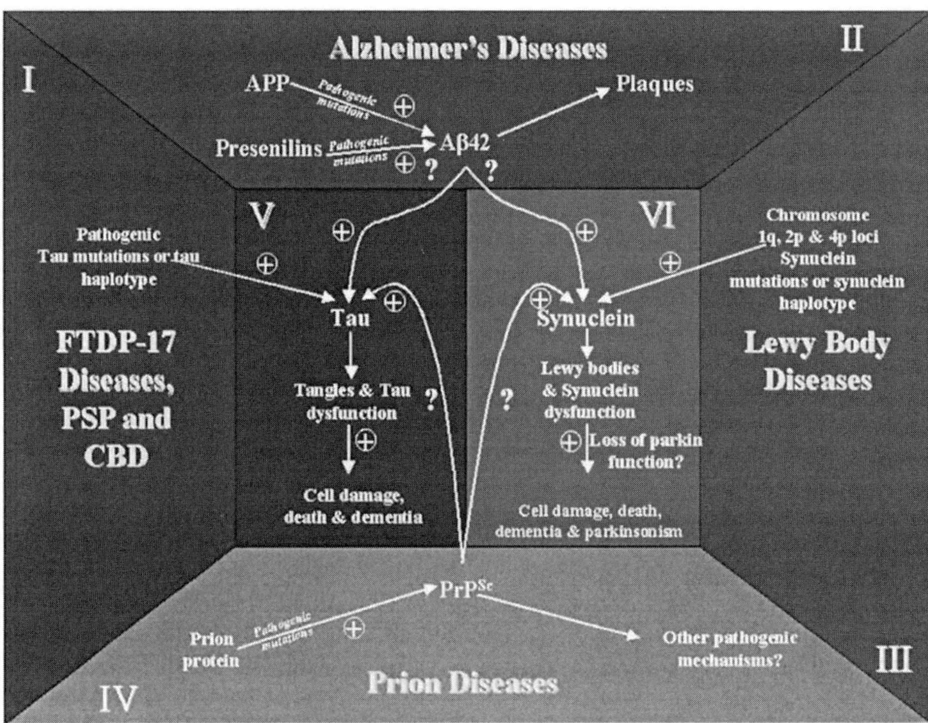

Fig. 1. Diagram outlining the relationships between the disease that constitute some of the tau- and synucleinopathies (adapted from ref. *26*).

variant and the cortical variant, tau haplotype predisposes to disease *(12–15)*. This means that genetic variability, either in expression levels or in alternate splicing contributes to the risk of disease.

PD and LBD *(16)* are the most common variants of Lewy body disease; in both cases, the movement disorder variant and the dementia variant, synuclein haplotype contributes to disease risk (*17,18* and Farrer, Dickson, and Hardy, unpublished data).

At one level, these data are not surprising. They suggest that part of the risk for depositing either tau or α-synuclein is the amount of the protein produced by the depositing neuron.

4. BOTH PATHOLOGIES CAN OCCUR AS SECONDARY EVENTS IN AD (Aβ PATHOLOGY) OR PD (PRION PROTEIN^{Sc} PATHOLOGY)

The wealth of genetic and cell biological data points to Aβ as the primary pathogenic molecule in AD *(19)*. Tangles are an invariant pathology of AD (their presence is required for the diagnosis); thus, tau pathology is clearly a secondary event in this disorder *(20)*. However, Lewy bodies are also a common pathology in AD *(21)*, even in those cases with amyloid precursor protein (APP) and presenilin mutations *(22,23)*. Thus, Lewy body formation must also be a secondary event in these conditions. Tantalizingly, it seems likely that tau and α-synuclein pathologies are alternates to each other in AD *(21)*.

Similarly, some cases of hereditary PD have tangles *(24)*, and those same cases can also have Lewy bodies, suggesting that essentially the same mechanisms can apply in PD.

5. CONCLUSIONS AND SYNTHESIS

The remarkable parallels between the tau- and synucleinopathies can be synthesized into a single simplified diagram of pathogenesis (Fig. 1) (adapted from ref. *26*). In this synthesis, the tau–tangle route to cell death and the synuclein–Lewy body route to cell death are envisioned as alternatives to each other, which can be initiated by rather similar external etiologies (Aβ, or prion protein^{Sc} and presumably other factors, too), or they can be initiated directly by mutations within the cognate molecules themselves. While outlining a set of relationships such as this is intellectually satisfying, it also has therapeutic implications. Therapies aimed at blocking the tau pathway to cell death, for example, may have a wider therapeutic benefit, but may also lead to an initiation of the synuclein pathway.

In addition, this pathogenic diagram may help us develop a partial understanding of selective vulnerability. Clearly some neurons (such as cortical pyramidal neurons) have a predilection, presumably because of the amount of tau expression, for developing tangles, whereas others (such as nigral neurons) have a predilection for developing Lewy bodies. In the diseases where tangles of Lewy bodies are a secondary consequence of other pathologies, such as in AD or PD, the anatomy of the tau and synuclein pathology will also be influenced by the distribution of the primary pathology. Thus, in the primary tau- and synucleinopathies, the distribution of pathology is likely to be determined largely by factors intrinsic to the tau and synuclein proteins (expression levels and degradation pathways) whereas in the secondary tau- and synucleinopathies, the distribution of the initiating lesions will also affect the selective vulnerability to cell loss.

REFERENCES

1. Goedert, M., Wischik, C.M., Crowther, R.A., Walker, J.E., and Klug, A. (1988) Cloning and sequencing of the cDNA encoding a core protein of the paired helical filament of Alzheimer disease: identification as the microtubule-associated protein tau. *Proc. Natl. Acad. Sci. USA* **85,** 4051–4055.
2. Spillantini, M.G., Schmidt, M.L., Lee, V.M.Y., Trojanowski, J.Q., Jakes, R., and Goedert, M. (1977) Alpha-synuclein in Lewy bodies. *Nature* **388,** 839–840.
3. Poorkaj, P., Bird, T.D., Wijsman, E., et al. (1998) Tau is a candidate gene for chromosome 17 frontotemporal dementia. *Ann. Neurol.* **43,** 815–825.
4. Hutton, M., Lendon, C.L., Rizzu, P., et al. (1998) Association of missense and 5'-splice-site mutations in tau with the inherited dementia FTDP-17. *Nature* **393,** 702–705.
5. Foster, N.L., Wilhelmsen, K., Sima, A.A.F., et al. (1997) Frontotemporal dementia and parkinsonism linked to chromosome 17: a consensus conference. *Ann. Neurol.* **41,** 706–715.
6. Polymeropoulos, M.H., Lavedan, C., Leroy, E., et al. (1997) Mutation in the alpha-synuclein gene identified in families with Parkinson's disease. *Science* **276,** 2045–2047.
7. Kruger, R., Kuhn, W., Muller, T., et al. (1998) Ala30Pro mutation in the gene encoding alpha-synuclein in Parkinson's disease. *Nat. Genet.* **18,** 106–108.
8. Muenter, M.D., Forno, L.S., Hornykiewicz, O., et al. (1998) Hereditary form of parkinsonism-dementia. *Ann. Neurol.* **43,** 768–781.
9. Farrer, M., Gwinn-Hardy, K., Muenter, M., et al. (1999) A chromosome 4p haplotype segregating with Parkinson's disease and postural tremor. *Hum. Mol. Genet.* **8,** 81–85.
10. Sergeant, N., Wattez, A., and Delacourte, A. (1999) Neurofibrillary degeneration in progressive supranuclear palsy and corticobasal degeneration: tau pathologies with exclusively "exon 10" isoforms. *J. Neurochem.* **72,** 1243–1249.
11. Buee, L., Bussiere, T., Buee-Scherrer, V., Delacourte, A., Hof, P.R., et al. (2000) Tau protein isoforms, phosphorylation and role in neurodegenerative disorders. *Brain Res. Rev.* **33,** 95–130.
12. Conrad, C., Andreadis, A., Trojanowski, J.Q., et al. (1997) Genetic evidence for the involvement of tau in progressive supranuclear palsy. *Ann. Neurol.* **41,** 277–281.
13. Baker, M., Litvan, I., Houlden, H., et al. (1999) Association of an extended haplotype in the tau gene with progressive supranuclear palsy. *Hum. Mol. Genet.* **8,** 711–715.
14. Di Maria, E., Tabaton, M., Vigo, T., et al. (2000) Corticobasal degeneration shares a common genetic background with progressive supranuclear palsy. *Ann. Neurol.* **47,** 374–347.
15. Houlden, H., Baker, M., Morris, H.R., et al. (2001) Corticobasal degeneration and progressive supranuclear palsy share a common tau haplotype. *Neurology* **56,** 1702–1706.
16. Okazaki, H., Lipkin, L.E., and Aronson, S.M. (1961) Diffuse intracytoplasmic ganglionic inclusions (Lewy type) associated with progressive dementia and quadriparesis in flexion. *J. Neuropathol. Exp. Neurol.* **20,** 237–244.
17. Kruger, R., Vieira-Saecker, A.M., Kuhn, W., et al. (1999) Increased susceptibility to sporadic Parkinson's disease by a certain combined alpha-synuclein/apolipoprotein E genotype. *Ann. Neurol.* **45,** 611–617.
18. Farrer, M., Maraganore, D.M., Singleton, A., et al. (2001) α-Synuclein gene haplotypes are associated with idiopathic parkinson's disease. *Hum. Mol. Genet.* **15,** 1847–1891.
19. Hardy, J. (1997) Amyloid, the presenilins and Alzheimer's disease. *Trends Neurosci.* **20,** 154–159.
20. Hardy, J., Duff, K., Hardy, K.G., Perez-Tur, J., and Hutton, M. (1998) Genetic dissection of Alzheimer's disease and related dementias: amyloid and its relationship to tau. *Nat. Neurosci.* **1,** 355–358.

21. Hansen, L.A., Masliah, E., Galasko, D., and Terry, R.D. (1993) Plaque-only Alzheimer disease is usually the Lewy body variant, and vice versa. *J. Neuropathol. Exp. Neurol.* **52,** 648–654.
22. Lantos, P.L., Luthert, P.J., Hanger, D., Anderton, B.H., Mullan, M., and Rossor, M. (1992) Familial Alzheimer's disease with the amyloid precursor protein position 717 mutation and sporadic Alzheimer's disease have the same cytoskeletal pathology. *Neurosci. Lett.* **137,** 221–224.
23. Lippa, C.F., Fujiwara, H., Mann, D.M., et al. (1998) Lewy bodies contain altered alpha-synuclein in brains of many familial Alzheimer's disease patients with mutations in presenilin and amyloid precursor protein genes. *Am. J. Pathol.* **153,** 1365–1370.
24. Hsiao, K., Dlouhy, S.R., Farlow, M.R., et al. (1992) Mutant prion proteins in Gerstmann-Straussler-Scheinker disease with neurofibrillary tangles. *Nat. Genet.* **1,** 68–71.
25. Piccardo, P. and Ghetti, B. (1998) Lewy bodies in the Indiana prion kindred. *Neurobiol. Aging* S4 19 S724.
26. Hardy, J. (1999) Pathways to primary neurodegenerative disease. *Mayo Clin. Proc.* **74,** 835–837.

20

Prevalence, Incidence, and Risk Factors for Dementia in Parkinson's Disease

Gilberto Levy, MD and Karen Marder, MD, MPH

1. INTRODUCTION

Dementia in patients with idiopathic Parkinson's disease (PD) increases functional impairment both directly, through the limitations imposed by cognitive impairment, and indirectly, due to increased susceptibility to the psychiatric side effects of dopaminergic and anticholinergic therapy, leading to restricted medication use and increased motor impairment. Cognitive impairment in PD has been shown to affect quality of life *(1)* and contribute to caregiver distress *(2)*, and has been associated with nursing home placement *(3)*. The development of dementia is also associated with reduced survival in patients with PD *(4)*.

2. PREVALENCE

Previous reviews have highlighted the wide variation in prevalence estimates of dementia in PD, ranging from under 10% to more than 80% *(5–8)*. The main factors that account for this variation are the accuracy of the diagnosis of idiopathic PD, the definition or diagnostic criteria for dementia, the means of assessing cognitive impairment, and the source of PD patients (community-based vs hospital-based).

2.1. *Diagnosis of PD*

The prevalence estimates of dementia in PD may vary depending on how often patients with other diseases are misdiagnosed as having PD. In a clinicopathological study of 100 cases, the diagnostic accuracy of clinically diagnosed PD was 76%; after retrospective application of the UK Parkinson's Disease Society Brain Bank clinical diagnostic criteria, the diagnostic accuracy improved to 82% *(9)*. The most frequent pathological diagnoses in cases clinically misdiagnosed as PD were progressive supranuclear palsy, multiple system atrophy, Alzheimer's disease (AD), and vascular disease. The presence of cases of progressive supranuclear palsy, vascular parkinsonism, or primarily dementing disorders, such as AD or dementia with Lewy bodies, in a sample of clinically diagnosed PD might be expected to increase prevalence estimates of dementia.

The influence of the accuracy of the clinical diagnosis of idiopathic PD on prevalence estimates is illustrated by a study by Aarsland et al. *(10)*, in which PD patients were classified as definite, probable, and possible clinical idiopathic PD, taking into account atypical clinical features. Among patients with definite PD 16.3% had dementia, whereas 35.1% of the probable PD group, and 54.3% of the possible PD group had dementia. In a study by Martilla and Rinne *(11)*, among PD patients with systemic clinical

From: *Mental and Behavioral Dysfunction in Movement Disorders*
Edited by: M-A. Bédard et al. © Humana Press Inc., Totowa, NJ

Table 1
Prevalence of Dementia in PD in Studies Using Formal Cognitive Evaluation

Investigator (yr) (reference)	Cognitive evaluation	DSM-III-R criteria	Prevalence % (n)
Hospital-based samples			
Celesia and Wanamaker (1972) *(18)*	Standardized mental state examination.	No	40 (153)
Loranger et al. (1972) *(94)*	Wechsler Adult Intelligence Scale.	No	36.5 (63)
Martin et al. (1973) *(17)*	Standardized mental state examination.	No	81 (100)
Lieberman et al. (1979) *(95)*	Standardized mental state examination.	No	32 (520)
Mindham et al. (1982) *(27)*	Standardized mental state examination.	No	20 (40)
Hershey (1982) *(14)*	Cognitive Capacity Screening Examination.	No	45 (22)
Piccirilli et al. (1984) *(50)*	Neuropsychological battery.	No	33 (70)
Taylor et al. (1985) *(19)*	Neuropsychological battery.	No	8 (100)
Oyebode et al. (1986) *(20)*	Neuropsychological battery.	No	7 (43)
Huber and Paulson (1986) *(96)*	Mini-Mental State.	No	33 (48)
Boyd et al. (1991) *(25)*	Neuropsychological battery.	No	31 (47)
Pillon et al. (1991) *(97)*	Neuropsychological battery.	No	18 (164)
Community-based samples			
Mjones (1949) *(98)*	Standardized mental state examination.	No	40 (194)
Marttila and Rinne (1976) *(11)*	Standardized mental state examination.	No	29 (444)
Ebmeier et al. (1991) *(99)*	Mini-Mental State.	Yes	23.3 (157)
Mayeux et al. (1992) *(40)*[a]	Neuropsychological battery.	Yes	41.3 (179)
Tison et al. (1995) *(100)*	Neuropsychological battery.	Yes	17.6 (60)
Marder et al. (1995) *(34)*[a]	Neuropsychological battery.	Yes	37.3 (279)
Aarsland et al. (1996) *(10)*	Mini-Mental State.	Yes	27.7 (245)

[a]Results of the same study reported after different periods of recruitment.

signs of arteriosclerosis (n = 124), dementia was present in 56.4%, while among those without signs of arteriosclerosis (n = 319), 18.2% were demented. Rather than implying a contribution of vascular mechanisms to dementia in PD, these results may be related to a higher frequency of vascular parkinsonism among patients with clinical signs of arteriosclerosis *(12)*. Misdiagnosis can also potentially lead to false associations of clinical characteristics with increased prevalence of dementia. Sroka et al. *(13)* subdivided PD cases into typical and atypical, the latter defined as parkinsonism that has signs unrestricted to the extrapyramidal system (e.g., pyramidal tract, brainstem, or cerebellar signs) and/or unusual evolution of the disease. The frequency of dementia in the atypical (n = 22) and typical (n = 71) cases was, respectively, 68 and 15%. Although patients were considered to have idiopathic PD *(14)*, one might expect the accuracy of the clinical diagnosis of PD to be further reduced among the atypical cases *(15)*.

2.2. *Diagnostic Criteria for Dementia*

The influence of the definition of dementia on prevalence estimates of dementia in PD is illustrated by several studies (Table 1). The broad range of prevalence estimates may be reduced if strict Diagnosis and Statistical Manual of Mental Disorders (DSM)-III-R criteria *(16)* are applied to studies with high prevalence estimates. Martin et al. *(17)* using a rating for the severity of intellectual impairment classified impairment as mild, moderate, and severe. Although 81 out of 100 PD patients were considered to have intellectual impairment, 58% of the sample had mild impairment that would probably not meet DSM-III-R criteria for dementia, leaving 23% with moderate to severe intellectual impairment. In a study by Celesia and Wanamaker *(18)*, 40% of 153 patients were considered to be demented, and 24% had moderate or severe impairment, while in a study by Marttila and Rinne *(11)*, 29% of 444 patients were demented, and only 13.8% had moderate or severe impairment. In these two studies, mild impairment did not require memory disturbance, unlike moderate and severe impairment, and, therefore, would not meet DSM-III-R criteria for dementia.

In two studies with particularly low estimates of dementia, stringent neuropsychological criteria for the diagnosis of dementia were employed. Taylor et al. *(19)* reported a frequency of 8% of dementia in 100 PD patients, defined as a Wechsler Adult Intelligence Scale-Revised (WAIS-R) verbal intelligence quotient (IQ) more than one standard deviation below that estimated by a test of premorbid intellectual function, global memory impairment measured by the Wechsler memory scale, the Rey auditory verbal learning test, and a test of delayed recognition, and anomia on a list of 14 common objects. All these conditions had to be met. In a study of Oyebode et al. *(20)*, 7% of 43 patients were considered to have "cognitive deficits typical of senile dementia of Alzheimer's type," including evidence of a significant decline in general intelligence and impairment in secondary memory, shown through impaired performance on an information–orientation scale or on a test of verbal recognition. The low prevalence estimates in these studies may be partly explained by the fact that recognition memory is relatively spared in PD dementia as compared to AD *(21)*, and naming impairment is not an early manifestation of the dementing process in PD *(22)*.

More recent studies of the prevalence of dementia in PD have adopted DSM-III-R criteria *(16)* for the diagnosis of dementia (Table 1). This definition requires a "loss of intellectual abilities of sufficient severity to interfere with social or occupational functioning," memory impairment, and either impairment of abstract thinking, impaired judgment, disturbances of higher cortical function, or personality change. Pirozzolo et al. *(23)* demonstrated cognitive impairment in 93% of PD patients when compared with age- and education-matched controls on neuropsychological measures, arguing that the continuous distribution of cognitive deficits rendered it difficult to make a clear distinction between demented and nondemented PD patients. On the other hand, their findings underscore the potentially large effect of the definition of dementia on prevalence estimates and may be seen as an argument in favor of the utilization of standard criteria for dementia that allow the comparison of different studies.

2.3. Assessment of Cognitive Impairment

In published studies reporting the prevalence of dementia in PD, nonstandardized clinical examination, standardized mental state examination consisting of tests of cognitive function derived from those used in clinical practice, screening cognitive tests such as the Mini-Mental State (MMS) *(24)*, and neuropsychological test batteries have been employed. The influence of the cognitive assessment on prevalence estimates is demonstrated in a study by Boyd et al. *(25)*, in which 31% of PD patients were considered to be demented using a discrepancy of over 10 points between the predicted National Adult Reading Test (NART) verbal IQ and the WAIS verbal IQ, and only 6.8% were demented using a MMS score below 24. Although time-consuming, the neuropsychological battery provides the most comprehensive and objective evaluation of cognitive impairment, including the evaluation of different cognitive domains. According to a review by Cummings et al. *(6)*, investigations using clinical examination found, on average, lower estimates of dementia in PD (30%) than investigations using a structured examination (40.5%), including standardized mental state examinations and screening cognitive tests, and those using neuropsychological testing (69.9%).

2.4. Source of PD Sample

The source of the PD sample is likely to influence the estimates of prevalence of dementia, as hospital or neurology clinic patients may not be representative of the general PD population. They may come to attention because of more severe disease, atypical features, and family history, and they may also differ from the PD population in demographic characteristics, such as age and education. Table 1 lists those studies providing information on prevalence of dementia based on formal cognitive evaluation by standardized mental state examination, screening cognitive test, or neuropsychological battery.

Overall, the estimates range from 7–81%. However, in community-based studies using DSM-III-R criteria for dementia, the variability in prevalence estimates is smaller, ranging from 17.6–41.3%.

3. INCIDENCE AND ASSOCIATION WITH INCREASED MORTALITY

Incidence is a more meaningful measure of the frequency of dementia in PD because dementia may reduce survival. This means that demented PD patients may be less likely to be represented in prevalence surveys *(4,26)*. Incidence studies may also provide a better measure of the magnitude of PD dementia than prevalence studies by improving diagnostic accuracy, i.e., by decreasing misdiagnosis of primarily dementing disorders, such as AD or dementia with Lewy bodies, as PD dementia.

Evidence that dementia was associated with reduced survival in PD was provided in a study by Mindham et al. *(27)*, in which demented PD patients were more likely to die during the 3-yr follow-up period than nondemented PD patients. In a community-based study in Aberdeen, Scotland, a 10-question mental status questionnaire was the most important predictor of mortality out of 65 demographic and clinical variables *(28)*. Piccirilli et al. *(29)* followed 34 PD patients with intellectual impairment matched by age, gender, disease duration, and disease severity to 34 patients without intellectual impairment for 7 yr; 33.3% of those with intellectual impairment and 12.5% of those without intellectual impairment died during follow-up, and a significantly higher percentage of deaths were observed in patients with more severe dementia. Roos et al. *(30)* demonstrated that patients who developed dementia had a significantly worse survival rate than patients of similar age and disease duration without dementia.

We have shown that demented patients matched by age and disease duration to nondemented PD patients had significantly decreased survival *(4)*. In a subsequent analysis, dementia contributed to increased mortality only in those with less severe disease, as measured by extrapyramidal signs; in those patients with a high extrapyramidal signs total score, the presence of dementia did not add to the magnitude of the risk of death *(31)*. Since severity of extrapyramidal signs is associated with both dementia and mortality in PD *(31)*, it is possible that the association of dementia with mortality in PD is confounded by disease severity, as measured by extrapyramidal signs. In order to address this question, we have recently performed an analysis in a cohort of 180 nondemented PD patients followed annually with neurological and neuropsychological evaluations, using Cox proportional hazards models with time-dependent covariates. In this analysis, we found that the development of dementia significantly increased the risk of death by about two times, after controlling for the total Unified Parkinson's Disease Rating Scale (UPDRS) *(32)* motor score at each study visit. The increased risk of death associated with dementia did not change after adjusting for depressive symptoms or hallucinations. These findings support an independent effect of dementia on mortality in PD (unpublished data).

Incidence rates of dementia have been estimated in both hospital-based and community-based studies using DSM-III-R criteria *(26,33–37)*. Overall, incidence rates of dementia in PD ranged from 42.6–112.5/1000 person-yr of observation (Table 2), but the two highest estimates (95.3 and 112.5/1000 person-yr) were obtained in the two community-based studies *(34,37)*. Although the incidence rates in these two longitudinal community-based studies were similar, because the incidence of dementia in the control groups of individuals without PD differed, the relative risk of developing dementia in the PD groups after adjustment for age, gender, and education was 1.7- *(34)* and 5.9-fold *(37)*. In a follow-up study based on Dutch nationwide morbidity registers, the relative risk of developing dementia in patients with PD was 3.0 *(38)*, an estimate similar to that reported in a study based on medical records from Rochester, Minnesota *(39)*.

4. RISK FACTORS

The study of risk factors for dementia in PD may be useful in several ways. First, knowledge of antecedent clinical features associated with an increased risk of developing dementia in patients with PD may provide useful prognostic information for clinicians and families. Second, since clinicopathologic studies have suggested that concomitant AD pathology may account for the presence of demen-

Table 2
Incidence of Dementia in PD

Investigator (yr) (reference)	Sample	Incidence rate (/1000 person-yr) (n)
Mayeux et al. (1990) *(26)*	Hospital-based	69 (249)
Biggins et al. (1992) *(33)*[a]	Hospital-based	47.6 (82)
Marder et al. (1995) *(34)*	Community-based	112.5 (140)
Mahieux et al. (1998) *(35)*	Hospital-based	67.2 (81)
Hughes et al. (2000) *(36)*[a]	Hospital-based	42.6 (83)
Aarsland et al. (2001) *(37)*	Community-based	95.3 (130)

[a]Results of the same study reported after different follow-up periods.
All studies diagnosed dementia according to DSM-III-R criteria.

tia in PD, the investigation of the association of AD risk factors with dementia in PD may help clarify to what extent concomitant AD is etiologically related to the development of dementia in PD. Third, the investigation of genetic and environmental risk factors may promote understanding of etiopathogenetic mechanisms and suggest potential preventive measures to the development of dementia in the setting of PD.

4.1. Demographic and Clinical Risk Factors

4.1.1. Demographic Risk Factors

Age has been consistently associated with dementia in PD in several different studies. Mayeux et al. *(26)* have shown that age-specific incidence rates for dementia in a clinic-based sample of PD increased with age, the cumulative incidence of dementia reaching 65% by age 85. In another study by the same investigators of a population-based sample, the age-specific prevalence of dementia in PD ranged from 12.4% in the group 50–59 yr old to 68.7% in the group >80 yr old *(40)*. In several subsequent longitudinal studies, the association of age with dementia in PD has been demonstrated *(33,34,36,37,41, 42)*. Although age at baseline evaluation and age at onset of disease tend to be highly correlated, age at onset was not a significant independent predictor of incident dementia in the investigation by Marder et al. *(34)*, and two additional studies have recently shown that only age at baseline evaluation was significantly associated with dementia when both variables were considered in multivariate analyses *(36,37)*, suggesting that current age may be a more important predictor of dementia in PD.

Gender and education may also influence the occurrence of dementia in PD. Some studies have reported a higher frequency of dementia in PD in males *(36,38,43–46)*, but this association has not been demonstrated in other studies *(37,40,47,48)*. The lack of consistency and the possibility of bias and confounding accounting for this relationship must be taken into consideration *(36,44)*. In one investigation, lower education was significantly associated with dementia in PD in a highly educated outpatient clinic sample *(45)*. Given the association of lower education with AD, this could support a nonspecific effect of education in the expression of cognitive impairment *(49)*.

4.1.2. Antecedent Clinical Features

Although duration of disease tends to be longer in demented as compared to nondemented PD patients *(33)*, disease duration has not emerged as a significant predictor of dementia in multivariate analyses *(36,37,41)*, suggesting that differences in disease duration in univariate analyses may be related to patients with longer disease duration being older or having more severe disease. Of all clinical features of PD, severity of extrapyramidal signs has been most consistently associated with dementia, which has been seen as evidence in favor of the contribution of the subcortical pathology that underlies the motor manifestations of the disease to the development of dementia in PD *(34,36,37,41,48,50–52)*.

Since some of the motor impairment in PD has been attributed to nondopaminergic mechanisms, as indicated by specific signs being relatively refractory to levodopa therapy, especially in middle and late stages of the disease *(53)*, we have explored the association of two subscores of the UPDRS *(32)*, representing predominantly dopaminergic (including facial expression, tremor, rigidity, and bradykinesia) and nondopaminergic (including speech and axial impairment) deficiency, with incident dementia in PD. When both subscores were included in a multivariate model, the subscore representing predominantly nondopaminergic deficiency, but not the subscore representing predominantly dopaminergic deficiency, was associated with incident dementia in PD *(54)*. In this and other studies, when specific domains of motor impairment were analyzed, speech, bradykinesia, and gait and balance impairment were associated with dementia in PD *(48,50,54–56)*, which is consistent with the finding of many studies *(30,43,55,57–59)* that the predominance of tremor is a predictor of benign clinical course.

In one study, bilateral as compared to unilateral disease onset was associated with memory impairment and low MMS scores an average of 9 yr later *(60)*. However, this finding must be interpreted cautiously in light of the fact that asymmetrical onset is one of the features that improve the accuracy in terms of positive predictive value of the clinical diagnosis of idiopathic PD *(15)*. In further support of the idea that nondopaminergic deficiency may underlie the development of dementia in PD, several studies have demonstrated an association of lower or decreasing response to levodopa treatment with cognitive decline or dementia in PD *(50,61,62)*.

Psychiatric symptoms have been associated with dementia in PD. In a study by Starkstein et al. *(63)*, patients with major depression showed a significantly greater cognitive decline than patients with minor depression or no depression. Stern et al. *(41)* reported a threefold increased risk of dementia in PD patients with depression as defined by DSM-III criteria. In two other studies, the presence of depressive symptoms on the Hamilton Depression Rating Scale *(64)* (17-item questionnaire, score range: 0–52), as defined by a score >6 *(65)* or >10 *(34)*, was associated with cognitive decline or dementia in PD. However, the association of depressive symptoms with dementia in PD has not been replicated in two longitudinal studies using the Montgomery and Asberg Depression Rating Scale *(66)* (10-item questionnaire, score range: 0–60). Hughes et al. *(36)* found no significant difference in depressive symptoms in PD patients with and without dementia, using either a lower (>6) or a higher (>19) cut-off in the Montgomery and Asberg Depression Rating Scale, while Aarsland et al. *(37)* found that neither major depression nor a score ≥6 were predictors of dementia in PD. In other studies, an association of levodopa-induced psychiatric side-effects, such as psychosis and confusional states, with intellectual deterioration or dementia in PD has been reported *(41,43,51,67,68)*.

4.1.3. Neuropsychological Predictors

Since cognitive impairment is part of the definition of dementia, worse performance on neuropsychological tests is to be expected to increase the risk of dementia in PD and other dementing disorders. However, the pattern of early cognitive impairment that is predictive of dementia in each disorder differs and may provide useful prognostic clinical information.

Few studies have examined the neuropsychological predictors of dementia in PD. In a study by Jacobs et al. *(69)*, baseline performance on two verbal fluency tasks (letter fluency and category fluency) was associated with incident dementia in PD patients. We have recently reexamined the pattern of cognitive impairment associated with incident dementia in an expanded cohort of PD patients with a longer duration of follow-up, including almost twice the number of incident dementia cases as reported in our previous analysis *(69)*. In addition to impairment in tests suggestive of executive dysfunction (letter fluency and Identities and Oddities of the Mattis Dementia Rating Scale), we found that impairment in verbal memory tests (total immediate recall and delayed recall of the Selective Reminding Test) was predictive of dementia in PD *(70)*. In another prospective study, the Picture Completion subtest of the WAIS-R, the interference section of the Stroop test, and letter fluency were independent predictors of incident dementia in PD *(35)*.

In the previous studies, results were considered to be different from the neuropsychological pattern characteristic of the preclinical stages of AD and were interpreted as suggesting the presence of executive cognitive dysfunction (e.g., deficits in planning, mental set, and mental shift) in the incipient stages of dementia in PD *(35,69)*. Based on these findings and on the association of impairment on a battery of tasks exploring higher order motor abilities (Luria tests) with dementia in PD *(71)*, Piccirilli et al. *(72)* suggested that early frontal impairment affecting performance on motor and cognitive tasks was a predictor of dementia in PD.

4.2. Environmental and Genetic Risk Factors

4.2.1. Environmental Risk Factors

Few studies have explored the association of environmental risk factors with PD dementia. In a case-control study investigating the association of toxic and occupational exposures, as well as personal habits with dementia in PD, we did not find significant differences in exposure to pesticides (roach or ant sprays) or chemicals (organophosphates, toluene, xylene) between demented and nondemented PD patients *(44)*. In a study by Glatt et al. *(45)*, no significant independent effects were observed for pesticides exposure, rural living, and well water exposure on the risk for dementia in PD.

In both previous case-control studies, smoking, alcohol consumption, and head injury did not emerge as putative risk factors for PD dementia *(44,45)*. In another case-control study, frequency of smoking was 38% among demented and 27% among nondemented PD patients, but there was no significant difference between the groups *(73)*. However, Ebmeier et al. *(48)* reported a fourfold significantly increased risk for dementia in PD during follow-up in those having a history of smoking. In another longitudinal study, we found that patients who had ever smoked had a twofold significantly increased risk of dementia compared to nonsmokers, while current smokers at baseline evaluation had a 4.5 times increased risk of dementia compared to nonsmokers *(74)*.

4.2.2. Genetic Risk Factors

Because of the association of the APOE-ε4 allele with AD, we and others have examined the association of APOE4 genotype with PD dementia. With the exception of one study *(75)*, no increased frequency of APOE-ε4 allele was found in PD dementia as compared to PD without dementia or controls *(76–79)*. On the other hand, two recent epidemiologic studies have reported an increased risk of PD dementia in carriers of the APOE-ε2 allele *(46,80)*.

Two studies with neuropathological confirmation of the diagnosis of PD assessed the association of APOE-ε4 allele with the concomitant pathological diagnosis of AD. Egensperger et al. *(81)* found similar frequencies of APOE-ε4 allele frequency in PD with concomitant AD, PD without concomitant AD, and controls, while Mattila et al. *(82)* found the APOE allele frequency to be significantly increased in PD with concomitant AD (29.4%) as compared to PD without concomitant AD (13.6%) and controls (14.4%). In addition, a gene–gene interaction of the APOE-ε4 allele and a common polymorphism of the gene encoding dipeptidyl carboxypeptidase1 (also known as angiotensin I converting enzyme) was associated with concomitant AD pathology in PD *(83)*. Because the relationship between concomitant AD on a pathological basis and PD dementia is not clear, the results of these pathological studies cannot be easily extrapolated to PD dementia.

Besides APOE genotype, we have examined the association between cytochrome P_{450} mono-oxygenase gene (CYP2D6) polymorphisms and PD in a case-control study of 121 PD patients, 39 of whom were demented, and 138 controls. No association between any of the CYP2D6 polymorphisms and PD or PD with dementia was observed *(84)*. Hubble et al. *(85)* examined the frequencies of the CYP2D6 29B+ poor metabolizer allele and monoamino oxidase B (MAOB) allele 1 in PD patients with and without dementia. Although no association of these candidate gene markers with PD dementia was observed, a gene–toxin interaction of the CYP2D6 29B+ allele and pesticide exposure was significantly associated with dementia in PD.

Table 3
Risk Factors for Dementia in PD

Demographic
Age *(26,33,34,36,37,40–42)*[a].
Male gender *(36 38,43–46)*.
Lower education *(45)*.
Clinical
Severity of extrapyramidal signs *(34,36,37,41,48,50,51)*.[a]
Lower or decreasing response to levodopa *(50,61,62)*.
Bilateral onset *(60)*.
Depressive symptoms or major depression *(34,41,63,65)*.
Levodopa-induced psychosis or confusional states *(41,43,51,67,68)*.
Neuropsychological
Executive dysfunction *(35,69,70)*.
Verbal memory impairment *(70)*.
Environmental and genetic
Smoking *(48,74)*.
APOE-ε2 *(46,80)*.
Gene-toxin interaction of the CYP2D6 29B+ allele and pesticide exposure *(85)*.
Other
Family history of dementia or Alzheimer's disease *(44,87)*.
Estrogen replacement therapy (inverse association) *(89)*.

[a]Consistently shown in several studies.

4.3. *Other Risk Factors*

Heston et al. *(86)* performed a family study in 12 PD patients selected from 304 autopsy cases with dementia. Although seven cases of PD among first-degree relatives in six families were observed, only one PD case was demented, leading the authors to conclude that "there was no independent genetic segregation of Parkinson's disease and dementia as would be expected if the two conditions were associated with different unlinked genes." In a pilot case-control study, a family history of dementia in first-degree relatives of PD patients was reported in 30% of the demented group and 5.6% of the non-demented group *(44)*. We also found a threefold increased risk of AD in siblings of demented PD patients compared to siblings of controls, supporting the possibility of aggregation of AD and PD dementia *(87)*. Mickel et al. *(88)* observed no increased risk of AD among relatives of demented PD patients compared with relatives of nondemented PD patients, but there were only 15 demented PD patients in this study.

In further support of a common etiology for PD dementia and AD, we reported an inverse association between estrogen replacement therapy and PD dementia compared to nondemented PD patients (odds ratio [OR]: 0.22; 95% confidence interval [CI]: 0.05–1.0) and controls (OR: 0.24; 95% CI: 0.07–0.78) *(89)*. Salganik and Korczyn *(73)* evaluated the association of cardiovascular risk factors with PD dementia using a case-control design. Hypertension, but not diabetes mellitus or coronary heart disease, was significantly associated with dementia in PD. However, in a longitudinal cohort study, no increased risk for dementia in PD was observed for patients reporting either hypertension or diabetes mellitus *(74)*.

5. CONCLUSION

Clinical-pathological series have suggested that dementia in PD may be heterogeneous, involving either only subcortical pathology or subcortical pathology and additional cortical Lewy bodies and/or AD pathology *(90–93)*. The fact that the biological basis of dementia in PD has not been clearly defined stems in part from the paucity of longitudinal studies in which autopsy material is available.

The study of risk factors for PD dementia may help clarify the biological basis of dementia in PD as a group and, eventually, define from a clinical standpoint subgroups with different pathological substrates. Only two risk factors, age and severity of extrapyramidal signs, have been consistently associated with dementia in PD in several different studies (Table 3). Because inconsistent findings must be interpreted cautiously and case-control studies are particularly prone to methodological biases, further studies using a longitudinal design are needed to evaluate putative risk factors for dementia in PD.

REFERENCES

1. Schrag, A., Jahanshahi, M., and Quinn, N. (2000) What contributes to quality of life in patients with Parkinson's disease? *J. Neurol. Neurosurg. Psychiatry* **69,** 308–312.
2. Aarsland, D., Larsen, J.P., Karlsen, K., Lim, N.G., and Tandberg, E. (1999) Mental symptoms in Parkinson's disease are important contributors to caregiver distress. *Int. J. Geriatr. Psychiatry* **14,** 866–874.
3. Aarsland, D., Larsen, J.P., Tandberg, E., and Laake, K. (2000) Predictors of nursing home placement in Parkinson's disease: a population-based, prospective study. *J. Am. Geriatr. Soc.* **48,** 938–942.
4. Marder, K., Leung, D., Tang, M., et al. (1991) Are demented patients with Parkinson's disease accurately reflected in prevalence surveys? A survival analysis. *Neurology* **41,** 1240–1243.
5. Brown, R.G. and Marsden, C.D. (1984) How common is dementia in Parkinson's disease? *Lancet* **2,** 1262–1265.
6. Cummings, J.L. (1988) Intellectual impairment in Parkinson's disease: clinical, pathologic, and biochemical correlates. *J. Geriatr. Psychiatry Neurol.* **1,** 24–36.
7. Dubois, B., Boller, F., Pillon, B., and Agid, Y. (1991) Cognitive deficits in Parkinson's disease, in *Handbook of Neuropsychology* (Boller, F. and Grafman, J., eds.), Elsevier Science Publishers, New York, pp. 195–240.
8. Marder, K. and Mayeux, R. (1991) The epidemiology of dementia in patients with Parkinson's disease. *Adv. Exp. Med. Biol.* **295,** 439–445.
9. Hughes, A.J., Daniel, S.E., Kilford, L., and Lees, A.J. (1992) Accuracy of clinical diagnosis of idiopathic Parkinson's disease: a clinico-pathological study of 100 cases. *J. Neurol. Neurosurg. Psychiatry* **55,** 181–184.
10. Aarsland, D., Tandberg, E., Larsen, J.P., and Cummings, J.L. (1996) Frequency of dementia in Parkinson disease. *Arch. Neurol.* **53,** 538–542.
11. Marttila, R.J. and Rinne, U.K. (1976) Dementia in Parkinson's disease. *Acta Neurol. Scand.* **54,** 431–441.
12. Winikates, J. and Jankovic, J. (1999) Clinical correlates of vascular parkinsonism. *Arch. Neurol.* **56,** 98–102.
13. Sroka, H., Elizan, T.S., Yahr, M.D., Burger, A., and Mendoza, M.R. (1981) Organic mental syndrome and confusional states in Parkinson's disease. Relationship to computerized tomographic signs of cerebral atrophy. *Arch. Neurol.* **38,** 339–342.
14. Hershey, L.A. (1982) Organic mental syndrome in Parkinson's disease. *Arch. Neurol.* **39,** 456–457.
15. Hughes, A.J., Ben Shlomo, Y., Daniel, S.E., and Lees, A.J. (1992) What features improve the accuracy of clinical diagnosis in Parkinson's disease: a clinicopathologic study. *Neurology* **42,** 1142–1146.
16. American Psychiatric Association (1987) *Diagnostic and Statistical Manual of Mental Disorders,* American Psychiatric Press, Washington, DC.
17. Martin, W.E., Loewenson, R.B., Resch, J.A., and Baker, A.B. (1973) Parkinson's disease. Clinical analysis of 100 patients. *Neurology* **23,** 783–790.
18. Celesia, G.G. and Wanamaker, W.M. (1972) Psychiatric disturbances in Parkinson's disease. *Dis. Nerv. Syst.* **33,** 577–583.
19. Taylor, A., Saint-Cyr, J.A., and Lang, A.E. (1985) Dementia prevalence in Parkinson's disease. *Lancet* **1,** 1037.
20. Oyebode, J.R., Barker, W.A., Blessed, G., Dick, D.J., and Britton, P.G. (1986) Cognitive functioning in Parkinson's disease: in relation to prevalence of dementia and psychiatric diagnosis. *Br. J. Psychiatry* **149,** 720–725.
21. Helkala, E.L., Laulumaa, V., Soininen, H., and Riekkinen, P.J. (1988) Recall and recognition memory in patients with Alzheimer's and Parkinson's diseases. *Ann. Neurol.* **24,** 214–217.
22. Stern, Y., Tang, M.X., Jacobs, D.M., et al. (1998) Prospective comparative study of the evolution of probable Alzheimer's disease and Parkinson's disease dementia. *J. Int. Neuropsychol. Soc.* **4,** 279–284.
23. Pirozzolo, F.J., Hansch, E.C., Mortimer, J.A., Webster, D.D., and Kuskowski, M.A. (1982) Dementia in Parkinson disease: a neuropsychological analysis. *Brain Cogn.* **1,** 71–83.
24. Folstein, M.F., Folstein, S.E., and McHugh, P.R. (1975) "Mini-mental state." A practical method for grading the cognitive state of patients for the clinician. *J. Psychiatr. Res.* **12,** 189–198.
25. Boyd, J.L., Cruickshank, C.A., Kenn, C.W., et al. (1991) Cognitive impairment and dementia in Parkinson's disease: a controlled study. *Psychol. Med.* **21,** 911–921.
26. Mayeux, R., Chen, J., Mirabello, E., et al. (1990) An estimate of the incidence of dementia in idiopathic Parkinson's disease. *Neurology* **40,** 1513–1517.
27. Mindham, R.H., Ahmed, S.W., and Clough, C.G. (1982) A controlled study of dementia in Parkinson's disease. *J. Neurol. Neurosurg. Psychiatry* **45,** 969–974.
28. Ebmeier, K.P., Calder, S.A., Crawford, J.R., Stewart, L., Besson, J.A., and Mutch, W.J. (1990) Parkinson's disease in Aberdeen: survival after 3.5 years. *Acta Neurol. Scand.* **81,** 294–299.
29. Piccirilli, M., D'Alessandro, P., Finali, G., and Piccinin, G.L. (1994) Neuropsychological follow-up of parkinsonian patients with and without cognitive impairment. *Dementia* **5,** 17–22.

30. Roos, R.A., Jongen, J.C., and van der Velde, E.A. (1996) Clinical course of patients with idiopathic Parkinson's disease. *Mov. Disord.* **11,** 236–242.
31. Louis, E.D., Marder, K., Cote, L., Tang, M., and Mayeux, R. (1997) Mortality from Parkinson disease. *Arch. Neurol.* **54,** 260–264.
32. Stern, M.B. (1988) The clinical characteristics of Parkinson's disease and parkinsonian syndromes: diagnosis and assessment, in *The Comprehensive Management of Parkinson's Disease* (Stern, M.B. and Murtig, M.I., eds.), PMA Publishing Corp., New York, pp. 3–50.
33. Biggins, C.A., Boyd, J.L., Harrop, F.M., et al. (1992) A controlled, longitudinal study of dementia in Parkinson's disease. *J. Neurol. Neurosurg. Psychiatry* **55,** 566–571.
34. Marder, K., Tang, M.X., Cote, L., Stern, Y., and Mayeux, R. (1995) The frequency and associated risk factors for dementia in patients with Parkinson's disease. *Arch. Neurol.* **52,** 695–701.
35. Mahieux, F., Fenelon, G., Flahault, A., Manifacier, M.J., Michelet, D., and Boller, F. (1998) Neuropsychological prediction of dementia in Parkinson's disease. *J. Neurol. Neurosurg. Psychiatry* **64,** 178–183.
36. Hughes, T.A., Ross, H.F., Musa, S., et al. (2000) A 10-year study of the incidence of and factors predicting dementia in Parkinson's disease. *Neurology* **54,** 1596–1602.
37. Aarsland, D., Andersen, K., Larsen, J.P., Lolk, A., Nielsen, H., and Kragh-Sorensen, P. (2001) Risk of dementia in Parkinson's disease: a community-based, prospective study. *Neurology* **56,** 730–736.
38. Breteler, M.M., de Groot, R.R., van Romunde, L.K., and Hofman, A. (1995) Risk of dementia in patients with Parkinson's disease, epilepsy, and severe head trauma: a register-based follow-up study. *Am. J. Epidemiol.* **142,** 1300–1305.
39. Rajput, A.H., Offord, K.P., Beard, C.M., and Kurland, L.T. (1987) A case-control study of smoking habits, dementia, and other illnesses in idiopathic Parkinson's disease. *Neurology* **37,** 226–232.
40. Mayeux, R., Denaro, J., Hemenegildo, N., et al. (1992) A population-based investigation of Parkinson's disease with and without dementia. Relationship to age and gender. *Arch. Neurol.* **49,** 492–497.
41. Stern, Y., Marder, K., Tang, M.X., and Mayeux, R. (1993) Antecedent clinical features associated with dementia in Parkinson's disease. *Neurology* **43,** 1690–1692.
42. Hely, M.A., Morris, J.G., Reid, W.G., et al. (1995) Age at onset: the major determinant of outcome in Parkinson's disease. *Acta Neurol. Scand.* **92,** 455–463.
43. Guillard, A. and Chastang, C. (1978) Maladie de Parkinson. Les facteurs de pronostic a long terme. *Revue Neurologique* **134,** 341–354.
44. Marder, K., Flood, P., Cote, L., and Mayeux, R. (1990) A pilot study of risk factors for dementia in Parkinson's disease. *Mov. Disord.* **5,** 156–161.
45. Glatt, S.L., Hubble, J.P., Lyons, K., et al. (1996) Risk factors for dementia in Parkinson's disease: effect of education. *Neuroepidemiology* **15,** 20–25.
46. Ramakrishnan, R., Zareparsi, S., Gancher, S., Camicioli, R., Nutt, J., and Payami, H. (2001) Risk factors for Parkinson's dementia: age, male gender, and apolipoprotein e2. *Neurology* **56,** A113.
47. Diamond, S.G., Markham, C.H., Hoehn, M.M., McDowell, F.H., and Muenter, M.D. (1990) An examination of male-female differences in progression and mortality of Parkinson's disease. *Neurology* **40,** 763–766.
48. Ebmeier, K.P., Calder, S.A., Crawford, J.R., Stewart, L., Besson, J.A., and Mutch, W.J. (1990) Clinical features predicting dementia in idiopathic Parkinson's disease: a follow-up study. *Neurology* **40,** 1222–1224.
49. Katzman, R. (1993) Education and the prevalence of dementia and Alzheimer's disease. *Neurology* **43,** 13–20.
50. Piccirilli, M., Piccinin, G.L., and Agostini, L. (1984) Characteristic clinical aspects of Parkinson patients with intellectual impairment. *Eur. Neurol.* **23,** 44–50.
51. Elizan, T.S., Sroka, H., Maker, H., Smith, H., and Yahr, M.D. (1986) Dementia in idiopathic Parkinson's disease. Variables associated with its occurrence in 203 patients. *J. Neural Transm.* **65,** 285–302.
52. Giladi, N., Treves, T.A., Paleacu, D., et al. (2000) Risk factors for dementia, depression and psychosis in long-standing Parkinson's disease. *J. Neural Transm. (Budapest)* **107,** 59–71.
53. Agid, Y., Graybiel, A.M., Ruberg, M., et al. (1990) The efficacy of levodopa treatment declines in the course of Parkinson's disease: do nondopaminergic lesions play a role? *Adv. Neurol.* **53,** 83–100.
54. Levy, G., Tang, M.X., Cote, L.J., et al. (2000) Motor impairment in PD: relationship to incident dementia and age. *Neurology* **55,** 539–544.
55. Zetusky, W.J., Jankovic, J., and Pirozzolo, F.J. (1985) The heterogeneity of Parkinson's disease: clinical and prognostic implications. *Neurology* **35,** 522–526.
56. Marder, K., Tang, M., Hemenegildo, N., et al. (1993) A factor analysis of extrapyramidal signs as risk factors for dementia in Parkinson's disease. *Mov. Disord.* **8,** 409.
57. Hoehn, M.M. and Yahr, M.D. (1967) Parkinsonism: onset, progression and mortality. *Neurology* **17,** 427–442.
58. Jankovic, J., McDermott, M., Carter, J., et al. (1990) Variable expression of Parkinson's disease: a base-line analysis of the DATATOP cohort. The Parkinson Study Group. *Neurology* **40,** 1529–1534.
59. Hershey, L.A., Feldman, B.J., Kim, K.Y., Commichau, C., and Lichter, D.G. (1991) Tremor at onset. Predictor of cognitive and motor outcome in Parkinson's disease? *Arch. Neurol.* **48,** 1049–1051.
60. Viitanen, M., Mortimer, J.A., and Webster, D.D. (1994) Association between presenting motor symptoms and the risk of cognitive impairment in Parkinson's disease. *J. Neurol. Neurosurg. Psychiatry* **57,** 1203–1207.
61. Portin, R. and Rinne, U.K. (1987) Predictive factors for cognitive deterioration and dementia in Parkinson's disease. *Adv. Neurol.* **45,** 413–416.

62. Caparros-Lefebvre, D., Pecheux, N., Petit, V., Duhamel, A., and Petit, H. (1995) Which factors predict cognitive decline in Parkinson's disease? *J. Neurol. Neurosurg. Psychiatry* **58,** 51–55.
63. Starkstein, S.E., Mayberg, H.S., Leiguarda, R., Preziosi, T.J., and Robinson, R.G. (1992) A prospective longitudinal study of depression, cognitive decline, and physical impairments in patients with Parkinson's disease. *J. Neurol. Neurosurg. Psychiatry* **55,** 377–382.
64. Hamilton, M. (1960) A rating scale for depression. *J. Neurol. Neurosurg. Psychiatry* **23,** 56–62.
65. Starkstein, S.E., Bolduc, P.L., Mayberg, H.S., Preziosi, T.J., and Robinson, R.G. (1990) Cognitive impairments and depression in Parkinson's disease: a follow up study. *J. Neurol. Neurosurg. Psychiatry* **53,** 597–602.
66. Montgomery, S.A. and Asberg, M. (1979) A new depression scale designed to be sensitive to change. *Br. J. Psychiatry* **134,** 382–389.
67. Guillard, A., Chastang, C., and Fenelon, G. (1986) Etude a long terme de 416 cas de maladie de Parkinson. Facteurs de pronostic et implications therapeutiques. *Revue Neurologique* **142,** 207–214.
68. Friedman, A. and Barcikowska, M. (1994) Dementia in Parkinson's disease. *Dementia* **5,** 12–16.
69. Jacobs, D.M., Marder, K., Cote, L.J., Sano, M., Stern, Y., and Mayeux, R. (1995) Neuropsychological characteristics of preclinical dementia in Parkinson's disease. *Neurology* **45,** 1691–1696.
70. Levy, G., Jacobs, D.M., Tang, M.X., et al. (2002) Memory and executive function impairment predict dementia in Parkinson's disease. *Mov. Disord.,* in press.
71. Piccirilli, M., D'Alessandro, P., Finali, G., Piccinin, G.L., and Agostini, L. (1989) Frontal lobe dysfunction in Parkinson's disease: prognostic value for dementia? *Eur. Neurol.* **29,** 71–76.
72. Piccirilli, M., D'Alessandro, P., Finali, G., and Piccinin, G. (1997) Early frontal impairment as a predictor of dementia in Parkinson's disease. *Neurology* **48,** 546–547.
73. Salganik, I. and Korczyn, A. (1990) Risk factors for dementia in Parkinson's disease. *Adv. Neurol.* **53,** 343–347.
74. Levy, G., Tang, M.X., Cote, L.J., et al. (2002) Do risk factors for Alzheimer's disease predict dementia in Parkinson's disease? An exploratory study. *Mov. Disord.* **17,** 250–257.
75. Arai, H., Muramatsu, T., Higuchi, S., Sasaki, H., and Trojanowski, J.Q. (1994) Apolipoprotein E gene in Parkinson's disease with or without dementia. *Lancet* **344,** 889.
76. Marder, K., Maestre, G., Cote, L., et al. (1994) The apolipoprotein epsilon 4 allele in Parkinson's disease with and without dementia. *Neurology* **44,** 1330–1331.
77. Koller, W.C., Glatt, S.L., Hubble, J.P., et al. (1995) Apolipoprotein E genotypes in Parkinson's disease with and without dementia. *Ann. Neurol* **37,** 242–245.
78. Inzelberg, R., Chapman, J., Treves, T.A., et al. (1998) Apolipoprotein E4 in Parkinson disease and dementia: new data and meta-analysis of published studies. *Alzheimer Dis. Assoc. Disord.* **12,** 45–48.
79. Whitehead, A.S., Bertrandy, S., Finnan, F., Butler, A., Smith, G.D., and Ben Shlomo, Y. (1996) Frequency of the apolipoprotein E epsilon 4 allele in a case-control study of early onset Parkinson's disease. *J. Neurol. Neurosurg. Psychiatry* **61,** 347–351.
80. Harhangi, B.S., de Rijk, M.C., van Duijn, C.M., Van Broeckhoven, C., Hofman, A., and Breteler, M.M. (2000) APOE and the risk of PD with or without dementia in a population-based study. *Neurology* **54,** 1272–1276.
81. Egensperger, R., Bancher, C., Kosel, S., Jellinger, K., Mehraein, P., and Graeber, M.B. (1996) The apolipoprotein E epsilon 4 allele in Parkinson's disease with Alzheimer lesions. *Biochem. Biophys. Res. Commun.* **224,** 484–486.
82. Mattila, P.M., Koskela, T., Roytta, M., et al. (1998) Apolipoprotein E epsilon4 allele frequency is increased in Parkinson's disease only with co-existing Alzheimer pathology. *Acta Neuropathol.* **96,** 417–420.
83. Mattila, K.M., Rinne, J.O., Roytta, M., et al. (2000) Dipeptidyl carboxypeptidase 1 (DCP1) and butyrylcholinesterase (BCHE) gene interactions with the apolipoprotein E epsilon4 allele as risk factors in Alzheimer's disease and in Parkinson's disease with coexisting Alzheimer pathology. *J. Med. Genet.* **37,** 766–770.
84. Wilhelmsen, K., Mirel, D., Marder, K., et al. (1997) Is there a genetic susceptibility locus for Parkinson's disease on chromosome 22q13? *Ann. Neurol.* **41,** 813–817.
85. Hubble, J.P., Kurth, J.H., Glatt, S.L., et al. (1998) Gene-toxin interaction as a putative risk factor for Parkinson's disease with dementia. *Neuroepidemiology* **17,** 96–104.
86. Heston, L.L. (1980) Dementia associated with Parkinson's disease: a genetic study. *J. Neurol. Neurosurg. Psychiatry* **43,** 846–848.
87. Marder, K., Tang, M.X., Alfaro, B., et al. (1999) Risk of Alzheimer's disease in relatives of Parkinson's disease patients with and without dementia. *Neurology* **52,** 719–724.
88. Mickel, S.F., Broste, S.K., and Hiner, B.C. (1997) Lack of overlap in genetic risks for Alzheimer's disease and Parkinson's disease. *Neurology* **48,** 942–949.
89. Marder, K., Tang, M.X., Alfaro, B., et al. (1998) Postmenopausal estrogen use and Parkinson's disease with and without dementia. *Neurology* **50,** 1141–1143.
90. Hughes, A.J., Daniel, S.E., Blankson, S., and Lees, A.J. (1993) A clinicopathologic study of 100 cases of Parkinson's disease. *Arch. Neurol.* **50,** 140–148.
91. Mattila, P.M., Rinne, J.O., Helenius, H., Dickson, D.W., and Roytta, M. (2000) Alpha-synuclein-immunoreactive cortical Lewy bodies are associated with cognitive impairment in Parkinson's disease. *Acta Neuropathol.* **100,** 285–290.
92. Hurtig, H.I., Trojanowski, J.Q., Galvin, J., et al. (2000) Alpha-synuclein cortical Lewy bodies correlate with dementia in Parkinson's disease. *Neurology* **54,** 1916–1921.
93. Jellinger, K. (2000) Morphological substrates of mental dysfunction in Lewy body disease: an update, in *Advances in Dementia Research* (Jellinger, K., Schmidt, R., and Windisch, M., eds.), Springer-Verlag, New York, pp. 185–212.

94. Loranger, A.W., Goodell, H., McDowell, F.H., Lee, J.E., and Sweet, R.D. (1972) Intellectual impairment in Parkinson's syndrome. *Brain* **95,** 405–412.
95. Lieberman, A., Dziatolowski, M., Kupersmith, M., et al. (1979) Dementia in Parkinson disease. *Ann. Neurol.* **6,** 355–359.
96. Huber, S.J. and Paulson, G.W. (1986) Relationship between primitive reflexes and severity in Parkinson's disease. *J. Neurol. Neurosurg. Psychiatry* **49,** 1298–1300.
97. Pillon, B., Dubois, B., Ploska, A., and Agid, Y. (1991) Severity and specificity of cognitive impairment in Alzheimer's, Huntington's, and Parkinson's diseases and progressive supranuclear palsy. *Neurology* **41,** 634–643.
98. Mjones, H. (1949) Paralysis agitans. A clinical and genetic study. *Acta Psychiat. Neurol.* **54(Suppl.),** 1–195.
99. Ebmeier, K.P., Calder, S.A., Crawford, J.R., Stewart, L., Cochrane, R.H., and Besson, J.A. (1991) Dementia in idiopathic Parkinson's disease: prevalence and relationship with symptoms and signs of parkinsonism. *Psychol. Med.* **21,** 69–76.
100. Tison, F., Dartigues, J.F., Auriacombe, S., Letenneur, L., Boller, F., and Alperovitch, A. (1995) Dementia in Parkinson's disease: a population-based study in ambulatory and institutionalized individuals. *Neurology* **45,** 705–708.

21

Neuropsychiatric Co-Morbidity in Dementia With and Without Movement Disorders

Clive G. Ballard, MD and Alan Thomas, PhD

1. INTRODUCTION

Classification of neuropsychiatric features has been problematic, with a number of different terminologies and meanings employed. Within the context of parkinsonism and dementia, the most important individual symptoms are psychosis (particularly visual hallucinations), mood disorders, and fluctuating cognition (FC); the current review focuses on these areas. Parkinsonism occurs in the majority of patients suffering from dementia with Lewy bodies (DLB), which, therefore, forms the core of the article. Parkinsonism does, however, arise in all dementias, and a brief discussion of the relationship between parkinsonism and neuropsychiatric features in Alzheimer's disease (AD) and vascular dementia (VaD) is hence included.

2. DLB–PARKINSON'S DISEASE DEMENTIA

DLB was first reported in the 1960s when it was thought to be a rare variant of dementia. Since the late 1980s, the development of anti-ubiquitin staining in conjunction with a series of representative hospital-based postmortem studies and the subsequent development of α-synuclein strains, indicated that it was, in fact, the second most common cause of neurodegenerative dementia, after AD, accounting for 15–20% of all late-onset dementias *(1)*. Although it is clear that DLB is an important and common condition, these prevalence rates need to be interpreted within context. The majority of cohorts come from specialist centers, and in addition, there is an inevitable bias towards undertaking postmortem examinations on these cases because they are often difficult to diagnose clinically and have an interesting symptom profile.

Lewy Body disease is considered to be a spectrum disorder, in the interface between the clinicopathological syndromes of Parkinson's disease (PD) and AD. There are, however, key differences. In PD, the Lewy bodies are mainly found in the substania nigra of the brainstem, whereas Lewy bodies are present throughout the brainstem and in a number of cortical areas in DLB *(2)*. In addition, 75–90% of DLB patients have many of the neuropathological features of AD, including senile plaques and neurofibrilliary tangles *(3)*; although typically, the burden of tangle pathology is less than that which is seen in "pure" AD. Although some of the clinical characteristics of DLB can be interpreted within the context of the overlap of two pathological substrates, it is the distinct clinical profile of DLB, with the combination of Parkinson's, neuropsychiatric features, FC, and severe neuroleptic sensitivity reactions, which makes it a clinically important and meaningful entity. This has led to the development of

From: *Mental and Behavioral Dysfunction in Movement Disorders*
Edited by: M-A. Bédard et al. © Humana Press Inc., Totowa, NJ

operationalized criteria for the diagnosis of the clinical syndrome *(1)*. In order for a diagnosis of DLB to be attributed, the patient must have a dementia syndrome and present with at least two of these three core features: (*i*) fluctuating of cognition with variations in attention and alertness; (*ii*) recurrent well-formed and detailed visual hallucinations; and (*iii*) spontaneous motor features of parkinsonism.

Parkinsonism is a core symptom of DLB with a frequency of 65–70% *(4)*.

2.1. Neuropsychiatric Symptoms

2.1.1. FC

Variation in cognitive performance is commonly observed in all the major late onset dementias. It is frustrating to caregivers and has a major impact upon the patient's ability to reliably perform every day activities. FC may present in several ways, which has often been previously described as "sundowning" or "intermittent delirium," depending upon the severity and diurnal pattern. In most prospective studies, FC occurs in 80% or more of people suffering from DLB, 30–50% of individuals with VaD, and 20% of people with AD *(5,6)*, although FC can be difficult to identify, particularly from case note review.

Recent studies in Newcastle have demonstrated that the severity of FC can be judged by experienced clinicians and is highly correlated with variability in performance on computer-based attentional tasks *(6)*. The variation can be detected over very short periods of time (on a second-to-second basis), suggesting that FC as observed clinically, is based on a dysregulation of continuously active arousal systems. The same phenomenon can also be identified by recording unstable patterns of electroencephalography (EEG) activity in the resting state, episodic slow wave activity; illustrating the close relationship between FC and episodes of impaired consciousness in these patients *(5)*. Although requiring replication from other groups, this strongly indicates that FC can be identified with a structured approach to assessment, although case note evaluations of FC are probably of little value.

Key reviews *(7)*, have concluded that these impairments of consciousness probably relate to deficits in the ascending cholinergic system, which maintain a consistent conscious level through pathways from the reticular activating system, to the reticular nucleus of the thalamus, projecting to the cortex. The hypothesized link between impaired consciousness and the cholinergic system receives support from preliminary case studies, in which "delirious episodes" in DLB patients were substantially improved by cholinesterase therapy *(8)*. This raises potentially important therapeutic issues.

2.1.2. Psychotic Symptoms

Psychotic symptoms are important in people with dementia, as they cause distress *(9)*, are problematic for caregivers *(10)*, and accelerate the need for institutional care *(11)*. Within the context of dementia, Burns et al. *(12)* classified psychosis into three main categories: delusions, hallucinations, and delusional misidentification. Delusions were defined as false unshakable ideas or beliefs that are held with extraordinary conviction and subjective certainty. They also had to be reiterated on at least two occasions more than 1 wk apart; this latter stipulation was designed to minimize overlap with confabulation and delirium. Hallucinations were described as precepts in the absence of a stimulus and had to be directly reported by either the patient or indirectly via an informant to be classified as a psychotic presentation (i.e., they could not be inferred from observed behaviors). Delusional misidentification, included the Capgras syndrome (the belief that a person, object, or environment has been replaced by a double or replica), delusional misidentification of visual images (whereby figures on television or in photographs are thought to exist in the real environment), delusional misidentification of mirror images (one's reflection is perceived as the image of a separate person), and the phantom boarder delusion (believing that strangers are living in or visiting the house). This theoretical classification system is supported by empirical evidence from a principal components analysis of a detailed list of individual symptoms *(13)*.

The most common forms of hallucinations are visual, in contrast to functional psychosis where auditory hallucinations predominate. In DLB, visual hallucinations are most commonly of people, children, and animals; but birds, insects, inanimate objects, undefined shapes, smoke, and fire are sometimes reported *(14)*. The hallucinations are usually of normal size, often move, and are almost always of complete forms. The majority of these characteristics are very similar to the presentation of visual hallucinations in either AD or Parkinson's disease, although unusually, patients with DLB commonly also experience concurrent hallucinations (usually of hallucinated figures) in the auditory modality *(14)*.

Diagnosing delusions in the presence of dementia can also be difficult. The majority of delusional beliefs are simple, and the type of complex elaborate delusional symptoms seen in functional psychosis are extremely rare, and are confined to a small number of people in the early stages of the dementia process *(12)*. The crux of the issue is to be able to distinguish people who make confabulations or assumptions that can be entirely explained as a result of impairments in higher cognitive functions, from those who are experiencing delusions. For example, does a person who does not remember leaving a handbag elsewhere, and suggests that someone may have stolen it, have a delusion? This is where the standard operationalized definition of a delusion and the additions made by Burns et al. *(12)*, are particularly helpful. A delusion has to be an unshakeable belief, hence in the example given, if an alternative explanation is put to the person that they may have forgotten their handbag and they accept this as a plausible explanation, they are not experiencing a delusion. The additional stipulation by Burns et al., that a delusion must be repeated, is helpful in distinguishing delusions from confabulation. In the example given, if a person had made a onetime suggestion on one occasion that a handbag had been stolen, even if held with conviction this would be a confabulation. If similar beliefs were reiterated over a period of time, they would be delusional. The most common individual symptoms are delusions of reference, the belief that other people are talking about the person, delusions of theft or possessions being hidden, and the phantom boarder delusion, believing that strangers are visiting or living in the house.

It is estimated that at least 80% of DLB patients experience some form of psychotic symptoms *(2,3,4,15–22)*, such as visual hallucinations, auditory hallucinations, delusions, or delusional misidentification. Visual hallucinations are the most common individual symptom, with a prevalence rate in excess of 60% in most prospective studies (Table 1). The person with DLB typically sees people, children, or animals of normal size, sometimes with accompanying auditory hallucinations.

2.1.2.1. Outcome of Psychotic Symptoms

Although visual hallucinations are typically described as persistent or recurrent in the consensus clinical criteria for DLB, there have been few longitudinal studies. Preliminary data from a small DLB cohort did provide some support for the persistence of visual hallucinations in these patients *(23)*. More recently in a larger more systematic study, we have confirmed the persistence of visual hallucinations over 1 yr of prospective follow-up in DLB patients, with visual hallucinations persisting for 1 yr in 77% of DLB patients, but only 26% of AD patients *(24)*. Delusions, delusional misidentification, and auditory hallucinations all persisted for the year of follow-up in approx 40% of both DLB and AD patients who experienced these symptoms at baseline.

2.2. Mood Disorders

Depression is important in the context of dementia, as it has a significant detrimental impact upon cognitive function *(25)*, and results in excess disability in the activities of daily living *(25)*, causes distress to patients *(26)*, is burdensome to their caregivers *(10)*, and reduces the life expectancy of the person with dementia *(27)*. Although the reported frequency of depression in DLB varies from 14–50% *(22)*, prospective studies indicate that clinically significant depression probably occurs in at least 30% of patients *(19,22)*, with some studies indicating a significantly higher frequency in DLB than AD *(22)*. Similarly to the picture in AD patients, depression is usually characterized by brief episodes that resolve spontaneously, with only 8 out of 69 (12%) of depressed DLB patients remaining depressed for 1 yr

Table 1
Key Studies Comparing DLB and AD

	No. of patients		% of subjects: Visual hallucinations		Fluctuating confusion		Parkinsonism	
Study	DLB	AD	DLB	AD	DLB	AD	DLB	AD
Byrne et al. *(15)*	15 (26%)	0	40%	0	80%	0	40%	—
Hansen et al. *(3)*	(33%)	—	—	—	—	—	—	—
McKeith et al. *(16)*	21[a]	37	48%	16%	86%	19%	62%	22%
McKeith et al. *(17)*	20[a]	21	80%	19%	90%	5%	85%	19%
Ballard et al. *(18)*	56[b]	0	16%	0	—	—	—	—
Galasko et al. *(4)*	38 (19%)	26 (13%)	32%	11%	—	—	46%	19%
Klakta et al. *(19)*	28 (25%)	58 (52%)	61%	35%	—	—	—	—
Weiner et al. *(20)*	24 (30%)	55 (69%)	64%	21%	—	—	—	—
Ala et al. *(21)*	39 (21%)	60 (19%)	23%	3%	—	—	41%	5%
Ballard et al. *(22)*	40[c]	40	65%	25%	75%	25%	61%	33%

[a]Brain Bank cases.
[b]Taken from dementia care register.
[c]Matched cases.

of prospective follow-up *(24)*. Anxiety has been studied very little in AD, but the prevalence is probably in excess of 40% *(22)*.

2.3. *Biological Basis*

Autopsy studies have identified more extensive reductions of presynaptic cholinergic activity in DLB compared to AD *(28)* and greater cholinergic deficits in the cortex of hallucinating compared to nonhallucinating patients, together with a relative overactivity of the serotonin (5-HT) system *(29)*. Specifically, two independent studies from Newcastle using different case series *(29,30)* reported an association between hallucinations and reduced cholinergic activity in the visual association areas (the data from Ballard et al. *[30]* are summarized in Table 2). This, together with the favorable treatment response of visual hallucinations to cholinesterase inhibitor therapy *(31)*, provides convincing evidence that cholinergic deficits in key brain areas are the main substrate of visual hallucinations in these patients. Delusions have been less studied, but were associated with increased muscarinic M1 receptor binding in a recent report *(30)*. An involvement of this cholinergic receptor is consistent with clinical evidence that the muscarinic agonist xanomeline relieves this symptom in AD *(32)*, although the finding must be considered as preliminary and requires replication. One preliminary study has examined the neurochemical associations of depression, indicating that DLB patients with major depression had a relative preservation of 5-HT re-uptake sites, compared to those without *(33)*. The associations of other neuropsychiatric features await evaluation.

2.4. *Treatment of Neuropsychiatric Features*

Good general principles of clinical practice are important in the management of neuropsychiatric symptoms arising in the context of dementia. Not all symptoms are distressing or impact upon the care of the individual patient, hence a clinical decision should be made regarding the need for intervention. If an intervention is considered appropriate, the quality of care available and the environment should be optimized as far as possible. In addition, psychosocial or environmental management approaches can

Table 2
A Comparison of Pirenzepine Binding and ChAT in Brodmann Area 36 Between DLB Patients with and without Visual Hallucinations and Delusions

	BA 36				
	VH present (n = 12)	VH absent (n = 5)	Statistical evaluation	Delusions present (n = 14)	Delusions absent (n = 7)
ChAT	1.7 ± 0.6	2.5 ± 0.7	T = 2.5, p = 0.02[a]	1.9 ± 0.6	1.9 ± 0.8
Pirenzepine	122.3 ± 31.6	106.3 ± 44.8	T = 0.9, p = 0.38	131.0 ± 31.4	93.5 ± 27.7

[a]In an analysis of variance (ANOVA) analysis, significant associations were identified between VH and/or delusions and BA 36, but not with BA 7 or BA 20.

Abbreviations: BA, Brodmann area; VH, visual hallucinations.

be very effective and are often the most appropriate first line intervention strategy. Having said this, psychiatric symptoms are more intense, more distressing *(34)*, and more persistent *(24)* in DLB patients than those with AD, and are, therefore, more likely to require pharmacological treatment.

In AD, the pharmacological management option of choice for psychiatric or behavioral disturbances would be neuroleptic treatment *(35)*. In DLB patients however, McKeith et al. *(17)* reported severe sensitivity reactions in 50% of patients suffering from DLB exposed to neuroleptic agents in an autopsy study. These reactions were characterized by cognitive decline, increased parkinsonism, drowsiness, and features of the neuroleptic malignant syndrome; resulting in a threefold increase in mortality. Despite initial reports indicating the potential value of risperidone *(36,37)*, subsequent reports have suggested that severe neuroleptic sensitivity reactions are also frequent with risperidone *(38,39)*. Almost all severe neuroleptic sensitivity reactions arise within 2 wk of a new neuroleptic prescription or a dose change *(39)*. Although very preliminary studies indicate that both olanzapine *(40)* and quetiapine *(41)* may be better tolerated, the studies involve small numbers of patients in whom the diagnosis of DLB has not been verified. Given the potential severity of neuroleptic sensitivity reactions, the possibility of larger trials with atypical antipsychotic agents raises major ethical issues.

An alternative pharmacological treatment approach, based upon the neurochemical associations of key neuropsychiatric symptoms in DLB patients, would be to consider cholinergic enhancement. A number of reports have now been published evaluating the potential role of cholinesterase therapy in DLB patients. Most studies have measured cognitive and neuropsychiatric outcomes and have not focused specifically on psychiatric symptoms. A pilot study evaluated tacrine in patients with Parkinson's disease dementia (PDD) *(42)*. The seven patients all had severe PD had suffered a confusional state exacerbated by dopaminergic drugs, and had Mini-Mental State Examination (MMSE) scores in the range 15–21. All seven patients benefited, with reductions in their hallucinatory experiences and improved cognition (orientation, attention, visuospatial awareness, and mean improvement in MMSE 7.1). Surprisingly, motor ability also improved (Unified Parkinson's Disease Rating Scale [UPDRS] mean scores pre- and posttreatment 79.3 and 29.6, p = 0.0001), which is an important observation with respect to the potential value of cholinesterase inhibitors in the management of DLB, where the exacerbation of parkinsonism is a potential concern.

The first trial to directly evaluate cholinesterase inhibitor therapy in DLB patients, involved a direct comparison of DLB and AD patients treated with tacrine *(43)*. Seventy-five patients were enrolled in the study, but only 39 completed the treatment period. Overall, 11 of the 20 AD patients and 11 of the 19 DLB patients were considered to be "responders," suggesting a similar efficacy of cholinesterase inhibitors in the two conditions. Subsequently, a number of case reports and case series of DLB patients treated with cholinesterase inhibitors have appeared in the literature. Kaufer et al. *(8)* reported two cases of clinically diagnosed DLB with prominent psychotic symptoms, and fluctuating levels of conscious-

Table 3
Summary of Case Studies and Trials of Cholinesterase Therapy for the Treatment of DLB

Study	Design	No. of DLB patients	Cholinesterase inhibitor used	Summary of outcome
Lebert et al. *(43)*	DLB–AD comparison	19	Tacrine	11 out of 19 "responders," comparable to AD.
Kaufer et al. *(8)*	Case series	2	Donepezil	Marked improvement of psychosis and fluctuating confusion.
Shea et al. *(44)*	Case series	9	Donepezil	Hallucinations improved in 8 patients and cognition in 7. Worsening parkinsonism in 3 people.
Aarsland et al. *(45)*	Case report	1	Donepezil	Marked improvement of cognition.
Ferguson and Howard *(46)*	Case series	2	Donepezil	Substantial improvement of behavior, cognition, and overall functioning, preventing the need for institutional care.
McKeith et al. *(31)*	Double-blind placebo-controlled trial	124	Rivastigmine	Significant improvement in in BPSD and cognition.

BPSD, behavioral and psychological symptoms of dementia.

ness or attention experienced substantial symptom resolution within 1 mo on donepezil therapy, and symptom control continued for the following year of treatment. In a larger series of nine consecutive patients with clinically diagnosed DLB treated with donepezil over a mean of 12 wk, hallucinations improved in eight, cognition in seven, and overall function was improved or maintained in six cases. In three of the nine cases, parkinsonian features deteriorated but subsequently responded to dopamine agonist therapy *(44)*. Aarsland et al. *(45)* reported the interesting case of a 71-yr-old woman with DLB symptoms for 2 yr, who experienced a remarkable improvement early in a 19-wk course of donepezil, benefits which were sustained. Baseline scores of 23/30 and 120/144 for the MMSE and UPDRS, respectively, improved to 28/30 and 143/144 after 19 wk of treatment. In two further elderly patients with a clinical diagnosis of DLB, substantial improvements in behavioral and cognitive function were seen with resolution of psychotic symptoms *(46)* in just 2 wk of donepezil treatment. The improvements in overall function avoided the need for continuing care in one case and institutional care in the other patient. These reports are summarized in Table 3.

Obviously, case reports need to be interpreted with caution. There is no confirmation of diagnostic accuracy, and there is an inevitable bias towards the publication of cases with favorable outcomes. Nonetheless, these cases do provide some important anecdotal evidence of the potential value of cholinesterase inhibitor therapy in DLB patients and suggest that treatment is safe, without severe exacerbation of parkinsonism.

The first double-blind placebo-controlled trial of cholinesterase inhibitor therapy for the treatment of DLB has now been published *(31)*. One hundred twenty-four patients in 18 centers in Europe participated. Patients were randomized to rivastigmine or placebo for 20 wk. Primary outcome measures were the Neuropsychiatric Inventory (NPI) for behavioral and psychological symptoms of dementia (BPSD) symptoms and the computerized Cognitive Drug Research (CDR) battery for cognitive

Table 4
Relationship Between Parkinsonism and Neuropsychiatric Features in DLB ($N = 95$)

	Significant parkinsonism ($n = 73$)	No parkinsonsim ($n = 22$)	Statistical evaluation
Depression	14 (19%)	5 (23%)	χ^2 0.1, $p = 0.72$
Anxiety	41 (56%)	8 (36%)	χ^2 1.9, $p = 0.17$
Impaired consciousness	58 (80%)	11 (50%)	χ^2 8.4, $p = 0.015$[a]
FC	73 (100%)	20 (91%)	χ^2 6.7, $p = 0.01$[a]
Delusions	44 (60%)	10 (46%)	χ^2 1.5, $p = 0.22$
Misidentification	37 (51%)	10 (46%)	χ^2 0.2, $p = 0.67$
Visual hallucinations	53 (73%)	16 (73%)	χ^2 0.0, $p = 0.99$
Auditory hallucinations	24 (33%)	12 (55%)	χ^2 3.4, $p = 0.03$[a]
MMSE	17.0 std 12.0	14.0 std 6.7	$t = 1.1$, $p = 0.27$
Yr of dementia	2.6 std 1.9	2.2 std 1.8	$t = 0.7$, $p = 0.47$
Yr of parkinsonism	3.4 std 1.3		

std, standard deviation.
[a]Statistically significant, $p < 0.05$.

function. Significant improvements in BPSD (total NPI improved in 61% patients on rivastigmine, compared with 28% placebo group; $p = 0.002$), and attentional performance were seen compared with placebo, and the active treatment was well-tolerated with no increase in adverse events requiring withdrawal, in comparison with the placebo group. Furthermore, there was no deterioration in parkinsonism in the treatment group.

The evidence certainly indicates that psychotic symptoms and cognition improve with cholinesterase therapy, and there is anecdotal evidence from some of the case reports suggesting that there may also be improvements in FC and impairments of consciousness. Given the potential hazards of neuroleptic treatment, many authorities would now recommend cholinesterase inhibitor therapy as a first-line treatment for psychotic symptoms in DLB patients, although corroboration from a second study is urgently needed before firm evidence-based practice guidelines can be developed. There are no trials evaluating antidepressant therapy in DLB. When concurrent major depression presents as a clinical management problem, cautious treatment with 5-HT re-uptake inhibitors is probably the best pragmatic course (hence avoiding antidepressants with pronounced anticholinergic properties), titrating dose against clinical response.

3. DLB PATIENTS WITH PARKINSONISM

The relationship between the presence of parkinsonism and the frequency of key neuropsychiatric features has not been examined in the published literature. From our own dementia case register in Newcastle, 73 (77%) of the DLB patients (clinically diagnosed using the international consensus criteria, with neuropathological verification of accuracy for the first 50 cases) experienced significant parkinsonism. There were very few differences between the profile of symptoms in those with and without parkinsonian features; although patients with parkinsonism were significantly less likely to experience auditory hallucinations and more likely to experience both FC and impaired consciousness (Table 4). A further logistic regression was undertaken to examine the associations of impaired consciousness with parkinsonism and to evaluate the potential confounding role of levadopa (L-dopa). Significant parkinsonism (Wald 3.4, $p = 0.05$) was entered into the equation, but L-dopa (Wald 1.6, $p = 0.2$) was not. The associations with impaired consciousness and FC may give some important clues as to the likely neuropathological substrates of these phenomena. In addition, there is no evidence of a link between parkinsonism and an increased tendency to experience either psychotic or mood symptoms.

4. PDD

PDD is a global category referring to all patients with PD who proceed to develop dementia. Those with PD for less than 1 yr before the emergence of cognitive deficits will probably meet the consensus clinical criteria for DLB. Some others will meet the criteria for DLB, except for a longer duration of parkinsonism. Pathologically, PD is characterized by neuronal cell loss and Lewy bodies in surviving neurons of the substantia nigra *(47)*. In addition, Lewy bodies are found in the cortex of nearly all PD patients *(47,48)*, particularly those with dementia. There will also be patients with concurrent AD and some individuals who experience cognitive impairments related more directly to the neurochemical deficits of PD. In reality, an overlap of these concurrent pathological processes will be the most common presentation. Although these issues will be reviewed in considerably more detail elsewhere, it is important to describe the heterogeneity of the PDD syndrome, as this creates considerable difficulties when interpreting neuropsychiatric data, which can be further compounded by the possible role of L-dopa and anticholinergic medications in exacerbating these syndromes.

An emerging literature in this field indicates that neuropsychiatric syndromes including delusions (5–10%), hallucinations (30%), and mood disorders, such as depression (20%), are frequent in patients with PD *(49)* and are even more frequent in PD patients with dementia. For example, Aarsland et al. *(50,51)* studied 235 patients with PD from a community register with a mean age of 74 and a mean duration of parkinsonism of 9 yr. Overall, 23 patients (10%) had hallucinations with insight, and 14 patients (6%) had psychosis with hallucinations or delusions. Older age, living in a care facility, and having cognitive impairment were associated with higher frequencies of psychotic symptoms. Higher doses of L-dopa were associated with vivid dreaming, but not with either hallucinations or delusions. More recently, the Stavanger group reported a the prevalence of psychosis in the 131 surviving patients from their original series *(52)*. Among the 48 patients with PDD, 9 (19%) experienced paranoid delusions, 12 (25%) experienced delusional misidentification, 24 (50%) had visual hallucinations, and 10 (21%) experienced auditory hallucinations. These frequencies were intermediate between the rates seen in DLB and PD without dementia *(53)*. There may be some specific phenomenological differences worthy of further consideration, for instance the Capgras syndrome occurred in 10% of DLB patients, but was not seen at all in patients with PDD *(53)*. In a comparison of PDD and AD patients, hallucinations were significantly more frequent in PDD (45%) than AD (19%), but there was no significant difference in the frequency of the other psychotic symptoms (delusions: PDD, 24%; AD 33%), again suggesting that hallucinations are characteristic of these patients.

From the same community PD cohort, major depression was diagnosed in 18 (8%) of patients *(54)*. Patients with depression were older at the time of examination, had a greater age at onset of PD, and had a lower score on the MMSE. Among patients living in nursing homes, the frequency of major depression was fourfold higher than among patients living at home (19.1 vs 4.9%). In a more recent report, 40% of PDD patients had significant depression and 31% had anxiety according to the NPI, which has slightly more lax criteria than those within the Diagnosis and Statistical Manual of Mental Disorders, fourth edition (DSM IV) which probably explains the relatively high absolute frequencies. Neither depression nor anxiety was significantly more frequent in PDD than AD *(52)*. FC has not been systematically evaluated in PDD, although very preliminary indications from ongoing studies suggest that significant fluctuation does occur.

In addition to the problems of interpretation relating to the pathological heterogeneity, referral bias is also an important consideration. For example, a meta-analysis of neuropsychiatric symptoms in DLB indicated a threefold higher frequency of visual hallucinations in patients presenting to a psychiatry clinic compared to those seen in a neurology setting *(18)*. Most studies indicate even lower frequencies of psychiatric symptoms in community cohorts. Therefore, although the studies of PDD are important in confirming the high frequency of visual hallucinations, it is difficult to make a direct comparison with DLB cohorts from different settings.

A further complicating factor is the potential role of L-dopa in triggering or exacerbating key neuropsychiatric symptoms particularly visual hallucinations and delusions. Early reports *(55–57)* and clinical experience indicate the potential of L-dopa to induce or aggravate psychotic symptomatology, whereas a number of more systematic studies in PD have failed to identify an association between L-dopa dose and the presence of psychosis *(50–52,58,59)*, and there is no evidence of an association between taking L-dopa (or the L-dopa dose) and the likelihood of experiencing either hallucinations or delusions in the context of DLB *(22)*. Furthermore, Goetz et al. *(60)* were unable to induce hallucinations in PD patients with the intravenous (IV) administration of L-dopa. Contrary evidence, however, comes from a recent autopsy study *(30)*. Visual hallucinations only occurred in patients taking L-dopa, although not all patients taking L-dopa had visual hallucinations, and the differences in choline acetyltransferase (ChAT) between hallucinating and nonhallucinating were similar in the patients not taking L-dopa, which does provide some support to the notion that L-dopa may increase vulnerability to visual hallucinations in DLB patients. While it is difficult to resolve this issue completely in the absence of placebo controlled data, the overall weight of evidence is consistent with the findings from cliniconeurochemical studies, indicating that cholinergic deficits are the main substrate of psychosis in these patients.

Progress in this area has been hampered to some degree by the arbitrary cutoff stipulating that a diagnosis of DLB can only be made when the dementia begins within 1 yr of the onset of the parkinsonism. Future studies need to empirically examine the relationship between both the clinical presentations and the neuropathological–neurochemical substrates of DLB and PDD and how these relate to the frequency and course of neuropsychiatric symptoms. It should, however, also be considered that duration of parkinsonism may not be the only important factor, and there may also be qualitative differences, for example, parkinsonism is more symmetrical in DLB *(61)*, and single-photon emission tomography (SPECT) studies have suggested key differences between DLB and PD in the pattern of loss of dopamine receptors in the caudate and putamen *(62)*.

5. AD

Meta-analyses of standardized studies conducted in clinical settings *(26,63)* indicate a mean prevalence of 31% for delusions, 21% for hallucinations, and 20% for major depression. The rates are lower in community studies *(64)*. Although less studied, anxiety symptoms are also frequent (prevalence range 17–38%) *(22,65–68)*. Periods of FC and/or impaired consciousness, characterized by changes in arousal ranging from episodes of lucidity, to reduced awareness and even stupor; although characteristic of DLB, occur in 20–30% of AD sufferers *(5,6)*.

5.1. Patients with Parkinsonism in the Context of AD

Within the Newcastle case register, 14 (9%) of the patients with an operationalized clinical diagnosis of AD (National Institute of Neurological and Communicative Disorders and Stroke/Alzheimer's Disease and Related Disorders Association [NINCDS/ADRDA] criteria) had significant parkinsonism. There were no significant differences in the frequencies of neuropsychiatric symptoms between patients with and without parkinsonism, but impairment of consciousness (36 vs 19%) and FC (64 vs 38%) did appear to be more frequent in the parkinsonian patients (Table 5).

6. VaD

Spontaneous parkinsonism is occasionally seen in patients with (VaD), with frequencies between 2 and 10% described in the literature depending upon the severity of the cognitive impairment. Although psychotic symptoms are common in VaD patients, (ranges: delusions 8–50%, visual hallucinations 13–25%, and delusional misidentification 26–27%) *(34,64,68–80)* have indicated a lower prevalence of key psychotic symptoms in VaD patients compared to those with AD. Prevalence estimates for depression in VaD vary from 8–66% (mean 32%) *(25,34,64,68,75,76,78,81–85)*. Six comparative

Table 5
Relationship Between Parkinsonism and Neuropsychiatric Features in AD (N = 162)

	Significant parkinsonism (n = 14)	No parkinsonsim (n = 148)	Statistical evaluation
Depression	2 (14%)	16 (11%)	χ^2 0.2, $p = 0.69$
Anxiety	6 (43%)	75 (51%)	χ^2 0.3, $p = 0.58$
Impaired consciousness	5 (36%)	28 (19%)	χ^2 2.2, $p = 0.14$
FC	9 (64%)	56 (38%)	χ^2 3.1, $p = 0.06$
Delusions	6 (43%)	45 (30%)	χ^2 0.9, $p = 0.34$
Misidentification	3 (21%)	29 (16%)	χ^2 0.0, $p = 0.87$
Visual hallucinations	4 (29%)	23 (16%)	χ^2 1.6, $p = 0.21$
Auditory hallucinations	2 (14%)	9 (6%)	χ^2 1.3, $p = 0.24$
MMSE	13.3 std 7.6	16.1 std 5.8	$t = 1.6$, $p= 0.12$
Yr of dementia	2.4 std 1.0	3.1 std 2.1	$t = 1.2$, $p = 0.23$
Yr of parkinsonism		2.3 std 1.6	

std, standard deviation.

studies have reported significantly higher prevalence rates of depression in VaD compared to AD (Table 6). Although there are a paucity of longitudinal studies, a preliminary report did indicate that depression was significantly less likely to resolve over 1 yr of follow-up in VaD patients compared to those with AD *(86)*. Anxiety has received considerably less focus than depression in VaD, although two recent studies have been reported. In the first study, anxiety symptoms were identified in 71% of 92 VaD patients from a hospital dementia case register *(68)*. A much lower frequency of 19% was, however, reported in a population sample of VaD patients *(64)*. Fluctuating confusion is one of the diagnostic elements for VaD and is a key item in the Hachinski scale. Although FC has been described in up to 45% of VaD patients, the pattern is very different to that seen in DLB, with intermittent periods of confusion rather than second-to-second variability in cognitive performance *(5,6)*.

6.1. Relationship Between Parkinsonism and Neuropsychiatric Features in VaD Patients

Within the Newcastle case register, eight (11%) of the patients with an operationalized clinical diagnosis of VaD (NINCDS AIRENS criteria). There were no differences in the frequencies of neuropsychiatric features between patients with and without parkinsonism (Table 7). This, perhaps, implies a different mechanism of FC and/or impaired consciousness in vascular and neurodegenerative dementias.

7. CONCLUSION

Neuropsychiatric symptoms, including FC and/or impaired consciousness, psychosis, and mood disorders, are frequent and important in DLB and PDD. In both DLB and AD, the presence of parkinsonism is associated with an increased frequency of impaired counsciousness, which may give important neuroanatomical clues to the key areas involved. Accumulating evidence indicates a predominantly cholinergic basis for visual hallucinations and delusions in DLB, with treatment trials supporting the value of cholinergic enhancement in these patients. Although there has been enormous progress in this field over the last few years, further work is needed to examine the frequency and basis of neuropsychiatric features in the continuum between DLB and PDD, to determine the mechanisms of FC and/or impaired consciousness and to examine the basis and treatment of mood disorders in these individuals.

REFERENCES

1. McKeith, I.G., Galasko, D., Kosaka, A., et al. (1996) Consensus guidelines for the clinical & pathological diagnosis of dementia with Lewy bodies (DLB): report of the Consortium on DLB International Workshop. *Neurology* **47**, 1113–1124.

Table 6
Frequency of Psychosis and Depression in VD

Study	Sample origins	Psychosis criteria	Dep criteria	N VaD	Mean age	% Dep	% VH	% Dels	% Mis	Psychosis overall
Cummings et al. *(69)*	Clinical	DSM 111	DSM 111	15	70	27				40
Ballard et al. *(70,81)*	Clinical	Burns	CAMDEX	14	78	21				9
Flynn et al. *(71)*	Clinical	BEHAV-AD		14	69			50		
Morriss et al. *(74)*	NH	DSM 111R		27	80			19		
Corey-Bloom et al. *(75)*	Clinical	DSM 11R	DSM IIIR	443*	78	39	22	37		
Ballard et al. *(34)*	Clinical	Burns	RDC	20	80	45	25	50	27	70
Binnetti et al. *(77)*	Clinical	DSM 111R		32	76			22		
Rovner et al. *(78)*	NH	GMS PGBRS	GMS PGBRS	9	79	44				11
Hope et al. *(79)*	Com	PBE	PBE	22	No significant differences in frequency between VaD and AD patients.					
Ballard et al. *(68)*	Clinical	Burns	DSM IIIR	92	79	19	22	36	26	
Chandler and Chandler *(80)*	NH	DSM III	DSM III	3	80	66				33
Lyketsos et al. *(64)*	Com	NPI	NPI	62	84	32	13	8		
Sultzer et al. *(76)*	Clinical	NBS	HDRS	28	70	> in VaD	No significant differences in scores between VaD and AD.			
Verhey et al. *(82)*	Clinical		DSM IIIR	43	74	9				
Greenwald et al. *(25)*	Clinical		DSM III	54	75	20				
Reding et al. *(85)*	Clinical		DSM III	26		8				
Newman et al. *(83)*	Com		DSM IIIR	140	>70	21				

Abbreviations: PGBRS, psychogeriatric behavioral rating scale; NBS, neurobehavioral scale; HDRS, Hamilton depression rating scale; NPI, neuropsychiatric inventory; GMS, Geriatric mental state schedule; PBE, present behavioural examination; Burns, criteria developed by Burns et al., 1990; Com, community; NH, nursing home; Dep, depression; VH, visual hallucination; Mis, delusional misidentification; Del, delusion; N, number; AD, Alzheimer's disease; VaD, vascular dementia; sample of mixed AD/VaD cases.

Table 7
Relationship Between Parkinsonism and Neuropsychiatric Features in VaD ($N = 72$)

	Significant parkinsonism ($n = 8$)	No parkinsonsim ($n = 64$)	Statistical evaluation
Depression	2 (25%)	9 (14%)	χ^2 0.7, $p = 0.42$
Anxiety	3 (38%)	40 (63%)	χ^2 1.8, $p = 0.17$
Impaired consciousness	4 (50%)	20 (31%)	χ^2 1.1, $p = 0.29$
FC	4 (50%)	38 (59%)	χ^2 0.3, $p = 0.61$
Delusions	4 (50%)	19 (30%)	χ^2 1.3, $p = 0.25$
Misidentification	1 (13%)	13 (20%)	χ^2 0.3, $p = 0.60$
Visual hallucinations	1 (13%)	11 (17%)	χ^2 0.1, $p = 0.73$
Auditory hallucinations	2 (25%)	4 (7%)	χ^2 3.3, $p = 0.07$
MMSE	10.3 std 4.6	18.4 std 5.6	$t = 2.4$, $p = 0.02^a$
Yr of dementia	2.0 std 0.7	2.7 std 2.0	$t = 0.8$, $p = 0.42$
Yr of parkinsonism	7.8 std 11.4		

std, standard deviation.
[a]Statistically significant, $p < 0.05$.

2. Perry, R.H., Irving, D., Blessed, G., et al. (1990) A clinically and pathologically distinct form of Lewy body dementia in the elderly. *J. Neurol. Sci.* **95,** 119–139.
3. Hansen, L., Salmon, D., Galasko, D., et al. (1990) The Lewy body variant of Alzheimer's disease: a clinical and pathological entity. *Neurology* **40,** 1–8.
4. Galasko, D., Katzman, R., Salmon, D.P., et al. (1996) Clinical and neuropathological findings in Lewy body dementia. *Brain Cogn.* **31,** 166–175.
5. Walker, M.P., Ayre, G.A., Cummings, J.L., et al. (2000) Quantifying fluctuation in dementia with Lewy bodies, Alzheimer's disease and vascular dementia. *Neurology* **54,** 1616–1625.
6. Walker, M.P., Ayre, G.A., Cummings, J.L., et al. (2000) The clinician assessment of fluctuation and the one day fluctuation assessment scale: two methods to assess fluctuating confusion in dementia. *Br. J. Psychiatry* **177,** 252–256.
7. Perry, E.K., Walker, M.P., Grace, J., et al. (1999) Acetylcholine in mind: a neurotransmitter correlate of consciousness. *Trends Neurosci.* **22,** 273–280.
8. Kaufer, D.I., Catt, K.E., Lopez, E.L., et al. (1998) Dementia with Lewy bodies: response of delirium like features to Donepezil. *Neurology* **51,** 1512.
9. Gilley, D.W., Whaler, M.E., Wilson, R.S., and Bennett, D.A. (1991) Hallucinations and associated factors in Alzheimer's disease. *J. Neuropsychiatry Clin. Neurosci.* **3,** 371–376.
10. Rabins, P.V., Mace, N.L., and Lucas, M.J. (1982) The impact of dementia on the family. *J. Am. Med. Assoc.* **248,** 333–335.
11. Steele, C., Rovner, B., Chase, G.A., and Folstein, M. (1990) Psychiatric symptoms and nursing home placement of patients with Alzheimer's disease. *Am. J. Psychiatry* **147,** 1049–1051.
12. Burns, A., Jacoby, R., and Levy, R. (1990) Psychiatric phenomena in Alzheimer's disease. I: disorders of thought content and II: disorders of perception. *Br. J. Psychiatry* **157,** 72–86.
13. Ballard, C., Bannister, C., Patel, A., et al. (1995) Classification of psychotic symptoms in dementia sufferers. *Acta Psychiatr. Scand.* **92,** 63–68.
14. Ballard, C., McKeith, I., Harrison, R., et al. (1997) Aspects of dementia: a detailed phenomenological comparison of complex visual hallucinations in dementia with Lewy bodies and Alzheimer's disease. *Int. Psychogeriatrics* **9,** 381–388.
15. Byrne, E.J., Lennox, G., and Lowe, J. (1989) Diffuse Lewy body disease, clinical features in 15 cases. *J. Neurol. Neurosurg. Psychiatry* **52,** 709–717.
16. Mckeith, I.G., Perry, R.H., Fairbairn, A.F., et al. (1992) Operational criteria for senile dementia of Lewy body type. *Psychol. Med.* **22,** 911–922.
17. McKeith, I., Fairbairn, A., Poerry, R., et al. (1992) Neuroleptic sensitivity in patients with senile dementia of Lewy body type. *BMJ* **305,** 673–678.
18. Ballard, C.G., Lowery, K., Harrison, R., et al. (1996) Non-cognitive symptoms, in *Dementia with Lewy Bodies* (Perry, R.H., McKeith, I.G., and Perry, E.K., eds.), Cambridge University Press, New York, pp. 67–84.
19. Klakta, L.A., Louis, E.D., and Schiffer, R.B. (1996) Psychiatric features in diffuse Lewy body disease: findings in 28 pathologically diagnosed cases. *Neurology* **47,** 1148–1152.
20. Weiner, W.F., Risser, R.C., Cullum, C.M., et al. (1996) Alzheimer's disease and its Lewy body variant: a clinical analysis of post-mortem verified cases. *Am. J. Psychiatry* **153,** 1269–1273.
21. Ala, T.A., Yang, K.H., Sung, J.H., et al. (1997) Hallucinations and signs of parkinsonism help distinguish patients Alzheimer's disease at presentation: a clinico-pathological study. *J. Neurol. Neurosurg. Psychiatry* **62,** 16–21.

22. Ballard, C., Holmes, C., McKeith, I., et al. (1999) Psychiatric morbidity in dementia with Lewy bodies: a prospective clinical and neuropathological comparative study with Alzheimer's disease. *Am. J. Psychiatry* **156,** 1039–1045.
23. Ballard, C.G., O'Brien, J., Coope, B., Fairbairn, A., Abid, F., and Wilcock, G. (1997) A prospective study of psychotic symptoms in dementia sufferers. *Int. Psychogeriatrics* **9,** 57–64.
24. Ballard, C.G., O'Brien, J., Swann, A.G., Thompson, P., Neill, D., and McKeith, I.G. (2001) The natural history of psychosis and depression in dementia with Lewy bodies. *J. Clin. Psychiatry* **62,** 46–49.
25. Greenwald, B.S., Kramer-Ginsberg, E., Marin, D.B., et al. (1989) Dementia with co-existent major depression. *Am. J. Psychiatry* **146,** 1472–1478.
26. Burns, A. (1991) Affective symptoms in Alzheimer's disease. *Int. J. Geriatr. Psychiatry* **6,** 371–376.
27. Burns, A., Lewis, G., Jacoby, R., and Levy, R. (1991) Factors affecting survival in Alzheimer's disease. *Psychol. Med.* **21,** 363–370.
28. Perry, E.K., Court, J.A., Johnson, M., et al. (1993) Autoradiographic comparison of cholinergic and other transmitter receptors in the normal human hippocampus. *Hippocampus* **3,** 307–315.
29. Perry, E.K., Marshall, E., Kerwin, J., et al. (1990) Evidence of a monoaminergic-cholinergic imbalance related to visual hallucinations in Lewy body dementia. *J. Neurochem.* **55,** 1454–1456.
30. Ballard, C., Piggott, M., Johnson, M., et al. (2000) Delusions associated with elevated muscarinic binding in dementia with Lewy bodies. *Ann. Neurol.* **48,** 868–876.
31. McKeith, I., Del Ser, T., Spano, P., et al. (2000) Efficacy of rivastigmine in dementia with Lewy bodies: a randomized double blind placebo controlled international study. *Lancet* **356,** 3031–3036.
32. Bodick, N.C., Offen, W.W., Shannon, H.E., et al. (1997) The selective muscarinic agonist xanomeline improves both the cognitive deficits and behavioural symptoms of Alzheimer's disease. *Alzheimer Dis. Assoc. Disord.* **11(Suppl. 4),** S16–S22.
33. Ballard, C.G., Piggott, M.A., Perry, E.K., et al. (2001) A positive association between 5HT re-uptake binding sites and depression in dementia with Lewy bodies. *J. Affect. Disord.,* in press.
34. Ballard, C., Saad, K., Patel, A., et al. (1995) The prevalence and phenomenology of psychotic symptoms in dementia sufferers. *Int. J. Geriatr. Psychiatry* **10,** 477–485.
35. Ballard, C.G. and O'Brien, J. (1999) Pharmacological treatment of behavioural and psychological signs in Alzheimer's disease: how good is the evidence for current pharmacological treatments? *BMJ* **319,** 138–139.
36. Lee, H., Cooney, J.M., and Lewer, B.A. (1994) Case report: the use of risperidone, an atypical neuroleptin Lewy body disease. *Int. J. Geriatr. Psychiatry* **9,** 415–417.
37. Allen, R.L., Walker, Z., D'Ath, P.J., et al. (1995) Risperidone for psychotic and behavioural symptoms in Lewy body dementia. *Lancet* **346,** 185.
38. McKeith, I.G., Ballard, C.G., and Harrison, R.W.S. (1995) Neuroleptic sensitivity to risperidone in Lewy body dementia. *Lancet* **346,** 699.
39. Ballard, C., Grace, J., McKeith, I., and Holmes, C. (1998) Neuroleptic sensitivity in dementia with Lewy bodies and Alzheimer's disease. *Lancet* **351,** 1032–1033.
40. Walker, Z., Grace, J., Overshot, R., et al. (1999) Olanzapine in dementia with Lewy bodies: a clinical study. *Int. J. Geriatr. Psychiatry* **14,** 459–466.
41. Parsa, M.A., Greenway, H.M., and Bastani, B. (2000) Quetiapine for the treatment of psychosis in Lewy body disease. *Neurology* **54(Suppl. 3),** A451.
42. Hutchinson, M. and Fazzini, E. (1996) Cholinesterase inhibitors in Parkinson's disease. *J. Neurol. Neurosurg. Psychiatry* **61,** 324–325.
43. Lebert, F., Pasquier, F., Souliez, L., et al. (1998) Tacrine efficacy in Lewy body dementia. *Int. J. Geriatr. Psychiatry* **13,** 516–519.
44. Shea, C., MacKnight, C., and Rockwood, R. (1998) Donepezil for treatment of dementia with Lewy bodies: a case series of nine patients. *Int. Psychogeriatr.* **10,** 229–239.
45. Aarsland, D., Bronnick, K., and Karlsen, K. (1999) Donepezil for dementia with Lewy bodies: a case study. *Int. J. Geriatr. Psychiatry* **14,** 69–72.
46. Fergusson, E. and Howard, R. (2000) Donepezil for the treatment of psychosis in dementia with Lewy bodies. *Int. J. Geriatr. Psychiary* **15,** 280–281.
47. Hughes, A.J., Daniel, S.E., Blankson, S., and Lee, A.J. (1993) A clinico-pathologic study of 100 cases of Parkinson's disease. *Arch. Neurol.* **50,** 140–148.
48. De Vos, R.A.I., Jansen, E.N.H., Stam, F.C., Ravis, R., and Swaab, D.F. (1995) Lewy body disease: clinico-pathological correlations in 18 consecutive cases of Parkinson's disease with and without dementia. *Clin. Neurol. Neurosurg.* **97,** 13–22.
49. Friedman, J.H. (2001) Atypical antipsychotics and the treatment of psychosis in Parkinson's disease. Education Program Syllabus 3BS.003, American Academy Neurology 53rd Annual Meeting, Philadelphia.
50. Aarsland, D., Larsen, J.P., Lim, N.G., et al. (1999) Range of neuropsychiatric disturbances in patients with Parkinson's disease. *J. Neurol. Neurosurg. Psychiatry* **67,** 492–496.
51. Aarsland, D., Larsen, J.P., Cummings, J.L., and Laake, K. (1999) Prevalence and clinical correlates of psychosis in Parkinson's disease. A community based study. *Arch. Neurol.* **56,** 595–601.
52. Aarsland, D., Cummings, J.L., and Larsen, J.P. (2001) Neuropsychiatric differences between Parkinson's disease with dementia and Alzheimer's disease. *Int. J. Geriatr. Psychiatry* **16,** 184–191.
53. Aarsland, D., Ballard, C., Larsen, J.P., and McKeith, I. (2001) A comparative study of psychiatric symptoms in dementia with Lewy bodies and Parkinson's disease with and without dementia. *Int. J. Geriatr. Psychiatry* **16,** 528–536.

54. Tandeberg, E., Larsen, J.P., Aarsland, D., and Cummings, J.L. (1996) The occurrence of depression in Parkinson's disease. A community based study. *Arch. Neurol.* **53,** 175–179.
55. Celesia, G.C. and Barr, A.N. (1970) Psychosis and psychiatric manifestations of levodopa therapy. *Arch. Neurol.* **23,** 193–2000.
56. Goodwin, F.K. (1971) Psychiatric side effects of levodopa in men. *JAMA* **218,** 1915–1921.
57. Jenkins, R.B. and Groh, R.H. (1970) Mental symptoms in parkinsonian patients treated with L-Dopa. *Lancet* **2,** 177–180.
58. Goetz, C.G., Vogel, C., Tanner, C.M., and Stebbins, G.T. (1998) Early dopaminergic drug-induced hallucinations in parkinsonian patients. *Neurology* **51,** 811–814.
59. Haeske-Dewick, H.C. (1995) Hallucinations in Parkinson's disease: characteristics and associated clinical features. *Int. J. Geriatr. Psychiatry* **10,** 487–495.
60. Goetz, C.G., Pappert, E.J., Blasucci, L.M., et al. (1998) Intravenous levodopa in hallucinating Parkinson's disease patients: high dose challenge does not precipitate hallucinations. *Neurology* **50,** 515–517.
61. Gnanalingham, K.K., Byrne, E.J., Thornton, A., Sambrook, M.R., and Bannister, P. (1997) Motor and cognitive function in Lewy body dementia: comparison with Alzheimer's and Parkinson's diseases. *J. Neurol. Neurosurg. Psychiatry* **62,** 243–252.
62. Walker, Z., Costa, D.C., Ince, P., McKeith, I.G., and Katona, C.L. (1999) In-vivo demonstration of dopaminergic degeneration in dementia with Lewy bodies. *Lancet* **354,** 646–647.
63. Ballard, C., Ayre, G., and Gray, A. (1999) Psychotic symptoms and behavioural disturbances in dementia: a review. *Rev. Neurol.* **155(Suppl. 4),** 44–52.
64. Lyketsos, C.G., Steinberg, M., Tschanz, J.T., Norton, M.C., Steffens, D.C., and Breitner, J.C. (2000) Mental and behavioural disturbances in dementia: findings from the Cache County study on memory in aging. *Am. J. Psychiatry* **157,** 708–714.
65. Wands, K., Merskey, H., Hachinski, V.C., Fishman, M., Fox, F., and Boniferro, M. (1990) A questionnaire investigation of anxiety and depression in early dementia. *J. Am. Geriatr. Soc.* **36,** 535–538.
66. Ballard, C.G., Patel, A., and Mohan, R. (1994) Anxiety in dementia sufferers. *Ir. J. Psychol. Med.* **11,** 108–111.
67. Ballard, C.G., Boyle, A., Bowler, C., and Lindesay, J. (1996) Anxiety disorders in dementia sufferers. *Int. J. Geriatr. Psychiatry* **11,** 987–990.
68. Ballard, C., Neill, D., O'Brien, J., McKeith, I.G., Ince, P., and Perry, R. (2000) Anxiety, depression and psychosis in vascular dementia: prevalence and associations. *J. Affect. Disord.* **59,** 97–106.
69. Cummings, J.L., Miller, B., Hill, M.A., et al. (1987) Neuropsychiatric aspects of multi-infarct dementia and dementia of the Alzheimer type. *Arch. Neurol.* **44,** 389–393.
70. Ballard, C.G., Mohan, R., Handy, S., Bannister, C., Davis, R., and Todd, N. (1991) Paranoid features in the elderly with dementia. *Int. J. Geriatr. Psychiatry* **6,** 155–157.
71. Flynn, F.G., Cummings, J.L., and Gornbein, J. (1991) Delusions in dementia syndromes: investigation of behavioural and neuropsychological correlates. *J. Neuropsychiatry Clin. Neurosci.* **3,** 364–370.
72. Berrios, G.E. and Brook, P. (1985) Delusions and the psychopathology of the elderly with dementia. *Acta Psychiatry Scand.* **72,** 296–301.
73. Birkett, D.P. (1972) The psychiatric differentiation of senility and arteriosclerosis. *Br. J. Psychiatry* **120,** 321–325.
74. Morriss, R.T., Rovner, B.W., Folstein, M.F., et al. (1990) Delusions in newly admitted residents of nursing homes. *Am. J. Psychiatry* **147,** 299–302.
75. Corey-Bloom, J., Galasko, D., Hofstetter, B., Jackson, J.E., and Thal, L.J. (1993) Clinical features distinguishing large cohorts with possible AD, probable AD and mixed dementia. *J. Am. Geriatr. Soc.* **41,** 31–37.
76. Sultzer, D.L., Levin, H.S., Mahler, M.E., et al. (1993) A comparison of psychiatric symptoms in vascular dementia and Alzheimer's disease. *Am. J. Psychiatry* **150,** 1806–1812.
77. Binetti, G., Bianchetti, A., Padovani, A., et al. (1993) Delusions in Alzheimer's disease and multi-infarct dementia. *Acta Neurol. Scand.* **88,** 5–9.
78. Rovner, B.W., Kajonck, S., Filipp, L., et al. (1986) Prevalence of mental illness in a community nursing home. *Am. J. Psychiatry* **143,** 1446–1449.
79. Hope, T., Keene, J., Fairburn, C., McShane, R., and Jacoby, R. (1997) Behavioural changes in dementia 2: are there behavioural syndromes? *Int. J. Geriatr. Psychiatry* **12,** 1074–1078.
80. Chandler, J.D. and Chandler, J.E. (1988) The prevalence of neuropsychiatric disorders in a nursing home population. *J. Geriatr. Psychiatry Neurol.* **1,** 71–76.
81. Ballard, C.G., Cassidy, G., Bannister, C., and Mohan, R. (1993) Prevalence, symptom profile and aetiology of depression in dementia sufferers. *J. Affect. Disord.* **29,** 1–6.
82. Verhey, F.R.J., Rozendaal, N., Ponds, W.H.M., and Jolks, J. (1993) Dementia, awareness and depression. *Int. J. Geriatr. Psychiatry* **8,** 851–856.
83. Newman, S.C. (1999) The prevalence of depression in Alzheimer's disease and vascular dementia in a population sample. *J. Affect. Disord.* **52,** 169–176.
84. Hargrave, R., Geck, L.C., Reed, B., and Mungas, D. (2000) Affective behavioural disturbances in Alzheimer's disease and ischaemic vascular disease. *J. Neurol. Neurosurg. Psychiatry* **68,** 41–46.
85. Reding, M., Haycox, J., and Blass, J. (1985) Depression in patients referred to a dementia clinic. *Arch. Neurol.* **42,** 894–896.
86. Ballard, C.G., Patel, A., Solis, M., Lowe, K., and Wilcock, G. (1996) A one-year follow-up study of depression in dementia sufferers. *Br. J. Psychiatry* **168,** 287–291.

22

Neurotransmitter Correlates of Neuropsychiatric Symptoms in Dementia with Lewy Bodies

Elaine K. Perry, BSc, PhD, DSc, **Margaret A. Piggott,** BSc, PhD, **Mary Johnson, Clive G. Ballard,** MD, MRCPsych, **Ian G. McKeith,** MD, FRCPsych, **Robert Perry,** PRCP, FRCPath, **and David Burn** MD, MRCP

1. INTRODUCTION

Dementia with Lewy bodies (DLB) is the second most common cause of dementia in the elderly after Alzheimer's disease (AD). The consensus clinical diagnostic criteria have been shown to be effective in terms of specificity and sensitivity in prospectively evaluated cohorts of DLB and AD patients *(1)*. The criteria include, in addition to progressive cognitive impairment, as in AD, the presence of visual hallucinations, fluctuations in cognition and attention, and extrapyramidal features; two of these three additional symptoms are required for the diagnosis of probable DLB.

The neuropathological diagnosis depends on the identification of Lewy bodies in the cortex and brainstem, with cortical densities being highest in archicortical areas, such as entorhinal and anterior cingulate, and higher than in Parkinson's disease (PD) without dementia. Lewy bodies, Lewy neurites, and most recently described, neuronal inclusion bodies are best identified using α-synuclein immunohistochemistry, although such features may also be evident in AD *(2)*. Whether DLB and PD plus dementia are identical or distinct disease categories is still a matter of debate.

Because cognitive function and the neuropsychiatric symptoms in DLB fluctuate, and no relation has been found between clinical symptoms and Lewy body pathology *(3,4)*, functional abnormalities are likely to be important. As in AD and PD, a variety of neurotransmitter systems are affected in DLB, and these are the current targets of useful symptomatic therapy. This chapter focuses on neurotransmitter correlates of key neuropsychiatric symptoms identified in a prospectively assessed cohort of DLB patients *(1)* and sets these findings in the context of neurochemical correlates reported in retrospectively assessed cohorts of DLB compared to AD and PD.

A summary of cholinergic and monoaminergic neurochemical activities in DLB, and comparisons with AD and PD are provided in Table 1. In addition, the relation between sleep abnormalities, increasingly considered as important, early manifestation of Lewy body disorders, and the multiple transmitter systems implicated are discussed in the final section.

From: *Mental and Behavioral Dysfunction in Movement Disorders*
Edited by: M-A. Bédard et al. © Humana Press Inc., Totowa, NJ

Table 1
Neurotransmitter Activities in DLB, Compared with AD and PD[a]

	DLB	AD	PD
I Cholinergic system			
ChAT	DLB	AD	PD
Cerebral cortex	↓↓	↓	↓[b]
Hippocampus	↓	↓↓	↓
Striatum	↓	↓	→
Thalamus	↓	→/↓	→
AChE			
Cortex	↓↓[c]	↓	↓
BuChE			
Cortex	→	↑	
VAChT			
Cortex		↓	↓[b,c]
Muscarinic receptors			
M1			
Cortex	↑	→	↑[b]
Striatum	↓	↑	→
M2			
Cortex		↓	
Nicotinic receptors			
α-BT binding (α-7)			
Cortex	→/↓	→	
Thalamus	↓	↓	
High affinity agonist site (α-4/α-3)			
Cortex	↓	↓	↓
Striatum	↓	→/↓	↓↓
Thalamus	→/↓	→/↓	→
II Monoaminergic systems			
Dopaminergic	DLB	AD	PD
Presynaptic			
Dopamine			
Striatum	↓	→	↓↓
Cortex	↓	→	↓
Dopamine transporter			
Striatum	↓[3]	→	↓↓[c]
Cortex	→		↓
Receptors			
D1 receptor[d]	→		→
D2 receptor[d]	↓	→	↑/→
D3 receptor[d]	→/↓		→
Serotonergic			
Presynaptic			
Serotonin			
Striatum	↓		↓
Cortex	↓	↓	↓
Serotonin transporter			
Cortex	↓	↓	↓
Receptors			
5-HT_{2A} receptor			
Cortex	→/↓	↓	↓
Noradrenergic			
Noradrenaline			
Striatum	↓		↓↓
Cortex		↓	
MAO-B		↑	

[a]Summary of neurochemical findings, modified and updated from McKeith, et al. *Fifth Generation Progress in Psychopharmacology,* 2002, pp. 1301–1315. Lippincott, Williams & Wilkins, Philadelphia.

[b]Denotes more extensive in PD plus dementia.

[c]Alteration reported using PET or SPECT neuroimaging.

[d]Striatal activities.

Abbreviations: AChE, acetylcholinesterase; BuChE, butyrylcholinesterase; VAChT, vesicular acetylcholine transporter; MAO-B, monoamine oxidase B.

2. THE CHOLINERGIC SYSTEM

2.1. *Cholinergic Abnormalities*

The cholinergic system is affected in DLB to a greater extent than in AD (Table 1). Recent reports on lower cortical choline acetyltransferase (ChAT) in the cortex, measured at autopsy, include those of Lippa et al. *(5)* and Tiraboschi et al. *(6)*. Using N-[^{11}C] methylpiperidin-4-yl acetate (a cholinesterase inhibitor) and positron emission tomography (PET) imaging in vivo, Shinotoh et al. *(7)* have also detected significantly greater reductions in DLB compared with AD. Not only are neocortical presynaptic activities reduced to a greater extent than AD, but there are also losses in DLB of cholinergic activity in the basal ganglia, including the striatum *(8)*, and in the pedunculopontine pathway that projects to such areas as the thalamus *(9)*.

Cortical ChAT reductions in DLB have been shown to correlate with cognitive function *(10,11)*. The cortical cholinergic deficit in DLB is, however, independent of the extent of Alzheimer-type pathology, although this pathology is associated with more severe cognitive impairment *(11)*. This observation, together with the fact that cognitive impairment in AD is often more severe than in DLB, despite the greater cholinergic deficit in the latter, suggests that loss of cholinergic function in the cortex is not sufficient alone to account for cognitive impairment in AD or in DLB with concomitant Alzheimer-type pathology. It has been suggested that the striatal cholinergic deficiency may contribute to the lesser degree of extrapyramidal symptoms (EPS) seen in DLB compared to PD, in which striatal cholinergic activity is normal. However, this has not yet been supported by clinical–pathological correlations, and it is likely that less extensive substantia nigra neuronal loss is also responsible of the reduced severity of EPS. The loss of thalamic cholinergic activity, which occurs particularly in the reticular formation, is likely to reflect degeneration of pedunculopontine neurons, which no doubt occurs in DLB as in PD *(12)*. Whether this relates to attentional dysfunction and/or disturbances in consciousness, which are more extensive in DLB compared with AD, remains to be established.

The pedunculopontine nucleus (PPN) is thought to be equivalent to the mesencephalic locomotor region, an area known to modulate spinal locomotion oscillators. Optimal sites for the induction of locomotion appear to be within the cholinergic neurons in the pars compacta of the PPN (PPNc) *(12)*. Approximately 50% of the large cholinergic neurons of the lateral part of the PPNc degenerate in PD. Cell loss within the PPNc in DLB is, therefore, likely to contribute towards the observed postural instability, gait disturbance, and falls.

In contrast to AD and similar to PD plus dementia, muscarinic M1 receptor binding in DLB is elevated *(13)*, a finding that has recently been confirmed by immunoabsorption studies *(14)*. M1 receptors are also not uncoupled to the same extent as in AD *(9)*. Nicotinic receptor changes include in the cortex a loss of the high affinity agonist binding site (reflecting the α-3 and α-4 subunits), but no change in the α-7 subunit or α-bungarotoxin (BT) binding *(13,15)*. In the thalamus, by contrast, there is little change in nicotine binding but a highly significant reduction in α-BT binding in the reticular nucleus *(16)*. Similar nicotinic receptor abnormalities occur in AD and, as far as has been investigated, in PD. In the striatum, there is a greater loss of nicotine binding in PD than in DLB, in keeping with the more extensive reduction in basal ganglia dopaminergic projections, but no loss in neuroleptic-free AD patients *(17)*. Although loss of cortical high affinity nicotinic receptor binding in AD has been related to synapse loss, as measured by synaptophysin levels *(18)*, synaptophysin loss only occurs in DLB when the pathology includes that of the Alzheimer type *(19)*.

2.2. *Clinical Correlates*

Originally, in a retrospectively assessed cohort of DLB patients, it was determined that cortical ChAT is reduced to a greater extent in patients with, as opposed to without, hallucinations *(20)*. In the more recent prospectively assessed series of patients, the same significant trend was observed, and it was also noted that the majority of patients experiencing hallucinations were receiving levadopa (L-dopa) therapy, whereas patients without hallucinations were not *(21)*. This suggests that hallucinations in DLB may be associated with combined low cholinergic activity and L-dopa medication.

In PD, visual hallucinations are associated with greater age and duration of disease, cognitive impairment, depression of mood, and sleep disturbance *(22,23)*. The occurrence of hallucinations in PD does not, however, seem to relate to either dose or duration of antiparkinsonian medication *(23)*. Nevertheless, the vast majority of patients with PD who develop hallucinations are taking dopaminergic therapies, so a facilitatory role for these agents is highly likely. Furthermore, and of direct relevance to DLB, patients with PD and dementia who are at risk for psychosis have atrophy of the nucleus basalis and a central cholinergic deficiency *(24)*.

In the prospective DLB cohort, the nicotinic receptor, measured using α-BT binding (α-7 subunit) was also lower in hallucinating compared with nonhallucinating patients *(15)*. This nicotinic receptor has not previously been implicated in psychosis, and it remains to be determined whether nicotinic antagonist agents blocking the α-7 subtype can induce hallucinations. The same receptor subtype was also associated with the symptom of delusional misidentification *(15)*. This involves misinterpreting images such as television images or mirror images. In patients with this symptom α-BT binding was again lower than in those without.

In the prospectively assessed cohort, an elevation in the muscarinic M1 subtype was detected using the radioligand pirenzepine in the group as a whole. In a comparison between subgroups of DLB with and without delusions, there was no difference in medication using agents with anticholinergic effects or in L-dopa treatment. The subgroups were also matched for age and severity of cognitive impairment. ChAT activity and nicotinic receptor binding was similar in the two groups. The muscarinic M1 receptor was, however, more elevated in individuals with delusions than those without *(21)*. This suggests that delusions may be associated with a loss of presynaptic cholinergic activity and a consequent, perhaps hypercompensatory, elevation in the M1 receptor subtype. Cholinergic therapy, which reduces delusions *(25)* is likely to be associated with a reduction in M1 receptors, a prediction that could be verified using single-photon emission computerized tomography (SPECT) imaging.

The associations between the neuropsychiatric symptoms and disturbances in cholinergic neurotransmission discussed above are likely to be relevant to pharmacotherapy. In a recent multicenter trial of the cholinesterase inhibitor rivastigmine, there were significant reductions in delusions and hallucinations over a 20-wk period in the group receiving rivastigmine, compared with those on placebo *(25)*. The other symptoms which improved markedly and significantly with rivastigmine were apathy and agitation, although these particular clinical features have not been assessed in the prospective DLB series under discussion. In an open label trial of donepezil in AD, Kaufer et al. *(26)* observed the greatest improvement in a 20-item measure of caregiver-rated treatment response, in general awareness, in which improvement correlated with reduced apathy ratings. It is relevant in this context that cholinergic function has been hypothesized to underpin mechanisms of conscious awareness (ref. *27*).

Another symptom not formally assessed in the rivastigmine clinical trial was fluctuations in attention or cognition. These occur in conjunction with various disturbances in consciousness, which include, at one extreme, episodes of stupor and unresponsiveness and other features such as the patient appearing to be unresponsive to external stimuli while still awake for periods of varying times, general clouding of consciousness, variability in cognitive function of over 50% from day-to-day, and variability in attentional performance. Variations in attention correlate with fluctuations in quantitative electroencephalography (EEG), and both EEG and fluctuations in attention occur across time spans as short as 90 s *(28)*. Since objective measurements, such as fluctuations in vigilance accuracy and EEG, relate to clinical evaluations of disturbances in consciousness, the latter can be considered a valid measure of this symptom. In the prospective DLB cohort, clinically assessed disturbances in consciousness did not relate to presynaptic cholinergic activities or to the muscarinic M1 receptor, but there was a significant relationship in temporal cortex with the nicotinic receptor subtype binding agonists with high affinity. Epibatidine binding to nicotinic receptors was reduced in many areas of the cortex in the DLB group overall, but in temporal association cortex the receptor was reduced to a lesser extent in patients experiencing disturbances in consciousness compared with those not affected (Ballard et al., in preparation). This suggests that there may be a subgroup of neurones expressing the high affinity nicotinic receptor subtype (which includes predominantly the α-3 and α-4 combined with β-2 subunits), which may be lost in those patients experiencing this symptom, leaving intact a subpopulation, which in itself, may be destabilizing by, for example, creating an imbalance between γ-amino butyric acid (GABA) and glutamate transmission.

Anatomical, physiological, and pathological evidence suggests that acetylcholine is an important neural correlate of consciousness *(27)*. The nicotinic receptor has, for example, been implicated in conscious awareness on account of its involvement in the mechanisms of general anaesthesia. Volatile inhalational anaesthetic agents interact with the α-4 β-2 receptor with high affinity at clinically relevant doses *(28)*. Muscarinic antagonists at progressively higher doses induce attentional deficits, hallucinations, and loss of consciousness (reviewed in ref. *28*). The broad spectrum of cognitive and neuropsychiatric symptoms in DLB, and multifactorial responsiveness to cholinergic therapy may, therefore, be related to a central role of acetylcholine, in both the cortex and thalamus, in conscious awareness.

3. THE DOPAMINERGIC SYSTEM

3.1. Dopaminergic Abnormalities

In the basal ganglia, the dopaminergic system is affected in DLB, though generally to a lesser extent than in PD. The presynaptic dopaminergic transporter or reuptake site, is significantly reduced in the posterior putamen in DLB *(29)*, whereas in PD, the loss is apparent at all rostrocaudal striatal levels. Dopamine turnover (ratio of homovanillic acid to dopamine) in the striatum is not increased in DLB as it is in PD *(29)*. The dopaminergic D2 receptor subtype in the striatum is reduced in DLB, but is not reduced in PD; at early stages of PD this receptor is up-regulated. This distinction suggests that there may be intrinsic striatal neuropathology in DLB involving a subpopulation of dopamine receptive neurons. Consistent with this is the finding of reduced striatal muscarinic M1 receptors, which tend to localize to D2-bearing neurons in DLB (Piggott et al., unpublished). In a recent study of striatal dopaminergic activities in a group of patients described as AD with Lewy bodies *(30)*, a loss not only of D2 but also D3 receptor binding, and elevation in D1 compared to AD without Lewy bodies was reported in the striatum. The reduction in the striatal dopamine uptake site, apparent in DLB postmortem has also been detected in vivo and found to be a distinguishing feature compared with AD *(31)*.

3.2. Clinical Correlates

No doubt these dopaminergic deficits in DLB and distinctions from PD and AD relate to extrapyramidal dysfunction, which in some respects may differ between PD and DLB and, although also occurring in AD, are not thought to be a core clinical feature of AD. Prospective evaluation of EPS in DLB, PD, and AD cohorts and correlation with basal ganglia neurotransmission is currently underway.

One of the distinguishing features of DLB, as compared to PD and AD, is the extreme sensitivity of patients to neuroleptic medication. This feature has been related, in a retrospectively assessed DLB cohort, to striatal D2 receptor binding, which is lower in DLB patients affected by neuroleptic sensitivity compared to those tolerant of the medication *(32)*. Sensitivity to D2 antagonists may, therefore, relate to an inability to up-regulate the receptor.

In a recent survey of dopaminergic markers in the cortex in the prospectively assessed DLB cohort, the dopamine transporter was assessed using mazindol binding, the D2 receptor using epidepride binding, and also the D1 receptor binding was evaluated. The only significant changes in the cerebral cortex among these markers were a moderate increase in the dopamine transporter, and a significant reduction in D2 receptor binding, which was not apparent in AD (Piggott et al., in preparation). Cortical dopaminergic abnormality in DLB was not associated with hallucinations, delusional misidentification, or fluctuations in consciousness. However, there was a relationship between the D2 receptor with auditory hallucinations. In Brodmann areas 20 and 22 in the temporal lobe, the reduction in D2 receptor binding was not as great in neuroleptic-free patients experiencing auditory hallucinations, compared with those who were not experiencing auditory hallucinations. It is of interest that the only symptom that related to dopaminergic markers in the cortex in DLB was auditory hallucinations, since this is one of the symptoms of psychosis in DLB that most closely resembles those in schizophrenia, in that dopaminergic dysregulation has long been implicated

4. THE SEROTONERGIC SYSTEM

As in the basal nucleus of Meynert and substantia nigra, there is also in DLB α-synuclein pathology (Lewy bodies, neuritis, and inclusion bodies) in the serotonergic raphé nuclei including dorsal raphé. There is, in both the striatum and the cortex, an extensive loss of the serotonin (5-HT) transporter or reuptake site (Piggott et al., unpublished observation). Cyanoimipramine binding to the transporter was examined in prospectively assessed patients and found to relate to depression, but not to any of the other neuropsychiatric symptoms discussed above. In patients with depression, the transporter was paradoxically less reduced than in patients without depression (Ballard et al., in preparation). There is some evidence that depression may be associated with compensatory regenerative activity in 5-HT neurons, and the finding of higher transporter binding in depressed compared to nondepressed patients may be consistent with such a concept. Of relevance is the finding of increased α-2-adrenergic receptor binding in locus coeruleus projection areas, such as frontal cortex in DLB, and the proposition that noradrenergic reinnervation and up-regulation may lower the threshold for increased agitation *(33)*.

The finding of relatively spared 5-HT transporter sites in DLB with depression contrasts with recent PET studies in depressed and nondepressed PD patients using 11C-WAY 100635, a ligand for the 5-HT_1 receptor *(34)*. In this study, there were similar reductions in binding potential in the raphé nuclei in both groups of patients, a finding likely to reflect either presynaptic 5-HT_1 receptor dysfunction or loss or serotonergic cell bodies. In the depressed but not nondepressed PD group, there was an additional reduction in cortical 5-HT_1 receptor binding, suggestive of postsynaptic receptor loss or dysfunction. 5-HT turnover in autopsy cortex (the ratio of 5-hydroxyindole acetic acid [5-HIAA] to 5-HT) was previously reported in a retrospectively assessed DLB series to be associated with hallucinations; turnover being relatively higher in comparison to cholinergic activity in hallucinating individuals *(20)*.

5. SLEEP ABNORMALITIES

Sleep abnormalities are increasingly considered to be an important symptom in PD and DLB and may predate the onset of other clinical features. In PD, rapid eye movement (REM) behavior disorder (RBD) is said to occur in 15% of all patients, and this interference with the maintenance of REM sleep atonia also occurs in DLB *(35,36)*. Furthermore, up to 40% of patients with RBD may eventually develop PD. In one retrospective clinicopathological study, 31 patients with RBD and degenerative dementia demonstrated a significantly different pattern of cognitive performance from 31 patients with AD. Significantly, the majority of patients with RBD met criteria for possible or probable DLB *(37)*.

In DLB, increased daytime sleepiness, sleep fragmentation, and nightmares have been described *(38)*. In DLB, compared with AD patients, significantly more limb movements during sleep, unpleasant dreams and confusion on waking were apparent *(38)*. In six DLB patients treated with rivastigmine compared to six untreated, there was a trend towards normalization of sleep patterns. This preliminary finding suggests there is a cholinergic component of sleep disturbances in DLB.

Pappert et al. *(39)* demonstrated a close association between the occurrence of hallucinations in PD and altered dream phenomena but not sleep fragmentation. In another study, compared with nonhallucinating PD patients, patients with hallucinations had a lower sleep efficiency, a reduced total REM sleep time and a reduced REM percentage. In 1922, Lhermitte *(40)* stressed the similarity between

Table 2
Alterations in Neurotransmitter Activities Through Sleep–Wake, Non-REM/REM Cycles

	ACh NBM	ACh PDP	DA VTA	NE LC	5-HT Raphé	HIS Hypothal	Orexin
Awake	++	++	+	+	+	+	+
Non-REM sleep	+	–	+	+/–	+/–	–	–
REM sleep	++	++	+	–	–	–	?

Abbreviations: ACh, acetylcholine; DA, dopamine; HIS, histamine; 5-HT, serotonin; Hypothal, hypothalamus; LC, locus coeruleus; NBM, nucleus basalis; PDP, pedunculopontine nucleus; VTA, ventral tegmental area.

dreams and peduncular hallucinosis and suggested that, in the latter condition, hallucinations might arise from a dysfunction of sleep–wake mechanisms secondary to the peduncular lesion.

Mechanisms involved in controlling sleep onset and duration, imitation and density of REM sleep, and dreaming directly involve alterations in neurotransmission (reviewed in ref. *41*) (see also Table 2). There is a progressive reduction in noradrenergic and 5-HT activity from sleep onset through non-REM sleep to REM onset, when these neurons are silent. In contrast, dopaminergic transmission in the ventral tegmental area is constant throughout the sleep–wake cycle. Cholinergic transmission in the nucleus basalis of Meynert is most active during waking and REM sleep and less active during non-REM sleep, whereas pedunculopontine cholinergic activity is absent during non-REM, but maximal during REM sleep. Many other transmitter systems are involved in, or affected during, the sleep–wake cycle, notably adenosinergic and orexinergic transmission. Hypothalmic orexin neurons are active during waking and inactive during sleep. Adenosine levels increase during waking and inhibitory effects on the basal forebrain neurons via A2A receptors are thought to trigger sleep onset *(42)*.

In attempting to understand mechanisms responsible for sleep abnormalities in DLB, orexin or adenosinergic transmission have not specifically been evaluated, but there are clearly abnormalities in all of the other transmitter systems implicated (Table 2). These abnormalities included α-synuclein pathology in the relevant subcortical nuclei and neurochemical abnormalities in the respective target areas. Linking these abnormalities to the various sleep disturbances in DLB is speculative at this stage. Daytime sleepiness could relate to impaired cholinergic transmission in the basal forebrain and/or reductions in serotonergic and noradrenergic transmission. RBD, during which the normal inhibition of movement is disrupted, could relate to brainstem cholinergic pathology. Cholinergic (and glutamate) neurons in the PPN play a critical role in maintaining the atonia that accompanies REM sleep. However, recent evidence on reductions in the dopamine transporter, detected using SPECT, in idiopathic RBD, together with responsiveness of RBD in PD to L-dopa, implicates striatal dopaminergic activity *(43–45)*. As in schizophrenia, it has been proposed that some of the neuropsychiatric symptoms in DLB, such as hallucinations or delusions could involve disruption of the mechanisms controlling dreaming with intrusion of dream mentation into the waking state.

5. CONCLUSION

It is likely, on the basis of the evidence summarized above and because of fluctuating symptoms in DLB, that disturbances in neurotransmission are an important pathological correlate of neuropsychiatric features. In prospectively assessed cases, visual hallucinations are associated with lower ChAT and the nicotinic α-7 receptor. Delusions relate to higher muscarinic M1 receptor, disturbances in consciousness to relatively preserved high affinity nicotinic receptor, and depression to relatively preserved 5-HT transporter. Therapeutically, cholinesterase inhibitors are effective in relieving hallucinations and delusions and other important symptoms, such as apathy. Neuroleptic agents are not the most appropriate antipsychotic agents for DLB patients, on account of the risk of increasing parkinsonism, and it

Table 3
Cholinergic Therapy in DLB

Rationale
Symptoms not related to LB pathology.
Fluctuations suggest functional correlates.
Symptoms characteristically anticholinergic.
Cholinergic correlates of cognitive and neuropsychiatric symptoms.
Neurofibrillary tangles minimal.
Cholinergic abnormalities more extensive and/or widespread compared with AD.
M1 receptors (cortex) functional—up-regulated and coupled.
Acetylcholinesterase inhibitors (ChEIs) reduce neuropsychiatric symptoms and improve cognitive function.
ChEIs do not induce extrapyramidal effects.
Disease stabilizing effects of ChEIs.
Neuroprotective role of nicotinic receptors in basal ganglia.

is likely that cholinergic drugs may emerge as a safer antipsychotic option. The possibility that such drugs may exacerbate syncope needs, however, to be evaluated. The rationale for cholinergic therapy in DLB is summarized in Table 3.

Cholinergic therapy may not only be of symptomatic benefit in DLB, but may also be disease stabilizing. Accumulating evidence in animal models suggest nicotinic receptor stimulation protects dopaminergic neurons from age-related changes, and in the human brain, substantia nigra neuron numbers are higher in individuals chronically exposed to nicotine (tobacco users) *(46)*. Evaluation of the extent of basal ganglia and cortical pathology in patients treated with different cholinesterase inhibitors and comparison with untreated patients is a worthwhile future objective.

ACKNOWLEDGMENTS

We acknowledge the research program support of the Medical Research Council and are grateful to Lorraine Hood for the preparation of this manuscript.

REFERENCES

1. McKeith, I.G., Ballard, C.G., Perry, R.H., et al. (2000) Prospective validation of consensus criteria for the diagnosis of dementia with Lewy bodies., *Neurology* **54,** 1050–1058.
2. Mukaetova-Ladinska, E.B., Hurt, J., Jakes, R., Xuereb, J., Honer, W.G., and Wischik, C.M. (2000) Alpha-synuclein inclusions in Alzheimer and Lewy body diseases. *Neuropathol. Exp. Neurol.* **59,** 408–417.
3. Gomez-Tortosa, E., Irizarry, M.C., Gomez-Isla, T., and Hyman, B.T. (2000) Clinical and neuropathological correlates of dementia with Lewy bodies. *Ann. NY Acad. Sci.* **920,** 9–15.
4. Stern, Y., Jacobs, D., Goldman, J., et al. (2001) An investigation of clinical correlates of Lewy bodies in autopsy-proven Alzheimer disease. *Neurology* **58,** 460–465.
5. Lippa, C.F., Smith, T.W., and Perry, E. (1999) Dementia with Lewy bodies: choline acetyltransferase parallels nucleus basalis pathology. *J. Neural. Transm.* **106,** 25–35.
6. Tiraboschi, P., Hansen, L.A., Alford, M., et al. (2000) Cholinergic dysfunction in diseases with Lewy bodies. *Neurology* **54,** 407–411.
7. Shinotoh, H., Aotsuka, A., Ota, T., et al. (2001) Brain cholinergic function in dementia with Lewy bodies and Alzheimer's disease measured by PET [abstracts]. *Proc. 5th Int. Conference on Progress in AD/PD* p.74.
8. Langlais, P.J., Thal, L., Hansen, L., Galasko, D., Alford, M., and Masliah, E. (1993) Neurotransmitters in basal ganglia and cortex of Alzheimer's disease with and without Lewy bodies. *Neurology* **43,** 1927–1934.
9. Perry, E.K., Court, J.A., Goodchild, R., et al. (1998) Clinical neurochemistry: developments in dementia research based on brain bank material. *J. Neural. Transm.* **105,** 915–933.
10. Perry, R.H., Irving, D., Blessed, G., et al. (1990) Senile dementia of Lewy body type. A clinically and neuropathologically distinct form of Lewy body dementia in the elderly. *J. Neurol. Sci.* **95,** 119–139.

11. Samuel, W., Alford, M., Hofstetter, C.R., and Hansen, L. (1997) Dementia with Lewy bodies versus pure Alzheimer disease: differences in cognition, neuropathology, cholinergic dysfucntion, and synapse density. *J. Neuropathol. Exp. Neurol.* **56,** 499–508.
12. Pahapill, P.A. and Lozano, A.M. (2000) The pedunculopontine nucleus and Parkinson's disease. *Brain* **123,** 1767–1783.
13. Perry, E.K., Smith, C.J., Court, J.A., et al. (1990) Cholinergic, nicotinic and muscarinic receptors in dementia of Alzheimer, Parkinson and Lewy body types. *J. Neural. Transm.* **2,** 149–158.
14. Shiozaki, K., Iseki, E., Uchiyama, H., et al. (1999) Alterations of muscarinic acetylcholine receptor subtypes in diffuse Lewy body disease: relation to Alzheimer's disease. *J. Neurol. Neurosurg. Psychiatry* **67,** 209–213.
15. Court, J.A., Ballard, C.G., Piggott, M.A., et al. (2001) Visual hallucinations are associated with lower α-bungarotoxin binding in dementia with Lewy bodies. *Pharmacol. Biochem. Behav.* **70,** 571–579.
16. Court, J., Spurden, D., Lloyd, S., et al. (1999) Neuronal nicotinic receptors in dementia with Lewy bodies and schizophrenia: alpha-bungarotoxin and nicotine binding in the thalamus. *J. Neurochem.* **73,** 1590–1597.
17. Court, J., Piggott, M., Lloyd, S., et al. (2000) Nicotine binding in human striatum: elevation in schizophrenia and reductions in dementia with Lewy bodies, Parkinson's disease, and in relation to neuroleptic medication. *Neuroscience* **98,** 79–87.
18. Sabbagh, M.N., Corey-Bloom, J., Alford, M., et al. (1998) Correlation of nicotinic receptor binding with clinical and neurochemical markers in Alzheimer's disease and dementia with Lewy bodies. *Neurobiol. Aging* **19,** S207.
19. Hansen, L.A., Daniel, S.E., Wilcock, G.K., et al. (1998) Frontal cortical synaptophysin in Lewy body diseases: relation to Alzheimer's disease and dementia. *J. Neurol. Neurosurg. Psychiatry* **64,** 653–656.
20. Perry, E.K., Marshall, E., Kerwin, J., et al. (1990) Evidence of a monoaminergic: cholinergic imbalance related to visual hallucinations in Lewy body dementia. *J. Neurochem.* **55,** 1454–1456.
21. Ballard, C., Piggott, M., Johnson, M., et al. (2000) Delusions associated with elevated muscarinic binding in dementia with Lewy bodies. *Ann. Neurol.* **48,** 868–876.
22. Barnes, J. and David, A.S. (2001) Visual hallucinations in Parkinson's disease: a review and phenomenological survey. *J. Neurol. Neurosurg. Psychiatry* **70,** 727–733.
23. Holroyd, S., Currie, L., and Wooten, G.F. (2001) Prospective study of hallucinations and delusions in Parkinson's disease. *J. Neurol. Neurosurg. Psychiatry* **70,** 734–738.
24. Nakano, I. and Hirano, A. (1984) Parkinson's disease: neuron loss in the nucleus basalis without concomitant Alzheimer's disease. *Ann. Neurol.* **15,** 415–418.
25. McKeith, I., Del Ser, T., Spano, P., et al. (2000) Efficacy of rivastigmine in dementia with Lewy bodies: a randomised double-blind, placebo-controlled international study. *Lancet* **356,** 2031–2036.
26. Kaufer, D. (1998) Beyond the cholinergic hypothesis: the effect of metrifonae and other cholinesterase inhibitors on neuropsychiatric symptoms in Alzheimer's disease. *Dement. Geriatr. Cogn. Disord.* **9,** 8–14.
27. Perry, E., Walker, M., Grace, J., and Perry, R. (1999) Acetylcholine in mind: a neurotransmitter correlate of consciousness? *Trends Neurosci.* **22,** 273–280.
28. Walker, M.P., Ayre, G.A., Cummings, J.L., et al. (2000) Quantifying fluctuation in dementia with Lewy bodies, Alzheimer's disease and vascular dementia. *Neurology* **54,** 1616–1625.
29. Piggott, M.A., Marshall, E.F., Thomas, N., et al. (1999) Striatal dopaminergic markers in dementia with Lewy bodies, Alzheimer's and Parkinson's diseases: rostrocaudal distribution. *Brain* **122,** 1449–1468.
30. Sweet, R.A., Hamilton, R.L., Healy, M.T., et al. (2001) Alterations of striatal dopamine receptor binding in Alzheimer disease are associated with Lewy body pathology and antemortem psychosis. *Arch. Neurol.* **58,** 466–472.
31. Hu, X.S., Okamura, N., Arai, H., et al. (2000) 18F-fluorodopa PET study of striatal dopamine uptake in the diagnosis of dementia with Lewy bodies. *Neurology* **55,** 1575–1577.
32. Piggott, M.A., Perry, E.K., Marshall, E.F., et al. (1998) Nigrostriatal dopaminergic activities in dementia with Lewy bodies in relation to neuroleptic sensitivity: comparisons with Parkinson's disease. *Biol. Psychiatry* **44,** 765–774.
33. Leverenz, J.B., Miller, M.A., Dobie, D.J., Peskind, E.R., and Raskind, M.A. (2001) Increased alpha 2-adrenergic receptor binding in locus coeruleus projection areas in dementia with Lewy bodies. *Neurobiol. Aging* **22,** 555–561.
34. Doder, M., Rabiner, E.A., Turjanski, N., Lees, A.J., and Brooks, D.J. (2000) Brain serotonin 1A receptors in Parkinson's disease with and without depression measured by positron emission tomography with 11C-WAY 100635. *Mov. Disord.* **15,** 213.
35. Wetter, T.C., Trenkwalder, C., Gershanik, O., and Hogl, B. (2001) Polysomnographic measures in Parkinson's disease: a comparison between patients with and without REM sleep disturbances. *Wien. Klin. Wochenschr.* **113,** 249–253.
36. Boeve, B.F., Silber, M.H., Ferman, T.J., et al. (1998) REM sleep behaviour disorder and degenerative dementia: an association likely reflecting Lewy body disease. *Neurology* **51,** 363–370.
37. Ferman, T.J., Boeve, B.F., Smith, G.E., et al. (1999) REM sleep behaviour disorder and dementia: cognitive differences when compared with AD. *Neurology* **52,** 951–957.
38. Grace, J.B., Walker, M.P., and McKeith, I.G. (2000) A comparison of sleep profiles in patients with Dementia with Lewy bodies and Alzheimer's disease. *Int. J. Geriatr. Psychiatry* **15,** 1028–1033.
39. Pappert, E.J., Goetz, C.G., Niederman, F.G., Raman, R., and Leurgans, S. (1999) Hallucinations, sleep fragmentation, and altered dream phenomena in Parkinson's disease. *Mov. Disord.* **14,** 117–121.
40. Lhermitte, J. (1922) Syndrome de la calotte du pédoncule cérébral. Les troubles psycho-sensoriels dans les lésions du mésencéphale. *Rev. Neurol. (Paris)* **38,** 1359–1365.
41. Perry, E.K. and Piggott, M.A. (2000) Neurotransmitter mechanisms of dreaming: implication of modulatory systems based on dream intensity. *Behav. Brain Sci.* **20,** 990–992.

42. Porkka-Heiskanen, T., Strecker, R.E., and McCarley, R.W. (2000) Brain site-specificity of extracellular adenosine concentration changes during sleep deprivation and spontaneous sleep: an in vivo microdialysis study. *Neuroscience* **99,** 507–517.
43. Eisensehr, I., Linke, R., Noachtar, S., Schwarz, J., Gildehaus, F.J., and Tatsch, K. (2000) Reduced striatal dopamine transporters in idiopathic rapid eye movement sleep behaviour disorder. Comparison with Parkinson's disease and controls. *Brain* **123,** 1155–1160.
44. Albin, R.L., Koeppe, R.A., Chervin, R.D., et al. (2000) Decreased striatal dopaminergic innervation in REM sleep behaviour disorder. *Neurology* **55,** 1410–1412.
45. Miyamoto, M., Miyamoto, T., Takekawa, H., Kubo, J., and Hirata, K. (2001) Parasomnia as an occasion for the diagnosis of Parkinson's disease. *Psychiatr. Clin. Neurosci.* **55,** 273–274.
46. Perry, E., Martin-Ruiz, C., Lee, M., et al. (2000) Nicotinic receptor subtypes in human brain ageing, Alzheimer and Lewy body diseases. *Eur. J. Pharmacol.* **393,** 215–222.

23

Acetylcholinesterase Inhibitors in the Treatment of Dementia in Parkinson's Disease

Amos D. Korczyn, MD, MSc **and Nir Giladi,** MD

1. DEMENTIA IN PARKINSON'S DISEASE

Much after James Parkinson made the optimistic statement that "the senses are not affected" *(1)*, a huge amount of data accumulated to demonstrate that dementia is quite common in advanced Parkinson's disease (PD) (see Chapters 17, 18, and 20 of this book), whereas more subtle neuropsychological changes are also present in earlier stages *(2,3)* (see also Chapters 6 to 9 of this book). The mechanisms underlying the cognitive decline in PD are still not completely clear *(4–6)*, but it is a major factor in the development of disability and dependency of the patients on the caregivers. The dementia of PD, thus, has a grave impact on the quality of life of the patients and their caregivers (see Chapter 37 of this book), as well as a negative effect on their survival *(7,8)* (see also Chapter 40 in this text).

Dementia is probably the leading cause for institutionalizations of PD patients. Early in the course of PD, executive dysfunction may predominate, although later on, memory is more significantly affected as well as other cortical symptoms, and the differences with other dementias, particularly Alzheimer's disease (AD), becomes quantitative rather than qualitative.

The neuropsychological differences between AD and movement disorders, and particularly Huntington's disease (HD), led to a distinction between "cortical" and "subcortical" dementias (see Chapter 17 of this book). As much as these differences apply to AD and HD, their application to PD causes great practical difficulties *(9–11)*. In reality, there is a significant overlap between the cortical and subcortical dementias, meaning that the two syndromes are more similar than different, and no study has been able to identify markers that can absolutely differentiate the dementias of AD and PD.

This difficulty is reflected by neuropathological overlaps (see Chapters 18 and 19). Rather than being a subcortical dementia, brains of demented PD patients contain significant amounts of cortical Lewy bodies *(12)* and amyloid plaques in the cortex *(13)*. The degeneration of the nucleus basalis of Meynert (nbM), which was initially thought to be unique to AD, is in fact shared in PD as well *(14–16)*. This is frequently accompanied by neuronal loss in the cholinergic septal nuclei and the dopaminergic ventral tegmental area as well *(17,18)*. On the other hand, AD patients frequently have subcortical pathology, particularly white matter lesions *(19)*. Furthermore, the two diseases affect elderly people, and age-associated changes, including vascular lesions, are common to both.

Other similarities between demented patients with PD and AD consist of neurophysiological changes, including electroencephalography (EEG) slowing, which is well known in AD, but also occurs in demented patients with PD *(20,21)*.

From: *Mental and Behavioral Dysfunction in Movement Disorders*
Edited by: M-A. Bédard et al. © Humana Press Inc., Totowa, NJ

Table 1
Clinical Characteristics of 28 PD Patients Included in the Study

Mean age (yr)	75 ± 4.6
Mean duration of symptoms (yr)	7.0± 5.3
Mean Hoehn and Yahr stage "off"	3.1 ± 0.7
Mean L-dopa dose (mg/d)	670 ± 340
Mean UPDRS total score	67.5 ± 12
Mean MMSE total score	19.5 ± 4.7
Mean ADAS-cog total score	28.3 ± 10.5

UPDRS, Unified Parkinson's disease rating scale; MMSE, Mini Mental State Examination; ADAS-cog, Alzheimer's disease Assessment Scale.

2. TREATMENT OF DEMENTIA IN PD

The treatment of AD is currently based primarily on the "cholinergic theory," which maintains that the degeneration of the nbM and possibly other subcortical cholinergic nuclei is responsible for the cognitive deficit. Consequently, attempts were made to correct these deficiencies with either cholinesterase inhibitors (ChEIs) or direct muscarinic agonists *(22–25)*. Although these treatments are partially successful at best, they are presently widely used. However, since the cholinergic deficits are not unique to AD, but occur also in PD, it is reasonable to study the effects of the same drugs in the dementia of PD. The concentration and attention deficits frequently affecting PD patients in the initial stages of the disease may be particularly responsive to cholinergic stimulation. Although it may improve cognition, the enhanced cholinergic tone could, theoretically, also lead to exacerbation of the extrapyramidal features of the disease *(26)*. Treatment should, therefore, proceed carefully with special attention to the motor manifestations of the disease.

Demented patients in general, and those with PD in particular, manifest quite severe behavioral symptoms including depression, anxiety, and psychosis *(27)*. The latter is particularly troublesome, being disruptive to the surrounding and requires treatment. The psychotic manifestations that are commonly associated with dementia respond to atypical neuroleptics and particularly clozapine *(28)*.

Further encouragement to the use of ChEIs in PD with dementia derives from experience with diffuse Lewy body disease (LBD) *(29,30)*. In a recently published study, McKeith et al. were able to demonstrate that the ChEI rivastigmine is quite safe and, more importantly, beneficial in dementia with Lewy bodies (DLB), improving various cognitive functions, most particularly concentration and delusions *(31)*. Notably, however, the definition of DLB is arbitrary rather than theoretical. In practice, the distinction is difficult in many cases and incomplete even by pathological criteria. This is not surprising because cortical Lewy bodies (almost) always occur on the background of cortical senile plaques, which are characteristic of AD. It is quite easy to ascribe to the "continuum theory," according to which patients with AD constitute one extreme, those with PD the other, and DLB cases are a combination.

Based on the encouraging results with ChEIs in DLB and the few small open trials that have suggested that ChEIs can improve cognitive functions in patients with PD and dementia *(32)*, we have recently published a study assessing the effect of rivastigmine in demented PD patients. We assessed the effect of rivastigmine on cognitive functions and other clinical features in an open trial for 26 wk and 8 wk of washout in 28 *(33)* consenting patients with PD and dementia (Table 1). PD was diagnosed according to published clinical criteria (18). All patients had at least 2 yr of PD symptoms and a clear response to levodopa (L-dopa) for more than 1 yr. Patients who fulfilled the Diagnosis and Statistical Manual of Mental Disorders, fourth edition (DSM IV) criteria for dementia *(34)* and scored less than 26 and more than 12 points on the Mini-Mental State Examination (MMSE) *(35)* performed during

Table 2
ADAS-cog Scores

Subcategories	Baseline	Wk 12	Wk 26	Wk 34	$p <$
Total	30.8 ± 12.8	23.6 ± 10.5	23.5 ± 15.0	25.9 ± 19.4	0.002
Word recall	6.6 ± 1.4	6.5 ± 1.3	6.2 ± 1.9	7.0 ± 1.8	N.S.
Naming	3.5 ± 2.2	2.8 ± 3.0	2.7 ± 3.2	3.0 ± 3.0	N.S.
Commands	1.9 ± 1.4	1.5 ± 1.3	1.8 ± 1.2	2.0 ± 1.5	N.S.
Construction	41.6 ± 30.1	31.2 ± 24.7	33.3 ± 24.1	35.7 ± 25.7	N.S.
Ideational	1.0 ± 1.3	0.7 ± 0.9	0.9 ± 1.2	0.8 ± 1.3	N.S.
Orientation	2.0 ± 1.9	1.7 ± 1.4	1.6 ± 1.9	1.8 ± 2.1	N.S.
Recognition	42.6 ± 24.6	26.7 ± 17.3	25.9 ± 22.8	24.3 ± 27.2	0.02
Language	0.6 ± 1.1	0.5 ± 1.1	0.5 ± 1.1	0.7 ± 1.3	N.S.
Comprehension	0.9 ± 1.0	1.0 ± 2.0	0.6 ± 0.8	1.0 ± 1.5	N.S.
Word finding	0.7 ± 0.8	0.3 ± 0.6	0.2 ± 0.7	0.4 ± 1.2	0.05
Remembering instructions	34.2 ± 19.1	19.1 ± 18.2	19.0 ± 22.9	17.0 ± 29.9	0.005
Concentration	1.1 ± 1.0	0.6 ± 0.9	0.2 ± 0.4	0.4 ± 0.8	0.003

N.S., not significant.

the "on" state in two consecutive sessions, at least 2 wk apart, were eligible for this study. We excluded from this study patients if significant cognitive changes appeared during the first year of their illness and those who developed psychotic features prior to L-dopa treatment or during the first year after L-dopa was introduced, as well as those with significant depression.

Patients were assessed by means of the Unified Parkinson's Disease Rating Scale (UPDRS) *(36)*, the Alzheimer's Disease Assessment Scale (ADAS-cog) *(37)*, and the MMSE. During the study, no change in antiparkinsonian medication was made for the first 12 wk, and afterwards, only six patients needed a change in their antiparkinsonian medications.

Rivastigmine was given openly at an initial dose of 1.5 mg twice daily and was increased after 4 wk to 3 mg twice daily, after 8 wk to 4.5 mg twice daily, and after 12 wk to a maximal dose of 6 mg twice daily. Mean rivastigmine dose at wk 12 was 7.3 ± 3.3 mg/d (n = 26) and 7.5 ± 3.5 mg/d at wk 26 (n = 20). Patients who developed side effects at any stage were either left on the same dose for an additional 2 wk or had their daily dose reduced to the previous level. Between wk 12 and 26 of the trial, we tried to keep the dose of rivastigmine constant at the maximal tolerated dose. At wk 26, rivastigmine was tapered down over a period of 2 wk and discontinued. Final assessment was performed 6 wk later (34 wk from baseline).

The total score on the ADAS-cog significantly improved over the study period ($p < 0.002$) (Table 2). The subscores that improved significantly from baseline on wk 26 were those of remembering instructions, concentration, and recognition. The total MMSE score showed some slight and not significant improvement at wk 26 compared to baseline (20.5 ± 5.1 vs 21.9 ± 5.4, respectively) (Table 3). However, we observed a significant improvement in the subscore of attention from the MMSE at wk 26.

The total UPDRS score showed a trend towards improvement from baseline (67.5 ± 12) to week 26 (64.3 ± 13.8) (Table 4). In the UPDRS, the only part that showed statistically significant change was part 1 (mental), while the activity of daily living (ADL) and the motor part showed nonsignificant changes.

A list of adverse events is given in Table 5, showing mainly cholinergic effects. Increased salivation (in 46% of patients) and worsening of tremor (in 39%) were the most frequent adverse events. Overall, 17 patients experienced side effects, but only 11 of them had to decrease the rivastigmine daily dose. Those patients who did have side effects usually had more than one. Eight patients discontinued rivastigmine for various reasons, mostly associated with therapy.

Table 3
MMSE Scores

Subcategories	Baseline $n = 28$	Wk 26 $n = 20$	Wk 34 $n = 20$	$p <$
Total	20.5 ± 5.1	21.9 ± 5.4	20.7 ± 7.4	N.S.
Orientation	8.0 ± 1.5	8.2 ± 2.2	7.6 ± 2.5	N.S.
Immediate memory	2.9 ± 0.5	3.0 ± 0.0	2.7 ± 0.7	N.S.
Attention	2.6 ± 1.7	3.7 ± 1.4	3.4 ± 1.8	0.002
Delayed recall	1.1 ± 1.2	1.2 ± 1.1	1.0 ± 1.0	N.S.
Language	6.2 ± 1.4	5.8 ± 2.2	6.3 ± 1.7	N.S.
Praxis	0.4 ± 0.5	0.4 ± 0.5	0.4 ± 0.5	N.S

N.S., not significant.

Table 4
UPDRS Scores

UPDRS	Baseline	Wk 12	Wk 26	Wk 34	p
Mean rivastigmine dose (mg/d)		7.2 ± 3.3	7.5 ± 3.5	none	
Total	67.5 ± 12	64.1 ± 12.5	64.3 ± 13.8	65.0 ±13.7	<0.06
Mental	6.2 ± 2.1	5.3 ± 2.0	4.4 ± 2.5	5.7 ± 3.0	<0.01
ADL	17.4 ± 5.4	16.3 ± 4.0	16.2 ± 5.3	17.9 ± 8.9	N.S.
Motor	43.9 ± 6.1	42.9 ± 6.7	43.6 ± 7.9	44.4 ± 9.7	N.S.

ADL, activity of daily living; N.S., not significant.

The rationale to try ChEIs for dementia in PD was based not only on the possible contribution of acetylcholine deficiency to the cognitive impairment in PD, but also on the possibility that some PD patients who develop dementia also have AD pathological changes *(37)*. From the pathological point of view, a pure PD can be seen in young onset patients, whereas aging is the most significant risk factor for PD dementia, supporting the concept of co-morbidity.

The effects of rivastigmine on attention in the subsections of the MMSE and the ADAS-cog (concentration, remembering instructions, and recognition) are of interest, because attention deficit is one of the hallmarks of subcortical dementia seen in PD. Such a specific effect on one cognitive modality is consistent with the suggestion that attention is directly associated with cholinergic activity. This effect of ChEIs on attention has also been reported in AD and particularly when rivastigmine was given to patients with DLB *(38)*.

One could expect that giving cholinergic drugs to PD patient might impair the dopaminergic–cholinergic relationships in the basal ganglia and cause motor deterioration *(26)*. As reflected by the ADL and motor parts of the UPDRS, we did not observe significant exacerbation of parkinsonism by rivastigmine in most cases. Nevertheless, tremors increased in 11 patients, necessitating a dose reduction in 8 patients, while in 3 cases, motor symptoms deteriorated, causing withdrawal from the study. It is possible that the design of the study, allowing dose reduction of rivastigmine, masked the full expression of these motor side effects.

Peripheral and central cholinergic side effects were reported in about half of the study population. Interestingly, neither peripheral cholinergic side effects nor increased tremor were reported as frequent side effects in patients with AD treated with rivastigmine *(24)*. It might well be that these side effects are disease-specific. Psychosis or confusion precipitated by ChEIs are probably as common in PD as

Table 5
Adverse Events (A/E)

Adverse event	No. of patients	Mean rivastigmine dose	Relation to drug
Increased salivation	13	6	Probable
Increased tremor	11	5.3	Possible
Confusion	4	5.2	Possible
Hallucinations	2	4.5	Possible
Nausea	2	9	Probable
General weakness	2	7.5	Possible
Hyperhydrosis	2	4.5	Probable
Diarrhea	2	6	Probable
Falls	1	6	Possible
Urinary tract infection	2	4.5	Unlikely

Overall, 17 patients had A/E. Most patients had more than one A/E.
In 11 patients, rivastigmine dose was reduced because of A/E.
Dose = mg/d

in AD, whereas there was a surprisingly low frequency of gastrointestinal side effects (nausea, diarrhea) among the PD patients, possibly reflecting habituation to these dopaminergically mediated side effects since all patients were on long-term L-dopa.

Previous studies of rivastigmine in AD proved the drug to be safe in elderly subjects, including those with coronary artery disease. However, one of our patients died suddenly at wk 22 and another developed an acute myocardial infarction. We could not associate the death to the rivastigmine treatment, especially when it happened at such an advanced stage of the study with no earlier warnings. However, this observation should be kept in mind in future studies to assess whether PD patients are more sensitive to rivastigmine than AD patients.

The open label design of the study and its relatively small size are important to note. A placebo or training effect is a theoretical explanation for some of the current results. However, the specific and consistent changes in cognitive subscores are difficult to attribute to a pure placebo effect.

It is possible that some of our patients were actually suffering from DLB, a disorder that has already been shown to respond significantly to rivastigmine treatment. Although none of our patients fulfilled the criteria for dementia with DLB *(39)*, no fully reliable criteria are available to exclude DLB cases, and as long as there is no biological marker that can differentiate the two, this possibility is hard to dismiss. It is also possible that some of our patients had coexistent AD, which could have contributed to their good response.

Despite those limitations, this subgroup of patients with PD and dementia gained significant clinical benefit from rivastigmine, which could also be shown by neuropsychological tests. These preliminary findings show the potential of cholinergic enhancement in the treatment of the cognitive dysfunction in various movement disorders and particularly PD. Future studies should explore the various drugs available and identify the patients or clinical manifestations most likely to respond to these pharmacological manipulations.

3. CONCLUSION

Cognitive decline occurs commonly in PD and causes significant disability and burden on patients and caregivers. However, the recent introduction of ChEIs to the treatment of AD may be extended to other neurodegenerative disorders. In particular, it is logical to try these therapies in PD, because of the cholinergic deficits that occur in PD as well. Our preliminary studies with rivastigmine have supported an intensive study of ChEIs in the cognitive decline associated with PD.

REFERENCES

1. Parkinson, J. (1817) *An Essay on the Shaking Palsy.* Sherwood, Neeley and Jones, London.
2. Lees, A.R. and Smith, E. (1983) Cognitive deficits in the early stages of Parkinson's disease. *Brain* **106,** 257–270.
3. Levin, B.E. and Katzen, H.L. (eds.) (1995) Early cognitive changes and nondementing behavioural abnormalities in Parkinson's disease, in *Behavioural Neurology of Movement Disorders,* vol. 65 (Weiner, W.J. and Lang, A.E., eds.), Raven Press, New York.
4. Aarsland, D., Tandberg, E., Larsen, J., and Cummings, J. (1996) Frequency of dementia in Parkinson's disease. *Arch. Neurol.* **53,** 538–542.
5. Albin, R.L., Young, A.B., and Penney, J.B. (1989) The functional anatomy of basal ganglia disorders. *Trends Neurosci.* **12,** 366–375.
6. Korczyn, A.D. (1990) Dementia in Parkinson's disease. Basic, clinical and therapeutic aspects and Alzheimer's and Parkinson's diseases. *Adv. Behav. Biol.* **2,** 177–180.
7. Nussbaum, M., Treves, T.A., Inzelberg, R., Rabey, J.M., and Korczyn, A.D. (1998) Survival in Parkinson's disease: the effect of dementia. *Parkinsonism and Related Disorders* **4,** 179–181.
8. Giladi, N., Treves, T.A., Paleacu, D., et al. (2000) Risk factors for dementia, depression and psychosis in long-standing Parkinson's disease. *J. Neural. Transm.* **107,** 59–71.
9. Mildworf, B., Treves, T.A., and Korczyn, A.D. (1993) Differentiation of memory deficits in Alzheimer's disease and in Parkinson's disease with dementia. *Neurology* **43,** A172–A172.
10. Massman, P.J., Delis, D.C., Butters, N., Levin, B.E., and Salmon, D.P. (1990) Are all subcortical dementia alike? Verbal learning and memory in Parkinson's disease and Huntington's patients. *J. Clin. Exp. Neuropsychol.* **12,** 729–744.
11. Aarsland, D., Cummings, J., and Larsen, J. (2001) Neuropsychiatric differences between Parkinson's disease with dementia and Alzheimer's disease. *Int. J. Geriatr. Psychiatry* **16,** 184–191.
12. Hurtig, H.I., Trojanowski, J.Q., Galvin, J., et al. (2000) Alpha-synuclein cortical Lewy bodies correlate with dementia in Parkinson's disease. *Neurology* **54,** 1916–1921.
13. Jellinger, K. (1994) Structural basis of dementia in Parkinson's disease, in *Dementia in Parkinson's Disease* (Korczyn, A.D., ed.), Monduzzi Editore, Milan, Italy.
14. Nakano, I. and Hirano, A. (1984) Parkinson's disease: neuron loss in the nucleus basalis without concomitant Alzheimer's disease. *Ann. Neurol.* **15,** 415–418.
15. Perry, E.K., Curtis, M., Dick, D.J., et al. (1985) Cholinergic correlates of cognitive impairment in Parkinson's disease: comparisons with Alzheimer's disease. *J. Neurol. Neurosurg. Psychiatry* **48,** 412–421.
16. Whitehouse, P.J., Martino, A.M., Marcus, K.A., et al. (1988) Reductions in acetylcholine and nicotine binding in several degenerative diseases. *Arch. Neurol.* **45,** 722–724.
17. Dubois, B. and Pillon, B. (1995) Do cognitive changes of Parkinson's disease result from dopamine depletion? *J. Neural. Transm.* **45,** 27–34.
18. Hughes, A., Daniel, S., Kilford, L., and Lees, A. (1992) Accuracy of clinical diagnosis of idiopathic Parkinson's disease—a clinico pathological study of 100 cases. *J. Neurol. Neurosurg. Psychiatry* **55,** 181–184.
19. Hirono, N., Kitagaki, H., Kazui, H., Hashimoto, M., and Mori, E. (2000) Impact of white matter changes on clinical manifestation of Alzheimer's disease: a quantitative study. *Stroke* **31,** 2182–2188.
20. Neufeld, M.Y., Blumen, S., Aitkin, I., Parmet, Y., and Korczyn, A.D. (1994) EEG frequency analysis in demented and non-demented parkinsonian patients. *Dementia* **5,** 23–28.
21. Neufeld, M.Y., Inzelberg, R., and Korczyn, A.D. (1998) EEG in demented and non-demented parkinsonian patients. *Acta Neurol. Scand.* **78,** 1–5.
22. Wilcock, G.K., Lilienfeld, S., and Gaens, E. (2000) Efficacy and safety of galantamine in patients with mild to moderate Alzheimer's disease: multicentre randomised controlled trial. *BMJ* **321,** 1445–1449.
23. Rogers, R.D., Sahakian, B.J., Hodges, J.R., Polkey, C.E., Kennard, C., and Robins, T.W. (1998) Dissociating executive mechanisms of task control following frontal lobe damage and Parkinson's disease. *Brain* **121,** 815–842.
24. Corey-Bloom, J., Anand, R., and Veach, J. (1998) A randomized trial evaluating the efficacy and safety of ENA 713 (rivastigmine tartrate), a new acetylcholinesterase inhibitor, in patients with mild to moderately severe Alzheimer's disease. *Int. J. Geriatr. Psychopharmacol.* **1,** 55–65.
25. Korczyn, A.D. (2000) Muscarinic M_1 agonists in the treatment of Alzheimer's disease. *Exp. Opin. Invest. Drugs* **9,** 2259–2267.
26. Duvoisin, R.C. (1967) Cholinergic-anticholinergic antagonism in Parkinsonism. *Arch. Neurol.* **17,** 124–136.
27. Korczyn, A.D. (2001) Neuropsychiatric manifestations in Parkinson's disease, in *Parkinson's Disease: Advances in Neurology,* vol. 86 (Calne, D.C.S., ed.), Lippincott Williams & Williams, Philadelphia, pp. 395–404.
28. Korczyn, A.D. (2001) Hallucinations in Parkinson's disease. *Lancet* **358,** 1031–1032.
29. Levy, R., Eagger, S., Griffiths, M., et al. (1994) Lewy bodies and response to tacrine in Alzheimer's disease. *Lancet* **343,** 176.
30. Wilcock, G.K. and Scott, M.I. (1994) Tacrine for senile dementia of Alzheimer's or Lewy body type. *Lancet* **344,** 544.
31. McKeith, I., Del Ser, T., Spano, P., et al. (2000) Efficacy of rivastigmine in dementia with Lewy bodies: a randomized, double-blind, placebo-controlled international study. *Lancet* **356,** 2031–2036.
32. Hutchinson, M. and Fazzini, E. (1996) Cholinesterase inhibitors in Parkinson's disease. *J. Neurol. Neurosurg. Psychiatry* **61,** 324–325.

33. Giladi, N., Shabtai, H., Benbunan, B., et al. (2001) The effect of treatment with rivastigmin (Exelon) on cognitive functions of patients with dementia and Parkinson's disease. *Neurology* **56,** A128.
34. American Psychiatric Association. (1994) *Diagnostic and Statistical Manual of Mental Disorders*, American Psychiatric Association, Washington, DC.
35. Folstein, M., Folstein, S., and McIlughs, P. (1975) The mini mental state: a practical method for grading the cognitive state of patients for the clinician. *J. Psychiatric Res.* **12,** 189–198.
36. Fahn, S., Elton, R., and Members-of-the-UPDRS-Development-Committee. (1987) *Recent Developments in Parkinson's Disease,* vol. 2 (Fahn, S., Marsden, C.D., Calne, D.B., and Goldstein, M., eds.), Macmillan Health Care Information, Florham Park, N.J., pp. 153–163.
37. Rosen, W., Mohs, R., and Davis, K. (1984) A new rating scale for Alzheimer's disease. *Am. J. Psychiatry* **141,** 1356–1364.
38. McKeith, I.G., Grace, J.B., Walker, Z., et al. (2000) Rivastigmine in the treatment of dementia with Lewy bodies: preliminary findings from an open trial. *Int. J. Geriatr. Psychiatry* **15,** 387–392.
39. McKeith, I.G., Galasko, D., Kosaka, K., Perry, E., Dickson, D., and Hansel, L. (1996) Consensus guide-lines for the clinical and pathological diagnosis of dementia with Lewy bodies (DLB): report of the consortium on DLB international workshop. *Neurology* **47,** 1113–1124.

VI
Neuropsychiatric Aspects of Movement Disorders

24
Mood Disorders and the Globus Pallidus

Edward C. Lauterbach, MD, FANPA, FAPA

1. INTRODUCTION

Mood disorders, including mania and depression, have been linked to abnormal cortical metabolism. For example, studies of patients with primary depressive disorders have consistently demonstrated frontal dysfunction *(1)*. These frontal areas project to subcortical areas, traversing distinct functionally segregated parallel corticostriatopallidothalamocortical (CSPTC) circuits, which project back to the frontal lobe *(2)*. Information processed in these CSPTC pathways can profoundly influence frontal function in a manner consistent with observed depressive pathophysiology *(3,4)*. Because the globus pallidus (GP) is positioned at the heart of CSPTC circuitry, the relation of the pallidum to depressive disorders is worth considering. Consequently, this chapter explores this relationship from hodological and clinical perspectives.

2. HODOLOGY

CSPTC circuits have been reviewed in more depth elsewhere *(2,5,6)* and are only briefly summarized here. Instead, CSPTC circuit subsystems are considered, including direct and indirect basal ganglia pathways and specific pallidal systems. Second, dopaminergic modulation and the anatomical organization of associative and limbic CSPTC circuits as they traverse the pallidum are explored. Third, pallidal influences over associative and limbic CSPTC circuits at pallidal and striatal levels are reviewed. Fourth, seven CSPTC circuits implicated in mood disorders are detailed. Finally, evidence of CSPTC integration of associative and limbic information is considered. Hodological relations regard the primate literature unless otherwise indicated.

2.1. CSPTC Circuit Subsystems

2.1.1. Direct and Indirect Pathways

CSPTC circuits utilize *direct* and *indirect* pathways. The direct pathway involves projections from striatum (Str), including caudate nucleus (CN), ventral striatum (VS), nucleus accumbens (NA), and putamen (Put), to the internal GP segment (GPi) and substantia nigra pars reticulata (SNpr), then from GPi/SNpr to thalamus (Th). The indirect pathway projects from the Str to the external GP segment (GPe), which in turn projects to GPi/SNpr *(7)* and subthalamic nucleus (STN) *(6,8)*; STN then projects to GPi/SNpr, and GPi projects to Th. Th then completes the CSPTC circuit with projections to frontal cortex and, through centromedial-parafascicular (CM-PF) nuclei of Th, to Str. VS representing limbic cortical areas projects substantially to the ventral pallidum (VP) situated just ventral to the anterior commissure; the VP also appears to involve direct and indirect pathways from Str, and both

From: *Mental and Behavioral Dysfunction in Movement Disorders*
Edited by: M-A. Bédard et al. © Humana Press Inc., Totowa, NJ

substance P and enkephalin are present in this pallidal region *(9)*. Rostral (*r*), anterior (*a*), ventral (*v*), and medial (*m*) Str tend to project more through the direct pathway, whereas caudal (*c*), posterior (*p*), dorsal (*d*), and lateral (*l*) Str tend to more often utilize the indirect pathway *(10)*. Corticostriatal, subthalamopallidal, and thalamocortical neurons of CSPTC circuits release glutamate, which is an excitatory neurotransmitter, whereas striatal and pallidal projections release γ-amino butyric acid (GABA), which is an inhibitory neurotransmitter. Striatopallidal neurons in the direct pathway release GABA colocalized with substance P, whereas those in the indirect pathway release GABA colocalized with enkephalin.

2.1.2. *Pallidosubthalamopallidal Relations*

Retrograde labeling studies have revealed two different clusters of GPe neurons that project to single GPi neurons *(7)*. The STN also receives direct cortical input, and single STN neurons project to both GPe and GPi in related functional domains *(7)*. GPi neurons appear to be innervated by interconnected GPe and STN neurons *(8)*.

2.1.3. *Pallidothalamic Relations*

Aside from well-known projections of GPi to Th, observations in primates indicate that GPe projects directly to the reticular nucleus (Ret) of Th *(7,9)*. *V* GPi projects to the CM-PF border, *pm* ventral anterior/ventrolateral (VA/VL) Th, and *l* magnocellular (mc) region (bilaterally) and *m* small-celled region (unilaterally) of the lateral habenula (LHAB) *(11)*. *D* GPi projects to parafascicular thalamic nucleus (PF), *al* VA/VL, and *l* LHABmc *(11)*. PF, in turn, projects to CN areas receiving prefrontal cortical input. Close inspection of associative territory GPi projections to *l* Th and Th central complex revealed axonal branching with widespread distribution throughout the nucleus lateralis oralis and PF, without any clear topographic organization *(12)*. Thus, pallidal projections can both specifically and diffusely regulate widespread neural systems.

2.2. *Dopaminergic Modulation and Anatomical Organization of CSPTC Circuits*

2.2.1. *Dopaminergic Modulation of CSPTC Circuits*

CSPTC circuit processing is modulated by dopamine (DA). VS and NA receive DA projections from the ventral tegmental area (VTA), whereas CN and Put receive DAergic projections from the substantia nigra pars compacta (SNpc). Direct pathway CN and Put neurons are primarily modulated by excitatory DA D1 receptors, and indirect pathway CN and Put neurons are primarily modulated by inhibitory DA D2 receptors. Ventral tier SNpc neurons project to Str striosomes, whereas dorsal tier SNpc neurons project to Str matrix *(13)*. Other inputs to striosomes include prefrontal, temporal, orbitofrontal, and insular cortices, and midline Th nuclei; striosomes then project back to ventral tier SNpc. Neocortical areas and CM-PF project to the Str matrix, which, in addition to CSPTC projections, projects to ventral tier SNpc *(13)*.

2.2.2. *Anatomical Organization of Associative and Limbic CSPTC Circuits Traversing the Pallidum*

Association cortex projects principally to CN and *r* Put, whereas limbic cortices, amygdala, and hippocampus project to VS *(7)*. Other inputs to Str include DAergic SNpc, serotonergic raphe, glutamatergic thalamic, GABAergic, cholinergic, and somatostatin-positive interneuron projections *(7)*. *Associative* CN and *vm* Put project to *dm* GPe and *d* GPi, *limbic* VS projects to *rm* polar GPi (*rm* GPi), and *sensorimotor* postcommissural Put projects to the *vl* GPe and *vl* GPi *(14)*. Specifically, *d* GPi receives Str information representing *dl* prefrontal cortex (DLPFC), *dm* prefrontal cortex, *p* parietal cortex, and frontal eye fields; *rm* GPi receives Str information representing cingulate cortex, *m* orbitofrontal cortex (MOFC), temporal polar cortex, and amygdala *(5,15,16)*. *R*, *c*, *v*, and *d* Str project to *r*, *c*, *v*, and *d* GP, respectively *(16)*. *Vm* Put also projects to VP, whereas *rv* Str (including NA) also projects to *vm* GPe and *vm* GPi *(16)*. In addition to the connections described above in Subheading 2.1.3., *v* GPi projects to midbrain tegmentum, pedunculopontine nucleus (PPN), *l* and *p* hypothalamus, *d* raphe nucleus, and the parabrachial nuclei associated with autonomic function *(11)*. Thus, the pallidum is positioned to both receive information from and influence widespread limbic and associative cortical and subcortical structures.

2.3. Pallidal Influences over Associative Limbic CSPTC Circuits

2.3.1. VP Pallidopallidal and Limbic-Associative Interfaces

VP projects to both GPe and GPi *(9,17)*, affording the opportunity for VP to influence limbic, associative, and sensorimotor domains of GPe and GPi. The VP-GPi pathway may have functional significance in Parkinson's disease (PD), where GPi stimulation may activate VP neurons, which may subsequently inhibit GPi neurons *(18)*. Limbic and associative dysfunction is evident in depression, a condition in which GP hypermetabolism has been observed *(19,20)*. GP hypermetabolism at 1 wk of treatment is among the earliest correlates of antidepressant response and is followed by hypometabolism at 6 wk of treatment *(21)*. Pallidopallidal control of limbic and associative circuits may, therefore, play a critical role in mood disorder physiology and its treatment.

2.3.2. Pallidostriatal Pathways and Limbic-Associative Interfaces

VP and *d* GPe pallidostriatal neurons project diffusely to Str, affording three ways in which large widespread areas of Str can be influenced by discrete pallidal loci: (*i*) directly from VP and GPe (to Str limbic and association territory); (*ii*) by VP projections to SNpc, then to Str; (*iii*) by VP projections to SNpc or STN, projecting back to VP or GPe, then to Str *(22)*. Pallidostriatal pathways may, therefore, vitally influence mood disorder pathophysiology.

2.4. Seven Prefrontal CSPTC Linked to Mood Disorders

Seven prefrontal CSPTC circuits with pallidal relays have been implicated in mood disorder pathophysiology, including those subserving the DLPFC, anterior cingulate area (ACA), subgenual prefrontal (SGPFC), MOFC, lateral orbitofrontal (LOFC), parietal, and temporal cortical areas. The preponderance of data suggest hypometabolism of DLPFC, ACA, and parietal areas in depression *(23–25)*. Further, there are data indicating SGPFC hypometabolism *(26)* and orbitofrontal cortex (OBFC) hypermetabolism *(27)* in depression, although there is also evidence of OBFC hypometabolism *(28)*, especially in medication-refractory depressed patients *(29)*. In mania, more limited data suggest global cortical hypermetabolism relative to depressive baseline *(30)*, especially in SGPFC *(26)*. Taken together, these data indicate involvement of DLPFC, ACA, SGPFC, MOFC, LOFC, parietal, and temporal CSPTC circuits in mood disorders. The bulk of the evidence regarding white matter and gray matter hyperintensities, as seen on magnetic resonance imaging (MRI), supports these suppositions *(31)*, indicating that interruptions of CSPTC circuits subserving these cortical areas are associated with mood disorders. These seven prefrontal CSPTC circuits emanate from associative and limbic striatal territory.

2.4.1. The DLPFC CSPTC Circuit

DLPFC Brodmann area (BA) 9 glial and neuronal depletion has been demonstrated in major depression *(32)*, and increased DLPFC BAs 9 and 46 metabolism after 6 wk of treatment has been correlated with antidepressant response *(21)*. DLPFC BAs 9 and 46 projects to associative *dl* head of CN (CNh). *Dl* CNh representing BAs 9 and *d* 46, in turn, projects to *plmd* GPe and *plmd* GPi *(2,5,6,14)*. *Plmd* GPe then projects to *plmd* GPi and *plmv* STN, which in turn projects to *plmd* GPi. *Plmd* GPi then projects to thalamic parvocellular mediodorsal nucleus (MDpc), parvocellular ventral anterior (VApc), *d* ventrolateral (VLd), magnocellular ventral anterior (VAmc), pars caudalis of ventral lateral (VLcr), *rd* PF, and the *dc* two-thirds of CM-PF, areas in common with projection fields of limbic (ACA CSPTC territory) and other associative (LOFC CSPTC territory) pallidal projections *(15,33)*. MDpc projects back to DLPFC. *Plmd* GP can, therefore, influence DLPFC and, perhaps, ACA and LOFC physiology in mood disorders.

2.4.2. The ACA CSPTC Circuit

ACA electrical stimulation can produce laughter with merriment *(34,35)*. ACA BA 24b reduced neural size and glial density is seen in major depression *(36)*, and increased metabolism of 24b after 6 wk of treatment correlates with antidepressant response *(21)*. ACA BA 24a,b,c projects to limbic VS, which also receives input from MOFC, limbic and paralimbic cortices, hippocampus, amygdala, entorhinal cortex, and superior and inferior temporal cortices *(5,37)*. VS projects to VP, *vrm* GPe, and *vrm* GPi *(5,14,16,17)*. The VS components *v* CN and *d* NA project enkephalinergic fibers to *d* VP and *l* VP, whereas *v* NA and *v* Put project substance P fibers to *v* VP and *m* VP *(17)*. "VP complex" components *r* GPe, *m* VP, and *vl* VP project to *m* MDmc; *m* VP and *vm* VP project to midline nuclei, and *vm* VP projects to *d* Th *(17)*. There is also evidence of projection to VApc, VLd, *rd* PF, and *dc* CM-PF, areas which also receive DLPFC- and LOFC-related pallidal projections *(15)*. VP itself projects to GPe, GPi, SNpr, STN, Th nuclei including anteroventral (AV), anteromedial (AM), MD, Ret, LHAB, *l* and *m* hypothalamus, bed nucleus of the stria terminalis (BNST), preoptic area, central gray, SNpc, VTA, and PPN *(9,17)*. Reciprocal projections exist between VP and STN, VP and *l* hypothalamus, VP and GPe, and VP and GPi *(17)*. Each domain of the "VP complex" (*r* polar GPe, *rm* GPi, and subcommissural VP) projects to LHAB *(17)*. Projections to SNpc dorsal tier suggest limbic VP can modulate *d* Str association territory *(17)*. Input to AV/AM comes from the ipsilateral *m* mamillary nucleus, deep layers of subicular cortex via the fornix, and noradrenergic cell bodies *(33)*. Ret receives input from hippocampus and midline Th nuclei receive hypothalamic (especially periventricular nucleus), amygdalal, lateral septal, periaqueductal gray, parabrachial nuclear, solitary tract nuclear, coeruleal, raphe, and reticular formation projections *(33)*. Th nuclei projecting to ACA include *l* MD (MDpc, MDdc), midline and *r* intralaminar (CL, Pc, PF), AV, and AM, as well as *m* VM, anterodorsal (AD), pulvinar, and laterodorsal *(33)*. The VP can, therefore, directly and indirectly influence limbic and associative cortical and subcortical physiology in mood disorders.

2.4.3. The SGPFC CSPTC Circuit

Two different SGPFC areas, involving BAs 24 and 25, may operate differentially in mood disorders. Subgenual BA 24 shows evidence of glial depletion in major depression and bipolar depression *(38, 39)*. Left subgenual BA 24 was associated with marked hypometabolism in depression and hypermetabolism in mania in a single patient *(26,38)*. In contrast, reduced BA 25 metabolism after 6 wk of treatment has correlated with antidepressant response; nonresponders showed no change *(21)*. BA 24 is connected to the NA, *m* Th nuclei, amygdala, *l* hypothalamus, and brainstem serotonergic, noradrenergic, and dopaminergic nuclei, and has been suggested to play a heuristic role in pathological guilt and anxiety in depression and rapid shifts between euphoria and anger in mania *(26)*. The VP has direct or indirect connections to many of these same structures. BA 25 has only recently been studied in primates and has been found to project to *m* CN, midline and MD Th, and amygdala (lateral parvocellular basal accessory and magnocellular basal nuclei) *(40)*. Inputs to specific pallidothalamic sites await identification, but it is likely that this area of *m* CN projects either to *rm* GPi or *mdm* GPi, similar to ACA or MOFC CSPTC circuits. Consequently, VP and GPi likely influence SGPFC physiology in mood disorders.

2.4.4. The MOFC CSPTC Circuit

Right MOFC subcortical hyperintensities correlate with depressive severity in late-onset depression *(41)*, and *r* and *p* OBFC BA 10, 47 appear to be glially and neuronally depleted in major depression *(32)*. Medial prefrontal cortex (MPFC)-MOFC (Walker's areas 10–14, 24, and 25) receives input from the *vm* basal amygdaloid nucleus, and MPFC-MOFC projects to *r* Str, to *central* VP and *rm* GPi, then to *dm* and *vl* MDmc, and back to MPFC-MOFC *(38)*. The MPFC-MOFC also projects to the hypothalamus and periaqueductal gray and has been suggested to provide frontal cortical influence over autonomic and endocrine function, guide behavior (including eating behavior), and regulate mood *(38)*. The VP and GPi may, therefore, mediate certain clinical features of mood disorders.

2.4.5. The LOFC CPSTC Circuit

Both OBFC and amygdalal hypermetabolism have been observed in primary depression *(27)*. LOFC is linked to MOFC by corticocortical connections, and is thought to integrate viscerosensory information with affective signals because it receives projections from the ventrolateral basal amygdaloid nucleus, entorhinal and perirhinal cortex, and subiculum, and it receives sensory input, including olfactory, gustatory, visceral, somatic sensory, and visual afferents *(38)*. The LOFC (BA 12, Walker's Areas 10–13) circuit projects to central *r* Str and *vm* CNh (*vm* CNh also receives input from ACA and superior and inferior temporal cortices *[5]*), then to *ammd* GPe, *ammd* GPi, and *l* VP, followed by *vl* MDmc, and back to LOFC *(5,6,14,38)*. *Ammd* GPe projects to *ammd* GPi and *ammv* STN, which in turn projects to *ammd* GPi. There is also evidence of *amd* GPi projection to VApc, VLd, rd PF, and dc CM-PF, areas in common with projection fields of limbic (ACA CSPTC territory) and associative (DLPFC CSPTC territory) pallidal projections *(15)*. VP, GPe, and GPi may therefore help mediate LOFC physiology in mood disorders.

2.4.6. Parietal CSPTC Circuit

Left temporoparietal hypoperfusion has been observed in rapid cycling bipolar disorder in a study of three subjects *(24)*. Depression has been associated with left parietal hypoperfusion in primary depression *(24)* and with right parietal lesions in post-stroke depression *(42)*. Increased inferior parietal BA 40 metabolism has been correlated with response of depression to fluoxetine at both 1 and 6 wk of treatment *(21)*. Posterior parietal cortex provides input to the DLPFC circuit *(5)*. Although the circuitry is yet to be defined, data also support the existence of a specific CSPTC circuit projecting to parietal cortex *(2)*. The GP may, therefore, influence parietal physiology in mood disorders.

2.4.7. Temporal CSPTC Circuit

Increased medial temporal BA 37 and hippocampal metabolism were present after 1 wk of treatment in patients with depression responding to fluoxetine; with continued treatment, hypometabolism of these areas developed *(21)*. Primary mania has been related to temporal lobe lesions, abnormal temporal volume and density, reduced right-compared-to-left hippocampal volume, and reduced right basal temporal cortical blood flow *(23,24)*. Superior and inferior temporal cortices provide input to ACA and LOFC circuits, and hippocampus and entorhinal cortex provide input to the ACA circuit *(5)*. More recently, there are data indicative of a specific CSPTC circuit projecting to temporal cortex *(2)*. The GP may, therefore, influence temporal physiology in mood disorders.

2.5. CSPTC Integration of Associative and Limbic Information

Although CSPTC circuits process information in a parallel functionally-segregated manner, there is anatomic evidence of integration through convergent projections from different territories to the same area of target structure, and divergent projections from a single territory to multiple territories in specific target structures. Convergences include: cortical projections from different lobes onto a single associative *Str* territory *(7)*, different Str territories onto the same *GP* region *(7,15,17)*, GPe and STN onto *GPi (13)*, associative and limbic GPi onto common *Th* nuclei (VApc, VAdc, CM-PF), *SN*, and *LHAB (15,17)*, and associative and limbic Th on *ACA (33)*. Divergences include single *cortical* area projections to CN and *v* Put *(7)*, *SN* projections to associative and limbic Str *(15,19)*, reciprocal projections between direct and indirect *Str* neurons *(17)*, single *Str* projections to different elongated bands within GPe and within GPi *(43,44)*, *limbic Str* to limbic VP, associative SNpr, and motor SNpc *(45, 46)*, *limbic VP* to *d* SNpc, *d* GPe, and *d* GPi *(19)*, single *GPe* projections to multiple STN neurons *(17)*, including limbic and motor regions *(45,46)*, *STN* projections to both GPe and GPi *(17)*, and *dl PF* projections to both associative and limbic Str *(15,19)*. Data from rat studies indicate that some single GPe neurons respond to either frontal or nonfrontal cortical stimulation that can facilitate, inhibit, or alter GPe discharge patterns *(47,48)*. Integration of different functional territories through convergences and divergences may provide a basis for simultaneous disturbances of mood, vegetative, motivational, cognitive, mnesic, behavioral, and perceptual functions in mood disorders *(33)*.

2.6. *Pallidal Control over Mood Disorder Substrates*

In light of the hodological relationships just summarized, the GP is positioned at the heart of CSPTC circuitry, receives information from associative and limbic areas demonstrated to be abnormal in mood disorders, exerts influences over associative and limbic thalamocortical projections to these same areas, and may be involved in integrating this information to influence widespread limbic and associative cortical and subcortical structures associated with mood disorders symptoms. These hodological relationships thus provide a compelling rationale for pondering clinical data regarding the pallidum and mood disorders.

3. CLINICAL CONSIDERATIONS

Clinical evidence also links the pallidum to mood disorders. The literature of MRI hyperintensities, diseases primarily and secondarily affecting the GP, focal GP lesions, pallidotomy, pallidal deep brain stimulation (DBS), and neurosurgical GP stimulation investigations was searched. The findings from these studies are detailed and interpretations are considered.

3.1. *MRI Subcortical Hyperintensities*

Studies that specifically address pallidal hyperintensities on MRI have not been apparent in earlier reviews of the literature *(23–25)*. A MEDLINE database literature search using the search terms "subcortical hyperintensit(ies)" and "globus pallidus" revealed only five citations. Only two studies specifically addressed pallidal hyperintensities in mood disorders.

Iidaka and colleagues retrospectively evaluated the prevalence and severity of signal hyperintensities in 30 elderly depressed patients, and 30 age-, gender-, and cerebrovascular risk factor-matched controls, on T2 weighted and proton density images *(49)*. Etat crible (dilated perivascular spaces) was excluded from consideration. Elderly depressed patients had more lenticular (putaminal and pallidal) (57 vs 27%), frontal (87 vs 57%), and pontine (33 vs 7%) hyperintensities than controls, and there was greater third ventricle dilatation in depressed subjects than in controls after adjusting for cerebrovascular risk factors. This study specifically rated lenticular hyperintensities, in contrast to previous studies. Inter-rater reliability for the lenticular ratings was 0.57, using a generalized κ. Overall, subjects with depression had twice as many lenticular and five times as many pontine hyperintensities as controls.

The other study examined white matter hyperintensities and basal ganglia volumes in 30 patients with bipolar disorder compared with age-, gender-, race-, and education-matched controls *(50)*. The authors found more frontal hyperintensities in bipolar disorder, and larger CN volume in male subjects with bipolar disorder.

Because studies evaluating the pallidum may not have been indexed under the term "globus pallidus," a second search was conducted using the terms "mood disorder," "magnetic resonance imaging," and "stroke" or "hyperintensity," producing 106 citations. None of these studies specifically examined pallidal hyperintensities, but two looked at pallidal volume. In one study, there was no difference in pallidal volume on MRI in 24 patients with bipolar disorder compared to controls matched for age, gender, race, height, handedness, and education *(51)*. The other was a postmortem study involving blinded planimetric volumetry of 1-mm slices of Put, CN, NA, GPe, and GPi in eight patients with mood disorders (four with major depression, two bipolar, two schizoaffective disorder) compared to eight age- and gender-matched controls *(52)*. Inter-rater and test-retest reliabilities ranged between $r = 0.95$–0.99. Volumetry revealed reduced volumes for bilateral GPe, left NA, and right Put in depressed patients relative to controls.

Thus, only one study has specifically examined lenticular hyperintensities, finding twice as many in patients with depression as in controls *(49)*, but Put was also included in the region of interest.

Table 1
Diseases Primarily Involving the GP

Autosomal dominant early-onset rapidly progressive familial parkinsonism with striatopallidal gliosis	
Bhatia et al., 1993 *(64)*	2 (100%) of 2 patients had depression.
Pallidal degeneration (e.g., carbon monoxide-induced)	
Meucci et al., 1989 *(65)*	Hypomanic thought disorder associated with *rad* GPi lesion.
Strub, 1989 *(66)*	Manic syndrome was followed by apathy syndrome resembling depression after bilateral GPi lesions.
Grinker, 1926 *(67)*	Apathy syndrome resembling depression in *r* and *dm* pallidal lesion.
LaPlane et al., 1989 *(54)*	Apathy syndrome resembled depressive symptoms and metabolism.
Mimura et al., 1999 *(68)*	24 (15.3%) of 156 patients had depression on 33-yr follow-up.
Lenticular nucleus lesions	
Bhatia and Marsden, 1994 *(69)*	Abulia (apathetic syndrome resembling depression) occurred in 10% (unilateral) and 24% (bilateral) of patients with pallidal lesions in cases reported in the literature. Disinhibition was associated with CN but not with pallidal lesions.
Pallidal stroke	
Starkstein et al., 1987 *(70)*	2 (67%) of 3 patients with left pallidal lesions had depressive disorders. 1 (50%) of 2 patients with right pallidal lesions had depressive disorder. Left pallidal lesions in major depression twice the rate of nondepressed. Right pallidal lesions in major depression four times the rate of nondepressed.
Herrmann et al., 1995 *(71)*	6 (67%) of 9 patients with major depression and left hemisphere stroke had pallidal lesions.

Diseases primarily, but not exclusively, neuropathologically affecting the GP.

Bilateral reduced GPe volume was found in a postmortem study of mood disorder subjects with primarily major depression *(52)*. In vivo MRI studies in patients with bipolar disorder, however, have not demonstrated substantial pallidal findings *(50,51)*.

3.2. Diseases Involving the Globus Pallidus

Table 1 shows the relations of mood disorders to diseases wherein neuropathology primarily involves the pallidum. Table 2 indicates relations to diseases which secondarily involve the GP either pathologically or physiologically. In primary pallidal diseases, strong associations between GP lesions and depression have been observed in a limited number of stroke patients. Among conditions that secondarily involve the pallidum, high rates of mania and depression have also been observed, linking depression to GPe lesions and mania to GPe overactivity, as in Huntington's disease *(46)*. High rates of mania and depression and behavioral disorders resembling these mood disorders are common in Fahr's syndrome. Apathy syndromes have also been identified in patients with pallidal lesions, and LaPlane has documented nosologic and metabolic similarities of apathy to depression *(53,54)*. Thus, pallidal disinhibition and overactivity appear to be associated with mania, while pallidal (especially GPe) lesions and underactivity appear to be associated with depression. More rarely, *r* GPi lesions have also been associated with manic symptoms. The above findings are consistent with previous models of mania *(55)* and depression *(3,4)*.

3.3. Focal GP Lesion Studies

A MEDLINE search was conducted using the terms "major depression" and "globus pallidus," and produced only five citations. Only two studies specifically addressed the relation of the globus pallidus to depression.

In the first study, we reviewed 10,000 MRI scans, searching for subjects with solitary focal lacunar infarctions limited to the pallidum, Put, CN, Th, STN, SN, or cerebellum *(3)*. We found 120 scans

Table 2
Diseases Secondarily or Nonspecifically Affecting the GP

Aphasia	
Herrmann et al,. 1993 *(72)*	GPe lesions in all subjects with major depression.
Fahr's syndrome	
Lauterbach et al., 1998 *(73)*	Mania prevalence 31%.
Konig et al., 1989 *(74)*	Depressive disorder prevalence 37%.
Martinelli et al., 1993 *(75)*	All cases of Fahr's attended by depression in one family.
Huntington's disease	
Lauterbach et al., 1998 *(73)*	Mania prevalence 10%. Depression prevalence 30–40%.
Idiopathic dystonia	
Lauterbach et al., 2000 *(76)*	Bipolar disorder prevalence 18%. Major depression prevalence 29%.
Parkinson's disease	
Slaughter et al., 2001 *(77)*	Major depression prevalence 24.8%.
Postencephalitic encephalitis lethargica	
Cheyette and Cummings, 1995 *(78)*	Depression frequently observed.
Progressive supranuclear palsy	
Cambier et al., 1985 *(79)*	Depression or irritable outbursts in 5 of 10 patients.
Vascular dementia	
Cummings, 1994 *(80)*	Depression is frequent and apathy ubiquitous in this dementia, which is often associated with pallidal infarcts.
Wilson's disease	
Lauterbach et al., 1998 *(73)*	Manic symptom prevalence 5–13%, depression prevalence 27%.
Cerebrovascular disease	
Vataja et al., 2001 *(81)*	GP lesions in 54% (left 27%, right 27%) of 109 patients with mixed-stroke lesions and depression; logistic regression correlates involved left internal capsule genu lesions, left or right GP lesions, and right occipital lobe infarct volume.

Diseases secondarily affecting the GP, either neuropathologically or neurophysiologically.

meeting this inclusion criterion. Scans were then examined to exclude clinically apparent cortical atrophy and periventricular white matter hyperintensities, reducing the number to 93 subjects. Subjects were then invited to participate, but were blind to the psychiatric nature of the study. Forty-five subjects agreed to participate, 23 refused, 11 had died, and 14 could not be contacted. MRI scans were evaluated blindly with respect to clinical condition, and clinical assessments were undertaken in a manner that was blind to MRI findings. Nine (20%) subjects met criteria for the Diagnostic and Statistical Manual of Mental Disorders, third edition (DSM-III) major depression ascertained by the Diagnostic Interview Schedule (DIS) interview. Each subject also met DSM-III-revised (DSM-III-R) and DSM-IV criteria ascertained by the Structured Clinical Interview for DSM (SCID). All subjects were right-handed, had pallidothalamic lesions (eight pallidal, one thalamic), and had secondary depression (no subject had ever experienced a mood disorder prior to infarction). Two additional subjects had secondary forme fruste major depression, both with midbrain nigrotegmental lesions. Of the three subjects with secondary mania, each had a cerebellar lesion. Secondary major depression after these subcortical infarcts was several-fold greater than in age-, gender-, and race-matched normal population controls drawn from the Epidemological Catchment Area study (odds ratio 3.50, 95% confidence interval [CI] 1.04–12.12, $p = 0.02$). We suggested that GPe lesions which disinhibit GPi inhibition of stimulatory glutamatergic thalamocortical projections to left DLPFC might account for secondary major depression; nigrotegmental lesions disrupting DA projections to Str might have led to a more mild, physiological disinhibition of GPi, perhaps accounting for milder, forme fruste secondary depression. The possibility of impaired parietofrontal interaction due to such lesions was also considered.

In the second study, we compared nine subjects with secondary major depression to 22 controls with subcortical lesions lacking life histories of any mood disorder *(4)*. All subjects were drawn from the first study. We sought correlations between depression and the location of the lesion within the pallidum. Pallidal lesions were found in 8 (89%) subjects with secondary major depression and 13 (59%) controls. Left *p* pallidal lesions occurred in four (44%) subjects with secondary major depression vs two (9%) controls ($p = 0.04$). Demographic and other factors (age, sex, race, salary, social class, retirement status, education, marital status, family history of depression, past medical history, and mental status score) did not differ between subjects and controls. These findings were consistent with *p* GPe lesions leading to increased GPi GABAergic inhibition of MDpc thalamocortical facilatatory projections to *d* and *m* prefrontal association cortices, with a lesser likelihood of GPi lesions disinhibiting MDmc projections to OBFC areas which, in turn, inhibit MDpc thalamocorticals and *d* and *m* prefrontal association cortices.

In summary, of the two studies specifically looking at depression as an outcome of focal disease limited to the pallidum, several findings were apparent: (*i*) depression was more common than expected and was associated with pallidal lesions; (*ii*) pallidal lacunar infarcts were 1.5 times more common in subjects with secondary depression than in controls; (*iii*) depression occurred in 67% of patients with left GP lesions, a rate nearly identical to the pallidal stroke study findings of Starkstein et al. (Table 1); (*iv*) left *p* pallidal lesions were nearly five times more common in subjects with secondary depression than in controls; (*v*) these findings were consistent with GPe and midbrain lesions leading to increased GPi-mediated inhibition of *d* prefrontal thalamocortical neurons, GPi lesions leading to disinhibition of *v* prefrontal thalamocortical neurons, and possible parietal dysfunction.

3.4. Pallidotomy and Pallidal DBS

Pallidotomy and pallidal DBS are thought to relieve pallidal inhibition on thalamic neurons. Laitinen considered posteroventral pallidotomy to spare GPi, but reduced its activity by lesioning neurons lateral to it *(56)*. Table 3 summarizes results of pallidotomy, and Table 4 summarizes findings in pallidal DBS and investigational neurosurgical intraoperative pallidal stimulation. Pallidotomy and DBS both tend to improve depression scores on the Beck Depression Inventory at a 3 to 6-mo follow-up. It is apparent however that, in some series, a fair number of patients can also become depressed after pallidotomy, ranging between 1–50% in different pallidotomy series, especially after left-sided pallidotomy. Manic symptoms have also been observed in about 6% in pallidotomy series, especially with right-sided pallidotomy and with high levels of DBS.

3.5. Neurosurgical Brain Stimulation

Neurosurgical intraoperative stimulation experiments suggest that multiple circuits distributed throughout GPe and GPi may mediate specific depressive symptoms (Table 4). These investigations indicate that stimulation of GPe and GPi can each evoke depressive symptomatology. Convergent and divergent pallidal projections to the thalamus from these circuits may help explain observations that stimulation in diverse sites (Table 4) can evoke identical complex behaviors *(57)*. Electrophysiological evidence of profusely branched GPi projections to CM and VA/VL (including L.po, Z.o., and V.o.a. of Hassler) and GPe projections to VA and Ret *(58,59)* is consistent with microscopic evidence of widespread diffusely branched nontopographic GPi projections to lateral Th and PF *(12)*. Stimulation of GPi, but not GPe, has been noted to produce positive field potentials in Th V.o.a. of Hassler (the *a* basal aspect of VL of Olszewski) and in Z.o. (superior VL of Olszewski) in squirrel monkeys *(59)*, and stimulation of *a* and *p* V.o.a. and other Th nuclei correlates with depressive mood symptoms in

Table 3
Pallidotomy and Mood Disorders

Krayenbuhl et al., 1960 *(82)*	Of 28 patients with unilateral pallidotomy and contralateral thalamotomy: 21.4% of left pallidotomies developed apathy and crying; 27.3% of left GPi pallodotomies developed apathy and crying; 6.25% of right pallidotomies exhibited loud speech, and 6.25% apathy; 7.1% right GPi pallidotomies had apathy.
Dogali et al., 1995 *(83)*	Of 18 patients, 1 (5.6%) developed transient sexual disinhibition.
Sutton et al., 1995 *(84)*	Of 5 patients, 2 (40%) had a dramatic worsening of presurgical depression.
Hariz and DeSalles, 1997 *(85)*	Of 14 patients, 1 (7.1%) developed depression and 2 (14.3%) suffered fatigue and hypersomnolence at 15-yr follow-up.
Hariz and DeSalles, 1997 *(85)*	Of 138 consecutive patients, 1 (0.72%) developed depression, and 2 (1.45%) developed fatigue and hypersomnolence.
Masterman et al., 1998 *(86)*	32 patients showed improved depression on BDI at 3–6 mo.
Perrine et al., 1998 *(87)*	28 patients had no change in depression scores, but 1 (3.6%) developed depression.
Bezerra, 1999 *(88)*	Of 17 patients with left-sided pallidotomy, 5 (29.4%) evolved major depression; 0 (0%) of 13 with right-sided pallidotomy had depression.
Ghika et al., 1999 *(89)*	Of 4 subjects, 2 (50%) developed depression, and another had an abulic syndrome resembling depression at 3–6 mo.
Straits-Troster et al., 2000 *(90)*	23 patients had improved depression on BDI at 3 mo.
Hariz and Bergenheim, 2001 *(91)*	5 (38.5%) of 13 posteroventral pallidotomy patients were depressed at 10 yr, vs 2 (15.4%) in preoperative period.

Mood disorder findings after pallidotomy. BDI refers to Beck Depression Inventory.

humans *(57)*. Sadness with motor inhibition or excitation was noted with stimulation of *d* V.o.a. or *v* V.o.a., respectively. Tiredness resulted from stimulation of the Ret near VA (Olszewski). Sadness and tiredness could both be elicited from V.o.a. and V.o.p. V.o.a. (Hassler 1959) appears to correspond to the *p* VApc and *a* VAdc nuclei of the Ilinskys, and Z.o. to VLd *(60)*; as reviewed under Subheading 2. above, these nuclei project to DLPFC, ACA, LOFC, and possibly other cortical areas involved in mood disorders. Consequently, multiple GPe and GPi sites linked to thalamic nuclei receiving pallidal projections from depression-related CSPTC circuits may mediate depressive symptoms and their pathophysiological correlates.

Euphoria, on the other hand, has been induced by stimulation of associative and limbic CN, but not GP *(57)*, consistent with pallidal sparing in mania associated with diseases secondarily affecting the GP. Preservation of GPe and GPi projections to thalamocortical neurons may, therefore, be critical to the expression of manic symptoms and pathophysiological correlates.

3.6. *Differential Regional Pallidal Effects*

In closing our review of findings, it is important to note that pallidal components (GPe and GPi) are not unitary in effect, but effects instead vary by region. The literature indicates: (*i*) that differences exist between left vs right, *d* vs *v*, and *a* vs *p* pallidal circuits; (*ii*) unilateral stimulation can produce bilateral effects; and (*iii*) neurotransmitters can exert opposing effects on different pallidal neurons. Although depressive dysmetabolisms and pallidal perturbations are more commonly left-sided, right-sided abnormalities have also been observed in primary depression *(20)* and secondary depression (Tables 1, 3, and 4). In a study of GPi DBS, *d* DBS ameliorated parkinsonism and induced dyskinesia whereas *pv* DBS ameliorated levodopa dyskinesia and induced parkinsonism *(61)*. An anteroposterior distinction is evident in *ad* pallidotomy efficacy for rigidity but not for hypokinesia or tremor *(62)*, in contrast to *pv* pallidotomy *(56)*. Unilateral GPi DBS has been observed to ameliorate dyskinesias

Table 4
Pallidal Therapeutic and Experimental Stimulation: Effects on Mood Disorders

Therapeutic Pallidal Stimulation	
Troster et al., 1997 *(92)*	9 DBS patients had a trend toward less depression at 3 mo, but 1 (11%) had worsened depression, and 2 (22.2%) had fatigue and inertia.
Ardouin et al., 1999 *(93)*	13 DBS patients had mildly improved mood on BDI at 3–6 mo; 5 patients had a nonsignificant worsening of BDI scores.
Ghika et al., 2000 *(94)*	High levels of DBS stimulation are associated with reversible emotional disturbances.
Miyawaki et al., 2000 *(95)*	Unilateral left or right DBS each resulted in mania in a single patient.
Straits-Troster et al., 2000 *(96)*	9 DBS patients displayed improved mood on BDI at 3 mo.
Experimental pallidal stimulation	
Schaltenbrand and Wahren, 1977 *(57)*	*rm* GPe and multiple other sites in *m* GPe induce sadness; *lm* GPi and *dm*, *d*, and *r* GPe induce tiredness.

Mood disorder findings after pallidal therapeutic DBS and during intraoperative neurosurgical experimental pallidal stimulation. BDI refers to Beck Depression Inventory.

bilaterally *(61)*. Furthermore, differential pallidal response to a given neurotransmitter has been noted. In contrast to expected inhibition, a minority of rat pallidal (GPe) neurons were excited by met-enkephalin *(63)*. These regional pallidal effects are compatible with several possibilities: (*i*) two opposing pallidal regions may be associated with depression, one correlating with DLPFC hypometabolism and the other with OBFC hypermetabolism; (*ii*) activation of GPi may mediate depression in one circuit, whereas inhibition of GPi may mediate depression in another circuit; and (*iii*) similar pallidal physiological states may mediate depression and mania in different circuits.

4. CONCLUSION

Hodological studies in primates reveal that the GP, especially *d* and *rm* GPe and GPi, as well as VP, may serve as a substrate for mood circuits. Lesions of these pallidal regions would, therefore, be expected to produce dysfunction in CSPTC circuits relevant to depression, presumably leading to depressive illness.

Clinical evidence reviewed above suggests that this is so, although not universally. Studies in patients with pallidal disturbances relate *p* GPe and, occasionally, *rm* GPi lesions to depression. As reviewed above, lenticular hyperintensities were twice as common in elderly depressives as in controls, and GPe volumes were reduced in patients with depressive disorders. Among diseases primarily involving the pallidum in limited series, 67% of left and 50% of right pallidal strokes were associated with major depression, and 67% of patients with depression and left hemispheric lesions had pallidal lesions. In the two studies actually looking at pallidal lesions, depression occurred in 67% of patients with left pallidal lesions, and 89% of patients with depression after stroke had pallidal lesions. Lesion location was consistent with GPe associative territory. Depression, and phenotypically similar apathy, are well documented concomitants of CO-induced *dm* pallidal degeneration. Diseases secondarily affecting the pallidum are associated with only half the rate of major depression observed in primary pallidal disease. Pallidotomy and pallidal DBS have been associated with mild improvements in depression in most patients, but also with severe depression in up to 50% of patients in some series. Neurosurgical investigations indicate that limbic and associative territory GPe and GPi stimulation is linked to depressive symptoms. Thus, pallidal disturbances in associative and limbic territories linked to the seven CSPTC circuits discussed above are associated with depression. *P* GPe and *r* GPi lesions are consistent with associative cortical hypometabolism and paralimbic cortical hypermetabolism in primary major depression. These pathophysiological observations are consistent with models of depression previously offered in the literature *(3,4,28)*.

Clinical data suggest that disinhibition of GP related to SGPFC BA 24, parietal, temporal, and other CSPTCs is associated with mania. These data, although scant, suggest excessive GPe activity and occasional GPi lesions in these CSPTC circuits. Although mania has been observed in Fahr's syndrome and, occasionally, after CO-induced *rad* GPi lesions and pallidal DBS, mania occurs more commonly in striatal disease and after thalmic stimulation. These pallidal disturbances are consistent with SGPFC BA 24 and associative CSPTC hypermetabolism observed in primary mania *(26,30)*.

Considering the quality of the data and the specificity of GP lesions for the pallidum across various data types, the evidence best supports an association of depression with left GPe lesions in associative territory. Manic behavior has been associated with primarily limbic GPi lesions. In diseases secondarily affecting the GP, GPe disinhibition has been associated with mania. It is also apparent that *vp* GP pallidotomy lesions and DBS stimulation are associated with mood disorders, and depression is more common with left-sided procedures, while mania is more common with right-sided procedures. Thus, based on these limited data, one might preliminarily hypothesize that left *d* GPe lesions are associated with depression, whereas right *r* GPi lesions and GPe disinhibition are associated with mania. Enthusiasm for these conclusions must be tempered, however, by anatomical and experimental stimulation evidence indicating multiple heuristic mood circuit projections distributed throughout the pallidum. There is also clinical evidence indicating associations of depressive symptoms with right GP lesions, GPe disinhibition, *rm* GPe intraoperative stimulation, right GPi pallidotomy, and both *rm* and *d* GPi intraoperative stimulation; furthermore, mild improvement in depressive mood is often observed after pallidotomy and pallidal DBS. Similarly, mania has been associated with *rad* GPi lesions and left DBS in single cases.

Thus, taken together, these data support the notion of multiple pallidal mood circuits, which may operate differentially, but with primary circuits for depression (reduced left *d* GPe inhibition on *d* GPi resulting in inhibition of *p* VApc, *a* VAdc, VLd, and *dc* CM-PF, and reduced left DLPFC, ACA, SGPFC BA 24, and parietal activation) and mania (right disinhibition of *r* GPe with increased inhibition of *r* GPi and disinhibition of MD, midline, and *r* intralaminar Th nuclei, with activation of SGPFC BA 24, and perhaps other cortical areas *[30]*). Two studies *(19,20)* have revealed increased pallidal, Str (VS, Put) and Th metabolism in depression, one finding this in both unipolar and bipolar depression before correcting for whole slice metabolism *(19)*; these findings are consistent with this depressive primary circuit in the context of overactive Str inhibition of GPe, reducing GPe inhibition on GPi, increasing GPi inhibition on Th, reducing Th stimulation of cortex in primary depression *(3,4)*. Secondary circuits may involve *rm* GPi dysfunction leading to OBFC and SGPFC BA 25 stimulation in depression, and in mania left GPi dysfunction leading to increased ACA and SGPFC BA 24 stimulation or reduced temporal BA 37 and hippocampal activation. Finally, based on experimental stimulation findings discussed above, there may well be other subsidiary circuits that mediate specific mood disorder symptomatologies, accounting for the diversity of findings reviewed above. Integrated converging and diverging pallidal projections provide the opportunity for discrete pallidal dysfunctions to influence widespread cortical areas consistent with findings from functional imaging studies in mood disorders.

An indication of the potential impact of GP regulation of Th can be seen in the potential importance of Th nuclei to mood disorder symptomatology. AV/AM, VA, MD, midline, and intralaminar Th nuclei have been suggested to regulate mnestic, motor, motivational, and emotional components of behavior *(33)*. Intrinsic to mood disorders, each of these receive projections from the VP complex, and VA, MD, and midline nuclei receive converging DLPFC, ACA, and SGPFC BA 24 territory pallidal projections. More specifically, VP projections to Ret, AV/AM, and MD have been suggested to pertain to rapid eye movement (REM) sleep and attention, motivation, and memory, respectively *(9)*, each disturbed in depression and mania. If cognitive and limbic information carried by pallidal projections can be integrated at convergences (e.g., VApc and VLd), and then disseminated at divergences (e.g., DLPFC and supplementary motor area), this might account for the expression of psychomotor disturbances of thinking and movement observed in mood disorders. Pallidal projections to hypothalamus, LHAB, BNST, monoaminergic nuclei, central gray, and reticular formation might account for remaining mood disorder symptoms. Integration through convergences and divergences might further explain mood disorder physiopathological concomitants observed in functional imaging studies.

The suppositions above rest upon limited data. White matter hyperintensities are often diffusely scattered, and it is difficult to evaluate the effect of lesions on single CSPTC circuits. Interpretation of lenticular hyperintensities is limited by putaminal inclusion. The meaning of reduced pallidal volumes remains to be interpreted. Conclusions drawn from data relating to diseases, which primarily and secondarily involve the pallidum, are hampered by involvement of extra-pallidal structures. Stroke data are more convincing, but suffer the same limitations and involve a small number of patients. Studies of focal solitary lesions confined to the pallidum are compelling but, to date, involve only a limited number of subjects. Cases reported in the pallidotomy and DBS literature are essentially anecdotal. Although the quality of the data is beset by these limitations, the direction of the findings across data types is suggestive of an important relationship between the pallidum and mood disorders. Nevertheless, much more data are needed from studies designed to minimize these limitations.

REFERENCES

1. Mayberg, H.S. (2000) Depression and frontal-subcortical circuits, in *Frontal-Subcortical Circuits in Psychiatric and Neurological Disorders* (Lichter, D.G. and Cummings, J.L., eds.), Guilford, New York, pp. 177–206.
2. Middleton, F.A. and Strick, P.L. (2001) A revised neuroanatomy of frontal-subcortical circuits, in *Frontal-Subcortical Circuits in Psychiatric and Neurological Disorders* (Lichter, D.G. and Cummings, J.L., eds.), Guilford, New York, pp. 45–58.
3. Lauterbach, E.C., Jackson, J.G., Price, S.T., Wilson, A.N., Kirsh, A.D., and Dever, G.E.A. (1997) Clinical, motor, and biological correlates of depressive disorders after focal subcortical lesions. *J. Neuropsychiatry Clin. Neurosci.* **9,** 259–266.
4. Lauterbach, E.C., Jackson, J.G., Wilson, A.N., Dever, G.E.A., and Kirsh, A.D. (1997) Major depression after left posterior globus pallidus lesions. *Neuropsychiatry Neuropsychol. Behav. Neurol.* **10,** 9–16.
5. Alexander, G.E., DeLong, M.R., and Strick, P.L. (1986) Parallel organization of functionally segregated circuits linking basal ganglia and cortex. *Annu. Rev. Neurosci.* **9,** 357–381.
6. Mega, M.S. and Cummings, J.L. (1994) Frontal-subcortical circuits and neuropsychiatric disorders. *J. Neuropsychiatry Clin. Neurosci.* **6,** 358–370.
7. Smith, Y., Bevan, M.D., Shink, E., and Bolam, J.P. (1998) Microcircuitry of the direct and indirect pathways of the basal ganglia. *Neuroscience* **86,** 353–387.
8. Shink, E., Bevan, M.D., Bolam, J.P., and Smith, Y. (1996) The subthalamic nucleus and the external pallidum: two tightly interconnected structures that control the output of the basal ganglia in monkey. *Neuroscience* **73,** 335–357.
9. Parent, A., Pare, D., Smith, Y., and Steriade, M. (1998) Basal forebrain cholinergic and noncholinergic projections to the thalamus and brainstem in cats and monkeys. *J. Comp. Neurol.* **277,** 281–301.
10. Parent, A., Smith, Y., Filion, M., and Dumas, J. (1989) Distinct afferents to internal and external pallidal segments in the squirrel monkey. *Neurosci. Lett.* **96,** 140–144.
11. DeVito, J.L. and Anderson, M.E. (1982) An autoradiographic study of efferent connections of the globus pallidus in *Macaca mulatta. Exp. Brain Res.* **46,** 107–117.
12. Arecchi-Bouchhioua, P., Yelnik, J., Francois, C., Percheron, G., and Tande, D. (1997) Three-dimensional morphology and distribution of pallidal axons projecting to both the lateral region of the thalamus and the central complex in primates. *Brain Res.* **754,** 311–314.
13. Masterman, D.L. and Cummings, J.L. (1997) Frontal-subcortical circuits: the anatomic basis of executive, social and motivational behaviors. *J. Psychopharmacol.* **11,** 107–114.
14. Shink, E., Sidibe, M., and Smith, Y. (1997) Efferent connections of the internal globus pallidus in the squirrel monkey: II. Topgraphy and synaptic organization of pallidal efferents to the pedunculopontine nucleus. *J. Comp. Neurol.* **382,** 348–363.
15. Sidibe, M., Bevan, M.D., Bolam, J.P., and Smith, Y. (1997) Efferent connections of the internal globus pallidus in the squirrel monkey: I. Topography and synaptic organization of the pallidothalamic projection. *J. Comp. Neurol.* **382,** 323–347.
16. Francois, C., Yelnik, J., Percheron, G., and Fenelon, G. (1994) Topographic distribution of the axonal endings from the sensorimotor and associative striatum in the macaque pallidum and substantia nigra. *Exp. Brain Res.* **102,** 305–318.
17. Haber, S.N., Lynd-Balta, E., and Mitchell, S.J. (1993) The organization of the descending ventral pallidal projections in the monkey. *J. Comp. Neurol.* **329,** 111–128.
18. Wu, Y.R., Levy, R., Ashby, P., Tasker, R.R., and Dostrovsky, J.O. (2001) Does stimulation of the GPi control dyskinesia by activating inhibitory axons? *Mov. Disord.* **16,** 208–216.

19. Buchsbaum, M.S., Wu, J., De Lisi, L.E., et al. (1986) Frontal cortex and basal ganglia metabolic rates assessed by positron emission tomography with [^{18}F]2-deoxyglucose in affective illness. *J. Affect. Disord.* **10,** 137–152.
20. Machale, S.M., Lawrie, S.M., Cavanaugh, J.T., et al. (2000) Cerebral perfusion in chronic fatigue syndrome and depression. *Br. J. Psychiatry* **176,** 550–556.
21. Mayberg, H.S., Brannan, S.K., Tekell, J.L., et al. (2000) Regional metabolic effects of fluoxetine in major depression: serial changes and relationship to clinical response. *Biol. Psychiatry* **48,** 830–843.
22. Spooren, W.P.J.M., Lynd-Balta, E., Mitchell, S., and Haber, S.N. (1996) Ventral pallidostriatal pathway in the monkey: evidence for modulation of basal ganglia circuits. *J. Comp. Neurol.* **370,** 295–312.
23. Soares, J.C. and Mann, J.J. (1997) The anatomy of mood disorders—review of structural neuroimaging studies. *Biol. Psychiatry* **41,** 86–106.
24. Soares, J.C. and Mann, J.J. (1997) The functional neuroanatomy of mood disorders. *J. Psychiatr. Res.* **31,** 393–432.
25. Dougherty, D. and Rauch, S.L. (1997) Neuroimaging and neurobiological models of depression. *Harv. Rev. Psychiatr.* **5,** 138–159.
26. Drevets, W.C., Price, J.L., Simpson, J.R. Jr., et al. (1997) Subgenual prefrontal cortex abnormalities in mood disorders. *Nature* **386,** 824–827.
27. Drevets, W.C. (1998) Funcional neuroimaging studies of depression: the anatomy of melancholia. *Annu. Rev. Med.* **49,** 341–361.
28. Mayberg, H.S. (1997) Limbic cortical dysregulation: a proposed model of depression. *J. Neuropsychiatry Clin. Neurosci.* **9,** 471–481.
29. Mayberg, H.S., Lewis, P.J., Regenold, W., and Wagner, H.N. Jr. (1994) Paralimbic hypoperfusion in unipolar depression. *J. Nucl. Med.* **35,** 929–934.
30. Baxter, L.R. Jr., Phelps, M.E., Maziotta, J.C., et al. (1985) Cerebral metabolic rates for glucose in mood disorders. Studies with positron emission tomography and fluorodeoxyglucose F 18. *Arch. Gen. Psychiatry* **42,** 441–447.
31. Campbell, J.J. III and Coffey, C.E. (2001) Neuropsychiatric significance of subcortical hyperintensity. *J. Neuropsychiatry Clin. Neurosci.* **13,** 261–288.
32. Rajkowska, G., Miguel-Hidalgo, J.J., Wei, J., et al. (1999) Morphometric evidence for neuronal and glial prefrontal pathology in major depression. *Biol. Psychiatry* **45,** 1085–1098.
33. Bentivoglio, M., Kultas-Ilinsky, K., and Ilinsky, I. (1993) Limbic thalamus: structure, intrinsic organization, and connections, in *Neurobiology of Cingulate and Limbic Thalamus: a Comprehensive Handbook* (Vogt, B.A. and Gabriel, M., eds.), Birkheauser, Boston, pp. 71–122.
34. Talairach, J., Bancaud, J., Geier, S., et al. (1973) The cingulate gyrus and human behavior. *EEG Clin. Neurophysiol.* **34,** 45–52.
35. Arroyo, S., Lesser, R.P., Gordon, B., et al. (1993) Mirth, laughter and gelastic siezures. *Brain* **116,** 757–780.
36. Cotter, D., Mackay, D., Landau, S., Kerwin, R., and Everall, I. (2001) Reduced glial cell density and neuronal size in the anterior cingulate cortex in major depressive disorder. *Arch. Gen. Psychiatry* **58,** 545–553.
37. Nakano, K., Kayahara, T., Ushiro, H., and Hasegawa, Y. (1995) Some aspects of basal ganglia-thalamocortical circuity and dexcending outputs of the basal ganglia, in *Age-Related Dopamine-Dependent Disorders* (Segawa, M. and Nomura, Y., eds.), (*Monogr. Neural Sci.* **14**), Karger, Basal, pp. 134–146.
38. Price, J.L. (1999) Prefrontal cortical networks related to visceral function and mood. *Ann. NY Acad. Sci.* **877,** 383–396.
39. Ongur, D., Drevets, W.C., and Price, J.L. (1998) Glial reduction in the subgenual prefrontal cortex in mood disorders. *Proc. Natl. Acad. Sci. USA* **95,** 13,290–13,295.
40. Freedman, L.J., Insel, T.R., and Smith, Y. (2000) Subcortical projections of area 25 (subgenual cortex) of the macaque monkey. *J. Comp. Neurol.* **421,** 172–188.
41. MacFall, J.R., Payne, M.E., Provenzale, J.E., and Krishnan, K.R.R. (2001) Medial orbital frontal lesions in late-onset depression. *Biol. Psychiatry* **49,** 803–806.
42. Robinson, R.G. (1998) *The Clinical Neuropsychiatry of Stroke*, Cambridge University Press, Cambridge.
43. Parent, A., Charara, A., and Pinault, D. (1983) Single striatofugal axons arborizing in both pallidal segments and in the substantia nigra in primates. *Brain Res.* **278,** 11–27.
44. Yelnik, J., Francois, C., Percheron, G., and Tande, D. (1996) A spatial and quantitative study of the striatopallidal connection in the monkey. *Neuroreport* **7,** 985–988.
45. Joel, D. and Weiner, I. (1994) The organization of the basal ganglia-thalamocortical circuits: open interconnected rather than closed segregated. *Neurosciences* **63,** 363–379.
46. Joel, D. (2001) Open interconnected model of basal ganglia-thalamocortical circuitry and its relevance to the clinical syndrome of Huntington's disease. *Mov. Disord.* **16,** 407–423.
47. Toan, D.L. and Schultz, W. (1985) Responses of rat pallidum cells to cortex stimulation and effects of altered dopaminergic activity. *Neuroscience* **15,** 683–694.
48. Chudler, E.H., Sugiyama, K., and Dong, W.K. (1995) Multisensory convergence and integration in the neostriatum and globus pallidus of the rat. *Brain Res.* **674,** 33–45.
49. Iidaka, T., Nakajima, T., Kawamoto, K., et al. (1996) Signal hyperintensities on brain magnetic resonance imaging in elderly depressed patients. *Eur. Neurol.* **36,** 293–299.
50. Aylward, E.H., Robert-Twillie, J.V., Barta, P.E., et al. (1994) Basal ganglia volumes and white matter hyperintensities in patients with bipolar disorder. *Am. J.Psychiatry* **151,** 687–693.
51. Strakowski, S.M., Delbello, M.P., Sax, K.W., et al. (1999) Brain magnetic resonance imaging of structural abnormalities in bipolar disorder. *Arch. Gen. Psychiatry* **56,** 254–260.

52. Baumann, B., Danos, P., Krell, D., et al. (1999) Reduced volume of limbic system—affiliated basal ganglia in mood disorders; preliminary data from a postmortem study. *J. Neuropsychiatry Clin. Neurosci.* **11,** 71–78.
53. LaPlane, D., Boulliat, J., Baron, J.C., Pillon, B., and Baulac, M. (1988) Obsessive-compulsive behavior caused by bilateral lesions of the lenticular nuclei. A new case. *Encephale* **14,** 27–32.
54. LaPlane, D., Levasseur, M., Pillon, B., et al. (1989) Obsessive-compulsive and other behavioural changes with bilateral basal ganglia lesions: a neuropsychological, magnetic resonance imaging and positron tomography study. *Brain* **112,** 699–725.
55. Lauterbach, E.C., Spears, T.E., and Price, S.T. (1992) Bipolar disorder in idiopathic dystonia: clinnical features and possible neurobiology. *J. Neuropsychiatry Clin. Neurosci.* **4,** 435–439.
56. Laitinen, L.V. (1993) Ventroposterolateral pallidotomy. *Stereotact. Funct. Neurosurg.* **62,** 41–52.
57. Schaltenbrand, G. and Wahren, W. (1977) *Atlas for Stereotaxy of the Human Brain, 2nd ed.*, Year Book Medical Publishers, Chicago.
58. Harnois, C. and Filion, M. (1982) Pallidofugal projections to thalamus and midbrain: a quantitative antidromic activation study in monkeys and cats. *Exp. Brain Res.* **47,** 277–285.
59. Yamamoto, T., Hassler, R., Huber, C., Wagner, A., and Sasaki, K. (1983) Electrophysiologic studies on the pallido- and cerebellothalamic projections in squirrel monkeys (*Saimiri sciureus*). *Exp. Brain Res.* **51,** 77–87.
60. Percheron, G., Francois, C., Talbi, B., Meder, J.F., Fenelon, G., and Yelnik, J. (1993) The primate motor thalamus analysed with reference to subcortical afferent territories. *Stereotact. Funct. Neurosurg.* **60,** 32–41.
61. Bejjani, B., Damier, P., Arnulf, I., et al. (1997) Pallidal stimulation for Parkinson's disease. Two targets? *Neurology* **49,** 1564–1569.
62. Cooper, I.S. and Bravo, G. (1958) Chemopallidectomy and chemothalamectomy. *J. Neurosurg.* **15,** 244–250.
63. Frey, J.M. and Huffman, R.D. (1985) Effects of enkephalin and morphine on rat globus pallidus neurons. *Brain Res. Bull.* **14,** 251–259.
64. Bhatia, K.P., Daniel, S.E., and Marsden, C.D. (1993) Familial parkinsonism with depression: a clinicopathological study. *Ann. Neurol.* **34,** 842–847.
65. Meucci, G., Rossi, G., and Mazzoni, M. (1989) A case of transient choreoathetosis with amnesic syndrome after acute monoxide poisoning. *Ital. J. Neurol. Sci.* **10,** 513–517.
66. Strub, R.L. (1989) Frontal lobe syndrome in a patient with bilateral globus pallidus lesions. *Arch. Neurol.* **46,** 1024–1027.
67. Grinker, R.R. (1926) Parkinsonism following carbon monoxide poisoning. *J. Nerv. Ment. Dis.* **64,** 18–28.
68. Mimura, K., Harada, M., Sumiyoshi, S., et al. (1999) [Long-term follow-up study on sequelae of carbon monoxide poisoning; serial investigation 33 years after poisioning.] *Seishin Shinkeigaku Zasshi* **101,** 592–618.
69. Bhatia, K.P. and Marsden, C.D. (1994) The behavioural and motor consequences of focal lesions of the basal ganglia in man. *Brain* **117(Pt. 4),** 859–876.
70. Starkstein, S.E., Robinson, R.G., and Price, T.R. (1987) Comparison of cortical and subcortical lesions in the production of post-stroke mood disorders. *Brain* **110,** 1045-1059.
71. Herrmann, M., Bartels, C., Schumacher, M., and Wallesch, C.-W. (1995) Poststroke depression: is there a pathoanatomic correlate for depression in the postacute state of stroke? *Stroke* **26,** 850–856.
72. Herrmann, M., Bartel, C., and Wallesch, C.W. (1993) Depression in acute and chronic aphasia: symptoms, pathoanatomical-clinical correlations and functional implications. *J. Neurol. Neursurg. Psychiatry* **56,** 672–678.
73. Lauterbach, E.C., Cummings, J.L., Duffy, J., et al. (1998) Neuropsychiatric correlates and treatment of lenticulostriatal diseases: a review of the literature and overview of research opportunities in Huntington's, Wilson's, and Fahr's diseases. *J. Neuropsychiatry Clin. Neurosci.* **10,** 249–266.
74. Konig, P. (1989) Psychopathological alterations in cases of symmetrical basal ganglia sclerosis. *Biol. Psychiatry* **25,** 459–468.
75. Martinelli, P., Guiliani, S., Ippoliti, M., Martinelli, A., Sforza, A., and Ferrari, S. (1993) Familial idiopathic strio-pallido-dentate calcifications with late onset extrapyramidal syndrome. *Mov. Disord.* **8,** 220–222.
76. Lauterbach, E.C. (2000) Dystonia, in psychiatric management, in *Neurological Disease* (Lauterbach, E.C., ed.), American Psychiatric Press, Inc., Washington, D.C., pp. 179–218.
77. Slaughter, J.R., Slaughter, K.A., Nichols, D., Holmes, S.E., and Martens, M.P. (2001) Prevalence, clinical manifestations, etiology, and treatment of depression in Parkinson's disease. *J. Neuropsychiatry Clin. Neurosci.* **13,** 187–196.
78. Cheyette, S.R. and Cummings, J.L. (1995) Encephalitis lethargica: lessons for contemporary neuropsychiaty. *J. Neuropsychiatry Clin. Neurosci.* **7,** 125–134.
79. Cambier, J., Masson, M., Viader, F., Limodin, J., and Strube, A. (1985) Frontal syndrome of progressive supranuclear palsy. *Rev. Neurol. (Paris)* **141,** 528–536.
80. Cummings, J.L. (1994) Vascular subcortical dementias: clinical aspects. *Dementia* **5,** 177–180.
81. Vataja, R., Pohjasvaara, T., Leppavuori, A., et al. (2001) Magnetic resonance imaging correlates of depression after ischemic stroke. *Arch. Gen. Psychiatry* **58,** 925–931.
82. Krayenbuhl, H., Wyss, O.A.M., and Yasargil, M.G. (1960) Bilateral thalamotomy and pallidotomy as treatment for bilateral parkinsonism. *J. Neurosurg.* **18,** 429–444.
83. Dogali, M., Fazzini, E., Kolodny, E., et al. (1995) Stereotactic ventral pallidotomy for Parkinson's disease. *Neurology* **45,** 753–761.
84. Sutton, J.P., Couldwell, W., Lew, M.F., et al. (1995) Ventroposterior medial pallidotomy in patients with advanced Park-inson's disease. *Neurosurgery* **36,** 1112–1117.
85. Hariz, M.I. and DeSalles, A.A. (1997) The side effects and complications of posteroventral pallidotomy. *Acta Neurochir. Suppl. (Wien.)* **68,** 42–48.

86. Masterman, D., DeSalles, A., Baloh, R.W., et al. (1998) Motor, cognitive, and behavioral performance following unilateral ventroposterior pallidotomy for Parkinson disease. *Arch. Neurol.* **55,** 1201–1208.
87. Perrine, K., Dogali, M., Fazzini, E., et al. (1998) Cognitive functioning after pallidotomy for refractory Parkinson's disease. *J. Neurol. Neurosurg. Psychiatry* **65,** 150–154.
88. Bezerra, M.L.S., Martinez, J.-V.L., and Nasser, J.A. (1999) Transient acute depression induced by high-frequency deep-brain stimulation. *N. Engl. J. Med.* **341,** 1003.
89. Ghika, J., Ghika-Schmid, F., Fankhauser, H., et al. (1999) Bilateral contemporaneous posteroventral pallidotomy for the treatment of Parkinson's disease: neuropsychological and neurological side effects. Report of four cases and review of the literature. *J. Neurosurg.* **91,** 313–321.
90. Straits-Troster, K., Fields, J.A., Wilkinson, S.B., et al. (2000) Health-related quality of life in Parkinson's disease after pallidotomy and deep brain stimulation. *Brain Cogn.* **42,** 399–416.
91. Hariz, M.I. and Bergenheim, A.T. (2001) A 10-year follow-up review of patients who underwent Leksell's posteroventral pallidotomy for Parkinson disease. *J. Neurosurg.* **94,** 552–558.
92. Troster, A.I., Fields, J.A., Wilkinson, S.B., et al. (1997) Unilateral pallidal stimulation for Parkinson's disease: neurobehavioral functioning before and 3 months after electrode implantation. *Neurology* **49,** 1078–1083.
93. Ardouin, C., Pillon, B., Peiffer, E., et al. (1999) Bilateral subthalamic or pallidal stimulation for Parkinson's disease affects neither memory nor executive functions: a consecutive series of 62 patients. *Ann. Neurol.* **46,** 217–223.
94. Ghika, J., Ghika-Schmid, F., and Vingerhoets, F. (2000) Bilateral pallidotomy (letter). *J. Neurosurg.* **92,** 509.
95. Miyawaki, E., Perlmutter, J.S., Troster, A.I., Videen, T.O., and Koller, W.C. (2000) The behavioral complications of pallidal stimulation: a case report. *Brain Cogn.* **42,** 417–434.
96. Straits-Troster, K., Fields, J.A., Wilkinson, S.B., et al. (2000) Health-related quality of life in Parkinson's disease after pallidotomy and deep brain stimulation. *Brain Cogn.* **42,** 399–416.

25

Cortical-Limbic-Striatal Dysfunction in Depression

Converging Findings in Basal Ganglia Diseases and Primary Affective Disorders

Taresa L. Stefurak, MSc, MD, FRCPC and Helen S. Mayberg, MD, FRCPC

1. INTRODUCTION

There is growing evidence that a complex functional–anatomical network subserves mood regulation and emotional processing under both normal and pathological conditions *(1–9)*. Normal emotions are multidimensional processes involving the expression of interactive, but distinct behavioral elements, e.g., feelings and moods, arousal and somatic states, cognitive evaluations and interpretations—all integral to any specific emotional state. The basic nature of these behaviors suggests a certain neurolocalization, although the specifics have not been completely characterized *(1,2,4,5,10)*. Given that normal circuits mediating these behaviors are not yet fully understood, a meaningful biological construct of "emotion disorders" must anticipate distinct neuroanatomical pathways for each of these component behaviors, as well as accommodate a system where these separate pathways are able to differentially interact in the expression of various pathological emotional states *(2,7,11)*.

Critical involvement of cortical-limbic, cortical-cortical, and frontal-striatal pathways have all been postulated to explain the stereotypic combination of mood, motor, somatic, and cognitive behaviors seen across different affective disorder diagnoses. These working disease models are based on converging behavioral, chemical, anatomical, and physiological studies in animals and humans *(2,12–18)* where associations between specific regions and various aspects of motivational and affective behaviors have all been described. The basal ganglia are repeatedly implicated in these models *(12,19,20)* with a specific role in the integration of emotions with cognitive and motor behaviors *(21–23)*.

Further support for the hypothesis that frontal-striatal pathways serve a critical role in a more complex emotion processing network is the spectrum of mood and behavioral disorders (depression, anxiety, obsessive compulsions, mania, bipolar) seen with almost all diseases involving the basal ganglia, including focal strokes, parkinsonism, Huntington's disease (HD), Tourrette's, and Wilson's disease, to name a few *(24)*. Localization of the specific focal lesion and degenerative process has provided an important first step in linking striatal integrity to mood and affective regulation *(9,25)*. The lesion approach, however, has not proven adequate to fully define biological mechanisms mediating common behavioral phenomena across disorders, since divergent emotional states can also be associated with seemingly comparable lesions. Resolution of this apparent contradiction has required the evolution from static evaluation of lesions to a more integrated view of the lesion in context of specific pathways in both resting and provoked states. Delineation of function interactions between frontal,

From: *Mental and Behavioral Dysfunction in Movement Disorders*
Edited by: M-A. Bédard et al. © Humana Press Inc., Totowa, NJ

limbic, and striatal regions previously implicated in emotional processing is an ongoing area of active research.

2. PARKINSON'S DISEASE: A MODEL SYSTEM TO STUDY EMOTION

Parkinson's disease (PD) is a particularly compelling index disease to explore the role of striatal pathways in disorders affecting mood and emotional processing. Although depression is the most prevalent of the neuropsychiatric symptoms seen in Parkinson's *(26,27)*, behavioral disturbances in these patients span the emotional spectrum ranging from apathy and depression to generalized anxiety and psychosis *(28–31)*. In addition to fairly stereotypic syndromes, PD patients also show profound lability in mood, often in the setting of little to no external provocation *(32–34)*. As dysfunction in emotional processing and mood regulation is a hallmark of all affective disorders, systematic examination of patients with PD would appear to provide a unique opportunity to define the role of basal ganglia dysfunction in these behaviors more generally. To this end, relationships between specific cortical-basal ganglia pathways and stereotypic mood, motor, cognitive, and somatic symptoms seen in PD and other secondary mood disorders can be critically compared to primary affective disorder patients.

2.1. *Neuropsychiatric Phenomenology*

The clinical characterization of all movement disorders, typified by PD, now includes behavioral features, in addition to classic motor system dysfunction. Neuropsychiatric symptoms including depression, psychosis, and anxiety, occur in up to 60% of Parkinson's patients, with 45% of patients suffering from two or more different class of symptoms *(28)* (see Chapters 27 and 28 of this book). Pharmacological treatments are available, but tend to be empiric, as neither the mechanism of these symptoms nor their relationship to primary motor and cognitive features of the illness are well established *(35–37)*. Most published studies have focused on specific psychiatric diagnoses, such as major depression, generalized anxiety disorder, or obsessive–compulsive disorder, with reported incidence rates up to 40% *(27,36,38–41)*. Few population studies have characterized the full range of behavioral syndromes observed, although recent studies have described at least one psychiatric symptom in 61% of a large PD population *(28,42)*. Although it is often argued that the long duration of illness (seen in many samples of this type) can bias the apparent neuropsychiatric prevalence, these types of symptoms, particularly depression, can affect patients at any stage of illness *(28,43,44)* and commonly predate the onset of motor symptoms *(45)*. Furthermore, although it is suggested that depression is a natural psychological response to a progressive neurodegenerative disease, several lines of evidence argue the contrary. Depression does not appear to be merely a reaction to physical impairment or disability, as rates of psychiatric symptoms are unrelated to disease stage *(46)*. Others go further to argue that living with PD as a chronic illness actually has little influence in and of itself, because the incidence of depression is greater in PD than in other motor disabling illnesses, with personal attitude the key to perceiving disability *(47,48)*. In addition, depression is as common in recent onset PD as in more advanced stages *(49,50)* and as previously stated, may even antedate motor symptoms by years *(45)*. A retrospective review of Parkinson's patients found higher prevalence of a psychiatric history than age-matched healthy control populations leading to the somewhat unexpected conclusion that a previous psychiatric history of depression or generalized anxiety disorder may actually increase the risk of developing PD two- to threefold up to 20 yr in the future *(51)*.

Although the criteria for the formal diagnosis of a major depressive episode are the same for primary and secondary depressions, PD patients show several distinctive features. Sad mood, anxiety, and somatic complaints are more commonly reported than self-blame symptoms such as guilt and suicide *(27, 39,52)*. Anxiety disorders more commonly precede the onset of parkinsonism in familial PD than in idiopathic PD *(53)*, suggesting that these neuropsychiatric features may actually define subtypes of clinical PD groups. Additional studies also support clustering of neuropsychiatric symptoms such as apathy with anxiety, as well as agitation with delusions and psychosis, again suggesting common neurobiological mechanisms *(28,44)*.

2.2. *Mood–Motor–Cognitive Interactions*

The prominent bradykinesia, hypomimia, and general appearance and demeanor of PD patients has contributed in the past to the under recognition of co-morbid mood symptoms, often masking the diagnosis of a major depression *(54)*. This interplay between emotions and motor behaviors is also seen with other movement disorders such as tics, tremors, and dyskinesias *(55)*. The mood–motor link is further observed in primary psychiatric disorders, characteristically manifesting as psychomotor retardation, although motor agitation is also described and may additionally be seen as a side effect of certain classes of antidepressants *(56–58)*. Motor retardation in melancholic depression is phenomenologically similar to the bradykinesia of PD *(29)*. Primary depressed patients perceive these signs of motor slowness as a difficulty translating thought-to-action with motor symptom recovery occurring in parallel to improved mood *(59,60)*. Primary depressed patients also display the characteristically parkinsonian reliance on cueing to initiate movements *(61)*. PD patients additionally experience fluctuations in both mood and motor symptoms, although the lack of reproducible, temporal concordance continues to foster debate regarding their biological basis *(62,63)*. Although initially attributed to chemical variations in medical levodopa (L-dopa) therapy *(64–66)*, surgical treatments that clinically improve motor symptoms can also evoke changes in mood state *(67–71)*.

In addition to mood–motor deficits, PD and primary depression share a similar cognitive profile. Cognitive impairment is seen in both groups and generally involves "frontal behaviors," including mental flexibility, switching set, attending to tasks, generating and accounting new memories, and formulating lists *(72–77)*. These types of cognitive symptoms, like other neuropsychiatric complaints may also predate motor symptoms and may be risk markers for the development of PD *(43–45,78)*. Subtle changes in these symptoms, presenting in the early stages of the disease, may be attenuated by parkinsonian treatment *(79–81)*. Disruption of prefrontal striatal pathways, as well as regional depletion of norepinephrine and acetylcholine are all proposed mechanisms *(9,12,82–84)*.

The relationship between mood, motor, and cognition in PD is further revealed by studies demonstrating more pronounced deterioration in cognitive performance, particularly frontal task, in depressed patients *(85)*, with depression being a poor prognostic indicator for cognitive decline long term *(43)*. The reverse interaction is also seen, in that the presence of dementia is a risk factor for development of neuropsychiatric symptoms *(28)*. Evidence of a more direct influence of emotions on specific cognitions is suggested by performance on tests such as the emotional Stroop task, where the extent to which PD patients slow their response to negative emotional stimuli correlates with motor impairment *(86)*. Although further studies are required, this specific defect may also identify PD patients at risk for depression *(87,88)*.

2.3. *Neurochemical Mechanisms*

The search for biological mechanisms mediating both primary and PD depression has centered on neurochemistry, fostered in large part by the success of pharmacological interventions used to ameliorate symptoms. Postmortem studies of neurotransmitters and their associated receptors have provided critical clues, corroborated by in vivo blood, urine, cerebrospinal fluid (CSF), and functional imaging studies *(89–97)*. Overall, these studies suggest common monoaminergic etiologies. Pathological loss of dopamine (DA)-producing cells and therapeutic motor response to dopaminergic agents has defined dopamine as fundamental in the pathogenesis of PD and, by association, the depression in PD. In contrast, serotonin has emerged as the leading candidate in studies of primary depression *(98)*. Although each disorder is weighted toward a specific neurochemical pathway, there is clear overlap, with the likely involvement of multiple neurotransmitters, peptides, and second messenger systems.

In support of a crucial serotonin defect is the demonstration of reduced levels of the major serotonin metabolite 5-hydroxindoleacetic acid (5-HIAA) in CSF of patients with PD as compared to controls *(99)*, and these levels were further reduced in depressed PD patients compared to those without co-morbid depression *(78,99)*. Changes in serotonin levels in CSF, brainstem, and cortical concentrations *(100)*, and the various receptor subtypes, have also been reported in primary depression with regionally specific involvement of cingulate and ventral frontal cortex *(98,101)*. Paulus and Jellinger *(102)* reported that depressed PD patients had more severe neuronal loss in the serotonergic-producing dorsal raphe nucleus than nondepressed PD patients. Both primary depression and PD depressed patients have a higher incidence of the short allele of serotonin transporter *(103–105)*.

Although much of the literature focuses on serotonin, DA has also been considered in the pathogenesis of primary depression based on changes in dopamine metabolites levels, receptor number and affinity, and receptor allele predilections *(106,107)*. Although, overall clinical depression severity has been correlated with DA metabolism *(108)*, the most compelling evidence demonstrates correlations between DA changes and specific depressive symptoms, particularly psychomotor speed. Recent assessment of presynaptic DA function by using positron emission tomography (PET) and 6-[^{18}F] fluoro-dopa revealed decreased uptake in the left caudate of unipolar depressed patients with psychomotor retardation in comparison to controls *(109)*. A similar association has been postulated for depression in PD. Treatment studies with DA-enhancing agents also support this hypothesis. Methylphenidate does have mood-enhancing properties and has been shown to be clinical useful in treating some depressed patients, particularly those with co-morbid medical illness, psychomotor slowing, and low energy *(110)*. However, dopaminergic stimulation alone does not generally alleviate the mood, vegetative, or cognitive symptoms, and these patients generally require typical antidepressants to achieve clinical remission. The more selective involvement of the mesolimbic and mesocortical dopamine systems has also been proposed *(111)*, although clinical studies show little support for global changes in depressive symptoms using L-dopa or DA agonists, even in the depression of PD *(112,113)*. It is, nonetheless, notable that preferential degeneration of the ventral tegmental area (VTA) has been described in case studies of PD patients with prominent mood and behavioral symptoms, although the data is limited *(114)*. On the other hand, L-dopa therapy in PD is well-associated with mood fluctuations, described as mania, but also as anxiety or depressive symptoms, which parallel motor fluctuations *(62,115)*, although they are not necessarily temporally concordant. Mood fluctuations have also been linked to parallel shifts in plasma L-dopa levels *(63,65,116)*, but mood shifts often precede both DA level changes and changes in motor symptoms, which are also known to positively correlate to DA levels *(33)*. Furthermore, mood fluctuations can occur even in early disease when endogenous DA availability and stores are thought to be reasonably stable (albeit reduced) and may disappear as the duration and treatment of disease progresses *(33)*. Additional evidence suggesting a specific role for DA in mood modulation is the observation that mood worsens in many patients who experience motor fluctuations even when the baseline mood itself is not considered low *(34)*.

Despite the evidence of multiple monoamine abnormalities, no single neurotransmitter defect fully explains of the spectrum of symptoms seen in either primary depression or PD depression. The chemical markers identified to date must still be interpreted in the context of multiple receptor subtypes, second messenger effects, and the functional anatomical network in which they reside. With serotonin, brainstem neurons project diffusely throughout cortex with little anatomical specificity *(117)*. Depressive symptoms, on the other hand have been repeatedly localized to specific regions of frontal, cingulate, and basal ganglia in both primary and secondary depressions. Interestingly, regions of orbital frontal cortex with serotonin transporter and metabolite abnormalities show a reasonably selective pattern of efferent projections back to dorsal raphe, providing an important chemical–anatomical link *(16,103,105)*. Dopaminergic projections from the VTA also show regional specificity for the orbital frontal cortex, cingulate, and anterior striatal regions identified in both the postmortem and functional neuroimaging studies *(118–122)*. Serotonin–DA interactions within these regions would provide a potential explanation integrating many of these findings, a hypothesis supported by a single-photon emission computerized tomography (SPECT) study demonstrating D2-receptor changes in the striatum and anterior cingulate in primary depressed patients treated with serotonin re-uptake inhibitors *(123)*.

2.4. *Anatomical Mechanisms*

A fundamental role for limbic structures in the regulation of mood and emotional states is well established *(3,15,124)*. Correlations between these regions and pathways mediating reward, motivational, and affect behaviors in animals are well documented *(6,124–128)*, with comparative studies further delineating pathways linking various "limbic" structures with widely distributed brainstem, striatal, paralimbic, and frontal sites *(12,14,20,129,130)*. The basal ganglia, with its rich reciprocal connections between all of these regions, is positioned as a likely interface between internal personal drives (mood and motivation) and responses to external stimuli, possibly through limbic motor-visceromotor pathways *(131)*.

Despite the apparent strong link of limbic regions to emotional behaviors, morphometric studies using computed tomography (CT) and magnetic resonance imaging (MRI) in primary affective disorders have not shown consistent structural involvement. Hippocampal atrophy is the best-replicated finding, but it is not specific to depression *(132–134)*. MRI studies report reductions in basal ganglia volume (caudate and putamen) in unipolar (UP) depression as well as bipolar (BP) disease *(135–137)*. Focal volume loss in ventral and dorsal medial frontal cortex in UP and BP patients has also been described *(138–141)*. No findings are consistently seen across studies.

In neurological depressions, classical lesion–deficits studies have identified three main etiological categories: (*i*) discreet lesions, as seen with trauma, ablative surgery, tumors, and focal seizures (reviewed in ref. *142*); (*ii*) conditions of neurodegeneration within an anatomical context best typified by the basal ganglia disorders *(24,26,90)*; and (*iii*) diseases with generalized or randomly distributed pathologies, such as Alzheimer's disease and multiple sclerosis *(143–145)*. CT and MRI studies in lesion patients demonstrate a high association of mood changes, with infarctions of the frontal lobe and basal ganglia, particularly those involving the head of the caudate *(146,147)*. Studies of frontal lobe stroke, trauma, and tumor patients additionally suggest the dorsolateral frontal lesions are more commonly associated with depression and depressive symptoms, while impulsiveness, mood lability, and mania are seen with ventral frontal lesions *(9)*. Plaques located within of the frontal, cingulate, and temporal lobes also correlate with depression in multiple sclerosis *(148,149)*. Across a spectrum of diseases, the consistent involvement of corticolimbic-striatal structures provides a basis for hypothesis-driven investigations of the integrity of pathways linking these regions using functional imaging techniques.

3. FUNCTIONAL IMAGING STUDIES

Functional imaging, i.e., PET, SPECT, and function MRI (fMRI), can complement structural imaging in that the consequences of anatomic or chemical lesions on global and regional brain function (metabolism, blood flow, transmitter) can be directly assessed. This approach has been an important tool for identifying previously unrecognized brain abnormalities and potential disease mechanisms. These methods additionally provide strategies to test how similar mood symptoms occur with anatomically or neurochemically distinct disease states, as well as why comparable lesions do not always result in comparable behavioral phenomena. Parallel studies of primary affective disorder and patients with neurological depressions provide complementary perspectives *(150)*.

3.1. *Resting State Studies in Primary and Secondary Depression*

Resting state studies of regional glucose metabolism (fluorine-18 deoxyglucose [FDG]-PET) or blood flow (cerebral blood flow [CBF] PET/SPECT) have been performed contrasting depressed and nondepressed patients to healthy controls. The repeated observation from independent studies of depression with degenerative and focal basal ganglia diseases, including PD, HD, and stroke *(122,151–154)*, is common abnormalities of paralimbic regions (ventral frontal, cingulate, and anterior temporal cortex hypometabolism) concordant with anatomical lesion–behavior findings. PET and SPECT studies in primary depression show a similar pattern with common involvement of frontal and cingulate regions and less consistently temporal lobe and striatum. Frontal abnormalities in primary and secondary depression localize to two known pathways: a prefrontal-striatal-thalamic path *(12,19)* and a frontolimbic path linking orbital frontal and anterior temporal cortex via the uncinate fasiculus *(155–157)*. Disease-specific disruption at different sites along these paths might best explain the presence of similar depressive symptoms in patients with different disease pathologies.

Identification of common frontolimbic patterns across different disease diagnoses has provided new insights regarding the localization of the "depression syndrome," but has done little to distinguish subtle differences in symptom profiles. While studies have repeatedly shown that frontal hypometabolism is strongly correlated with depression severity, the relationship of frontal abnormalities to specific symptoms is less clear *(122,158)*. For instance, although apathy, psychomotor slowing, and depressed mood are strongly intercorrelated behaviorally in patients with major depression *(31, 159,160)*, they can also occur independently, suggesting they may not colocalize to the same brain regions. This is particularly true in PD where bradyphrenia, considered a pathognomonic feature of the illness, occurs commonly without apathy or depression *(161)*. Similarly, primary affective disorder and PD patients may both show evidence of mood lability, either alone or as part of a major depressive episode, also suggesting separate but functional interactive regions or pathways.

This concept is exemplified by examination of resting state patterns seen in FDG-PET scans of UP depressed, PD depressed, and BP depressed patients. In BP, like UP and PD depression, bilateral prefrontal hypometabolism is evident *(7,121,162)* (see Fig. 1). Unlike UP, bilateral hypermetabolism of the globus pallidus (GP) and anterior insula is also seen. When BP, UP, and PD depressions are further compared, comparable increases in GP are seen in BP and UP; whereas common insula findings are seen only in PD and UP. One interpretation of these findings relates to the variation in clinical symptoms across the three groups. UP and PD share many somatic features, which might be circumstantially attributed to their common insular metabolic pattern thought to localize to this part of cortex *(163)*. Mood lability, most characteristic of BP, can also be seen in PD, but generally not UP. This lability may be reflected by the GP overactivity seen selectively in BP and PD, which is one of the few clinical features shared by these two populations other than the depression symptoms themselves. Additional evidence linking depression, mood lability, and basal ganglia function is provided by case studies describing acute onset of depression and mania following focal lesions of GP and caudate *(164–166)*, as well as with subcortical deep brain stimulation (DBS) for treatment of PD *(67,68,167)* (see below and Fig. 2).

These resting state findings help to define what may be critical components of our postulated "mood regulatory network." However, the functional dynamics of this system cannot be ascertained with this type of study. Examination of regional changes associated with antidepressant treatment is one approach, using changes in specific symptoms as an index of changes in specific regions and pathways. An alternative method is to use specific activation paradigms, whereby basal mood state is transiently altered. This method can be used to establish regions critical to normal emotional processing and experience as well as to assess alterations in patient populations. Both of these approaches provide additional perspectives to understanding the requisite brain regions modulating mood and emotional behaviors under various state conditions.

3.2. Treatment Studies

Studies of resting state changes in regional metabolism or blood flow with recovery from a major depressive episode report normalization of many regional abnormalities identified in the pretreatment state. Changes in cortical (prefrontal, ventral prefrontal, parietal), limbic-paralimbic (cingulate, amyg-

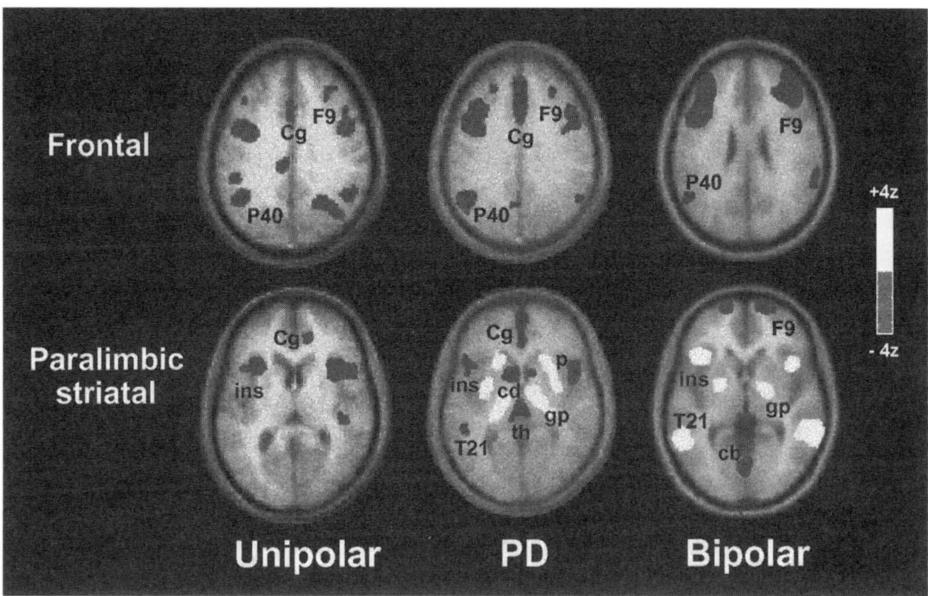

Fig. 1. Metabolic abnormalities in depression. FDG-PET studies in UP, PD, and BP. Axial slices at the level of frontal cortex and basal ganglia. black: areas of significant decreases in metabolism relative to controls; white: areas of significant increases in metabolism relative to controls. Bilateral prefrontal (F9) and parietal (P40) cortex, thalamus (thal) and anterior cingulate (Cg) hypometabolism is common to depressed patients with UP and BP and PD. Metabolic patterns in temporal (T21) and insular (ins) regions differentiate UP and PD from BP. Only PD and BP alone share hypermetabolism within the basal ganglia: putamen (p), caudate (cd), and globus pallidus (gp).

dala, insula, and subcortical [caudate–pallidum] areas have been described following various treatments, including medication, psychotherapy, sleep deprivation, electroconvulsive therapy (ECT), repetitive transcranial magnetic stimulation (rTMS), and ablative surgery. Normalization of frontal and anterior cingulate hypometabolism is the best-replicated finding *(168–172)*. Changes in limbic-paralimbic and subcortical regions are more variable and often involve changes that result in a new equilibrium state, which is distinct from the pattern of nondepressed healthy individuals *(171,173–176)*. Changes necessary for clinical recovery have not been determined, nor have clear distinctions been made between different modes of treatment.

A next step has been to consider differences associated with a good versus a poor response to a given treatment. Addressing this question, one study has reported distinct patterns of change at 1 wk and 6 wk of treatment with the serotonin re-uptake inhibitor fluoxetine, with the time course of metabolic changes reflecting the known temporal delay in clinical response *(171)*. Clinical improvement was associated with limbic-paralimbic and striatal decreases (subgenual cingulate, hippocampus, pallidum, insula) and brainstem and cortical increases (prefrontal, parietal, anterior–posterior cingulate). Failed response to fluoxetine was associated with a persistent 1-wk pattern (hippocampal and pallidal increases, posterior cingulate decreases) and absence of either subgenual cingulate or prefrontal changes. These findings suggest not only an interaction between limbic-paralimbic, striatal, and neocortical pathways, but also differences among patients in adaptation of specific target regions to chronic serotonergic modulation. Failure to induce the requisite adaptive changes was seen as a contributing cause of treatment nonresponse.

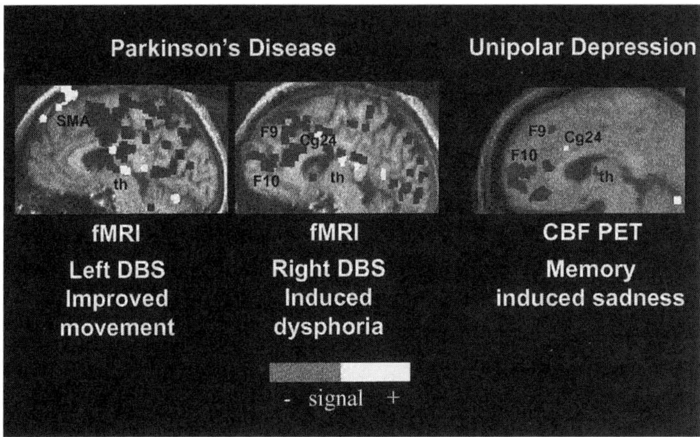

Fig. 2. Common medial frontal changes with transient sadness. fMRI and ^{15}O-water PET studies of transient dysphoria. Left and center images: fMRI study of a Parkinson's patient undergoing subthalamic DBS. Left-sided stimulation resulted in improvement in motor functioning and was associated with fMRI bold signal increases in striatum, thalamus (th), and primary motor cortex and a decrease in supplementary motor areas (SMA) (left image). Right-sided stimulation induced a transient dysphoric mood (center image) and decreases in medial frontal cortex (F10, 11) and increases in insula and anterior cingulate (Cg24) matching regional PET blood flow changes seen in mood induction in primary bipolar and unipolar patients (right image). Black: areas of fMRI or PET signal decrease; white: fMRI and PET increases.

In a new study of PD depression, in which patients were also treated for 6 wk with fluoxetine, comparable changes in dorsal cortical and ventral limbic-paralimbic regions have been identified *(177)*. Like UP depression, cortical increases (prefrontal and parietal) were seen in patients who responded to the treatment, and these increases resulted in the normalization of the pretreatment hypometabolic pattern. Clinical improvement was also associated with metabolic decreases in the subgenual cingulate and hippocampus, again identical to that seen in UP. These decreases were not found in PD patients who remained depressed, despite comparable treatment. In addition to these common changes, the PD depressed group showed a somewhat different pattern of changes in GP. While the change pattern again distinguished responders from nonresponders, the direction of change was the opposite of that seen in UP *(171)*. Decreased GP metabolism, with treatment, was seen in nonresponders, an effect not seen in responders who showed no difference pre- and posttreatment. This change pattern is of particular interest, as all PD depressed patients and all PD patients without depression show increased activity in this region at baseline. Whether these findings relate to a specific depression feature or reflect a disease-specific effect unique to PD is not yet clear. Given the other evidence, it is possible that these changes in the basal ganglia could relate to the presence of certain depressive features, possibly mood lability, and this remains a focus of ongoing studies.

3.3. Prognostic Markers

Published studies also demonstrate that pretreatment rostral (pregenual) cingulate metabolism may be useful in predicting response to pharmacotherapy *(7,178,179)*. Across published studies, hypermetabolism has been identified in eventual treatment responders; hypometabolism in nonresponders. A similar hypermetabolic pattern in a nearby region of the dorsal anterior cingulate has also been shown to predict good response to one night of sleep deprivation *(180)*. The involvement of rostral anterior cingulate is of particular significance, as this region has unique reciprocal connections, not only with the dorsal anterior cingulated, but also with other regions showing abnormalities in the depressed state (dorsal and ventral prefrontal, insula). The anterior cingulate is also implicated across configurations of direct and indirect frontal-striatal pathways *(12,19,21,181)*.

3.4. Behavioral Challenge Studies

Mood provocation studies offer a different perspective for examining the dynamics of these "functional networks," by use of acute changes in emotion rather than chronic changes in abnormally sustained mood states. These studies can define normal mood modulatory regions and pathways, as well as alternations in specific patient populations. Studies of recovered patients challenged with these types of emotional stress tests may help to explain abnormal mood modulation in patients who appear clinically well. A method to provoke emotional states in healthy populations has commonly employed recollection of past personal memories *(182–184)*. Pardo et al. *(185)* first described blood flow increases using PET in superior and inferior prefrontal cortex during spontaneous recollection of sad events. Subsequent studies using a variety of provocation methods identified additional changes involving insula, hypothalamus, cerebellum, amygdala, and basal ganglia studies *(10,186–191)*. Across studies, increases in midline limbic regions were most prominent. Frontal decreases reminiscent of resting state findings in clinically depressed patients have also been reported, but not consistently *(10,189–191)*. Timing of scans and the specific instructions appear to have a critical impact on both patterns and direction of regional changes.

One such study further examined the concordance of the localization of changes with transient normal sadness to resting-state abnormalities seen in depression and found that sadness mirrors changes associated with remission of depressive symptoms *(190)*. More specifically, shifts in negative mood states in both patients and healthy volunteers involve a nearly identical set of limbic (subgenual cingulate, anterior insula) and cortical (prefrontal, parietal, postcingulate) regions.

Other studies using this same paradigm of transient provoked sadness have been performed in recovered UP and BP depressed patients *(192,193)*. These studies have identified many areas of common change to those seen in healthy volunteers but also several interesting differences. In both UP and BP patients, sadness is associated with increases in GP, although to a greater degree in BP than UP. As previously discussed, increased activity is seen in this region in actively depressed BP patients at rest (without provocation), but not in depressed UP patients (see Fig. 1), suggesting that these regions may serve a critical role in acute mood shifts in affective disease, which is exaggerated even without provocation in BP patients. The GP change pattern seen with mood provocation would support the hypothesis that pallidal overactivity at rest may be a marker of instability or vulnerability in the mood regulatory system in certain clinical populations, in keeping with the phenomenology of symptoms seen in these groups.

4. FRONTAL-LIMBIC-STRIATAL DYSREGULATION: A WORKING MODEL OF DEPRESSION

The converging findings presented in this chapter have been formulated into a working model of depression and mood regulation involving cortical-limbic and frontal-striatal pathways (Fig. 3) *(7,194)*.

Brain regions with known anatomical interconnections that also show consistent and synchronized changes using PET in various behavioral states, transient sadness, baseline depressed, pre- and posttreatment (as described in previous sections of this chapter), have been grouped into two general compartments: dorsal cortical and ventral limbic. This dorsal-ventral segregation additionally defines those brain regions in which an inverse relationship is seen across experiments.

The dorsal-cortical compartment includes primarily neocortical elements and is postulated to mediate cognitive aspects of negative emotion such as apathy, psychomotor slowing, and impaired attention and executive function, based on complementary structural and functional lesion-deficit correlational studies *(122,195–198)*, symptom-specific treatment effects in depressed patients *(169,171,199)*, activation

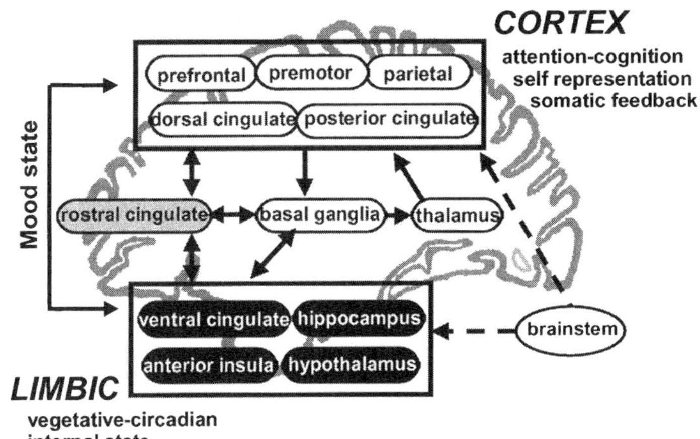

Fig. 3. Working model of depression. Regions with known anatomical interconnections that also show synchronized changes using PET in 3 behavioral states—normal transient sadness (controls), baseline depressed (patients), and posttreatment (patients)—form the basis of this schematic. Regions are grouped into 2 main compartments, cortical and limbic, both with known connections to subcortical targets, as delineated. The frontal-limbic (dorsal-ventral) segregation additionally identifies those brain regions where an inverse relationship is seen across the different PET paradigms. Sadness and depressive illness are both associated with decreases in dorsal neocortical regions (mainly prefrontal) and relative increases in ventral limbic areas (subgenual cingulate). The model, in turn, proposes that illness remission occurs when there is inhibition of the overactive limbic regions and activation of the previously hypofunctioning cortical areas (solid black arrows); an effect facilitated by various forms of treatment (dotted lines). Adapted from refs. *7* and *193*.

studies designed to explicitly map these behaviors in healthy volunteers *(190,191,200,201)*, and connectivity patterns in primates *(13,125,202–204)*.

The ventral-limbic compartment is composed predominantly of limbic and paralimbic regions known to mediate circadian, somatic, and vegetative aspects of depression, including sleep, appetite, libidinal, and endocrine disturbances, based on clinical and related animal studies *(6,129,163,205)*.

The rostral cingulate (rCg24a) is isolated from both the ventral and dorsal compartments based on its cytoarchitectural characteristics and reciprocal connections to both dorsal and ventral anterior cingulate *(130,206)*. Contributing to this position in the model are the observations that metabolism in this region uniquely predicts antidepressant response *(177,207)* and is also the principal site of aberrant response during mood induction in remitted depressed patients *(192)*. These anatomical and clinical distinctions suggest that the rostral anterior cingulate may serve an important regulatory role in the overall network by facilitating the interactions between the dorsal and ventral compartments *(208–210)*.

While there is no question that the model requires additional details, particularly regarding the contribution of specific frontal lobe and basal ganglia subregions, it provides a working platform to consider other behavioral elements relevant to depression, emotional processing, and the ongoing regulation of mood states.

4.1. *Testing the Model*

Final examples demonstrating the critical role of striatal regions in the modulation of mood and emotions is taken from the neurosurgical literature. Treatment of refractory depression has successfully utilized an approach whereby cingulotomy and/or subcaudate tractotomy is performed resulting in focal disruption of pathways linking frontal cortex to basal ganglia. Unfortunately, there is little data as to which pathways have been disrupted or the mechanisms by which these lesions impact functionality *(173,211)*. These deficiencies have been somewhat addressed in studies of subcortical DBS in the surgical treatment of PD, where PET and fMRI studies have been performed *(167,212, 214)*. Of specific relevance to the issues raised in this chapter is the growing number of cases of iatrogenic mood symptoms induced by DBS. Reports describe a spectrum of emotional changes from depression to mania and include stimulation of subthalamic nucleus, GP, and substantia nigra *(67,68)*.

We have studied a case of DBS stimulation in the region of the subthalamic nucleus (STN) that induced a transient temporally-concordant dysphoric mood in a woman with PD and a past history of major depression, in remission at the time of the implantation *(167)*. During initial programming, bilateral high frequency stimulation improved motor symptoms. Unexpectedly, right stimulation alone elicited several reproducible episodes of acute dysphoria accompanied by a constellation of unpleasant visceral sensations and negative feelings and memories, reminiscent of her previous experiences with depression. fMRI was performed during sequential individual electrode stimulation to map regions mediating these acute and transient behavior changes. Ipsilateral increases were seen in motor regions for right- and left-sided stimulation in a pattern previously reporting using PET *(212–214)* and paralleling contralateral motor improvement. Unique to right-sided stimulation with onset of mood symptoms were unique increases in anterior cingulate and anterior insula, as well as widespread decreases, in medial prefrontal cortex. Four weeks later, the mood disturbance had spontaneously resolved despite identical stimulation parameters. These medial frontal decreases and anterior cingulate increases correspond almost exactly to PET blood flow changes seen in mood induction experiments in both BP and UP remitted patients described above· *(192,193)* (see Fig. 2). They also correspond to the pattern of remote metabolic changes seen with subcortical infractions associated with a variety of cognitive and behavioral manifestations *(122,215,216)*.

This case study, considered in the context of other findings presented in this chapter, would suggest that the neural pathways mediating emotion have important sites of convergence within the basal ganglia. We hypothesize that as basal ganglia circuitry becomes disrupted with neurodegeneration in PD (possibly at the level of the GP), emotional control, and not just motor control, is affected. Striatal dysfunction in this setting would potentially impair emotional responses to external cognitive or affective stressors resulting in inappropriate or exaggerated behavior, which may manifest clinically as either mood lability or depression, an effect brought out in our patient with direct stimulation of this circuit. The extent to which electrode site and stimulation parameters contribute to these transient psychiatric symptoms with DBS requires careful further study. Likewise, studies are needed to determine to what extent individual patient factors, such as genetics *(104)*, personality *(217,218)*, or co-morbid psychiatric diagnoses, influence network functioning under baseline and stress conditions. Future studies will better define these dynamic functional–anatomical relationships between basal ganglia regions, mood lability, depression, and other behaviors in PD with clinical potential to enhance awareness and minimize potential risks and morbidity associated with PD and its treatments.

ACKNOWLEDGMENTS

We thank our collaborators, Stephen Brannan, Rob Mahurin, Diane Solomon, Mario Liotti, at the Research Imaging Center, and Anthony Lang, Jean Saint-Cyr, Peter Pahapill, David Mikulis, Andreas Lozano, and Stephanie Krueger at the University of Toronto for their significant contributions to the research discussed in this chapter. This work was support by National Institutes of Mental Health MH495533, the National Alliance for Research on Schizophrenia and Depression (NARSAD), the Charles A. Dana Foundation, The Sandra A. Rotman Program in Neuropsychiatry, and the Parkinson's Society of Canada.

REFERENCES

1. Heller, W., Nitschke, J.B., Elienne, M., and Miller, G. (1997) Patterns of regional brain activity differentiating types of anxiety. *J. Abnorm. Psychol.* **106,** 376–385.
2. Davidson, R. (2001) Toward a biology of personality and emotion. *Ann. NY Acad. Sci.* **935,** 191–207.
3. Damasio, A.R. (1994) *Descartes' Error*, GP Putnam's Sons, New York.
4. Lang, P.J. (1994) The varieties of emotional experience: a meditation on James-Lange theory. *Psychol. Rev.* **101,** 211–221.
5. Rolls, E.T. (1990) A theory of emotion, and its application to understanding the neural basis of emotion. *Cogn. Emotion* **4,** 161–190.
6. Maclean, P.D. (1990) *The Triune Brain in Evolution: Role in Paleocerebral Function*, Plenum, New York.
7. Mayberg, H.S. (1997) Limbic-cortical dysregulation: a proposed model of depression, in *The Neuropsychiatry of Limbic and Subcortical Disorders* (Salloway, S., Malloy, P., and Cummings, J.L., eds.), American Psychiatric Press, Washington, D.C., pp. 167–177.
8. Drevets, W.C. (2001) Neuroimaging and neuropsychological studies of depression: implication for the cognitive-emotional features of mood disorders. *Curr. Opin. Neurobiol.* **11,** 240–249.
9. Cummings, J.L. (1993) Frontal-subcortical circuits and human behavior. *Arch. Neurol.* **50,** 873–880.
10. Damasio, A.R., Grabowski, T.J., Bechara, A., et al. (2000) Subcortical and cortical brain activity during the feeling of self-generated emotions. *Nat. Neurosci.* **3,** 1049–1056.
11. Saxena, S., Brody, A., Schwartz, J., and Baxter, L. (1998) Neuroimaging and frontal-subcortical circuitry in obessive-compulsive disorder. *Br. J. Psychiatry* **35(Suppl.),** 26–37.
12. Alexander, G.E., Crutcher, M.D., and De Long, M.R. (1990) Basal ganglia-thalamocortical circuits: parallel substrates for motor, oculomotor, 'prefrontal' and 'limbic' functions. *Prog. Brain Res.* **85,** 119–146.
13. Carmichael, S.T. and Price, J.L. (1995) Limbic connections of the orbital and medial prefrontal cortex in macaque monkeys. *J. Comp. Neurol.* **363,** 615–641.
14. Carmichael, S.T. and Price, J.L. (1996) Connectional networks within the orbital and medial prefrontal cortex of macaque monkeys. *J. Comp. Neurol.* **371,** 179–207.
15. Mesulam, M.M. (1990) Large-scale neurocognitive networks and distributed processing for attention, language, and memory. *Ann. Neurol.* **28,** 597–613.
16. Nauta, W.J.H. (1986) Circuitous connections linking cerbral cortex, limbic system, and corpus striatum, in *The Limbic System: Functional Organization and Clinical Disorders* (Doane, R.K. and Livingston, K.E., eds.), Raven, New York, pp. 43–54.
17. Lang, P.J., Bradley, M.M., and Cuthbert, B.N. (1998) Emotion, motivation and anxiety: brain mechanisms and psychobiology. *Biol. Psychiatry* **44,** 1248–1263.
18. Garcia-Cairasco, N., Miguell, E., Rauch, S.L., and Leckman, J. (1997) Current controversies and future direction in basal ganglia research. Investigating basic neuroscience and clinical investigations. *Psychiatry Clin. N. Am.* **20,** 945–962.
19. Haber, S.N., Fudge, J.L., and McFarland, N.R. (2000) Striatonigrostriatal pathways in primates form an ascending spiral from the shell to the dorsolateral striatum. *J. Neurosci.* **20,** 2369–2382.
20. Graybiel, A. (1995) Building action repetoiries: memory and learning functions of the basal ganglia. *Curr. Opin. Neurobiol.* **5,** 733–741.
21. Kimura, M. and Graybiel, A. (1995) Role of basal ganglia in sensorimotor association learning, in *Functions of the Cortico-Basal Ganglia Loop* (Kimura, M. and Graybiel, A. M., eds.), Springer Verlag, New York, pp. 2–17.
22. Louilot, A., Taghzouti, K., Simon, H., and Le Moal, M. (1989) Limbic system, basal ganglia, and dopaminergic neurons. Executive and regulatory neurons and their role in the organization of behavior. *Brain Behav. Evol.* **33,** 157–161.
23. Schultz, W., Tremblay, L., and Hollerman, J.R. (2000) Reward processing in primate orbitofrontal cortex and basal ganglia. *Cerebral Cotex* **10,** 272–283.
24. Ghika, J. (2000) Mood and behavior in disorders of the basal ganglia, in *Behavior and Mood Disorders in Focal Brain Lesions* (Bogousslavsky, J. and Cummings, J.L., eds.), Cambridge University Press, Cambridge, pp. 122–201.
25. Robinson, R.G., Kubos, K.L., Starr, L.B., Rao, K., and Price, T.R. (1984) Mood disorders in stroke patients. Importance of location of lesion. *Brain* **107,** 81–93.
26. Cummings, J.L. (1992) Depression and Parkinson's disease: a review [see comments]. *Am. J. Psychiatry* **149,** 443–454.
27. Huber, S.J., Friedenberg, D.L., Paulson, G.W., and Shuttlesworth, F.C. (1990) The pattern of depressive symptoms varies with progression of Parkinson's disease. *J. Neurol. Neurosurg. Psychiatry* **53,** 275–278.
28. Aarsland, D., Larsen, J.P., Lim, N. G., et al. (1999) Range of neuropsychiatric disturbances in patients with Parkinson's disease. *J. Neurol. Neurosurg. Psychiatry* **67,** 492–496.
29. Fleminger, S. (1991) Left-sided Parkinson's disease has a greater incidence of anxiety and depression. *Psycholog. Med.* **21,** 629–638.
30. Fenelon, G., Mahieux, F., Huon, R., and Ziegler, M. (2000) Hallucinations in Parkinson's disease: prevalence, phenomenology and risk factors. *Brain* **123,** 733–745.
31. Starkstein, S.E., Mayberg, H.S., Preziosi, T.J., Andrezejewski, P., Leiguarda, R., and Robinson, R.G. (1992) Reliability, validity, and clinical correlates of apathy in Parkinson's disease. *J. Neuropsychiatry Clin. Neurosci.* **4,** 134–139.

32. Hardie, R., Less, A., and Stern, G. (1984) On-off fluctuations in Parkinson's disease: a clinical and enuropharmacological study. *Brain* **17,** 899–904.
33. Nissenbaum, H., Quinn, N., Brown, R.G., et al. (1987) Mood swings associated with the on-off phenomenon in Parkinson's disease. *Psychol. Med.* **17,** 899–904.
34. Lees, A.J. (1989) The on-off phenomenon. *J. Neurol. Neurosurg. Psychiatry* **52(Suppl.),** 29–37.
35. Juncos, J. (1999) Management of psychotic aspects of Parkinson's disease. *J. Clin. Psychiatry* **60(Suppl. 8),** 42–53.
36. Cummings, J.L. and Masterman, D.L. (1999) Depression in patients with Parkinson's disease. *Int. J. Geriatr. Psychiatry* **14,** 711–718.
37. Zesiewicz, T.A., Gold, M., Chari, G., and Hauser, R.A. (1999) Current issues in depression in Parkinson's disease. *Am. J. Geriatr. Psychiatry* **7,** 110–118.
38. Aarsland, D., Larsen, J.P., Cummins, J.L., and Laake, K. (1999) Prevalence and clinical correlates of psychotic symptoms in Parkinson disease: a community-based study. *Arch. Neurol.* **56,** 595–601.
39. Menza, M.A., Robertson-Hoffman, D.E., and Bonaspace, A.S. (1993) Parkinson's disease and anxiety: comorbidity with depression. *Biol. Psychiatry* **34,** 465–470.
40. Hollander, E., Cohen, I., Richards, M., Mullen, L., DeCaria, C., and Stern, Y. (1993) A pilot study of the neuropsychological obsessive-compulsive disorder and Parkinson's disease: basal ganglia disorders. *J. Neuropsychiatry Clin. Neurosci.* **5,** 104–107.
41. Richard, I.H., Schiffer, R., and Kurlan, R. (1996) Anxiety and Parkinson's disease. *J. Neuropsychiatry Clin. Neurosci.* **8,** 383–392.
42. Brown, R.G. and MacCarthy, B. (1990) Psychiatric morbidity in patients with Parkinson's disease. *Psychol. Med.* **20,** 383–392.
43. Starkstein, S.E., Preziosi, T.J., Forrester, A.W., and Robinson, R.G. (1990) Specificity of affective and autonomic symptoms of depression in Parkinson's disease. *J. Neurol. Neurosurg. Psychiatry* **53,** 869–873.
44. Tandberg, E., Larsen, J.P., Aarsland, D., Laake, K., and Cummings, J.L. (1997) Risk factors for depression in Parkinson's disease. *Arch. Neurol.* **54,** 625–630.
45. Santamaria, J., Tolosa, E., and Valles, A. (1986) Parkinson's disease with depression: a possible subgroup of idiopathic parkinsonism. *Neurology* **36,** 1130–1133.
46. Brown, R.G. and Jahanshahi, M. (1995) Depression in Parkinson's disease: a psychosocial viewpoint. *Adv. Neurol.* **65,** 61–84.
47. Shifren, K. (1996) Individual differences in the perception of optimism and disease severity: a study among individuals with Parkinson's disease. *J. Behav. Med.* **19,** 241–271.
48. Ehmann, T.S., Benniger, R.J., Gawel, M.J., and Riopelle, R.J. (1990) Depressive symptoms in Parkinson's disease: a comparison with control subjects. *J. Geriatr. Psych. Neurol.* **2,** 3–9.
49. Starkstein, S.E., Preziosi, T.J., Bolduc, P.L., and Robinson, R.G. (1990) Depression in Parkinson's disease. *J. Nerv. Ment. Dis.* **178,** 27–31.
50. Celesia, C.G. and Wannamaker, W.M. (1972) Psychiatric disturbances in Parkinson's disease. *Dis. Nerv. Syst.* **33,** 577–583.
51. Shiba, M., Bower, J.H., Maraganore, D.M., et al. (2000) Anxiety disorders and depressive disorders preceding Parkinson's disease: a case-control study. *Mov. Disord.* **15,** 669–677.
52. Brown, F.W., Golding, J.M., and Smith, G.R. Jr. (1990) Psychiatric comorbidity in primary care somatization disorder. *Psychosom. Med.* **52,** 445–451.
53. Lauterbach, E.C. and Duvoisin, R.C. (1991) Anxiety disorders in familial parkinsonism. *Am. J. Psychiatry* **148,** 274.
54. Standaert, D.G. and Stern, M.B. (1993) Updates on the management of Parkinson's disease. *Med. Clin. North Am.* **77,** 169–183.
55. Larmande, P., Palisson, E., Saikali, I., et al. (1993) Disparition de l'akinesies dans une maladia de Parkinson au cours d'un acces manigue. *Rev. Neurol.* **149,** 557–578.
56. Caligiuri, M.P. and Ellwanger, J. (2000) Motor and cognitive aspects of motor retardation in depression. *J. Affect. Disord.* **57,** 83–93.
57. Sobin, C., Mayer, L., and Eudicott, J. (1998) The motor agitation and retardation scale: a scale for the assessment of motor abnormalities in depressed patients. *J. Neuropsychiatry Clin. Neurosci.* **10,** 85–92.
58. Gill, H.S., Devane, L.C., and Risch, S.C. (1997) Extrapyramidal symptoms associated with cyclic antidepressant treatment: a review of the literature and consolidating hypothesis. *J. Clin. Psychopharmacol.* **17,** 377–389.
59. Dantchev, N. and Widlocher, D.J. (1998) The measurement of retardation in depression. *J. Clin. Psychiatry* **59(Suppl. 14),** 19–25.
60. Wolfe, J., Granholm, E., Butters, N., Saunders, E., and Janowsky, D. (1987) Verbal memory deficits associated with major affective disorders: a comparison of unipolar and bipolar patients. *J. Affect. Disord.* **13,** 83–92.
61. Rogers, M., Bradshaw, J., Phillips, J., et al. (2000) Parkinsonian motor characteristics in unipolar major depression. *J. Clin. Exp. Neuropsychol.* **22,** 232–244.
62. Richard, I.H., Justus, A.W., and Kurlan, R. (2001) Relationship between mood and motor fluctuations in Parkinson's disease. *J. Neuropsychiatry* **13,** 35–41.
63. Maricle, R.A., Nutt, J.G., and Carter, J.H. (1995) Mood and anxiety fluctuation in Parkinson's disease associated with levodopa infusion: preliminary findings. *Mov. Disord.* **10,** 329–332.
64. Saint-Cyr, J.A., Taylor, A.E., and Lang, A.E. (1993) Neuropsychological and psychiatric side effects in the treatment of Parkinson's disease. *Neurology* **43(12 Suppl. 6),** S47–S52.

65. Maricle, R., Nutt, J., Valentine, R., et al. (1995) Dose-response relationship of levodopa with mood and anxiety in fluctuating Parkinson's disease: a double-blind, placebo-controlled study. *Neurology* **45,** 1757–1760.
66. Menza, M., Sage, J., and Marshall, E. (1990) Mood changes and on-off phenomena in Parkinson's disease. *Mov. Disord.* **5,** 148–151.
67. Bejjani, B.P., Damier, P., Arnulf, I., et al. (1999) Transient acute depression induced by high-frequency deep-brain stimulation. *N. Engl. J. Med.* **340,** 1476–1480.
68. Miyawaki, E., Perlmutter, J.S., Troster, A.I., Videen, T.O., and Koller, W.C. (2000) The behavioral complication of pallidal stimulation: a case report. *Brain Cogn.* **42,** 417–434.
69. Trepanier, L.L., Kumar, R., Lozano, A.M., Lang, A.E., and Saint-Cyr, J.A. (2000) Neuropsychological outcome of GPi pallidotomy and GPi or STN deep brain stimulation in Parkinson's disease. *Brain Cogn.* **42,** 324–347.
70. Saint-Cyr, J.A., Trepanier, L.L., Kumar, R., Lozano, A.M., and Lang, A.E. (2000) Neurospychological consequences of chronic bilateral stimulation of subthalamic nucleus in Parkinson's disease. *Brain* **123,** 2091–2108.
71. Ardouin, C., Pillon, B., Peiffer, E., et al. (1999) Bilateral subthalamic or pallidal stimulation for Parkinson's disease affects neither memory nor executive functions: a consecutive series of 62 patients. *Ann. Neurol.* **46,** 217–223.
72. Mohr, E., Juncos, J., Cox, C., Litvan, I., Feido, P., and Chase, T.N. (1990) Selective deficits in cognition and memory in high functioning Parkinsonian patients. *J. Neurol. Neurosurg. Psychiatry* **53,** 603–606.
73. Zalla, T., Sirigu, A., Pillon, B., Dubois, B., Agid, Y., and Grafman, J. (2000) How patients with Parkinson's disease retrieve and manage cognitive events knowledge. *Cortex* **36,** 163–179.
74. Gauntlett-Gilbert, J., Roberts, R.C., and Brown, V.J. (1999) Mechanisms underlying attentional set-shifting in Parkinson's disease. *Neuropsychologia* **37,** 817–828.
75. Brown, R.G., Scott, L.C., Bench, C.J., and Dolan, R.J. (1994) Cognitive function in depression: its relationship to the presence and severity of intellectual decline. *Psychol. Med.* **24,** 829–847.
76. Flint, A.J., Black, S.E., Campbell-Taylor, I., Gailey, G.F., and Levinton, C. (1993) Abnormal speech articulation, psychomotor retardation, and subcortical dysfunction in major depression [see comments]. *J. Psychiatr. Res.* **27,** 309–319.
77. Calev, A., Korin, Y., Shapira, B., Kugelmass, S., and Lerer, B. (1986) Verbal and non-verbal recall by depressed and euthymic affective patients. *Psychol. Med.* **16,** 789–794.
78. Mayeux, R., Stern, Y., Rosen, J., and Leventhal, J. (1981) Depression, intellectual impairment, and Parkinson disease. *Neurology* **31,** 645–650.
79. Cooper, J.A., Sagar, H.J., Doherty, S.M., Jordan, N., Tidswell, P., and Sullivan, E.V. (1992) Different effects of dopaminergic and anticholinergic therapies on cognitive and motor function in Parkinson's disease. A follow-up study of untreated patients. *Brain* **115,** 1701–1725.
80. Ivory, S.J., Knight, R.G., Longmore, B.E., and Caradoc-Davies, T. (1999) Verbal memory in non-demented patients with idiopathic Parkinson's disease. *Neuropsychologia* **37,** 817–828.
81. Swainson, R., Rogers, R.D., Sahakian, B.J., Summers, B.A., Polkey, L.E., and Robbins, T.W. (2000) Probabilistic learning and reversal deficits in patients with Parkinson's disease or frontal or temporal lobe lesions: possible adverse effects of dopaminergic medication. *Neuropsychologia* **38,** 596–612.
82. Sagar, H.J. (1999) Clinicopathological heterogeneity and non-dopaminergic influences on behavior in Parkinson's disease. *Adv. Neurol.* **80,** 409–417.
83. Hu, M.T., Taylor-Robinson, S.D., Chaudhuri, K.R., et al. (2000) Cortical dysfunction in non-demented Parkinson's disease patients: a combined (31)P-MRS and (18)FDG-PET study. *Brain* **123,** 340–352.
84. Young, G. and McGlone, J. (1995) Cerebral localization, in *Clinical Neurology* (revised) Vol. 1 (Yoynt, R., ed.), Lippincott-Raven, Philadelphia, pp. 1–97.
85. Starkstein, S.E., Rabins, P.V., Berthier, M.L., Cohen, B.J., Folstein, M.F., and Robinson, R.G. (1989) Dementia of depression among patients with neurological disorders and functional depression. *J. Neuropsychiatry Clin. Neurosci.* **1,** 263–268.
86. Serra-Mestres, J. and Ring, H.A. (1999) Vulnerability to emotional negative stimuli in Parkinson's disease: an investigation using emotional stroop task. *Neuropsychiatry Neuropsychol. Behav. Neurol.* **12,** 52–57.
87. Willliams, J.M., Mathew, A., and Macleod, C. (1996) The emotional stroop task and psychopathology. *Psychol. Bull.* **120,** 3–24.
88. Moss, K., Bralley, B.P., Williams, R., and Matthewes, A. (1993) Subliminal processing of emotional information in anxiety and depression. *J. Abnorm. Psychol.* **102,** 304–311.
89. Graeff, F.G., Guimaraes, F.S., DeAndrade, T.G., and Deakin, J.F. (1996) Role of 5-HT in stress, anxiety, and depression. *Pharmacol. Biochem. Behav.* **54,** 129–141.
90. Mayberg, H.S. and Solomon, D.H. (1995) Depression in Parkinson's disease: a biochemical and organic viewpoint. *Adv. Neurol.* **65,** 49–60.
91. Schildkraut, J.J. (1965) The catecholamine hypothesis of affective disorders: a review of supporting evidence. *Am. J. Psychiatry* **122,** 509–522.
92. Maas, J.W., Fawcett, J.A., and Dekirmenjian, H. (1972) Catecholamine metabolism, depressive illness and drug response. *Arch. Gen. Psychiatry* **26,** 252–262.
93. Miyawaki, E., Meah, Y., and Koller, W.C. (1997) Serotonin, dopamine and motor effects in Parkinson's disease. *Clin. Neuropharmacol.* **20,** 300–310.
94. Haapaniemi, T., Ahonen, A., Torniaimen, P., Santaniemi, K., and Myllyla, V. (2001) [^{123}I] *B*-CIT SPECT demonstrates decreased brain dopamine and serotonin transporter level in untreated parkinsonian patients. *Mov. Disord.* **16,** 124–130.

95. Mayberg, H.S., Ross, C.A., Dannals, R.F., Wilson, A.A., Ravert, H.T., and Frost, J.J. (1991) Elevated mu opiate receptors measured by PET in patients with depression. *J. Cereb. Blood Flow Metab.* **11,** 821.
96. Drevets, W.C., Frank, E., Price, J.C., et al. (1999) PET imaging of serotonin 1A receptor binding in depression. *Biol. Psychiatry* **46,** 1375–1387.
97. Arango, V., Ernsberger, P., Marzuk, P. M., et al. (1990) Autoradiographic demonstration of increased serotonin 5-HT2 and b-adrenergic receptor binding sites in the brain of suicide victims. *Arch. Gen. Psychiatry* **47,** 1038–1047.
98. Arango, V., Underwood, M.D., Bakalian, M.J., et al. (1999) Reduction in serotonin transporter sites in prefrontal cortex is localized in suicide and widespread in major depression. *Soc. Neurosci. Abstr.* **25,** 1798.
99. Kostic, V.S., Dijuric, B.M., Covickovic-Sternic, N., Bumbasirevic, L., Nicolic, M., and Mrsulja, B.B. (1987) Depression and Parkinson's disease: possible role of serotonergic mechanism. *J. Neurol.* **234,** 94–96.
100. Koslow, S.H., Maas, J.W., Bowden, C.L., Davis, J.M., Hanin, I., and Javaid, J. (1983) CSF and urinary biogenic amines and metabolites in depression and mania. A controlled, univariate analysis. *Arch. Gen. Psychiatry* **40,** 999–1010.
101. Caldecott-Hazard, S., Morgan, D.G., DeLeon-Jones, F., Overstreet, D.H., and Janowsky, D. (1991) Clinical and biochemical aspects of depressive disorders: II. Transmitter/receptor theories. *Synapse* **9,** 251–301.
102. Paulus, W. and Jellinger, K. (1991) The neuropathological basis of different clinical subgroups of Parkinson's disease. *J. Neuropath. Exp. Neurol.* **50,** 743–755.
103. Mann, J.J., Huang, Y.Y., Underwood, M.D., et al. (2000) A serotonin transporter gene promoter polymorphism (5-HTTLPR) and prefrontal cortical binding in major depression and suicide. *Arch. Gen. Psychiatry* **57,** 729–738.
104. Menza, M.A., Palermo, B., DiPaola, R., Sage, J., and Ricketts, M. (1999) Depression and anxiety in Parkinson's disease: possible effect of genetic variation in the serotonin transporter. *J. Geriatr. Psych. Neurol.* **12,** 49–52.
105. Owens, M.J. and Nemeroff, U.B. (1994) Role of serotonin in the pathophysiology of depression: focus on the serotonin transport. *Clin. Chem.* **40,** 288–295.
106. Wilner, P. (1993) Dopamine and depression. *J. Neural. Trans. Gen. Sect.* **91,** 75–109.
107. Mann, J.J. and Kapur, S. (1995) A dopaminergic hypothesis of major depression. *Clin. Neuropharmacol.* **18(Suppl. 1),** S57–S65.
108. Lambert, G., Johansson, M., Agren, K., and Friberg, P. (2000) Reduced brain norepinephrine and dopamine release in treatment-refractory depressive illness. *Arch. Gen. Psychiatry* **57,** 787–793.
109. Martinot, M.-L.P., Bragulat, V., Artiges, E., et al. (2001) Decreased presynaptic dopaminate function in the left caudate of depressed patients with affective flattening and psychomotor retardation. *Am. J. Psychatry* **158,** 314–316.
110. Martin, W.R., Sloan, J.W., Sapira, J.D., and Jasinski, D.R. (1971) Physiologic, subjective, and behavioral effects of amphetamine, methamphetamine, ephedrine, phenmetrazine, and methylphenidate in man. *Clin. Pharmacol. Ther.* **12,** 245–258.
111. Fibiger, H.C. (1984) The neurobiological substrates of depression in Parkinson's disease: a hypothesis. *Can. J. Neurol. Sci.* **11(1 Suppl.),** 105–107.
112. Marsh, C.G. and Markham, C.H. (1973) Does levodopa alter depression and psychopathology in Parkinson's patients? *J. Neurol. Neurosurg. Psychiatry* **36,** 925–935.
113. Armin, S., Andreas, H., Hermann, W., Eckard, K., Wolfgang, G., and Otto, B. (1997) Pramipexole, a dopamine agonist, in major depression: antidepressant effects and tolerability in an open-label study with multiple doses. *Clin. Neuropharmacol.* **20(Suppl. 1),** S36–S45.
114. Torack, R.M. and Morris, J.C. (1988) The association of ventral tegmental area histopathology with adult dementia. *Arch. Neurol.* **45,** 497–501.
115. Nissenbaum, H., Quinn, N.P., Brown, R.G., Toone, B., Gotham, A.M., and Marsden, C.D. (1987) Mood swings associated with the "on-off" phenomenon in Parkinson's disease. *Psychol. Med.* **17,** 899–904.
116. Kulisevsky, J., Avila, A., Barbanoj, M., Antonijoan, R., Berthier, M.L., and Gironell, A. (1996) Acute effects of levodopa on neuropsychological performance in stable and fluctuating Parkinson's disease patients at different levodopa plasma levels. *Brain* **119,** 2121–2132.
117. Azmitia, E.C. and Gannon, P.J. (1986) The primate serotonergic system: a review of human and animal studies and a report on Macaca fascicularis, in *Advances in Neurology,* vol. 43 (Fahn, S., ed.), Raven, New York, pp. 407–468.
118. Glowinski, J., Tassin, J., and Thierry, A. (1984) The meso-cortico-prefrontal dopaminergic neurons. *TINS* **7,** 415–418.
119. Nauta, W. and Domesick, V. (1984) Afferent and efferent relationships of the basal ganglia, in *Functions of the Basal Ganglia* (O'Conner, M. and Evered, D., eds.), Pitman, London, pp. 3–29.
120. Simon, H., LeMoal, M., and Calas, A. (1979) Efferents and afferents of the ventral tegmental-A10 region studied after local injection of {3H}-leucine and horseradish peroxidase. *Brain Res.* **178,** 17–40.
121. Mayberg, H.S., Starkstein, S.E., Sadzot, B., et al. (1990) Selective hypometabolism in the inferior frontal lobe in depressed patients with Parkinson's disease. *Ann. Neurol.* **28,** 57–64.
122. Mayberg, H.S., Lewis, P.J., Regenold, W., and Wagner, H.N. Jr. (1994) Paralimbic hypoperfusion in unipolar depression. *J. Nucl. Med.* **35,** 929–934.
123. Larisch, R., Klimke, A., Vosberg, H., Loffler, S., Gaebel, W., and Muller-Gartner, H. W. (1997) In vivo evidence for the involvement of dopamine-D2 receptors in striatum and anterior cingulate gyrus in major depression. *Neuroimage* **5,** 251–260.
124. LeDoux, J.E. (1996) In search of an emotional system in the brain: leaping from fear to emotion and consciousness, in *The Cognitive Neurosciences* (Gazzaniga, M.S., ed.), MIT Press, Cambridge, MA, pp. 1049–1061.
125. Barbas, H. (1995) Anatomic basis of cognitive-emotional interactions in the primate prefrontal cortex. *Neurosci. Biobehav. Rev.* **19,** 499–510.

126. Dias, R., Robbins, T.W., and Roberts, A.C. (1996) Dissociation in prefrontal cortex of affective and attentional shifts. *Nature* **380,** 69–72.
127. Rolls, E.T. (1996) The orbitofrontal cortex. *Philos. Trans. R. Soc. Lond. B Biol. Sci.* **351,** 1433–1444.
128. Tremblay, L. and Schultz, W. (1999) Relative reward preference in primate orbitofrontal cortex [see comments]. *Nature* **398,** 704–708.
129. Mesulam, M.M. and Mufson, E.J. (1992) Insula of the old world monkey I, II, III. *J. Comp. Neurol.* **212,** 1–52.
130. Vogt, B.A. and Pandya, D.N. (1987) Cingulate cortex of the rhesus monkey: II. Cortical afferents. *J. Comp. Neurol.* **262,** 271–289.
131. Holstege, G. (1992) The emotional motor system. *Eur. J. Morphol.* **30,** 67–79.
132. Sheline, Y.I., Wang, P.W., Gado, M.H., Csernansky, J.G., and Vannier, M.W. (1996) Hippocampal atrophy in recurrent major depression. *Proc. Natl. Acad. Sci. USA* **93,** 3908–3913.
133. Sheline, Y.I. (2000) 3D MRI studies of neuroanatomic changes in unipolar major depression: the role of stress and medical comorbidity. *Biol. Psychiatry* **48,** 791–800.
134. Bremner, J.D., Randall, P., Scott, T.M., et al. (1995) MRI-based measurement of hippocampal volume in posttraumatic stress disorder. *Am. J. Psychiatry* **152,** 973–981.
135. Videbech, P. (1997) MRI findings in patients with affective disorders: a meta-analysis. *Acta Psychiatr. Scand.* **96,** 157–168.
136. Swayze, W.W., Andeasen, N.C., Alliger, R.J., Ehrhardt, J.C., and Yuh, W.T.C. (1992) Subcortical and temporal structures in affective disorders and schizophrenia: a magnetic resonance imaging study. *Biol. Psychiatry* **31,** 221–240.
137. Husain, M.M., McDaonald, W.M., Dovaisvanu, B.M., and et al. (1991) A magnetic resonance imaging study of putamen nuclei in major depression. *Pscyhol. Res.* **40,** 95–99.
138. Drevets, W.C., Price, J.L., Simpson, J.R. Jr., et al. (1997) Subgenual prefrontal cortex abnormalities in mood disorders. *Nature* **386,** 824–827.
139. Ongur, D., Drevets, W.C., and Price, J.L. (1998) Glial reduction in the subgenual prefrontal cortex in mood disorders. *Proc. Natl. Acad. Sci. USA* **95,** 13,290–13,295.
140. MacFall, J.R., Payne, M.E., Provenzale, J.E., and Krishnan, K.R. (2001) Medial orbital frontal lesions in late-onset depression. *Biol. Psychiatry* **49,** 803–806.
141. Rajkowska, G. (2000) Postmortem studies in mood disorders indicate altered numbers of neurons and glial cells. *Biol. Psychiatry* **48,** 766–777.
142. Starkstein, S.E. and Robinson, R.G. (1993) *Depression in Neurologic Diseases*, Hopkins University Press, Baltimore.
143. Goodstein, R.K. and Ferrell, R.B. (1977) Multiple sclerosis—presenting as depressive illness. *Dis. Nerv. Syst.* **38,** 127–131.
144. Hirono, N., Mori, E., Ishii, K., et al. (1998) Frontal lobe hypometabolism and depression in Alzheimer's disease. *Neurology* **50,** 380–383.
145. Cummings, J.L. and Victoroff, J.I. (1990) Noncognitive neuropsychiatric syndromes in Alzheimer's disease. *Neuropsych. Neuropsychol. Behav. Neurol.* **2,** 140–158.
146. Robinson, R.G. (1998) *The Clinical Neuropsychiatry of Stroke*, Cambridge University Press, Cambridge, UK.
147. Starkstein, S.E., Robinson, R.G., and Price, T.R. (1987) Comparison of cortical and subcortical lesions in the production of poststroke mood disorders. *Brain* **110,** 1045–1059.
148. Honer, W.G., Hurwitz, T., Li, D.K., Palmer, M., and Paty, D.W. (1987) Temporal lobe involvement in multiple sclerosis patients with psychiatric disorders. *Arch. Neurol.* **44,** 187–190.
149. Pujol, J., Bello, J., Deus, J., Cardoner, N., Marti-Vialta, J.L., and Capdevila, A. (2000) Beck depression inventory factors related to demyelinating lesions of the left arcuate fasiculus region. *Psychiatry Res. Neuroimag. Sect.* **99,** 151–159.
150. Mayberg, H.S. (1994) Functional imaging studies in secondary depression. *J. Psychiatr. Ann* **24,** 643–647.
151. Mayberg, H.S., Starkstein, S.E., Peyser, C.E., Brandt, J., Dannals, R.F., and Folstein, S.E. (1992) Paralimbic frontal lobe hypometabolism in depression associated with Huntington's disease. *Neurology* **42,** 1791–1797.
152. Mayberg, H.S., Starkstein, S.E., Sadzot, B., et al. (1990) Selective hypometabolism in the inferior frontal lobe in depressed patients with Parkinson's disease. *Ann. Neurol.* **28,** 57–64.
153. Jagust, W.J., Reed, B.R., Martin, E.M., Eberling, J.L., and Nelson-Abbott, R.A. (1992) Cognitive function and regional cerebral blood flow in Parkinson's disease. *Brain* **115,** 521–537.
154. Ring, H.A., Bench, C.J., Trimble, M.R., Brooks, D.J., Frackowiak, R.S., and Dolan, R.J. (1994) Depression in Parkinson's disease. A positron emission study. *Br. J. Psychiatry* **165,** 333–339.
155. Porrino, L.J., Crane, A.M., and Goldman-Rakic, P.S. (1981) Direct and indirect pathways from the amygdala to the frontal lobe in rhesus monkeys. *J. Comp. Neurol.* **198,** 121–136.
156. Papez, J.W. (1937) A proposed mechanism of emotion. *Arch. Neurol. Psychol.* **38,** 725–743.
157. Nauta, W.J. (1971) The problem of the frontal lobe: a reinterpretation. *J. Psychiatr. Res.* **8,** 167–187.
158. Bench, C.J., Friston, K.J., Brown, R.G., Scott, L.C., Frackowiak, R.S., and Dolan, R.J. (1992) The anatomy of melancholia—focal abnormalities of cerebral blood flow in major depression. *Psychol. Med.* **22,** 607–615.
159. Levy, M., Cummings, J.L., and Fairbanks, L.A. (1998) Apathy is not depression. *J. Neuropsychiatry Clin. Neurosci.* **10,** 314–319.
160. Marin, R.S., Biedrzycki, R.C., and Firinciogullari, S. (1991) Reliability and validity of the Apathy Evaluation Scale. *Psychiatry Res.* **38,** 143–162.

161. Rogers, D., Lees, A.J., Smith, E., Trimble, M., and Stern, G.M. (1987) Bradyphrenia in Parkinson's disease and psychomotor retardation in depressive illness. An experimental study. *Brain* **110,** 761–776.
162. Mayberg, H.S. (1994) Frontal lobe dysfunction in secondary depression. *J. Neuropsychiatry Clin. Neurosci.* **6,** 428–442.
163. Augustine, J.R. (1996) Circuitry and functional aspects of the insular lobe in primates including humans. *Brain Res. Brain Res. Rev.* **22,** 229–244.
164. Mendez, M.F., Adams, N.L., and Lewandowski, K.S. (1989) Neurobehavioral changes associated with caudate lesions. *Neurology* **39,** 399–454.
165. Bhatia, K.P. and Marsden, C.D. (1994) The behavioral and motor consequences of focal brain lesion of the basal ganglia in man. *Brain* **117,** 859–876.
166. Starkstein, S.E., Mayberg, H., Berthier, M.L., et al. (1990) Mania after brain injury: neuroradiological and metabolic findings. *Ann. Neurol.* **27,** 652–659.
167. Stefurak, T., Mikulis, D.J., Mayberg, H.S., et al. (2001) Deep brain stimulation associated with dysphoria and cortico-limbic changes detected by fMRI. *Mov. Disord.* **16(Suppl.),** S170.
168. Baxter, L.R. Jr., Schwartz, J.M., Phelps, M.E., et al. (1989) Reduction of prefrontal cortex glucose metabolism common to three types of depression. *Arch. Gen. Psychiatry* **46,** 243–250.
169. Buchsbaum, M.S., Wu, J., Siegel, B.V., et al. (1997) Effect of sertraline on regional metabolic rate in patients with affective disorder. *Biol. Psychiatry* **41,** 15–22.
170. Drevets, W.C., Videen, T.O., Price, J.L., Preskorn, S.H., Carmichael, S.T., and Raichle, M.E. (1992) A functional anatomical study of unipolar depression. *J. Neurosci.* **12,** 3628–3641.
171. Mayberg, H.S., Brannan, S.K., Tekell, J.L., et al. (2000) Regional metabolic effects of fluoxetine in major depression: serial changes and relationship to clinical response. *Biol. Psychiatry* **48,** 830–843.
172. Brody, A.L., Saxena, S., Silverman, D.H., et al. (1999) Brain metabolic changes in major depressive disorder from pre- to post-treatment with paroxetine. *Psychiatry Res.* **91,** 127–139.
173. Malizia, A.L. (1997) The frontal lobes and neurosurgery for psychiatric disorders. *J. Psychopharmacol.* **11,** 179–187.
174. Nobler, M.S., Oquendo, M.A., Kegeles, L.S., et al. (2001) Decreased regional brain metabolism after ect. *Am. J. Psychiatry* **158,** 305–308.
175. Teneback, C.C., Nahas, Z., Speer, A.M., et al. (1999) Changes in prefrontal cortex and paralimbic activity in depression following two weeks of daily left prefrontal TMS. *J. Neuropsychiatry Clin. Neurosci.* **11,** 426–435.
176. Kennedy, S.H., Evans, K.R., Kruger, S., et al. (2001) Changes in regional brain glucose metabolism measured with positron emission tomography after paroxetine treatment of major depression. *Am. J. Psychiatry* **158,** 899–905.
177. Stefurak, T., Mahurin, R., Soloman, D., Brannan, T., and Mayberg, H. (2001) Response specific regional metabolism changes with Fluoxetine treatment in depressed Parkinson's patients. *Mov. Disord.* **16(Suppl.),** S39.
178. Brannan, S.K., Mayberg, H.S., McGinnis, S., et al. (2000) Cingulate metabolism predicts treatment response: a replication. *Biol. Psychiatry* **47,** 107.
179. Pizzagalli, D., Pascual-Marqui, R.D., Nitschke, J.B., et al. (2001) Anterior cingulate activity as a predictor of degree of treatment response in major depression: evidence from brain electrical tomography analysis. *Am. J. Psychiatry* **158,** 405–415.
180. Wu, J., Buchsbaum, M.S., Gillin, J.C., et al. (1999) Prediction of antidepressant effects of sleep deprivation by metabolic rates in the ventral anterior cingulate and medial prefrontal cortex [published erratum appears in *Am. J. Psychiatry* 1999 Oct;156(10):1666]. *Am. J. Psychiatry* **156,** 1149–1158.
181. Swanson, L.W. (2000) Cerebral hemisphere regulation of motivated behavior. *Brain Res.* **886,** 113–164.
182. Brewer, D. and Doughtie, E.B. (1980) Induction of mood and mood shift. *J. Clin. Psychol.* **36,** 215–226.
183. Martin, M. (1990) On the induction of mood. *Clin. Psychol. Rev.* **10,** 669–697.
184. Goodwin, A.M. and Williams, J.M. (1982) Mood-induction research—its implications for clinical depression. *Behav. Res. Ther.* **20,** 373–382.
185. Pardo, J.V., Pardo, P.J., and Raichle, M.E. (1993) Neural correlates of self-induced dysphoria. *Am. J. Psychiatry* **150,** 713–719.
186. George, M.S., Ketter, T.A., Parekh, P.I., Herscovitch, P., and Post, R.M. (1996) Gender differences in regional cerebral blood flow during transient self-induced sadness or happiness. *Biol. Psychiatry* **40,** 859–871.
187. Schneider, F., Gur, R.E., Mozley, L.H., et al. (1995) Mood effects on limbic blood flow correlate with emotional self-rating: a PET study with oxygen-15 labeled water. *Psychiatry Res.* **61,** 265–283.
188. Lane, R.D., Reiman, E.M., Ahern, G.L., Schwartz, G.E., and Davidson, R.J. (1997) Neuroanatomical correlates of happiness, sadness, and disgust. *Am. J. Psychiatry* **154,** 926–933.
189. Gemar, M.C., Kapur, S., Segal, Z.V., Brown, G.M., and Houle, S. (1996) Effects of self-generated sad mood on regional cerebral activity: a PET study in normal subjects. *Depression* **4,** 81–88.
190. Mayberg, H.S., Liotti, M., Brannan, S.K., et al. (1999) Reciprocal limbic-cortical function and negative mood: converging PET findings in depression and normal sadness. *Am. J. Psychiatry* **156,** 675–682.
191. Liotti, M., Mayberg, H.S., Brannan, S.K., et al. (2000) Differential neural correlates of sadness and fear in healthy subjects: implications for affective disorders. *Biol. Psychiatry* **48,** 30–42.
192. Liotti, M., Mayberg, H., McGinnis, S., Brannan, S., and Jerabek, P. (2002) Unmasking disease-specific cerebral blood flow abnormalities: mood challenge in patients with remitted unipolar depression. *Am. J. Psychiatry* **159,** 1830–1840.
193. Kruger, S., Goldapple, K., Liotti, M., Houle, S., and Mayberg, H. (2001) Cerebral blood flow in bipolar measured by PET. Trait effects at baseline and after mood induction. *Biol. Psychiatry* **49,** S25.

194. Mayberg, H.S. (2000) Depression and subcortical circuits: the emerging role of prefrontal-limbic interactions, in *Frontal-Subcortical Circuits in Psychiatry and Neurology* (Lichter, D.G. and Cummings, J.L., eds.), Guilford Press, New York, pp. 177–206.
195. Bench, C.J., Friston, K.J., Brown, R.G., Frackowiak, R.S., and Dolan, R.J. (1993) Regional cerebral blood flow in depression measured by positron emission tomography: the relationship with clinical dimensions. *Psychol. Med.* **23,** 579–590.
196. Devinsky, O., Morrell, M.J., and Vogt, B.A. (1995) Contributions of anterior cingulate cortex to behaviour. *Brain* **118,** 279–306.
197. Dolan, R.J., Bench, C.J., Brown, R.G., Scott, L.C., and Frackowiak, R.S. (1994) Neuropsychological dysfunction in depression: the relationship to regional cerebral blood flow. *Psychol. Med.* **24,** 849–857.
198. Maddock, R.J. (1999) The retrosplenial cortex and emotion: new insights from functional neuroimaging of the human brain. *Trends Neurosci.* **22,** 310–316.
199. Bench, C.J., Frackowiak, R.S., and Dolan, R.J. (1995) Changes in regional cerebral blood flow on recovery from depression. *Psychol. Med.* **25,** 247–261.
200. Pardo, J.V., Fox, P.T., and Raichle, M.E. (1991) Localization of a human system for sustained attention by positron emission tomography. *Nature* **349,** 61–64.
201. George, M.S., Ketter, T.A., Parekh, P.I., Horwitz, B., Herscovitch, P., and Post, R.M. (1995) Brain activity during transient sadness and happiness in healthy women. *Am. J. Psychiatry* **152,** 341–351.
202. Mesulam, M.M. (1985) Patterns in behavioral neuroanatomy: association areas, the limbic system, and hemispheric specialization, in *Principles of Behavioral Neurology* (Mesulam, M.M., ed.), F.A. Davis, Philadelphia, pp. 1–70.
203. Morecraft, R.J., Geula, C., and Mesulam, M.M. (1993) Architecture of connectivity within a cingulo-fronto-parietal neurocognitive network for directed attention. *Arch. Neurol.* **50,** 279–284.
204. Petrides, M. and Pandya, D. (1994) Comparative architectonic analysis of the human and macaque frontal cortex, in *Handbook of Neuropsychology* (Boller, G.J., ed.), Elsevier Science Publishers, Amsterdam, pp. 17–58.
205. Neafsey, E.J. (1990) Prefrontal cortical control of the autonomic nervous system: anatomical and physiological observations. *Prog. Brain Res.* **85,** 147–165.
206. Vogt, B.A., Nimchinsky, E.A., Vogt, L.J., and Hof, P.R. (1995) Human cingulate cortex: surface features, flat maps, and cytoarchitecture. *J. Comp. Neurol.* **359,** 490–506.
207. Mayberg, H.S., Brannan, S.K., Mahurin, R.K., et al. (1997) Cingulate function in depression: a potential predictor of treatment response. *Neuroreport* **8,** i-ii.
208. Crino, P.B., Morrison, J.H., and Hof, P.R. (1993) Monoamine innervation of cingulate cortex, in *The Neurobiology of Cingulate Cortex and Limbic Thalamus: a Comprehensive Handbook* (Vogt, B.A. and Gabriel, M., eds.), Birkhauser, Boston, pp. 285–310.
209. Pandya, D.N. and Yeterian, E.H. (1996) Comparison of prefrontal architecture and connections. *Philos. Trans. R. Soc. Lond. B Biol. Sci.* **351,** 1423–1432.
210. Petrides, M. and Pandya, D.N. (1984) Projections to the frontal cortex from the posterior parietal region in the rhesus monkey. *J. Comp. Neurol.* **228,** 105–116.
211. Cosgrove, G.R. and Rauch, S.L. (1995) Psychosurgery. *Neurosurg. Clin. N. Am.* **6,** 167–176.
212. Ceballos-Baumann, A.O., Boecker, H., Bartenstein, P., et al. (1999) A positron emission tomographic study of subthalamic nucleus stimulation in Parkinson disease: enhanced movement-related activity of motor-association cortex and decreased motor cortex resting activity. *Arch. Neurol.* **56,** 997–1003.
213. Fukada, M., Mentis, M.J., Ma, Y., et al. (2001) Networks mediating the clinical effetcs of pallidal brain stimulation for Parkinson's disease. A PET study of resting-state glucose metabolism. *Brain* **124,** 1601–1609.
214. Limousin, P., Greene, J., Pollak, P., Rothwell, J., Benabid, A.L., and Frackowiak, R. (1997) Changes in cerebral activity pattern due to subthalamic nucleus or internal pallidum stimulation in Parkinson's disease. *Ann. Neurol.* **42,** 283–291.
215. Starkstein, S.E., Mayberg, H.S., Berthier, M.L., et al. (1990) Mania after brain injury: neuroradiological and metabolic findings. *Ann. Neurol.* **27,** 652–659.
216. Kwan, L.T., Reed, B.R., Eberling, J.L., et al. (1999) Effects of subcortical cerebral infarction on cortical glucose metabolism and cognitive function. *Arch. Neurol.* **56,** 809–814.
217. Menza, M.A., Golbe, L.I., Cody, R.A., and Forman, N.E. (1993) Dopamine-related personality traits in Parkinson's disease. *Neurology* **43,** 505–508.
218. Bienvenu, O.J., Nestadt, G., Samuels, J.F., Cosata, P., Howard, W.T., and Eaton, W.W. (2001) Phobic, panic and major depressive disorders and the five-factor model of personality. *J. Nerv. Ment. Disord.* **189,** 154–161.

26

Agitation and Apathy in Hyper- and Hypokinetic Movement Disorders

Irene Litvan, MD and Jaime Kulisevsky, MD

1. INTRODUCTION

Anatomical, neurophysiological, and neurochemical evidence supports the notion of parallel direct and indirect basal ganglia thalamocortical motor systems, the differential involvement of which accounts for the hypokinesia or hyperkinesia observed in basal ganglia disorders. In addition to the regulation of movement, the basal ganglia are involved in a variety of cognitive and behavioral functions, such as the generation and execution of context-dependent behaviors and the neural integration of motivational processes into behavioral output *(1–4)*. However, the role of the basal ganglia in neuropsychiatric behaviors is not well known. In this chapter, we briefly review the pathophysiology of hyper- and hypokinesia in diseases of basal ganglia origin trying to establish a parallel with the concepts of hyperactive and hypoactive neuropsychiatric behaviors in the same diseases. We propose that symptoms such as agitation are more frequent and severe in patients with hyperkinetic movement disorders than in those with a hypokinetic disease.

2. FRONTOSUBCORTICAL CIRCUITS: MOTOR AND BEHAVIORAL SYMPTOMS

Five frontosubcortical circuits unite regions of the frontal lobe (supplementary motor area, frontal eye fields, and dorsolateral prefrontal, orbitofrontal, and anterior cingulate cortices) with the striatum, globus pallidus, and thalamus in functional systems that mediate volitional motor activity, saccadic eye movements, executive functions, social behavior, and motivation *(1–4)*. Abnormalities within the interconnected corticostriatopallidothalamic circuitry have been proposed to contribute to the pathophysiology of many motor and neuropsychiatric disorders *(5–7)*. The "motor" loops of the frontosubcortical circuitry are known to be the locus of pathology in primary movement disorders manifested mainly by hyperkinesia, such as Huntington's disease (HD) and hemiballism, or by hypokinesia such as Parkinson's disease (PD) and progressive supranuclear palsy (PSP) *(2–4)*. Akinesia refers to slow or low amplitude movement. Hypokinetic movement disorders may be accompanied by more or less tremor and/or rigidity. Hyperkinesia refers to involuntary excessive movement, such as chorea, athetosis, ballismus, and tics.

Three major behavioral–cognitive syndromes occur after damage to the "complex" loops: (*i*) damage to the dorsolateral prefrontal circuit is associated with executive dysfunction; (*ii*) damage to the orbitofrontal circuit causes disinhibited, irritable, and labile behavior; and (*iii*) damage to the medial frontal–anterior cingulate circuit causes akinesia, apathy, and unconcern *(1–7)*. Accordingly, the complex or

From: *Mental and Behavioral Dysfunction in Movement Disorders*
Edited by: M-A. Bédard et al. © Humana Press Inc., Totowa, NJ

"limbic" loops have been proposed as the source of psychopathology in seemingly disparate forms of neuropsychiatric disorders such as schizophrenia, depression, Gilles de la Tourette Syndrome (GTS), or obsessive–compulsive disorder (OCD) *(4–7)*.

3. ARE THERE EQUIVALENT FORMS OF MOTOR AND BEHAVIORAL SYMPTOMS?

Interestingly, particular neuropsychiatric disturbances are accompanied by a seemingly equivalent pattern of observable motor behaviors. Agitation, for instance, is commonly referred as psychomotor agitation, denoting excessive motor activity associated with a feeling of inner tension, and depression is generally associated with a significant reduction in the production of movement *(6,7)*. Correspondingly, apathy, a psychological syndrome closely associated with depression, which has been defined as the absence or lack of feeling, emotion, interest, concern, and motivation *(8)*, can also be considered a hypoactive neuropsychiatric syndrome associated with specific aspects of brain damage, mainly characterized by decreased activity, lack of productivity, effort, and initiative *(9–11)*. Motor and behavioral abnormalities may occur together, and neuropsychiatric disturbances, such as apathy, depression, agitation, or irritability, are now recognized as part of both hyperkinetic and hypokinetic disorders classically described as exclusively or predominantly motor diseases *(5,12–16)*. Reasonably, an overlap of the anatomical models for these disorders *(7)* should correspond with the commonalties in the neuropsychiatric symptoms identified among many of these disorders (e.g., GTS, HD, PSP, or PD).

While episodes of hyperactive behaviors, such as mania, seems relatively frequent in patients with hyperkinetic movement disorders such as HD, Sydenham's chorea, postencephalitic parkinsonism, Wilson's disease, and GTS, they seem uncommon in patients with hypokinetic movement disorders such as PD or PSP *(17)*. It is noteworthy that in fluctuating patients with Parkinson's disease, agitated, even manic, swing states and dyskinetic movements mainly occur during "on" periods and were typically attributed to striatal and limbic dopaminergic overactivity *(18,19)*. In addition to the association of neuropsychiatric and motor symptoms in a number of basal ganglia disorders, there are also in the literature some interesting single cases showing the concordant coexistence of hyperkinetic motor symptoms with hyperactive behaviors and the reverse association appearing after discrete basal ganglia lesions *(20)*. For instance, we have reported the acute presentation of both hemiballism and mania in a patient with a small ischemic infarction of the right thalamus in whom the movement disorder and altered behavior occurred without other concomitant neurologic manifestations *(17)*. In almost 40% of the patients from a series with acquired OCD associated with structural brain lesions (which were exclusively found in frontal-limbic-basal ganglia circuits), OCD symptoms coexisted with a chronic tic disorder (motor or phonic) *(21)*. Another interesting example is the case of a patient who presented both parkinsonism and a bipolar disorder after a mesencephalic infarction with the particularity that hypokinetic symptoms and signs presented in coincidence with the depressive phases and totally reversed in coincidence with manic episodes *(22)*. However, despite many suggestions linking hyperkinesia with hyperactive behaviors and hypokinesia with hypoactive behaviors in patients with basal ganglia disorders *(7,23)*, to the best of our knowledge, this hypothesis had not been formally tested.

4. AGITATION AND APATHY IN MOVEMENT DISORDERS: A HYPOTHESIS-DRIVEN STUDY

We recently tested the hypothesis that, in addition to contrasting motor dysfunction patterns, hyperkinetic (e.g., GTS or HD) disorders also have contrasting patterns of neuropsychiatric symptoms, with greater frequency of hyperactive behaviors when compared to hypokinetic (e.g., PSP or PD) disorders *(24,25)*. We hypothesized that the predominance of hyperactive (e.g., agitation, irritation, euphoria, or anxiety) or hypoactive (e.g., apathy) behaviors would result from the differential involvement of the frontosubcortical circuits in analogy to the hyperkinesias or hypokinesia, which appears to rely on the differential involvement of the direct striatonigral and the indirect striatopallidal *(3,4)* output

Table 1
Demographic Data of Patients with HD, GTS, and PSP

	GTS (n = 26)	HD (n = 29)	PSP (n = 54)	Significance
Age (yr)	30.2 ± 2.2	43.8 ± 2.1	67.3 ± 1.4	PSP ≠ HD ≠ GTS[a]
Sex, male/female	21/5	14/15	32/22	n.s.
Education (yr)	10.6 ± 0.5	13.4 ± 0.4	14.0 ± 0.4	PSP and HD ≠ GTS[a]
Disease duration (yr)	20.3 ± 1.7	5.6 ± 1.6	4.4 ± 1.1	GTS ≠ both PSP and HD[a]
Mini-Mental State Examination score	28.7 ± 0.8	24.5 ± 0.8	27.2 ± 0.5	GTS and PSP ≠ HD[a]
Mattis Dementia Rating Scale score	NA	121.2 ± 3.5 (n = 28)	117.9 ± 2.4 (n = 49)	n.s.

Data are expressed as mean ± standard error of the mean (SEM).
[a]$p < 0.001$ (one-way [ANOVA]).
n.s., nonsignificant.
≠ indicates pairs of means that are significantly different (Tukey-Kramer); NA, not available.

pathways of the basal ganglia in these disorders *(23)*. Taking agitation and apathy as the opposite ends of abnormal hyperactive and hypoactive behavior, in a recent study *(25)*, we investigated whether patients with GTS manifesting tics and patients with HD manifesting chorea, showed a higher frequency of agitation and whether patients with PSP manifesting parkinsonism showed a contrasting pattern with greater apathy. Thereafter, we included a larger sample of patients with definite or probable PSP (n = 34) making a total of 109 patients (Table 1), who were reported elsewhere *(24,25)*. Clinical diagnosis of HD (n = 29) was made on the basis of positive family history of the disease, typical choreiform movements, and dementia, according to Diagnostic and Statistical Manual of Mental Disorders, Fourth Edition (DSM-IV) criteria, and were molecularly confirmed with expanded CAG repeat lengths in IT15 on chromosome 4. Chorea was scored according to the Unified HD Rating Scale *(26)*. The total chorea score, which was derived by adding all chorea items (e.g., face, upper and lower extremities, and trunk), was used to classify the patients into three subgroups: those with low (<12), medium *(12–19)*, and high (>19) total chorea scores. Diagnosis of GTS (n = 26) was established on the basis of the diagnostic criteria of the DSM-IV *(27)*. Patients with a history of childhood Attention Deficit Hyperactivity Disorder *(28)* were excluded. The phenomenology and severity of tics in GTS were scored according to the Yale Global Tic Severity Scale (YGTSS) *(29)*. The patients with PSP fulfilled the research criteria of the National Institute of Neurological Disorders and Stroke (NINDS)-Society for Progressive Supranuclear Palsy for the diagnosis of PSP (15 definite, eventually autopsy-confirmed, and 39 probable, who have an optimal [100%] positive predictive value according to clinicopathologic studies) *(30)*. Hypokinesia was scored by adding the motor items (i.e., speech, limb rigidity, and neck rigidity) assessed using the Unified Parkinson's Disease Rating Scale (UPDRS) *(31)*.

In all three groups, the overall degree of cognitive impairment was evaluated using the Mini-Mental State Examination *(32)*. Neuropsychiatric evaluation was carried out using the Neuropsychiatric Inventory (NPI), as previously described *(33)*, a caregiver-based rating scale of established validity and reliability *(33–35)*. The NPI contains 10 subscales designed to rate various psychiatric domains, in which scores are based on abnormal behaviors present in the past month. They include delusions, hallucinations, agitation, depression, anxiety, euphoria, apathy, disinhibition, irritability, and aberrant motor behavior. Since the GTS patients did not have caregivers, other informants (usually a first-degree relative) were interviewed. Briefly, screening questions for each behavior were posed first, and if a positive response was obtained for any of the ten behavioral domains, this aspect was then further explored

Table 2
NPI Composite Scores of Patients With GTS, HD, and PSP

Behavior	PSP (n = 54)	HD (n = 29)	GTS (n = 26)	Significance
Apathy	6.24 ± 0.5 (81)	2.28 ± 0.7 (34)	0.85 ± 0.7 (35)	PSP ≠ both HD and GTS[a]
Agitation	0.66 ± 0.4 (24)	1.66 ± 0.5 (45)	2.23 ± 0.5 (38)	GTS ≠ PSP[a]
Anxiety	0.43 ± 0.3 (17)	1.2 ± 0.3 (34)	4.12 ± 0.5 (50)	GTS ≠ both PSP and HD[a]
Irritability	0.91 ± 0.3 (20)	1.31 ± 0.4 (38)	2.30 ± 0.4 (42)	GTS ≠ PSP[a]
Euphoria	0	0.93 ± 0.5 (17)	1.61 ± 0.5 (42)	PSP ≠ both HD and GTS[a]
Disinhibition	2.61 ± 0.4 (57)	0.69 ± 0.3 (24)	1.35 ± 0.6 (31)	n.s.
Depression	0.96 ± 0.3 (24)	1.41 ± 0.4 (41)	3.00 ± 0.5 (61)	n.s.
Delusions	0.19 ± 0.2 (4)	0.66 ± 0.4 (10)	0.46 ± 0.3 (19)	n.s.
Abnormal motor behavior	0.61 ± .22 (7)	0.41 ± 0.3 (7)	0.43 ± 0.4 (12)	n.s.
Hallucinations	0.4 ± 0.03 (2)	0	0.08 ± 0.02 (15)	n.s.
Total NPI score	12.6 ± 1.7 (89)	10.6 ± 2.3 (83)	16.4 ± 2.5 (85)	n.s.

Patients data are expressed as mean ± SEM NPI composite scores (frequency of changes in percentage). The maximum composite score is 12.

*$p < 0.005$.

n.s., nonsignificant ($p > 0.005$, Bonferroni-Holm correction).

(GTS ≠ PSP) indicates pairs of means that are significantly different and the mean with a lower p value.

with scripted questions. The caregiver rated the behaviors using a 1 to 4 scale for frequency (1, occasionally; 2, often; 3, frequently; and 4, very frequently) and a 1 to 3 score for severity (1, mild; 2, moderate; and 3, marked). The composite score for each behavioral domain is the product of the frequency and severity subscores for that particular behavior (maximum, 12). The total score of the NPI is the sum of the subscale scores. The GTS patients were also administered the 17-item Hamilton Rating Scale for Depression *(36)* and obsessive–compulsive behavior was rated with the Leyton Obsessional Inventory *(37)*.

While there were no statistically significant differences between HD and PSP patients in years of formal education, PSP patients were significantly older than those with HD. Patients with GTS were significantly younger, had significantly fewer years of education, and longer symptom duration than both HD and PSP groups (Table 1). Most HD patients (79%) were not taking medications. The remaining patients received either a selective serotonin reuptake inhibitor (SSRI), or low dosages of a typical or an atypical neuroleptic. Among PSP patients, 41% were receiving levodopa with unclear or no motor benefit, 15 patients received antidepressants, and one patient was taking ritalin. Fourteen GTS (54%) patients received no medication, and 12 patients were receiving pharmacological treatments to control motor and phonic tics, associated conditions (i.e., depression, OCD, generalized anxiety disorder), or both. Medication included tetrabenazine, risperidone, tiapride, clonazepam, sertraline, clomipramine, alprazolam, and carbamazepine.

No significant differences were observed in the Mattis Dementia Rating Scale scores between PSP and HD patients. The GTS and PSP groups had significantly higher Mini-Mental State Examination scores than the HD group (Table 1). The NPI values of the patients are shown in Table 2, which also shows no significant differences between groups in the total NPI scores. However, as previously reported, patients with PSP exhibited significantly higher hypoactive behavioral scores than those with HD and GTS (Fig. 1). Conversely, both GTS and HD patients exhibited higher hyperactive behavioral scores than PSP patients, but these differences did not achieve the strict statistical significance level set in our study (0.005) (Fig. 1). Because depression is frequently observed in many neurologic conditions, and we did not attempt to separate reactive vs nonreactive depression, depression was not included as a hypoactive behavior.

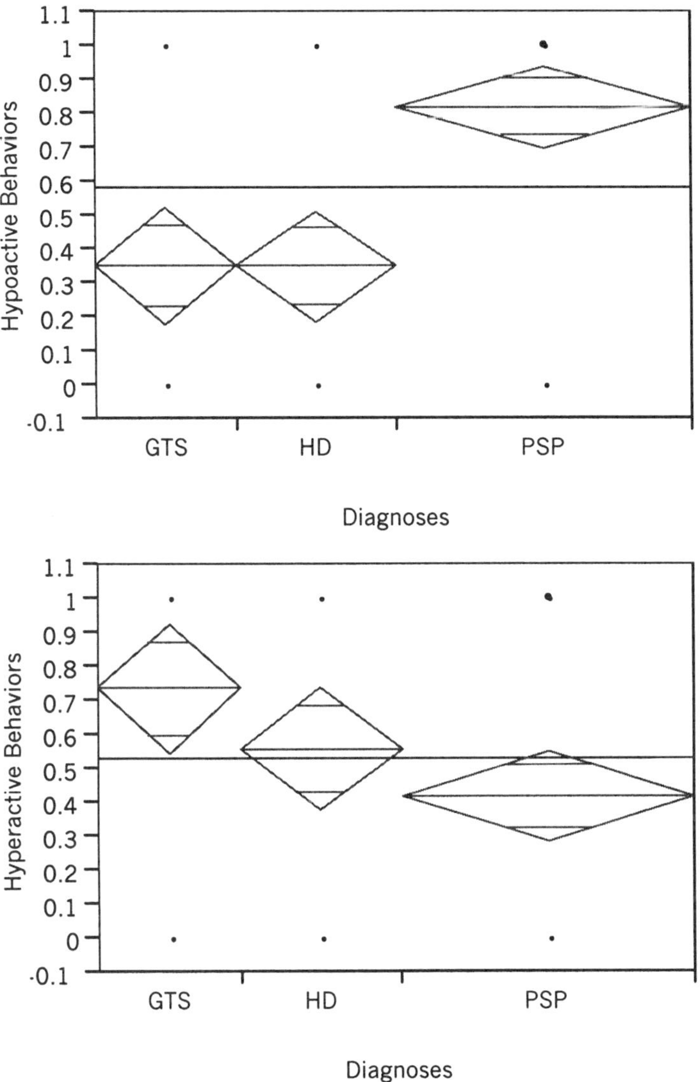

Fig. 1. Hyperactive and hypoactive behaviors in GTS, HD, and PSP. Patients with PSP had significantly higher hypoactive behaviors ($p < 0.0001$) than those with GTS and HD. According to the significance levels set in this study ($p \pm 0.005$; after Bonferroni correction), no significant differences in hyperactive behaviors across diseases ($p = 0.028$) were found.

On individual subscales, patients with GTS and HD had higher scores on the assessments of agitation (GTS significantly different from PSP), anxiety (GTS significantly different from both PSP and HD), and irritability (GTS significantly different from PSP), while patients with PSP had significantly higher apathy scores than both HD and GTS patients (Table 2 and Fig. 2). Patients with GTS exhibited more depression and euphoria than those with PSP, and those with PSP had higher disinhibition scores than those with HD. There was a significant association between the total HD motor scores and agitation in HD patients. Moreover, patients with higher chorea scores exhibited a hyperactive behavior more frequently (12 out of 18 patients [67%] in the group with higher and middle chorea scores) than those with the lower chorea scores (4 out of 11 patients [36%] in the group with the lowest chorea scores). The degree of chorea was also inversely associated with the total Mattis Dementia Rating

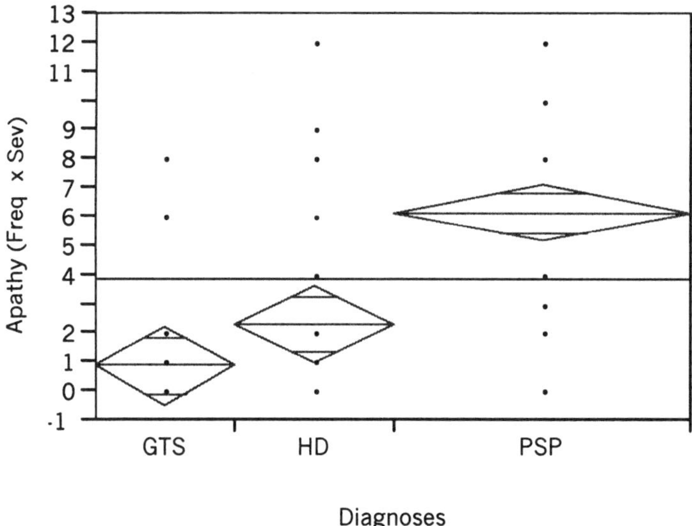

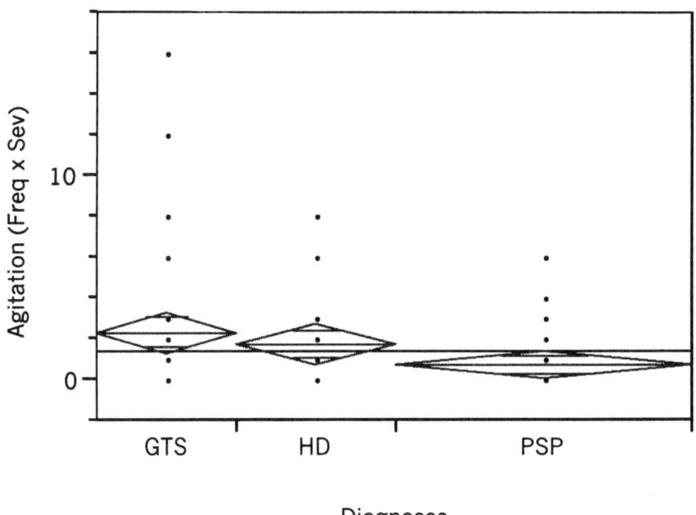

Fig. 2. NPI apathy and agitation composite scores in patients with GTS, HD, and PSP. Patients with PSP had significantly higher apathy scores ($p < 0.0001$) than those with GTS and HD. According to the significance levels set in this study ($p \pm 0.005$; after Bonferroni correction), there were no significant differences in the agitation composite scores across diseases ($p = 0.032$).

Scale score, indicating that chorea was worse in patients with a higher degree of dementia. In GTS patients, the complexity of the motor tics according to the YGTSS was strongly associated with the total NPI, anxiety, and agitation scores. In addition, the number and intensity of motor and phonemic tics tended to be or were associated with agitation. No association between the Leyton Obsessional Inventory and the NPI scores was found. The total motor scores of patients with PSP were inversely associated with the Mini-Mental State Examination total score. There was no relation between total PSP motor scores and apathy. Disease duration in PSP was strongly associated with the total and axial motor scores and inversely related with the Mini-Mental Status Examination scores, but were not related with the Mattis Dementia Rating Scale total score.

4.1. Agitation and Apathy in PSP, GTS, and HD

In accordance with the proposed hypotheses, we found that agitation predominated in patients with GTS and HD, whereas patients with PSP more frequently displayed apathy. However, some agitation and apathy occurred in both hypokinetic and hyperkinetic movement disorders, suggesting that motor and behavioral neuronal circuits may degenerate independently. This latter hypothesis is supported in PSP by the association between symptom duration and motor disability and the lack of an association between symptom duration and behavioral disturbances. These findings are in agreement with previous observations *(24,25)*. However, in this larger study, the frequency and severity of the agitation exhibited by the patients with HD was similarly higher, but not significantly different than that observed in patients with PSP. The considerable symptomatic overlap observed may be secondary to the disappearance during later disease stages of the relatively distinct anatomic involvement observed initially. In HD, for example, the orbitofrontal and anterior cingulate cortices, ventromedial caudate and subthalamic nuclei are affected to different degrees depending upon the stage of the disease.

Hyperactive behaviors such as agitation, OCD, mania, psychosis, and intermittent explosive disorder are all described in patients with HD and GTS *(38)*, as well as in those with other hyperkinetic disorders, such as neuroacanthocytosis, Sydenham's chorea, basal ganglia calcifications, Wilson's disease *(6,39–42)*, subcortical hyperkinetic movements disorders associated with stroke lesions *(20)*, and in the "on" (hyperkinetic) phase of PD *(18,19)*. In contrast, to the best of our knowledge, they are uncommon in untreated hypokinetic disorders. Although anxiety was more common and severe among patients with GTS, the two groups with hyperkinetic disorders (HD and GTS) shared the same pattern of behavior in virtually all subscales of the NPI.

We hypothesized that in GTS, as well as in HD *(24,25)*, hyperactive behaviors result from an excitatory subcortical output through the medial and orbitofrontal circuits to the pallidum, thalamus, and cortex. This may occur in parallel with the excitatory stimulation of premotor–motor and supplementary motor cortices, resulting either in tics or choreic movements. Functional neuroimaging studies in patients with GTS *(43–46)* and HD *(47–49)* suggest an altered relationship between limbic-related cortical regions and striatum mediating complex cognition and behaviors, with other nonlimbic cortical regions implicated in the generation of hyperkinetic movements. In fact, positron emission tomographic (PET) studies reveal decreased metabolic rates in basal ganglia (caudate and putamen in HD and ventral striatrum in GTS) that coexist with normal or increased metabolism in various cortical regions *(43–46)*. Our clinical findings of hyperactive behaviors in GTS and HD concur with previous speculations that disinhibited behavior and hyperkinesia in HD and GTS may result from an excitatory subcortical output through the medial and orbitofrontal circuits to the pallidum, thalamus, and cortex *(24,25)*. Although the biological basis for GTS is widely supported by genetic, biochemical, neuropharmacological, neuroimaging, and electrophysiological studies *(50–55)*, only a small number of GTS brains have been evaluated pathologically and histochemically *(54–56)*. However, clinical investigations suggest that the basal ganglia are a primary site of dysfunction in GTS. Our findings are consistent with this view. We found a significant association between the complexity of tics and the total NPI score. In addition, the intensity and number of tics had trends or were significantly associated with the agitation, irritability, and anxiety scores. Because the various hyperactive behaviors were significantly related in our patients with GTS, HD, and PSP, it is possible that they share common mechanisms. Although HD and GTS are inheritable conditions, which may show similar types of both hyperkinetic movements (tics and chorea) and associated psychiatric disorders (obsessive–compulsive spectrum disorders, depression, mania, psychosis, and personality changes) *(41,57,58)*, anxiety is not commonly described in psychiatric reports of patients with HD *(57)*. By contrast, the presence of severe nonOCD anxiety in the present study agree with previous data reporting a high prevalence of anxiety across the entire lifespan in GTS *(59–62)*, a finding that raises the possibility of increased susceptibility to anxiety in GTS patients *(63)*. We suggest that anxiety in GTS may be attributed to abnormal activity in some components of frontal-limbic-subcortical circuits (orbitofrontal cortex, amygdala, and ventral tegmental area) that are integral to the clinical expression of GTS (including stress sensitivity) *(64–70)* and, less frequently, of HD *(71)*.

On the other hand, in patients with PSP in whom apathy is usually present, it is hypothesized that this behavior is the consequence of hypostimulation of the frontosubcortical circuits resulting from pathologic changes on several subcortical and brainstem integrated nuclei (e.g., in the substantia nigra, striatum, and pallidum) that decrease dopaminergic stimulation of frontosubcortical circuits *(72–74)*. Supportive evidence that the frontosubcortical circuits are disconnected in PSP by prominent subcortical damage is provided by PET measures of glucose consumption (hypometabolism in the frontal cortex) and studies of the nigral dopaminergic system (decreased striatal dopamine D2 receptor uptake ratios) *(72–77)*. However, in PSP there are also cortical pathologic characteristics, such as increased number of neurofibrillary tangles in the anterior cingulate cortex, entorhinal cortex, and hippocampus, that could contribute to the behavioral abnormalities *(78–81)*. In fact, in patients with Alzheimer's disease, imaging studies reveal that apathy correlates with diminished perfusion in the anterior temporal, orbitofrontal, anterior cingulate, and dorsolateral prefrontal regions *(82–85)*. On the other hand, functional imaging studies also indicate an association between frontal cortex dysfunction and agitation *(86–90)*.

As shown, quantitative delineation of the neuropsychiatric symptoms by instruments such as the NPI, allow systematic investigation of the correlates and determinants of these symptoms. In this way, parallel with the functional imaging studies, a recent neuropathological study *(91)* using the NPI found that neurofibrillary tangle burden in the orbitofrontal and anterior cingulate cortex was significantly associated with agitation and apathy and had a trend to be associated with the anterior cingulate cortex of pathologically confirmed patients with Alzheimer disease.

Future functional neuroimaging and pathological studies should examine the relative contribution of different frontosubcortical circuits in apathy and hypokinesia and agitation and hyperkinesia in basal ganglia disorders such as HD, GTS, and PSP.

5. CONCLUSION

We have briefly reviewed the suggested links between hyper- and hypokinetic movement disorders and equivalent neuropsychiatric behaviors, such agitation and apathy. We examined and found that the pattern of behavioral disturbances (agitation) associated with hyperkinetic movement disorders (GTS and HD) with a proposed excitatory basal ganglia output differed from the profile of behavior (apathy) of a hypokinetic movement disorder with a proposed hypostimulation of basal ganglia circuits (PSP). Based on our findings *(24,25)* and those of the literature, and on the anatomical lesions known to occur in these movement disorders, we suggest that in hyperkinetic disorders, agitation is secondary to an excitatory subcortical output through the medial and orbitofrontal cortical circuits, while apathy in hypokinetic disorders is secondary to hypostimulation of the medial frontal circuit. Neuroimaging studies of patients with hypokinetic and hyperkinetic disorders, evaluating both neuropsychiatric and movement features, are necessary to further disentangle the role of the basal ganglia in neuropsychiatric behaviors.

ACKNOWLEDGMENTS

The authors acknowledge the significant contributions of Drs. Jane Paulsen, Marcelo L. Berthier, Jeffrey Cummings, and Michael Mega.

REFERENCES

1. Alexander, G.E., DeLong, M.R., and Strick, P.L. (1986) Parallel organization of functionally segregated circuits linking basal ganglia and cortex. *Ann. Rev. Neurosci.* **9,** 357–381.

2. Alexander, G.E. and Crutcher, M.D. (1990) Functional architecture of basal ganglia circuits: neural substrates of parallel processing. *Trends Neurosci.* **13,** 266–271.
3. Albin, R.L., Young, A.B., and Penney, J.B. (1995) The functional anatomy of disorders of the basal ganglia. *Trends Neurosci.* **18,** 63–64.
4. Feger, J. (1997) Updating the functional model of the basal ganglia. *Trends Neurosci.* **20,** 152–153.
5. Cummings, J.L., Diaz, C., Levy, M., Binetti, G., and Litvan, I. (1996) Neuropsychiatric syndromes in neurodegenerative diseases: frequency and significance. *Semin. Clin. Neuropsychiatry* **1,** 241–247.
6. Salloway, S. and Cummings, J.L. (1996) Subcortical structures and neuropsychiatric illness. *Neuroscientist* 66–75.
7. Cummings, J.L. (1995) Anatomic and behavioral aspects of frontal-subcortical circuits. *Ann. NY Acad. Sci.* **769,** 1–13.
8. Marin, R.S. (1991) Apathy: a neuropsychiatric syndrome. *J. Neuropsychiatry Clin. Neurosci.* **3,** 243–254.
9. Andersson, S., Krogstad, J., and Finset, A. (1999) Apathy and depressed mood in acquired brain damage: relationship to lesion localization and psychophysiological reactivity. *Psychol. Med.* **29,** 447–456.
10. Starkstein, S.E. and Manes, F. (2000) Apathy and depression following stroke. *CNS Spectrums* **5,** 43–50.
11. Levy, M.L., Cummings, J.L., Fairbanks, L.A., et al. (1998) Apathy is not depression. *J. Neuropsychiatry Clin. Neurosci.* **10,** 314–319.
12. Albert, M.L., Feldamn, R.G., and Willis, A.L. (1974) The "subcortical" dementia of progressive supranuclear palsy. *J. Neurol. Neurosurg. Psychiatry* **37,** 121–130.
13. Starkstein, S.E., Preziosi, T.J., Berthier, M.L., Bolduc, P.L., Mayberg, H.S., and Robinson, R.G. (1989) Depression and cognitive impairment in Parkinson's disease. *Brain* **112,** 1141–1153.
14. Robertson, M.M., Trimble, M.R., and Lees, A.J. (1988) The psychopathology of the Gilles de la Tourette's syndrome. A phenomenological analysis. *Br. J. Psychi*atry **152,** 383–390.
15. Chiu, H.F. (1995) Psychiatric aspects of progressive supranuclear palsy. *Gen. Hosp. Psychiatry* **17,** 135–143.
16. Litvan, I., Mega, M.S., Cummings, J.L., and Fairbanks, L. (1996) Neuropsychiatric aspects of progressive supranuclear palsy. *Neurology* **47,** 1184–1189.
17. Kulisevsky, J., Berthier, M.L., and Pujol, J. (1993) Hemiballismus and secondary mania following a right thalamic infarction. *Neurology* **43,** 1422–1424.
18. Nissembaum, H., Quinn, N.P., Brown, R.G., Toone, B., and Gotham, A.M. (1987) Mood swings associated with the 'on-off' phenomenon in Parkinson's disease. *Psychol. Med.* **17,** 899–904.
19. Menza, M.A., Sage J., Marshall, E., Cody, R., and Duvoisin, R. (1990) Mood changes and "on-off" phenomena in Parkinson's disease. *Mov. Disord.* **2,** 148–151.
20. Berthier, M.L., Kulisevsky, J., Gironell, A., and Fernández-Benitez, J.A. (1996) Poststroke bipolar affective disorder: clinical subtypes, concurrent movement disorders, and anatomical correlates. *J. Neuropsychiatry Clin. Neurosci.* **8,** 160–167.
21. Berthier, M.L., Kulisevsky, J., Gironell, A., and Heras, J.A. (1996) Obsessive-compulsive disorders associated with brain lesions: clinical phenomenology, cognitive function, and anatomic correlates. *Neurology* **47,** 353–361.
22. Kulisevsky, J., Avila, A., and Berthier, M.L. (1995) Bipolar affective disorder and unilateral parkinsonism after a brainstem infarction. *Mov. Disord.* **10,** 799–802.
23. DeLong, M.R. (1990) Primate models of movement disorders of basal ganglia origin. *Trends Neurosci.* **13,** 281–285.
24. Litvan, I., Paulsen, J.S., Mega, M.S., and Cummings, J. (1998) Neuropsychiatric behavioral assessment of patients with hyperkinetic and hypokinetic movement disorders. *Arch. Neurol.* **55,** 1313–1319.
25. Kulisevsky, J., Litvan, I., Berthier, M.L., Pascual-Sedano, B., Paulsen, J., and Cummings, J.L. (2001) Neuropsychiatric assessment of Gilles de la Tourette patients: a comparative study with other hyperkinetic and hypokinetic movement disorders. *Mov. Disord.* **16,** 1098–1104.
26. Huntington Study Group (1996). Unified Huntington's disease rating scale: reliability and consistency. *Mov. Disord.* **11,** 136–142.
27. American Psychiatric Association (1994) *Diagnostic and Statistical Manual of Mental Disorders.* Fourth Edition, American Psychiatric Association, Washington, DC.
28. Wodrich, D.L., Benjamin, E., and Lachar, D. (1997) Tourette's syndrome and psychopathology in a child psychiatric setting. *J. Am. Acad. Child Adolesc. Psychiatry* **36,** 1618–1624.
29. Leckman, J.F., Riddle, M.A., Hardin, M.T., et al. (1989) The Yale Global Tics Severity Scale (YGTSS): initial testing of a clinical-rated scale of tic severity. *J. Am. Acad. Child Adolesc. Psychiatry* **28,** 566–573.
30. Litvan, I., Agid, Y., Calne, D., et al. (1996) Clinical research criteria for the diagnosis of progressive supranuclear palsy (Steele-Richardson-Olszewski syndrome): report of the NINDS-SPSP International Workshop. *Neurology* **47,** 1–9.
31. Fahn, S., Elston, R.L., and members of the UPDRS development committee (1987) Unified Parkinson's Disease rating scale, in *Recent Developments in Parkinson's Disease,* vol. 2 (Fahn, S., Marsden, C.D., Goldstein, M., and Calne, D.B., eds.), MacMillan, New York, pp. 153–163.
32. Folstein, M.F., Folstein, S.E., and McHugh, P.R. (1975) 'Mini-mental state'. A practical method for grading the mental state of patients for the clinician. *J. Psychiatr. Res.* **12,** 189–198.
33. Cummings, J.L., Mega, M., Gray, K., Rosenberg-Thompson, S., Carusi, D.A., and Gornbey, P.H. (1994) The Neuropsychiatric Inventory: comprehensive assessment of psychopathology in dementia. *Neurology* **44,** 2308–2314.
34. Binetti, G., Mega, M.S., Magni, E., et al. (1998) Behavioral disturbances in Alzheimer's disease: a transcultural perspective. *Arch. Neurol.* **55,** 539–544.
35. Diaz-Olavarrieta, C., Cummings, J.L., Velásquez, J., and Garcia de la Cadena, C.J. (1999) Neuropsychiatric manifestations of multiple sclerosis. *J. Neuropsychiatry Clin. Neurosci.* **11,** 51–57.

36. Hamilton, M.A. (1960) A rating scale for depression. *J. Neurol. Neurosurg. Psychiatry* **23,** 56–62.
37. Robertson, J.R. and Mulhall, D. (1979) The clinical evaluation of obsessionality: a development of the Leyton Obsessional Inventory. *Psychol. Med.* **9,** 147–154.
38. Berthier, M.L., Kulisevsky, J., and Campos, V.M. (1998) Bipolar disorder in adult patients with Tourette's syndrome: a clinical study. *Biol. Psychiatry* **43,** 364–370.
39. Trautner, R.J., Cummings, J.L., Read, S.L., and Benson, D.F. (1988) Idiopathic basal ganglia calcification and organic mood disorder. *Am. J. Psychiatry* **145,** 350–353.
40. López-Villegas, D., Kulisevsky, J., Deus, J., et al. (1996) Neuropsychological alterations in patients with computed tomography-detected basal ganglia calcification. *Arch. Neurol.* **53,** 251–256.
41. Cummings, J.L. and Cunningham, K. (1992) Obsessive-compulsive disorder in Huntington's disease. *Biol. Psychiatry* **31,** 263–270.
42. Cummings, J.L. (1993) Frontal-subcortical circuits and human behavior. *Arch. Neurol.* **50,** 873–880.
43. Wright, C.I., Peterson, B.S., and Rauch, S.L. (1999) Neuroimaging studies in Tourette syndrome. *CNS Spectrums* **4,** 54–61.
44. Eidelberg, D., Moeller, J.R., Antonini, A., et al. (1997) The metabolic anatomy of Tourette's syndrome. *Neurology* **48,** 927–934.
45. Braun, A.R., Randolph, C., Stoetter, B., et al. (1995) The functional neuroanatomy of Tourette's syndrome: an FDG-PET study. II. Relationships between regional cerebral metabolism and associated behavioral and cognitive features of the illness. *Neuropsychopharmacology* **13,** 151–168.
46. Braun, A.R., Stoetter, B., Randolph, C., et al. (1995) The functional neuroanatomy of Tourette's syndrome: an FDG-PET study. II. Relationships between regional cerebral metabolism and associated behavioral and cognitive features of the illness. *Neuropsychopharmacology* **13,** 151–168.
47. Mayberg, H.S., Starkstein, S.E., Peyser, C.E., Brandt, J., Dannals, R.F., and Folstein, S.E. (1992) Paralimbic frontal lobe hypometabolism in depression associated with Huntington's disease. *Neurology* **42,** 1792–1797.
48. Antonini, A., Leenders, K.L., Spiegel, R., et al. (1996) Striatal glucose metabolism and dopamine D2 receptor binding in asymptomatic gene carriers and patients with Huntington's disease. *Brain* **119,** 2085–2095.
49. Andrews, T.C. and Brooks, D.J. (1998) Advances in the understanding of early Huntington's disease using the functional imaging techniques of PET and SPET. *Mol. Med. Today* **4,** 532–539.
50. Butler, I.J., Koslow, S.H., Seifert, W.E. Jr., Caprioli, R.M., and Singer, H.S. (1979) Biogenic amine metabolism in Tourette syndrome. *Ann. Neurol.* **6,** 37–39.
51. Cohen, D.J., Shaywitz, B.A., Young, J.G., et al. (1979) Central biogenic amine metabolism in children with the syndrome of chronic multiple tics of Gilles de la Tourette: norepinephrine, serotonin, and dopamine. *J. Am. Acad. Child Adolesc. Psychiatry* **18,** 320–341.
52. Nee, L.E., Caine, D.E., Polinsky, R.J., Eldridge, R., and Ebert, M.H. (1980) Gilles de la Tourette syndrome: clinical and family study of 50 cases. *Ann. Neurol.* **7,** 41–49.
53. Pauls, D.L. and Leckman, J.F. (1986) The inheritance of Gilles de la Tourette's syndrome and associated behaviors: evidence for autosomal dominant transmission. *N. Engl. J. Med.* **315,** 993–997.
54. Singer, H.S., Hahn, I.-H., and Moran, T.H. (1991) Abnormal dopamine uptake sites in post-mortem striatum from patients with Tourette's syndrome. *Ann. Neurol.* **30,** 558–562.
55. Swerdlow, N.R. and Young, A.B. (1999) Neuropathology in Tourette syndrome. *CNS Spectrums* **4,** 65–74.
56. Haber, S.N., Kowall, N.W., Vonsattel, J.P., Bird, D.E., and Richardson, E.P. Jr. (1986) Gilles de la Tourette's syndrome. A postmortem neuropathological and immunohistochemical study. *J. Neurol. Sci.* **75,** 225–241.
57. McHugh, P.R. and Folstein, M.F. (1975) Psychiatric syndromes of Huntington's chorea: a clinical and phenomenology study, in *Seminars in Psychiatry: Psychiatric Aspects of Neurologic Disease (*Benson, D.F., Blumer, D., eds., Greenblatt, M., series ed.), Grune and Stratton, New York, pp. 267–286.
58. De Marchi, N., Morris, M., Mennella, R., La Pia, S., and Nestadt, G. (1998) Association of obsessive-compulsive disorder and pathological gambling with Huntington's disease in an Italian pedigree: possible association with Huntington's disease mutation. *Acta Psychiatr. Scand.* **97,** 62–65.
59. Comings, D.E. and Comings, B.G. (1987) A controlled study of Tourette syndrome III: phobias and panic attacks. *Am. J. Hum. Genet.* **41,** 761–781.
60. Robertson, M.M., Channon, S., Baker, J., and Flynn, D. (1993) The psychopathology of Gilles de la Tourette's syndrome. A controlled study. *Br. J. Psychiatry* **162,** 114–117.
61. Robertson, M.M., Banerjee, S., Hiley, P.J., and Tannock C. (1997) Personality disorder and psychopathology in Tourette's syndrome: a controlled study. *Br. J. Psychiatry* **171,** 283–286.
62. Spencer, T., Biederman, J., Harding, M., Wilens, T., and Faraone, S. (1995) The relationship between tic disorders and Tourette's syndrome revisited. *J. Am. Acad. Child Adolesc. Psychiatry* **34,** 1133–1139.
63. Coffey, B., Frazier, J., and Chen, S. (1992) Comorbidity, Tourette syndrome, and anxiety disorders, in *Advances in Neurology,* vol. 58 (Chase, T.M, Friedhoff, A.J., and Cohen, D.J., eds.), Raven Press, New York, pp. 95–104.
64. Comings, D.E. (1994) Tourette syndrome: a hereditary neuropsychiatric spectrum disorder. *Ann. Clin. Psy*chiatry **6,** 235–237.
65. Leckman, J.F., Walker, D.E., and Cohen, D.J. (1993) Premonitory urges in Tourette's syndrome. *Am. J. Psychiatry* **153,** 98–102.
66. León, M., Berthier, M.L., and Kulisevsky, J. (1998) Self-touching tics in Tourette's syndrome induced by comorbid somatic and cognitive psychiatric symptoms. *Neurology* **50,** A46.

67. Berthier, M.L., Campos, V.M., and Kulisevsky, J. (1996) Echopraxia and self-injurious behavior in Tourette's syndrome: a case report. *Neuropsychiatry Neuropsychol. Behav. Neurol.* **9,** 280–283.
68. León, M., Berthier, M.L., Kulisevsky, J., and Campos, V.M. (1999) Reflex tics in Tourette's syndrome: "loose clothing" and the overestimation of somatosensory stimuli. *Neurology* **52,** A520–A521.
69. Devinsky, O. (1983) Neuroanatomy of Gilles de la Tourette's syndrome. Possible midbrain involvement. *Arch. Neurol.* **40,** 508–514.
70. Leckman, J.F. (1993) Tourette's syndrome, in *Obsessive-Compulsive-Related Disorders* (Hollander, E., ed.), American Psychiatric Press, Washington, DC, pp. 113–137.
71. Lucey, J.V., Costa, D.C., Adehesad, G., et al. (1997) Brain blood flow in anxiety disorders: OCD, panic disorder, and post-traumatic stress disorder on ^{99}Tc HMPAO single photon emission tomography (SPECT). *Br. J. Psychiatry* **171,** 346–350.
72. D'Antona, R., Baron, J.C., Samson, Y., et al. (1985) Subcortical dementia. Frontal cortex hypometabolism detected by positron tomography in patients with progressive supranuclear palsy. *Brain* **108,** 785–799.
73. Foster, N.L., Gilman, S., Berent, S., Morin, E.M., Brown, M.B., and Koeppe, R.A. (1988) Cerebral hypometabolism in progressive supranuclear plasy studied with positron emission tomography. *Ann. Neurol.* **24,** 399–406.
74. Blin, J., Baron, J.C., Dubois, B., et al. (1990) Positron emission tomography study in progressive supranuclear palsy. Brain hypometabolic pattern and clinico-metabolic correlations. *Arch. Neurol.* **47,** 747–752.
75. Brooks, D.J., Ibanez, V., Sawle, J.V., et al. (1990) Differing patterns of striatal 18F-dopa uptake in Parkinson's disease, multiple system atrophy, and progressive supranuclear palsy. *Ann. Neurol.* **28,** 547–555.
76. Brooks, D.J., Ibanez, V., Sawle, J.V., et al. (1992) Striatal D2 receptor status in patients with Parkinson's disease, striatonigral degeneration, and progressive supranuclear palsy, measured with 11C-raclopride and positron emission tomography. *Ann. Neurol.* 31, 184–192.
77. Brooks, D.J. (1994) PET studies in progressive supranuclear palsy. *J. Neural Transm. Suppl.* **42,** 119–134.
78. Hof, P.R., Delacourte, A., and Bouras, C. (1992) Distribution of cortical neurofibrillary tangles in progressive supranuclear palsy: a quantitative analysis of six cases. *Acta Neuropathol. (Berl.)* **84,** 45–51.
79. Verny, M., Duyckaerts, C., Agid, Y., and Hauw, J.J. (1996) The significance of cortical pathology in progressive supranuclear palsy: clinicopathological data in 10 cases. *Brain* **119,** 1123–1136.
80. Braak, H., Jellinger, K., Braak, E., and Bohl, J. (1992) Allocortical neurofibrillary changes in progressive supranuclear palsy. *Acta Neuropathol. (Berl.)* **84,** 478–483.
81. Brandel, J.P., Hirsch, E.C., Malessa, S., Duyckaerts, C., Cervera, P., and Agid, Y. (1991) Differencial vulnerability of cholinergic projections to the emdiodorsal nucleus of the thalamus in senile dementia af Alzheimer type and progressive supranuclear plasy. *Neuroscience* **41,** 25–31.
82. Craig, A.H., Cummings, J.L., Fairbanks, L., et al. (1996) Cerebral blood flow correlates of apathy in Alzheimer's disease. *Arch. Neurol.* **53,** 116–1120.
83. Ot, B.R., Noto, R.B., and Fogel, B.S. (1996) Apathy ands loss of insight in Alzheimer's disease: a SPECT imaging study. *J. Neuropsychiatry Clin. Neurosci.* **8,** 41–46.
84. Devinski, O., Morrel, M.J., and Vogt, V.A. (1995) Contribution of anterior cingulate cortex to behavior. *Brain* **118,** 279–306.
85. Migneco, O., Benoit, M., Koulibali, P.M., et al. (2001) Perfusion brain SPECT and statistical parametric mapping analysis indicate that apathy is a cingulated syndrome: a study in Alzheimer's disease and nondemented patients. *Neuroimage* **13,** 896–902.
86. Volkow, N.D. and Tancredi, L. (1987) Neural substrates of violent behavior: a preliminary study with positron emission tomography. *Br. J. Psychiatry* **151,** 668–673.
87. Amen, D.G., Stubblefield, M., Carmichael, B., and Thisted, R. (1996) Brain SPECT findings and aggressiveness. *Ann. Clin. Psychiatry* **8,** 129–137.
88. Goyer, P.F., Andreason, P.J., Semple, W.E., et al. (1994) Positron emission tomography and personality disorders. *Neuropsychopharmacology* **10,** 21–28.
89. Sultzer, D.L., Mahler, M.E., Mandelkern, M.A., et al. (1995) The relationship between psychiatric symptoms and regional cortical metabolism in Alzheimer's disease. *J. Neuropsychiatry Clin. Neurosci.* **7,** 476–484.
90. Hirono, N., Mega, M.S., Dinov, I.D., et al. (2000) Left frontotemporal hypoperfusion is associated with aggression in patients with dementia. *Arch. Neurol.* **57,** 861–866.
91. Tekin, S., Mega, M.S., Masterman, D.M., et al. (2001) Orbitofrontal and anterior cingulate cortex neurofibrillary tangle burden is associated with agitation in Alzheimer disease. *Ann. Neurol.* **49,** 355–361.

27

Diagnosis and Treatment of Depression in Parkinson's Disease

Vladimir S. Kostić, MD, PhD, Elka Stefanova, MD, PhD, Nataša Dragašević, MD, and Saška Potrebić, MD

1. INTRODUCTION

Depression and anxiety are the most common and frequently disabling psychiatric conditions that accompany Parkinson's disease (PD). Although James Parkinson, in his original report of six patients, wrote that the "senses and intellect being uninjured" *(1)*, he still used descriptions like "melancholy" and "unhappy sufferer." In early 1920s, some authors argued that "abnormal psychic functioning" was a part of the disease process and that "the mental set was always depressive" *(2)*. Nowadays, it is widely accepted that, despite discrepancies in patient selection, inconsistent definitions of depression, and different methods of assessment, a considerable risk of depression appears to accompany PD. Depressive symptoms in parkinsonian patients have been classified as "organic mood syndrome" in the Diagnostic and Statistical Manual of Mental Disorders, third edition, revised (DSM-IIIR) and as "mood disorder due to a general medical condition" in DSM-IV. Although the exact etiology of depression in PD is unclear, available evidence suggests that biochemical changes, psychosocial factors, and situational stressors may all contribute to its development *(3)*. Finally, although major depression (MD) may occur in PD, studies indicate that the majority of depressed parkinsonians have less severe forms such as minor depression, dysthymic disorder, and subsyndromal forms *(4–6)*.

Over the past decade, significant breakthroughs have been made in our capacity to treat depression. Yet, after an extensive literature search, Klaassen et al. *(7)* stated that "the disappointing conclusion of this review is that the question of how depression in PD should be treated cannot be answered authoritatively."

2. FREQUENCY OF DEPRESSION IN PD

Depression occurs more frequently in patients with PD than in age-matched population. Gotham and colleagues *(8)* reviewed 14 studies comprised of 1500 parkinsonian patients and estimated a mean depression prevalence of 46% (range: 20–90%). The mean frequency of depression associated with PD reported in 26 studies summarized in a more recent review of Cummings *(9)* was 43% (range 4–70%). The author noted that the lowest reported frequencies were found in studies that had been done before standardized psychiatric instruments were in general use. More recent studies revealed similar estimates of depression prevalence in PD. Starkstein et al. *(6)* compared the prevalence of MD and dysthymia in the classic tremor-dominant versus akinetic-rigid form of PD. No difference was found for dysthymia (classic PD: 31%; akinetic-rigid PD: 32%), but patients with the akinetic-rigid

From: *Mental and Behavioral Dysfunction in Movement Disorders*
Edited by: M-A. Bédard et al. © Humana Press Inc., Totowa, NJ

form of PD had a significantly higher prevalence of MD (38 vs 15%, respectively). Our experience is close to their findings. In 247 consecutive PD patients, blindly to the neurological data, we applied the standardized psychiatric instruments according to the DSM-IIIR and found that 63 (25.5%) of our patients met the criteria for MD and 42 (17%) for minor depression *(10)*. Applying DSM-IV criteria, Giladi et al. *(11)* identified depression in one-third of 172 consecutive patients with long-standing PD (mean symptom duration of 12 yr). In a study using the Geriatric Depression Scale, out of 102 patients with PD living at home, most of them being moderately to severely disabled (28% belonged to stage 4 and 5 of the Hoehn and Yahr staging system), moderate and severe depressive symptoms were found in 47% and 5%, respectively *(12)*. In one retrospective study, the incidence rate of depression in PD was 1.86%/yr, and the cumulative risk was 8.6%, suggesting that the incidence of depression was increased in PD in comparison to age-matched population *(13)*. In a recent survey of 80 consecutive PD patients, examined with the depression module of the Structured Clinical Interview for DSM-Depression to confirm or reject the DSM-IV diagnosis of depressive disorder, MD was diagnosed in 13 patients (16%), disthymic disorder in 18 patients (22%), whereas 6 patients were signed as "depressive disorder not otherwise specified" (7%).

Most studies have covered patients consecutively referred to tertiary or quaternary centers, and these results might be different from population-based studies. Therefore, Hantz et al. *(14)*, used the 30-item General Health Questionnaire and the Structured Clinical Interview for DSM-IIIR-Non-Patient Version to study 73 patients with PD, each living in the community, and found the lowest published rate of MD (2.7%). In another community-based study, comprising 245 patients with PD, only 7.7% met the criteria for MD *(4)*. Although this study also suggested that the prevalence of MD in PD was lower than previously reported, the authors observed a significant percentage of patients (45.5%) that experienced mild depressive symptoms. In a sample of 139 patients with PD from Rogaland County (Norway), Aarsland et al. *(15)* applied a caregiver-based structured interview and reported depression (38% of patients) and hallucinations (27%) to be the most common psychiatric problems. In a more recent, population-based study, 19.6% of 97 patients with PD had moderate to severe depression (Beck Depression Inventory [BDI] ≥ 18) *(16)*.

3. CHARACTERISTICS OF DEPRESSION IN PD

The profile of depression associated with PD is not the same as that described in patients with primary depression, which is characterized by greater anxiety and less self-punitive ideation (elevated levels of dysphoria and pessimism about the future, sadness, irritability, and suicidal ideation), but without, or at least with less, guilt, self-blame, feelings of failure, and punishment in depressed PD patients. The other subtle differences from idiopathic mood disorders include a relative lack of hallucinations and delusions and a low suicidal rate *(17)*. This pattern is also a frequent finding in older nonparkinsonian depressed patients.

There appears to be a special relationship between anxiety and depression in PD. Henderson et al. *(18)* found that depression in combination with symptoms of panic and/or anxiety occurred in 38% of PD patients and in only 8% of healthy spouse controls. Menza et al. *(19)* reported that 92% of PD patients with anxiety had a co-morbid depressive disorder, and vice versa, 67% of depressed parkinsonians also had an anxiety disorder diagnosis, most frequently the panic disorder, phobic disorder, and generalized anxiety disorder *(20)*. Surveys indicate that some PD patients develop anxiety before the parkinsonian motor signs *(21)*.

Risk factors for depression in PD, although questioned in some studies, include early-onset of parkinsonian features, a family history of PD, impaired cognition, the presence of psychosis, female gender, right-sided parkinsonism, and akinetic-rigid presentation of the disease *(22)*. Although the discussion of clinical correlates of depression in PD is beyond the scope of this manuscript, it is important to note that no association, or only modest correlation between the degree of physical impairment and the degree of depression in PD has been found *(9)*. Even then, the correlation was not sufficiently

Table 1
Symptom Criteria for MD

Two-week period of depressed mood or loss of interest or pleasure in activities.
Presence of five or more of the following:
- Depressed mood.
- Diminished interest or pleasure in activities.
- Weight change or appetite change.
- Sleep changes.
- Psychomotor agitation or retardation.
- Fatigue or loss of energy.
- Feelings of worthlessness or guilt.
- Difficulty concentrating.
- Thoughts of death or suicide.

Adapted from ref. *22a*.

strong to support motor disability as a primary determinant of depression in PD. Studies of PD suggest that depressive symptoms often precede those of motor dysfunction (in 15–25% patients) *(23)*, which favor hypothesis that depression in PD occurs as a primary consequence of neurodegeneration *(4)*.

4. DIAGNOSIS AND ASSESSMENT OF DEPRESSION IN PD

Even for the experienced clinician, the evaluation of depressive symptoms that accompany certain medical illness can be a diagnostic challenge. In one report, 103 nondemented PD patients were examined by neurologists, who were then asked to report their immediate impression of depression. These patients were then administered the BDI to determine whether depressive criteria were met. The two assessments agreed in only 35% *(24)*. In the DSM-IV, depressed mood (>2 wk) or anhedonia must be associated with at least five of nine symptoms (Table 1) in order to satisfy the criteria for a major depressive episode. These symptoms, in order to be considered in the diagnosis, cannot be due to a general medical condition, and, therefore, DSM-IV criteria technically exclude a diagnosis of MD or dysthymic disorder in PD. Zesiewicz et al. *(3)* stated that, nonetheless, the remaining DSM-IV criteria can be used to evaluate and classify the depression associated with PD and that they are widely accepted as a standardized method of evaluation. The DSM-IV divides depressive disorders into several categories, although such separation of problems into clear-cut groups is not always easy *(25)*. For instance, almost half of PD patients with depressive symptoms do not meet the criteria for MD or dysthymia and may be classified as "subsyndromal symptomatic depression" *(26)*. The diagnosis of depression in PD can be confounded by an overlap of the motor features of PD and the clinical features of depression. Namely, slowness, masked faces, sad appearance, fatigue, sleeplessness, weight loss, sweating, poor concentration, loss of energy, early morning waking, and increased urinary frequency were observed in both depressed and nondepressed PD patients. Such symptom overlap is a well-recognized diagnostic problem in PD and makes global assessments, solely based on an observer or self-rating, of doubtful validity *(8)*. Therefore, Valldeoriola et al. *(27)* suggest that weight change, sleep disturbances, motor retardation, and fatigue should be viewed with caution or completely excluded as the diagnostic criteria for depression in PD. However, some results, quite conversely, suggest that the occurrence of some of these signs (sleep problems, pain, and fatigue) in PD patients should indicate examination for the presence of depression. Starkstein et al. *(28)* reported that anorexia, pain, loss of libido, and sleep disturbances were very characteristic of depressed PD patients and uncommon in non-depressed parkinsonians. The prevalence of severe pain was twice as high in depressed in comparison with nondepressed parkinsonians *(29)*. Contrary to these data, Menza and Rosen *(30)* reported that although depression and anxiety correlated with some sleep measures, neither contributed significantly to the overall variance in sleep quality, favoring the disease process itself as a main contributor to sleep disturbances in PD *(31)*. Fatigue, a poorly understood symptom in PD, significantly correlated with depression, but not with the disease severity *(32)*, although many nondepressed patients also complained of fatigue. The available clinical data implicate that the occurrence of sleep disturbances, pain, or fatigue suggest that the diagnosis of depression in PD should be taken into consideration, primarily due to the fact that some of these symptoms withdraw readily after initiation of antidepressant therapy. In light of these data, Rabinstein and Shulman *(22)* suggested that a high index of suspicion is required to accurately identify depression in PD. Addressing the problem of symptom overlap, Hoogendijk and colleagues *(33)* formulated decision rules with which it is less difficult to attribute a symptom to either PD or MD. The first criterion was whether fluctuations of a depressive symptom coincided with fluctuations of motor symptoms and, the second one, whether the symptom was relieved by dopaminergic treatment. They proposed that positive answers suggested that the "depression" symptom probably had parkinsonian origin. By using this exclusion method, the authors observed decrease in the prevalence of the DSM-IIIR diagnosis of MD from 23 to 13% in PD patients. The somatic items "psychomotor retardation–agitation" and "loss of energy–fatigue," and to a certain degree "loss of interest," showed an overlap with PD symptoms. However, all of their nine excluded patients fitted the criteria for the DSM-IV category "mood disorder due to a general medical condition."

The same reasons of overlapping questioned the usefulness of clinical rating scales for quantification and diagnosis of depression. For instance, the use of the BDI in PD patients has been criticized, since several parkinsonian features could affect several of its items (body image, work inhibition, fatigability, and somatic preoccupation) *(34)*. Therefore, Cantello et al. *(34)* has consistently used a revised version of the BDI (shortened BDI), which omits these four items. However, Levin et al. *(35)* confirmed that these items on the BDI did not influence the validity of this measure of depression associated with PD. Conversely, Leentjens et al. *(36)* found that the psychometric properties of the BDI for parkinsonian population are not ideal and that the widely used standard cut-off scores are not appropriate for these patients. The authors suggested the additional use of diagnostic criteria. The same group *(37)* however, justified the use of the 17-item Hamilton Rating Scale for Depression (HDRS) and the Montgomery-Asberg Depression Rating Scale to measure depressive symptoms in both depressed and nondepressed PD patients, to diagnose depressive disorder in PD, and to dichotomize patient samples into depressed and nondepressed groups. The concurrent validity of both rating scales with the DSM-IV criteria for depressive disorder was high.

4.1. The Importance of Diagnosing Depression

Depression may have an impact on several aspects of PD, such as the basic parkinsonian symptomatology, response to drugs, cognition, sleep, fatigability, and appetite. Melamed *(23)* suggests that "in a patient with a more advanced illness who is optimally managed, a sudden motor deterioration without an obvious cause, … , may be a result of the development of depression." In a study of 101 patients with PD, those who were depressed showed reduced functional activity and increased motor disability than patients without depression *(5)*. On multiple regression analyses, depression predicted impaired social, role, and physical functioning in PD patients *(38)*. Moreover, a longitudinal study by Starkstein et al. *(39)* showed that those PD patients with initially associated MD compared to nondepressed patients or those with minor depression had significantly greater cognitive decline, as well as greater deterioration in Activities of Daily Living (ADLs) scores. Therefore, Tom and Cummings *(40)* suggested that "treatment of depression in patients with PD may significantly slow cognitive decline, deterioration in ADLs, and progression to the more advanced stages of the disease." There is an increased risk of morbidity and mortality from the coexisting medical condition *(17)*. Cognitive functions are also adversely affected by the coexistence of depression. In a prospective cohort study of nondemented patients with PD, the coexistence of depressive features was associated with a significantly greater risk of developing dementia *(41)*. In recent studies, depression in PD patients was the factor that explained the largest part of the experienced alterations of the quality of life *(42,43)*. Interestingly enough, the most commonly "accused" physical disability in PD made only a small contribution to the decrease in the health-related quality of life *(42)*. Therefore, to improve the quality of life in PD patients, it is necessary to make every effort for early recognition and successful treatment of depression *(43)*.

5. TREATMENT OF DEPRESSION IN PD

The effective treatment of depression in PD is often multifaceted and frequently involves one or more treatment modalities such as psychotherapy, medication, and, rarely, electroconvulsive therapy (ECT). In addition to initiating pharmacotherapy, a neurologist must be aware that a part of the depression in PD may be situational and that even a discrete support and guidance by the neurologist will have beneficial effects.

In selecting a pharmacological agent, attention should initially focus an individual patient's profile, the potential adverse effects, and the pharmacodynamic issues of both aging and polypharmacy. Menza et al. *(19)* found that 92% of PD patients who had anxiety also suffered from a concomitant depressive disorder, while 67% of the depressed PD patients experienced an anxiety disorder. The prevalence and serious consequences of co-morbid depression and anxiety in PD emphasizes the need for those antidepressant agents that can effectively treat both depression and anxiety disorders.

The majority of PD patients belong to the geriatric population. Aging is accompanied by physiological changes that produce higher concentrations of pharmacologically active drugs than would be achieved with the same dose in a younger individual. Therefore, psychotropic drugs in the elderly parkinsonians should be started at a dosage that is 25–50% of the standard adult dosage. Elderly depressed PD patients may show slower resolution of symptoms, and patience on both sides may be necessary. But, once the patient responds to pharmacotherapy, full dosage medication should be continued for at least 6 mo to 1 yr post-remission. The patient should be informed that an antidepressant medication must be maintained for two or more weeks before improvement can be expected. Parallel intake of other antiparkinsonian drugs, as well as this delayed antidepressive response, contribute to poor compliance as the major obstacle to successful long-term antidepressant treatment. Lasser et al. *(44)* suggest a "family approach" for improving compliance. Prior to declaring treatment failure, patients should receive 8–12 wk of the maximally tolerated dosage of a particular antidepressant, when the switch to an antidepressant from another class can be accomplished.

Despite the high frequency of depression in PD, surprisingly few studies have focused the issue of its optimal treatment. After an extensive literature search, Klaassen et al. *(7)* found only 12 controlled studies of treatment efficacy of antidepressants in PD with major methodological problems in the majority of them. Recently, in a survey of antidepressant drug use in PD, Richard and Kurlan *(45)* analyzed the answers of 49 investigators (caring for approx 23,140 PD patients) and found that they used selective serotonin (5-HT) re-uptake inhibitors (SSRIs) as the first-line therapy 51% of the time, tricyclic antidepressants 41% of the time, and other agents 8% of the time.

5.1. Depression and Antiparkinsonian Medication

The relationship between depression and antiparkinsonian therapy is controversial. Some authors described increased vulnerability to depression at times of rapid deterioration of motor symptoms: even in patients with daily fluctuations, greater depression was found during the "off" periods *(46)*. Anecdotal clinical observations that emotional status often changes predictably with levodopa administration were substantiated to a certain degree in a study that showed that at least momentary changes in depressive mood and anxiety may be a consequence of intracerebral dopamine (DA) depletion and repletion *(46)*. However, for the long-term, the response of depression to levodopa was generally disappointing. Yahr et al. *(47)* mentioned that in most of their patients who started to receive levodopa, a feeling of apathy and depression was replaced by one of well-being and renewed interest in family life. In contrast, Damasio et al. *(48)* observed that 13 out of 30 patients with PD were depressed 2 mo after starting levodopa therapy. Also, Marsh and Markham *(49)* found that levodopa may aggravate depression in some PD patients. Levodopa administration for up to 6 mo in dosages sufficient to improve motor function has only minor effects on cognitive function and induces only small decreases in scores of depression *(50)*. In a prospective study of 34 *de novo* patients with PD, Choi et al. *(51)* evaluated long-term effects of levodopa (6–28 mo of follow-up) and found that this therapy did not alter "parkinsonian depression." Therefore, it is widely accepted that for the long-term, levodopa is not an effective antidepressant in PD.

There is an interesting, although controversial, possibility of the relationship between anxiety and levodopa therapy in PD *(20)*. Vazquez et al. *(52)* found that panic attacks were related to levodopa therapy, which is in accordance with the observation that anxiety fluctuations may be an important component of levodopa-induced fluctuations. However, other studies failed to find significant correlation between anxiety and the levodopa dose, suggesting that the role of levodopa in anxiety accompanying PD is unlikely *(19)*.

In several studies dealing with MD, bromocriptine has had efficacy comparable with standard antidepressants *(53)* and appears useful in antidepressant-resistant depression *(54)* and in relapses during treatment with SSRIs *(55)*. In one study *(56)*, short-term high dose bromocriptine (85–220 mg/d) improved depression in ten PD patients. However, high doses of bromocriptine, besides dopaminergic, have been considered to stimulate other neurotransmitter systems. Pergolide, another ergot-derived DA agonist, has no effect on depression in PD *(57)*. In relation to the hypothesis implicating the DA system in modulation of mood, of some interest may be a report on a case of a PD patient who developed an acute episode of mania caused by a single subcutaneous injection of apomorphine (2 mg) *(58)*.

Some of the new, D_3 receptor-preferring agonists may have a potential effect on the depression that accompanies PD, presumably acting postsynaptically at D_3 receptors in the mesolimbic system. Pramipexole (mean daily dose 0.7 mg), used as an adjunct to antidepressants, was effective in 50% of patients with bipolar and in 40% of those with unipolar depression *(59)*. Experience from the open label studies has been confirmed in a double-blind randomized placebo-controlled parallel-group clinical trial that compared pramipexole, fluoxetine, and placebo in 174 patients with MD *(60)*. After 8 wk, pramipexole proved to be superior to placebo in alleviating symptoms of depression (dose of 1 mg/d has the best balance between efficacy and tolerability). Thus, the D_3 receptor-preferring agonists may offer PD patients a broader spectrum of antiparkinsonian efficacy than the traditional DA agonists.

Amantadine, originally introduced into pharmacotherapy as an antiviral compound, was shown to have multiple pharmacological effects on the central nervous system (CNS), including antiparkinsonian and, also, certain antidepressant properties. Flaherty and Bellur *(61)* reported that, among the side effects in a normal hospital employee population taking amantadine for influenza prophylaxis, was mood elevation. This is in accordance with the observation that the drug may alleviate depressive symptoms in elderly patients who do not meet the criteria for MD *(40)*. Amantadine appears to show significant antidepressant efficacy comparable to standard antidepressants in patients with Borna disease virus infection, with an explanation that such effect may be a result of its antiviral properties, although it may also act through several mechanisms suggested to be involved in mood regulation (i.e., as an N-methyl-D-aspartate receptor antagonist) *(62)*.

The rationale for the use of catechol-O-methyltransferase (COMT) inhibitors in PD is the possibility to prolong the pharmacological half-life of levodopa in the plasma and brain. However, studies in animal models of depression revealed their potential antidepressant properties *(63)*. This hypothesis was substantiated with promising results in one open study that enrolled 21 patients with major depressive disorder *(64)*. One possibility is that co-administration of COMT inhibitors and levodopa may have antidepressant effect through an increase in DA mechanisms. Another interesting possibility is that COMT inhibition by itself may induce increase in S-adenosyl-L methionine (SAM), whose decreased levels have been linked to depression *(65)*. Interestingly enough, in an open label study, Di Rocco et al. *(66)*, with 13 depressed PD patients who failed to benefit or had been unable to tolerate other antidepressants, showed that SAM administration may improve depression.

The possible effects of different types of surgery for PD on depressive symptoms that may accompany this disease are still far from being conclusive. Recently, Bejjani et al. *(67)* reported that although stimulation of the left subthalamic nucleus in one patient improved symptoms of PD, electrical stimulation through a second electrode positioned in the central region of the left substantia nigra induced a transient acute depression. Bezerra et al. *(68)* reported persistent MD that developed immediately after the left-sided pallidotomy in 5 out of 17 operated PD patients. Interestingly enough, the authors stated that "they were treated with an SSRI and improved markedly." Postoperative depression was also described after bilateral posteroventral pallidotomy *(69)*. However, Straits-Troster et al. *(70)* explored the multidimensional outcome of three neurosurgical interventions in PD (pallidotomy, pallidal, and thalamic deep brain stimulation), and 3 mo after surgery, all three groups showed significant mood improvement.

5.2. Tricyclic Antidepressants

Tricyclic antidepressants (TCAs), available for over three decades, have proved to be efficacious as both antidepressant and anxiolytic agents *(71)*. TCAs as a class are thought to be effective through re-uptake blockade of noradrenaline (NA) or 5-HT (or both) *(25)*.

In a limited number of studies, TCAs have been found to have beneficial effects on depression in PD *(72–76)*, and they might also have some antiparkinsonian effects. Out of 12 identified controlled studies of treatment efficacy for depression in PD, 5 utilized TCAs *(7)*. However, only one *(75)* was specifically designed to enroll patients who all had both PD and depression, while in the remaining studies, the number of depressed parkinsonians varied from 10–80% (mean: 41%). Clinical designs of these studies were mainly devoted to evaluation of the effects of TCAs on motor symptoms or headache control in PD *(7)*. The potentially most dangerous adverse effect of TCAs is a delay in cardiac conduction that may precipitate complete heart block. Among anticholinergic effects (dry mouth, blurred vision, constipation, urinary retention, precipitation of acute glaucoma, tremor) cognitive toxicity is most severe, with distracting confusion and delirium. TCAs can cause α-adrenergic blocking effects and, thereby, produce orthostatic hypotension. Antihistamine activity is linked to somnolence and fatigue, while 5-HT re-uptake blockade can lead to nausea, sexual dysfunction, and weight gain. These agents also have significant interactions with other drugs, such as monoamine oxidase inhibitors (MAOI) *(25)*.

For these reasons, the use of TCAs, especially in elderly and cognitively impaired parkinsonians is associated with severe limitations *(77)*. However, the use of the secondary amines (nortriptyline [initial nighttime dose of 20–40 mg] and desipramine [initial nighttime dose of 25–50 mg]) is recommended to minimize anticholinergic adverse effects, especially in PD patients whose depression is associated with restless agitation and insomnia *(22)*. These sedative properties are undesirable in anergic and withdrawn patients. Imipramine and desipramine may be recommended when depression is co-morbid with panic disorders, although in some patients, TCAs can exacerbate panic attacks *(70)*. Improvement of depressive symptoms in responders to desipramine or imipramine has been observed in some patients as early as the first week. Faster initial antidepressant effects occurring within 4–7 d have been described with amoxapine, but unfortunately, this agent produced extrapyramidal effects *(78)*.

5.3. SSRIs

The introduction of SSRIs has offered a new means for the treatment of depression in PD *(77)*. SSRIs have little impact on cognition, produce negligible anticholinergic (paroxetine may be an exception) and cardiovascular effects, and do not alter blood pressure, all of which make them particularly useful in elderly patients. They generally have a mild adverse effect profile, which includes weight

Table 2
Classification of Antidepressants with Potential Use in PD

Class	Generic name	Recommended dosage (mg/d)
Mixed 5-HT and NA reuptake inhibitors		
First-generation tricyclic antidepressants	Amitriptyline	75–300
	Clomipramine	100–250
	Doxepin	100–300
	Imipramine	100–300
	Trimipramine	100–300
Second-generation tricyclic antidepressants	Desipramine	100–300
	Nortriptyline	50–150
Tetracyclic antidepressant	Maprotiline	100–200
Triazolopyridines	Trazodone	150–400
MAOI		
Nonselective inhibitors of MAO-A and MAO-B	Phenelzine	60–90
	Tranylcypromine	20–60
	Selegiline[a]	30–60
Reversible inhibitors of MAO-A	Moclobemide	300–600
	Brofaromine	75–150
Selective 5-HT re-uptake inhibitors	Fluoxetine	20–60
	Sertraline	50–200
	Citalopram	20–80
	Fluvoxamine	100–300
	Paroxetine	20–50
5-HT and NA re-uptake inhibitors	Venlafaxine	75–350
5-HT_{2A} receptor antagonist	Nefazodone	200–600
	Trazodone	150–600
DA re-uptake inhibitor	Bupropion	200–450
Antagonist of α_2-receptors	Mirtazapine	14–45
NA re-uptake inhibitors	Reboxatine	Undetermined
	Viloxazine	100–400
GABAmimetics	Fengabine	900–1800

5HT, serotonin; NA, noradrenalin; GABA, γ-aminobutyric acid; DA, dopamine; MAO, monoamine oxidase.

[a]Loses its selectivity for MAO B in higher dosages.

loss, anorexia, somnolence, postural tremor, light-headedness, gastrointestinal disturbances, allergic reactions, and sexual dysfunction *(44)*. About 10–15% of particularly older patients experience "activating" effects (anxiety, restlessness, insomnia). Therefore, sertraline, due to its activating properties, may be helpful with morning dosing, while the more sedating paroxetine administered at bedtime. Each of the SSRIs (fluvoxamine, paroxetine, and fluoxetine, more than sertraline and citalopram) (Table 2) can potentially inhibit cytochrome P450 2D6 activity and, thus, affect metabolism of concomitantly administered medication. The shorter acting SSRIs (paroxetine, fluvoxamine) may be associated with a discontinuation syndrome, with tremor, nausea and vomiting, dysequilibrium, fatigue, myalgias, paresthesias, insomnia, anxiety, and diarrhea *(25)*. However, it seems that the benefit of SSRIs outweighs the potential problems due to adverse effects, and they are considered to be among the major treatment options for depression in PD *(22,40,77)*.

Paradoxically, in spite of these opinions, there are only few open label studies addressing the issues of their efficacy and tolerability in this clinical condition. Two open label studies suggested that sertraline reduced depression in PD patients, with additional beneficial effect on anxiety, without influencing motor function *(79,80)*. A 2-yr open label study with paroxetine found that 85% of depressed PD patients experienced a reduction in depressive symptoms *(81)*. In another open label study with paroxetine (20 mg/d) given to 33 nondemented depressed PD patients during 6 mo, Ceravolo et al. *(82)* reported significant improvement of depression, as evaluated by BDI and HDRS, without influence on parkinsonian symptoms. In only one patient was fully reversible worsening of tremor observed. However, paroxetine frequently may induce tremor as an adverse effect, with a prevalence of 1–2%. The dosages of SSRIs for depression in PD are the same as for depression in the general population. In a case report of a 55-yr-old depressed PD patient, depressive symptoms responded well to treatment with fluvoxamine (100 mg/d). Tryptophan depletion testing, which acutely lowers central 5-HT levels, caused a brief exacerbation of depression, which resolved again upon tryptophan repletion *(83)*. This "experiment" supports a serotonergic hypothesis for depression in PD *(84–86)*.

The major concern for the use of SSRIs in PD is that they may induce extrapyramidal symptoms and/or akathisia and aggravate parkinsonism. Several case reports described a reversible worsening of parkinsonism after 10–14 d (generally within the first month) of treatment with fluoxetine *(87,88)*, paroxetine *(89)*, and citalopram *(90)*. In a recent review, 127 reports of SSRI-induced movement disorders in nonparkinsonian subjects were identified, including 25 cases of parkinsonism *(91)*. One possible explanation is that SSRIs may inhibit metabolic production or release of DA. It has been shown that 5-HT_{2C} receptors exert a tonic suppressive influence on the activity of mesocortical DA pathways, as well as their mesolimbic and nigrostriatal counterparts *(92)*. Finally, fluoxetine at higher doses (40 mg/d) may reduce levodopa-induced dyskinesia in PD patients, supporting the idea that this drug has some antidopaminergic properties. Patients with PD, in whom DA levels are already reduced, may be particularly susceptible to such effects. However, clinical trials in PD patients failed to confirm significant worsening of extrapyramidal symptoms during the SSRIs use *(79,80)*. Montastruc et al. *(93)* found no changes in bradykinesia and rigidity in 14 nondepressed PD patients who were on fluoxetine for 1 mo. In two retrospective studies, worsening of motor symptoms was observed in only small number of PD patients treated with SSRIs *(94,95)*. In a recent prospective study comprising 65 depressed PD outpatients treated with paroxetine (10–20 mg/d) for at least 3 mo, 2 out of 52 patients who completed the study (3%) experienced worsening of parkinsonian symptoms *(96)*. In conclusion, although they should be used cautiously, at least during the first month of treatment, the SSRIs are regarded as the rational choice in the treatment of depression in PD *(3,22,40,77)*.

A reversible, but potentially dangerous condition known as the "serotonin syndrome" has been reported to occur in rare cases when SSRIs are given alone or in combination with MAOIs, leading to the recommendation against giving selegiline and an antidepressant (SSRI or TCA) simultaneously. The serotonin syndrome is a symptom complex of confusion, agitation, myoclonus, diaphoresis, hyperreflexia, diarrhea, tremor, shivering, incoordination, and fever (at least three of these symptoms have to be present for the diagnosis). Most cases of the serotonin syndrome are mild and respond to withdrawal of serotonergic drugs, but rare cases may be associated with seizures, coma, and rarely death. The interaction between selegiline and SSRIs is of special importance in PD, but it does not appear to occur with the typical daily dose of selegiline used in PD (10 mg/d). In PD patients who were treated with both selegiline and sertraline or paroxetine *(97)* or selegiline and fluoxetine *(98)*, no adverse effects were noted from the combinations. In a survey of Parkinson Study Group, a serotonin-like syndrome was reported in only 11 of 4568 patients (0.24%) receiving both selegiline and an SSRI, but this condition was considered serious in only two patients (0.04%) *(99)*.

5.4. MAOIs

Classical irreversible MAOIs, such as phenelzine and tranylcypromine, have been used since the 1950s to treat depression, but with time, their usage has been reduced to cases of treatment-resistant depression. The reasons for this reduction are their adverse reactions, particularly the potentially fatal interaction with tyramine-containing foods and some pharmacological agents, with a hyperdopaminergic crisis (e.g., severe hypertension, hyperpyrexia, tachicardia, and diaphoresis), which has been reported in as many as 8% of patients receiving MAOI *(100)*. In preliminary studies, nomiphensine and phenelzine showed antidepressant efficacy in PD patients *(101–103)*. Fahn and Chouinard *(104)* evaluated tranylcypromine, a drug that inihibits both MAOs, in 37 patients with PD, as a possible neuroprotective agent based on the hypothesis that inhibition of MAO-A and MAO-B may reduce the generation of hydrogen peroxide and the subsequent free radical species. Although their study was not focused on depression in PD, the authors simply stated that "depression lifted in all five patients who had this problem at the time tranylcypromine was initiated."

More recently, MAOIs that have specificity for one of the two different types of MAO have been developed. At dosages of <10 mg/d (dosages used in PD), selegiline, as an MAO-B inhibitor, is not associated with the catecholaminergic "cheese" reaction that may occur with MAO-A or combined MAO-A and MAO-B inhibitors. However, at dosages above 30 mg/d, selegiline loses its specificity and also inhibits MAO-A. Therefore, at these higher dosages, selegiline has the potential to cause a hypertension crisis if excessive dietary tyramine is consumed. Sunderland et al. *(105)* found that high-dose selegiline (60 mg/d), in a double-blind randomized cross-over study in comparison to placebo, induced significant improvement in the HDRS score (37.4% decrease), but not in subjective behavioral measures in 16 treatment-resistant older depressive patients. Another double-blind placebo-controlled study showed improvement of depression after 6 wk at 30 mg/d, while it was unchanged after 3 wk at 10 mg/d *(106)*. Therefore, the conclusion is that a higher dosage of selegiline (30–60 mg/d) appears to be necessary for effective treatment of depression *(107)*. These dosages are significantly higher than the dosage used in PD. However, in a multicenter double-blind randomized placebo-controlled trial, without specifying whether any patients met criteria for depression, the authors reported significant decrease in the HDRS scores after 3 mo of treatment with 10 mg/d of selegiline *(108)*. This may be in accordance with initially described features of selegiline as a "psychic energizer" and the findings that in untreated patients with mild PD selegiline enhanced a sense of well-being *(109)*.

Besides the already described syndrome induced by the combination of selegiline and fluoxetine, Ritter and Alexander *(110)* assessed the safety of combining selegiline with other antidepressants, found no selegiline drug interactions, and suggested that bupropion, TCAs, and trazodone, were reasonable choices in combination with this MAO-B inhibitor.

Moclobemide, a reversible inhibitor of MAO-A, is generally well-tolerated and, because it selectively binds to MAO-A, MAO-B is free to metabolize tyramine and, thus, there is no need for dietary restrictions. Moclobemide is also free from significant anticholinergic and orthostatic effects. Moclobemide has been found successful in treating both agitated and retarded forms of depression *(111)*, as well as in treating social phobia and panic disorders *(112)*. Takats et al. *(113)* reported its beneficial effects in the treatment of depression in PD. Jansen-Steur and Ballering *(114)* confirmed such antidepressant properties in PD patients with MD, but in the other branch of the study, the authors found that the combination of moclobemide (600 mg/d) and selegiline (10 mg/d), under tyramine restriction, had more pronounced efficacy on mood and cognitive performance than moclobemide monotherapy. In an open label study, we followed 17 PD patients with MD who were on optimal and stable dosage of antiparkinsonian medication during the preceding 6 mo. Administration of moclobemide (mean daily dosage 490 mg) caused significant and stable improvement in the course of a 3-mo follow-up (30–40% decrease in the HDRS score), which was worsened again 1 mo after moclobemide discontinuation (Fig. 1). No major side effects, and in particular, elevation of blood pressure, occurred during the co-administration of levodopa and moclobemide. Moreover, moclobemide exerts a mild antiparkinsonian effect in nondepressed PD patients *(115)*, without altering mood and cognitive measures. In 20 nondepressed patients with PD who developed levodopa-induced motor response fluctuations, we found that moclobemide (450 mg/d) as adjunct therapy moderately reduced "off" time duration by 27% *(116)*. Therefore, we suggested that moclobemide may be specially indicated in elderly or depressed fluctuating parkinsonian patients.

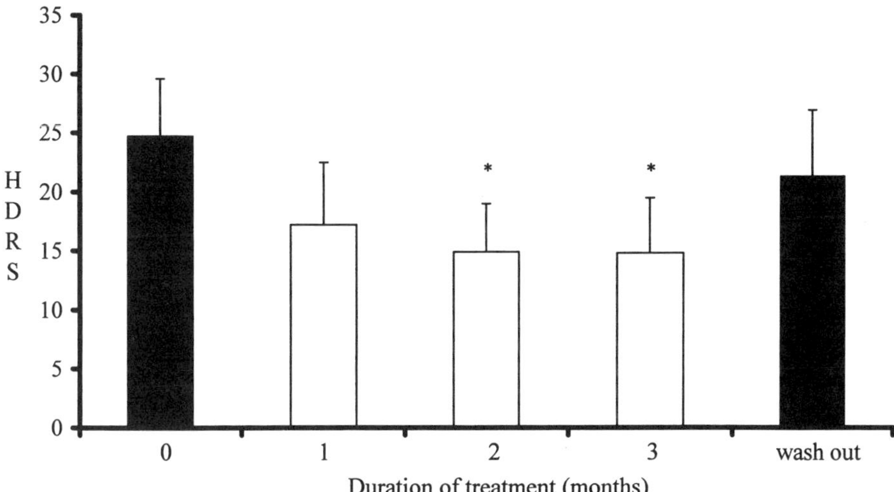

Fig. 1. HDRS scores before and in the course of 3-mo treatment (□) of 17 patients with PD and MD with moclobemide; the last column (■) present HDRS score 1 mo after moclobemide discontinuation. $*p < 0.05$.

5.5. *Newer Antidepressants*

Different agents collectively termed "newer antidepressants," such as buspirone, venlafaxine, nefazodone, and mirtazapine (Table 2), have appealing pharmacological profiles and may be beneficial in the treatment of depression that accompany PD, although controlled studies have not yet been carried out.

Buspiron has no effect on depression in PD patients *(117)* and although it has dopaminergic agonist effects similar to amfebutamone (bupropion), it worsens disability and anxiety ratings in nondepressed parkinsonians *(39)*. Bupropion, a monocyclic antidepressant, has a side effect profile similar to that of the SSRIs and is associated with an increased risk of seizures *(25)*. It showed limited efficacy in the treatment of depressive symptoms in PD *(118)* and was rather poorly tolerated by some patients. However, some authors still consider bupropion as "probably the first-line antidepressant… in PD" *(119)*, albeit without evidence. In only one case report, that on a 70-yr-old PD patient with drug-resistant depression, did Leentjens et al. *(120)* describe a quick and complete remission of depressive symptoms after bupropion administration.

Venlafaxine is specifically designed to produce antidepressant activity by blocking the re-uptake of both 5-HT and NA. Its pharmacological features include the possibility of a rapid response, efficacy for late-life depression, and efficacy in treating anxiety associated with depression and anxiety disorders *(121)*. It has a similar side effect profile to that of the SSRIs, but, also, the dose-related side effect of increased mean blood pressure *(25)*. Nefazodone, chemically related to trozodone, is a weaker 5-HT and NA re-uptake inhibitor, but a potent 5-HT_{2A} receptor antagonist *(121)*. The adverse effects include sedation, dizziness, nausea, and dry mouth. Reboxetine is the first selective NA re-uptake inhibitor to be introduced since the TCAs. Unfortunately, no guidelines or, at least, no preliminary studies are available for their administration in depressed PD patients.

Mirtazapine differs from other new dual-acting antidepressants by not being a re-uptake inhibitor. It directly enhances NA neurotransmission by the blockade of α_2-autoreceptors. The rapid increase in 5-HT synaptic levels by the blockade of α_2-heteroreceptors indirectly enhances 5-HT_{1A}-mediated neurotransmission, since mirtazapine blocks 5-HT_2 and 5-HT_3 receptors *(122)*. Mirtazapine is effective in all levels of severity of depressive illness, as well as in a broad range of symptoms associated with depression, including anxiety symptoms and sleep disturbances, with a potentially faster onset of overall therapeutic efficacy. Transient somnolence, hyperphagia, and weight gain are the most commonly reported adverse events, which may be attributed to the antihistaminic (H_1) activity of mirtazapine at low doses, since somnolence appears to be less frequent at higher doses *(123)*. The low potential for interaction with drugs that are metabolized by CYP2D6 make mirtazapine an important option for the treatment of MD in patients who require polytherapy. Mirtazapine has been shown to be efficacious in the elderly *(123)*. However, this interesting antidepressant has not been studied in depression accompanying PD. Instead, there is a report that mirtazapine reduces or eliminates parkinsonian tremor, action tremor, and levodopa-induced dyskinesia in five PD patients *(124)*.

5.6. *ECT*

Treatment with ECT should be considered for patients who do not respond to antidepressant agents, who are not able to wait for the response to psychoactive drugs, or who have cardiovascular conditions that put them at high risk of complications from antidepressant agents (e.g., heart block or orthostatic hypotension). ECT is also a treatment modality available for the therapy of depression in PD *(125)* with parallel and transient improvement in motor signs (rigidity and bradykinesia more than tremor) as well *(126)*. The favorable response for the extrapyramidal motor symptoms usually antedates the antidepressant response, but motor symptoms also relapse more quickly *(40)*. Patients may relapse into depressive episode from 1 wk to 6–12 mo after ECT *(125)*. Moellentine et al. *(127)* compared, in a retrospective study, the outcomes of 25 PD patients receiving ECT for psychiatric indications with outcomes of age- and sex-matched patients without neurological disease also receiving ECT for psychiatric indication. No difference in efficacy of ECT was found between the two groups. Although short-term efficacy rates for ECT exceed or are comparable to those of pharmacotherapy, studies on maintenance ECT remain sparse. Maintenance ECT proved to be beneficial in some nondepressed and nondemented patients with drug refractory PD or PD with intolerance to antiparkinsonian drugs or who relapsed after having responded to an initial course of ECT *(128)*. The antiparkinsonian and, possibly, antidepressant effects of ECT involve the dopaminergic and serotonergic mechanisms *(40)*.

Rubinstein and Shulman *(22)* stated that, despite all these data, ECT as a therapy for depression in PD is rarely appropriate, since intractable MD and suicidal ideation are rare in PD. Also, PD patients, especially those with cognitive impairment, are more susceptible to different ECT-related adverse effects, such as confusion or prolonged delirium *(125)*.

5.7. *Transcranial Magnetic Stimulation*

Transcranial magnetic stimulation, given as a single pulse (TMS) or as a train of repetitive stimuli (rTMS), causes cortical neurons just below the skull to depolarize in response to the electrical current generated in them by rapid oscillation in the magnetic field. Since the preliminary animal evidence suggests that rTMS is similar to electroconvulsive shock in animal models of depression, several groups investigated whether rTMS might have antidepressant activity. Early open studies used low frequency rTMS (0.3–1 Hz) over the cranial vertex and revealed some antidepressant effect. A number of sham-controlled studies showed that daily stimulation with both high-frequency rTMS (5–20 Hz) over the left dorsolateral prefrontal cortex (DLPFC) *(129)* and right prefrontal slow rTMS (0.5–1 Hz) have probable antidepressant effects *(130)*. The selection of this region for rTMS in depression was based on the imaging findings of abnormal prefrontal function in depression and the evidence that modulation of prefrontal function was linked to the efficacy of ECT *(131)*. In normal volunteers, high frequency rTMS over the left DLPFC transiently induced dysphoria, but elevated mood over the right DLPFC *(132)*. However, this effect of lateralization on mood in patients with MD has been found to be the opposite to lateralization findings in healthy volunteers. The explanation for lateralization findings in antidepressant efficacy of fast or slow frequency rTMS is based on the suggestion that mood disorders may result from a relative imbalance of frontal lobe function, wherein depression occurs with a

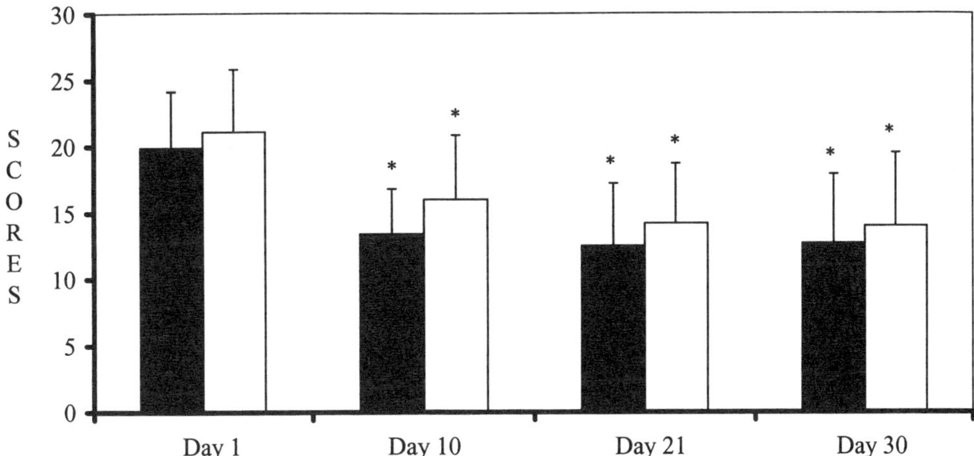

Fig. 2. HDRS (■) and BDI scale (□) scores before (Day 1) and after 10 consecutive days of slow repetitive (0.5 Hz) TMS (Day 10), as well as during the follow-up (Day 21 and Day 30) after finishing the stimulation protocol. $*p < 0.05$.

hypofunctioning left frontal lobe and the findings that both fast and slow frequency rTMS induce immediate cortical suppression, but only the fast frequency one produces subsequent cortical excitation.

In an open study that comprised 10 depressed PD patients, we found that daily sessions of slow rTMS (frequency 0.5 Hz; field intensity 10% above the motor threshold) over both prefrontal regions (100 stimuli per prefrontal region daily) during 10 consecutive days induced moderate, but significant, decrease in the HDRS (33–37%) and the BDI scores (24–34%), which persisted 3 wk after finishing the stimulation (Fig. 2). In parallel, we also observed mild improvement (18–20% on Unified Parkinson's Disease Rating Scale [UPDRS]) of motor symptoms, the effect already observed in previous studies *(133)*.

The rTMS shares many of the behavioral and biochemical actions of ECT and other antidepressant treatments. It acutely modulates DA and 5-HT content and turnover rates and chronically affects the intracellular mechanisms regulating neuroplasticity, modulates cortical β-adrenergic receptors, increases N-methyl-D-aspartate receptors in various brain regions, reduces frontal cortex 5-HT_2 receptors, and induces subsensitivity of presynaptic serotonergic autoreceptor activity, which was previously observed after other antidepressant treatments *(134)*.

Given the speed of antidepressant effects and motor improvement with rTMS, as well as the known and substantial delay in improvement with the common antidepressant medication, one of the potential strategies for rTMS use may be the role of "an augmentation agent to hasten clinical response in pharmacologically treated" patients with PD and depression *(134)*.

5.8. Sleep Deprivation

Patients with MD, in contrast to normal subjects, often show marked improvements in mood after a night of sleep loss, which are quickly extinguished after subsequent sleep. Abnormalities of rapid eye movement (REM) sleep are also frequently observed in patients with a major depressive disorder *(135)*. We also found significant shortening of REM sleep latency in depressed compared to nondepressed PD patients *(31)*. A special role for the REM sleep in depression is supported by the well-known REM sleep suppression effect of most antidepressants and by the antidepressant effect of selective REM deprivation by awakenings *(135)*. Therefore, several paradigms of sleep deprivation (selective

REM sleep deprivation, total sleep deprivation, early and late partial sleep deprivation) have been tested, and it has been suggested that sleep deprivation might improve depression *(136)*. Moreover, the preliminary observation suggests that combined therapy with total sleep deprivation plus paroxetine may be twice as successful at achieving rapid response in elderly depressed patients than conventional monotherapy with paroxetine or placebo *(137)*.

Total sleep deprivation may relieve the depressive symptoms in PD *(138)*. Bertolucci et al. *(139)* reported that total sleep deprivation for one night improved depression ratings by 26%, but also had beneficial effects on parkinsonian motor signs. Interestingly enough, such improvement in depression scores was sustained for 8 d. Future studies are needed to clarify this approach of doubtful clinical utility.

6. CONCLUSION

A significant proportion of PD patients suffer from depression. Depression in PD can lead to a significant reduction in functional abilities and cognitive measures and has a profound negative impact on a patient's sense of well-being and functioning. Therefore, early recognition and effective treatment of depressive symptoms should be of great benefit. Although only few placebo-controlled studies of antidepressant therapy in PD have been reported so far, there is no doubt that depression in PD is a treatable, albeit undertreated condition (in a survey of Richard and Kurlan *[45]*, only 26% of PD patients receive pharmacotherapy for depression). Presently, "there are no established first-choice antidepressant drugs for patients with PD" *(40)*, and, therefore, proposals for an algorithmic approach to the pharmacological treatment of these patients reflect more the author's position than the evidence-based conclusions. Unfortunately, until well-designed clinical trials have been performed, the selection of antidepressant medication in PD will be largely driven by the differences in the side effect profiles of the available drugs *(22)* and by the personal experience of the clinician, as well.

REFERENCES

1. Parkinson, J. (1817) *An Essay on the Shaking Palsy*, Sherwood, Neely and Jones, London.
2. Jackson, J.A., Free, G.B.M., and Pike, H.V. (1923) The psychic manifestations in paralysis agitans, *Arch. Neurol.* **10,** 680–684.
3. Zesiewicz, T.A., Gold, M., Chari, G., and Hauser, R.A. (1999) Current issues in depression in Parkinson's disease. *Am. J. Geriatr. Psychiatry* **7,** 110–118.
4. Tandberg, E., Larsen, J.P., Aarsland, D., and Cummings, J.L. (1996) The occurrence of depression in Parkinson's disease: the community based study. *Arch. Neurol.* **53,** 175–179.
5. Liu, C.-Y., Wang, S.-J., Fuh, J.-L., Lin, C.-H., Yang Y.-Y., and Liu, H.-C. (1997) The correlation of depression with functional activity in Parkinson's disease. *J. Neurol.* **244,** 493–498.
6. Starkstein, S.E., Petricca, G., Shemerinski, E., et al. (1998) Depression in classic versus akinetic-rigid Parkinson's disease. *Mov. Disord.* **13,** 29–33.
7. Klaassen, T., Verhey, F.R., Sneijders, G.H., Rozendaal, N., de Vet, H.C., and van Praag, H.M. (1995) Treatment of depression in Parkinson's disease: a meta-analysis. *J. Neuropsychiatry Clin. Neurosci.* **7,** 281–286.
8. Gotham, A.M., Brown, R.G., and Marsden, C.D. (1986) Depression in Parkinson's disease: a quantitative and qualitative analysis. *J. Neurol. Neurosurg. Psychiatry* **49,** 381–389.
9. Cummings, J.L. (1992) Depression in Parkinson's disease: a review. *Am. J. Psychiatry* **149,** 443–454.
10. Kostić, V.S., Filipović, S.R., Lečić, D., Momcilovic, D., Sokic, D., and Šternić, N. (1994) Effect of age at onset on frequency of depression in Parkinson's disease. *J. Neurol. Neurosurg. Psychiatry* **57,** 1265–1267.
11. Giladi, N., Treves, T.A., Paleacu, D., et al. (2000) Risk factors for dementia, depression and psychosis in long-standing Parkinson's disease. *J. Neural. Transm.* **107,** 59–71.
12. Caap-Ahlgren, M. and Dehlin, O. (2001) Insomnia and depressive symptoms in patients with Parkinson's disease—relationship to health-related quality of life. An interview study of patients living at home. *Arch. Gerontol. Geriatr.* **32,** 23–33.
13. Doonief, G., Mirabello, E., Bell, K., Marder, K., Stern, Y., and Mayeux, R. (1992) An estimate of the incidence of depression in idiopathic Parkinson's disease. *Arch. Neurol.* **49,** 305–307.
14. Hantz, P., Caradoc-Davies, G., Caradoc-Davies, T., Weatherall, M., and Dixon, G. (1994) Depression in Parkinson's disease. *Am. J. Psychiatry* **151,** 1010–1014.
15. Aarsland, D., Larsen, J.P., Lim, N.G., et al. (1999) Range of neuropsychiatric disturbances in patients with Parkinson's disease. *J. Neurol. Neurosurg. Psychiatry* **67,** 492–496.

16. Schrag, A., Jahanshahi, M., and Quinn, N.P. (2001) What contributes to depression in Parkinson's disease? *Psychol. Med.* **31,** 65–73.
17. Brown, R. and Jahanshahi, M. (1995) Depression in Parkinson's disease: a psychosocial viewpoint. *Adv. Neurol.* **65,** 61–84.
18. Henderson, R., Kurlan, R., and Kersun, J.M. (1992) Preliminary examination of the comorbidity of anxiety and depression in Parkinson's disease. *J. Neuropsychiatry Clin. Neurosci.* **4,** 257–264.
19. Menza, M.A., Robertson-Hoffman, D.E., and Bonapace, A.S. (1993) Parkinson's disease and anxiety: comorbidity with depression. *Biol. Psychiatry* **34,** 465–470.
20. Walsh, K. and Bennett, G. (2001) Parkinson's disease and anxiety. *Postgrad. Med. J.* **77,** 89–93.
21. Shiba, M., Bower, J.H., Maraganore, D.M., et al. (2000) Anxiety disorders and depressive disorders preceding Parkinson's disease: a case-control study. *Mov. Disord.* **15,** 669–677.
22. Rabinstein, A.A. and Shulman, L.M. (2001) Management of behavioral and psychiatric problems in Parkinson's disease. *Parkinsonism Rel. Disord.* **7,** 41–50.
22a. American Psychiatric Association. (1994) Diagnostic and statistical manual of mental disorders (4th ed.). Washington, DC, APA.
23. Melamed, E. (1997) Neurobehavioral abnormalities in Parkinson's disease, in *Movement Disorders: Neurologic Principles and Practice* (Watts, R.L. and Koller, W.C., eds.), McGraw-Hill, New York, pp. 257–262.
24. Shulman, L.M., Leifert, R., Singer, C., and Weiner, W.J. (1997) The diagnostic accuracy of neurologists for anxiety, depression, fatigue, and sleep disorders in Parkinson's disease [abstract]. *Mov. Disord.* **12,** 127.
25. Sutor, B., Rummans, T.A., Jowsey, S.G., et al. (1998) Major depression in medically ill patients. *Mayo Clin. Proc.* **73,** 329–337.
26. Starkstein, S.E., Preziosi, T.J., Bolduc, P.L., and Robinson, R.G. (1990) Depression in Parkinson's disease. *J. Nerv. Ment. Dis.* **178,** 27–31.
27. Vallderiolla, F., Nobbe, F.A., and Tolosa, E. (1997) Treatment of behavioral disturbances in Parkinson's disease. *J. Neural. Transm.* **51,** 175–204.
28. Starkstein, S.E., Preziosi, T.J., Forrester, A.W., and Robinson, R.G. (1990) Specificity of affective and autonomic symptoms of depression in Parkinson's disease. *J. Neurol. Neurosurg. Psychiatry* **53,** 869–873.
29. Marinković, Z., Kostić, V.S., Šternić, N., and Marinković, S. (1990) Pain in Parkinson's disease. *Serb. Arch.* **118,** 459–462.
30. Menza, M.A. and Rosen, R.C. (1995) Sleep in Parkinson's disease: the role of depression and anxiety. *Psychosomatics* **36,** 262–266.
31. Kostić, V.S., Šušić, V., Przedborski, S., and Šternić, N. (1991) Sleep EEG in depressed and nondepressed patients with Parkinson's disease. *J. Neuropsychiatry Clin. Neurosci.* **3,** 99–103.
32. Friedman, J. and Friedman, H. (1993) Fatigue in Parkinson's disease. *Neurology* **43,** 2016–2018.
33. Hoogendijk, W.J.G., Sommer, I.E.C., Tissingh, G., Deeg, D.J.H., and Wolters, E.C. (1998) Depression in Parkinson's disease. *Psychosomatics* **39,** 416—421.
34. Cantello, R., Gilli, M., Riccio, A., and Bergamasco, B. (1986) Mood changes associated with end-of-dose-deterioration in Parkinson's disease. *J. Neurol. Neurosurg. Psychiatry* **49,** 1182–1190.
35. Levin, B.E., Llabre, M.M., and Weiner, W.J. (1988) Parkinson's disease and depression: psychometric properties of the Beck Depression Inventory. *J. Neurol. Neurosurg. Psychiatry* **51,** 1401–1404.
36. Leentjens, A.F.G., Verhey, F.R.J., Luijckx, G.-J., and Troost, J. (2000) The validity of the Beck Depression Inventory as a screening and diagnostic instrument for depression in patients with Parkinson's disease. *Mov. Disord.* **15,** 1221–1224.
37. Leentjens, A.F.G., Verhey, F.R.J., Lousberg, R., Spitsbergen, H., and Wilmink, F.W. (2000) The validity of the Hamilton and Montgomery-Asberg Depression Rating Scales as screening and diagnostic instrument for depression in patients with Parkinson's disease. *Int. J. Geriatr. Psychiatry* **15,** 644–649.
38. Cole, S.A., Woodard, J.L., Juncos, J.L., Kogos, J.L., Youngstrom, E.A., and Watts, R.L. (1996) Depression and disability in Parkinson's disease. *J. Neuropsychiatry Clin. Neurosci.* **8,** 20–25.
39. Starkstein, S.E., Mayberg, H.S., Leiguarda, R., Preziosi, T.J., and Robinson, R.G. (1992) A prospective longitudinal study of depression, cognitive decline, and physical impairments in patients with Parkinson's disease. *J. Neurol. Neurosurg. Psychiatry* **55,** 377–382.
40. Tom, T. and Cummings, J.L. (1998) Depression in Parkinson's disease: pharmacological characteristics and treatment. *Drugs Aging* **12,** 55–74.
41. Marder, K., Tang, M.X., Cote, L., Stern, Y., and Mayeux, R. (1995) The frequency and associated risk factors for dementia in patients with Parkinson's disease. *Arch. Neurol.* **52,** 695–701.
42. Karlsen, K.H., Larsen, J.P., Tandberg, E., and Maeland, J.G. (1999) Influence of clinical and demographic variables on quality of life in patients with Parkinson's disease. *J. Neurol. Neurosurg. Psychiatry* **66,** 431–435.
43. Kuopio, A.-M., Martilla, R.J., Helenius, H., Toivonen, M., and Rinne, U.K. (2000) The quality of life in Parkinson's disease. *Mov. Disord.* **15,** 216–223.
44. Lasser, R., Siegel, E., Dukoff, R., and Sunderland, T. (1998) Diagnosis and treatment of geriatric depression. *CNS Drugs* **9,** 17–30.
45. Richard, I.H. and Kurlan, R. (1997) A survey of antidepressant drug use in Parkinson's disease. *Neurology* **49,** 1168–1170.
46. Maricle, R.A., Nutt, J.G., Valentine, R.J., and Carter, J.H. (1995) Dose-response relationship of levodopa with mood and anxiety in fluctuating Parkinson's disease: a double-blind, placebo-controlled study. *Neurology* **45,** 1757–1760.

47. Yahr, M.D., Duvoisin, R.C., Schear, M.J., Barrett, R.E., and Hoehn, M.M. (1969) Treatment of parkinsonism with levodopa. *Arch. Neurol.* **21,** 343–354.
48. Damasio, A.R., Antunes, J.L., and Macedo, C. (1970) L-dopa, parkinsonism, and depression. *Lancet* **2,** 611–612.
49. Marsh, G.G. and Markham, C.H. (1973) Does levodopa alter depression and psychopathology in parkinsonism patients? *J. Neurol. Neurosurg. Psychiatry* **36,** 925–935.
50. Growdon, J.H., Kieburtz, K., McDermott, M.P., Panisset, M., and Friedman, J.H. (1998) Levodopa improves motor function without impairing cognition in mild non-demented Parkinson's disease patients. Parkinson Study Group. *Neurology* **50,** 1327–1331.
51. Choi, C., Sohn, Y.H., Lee, J.H., and Kim, J.-S. (2000) The effect of long-term levodopa therapy on depression in de novo patients with Parkinson's disease. *J. Neurol. Sci.* **172,** 12–16.
52. Vazquez, A., Jimenez-Jimenez, F.J., Garcia-Ruiz, P., and Garcia-Urra, D. (1993) "Panic attacks" in Parkinson's disease: a long-term complication of levodopa therapy. *Acta Neurol. Scand.* **87,** 14–18.
53. Theohar, C., Fischer-Cornelssen, K., Akesson, H.O., Ansari, H., Gerlach, J., and Harper, P. (1981) Bromocriptine as antidepressant: double-blind comparative study with imipramine in psychogenic and endogenous depression. *Curr. Ther. Res.* **30,** 830–842.
54. Inoue, T., Tsuchiya, K., Miura, J., et al. (1996) Bromocriptine treatment of tricyclic and heterocyclic antidepressant-resistant depression. *Biol. Psychiatry* **40,** 151–153.
55. MacGrath, P.J., Quitkin, F.M., and Klein, D.F. (1995) Bromocriptine treatment of relapses seen during selective serotonin re-uptake inhibitor treatment of depression. *J. Clin. Psychopharmacol.* **15,** 289–291.
56. Jouvent, R., Abensour, P., Bonnet, A.M., Widlocher, D., Agid, Y., and Lhermitte, F. (1983) Antiparkinsonian and antidepressant effects of high doses bromocriptine. *J. Affect. Disord.* **5,** 141–145.
57. Factor, S.A., Molho, E.S., Podskalny, G.D., and Brown, D. (1995) Parkinson's disease: drug-induced psychiatric states. *Adv. Neurol.* **65,** 115–138.
58. Przedborski, S., Liard, A., and Hildebrand, J. (1992) Induction of mania by apomorphine in a depressed parkinsonian patient. *Mov. Disord.* **7,** 285–287.
59. Sporn, J., Gnaemi, S.N., Sambur, M.R., et al. (2000) Pramipexole augmentation in the treatment of unipolar and bipolar depression: a retrospective chart review. *Ann. Clin. Psychiatry* **12,** 137–140.
60. Corrigan, M.H., Denahan, A.Q., Wright, C.E., Ragual, R.J., and Evans, D.L. (2000) Comparison of pramipexole, fluoxetine, and placebo in patients with major depression. *Depression Anxiety* **11,** 58–65.
61. Flaherty, J.A. and Bellur, S.N. (1981) Mental side effects of amantadine therapy: its spectrum and characteristics in a normal population. *J. Clin. Psychiatry* **42,** 344–345.
62. Dietrich, D.E., Bode, L., Spannhuth, C.W., et al. (2000) Amantadine in depressive patients with Borna disease virus (BDV) infection: an open trial. *Bipolar Disord.* **2,** 65–70.
63. Moreau, J.L., Borgulya, J., Jenck, F., and Martin, J.R. (1994) Tolcapone: a potential new antidepressant detected in a novel animal model of depression. *Behav. Pharmacol.* **5,** 344–350.
64. Fava, M., Rosenbaum, J.F., Kolsky, A.R., et al. (1999) Open study of the catechol-O-methyltransferase inhibitor tolacapone in major depressive disorder. *J. Clin. Psychopharmacol.* **19,** 329–335.
65. Bresa, G.M. (1994) S-adenosyl-L-methionine as antidepressant: a meta analysis of clinical studies. *Acta Neurol. Scand.* **154(Suppl),** 7–14.
66. Di Rocco, A., Rogers, J.D., Brown, R., Werner, P., and Bottiglieri, T. (2000) S-adenosyl-methionine improves depression in patients with Parkinson's disease in an open-label clinical trial. *Mov. Disord.* **15,** 1225–1229.
67. Bejjani, B.-P., Damier, P., Arnulf, I., et al. (1999) Transient acute depression induced by high-frequency deep-brain stimulation. *N. Engl. J. Med.* **340,** 1476–1480.
68. Bezerra, M.L.S., Martinez, J.-V.L., and Nasser, J.A. (1999) Transient acute depression induced by high-frequency deep-brain stimulation [correspondence]. *N. Engl. J. Med.* **340,** 1003–1004
69. Ghika, J., Ghika-Schmid, F., Fankhauser, H., et al. (1999) Bilateral contemporaneous posteroventral pallidotomy for the treatment of Parkinson's disease: neuropsychological and neurological side effects. Report of four cases and review of the literature. *J. Neurosurg.* **91,** 313–321.
70. Straits-Toster, K., Fields, J.A., Wilkinson, S.B., et al. (2000) Health-related quality of life in Parkinson's disease after pallidotomy and deep brain stimulation. *Brain Cogn.* **42,** 399–416.
71. Bakish, D., Habib, R., and Hooper, C.L. (1998) Mixed anxiety and depression: diagnosis and treatment options. *CNS Drugs* **9,** 271–180.
72. Denmark, J.C., David, J.D.P., and McComb, S.G. (1961) Imipramine hydrochloride (Tofranil) in parkinsonism: a preliminary report. *Br. J. Clin. Pract.* **15,** 523–524.
73. Strang, R.R. (1965) Imipramine in treatment of parkinsonism: a double-blind placebo study. *BMJ* **2,** 33–34.
74. Laitinen, L. (1969) Desipramine in treatment of parkinson's disease: a placebo-controlled study. *Acta Neurol. Scand.* **45,** 109–113.
75. Andersen, J., Aabro, E., Gulmann, N., Hjelmsted, A., and Pedersen, H.E. (1980) Antidepressive treatment in Parkinson's disease. *Acta Neurol. Scand.* **62,** 210–219.
76. Indaco, A. and Carrieri, P.D. (1988) Amitryptiline in the treatment of headache in patients with Parkinson's disease. *Neurology* **38,** 1720–1722.
77. Cummings, J.L. and Masterman, D.A. (1999) Depression in patients with Parkinson's disease. *Int. J. Geriatr. Psychiatry* **14,** 711–718.
78. Cunningham, L.A. (1994) Depression in medically ill: choosing an antidepressant. *J. Clin. Psychiatry* **55(Suppl. A),** 98–100.

79. Meara, R.J., Bhowmick, B.K., and Hobson, J.P. (1996) An open uncontrolled study of the use of sertraline in the treatment of depression in Parkinson's disease. *J. Serotonin Res.* **4,** 243–249.
80. Hauser, R.A. and Zesiewicz, T.A. (1997) Sertraline for the treatment of depression in Parkinson's disease. *Mov. Disord.* **12,** 756–757.
81. Wittgens, W., Donath, O., and Trenckmann, U. (1997) Treatment of depressive syndromes in Parkinson's disease with paroxetine [abstract]. *Mov. Disord.* **12,** 128.
82. Ceravolo, R., Nuti, A., Piccinni, A., et al. (2000) Paroxetine in Parkinson's disease: effects on motor and depressive symptoms. *Neurology* **55,** 1216–1218.
83. McCance-Katz, E.F., Marek, K.L., and Price, L.H. (1992) Serotonergic dysfunction in depression associated with Parkinson's disease. *Neurology* **42,** 1813–1814.
84. Mayeux, R., Stern, Y., Sano, M., Williams, J.B., and Cote, L.J. (1988) The relationship of serotonin to depression in Parkinson's disease. *Mov. Disord.* **3,** 237–244.
85. Kostić, V.S., Djuričić, B.M., Šternić, N., Bumbaširević, L.J., Nikolić, M., and Mršulja, B.B. (1987) Depression and Parkinson's disease: possible role of serotonergic mechanisms. *J. Neurol.* **234,** 94–96.
86. Kostić, V.S., Lečić, D., Doder, M., Marinković, J., and Filipović, S. (1996) Prolactine and cortisol responses to fenfluramine in Parkinson's disease. *Biol. Psychiatry* **40,** 769–775.
87. Chouinard, G. and Sultan, S. (1992) A case of Parkinson's disease exacerbated by fluoxetine. *Hum. Psychopharmacol.* **7,** 63–66.
88. Jansen-Steur, E.N.H. (1993) Increase of Parkinson disability after fluoxetine medication. *Neurology* **43,** 211–213.
89. Jimenez-Jimenez, F.J., Tejeiro, J., Martinez-Junquera, G., et al. (1994) Parkinsonism exacerbated by paroxetine [letter]. *Neurology* **44,** 2406.
90. Linazasoro, G. (2000) Worsening of Parkinson's disease by citalopram. *Parkinsonism Rel. Disord.* **6,** 111–113.
91. Gerber, P.E. and Lynd, L.D. (1998) Selective serotonin-reuptake inhibitor-induced movement disorders. *Ann. Pharmacother.* **32,** 692–698.
92. Gobert, A., Rivet, J.-M., Lejeune, F., et al. (2000) Serotonin_{2C} receptors tonically suppress the activity of mesocortical dopaminergic and adrenergic, but not serotonergic, pathways: a combined dialysis and electrophysiological analysis in the rat. *Synapse* **36,** 205–221.
93. Montastruc, J.L., Fabre, N., and Blin, O. (1995) Does fluoxetine aggravate Parkinson's disease? A pilot prospective study. *Mov. Disord.* **10,** 355–356.
94. Caley, C.F. and Friedman, J.H. (1992) Does fluoxetine exacerbate Parkinson's disease? *J. Clin. Psychiatry* **53,** 278–282.
95. Richard, I.H., Maughn, A., and Kurlan, R. (1999) Do serotonin reuptake inhibitor worsen Parkinson's disease? A retrospective case series. *Mov. Disord.* **14,** 155–157.
96. Tesei, S., Antonini, A., Canesi, M., Zecchinalli, A., Mariani, C.B., and Pezzoli, G. (2000) Tolerability of paroxetine in Parkinson's disease: a prospective study. *Mov. Disord.* **15,** 986–989.
97. Toyama, S.C. and Iakono, R.P. (1994) Is it safe to combine a selective serotonin reuptake inhibitor with selegiline? *Ann. Pharmacother.* **28,** 405–406.
98. Waters, C.H. (1994) Fluoxetine and selegiline. *Can. J. Neurol. Sci.* **21,** 259–261.
99. Richard, I., Kurlan, R., Tanner, C., Factor, S., Hubble, J., Suchowersky, O., and Waters, C. (1997) Serotonin syndrome and the combined use of deprenyl and an antidepressant in Parkinson's disease: Parkinson Study Group. *Neurology* **48,** 1070–1077.
100. Keller, M.B. and Hanks, D.L. (1995) Anxiety symptom relief in depression treatment outcomes. *J. Clin. Psychiatry* **56(Suppl. 6),** 22–29.
101. Hoffman, W.F. (1985) Treatment of major depression and Parkinson's disease with combined phenelzine and amantadine [letter]. *Am. J. Psychiatry* **142,** 273.
102. Hargrave, R. and Ashford, J.W. (1992) Phenelzine treatment of depression in Parkinson's disease. *Am. J. Psychiatry* **149,** 1751–1752.
103. Brown, A.S. and Gershon, S. (1993) Dopamine and depression. *J. Neural. Transm.* **91,** 75–109.
104. Fahn, S. and Chouinard, S. (1998) Experience with tranylcypromine in early Parkinson's disease. *J. Neural. Transm.* **52(Suppl.),** 49–61.
105. Sunderland, T., Cohen, R.M., Molchan, S., et al. (1994) High-dose selegiline in treatment-resistant older depressive patients. *Arch. Gen. Psychiatry* **51,** 607–615.
106. Mann, J.J., Aarons, S.F., Wilner, P.J., et al. (1989) A controlled study of the antidepressant efficacy and side-effects of (-)-deprenyl: a selective monoamino oxidase inhibitor. *Arch. Gen. Psychiatry* **46,** 45–50.
107. Kuhn, W. and Muller, T. (1996) The clinical potential of deprenyl in neurologic and psychiatric disorders. *J. Neural. Transm.* **48,** 85–93.
108. Allain, H., Pollak, P., and Neukirch, H.C. (1993) Symptomatic effect of selegiline in de novo parkinsonian patients: the French Selegiline Multicenter Trial. *Mov. Disord.* **8(Suppl. 1),** S36–S40.
109. Parkinson Study Group. (1989) Effect of deprenyl on the progression of disability in early Parkinson's disease. *N. Engl. J. Med.* **321,** 1364–1371.
110. Ritter, J.L. and Alexander, B. (1997) Retropsective study of selegiline-antidepressant drug interactions and a review of the literature. *Ann. Clin. Psychiatry* **9,** 7–13.
111. Angst, J. and Stabl, M. (1992) Efficacy of moclobemide in different patient groups: a meta-analysis of studies. *Psychopharmacology* **106(Suppl.),** S109–S113.
112. Bakish, D., Saxena, B.M., Bowen, R., and D'Souza, J. (1993) Reversible monoamine oxidase A inhibitors in panic disorders. *Clin. Neuropharmacol.* **16(Suppl. 2),** 77–82.

113. Takats, A., Tarczy, N., Simo, M., Szombathely, E., Bodrogi, A., and Karpati, R. (1994) Moclobemide treatment in Parkinson's disease with depression. *New Trends Clin. Neuropharmacol.* **8,** 260.
114. Jansen-Steur, E.N.H. and Ballering, L.A.P. (1997) Moclobemide and selegiline in the treatment of depression in Parkinson's disease. *J. Neurol. Neurosurg. Psychiatry* **63,** 547–548.
115. Sieradzan, K., Channon, S., Ramponi, C., Stern, G.M., Lees, A.J., and Youdim, M.B.H. (1995) The therapeutic potential of moclobemide, a selective monoamine oxidase A inhibitor in Parkinson's disease. *J. Clin. Psychopharmacol.* **15(Suppl. 2),** 51–59.
116. Šternić, N., Kacar, A., Filipović, S., Svetel, M., and Kostić, V.S. (1998) The therapeutic effect of moclobemide, a reversible selective monoamine oxidase A inhibitor, in Parkinson's disease. *Clin. Neuropharmacol.* **21,** 93–96.
117. Silver, J.M. and Yudofski, S.C. (1992) Drug treatment of depression in Parkinson's disease, in *Parkinson's Disease: Neurobehavioral Aspects* (Huber, S.J. and Cummings, J.L., eds.), Oxford University Press, New York, pp. 240–254.
118. Goetz, C.G., Tanner, C.M., and Klawans, H.L. (1984) Bupropion in Parkinson's disease. *Neurology* **34,** 1092–1094.
119. Kanner, A.M. (2000) The treatment of depression in various neurological disorders. *Syllabi of AAN* **4TP.003,** 18–30.
120. Leentjens, A.F., Verhey, F.R., and Vreeling, F.W. (2000) Successful treatment of depression in a Parkinson disease patient with bupropion. *Ned. Tijdschr. Geneeskd.* **144,** 2157–2159.
121. Kent, J.M. (2000) SnaRIs, NaSSAs, and NaRIs: new agents for the treatment of depression. *Lancet* **355,** 911–918.
122. Gorman, J.M. (1999) Mirtazapine: clinical overview. *J. Clin. Psychiatry* **60(Suppl. 17),** 9–13.
123. Fawcett, J. and Barkin, R.L. (1998) Review of the results from the clinical studies on the efficacy, safety and tolerability of mirtazapine for the treatment of patients with major depression. *J. Affect. Disord.* **51,** 267–285.
124. Pact, V. and Giduz, T. (1999) Mirtazapine treats resting tremor, essential tremor, and levodopa-induced dyskinesias. *Neurology* **53,** 1154.
125. Douyon, R., Serby, M., Klutchko, B., and Rotrosen, J. (1989) ECT and Parkinson's disease revisited: a naturalistic study. *Am. J. Psychiatry* **146,** 1452–1455.
126. Faber, R. and Trimble, M. (1991) Electroconvulsive therapy in Parkinson's disease and other movement disorders. *Mov. Disord.* **6,** 293–303.
127. Moellentine, C., Rummans, T., Ahlskog, J.E., et al. (1998) Effectiveness of ECT in patients with parkinsonism. *J. Neuropsychiatry Clin. Neurosci.* **10,** 187–193.
128. Wengel, S.P., Burke, W.J., Pfeiffer, R.F., Roccaforte, W.H., and Paige, S.R. (1998) Maintenance electroconvulsive therapy for intractable Parkinson's disease. *Am. J. Geriatr. Psychiatry* **6,** 263–269.
129. George, M.S., Wassermann, E.M., Kimbrell, T.A., et al. (1997) Mood improvement following daily left prefrontal repetitive transcranial magnetic stimulation in patients with depression: a placebo-controlled crossover trial. *Am. J. Psychiatry* **154,** 1752–1756.
130. Klein, E., Kreinin, I., Chistyakov, A., et al. (1999) Therapeutic efficacy of right prefrontal slow repetitive transcranial magnetic stimulation in major depression: a double-blind controlled study. *Arch. Gen. Psychiatry* **56,** 315–320.
131. Nobler, M.S., Sackeim, H.A., Prohovnik, I., et al. (1994) Regional cerebral blood flow in mood disorders III: treatment and clinical response. *Arch. Gen. Psychiatry* **51,** 884–897.
132. Pascual-Leone, A., Catala, M.D., and Pascual, A.P. (1996) Lateralized effect of rapid-rate transcranial magnetic stimulation of prefrontal cortex on mood. *Neurology* **46,** 499–502.
133. Mally, J. and Stone, T.W. (1999) Therapeutic and "dose-dependent" effect of repetitive microelectroshock induced by transcranial magnetic stimulation in Parkinson's disease. *J. Neurosci. Res.* **57,** 935–940.
134. George, M.S., Lisanby, S.H., and Sackeim, H.A. (1999) Transcranial magnetic stimulation: applications in neuropsychiatry. *Arch. Gen. Psychiatry* **56,** 300–311.
135. Berger, M. and Riemann, D. (1993) Normal and abnormal REM sleep regulation: REM Sleep in depression—an overview. *J. Sleep Res.* **2,** 211–223.
136. Demet, E.M., Chicz-Demet, A., Fallon, J.H., and Sokolski, K.N. (1999) Sleep deprivation therapy in depressive illness and Parkinson's disease. *Prog. Neuropsychopharmacol. Biol. Psychiatry* **23,** 753–784.
137. Green, T.D., Reynolds, C.F., Mulsant, B.H., et al. (1999) Accelerating antidepressant response in geriatric depression: a post hoc comparison of combined sleep deprivation and paroxetine versus monotherapy with paroxetinem nortriptyline, or placebo. *J. Geriatr. Psychiatry Neurol.* **12,** 67–71.
138. Perry, W., Benbow, C., West, L., and Rockwell, E. (1993) Sleep deprivation in an elderly man with Parkinson's disease [letter]. *Am. J. Psychiatry* **150,** 350.
139. Bertolucci, P.H., Andrade, L.A., Lima, J.G., and Carlini, E.A. (1987) Total sleep deprivation and Parkinson's disease. *Arq. Neuropsiqiatr.* **45,** 224–230.

28

Diagnosis and Treatment of Hallucinations and Delusions in Parkinson's Disease

Dag Aarsland, MD, PhD and Jan Petter Larsen, MD, PhD

1. INTRODUCTION

Hallucinations and delusions in Parkinson's disease (PD) have attracted attention because they are common, have important clinical consequences both for patients, their families, and the health care system, and they are treatable. According to the Diagnostic and Statistical Manual of Mental Disorders, fourth edition (DSM IV) *(1)*, a delusion is a false belief based on incorrect inference about external reality that is firmly sustained despite what almost everyone else believes. Hallucination is a sensory perception that has the compelling sense of reality of a true perception, but that occurs without external stimulation of the relevant sensory organ. The person may or may not have insight in that he or she is having a hallucination. Psychotic symptoms such as hallucinations and delusions are the cardinal features of psychiatric disorders such as schizophrenia, schizo-affective disorder, delusional disorder, and brief psychotic disorder. Psychotic symptoms may also occur during the course of delirium or dementias and may be due to a range of other general medical and neurological conditions, including PD.

2. EPIDEMIOLOGY

Studies investigating the prevalence of hallucinations and delusions in PD have yielded large differences with prevalences ranging from 3–60% *(2)*. The methodological differences underlying such disparate findings include differences in: (*i*) case selection procedure; (*ii*) diagnostic accuracy of PD; (*iii*) study design; and (*iv*) diagnostic procedures for identification of psychotic symptoms. First, samples from movement disorder clinics will show prevalence of psychiatric symptoms that differ from samples from psychiatric or neuropsychiatric clinics or community-based samples. One major confounding factor is whether patients with dementia are included or not, since hallucinations are more common in PD patients with dementia than those without. Second, the accuracy of the clinical diagnosis of PD is suboptimal, and even experienced clinicians using established diagnostic criteria will have less than perfect diagnostic sensitivity and specificity *(3)*. Typically, PD samples may erroneously include patients with dementia with Lewy bodies (DLB), progressive supranuclear palsy (PSP), or Alzheimer's disease (AD) *(4,5)*. Because the prevalence of psychotic symptoms in PD differ from that in DLB *(6)*, PSP *(7)*, and AD *(8)*, inclusion of non-PD patients with parkinsonism will influence the reported prevalence. Third, because hallucinations are not always reported spontaneously *(9)*, retrospective chart reviews are likely to underestimate the prevalence of psychotic symptoms. Accordingly, prospective studies are needed. Fourth, the use of different definitions for psychotic symptoms and differ-ent diagnostic procedures influence the observed prevalence. Fenelon and coworkers included

From: *Mental and Behavioral Dysfunction in Movement Disorders*
Edited by: M-A. Bédard et al. © Humana Press Inc., Totowa, NJ

Table 1
Prevalence of Hallucinations in PD: Recent Studies

Authors (reference)	Year	Sample selection	*N*	Observation period	Instrument	Result
Sanchez-Ramos et al. *(10)*	1996	Movement disorder clinic	214	?	Questionnaire	26%
Naimark et al. *(11)*	1996	Alzheimer disease centers	101[a]	Current	Clinical examination	36%
Graham et al. *(12)*	1997	Movement disorder clinic	129	Ever	Qestionnaire	25%
Inzelberg et al. *(13)*	1998	Movement disorder clinic	121	Ever	Questionnaire	37%
Aarsland et al. *(14)*	1999	Population based	245	Past week	UPDRS thought disorder subscale	Current: 16% Ever: 26%
Fenelon et al. *(9)*	2000	PD clinic	216	Past 3 mo	Clinical interview	Minor: 26% Visual: 22%
Holroyd et al. *(15)*	2001	Movement disorder clinic	102	Past week	?	26.5%
Barnes and David *(16)*	2001	Community	182	Past 3 mo	Questionnaire	17.2%

[a]Only PD patients with dementia included.
UPDRS, Unified Parkinson's Disease Rating Scale.

minor forms of hallucinations and found higher prevalence than most previous studies *(9)*. The symptoms may fluctuate, and the time frame of interest, which typically vary from 1 wk to 3 mo prior to assessment, will thus influence the proportion of patients reporting that the symptoms have been present. Finally, some, but not all, studies exclude symptoms occurring during a delirium.

In 1991, Cummings rewiewed the literature and reported the approximate frequency of visual hallucinations to be 30%, whereas 10% had delusions *(2)*. These numbers were based mainly on reports of side effects in clinical trials of antiparkinsonian agents. More recent epidemiological studies have, nevertheless, confirmed the previous conclusions (Table 1). Although these studies vary according to sample selection, time frame, and diagnostic procedure to identify the psychotic symptoms, the prevalence of visual hallucinations have been found to be in the range of 16–26%. Auditory hallucinations are less common, but may occur in 8–10%, but are usually accompanied by visual hallucinations *(9, 13)*. Delusions have been less well studied, but seem to occur less commonly in PD, although a prevalence of 16% with delusions have been reported *(17)*.

Prospective, longitudinal studies of psychotic symptoms in PD are rare. This is unfortunate, since such studies are required to assess the course, incidence of, and potential risk factors and mechanisms for such symptoms. In a 6-yr prospective study, 10 of 100 PD patients had "mental symptoms other than dementia, i.e., agitation, hallucinations, and delusions" before treatment with levodopa, whereas 25 out of 41 patients (60%) had such symptoms after 6 yr of treatment *(18)*. Thus, the annual incidence of newly developing psychotic symptoms was around 4%. However, the sample was unusual with respect to a high baseline prevalence of dementia (56%). Given the strong association between dementia and hallucinations in PD, this would probably have a major impact on the reported incidence. Bell and coworkers *(19)* reported that 51 of 393 (13%) PD patients had psychosis at baseline, 15 (4%) unrelated to treatment. At follow-up nearly 5 yr later, none of the patients with nondrug-induced psychosis were still psychotic, and the authors conclude that nondrug-related psychotic symptoms in PD are transient. Nine new cases of nondrug-related psychosis had emerged *(19)*. In a recent prospective longitudinal study, hallucinations were persistent, and the frequency increased from 33 to 63% from baseline to the 4-yr follow-up evaluation *(20)*.

3. PHENOMENOLOGY

The typical hallucinations in PD are formed visual images of people or animals and occur daily or several days a week in most patients, and they generally last for a few seconds to 30 min usually with a sudden onset *(9,16)*. Fenelon and coworkers *(9)* reported that the hallucinations were more frequent in the evening or during the night in nearly 50% of the patients. Insight was retained in all patients without dementia, but only in 64% of demented patients. Minor forms of hallucinations, i.e., the sensation of the presence of a person, a sideways passage or illusions, were present in 25.5% of the patients, whereas formed hallucinations were found in an additional 22%. The hallucinations are often blurred, moving, and sometimes recurrent *(16)*. Auditory hallucinations are less common and are usually verbal or musical or consist of other noises *(9)*. The most common thought content of the delusions are delusions of theft and phantom boarder delusion (i.e., the delusion that unwelcomed guests are in the house) *(6)*. Most cross-sectional studies find a close relationship between psychotic symptoms and cognitive impairment and severity of parkinsonism *(16)*. However, in the only prospective, longitudinal study of hallucinations in PD, no relation between long-term severity of hallucinations and cognitive impairment and motor symptoms was found *(20)*. Several studies have also found a relationship between depression and hallucinations *(16)*.

Previous studies of psychotic symptoms in PD have usually not attempted to classify the symptoms according to psychiatric diagnostic entities. Based on a review of the literature, Peyser and coworkers *(21)* identified six psychotic syndromes occurring in PD patients: (*i*) hallucinations with preserved insight; (*ii*) medication-induced psychotic disorders in clear consciousness; (*iii*) delirium; (*iv*) schizophrenia-like psychotic disorders in clear consciousness and in the absences of medication treatment; (*v*) schizophrenia with subsequent development of PD; and (*vi*) other psychotic disorders. The latter three categories are rare *(15)*, and only 2% of patients with hallucinations were found to have a delirium in a recent study *(9)*. This classification scheme is heavily influenced by the DSM-IV, but it is difficult to rely simply on this and do justice to the phenomenology of the PD patients with psychotic phenomena *(15,21)*. For instance, the DSM-IV criteria include etiologic diagnostic criteria, such as "substance-induced psychotic disorder" and "psychotic disorder due to PD," but dis-entangling the etiologic role of antiparkinsonian medication treatment from the brain disease *per se* is a difficult problem, in particular in the case of an individual patient. In this respect, it is interesting that there are several reports of a schizophrenia-like illness in untreated PD patients (reviewed in ref. *21*). Furthermore, there seem to be a continuum of insight rather than clear categories of insight or no insight *(15)*. An additional category to consider is an affective psychotic syndrome, i.e., depression or mania associated with mood-congruent hallucinations or delusions. This is of particular importance, since several studies have reported an association between psychotic symptoms and depression *(16)* and since the treatment of psychotic depression differs from depression without psychosis *(22)*. Although the frequency of depressive psychosis in PD has not been formally studied, there is some evidence to suggest that it is uncommon *(23)*. The mere co-occurrence of visual hallucinations and depressive symptoms do not warrant the diagnosis psychotic depression, since the criteria of major depression have to be met, and the psychotic phenomena should usually be mood-congruent, i.e., the content of the hallucination or delusion is consistent with the depressive themes *(1)*.

4. CLINICAL CONSEQUENCES

Although hallucinations are frequently minor and pose little problems for the patient with PD *(9)*, there is much evidence showing that they may have severe clinical consequences for the patients themselves, their family, and for the society. Hallucinations in PD patients are associated with other emotional disturbances. More than a quarter of PD patients with hallucinations reported co-occurring anxiety *(9)*, and hallucinations are associated with more depressive symptoms *(24)*. In addition, PD patients with hallucinations have lower sleep efficiency and a reduced rapid eye movement (REM) sleep time and percentage *(25)*, as well as more daytime sleepiness *(26)*, and altered dream-phenomena *(27)*

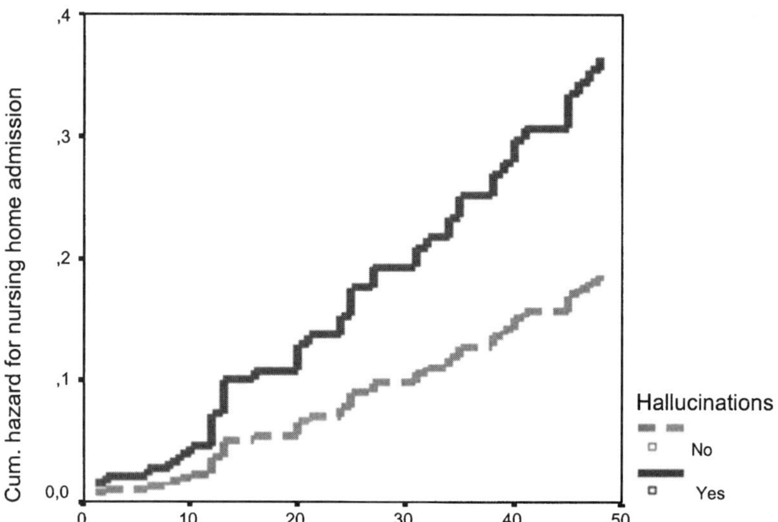

Fig. 1. Four-year cumulative risk for nursing home admission for patients with PD with (solid line) and without (dotted line) hallucinations. Hallucinations defined as UPDRS, thought disorder scale score equal to 2 or more. Cox regression curve, adjusted for age, dementia, and UPDRS activities of daily living (ADL) score. Copyright: American Geriatrics Society.

than those without hallucinations. Finally, in one case-control study, PD patients with hallucinations had a higher mortality rate than nonhallucinators *(28)*.

Spouses of home-dwelling PD patients perceive increased level of stress, lower quality of life, and more depression compared to healthy control subjects *(29)*, and the burden of spouses of PD patients is similar to that reported by spouses of patients with stroke and dementia *(30)*. To investigate which clinical features would be associated with caregiver stress, we investigated the relationships of the patients' motor, cognitive, and psychiatric disturbances to caregiver stress. In a multivariate regression model, the degree of psychiatric symptoms, such as depression, agitation, and delusions, were independent correlates of perceived caregiver stress in addition to cognitive and functional impairment *(29)*. Thus, psychotic symptoms in PD contribute to caregiver stress.

A considerable proportion of PD patients live in nursing homes *(31)*. Motor symptoms and associated functional impairment are two among many factors potentially contributing to the institutionalization of PD patients, but psychotic and other neuropsychiatric symptoms may also contribute. To identify the predictors of nursing home admission in PD, 178 community-dwelling patients were followed prospectively for 4 yr, and the time for nursing home admission was recorded *(32)*. Forty-seven (26%) patients were admitted to a nursing home. The presence of hallucinations at the baseline evaluation was a significant predictor of nursing home admission, independent of the effects of age, motor impairment, and dementia. The relative risk for institutionalization for patients with hallucinations was 2.0 (95% confidence interval 1.1–3.5) (Fig. 1) *(32)*. What are the mechanisms for this effect? Possibly, the psychotic symptoms, and associated anxiety and agitation, may lead to institutionalization secondary to the increased stress perceived by the caregiver. Another possibility is that hallucinations may be a marker of a more severe subtype of PD. PD patients with dementia, who frequently have hallucinations, have abundant cortical Lewy bodies, and share many clinical and pathological features of patients with DLB *(33)*. Hallucinations may, thus, signal the conversion from pure PD to DLB, with more marked behavioral changes and cognitive impairment in addition to the functional impairment caused by the motor symptoms of the disease, resulting in a higher risk for nursing home placement.

Table 2
Differential Diagnosis of Patients with Parkinsonism and Psychosis

Symptom presentation	PD	DLB	AD	NIP
Onset of parkinsonism	Early	Early/late	Late	Late
L-dopa response	Good	Vary	Unknown	Poor
Onset of psychosis	Late	Early	Late	Early
Dementia prevalence	25%	100%	100%	Vary
Pattern of cognitive	Executive	Executive	Memory	Vary
Dysfunction	Visuospatial	Visuospatial	Aphasia, apraxia	

Abbreviations: PD, Parkinson's disease; DLB, Dementia with Lewy bodies; AD, Alzheimer's disease; NIP, neuroleptic-induced parkinsonism; L-dopa, levadopa.

5. DIAGNOSIS

The two main issues with regard to the diagnosis of psychotic symptoms in PD are: (*i*) to identify, describe, and quantify the hallucinations and delusions in the patients with PD; and (*ii*) to establish the correct diagnosis in patients who present with psychotic symptoms and parkinsonism. It is important to identify psychotic symptoms because they have important clinical consequences, provide prognostic information, and are potentially treatable. The clinician should question the patient and caregiver for the presence of hallucinations, since they may not always spontaneously report them. The use of validated rating scales are recommended, and scales which take into account the commonly co-existing cognitive impairment should be used. A specific rating scale for assessing the psychotic symptoms in PD, the Parkinson Psychosis Rating Scale *(34)*, has been developed. The scale assesses visual hallucinations, illusions–misidentification, paranoid ideation, sleep disturbances, confusion, and sexual preoccupation. Inter-rater reliability and concurrent validity, as well as sensitivity to change, have been demonstrated *(34)*. The items are tailored towards the specific symptoms of psychosis occurring in PD patients and enables the important distinction between confusional and nonconfusional psychotic states. The Neuropsychiatric Inventory (NPI), designed for use in subjects with brain disease, is a structured caregiver-based interview that rates frequency and intensity of symptoms *(35)*. High reliability and validity have been established *(35)*. This instrument is useful both because cognitive impairment is accounted for by being caregiver-based and because important psychiatric and behavioral symptoms frequently associated with hallucinations and delusions are also assessed. The NPI has been widely used to assess psychopathology in patients with dementia and other brain diseases, thus allowing for comparison between diseases. However, not every patient has a reliable caregiver, and patients may not always tell their caregivers about their symptoms.

Neurologists and psychiatrists will frequently see elderly patients with parkinsonism and psychotic symptoms, and the differential diagnosis is not always straightforward. Co-occurrence of parkinsonism and psychotic symptoms may be present in several disorders, among the most common are PD, DLB, AD with psychosis and parkinsonism, and neuroleptic-induced parkinsonism. Although these disorders differ with regard to presentation and course of symptoms, the patients may appear clinically identical at cross-sectional evaluations, with cognitive impairment, hallucinations, and parkinsonism (Table 2). A careful history will usually reveal the correct diagnosis, however. PD patients typically have unilateral onset of parkinsonism, respond well to levodopa treatment, and cognitive and psychotic symptoms develop after several years of disease. Hallucinations occurring within the first 3 mo of starting levodopa indicate a diagnosis other than PD, either a co-morbid psychotic illness or an evolving parkinsonism-plus syndrome *(36)*. Conversely, DLB patients may present with hallucinations or dementia, although they may also present with parkinsonism *(37)*. Cross-sectionally, DLB patients may be clinically indistinguishable from PD patients with dementia, since the cognitive and psychiatric symptoms are rather similar *(6,38)*. Although generally stated that parkinsonism in DLB is mild, the severity and symptom pattern of parkinsonism is similar in DLB and PD *(39)*. Likewise, the response to antiparkinsonian agents in DLB patients may vary from none to good, although this has not yet been systematically studied. Patients with PSP, a neurological disorder characterized by progressive vertical supranuclear gaze palsy and parkinsonism with early postural instability, frequently develop cognitive symptoms similar to those observed in PD *(40)*. They may also develop psychotic symptoms, although less common than PD patients even among those treated with antiparkinson agents *(7)*. AD is characterized by progressive dementia with memory impairment, aphasia, agnosia, and apraxia. Hallucinations are less common, and delusions are more common in AD compared to PD patients with dementia *(8)*. Extrapyramidal symptoms occur in some patients with AD *(41)*, but usually occurs several years after disease onset. Traditional antipsychotic agents are widely used in elderly patients *(42)*. Since this population has a high risk for development of drug-induced parkinsonism, they may present with parkinsonism and a history of psychotic symptoms.

6 TREATMENT

6.1. General Management

Psychotic symptoms are usually considered to represent behavioral side-effects of antiparkinsonian drugs *(2)*, a view reflected in the use of terms such as drug-induced, dopaminomimetic, and dopaminergic-induced psychosis. However, studies before levodopa was introduced and recent studies suggest that drug treatment may not account for all cases of psychotic symptoms in PD. First, psychotic symptoms were described in PD before levodopa was introduced *(43)* and in untreated patients *(19)*. Second, most studies find that psychotic symptoms are not related to the dose, duration of treatment, or number of dopaminergic agents *(14–16)*. Third, hallucinations do not relate to levodopa plasma level or to sudden changes in plasma level *(44)*. Finally, although dopaminergic agents may induce psychotic symptoms in non-PD patients *(2)*, PSP patients treated with dopaminergic agents do not develop hallucinations *(7)*. Thus, dopaminergic agents may provide a neurochemical milieu with a high risk for psychosis in PD, but are not necessary or sufficient to cause psychosis. The association between duration and severity of disease, dementia, depression, sleep disturbance, visual disturbances, and psychotic symptoms (see review in ref. *16*) suggests a multifactorial etiology, including brain changes associated with the disease itself.

Neurochemical changes potentially contributing to hallucinations in PD include limbic dopaminergic hypersensitivity *(45)*, cholinergic deficits *(46)*, and serotonergic over-activity *(47)*. These hypotheses provide a background for a rational choice of symptomatic treatment, such as dopaminergic blocking agents (i.e., antipsychotics), cholinesterase inhibitors, and serotonin (5-HT) blocking agents. However, before symptomatic drug therapy is introduced, the following procedures should be considered (see Fig. 2):

1. Is treatment necessary? Hallucinations, particularly minor forms, are not always troublesome for patients or their caregivers, and treatment measures may not be indicated. Frequently, however, symptoms are distressing, and associated with delusions, anxiety and agitation, and possibly delirium, and treatment is mandatory.
2. Identify and treat causal factors. Psychotic symptoms, particularly when accompanied by a confusional state, can arise from a new medical illness or exacerbation of a preexisting chronic illness, from drug reactions (antiparkinson agents as well as other agents) or interaction, and from fever or trauma. Thus, a careful drug history and medical work-up is required, and potential contributing factors removed if possible.
3. Reduction of antiparkinsonian treatment. It is commonly stated that reduced daily dosage or number of antiparkinsonian treatments may reduce the severity or occurrence of psychotic symptoms in PD patients. Clinical experience and uncontrolled trials suggest that this strategy is effective *(18,48,49)*, although it has not yet been rigorously tested. If the symptoms have developed subsequent to introduction of a new drug, or to a dose increment, the first step should be to return to the previous regimen. It has been suggested that the side effects are more related to the number of drugs than to drug dose *(50)*. Accordingly, in patients taking more

than one antiparkinson drug, one should start by discontinuation of add-on drugs. Well-designed comparative studies providing insight into the differences in the frequency of hallucinations with different agents are not available. It is generally considered that anticholinergic agents, selegiline, and dopamine agonists should be withdrawn first *(2)*, then amantadine and catechol-O-methyl-transferase (COMT)-inhibitors, and finally levodopa is reduced *(50)*. Frequently, however, withdrawal or reduction of antiparkinsonian agents may cause worsening of parkinsonism. Since antipsychotic agents with low risk of worsening of parkinsonism (see Subheading 6.2.) are available, some authors find reduction of antiparkinsonian treatment to be an undesirable procedure, and instead recommend simply to add an atypical antipsychotic to the existing treatment regimen *(51)*.

6.2. *Atypical Antipsychotics*

The antipsychotic action of antipsychotic agents are highly correlated with their affinities for D2 receptors of the mesolimbic dopaminergic neurons *(52)*. Blockade of striatal D2 receptors leads to parkinsonism in non-PD patients and to severe worsening of parkinsonism in PD patients. In contrast, atypical antipsychotic agents have a low potential for extrapyramidal side effects in non-PD populations *(52)*. This may be due to the high 5-HT-2 occupancy, lower D2 occupancy, or a higher affinity to the D4 receptor limited to the mesocortical dopamine system compared to traditional antipsychotics. Open label case series suggest that clozapine, the first atypical antipsychotic agent, reduces psychotic symptoms with no or little worsening of parkinsonism in PD patients *(53)*. This preliminary evidence was confirmed in two placebo-controlled trials of clozapine *(54,55)*. In both studies, 60 PD patients with hallucinations received clozapine 6.25–50 mg/d (mean final daily dose 24.7 mg at wk 4 *[54]* or 36 mg at wk 3 *[55]*). Only nondemented patients with a Mini-Mental State Examination (MMSE) score greater than 20 were included in one *(55)*, whereas the mean MMSE scores were 21.7 (placebo group) and 23.8 (clozapine group) in the other study *(54)*. Significant improvements on clozapine compared to placebo were reported in both studies. Improvements were noted already after 1 wk *(55)*, and 48% of the clozapine and 11% of the placebo group achieved marked or full recovery *(54)*. No worsening of parkinsonism, and even improvement of tremor, was noted in one study *(54)*. In the other study, some worsening of parkinsonism was reported, although significant differences on the Unified Parkinson's Disease Rating Scale (UPDRS) were not found *(55)*. Clozapine has high affinity to muscarinic receptors, but cognition as measured with the MMSE did not change during treatment *(54,55)*. Sedation *(54,55)* and weight gain *(54)* were the only additional adverse events reported. Previous reports suggest that the most frequent side effects of clozapine are sedation, orthostatic hypotension, tachycardia, weight gain, hyperthermia, and drooling, which often disappear when doses are reduced *(53)*. Clozapine has been shown to induce agranulocytosis in 0.5–1%, and frequent white cell blood counts are required during treatment. Thus, clozapine treatment is cumbersome in PD patients with impaired mobility, and there is a need for alternative drugs.

The evidence for the use of the newer atypical antipsychotics risperidone, olanzapine, and quetiapine was reviewed by Friedman and Factor *(50)*. They reported eight studies with a total of 82 patients treated with risperidone, nine studies with 130 patients treated with olanzapine, and seven studies with 123 patients treated with quetiapine. On risperidone, 77% had improved psychosis, whereas 37% had worsening of parkinsonism. On olanzapine, improvement of psychosis was noted in 70%, and worsening of parkinsonism in 38% of patients. On quetiapine, 85% reported improved psychosis, and worsening of parkinsonism was found in only 13%. The authors concluded that clozapine is the only drug with confirmed benefit without worsening of parkinsonism, that risperidone is poorly tolerated with respect to worsening of parkinsonism, and that olanzapine will worsen parkinsonism in a majority of patients. It was suggested that quetiapine might prove to be as effective and better tolerated than clozapine. They recommend that if symptomatic treatment is needed, quetiapine should be the first choice, beginning with 12.5 mg at bedtime and then increasing by 12.5 mg every 4–7 d until 50 mg/d, and thereafter changes as indicated. Clozapine was recommended as the second-line choice, beginning at 6.25 mg at bedtime and increases by the same amount until psychosis remits or side effects occur. If olanzapine is used, starting dose should be 2.5 mg, with weekly increases as indicated *(50)*.

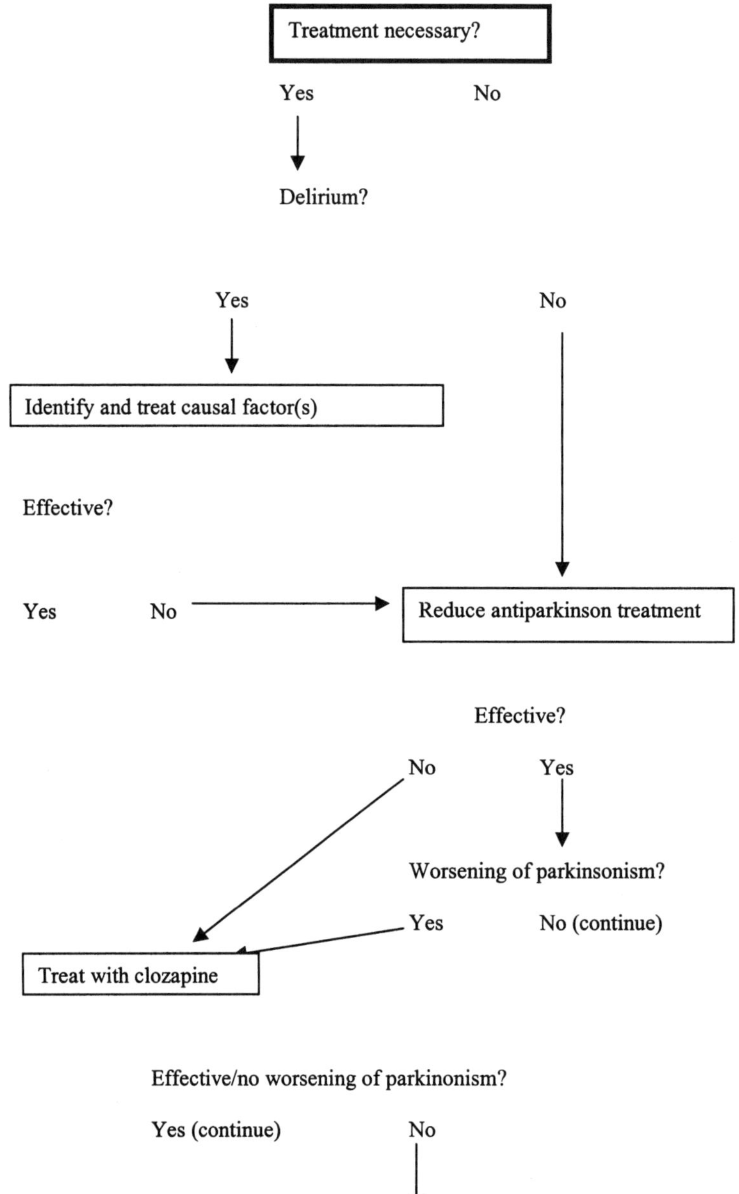

Fig. 2. Treatment algorithm of psychotic symptoms in PD.

Recent open label studies not included in this review are summarized in Table 3. Worsening of parkinsonism on olanzapine was reported in one *(56)* but not another study *(57)*. Two studies of quetiapine reported no worsening of parkinsonism *(51,58)*. In one trial of clozapine replacement by quetiapine, 12 of 15 patients were successfully switched to quetiapine *(59)*. Three patients dropped out, one due to increased dyskinesia and tremor, whereas none of the remaining 12 had significant worsening of parkinsonism 8 wk after clozapine discontinuation *(59)*. One study with risperidone reported no aggravation of parkinsonism in 16 patients *(60)*. In several studies, it was noted that the starting dose *(57, 60)* and titration rate *(59)* influence the effect on motor symptoms. Importantly, several reports show

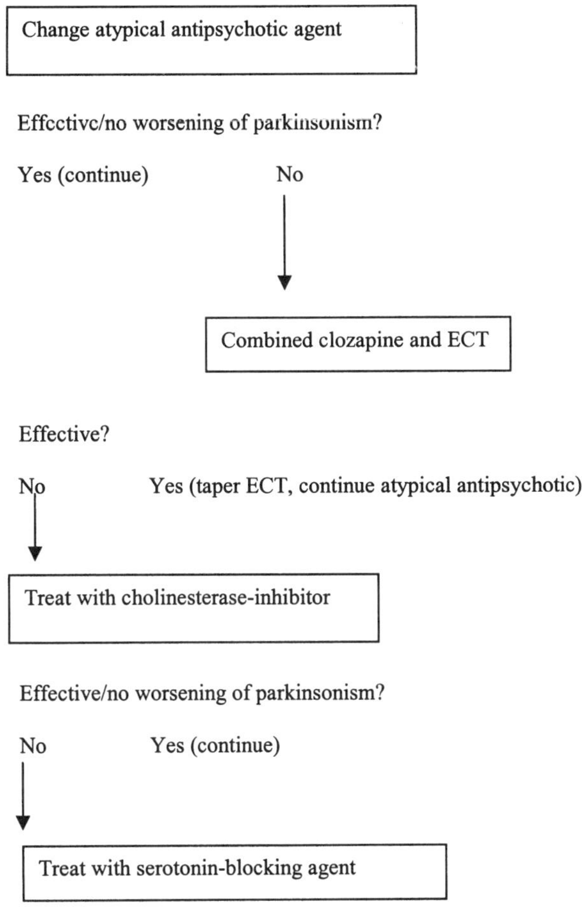

Fig. 2. (Continued)

that the clinical response and tolerability vary between patients, and switching from one antipsychotic to another may be attempted *(61)*.

Recently, three controlled studies of the newer atypical antipsychotics were reported. Olanzapine (2.5–7.5 mg/d) improved dyskinesias compared to placebo, but induced increases in "off"-time and parkinsonism *(62)*. In one of the first head-to-head comparison of two atypical antipsychotics, eight nondemented PD patients with hallucinations received clozapine (mean peak dose 25.8 mg/d) and seven received olanzapine (mean peak dose 11.4 mg/d) for 9 wk *(63)*. The study was stopped after 15 patients had completed the study because of worsening of parkinsonism in the olanzapine group. Whereas a modest improvement of UPDRS motor score was found in the clozapine group, statistically significant worsening was observed in the olanzapine group. Six of seven patients in the olanzapine group withdrew prior to 9 wk, due to aggravated parkinsonism. Improvement of psychotic symptoms was found in the clozapine but not the olanzapine group *(63)*. In a double-blind trial of low-dose risperidone (mean dose 1.2 mg/d) and clozapine (mean dose 62.5 mg/d), a greater degree of antipsychotic response was found on risperidone than on clozapine *(64)*. Motor symptoms improved somewhat on clozapine, but worsened slightly on risperidone *(64)*. These effects and between-group differences were not statistically significant, but the statistical power was low due to the low number of patients included.

Table 3
Summary of Recent Case Series of Atypical Antipsychotics in PD with Psychosis

Study (references)	Drug	*N*	Mean dose (mg/d)	Improved pychosis	Worsened parkinsonism
Gimenez-Roldan	Olanzapine	9	4.7	Improved	3/9
et al. *(56)*	Clozapine	9	16.9	Improved	Nonsignificant improvement
Aarsland et al. *(57)*	Olanzapine	21	4.5	12/15	No worsening
Goetz et al. *(63)*[a]	Olanzapine,	15	11.4	Nonsignificant improvement	Worsening
	Clozapine		25.8	Improved	No worsening
Targum and Abbott (52 wk) *(58)*	Quetiapine	11		6/11	No worsening
Fernandez *(61)*	Quetiapine[b]	15	62.5	12/15 no change from clozapine	1/15
Dewey and O'Suillebeabhain *(51)*	Quetiapine[c]	61	86	40	No worsening
Mohr et al. *(60)*	Risperidone	17	1.1	16/17	1/17
Ellis et al. *(64)*[a]	Risperidone	10	1.2	Improved	Worsening
	Clozapine		62.5	No improvement	Improvement

[a]Double-blind.
[b]Clozapine replacement.
[c]Retrospective.

Based on these studies, the conclusion was made that clozapine, and possibly quetiapine, have a more benign profile on motor symptoms in PD patients than olanzapine and risperidone *(50,65)*. The results should, however, be viewed carefully, since the doses used may not be directly comparable. A positron emission tomography (PET)-study with schizophrenic patients found that the amount required to occupy 50% of maximum D2 occupancy was 0.8 mg/d of risperidone, 3.2 mg/d of olanzapine, and 112 mg/d of clozapine *(66)*. The dose of a drug is, therefore, a central determinant of its receptor occupancy. Mean daily doses of 11.2 mg olanzapine and 25.8 mg clozapine were compared in PD patients *(63)*. Accordingly, these dosages may have different level of striatal D2 occupancy, which would influence the effect on motor symptoms. The studies reporting no worsening of olanzapine in PD patients used mean doses of 6.5 mg *(67)* and 4.5 mg *(57)*, considerably lower than in the Goetz et al. study *(63)*. However, since the design of that study permitted a clinical titration of the dose, it is possible that clozapine may be able to muster a greater clinical response with a lower level of D2 occupancy. This view is consistent with the findings of a much lower maximum D2 occupancy of clozapine (71%) compared to risperidone (91%) and olanzapine (92%) *(66)*, indicating that the fundamental mechanism of response of clozapine may be different from that of olanzapine and risperidone. The receptor profile of quetiapine is more similar to that of clozapine *(68)*. Adverse events other than worsening of parkinsonism may occur on these drugs. Clozapine and olanzapine, but not risperidone and quetiapine, have marked anticholinergic and antihistaminergic effects *(52)*. Although cognition do not seem to decline in most patients, some may nevertheless withdraw from treatment with these agents due to sedation and confusion *(53,57)*. On the other hand, the antihistaminergic sedative effect may induce a substantial benefit on sleep disorders *(53)*. Finally, the atypical antipsychotics have a marked α1-receptor blockade *(52)*, which may cause hypotension.

In summary, clozapine has demonstrated effect and tolerability in PD patients with psychotic symptoms and is recommended as the first-line treatment if symptomatic antipsychotic treatment is necessary in these patients. If nonresponse, side effects, or for practical reasons (i.e., blood sampling) clozapine cannot be used, one of the newer antipsychotics should be introduced, and there are good reasons to recommend quetiapine as the second-line choice (Fig. 2).

6.3. Other Treatments

Case reports indicate that electroconvulsive therapy (ECT) may improve hallucinations and delusions in PD patients with clear sensorium *(69)*. This is important, since unlike other antipsychotic therapies, ECT has been shown to improve parkinsonism *(70)*, an effect that can be maintained for several years *(71)*. ECT may be used as an adjunctive therapy in patients not responding to atypical antipsychotics *(69)*. ECT induces a range of changes in the brain. The antiparkinson effect is thought to be secondary to an enhancement of dopaminergic transmission *(72)*. ECT has a major impact on the 5-HT system as well, which might contribute to the observed antipsychotic effect. ECT may induce memory impairment and delirium, particularly in patients with brain disease and dementia *(73)*.

Levodopa administration causes flushing out of 5-HT from serotonergic nerve terminals, and overstimulation of serotonergic receptors in the limbic system may contribute to psychotic symptoms in PD *(47)*. This hypothesis is supported by the fact that hallucinogens are agonists at 5-HT-2 receptors. Thus, 5-HT receptor blockers represent a potential treatment strategy for PD patients with psychotic symptoms. In 15 of 16 PD patients, visual hallucinations improved markedly after treatment with the 5-HT-3 receptor blocker ondansetron. Delusions, confusion, and daily functioning improved as well *(47)*. No worsening of parkinsonism, mood, or cognition was noted. In one report, less favorable results were found, but this may be due to the use of somewhat lower dosages *(74)*.

Mianserin (mean dose 37 mg/d), a 5-HT-2 receptor blocker and α2-antagonist with antidepressive properties, markedly and rapidly improved visual hallucinations and other symptoms of delirium in 10 of 12 PD patients in an open label study *(75)*. A slight but statistically significant improvement of parkinsonism was reported. After withdrawal, the symptoms rapidly reemerged, but disappeared after restarting mianserin. The effect seems to be related to the immediate effect on the 5-HT-2 receptor, since the clinical improvement occurs within 1 wk. If this hypothesis holds true, mechanism of effect of atypical antipsychotics in PD patients may also be partially attributable to their antagonism at the 5-HT-2 receptor.

PD patients have marked disturbances of the cholinergic system *(76)*, most marked in those with dementia *(77)*. In DLB, an association between hallucinations and cholinergic deficit has been reported *(78)*. Accordingly, cholinergic agents may improve psychotic symptoms in DLB and PD. Hutchinson reported that the frequency of hallucinations was greatly reduced after treatment with a low dose of the cholinesterase inhibitor tacrine (80 mg/d) in seven patients with PD and dementia, and in five cases they were essentially eliminated *(79)*. Similarly, cholinesterase inhibitors have been found to improve hallucinations in DLB *(80)* and AD *(81)*. Theoretically, cholinergic agents could worsen parkinsonism. Surprisingly, however, such worsening has not been found, and even a slight improvement of motor symptoms has been reported *(79,82)*, possibly secondary to pharmacokinetic interaction causing an increased plasma concentration of levodopa *(83)*. Thus, cholinergic agents may improve psychotic symptoms in PD patients without worsening of parkinsonism, and they may also improve cognition *(82)*. Controlled trials of cholinesterase inhibitors for hallucinations in PD are needed.

7. CONCLUSIONS

Psychotic symptoms, in particular visual hallucinations, are common in patients with PD. Although occasionally mild and transient, many patients suffer from long-standing hallucinations accompanied by delusions and behavioral disturbances. Psychotic symptoms may, thus, be troublesome for the patients themselves and for their caregivers, force the clinicians to reduce antiparkinsonian therapy, and are important predictors for admission to nursing home. Fortunately, effective and well-tolerated treatments are becoming available. Although only two placebo-controlled trials exist, there is evidence that the atypical antipsychotic agent clozapine reduces psychotic symptoms without worsening of parkinsonism. Preliminary evidence also indicates that some of the newer antipsychotics are useful alternatives to clozapine. Finally, future studies will determine if nondopaminergic strategies, in particular cholinergic agents, can reduce psychotic symptoms in PD patients.

REFERENCES

1. American Psychiatric Association (1994) Diagnostic and Statistical Manual of Mental Disorders, 4th ed., American Psychiatric Association, Washington, DC.
2. Cummings, J.L. (1991) Behavioral complications of drug treatment of Parkinson's disease. *J. Am. Geriatr. Soc.* **39,** 718–716.
3. Gelb, D.J., Oliver, E., and Gilman, S. (1999) Diagnostic criteria for Parkinson's disease. *Arch. Neurol.* **56,** 33–39.
4. Litvan, I., MacIntyre, A., Goetz, C.G., et al. (1998) Accuracy of the clinical diagnoses of Lewy body disease, Parkinson's disease, and dementia with Lewy bodies. *Arch. Neurol.* **55,** 969–978.
5. Jellinger, K. (1999) Neuropathological correlates of mental dysfunction in Parkinson's disease: an update, in *Mental Dysfunction in Parkinson's Disease* (Wolters, E., Scheltens, P., Berendse, H.W., eds.), Academic Pharmaceutical Productions, Utrecht, The Netherlands, pp. 82–105.
6. Aarsland, D., Ballard, C., Larsen, J.P., and McKeith, I.G. (2001) A comparative study of psychiatric symptoms in dementia with Lewy bodies and Parkinson's disease with and without dementia. *Int. J. Geriatr. Psychiatry* **16,** 528–536.
7. Aarsland, D., Litvan, I., and Larsen, J.P. (2001) Neuropsychiatric symptoms of patients with progressive supranuclear palsy and Parkinson's disease. *J. Neuropsychiatry Clin. Neurosci.* **13,** 42–49.
8. Aarsland, D., Cummings, J.L., and Larsen, J.P. (2001) Neuropsychiatric differences between Parkinson's disease with dementia and Alzheimer's disease. *J. Int. Geriatr. Psychiatry* **16,** 184–191.
9. Fenelon, G., Mahieux, F., and Huon, R. (2000) Hallucinations in Parkinson's disease. Prevalence, phenomenology and risk factors. *Brain* **123,** 733–745.
10. Sanchez-Ramos, J.R., Ortoll, R., and Paulson, G.W. (1996) Visual hallucinations associated with Parkinson's disease. *Arch. Neurol.* **53,** 1265–1268.
11. Naimark, D., Jackson, E., Rockwell, E., et al. (1996) Psychotic symptoms in Parkinson's disease patients with dementia. *J. Am. Geriatr. Soc.* **44,** 296–299.
12. Graham, J.M., Grunewald, R.A., and Sagar, H.J. (1997) Hallucinations in idiopathic Parkinson's disease. *J. Neurol. Neurosurg. Psychiatry* **63,** 434–440.
13. Inzelberg, R., Kipervasser, S., and Korczyn, A.D. (1998) Auditory hallucinations in Parkinson's disease. *J. Neurol. Neurosurg. Psychiatry* **64,** 533–535.
14. Aarsland, D., Larsen, J.P., Cummings, J.L., and Laake, K. (1999) Prevalence and clinical correlates of psychosis in Parkinson's disease. *Arch. Neurol.* **56,** 595–601.
15. Holroyd, D., Currie, L., and Wooten, G.F. (2001) Prospective study of hallucinations and delusions in Parkinson's disease. *J. Neurol. Neurosurg. Psychiatry* **70,** 734–738.
16. Barnes, J. and David, A.S. Visual hallucinations in Parkinson's disease: a review and phenomenological survey. *J. Neurol. Neurosurg. Psychiatry* **70,** 727–733.
17. Aarsland, D., Larsen, J.P., Lim, N.G., et al. (1999) Range of neuropsychiatric disturbances in patients with Parkinson's disease. *J. Neurol. Neurosurg. Psychiatry* **67,** 492–496.
18. Sweet, R.D., McDowell, F.H., Feigenson, J.S., Loranger, A.W., and Goodel, H. (1976) Mental symptoms in Parkinson's disease during chronic treatment with levodopa. *Neurology* **26,** 305–310.
19. Bell, K., Dooneief, G., Marder, K., et al. (1991) Non-drug-induced psychosis in Parkinson's disease. *Neurology* **41 (Suppl. 1),** 191.
20. Goetz, C.G., Leurgans, S., Pappert, E.J., Raman, R., and Stemer, A.B. (2001) Prospective longitudinal assessment of hallucinations in Parkinson's disease. *Neurology* **57,** 2078–2082.
21. Peyser, C.E., Naimark, D., Zuniga, R., and Jeste, D. (1998) Psychoses in Parkinson's disease. *Semin. Clin. Neuropsychiatry* **3,** 41–50.
22. Small, G.W. and Salzman, C. (1998) Treatment of depression with new and atypical antidepressants, in *Clinical Geriatric Psychopharmacology, 3rd ed.* (Salzman, C., ed.), Williams & Wilkins, Baltimore, pp. 245–261.
23. Cummings, J.L. (1992) Depression and Parkinson's disease: a review. *Am. J. Psychiatry* **149,** 443–454.
24. Tandberg, E., Larsen, J.P., Aarsland, D., Laake, K., and Cummings, J.L. (1997) Risk factors for depression in Parkinson's disease. *Arch. Neurol.* **54,** 625–630.
25. Comella, C.L., Tanner, C.A., and Ristanovic, R.K. (1993) Polysomnographic sleep measures in non-demented Parkinson's disease patients with treatmentinduced hallucinations. *Ann. Neurol.* **34,** 710–714.
26. Tandberg, E., Larsen, J.P., and Karlsen, K. (1999) Excessive daytime sleepiniess and sleep benefit in Parkinson's disease: a community-based study. *Mov. Disord.* **14,** 922–927.
27. Pappert, E.J., Goetz, C.G., Niederman, F.G., et al. (1999) Hallucinations, sleep fragmentation, and altered dream phenomena in Parkinson's disease. *Mov. Disord.* **14,** 117–121.
28. Goetz, C.G. and Stebbins, G.T. (1995) Mortality and hallucinations in nursing home patients with advanced Parkinson's disease. *Neurology* **45,** 669–676.
29. Aarsland, D, Larsen, J.P., Karlsen, K., Lim, N.G., and Tandberg, E. (1999) Mental symptoms in Parkinson's disease are important contributors to caregiver distress. *Int. J. Geriatr. Psychiatry* **14,** 866–874.
30. Thommessen, B., Aarsland, D., Braekhus, A., Oksengaard, A.R., Engedal, K., and Laake, K. (2002) The psychosocial burden on spouses of the elderly with stroke, dementia and Parkinson's disease. *Int. J. Geriatr. Psychiatry* **17,** 78–84.
31. Larsen, J.P. and the Norwegian Study Group of Parkinson's Disease in the Elderly (1991) Parkinson's disease as community health problem: study in Norwegian nursing home. *BMJ* **303,** 741–743.
32. Aarsland, D., Larsen, J.P., Tandberg, E., and Laake, K. (2000) Predictors of nursing home placement in Parkinson's disease: a population-based, prospective study. *J. Am. Geriatr. Soc.* **48,** 938–942.

33. Hurtig, H.I., Trojanowski, J.Q., Galvin, J., et al. (2000) Alpha-synuclein cortical lewy bodies correlate with dementia in Parkinson's disease. *Neurology* **54,** 1916–1921.
34. Friedberg, G., Zoldan, J., Weizman, A., and Melamed, E. (1998) Parkinson Psychosis Rating Scale: a practical instrument for grading psychosis in Parkinson's disease. *Clin. Neuropharmacol.* **21,** 280–284.
35. Cummings, J.L., Mega, M., Gray, K., et al. (1994) The Neuropsychiatric Inventory: comprehensive assessment of psychopathology in dementia. *Neurology* **44,** 2308–2314.
36. Goetz, C.G., Vogel, C., Tanner, C.M., and Stebbins, G.T. (1998) Early dopaminergic drug-induced hallucinations in parkinsonian patients. *Neurology* **51,** 811–814.
37. McKeith, I.G., Galasko, D., Kosaka, K., et al. (1996) Consensus guidelines for the clinical diagnosis of dementia with Lewy bodies (DLB): report of the consortium on DLB international workshop. *Neurology* **47,** 1113–1124.
38. Aarsland, D., Salmon, D., Galasko, D., and Larsen, J.P. (2001) Cogntion in dementia with Lewy-bodies and Parkinson's disease. *Mov. Disord.* **16(Suppl. 1),** A524.
39. Aarsland, D., Ballard, C., McKeith, I., Perry, R.H., and Larsen, J.P. Comparison of extrapyramidal signs in Dementia with Lewy bodies and Parkinson's disease. *J. Neuropsychiatry Clin. Neurosci.*, in press.
40. Pillon, B., Dubois, B., Lhermitte, F., et al. (1986) Heterogeneity of cognitive impairment in progressive supranuclear palsy, Parkinson's disease, and Alzheimer's disease. *Neurology* **36,** 1179–1185.
41. Heyman, A., Fillenbaum, G.G., Gearing, M., et al. (1999) Comparison of Lewy body variant of Alzheimer's disease with pure Alzheimer's disease. *Neurology* **52,** 1839–1844.
42. Byerly, M.J., Weber, M.T., Brooks, D.L., Snow, L.R., Worley, L.A., and Lescouflair, E. (2001) Antipsychotic medications and the elderly. Effects on cognition and implications for use. *Drugs Aging* **18,** 45–61.
43. Mjønes, H. (1949) Paralysis agitans. A clinical and genetic study. *Acta. Psychiatr. Scand.* **54(Suppl. 54)**.
44. Goetz, C.G., Pappert, E.J., Blasucci, L.M., et al. (1998) Intravenous levodopa in hallucinating Parkinson's disease patients: high-dose challenge does not precipitate hallucinations. *Neurology* **50,** 515–517.
45. Moskowitz, C., Moses, H., and Klawans, H.L. (1978) Levodopa-induced psychosis: a kindling phenomenon. *Am. J. Psychiatry* **135,** 669–674.
46. Perry, E., Wlaker, M., Grace, J., and Perry, R. (1999) Acetylcholine in mind: a neurotransmitter correlate of consciousness? *Trends Neurosci.* **22,** 273–280.
47. Zoldan, Z., Friedberg, G., Livneh, M., and Melamed, M. (1995) Psychosis in advanced Parkinson's disease: treatment with ondansetron, a 5HT3 receptor antagonist. *Neurology* **45,** 1305–1308.
48. Goetz, C.G., Tanner, C.M., and Klawans, H.L. (1982) Pharmacology of hallucinations induced by long-term drug therapy. *Am. J. Psychiatry* **139,** 494–497.
49. Fischer, P., Danielczyk, W., Simanyi, M., and Streifler, M.B. (1990) Dopaminergic psychosis in advanced Parkinson's disease. *Adv. Neurol.* **53,** 391–397.
50. Friedman, J.H. and Factor, S.A. (2000) Atypical antipsychotics in the treatment of drug-induced psychosis in Parkinson's disease. *Mov. Disord.* **15,** 201–211.
51. Dewey, R.B. and O'Suillebeabhain, P.E. (2000) Treatment of drug-induced psychosis with quetiapine and clozapine in Parkinson's disease. *Neurology* **55,** 1753–1754.
52. Meltzer, H.Y. (2000) Antipsychotic and anticholinergic drugs, in *New Oxford Textbook of Psychiatry* (Gelder, M.G., Lopez-Ibor, J. Jr., and Andreassen, N.C., eds.), Oxford University Press, Oxford, pp. 1314–1326.
53. Auzu, P., Øzsancak, C., Hannequin, D., and Moore, N. (1996) Clozapine for the treatment of psychosis in Parkinson's disease: a review. *Acta Neurol. Scand.* **94,** 329–336.
54. The Parkinson Study Group. (1999) Low-dose clozapine for the treatment of drug-induced psychosis in Parkinson's disease. *N. Engl. J. Med.* **340,** 757–763.
55. The French Clozapine Parkinson Study Group. (1999) Clozapine in drug-induced psychosis in Parkinson's disease. *Lancet* **353,** 2041–2042.
56. Roldan-Gimenez, S., Mateo, D., Navarro, E., and Gines, M.M. (2001) Efficacy and safety of clozapine and olanzapine: an open-label study comparing two groups of Parkinson's disease patients with dopaminergic-induced psychosis. *Parkinsonism Relat. Disord.* **7,** 121–127.
57. Aarsland, D., Larsen, J.P., and Lim, N.G. (1999) Olanzapin for psychosis in patients with Parkinson's disease with and without dementia. *J. Neuropsychiatry Clin. Neurosci.* **11,** 393–394.
58. Targum, S.D. and Abbott, J.L. (2000) Efficacy of quetiapine in Parkinson's patients with psychosis. *J. Clin. Psychopharmacol.* **20,** 54–60.
59. Fernandez, H.H., Lannon, M.C., Friedman, J.H., and Abbott, B.P. (2000) Clozapine replacement by quetiapine for the treatment of drug-induced psychosis in Parkinson's disease. *Mov. Disord.* **15,** 579–581.
60. Mohr, E., Mendis, T., Hildebrand, K., and De Deyn, P.P. (2000) Risperdione in the treatment of dopamine-induced psychosis in Parkinson's disease: an open pilot trial. *Mov. Disord.* **15,** 1230–1237.
61. Fernandez, H. (2000) Quetiapine for l-dopa-induced psychosis in PD. *Neurology* **55,** 899.
62. Manson, A.J., Schrag, A., and Lees, A. (2000) Low-dose olanzapine for levodopa induced dyskinesias. *Neurology* **55,** 795–799.
63. Goetz, C.G., Blasucci, L.M., Leurgans, S., and Pappert, E.J. (2000) Olanzapine and clozapine. Comparative effects on motor function in hallucinating PD patients. *Neurology* **55,** 789–794.
64. Ellis, T., Cudkowicz, M.E., Sexton, P.M., and Growdon, J.H. (2000) Clozapine and risperidone treatment of psychosis in Parkinson's disease. *J. Neuropsychiatry Clin. Neurosci.* **12,** 364–369.
65. Richard, I.H. and Nutt, J. (2000) Worsening of motor function in Parkinson's disease. A "typical" response to "atypical" antipsychotic medications. *Neurology* **55,** 748–749.

66. Kapur, S., Zipursky, R.B., and Remington, G. (1999) Clinical and theoretical implications of 5-HT2 and D2 receptor occupancy of clozapine, risperidone, and olanzapine in schizophrenia. *Am. J. Psychiatry* **156,** 286–293.
67. Wolters, E.C., Jansen, E.N.H., Tuynman-Qua, H.G., and Bergamns, P.L.M. (1996) Olanzapine in the treatment of dopaminomimetic psychosis with Parkinson's disease. *Neurology* **47,** 1085–1087.
68. Green, B. (1999) Focus on quetiapine. *Curr. Med. Res. Opin.* **15,** 145–151.
69. Factor, S.A., Molho, E.S., and Brown, D. (1995) Combined clozapine and electroconvulsive therapy for the treatment of drug-induced psychosis in Parkinson's disease. *J. Neuropsychiatry Clin. Neurosci.* **7,** 304–307.
70. Andersen, K., Balldin, J., Gottfries, C.G., et al. (1987) A double-blind study of electroconvulsive therapy in Parkinson's disease with "on-off" phenomena. *Acta Neurol. Scand.* **76,** 191–199.
71. Aarsland, D., Larsen, J.P., Waage, Ø., and Langeveld, H. (1997) Maintenance ECT in Parkinson's disease. *Convuls. Ther.* **13,** 274–277.
72. Barkai, A., Durkin, M., and Nelson, D. (1990) Locapized alterations of dopamine receptor binding in rat brain by repeated electronvulsive shock: an autoradiographic study. *Brain Res.* **529,** 208–213.
73. Abrams, R. (1992) *Electroconvulsive Therapy, 2nd ed.* Oxford University Press, New York.
74. Eichhirn, T., Brunt, E., and Oertel, W.H. (1996) Ondansetron treatment of l-dopa-induced psychosis. *Neurology* **47,** 1608–1609.
75. Ikeguchi, K. and Kuroda, A. (1995) Mianserin treatment of patients with psychosis induced by antiparkinsonian drugs. *Eur. Arch. Psychiatry Clin. Neurosci.* **244,** 320–324.
76. Perry, E., Irving, D., Kerwin, J.M., et al. (1993) Cholinergic transmitter and neurotrophic activities in Lewy body dementia: similarity to Parkinson's and distinction from Alzheimer disease. *Alzheimer Dis. Assoc. Disord.* **7,** 69–79.
77. Kuhl, D.E., Minoshima, S., Fessler, J.A., et al. (1996) In vivo mapping of cholinergic terminals in normal aging, Alzheimer's disease, and Parkinson's disease. *Ann. Neurol.* **40,** 399–410.
78. Perry, E.K., Kerwin, J., Perry, R.H., Irving, D., Blessed, G., and Fairbairn, A. (1990) Cerebral cholinergic activity is related to the incidence of visual hallucinations in senile dementia of Lewy body type. *Dementia* **1,** 2–4.
79. Hutchinson, M. and Fazzini, E. (1996) Cholinesterase inhibition in Parkinson's disease. *J. Neurol. Neurosurg. Psychiatry* **61,** 324–326.
80. McKeith, I., Del Ser, T., Spano, P.F., et al. (2000) Efficacy of rivastigmine in dementia with Lewy bodies: a randomised, double-blind placebo-controlled international study. *Lancet* **356,** 2031–2036.
81. Kaufer, D., Cummings, J.L., and Christine, D. (1996) Effect of tacrine on behavioral symptoms in Alzheimer's disease: an open-label study. *J. Geriatr. Psychiatry Neurol.* **9,** 1–6.
82. Aarsland, D., Laake, K., Larsen, J.P., and Janvin, C. (2002) Donepezil treatment in Parkinson's disease with dementia: a double.blind, placebo-controlled crossover study. *Neuro. Nursing Psych.* **72,** 708–712.
83. Okereke, C.S., Kumar, D., Cullen, E.I., Pratt, R.D., and Hahne, W.F. (2001) Pharmacokinetics and safety of concurrent donepezil HCl and levodopa/carbidopa administration in subjects with Parkinson's disease. *Neurology* **56(Suppl. 3),** A457.

29

REM Sleep Behavior Disorder in Parkinson's Disease, Dementia with Lewy Bodies, and Multiple System Atrophy

Bradley F. Boeve, MD, Michael H. Silber, MBChB, Tanis J. Ferman, PhD, Joseph E. Parisi, MD, Dennis W. Dickson, MD, Glenn E. Smith, PhD, John Lucas, PhD, and Ronald C. Petersen, PhD, MD

1. REM SLEEP BEHAVIOR DISORDER

1.1. What is REM Sleep Behavior Disorder?

Rapid eye movement sleep behavior disorder (RBD) is characterized by loss of normal skeletal muscle atonia during rapid eye movement (REM) sleep with prominent motor activity and dreaming. The evolving literature and our clinical experience suggests RBD may not simply represent an interesting parasomnia, but rather reflect dysfunction in REM sleep control that has relevance for understanding certain neurodegenerative disorders. In this chapter, we first review the clinical and polysomnographic features of RBD, criteria for diagnosis of RBD, management of RBD, pathophysiologic underpinnings of RBD, and neuroimaging findings. We then view RBD in the context of certain neurodegenerative disorders. The window that RBD provides in understanding key features of REM sleep control as well as the clinical and pathophysiologic significance of REM sleep dyscontrol in neurodegenerative disorders become clear.

1.2. Clinical Features of RBD

The typical clinical features of RBD are listed in Table 1; details of these features can be found in several references *(1–9)*. Most patients with RBD have been male. The mean age of onset is between 50 and 65 yr, with a range of 20–80 yr. Patients often vocalize, ranging from mumbles and screaming, to intelligible speech, sometimes with swearing. Many spouses describe the violent behaviors and vocalizations being very different from the calm manner and speech patients usually exhibit during wakefulness. Movements can vary from single limb jerks to flurries of "shaking" or "tremoring" to complex behaviors such as punching, running, spiking a football, and so on. Although some may describe pleasant dream content, most patients view them as nightmares with spiders, snakes, dogs, bears, or burglers that chase or attack them or their relatives or friends. Patients typically describe the content of their dreams upon being awakened at the time of the behavior, although patients with significant dementia may not be able to describe their dreams. Some bedpartners have attempted to awaken

From: *Mental and Behavioral Dysfunction in Movement Disorders*
Edited by: M-A. Bédard et al. © Humana Press Inc., Totowa, NJ

Table 1
Typical Clinical Features of RBD

Male gender predilection.
Mean onset age 50–65 yr (range 20–80 yr).
Vocalizations, swearing, screaming.
Motor activity varies from simple limb jerks to complex motor behavior, with injuries to patient or bedpartner.
Dreams often involve chases or attacks by animals or humans.
Exhibited behaviors mirror dream content.
Behaviors tend to occur in latter half of the sleep period.
When associated with neurodegenerative disease, RBD often precedes dementia and/or parkinsonism by years or decades.

patients during an episode, and their comments and gestures become interwoven into the dream. These behaviors can lead to falling off or leaping from the bed, striking bedposts or nightstands, and injuries to patients and bedpartners can occur, sometimes leading to fractures or subdural hematomas. Some patients have been known to tie themselves to bedposts or erect padded panels between them and bedpartners to minimize injury. Because most REM sleep occurs in the latter half of the sleep period, RBD tends to occur in the early morning hours, although some may begin exhibiting RBD shortly after falling asleep if REM sleep drive is increased due to sleep deprivation, narcolepsy, or untreated obstructive sleep apnea (OSA). As is discussed later, RBD can occur in association with neurodegenerative disease, most often Parkinson's disease (PD), dementia with Lewy bodies (DLB), or multiple system atrophy (MSA). In many cases, RBD begins years to decades before parkinonism and/or dementia evolves. Our clinical experience also indicates that in some patients with RBD, particularly in those with coexisting PD, DLB, or MSA, the frequency and severity of dream enactment behavior gradually wanes over time.

The differential diagnosis of disruptive sleep behavior includes the non-REM parasomnias (somnambulism, night terrors, confusional arousals), nightmares, nocturnal panic attacks, nocturnal seizures, noctural wandering associated with dementia, and OSA. The history usually allows differentiation of these disorders from RBD. Somnambulism and nocturnal wandering associated with dementia tend to be less violent, not associated with tormenting dreams, involve walking away from the bed rather than leaping or jumping, involve more purposeful activity with a rumaging quality, and in somnambulism tend to occur in the first third of the night when most non-REM sleep occurs. Night terrors and confusional arousals also tend to occur early in the night, involve screaming or anxiety, are not usually associated with dreams, involve inconsistent or incoherent speech during or immediately following the behavior, and little recall after awakening. Nocturnal panic attacks involve extreme anxiety, tachycardia, diaphoresis, and immediate full awareness; dream enactment does not occur. Patients with nocturnal seizures tend to exhibit posturing or generalized tonic–clonic activity without associated dreams, may be incontinent, and are often somnolent or disoriented for minutes to hours following an episode. Patients with moderate to severe OSA can have features that are strongly suggestive of RBD, yet their "RBD" can be abolished with nasal continuous positive airway pressure (CPAP).

Eliciting a careful history often allows identification of the disorder, but when diagnostic clarification is necessary, particularly when the risk for injury is high, polysomnography with simultaneous video-polysomnographic (PSG) monitoring is warranted.

1.3. PSG Features of RBD

REM sleep is characterized by the following PSG findings: rapid eye movements, minimal to no electromyographic (EMG) tone, and mixed α- and θ-activity on electroencephalography (EEG) (Fig. 1A). The characteristic electrophysiologic finding in patients with RBD is elevated EMG tone on the submental or limb EMG derivations, otherwise known as REM sleep without atonia (RSWA). This usually takes the form of a pathologic accentuation of normal phasic twitches, although sometimes EMG tone is tonically increased (Fig. 1B). Simultaneous video/PSG recording is essential for evaluating patients with suspected RBD, as vocalizations and limb movements can be captured and viewed concurrently with PSG data. When vocalizations and/or limb movements emerge out of REM sleep, without associated epileptiform activity on the EEG derivations (as in Fig. 1B), the diagnosis of RBD is established. In our experience, violent and complex dream enactment behavior is encountered rather infrequently during a single night PSG recordings; rather, increased EMG tone during REM sleep and sparse limb jerks are the norm.

1.4. Diagnostic Criteria for RBD

The two published sets of diagnostic criteria for RBD are shown in Tables 2 and 3 *(5,10)*. As can be seen, RBD is characterized by both abnormal REM sleep behavior and abnormal REM sleep electromyography.

Clinicians must decide whom to refer to a sleep medicine specialist for polysomnography and, also, to which sleep disorder center for referral. We tend to recommend evaluations with sleep medicine clinicians and PSG in patients who have one or more of the following features: young age (and thus long-term medical therapy may be necessary), dream enactment behavior is frequent and severe enough to raise concerns about patient and bedpartner injury, diagnosis cannot be surmised with confidence by history alone, or a history suggestive of OSA is elicited (i.e., loud crescendo snoring, irregularities in snoring with snorts or gasps, observed apnea, daytime hypersomnolence). Determining the presence or absence of OSA is critical, as the drug of choice for RBD, clonazepam, can exacerbate untreated OSA; untreated OSA increases the risk of cardiovascular and cerebrovascular morbidity and affects cognitive functioning and quality of life. If further studies indicate that RBD may be helpful in establishing the precise diagnosis of patients with parkinsonism and/or dementia (as described in Subheading 2), PSG may be indicated in those clinical settings as well. Not all sleep disorder centers have staff with expertise in the evaluation of parasomnias, nor are all equipped with simultaneous video/PSG monitoring capabilities, thus referral to appropriate centers is necessary. The American Academy of Sleep Medicine (www.aasmnet.org) can be contacted for information regarding specialized accredited sleep disorders centers.

1.5. Management of RBD

The goals of therapy are to minimize the abnormal behavior and unpleasant dreams and, particularly, to minimize the potential for injury. All patients and their bedpartners should be counselled on simple steps to minimize injury, such as moving lamps, nightstands, and the like, away from the bed, and placing a mattress or cushion of some type on the floor adjacent to the bed (many patients use inexpensive foam rubber mattresses). Clonazepam has been the mainstay of medical therapy, usually effective at 0.25–0.5 mg/night, but doses above 1 mg nightly are necessary in some patients *(3,9)*. Recent experience with melatonin shows that doses ranging from 3–12 mg/night can be effective, either as sole therapy or in conjunction with clonazepam when either melatonin or clonazepam alone is ineffective *(11,12)*. Other drugs reported to improve RBD include donepezil *(13)*, levodopa *(14)*, carbamazepine *(15)*, triazolam *(9)*, and clozapine *(9)*.

It is not clear why clonazepam, melatonin, and other agents improve RBD. Clonazepam reduces phasic activity in REM sleep, and although clonazepam clearly improves both unpleasant dreams and dream enactment behavior in most patients, REM sleep without atonia is still evident in those who undergo PSG while taking the drug. Melatonin has been shown to decrease the percentage of REM sleep epochs without muscle atonia and decrease the number of stage shifts in REM sleep, suggesting it has a more direct mode of action on REM sleep pathophysiology, perhaps by restoring circadian modulation of REM sleep *(11)*.

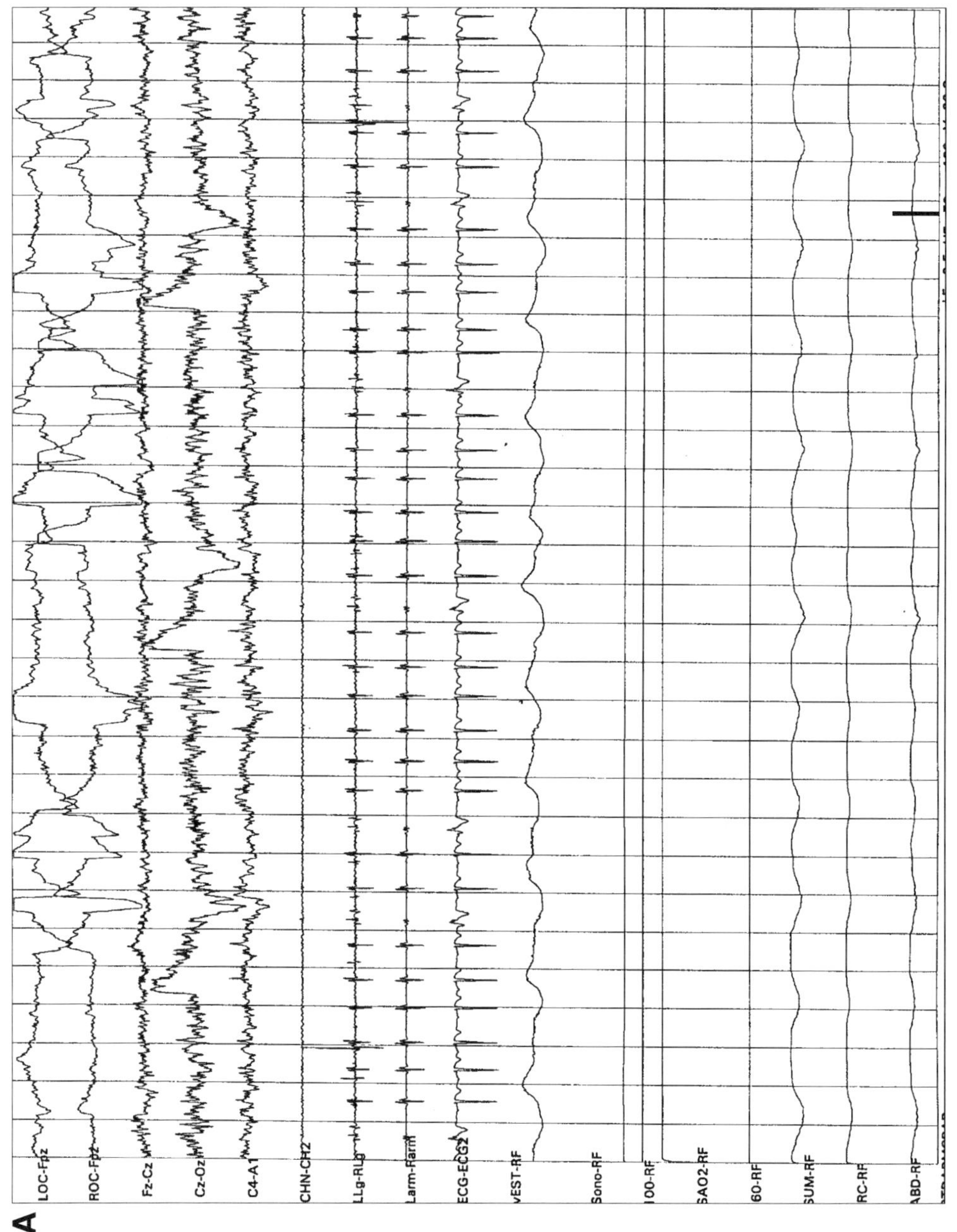
A
LOC-Fpz
ROC-Fpz
Fz-Cz
Cz-Oz
C4-A1
CHN-CH2
LLg-RLg
Larm-Rarm
ECG-ECG2
VEST-RF
Sono-RF
100-RF
SAO2-RF
60-RF
SUM-RF
RC-RF
ABD-RF

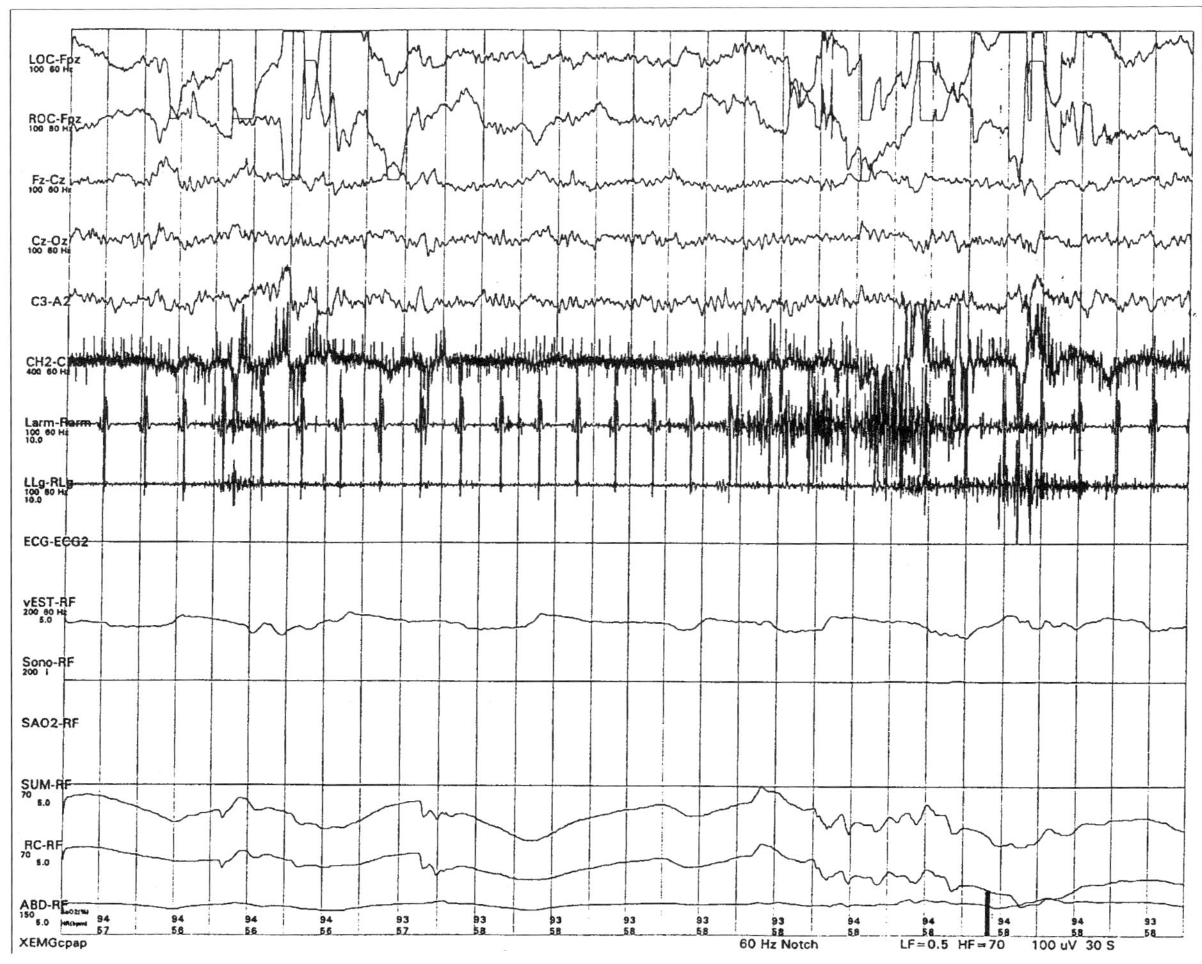

Fig. 1. Polysomnograms showing normal REM sleep (**A**) and RSWA, the electrophysiologic substrate for RBD (**B**). See text for details.

Table 2
Diagnostic Criteria for RBD

A. Patient has a complaint of violent or injurious behavior during sleep.
B. Limb or body movement is associated with dream mentation.
C. At least one of the following occurs:
   1. Harmful or potentially harmful sleep behaviors.
   2. Dreams appear to be "acted out."
   3. Sleep behaviors disrupt sleep continuity.
D. PSG monitoring demonstrates at least one of the following electrophysiologic measures during REM sleep:
   1. Excessive augmentation of chin EMG tone.
   2. Excessive chin or limb phasic EMG twitching, irrespective of chin EMG activity, and one or more of the following clinical features during REM sleep:
      a. Excessive limb or body jerking.
      b. Complex, vigorous, or violent behaviors.
      c. Absense of epileptic activity in association with the disorder.
E. The symptoms are not associated with mental disorders, but may be associated with neurologic disorders.
F. Other sleep disorders (e.g., sleep terrors or sleepwalking) can be present, but are not the cause of the behavior.

Minimal criteria: B plus C

Adapted with permission from ref. *10*.

Table 3
Diagnostic Criteria for RBD

A. History of problematic sleep behavior that is:
   1. Harmful or potentially harmful, or
   2. Disruptive of sleep continuity, or
   3. Annoying to self or bedpartner, and
   4. Any PSG abnormality listed (see below).
B. No history of problematic sleep behaviors but:
   1. Any PSG abnormality listed (see below) and
   2. Any videotaped behavioral abnormality listed (see below).

Minimum criteria: A or B

PSG
At least one of the following during REM sleep:
   1. Excessive augmentation of chin EMG tone.
   2. Excessive chin or limb EMG twitching, irrespective of chin EMG tone.

Videotaped behavioral abnormality
Record of at least one of the following during REM sleep:
   1. Excessive limb or body jerking.
   2. Complex movements.
   3. Vigorous or violent movements.

Adapted with permission from ref. *5*.

1.6. Pathophysiology of RBD

Studies in the cat have shown that there are two systems involved in normal REM sleep: one for generating muscle atonia and one for suppressing locomotor activity (Fig. 2A). Muscle atonia involves active inhibition by neurons in the nucleus reticularis magnocellularis (NRMC) in the medulla via the ventrolateral reticulospinal tract synapsing on the spinal motoneurons. NRMC neurons receive excitatory influences from the peri-locus coeruleus (peri-LC) region in the pons via the lateral tegmento-

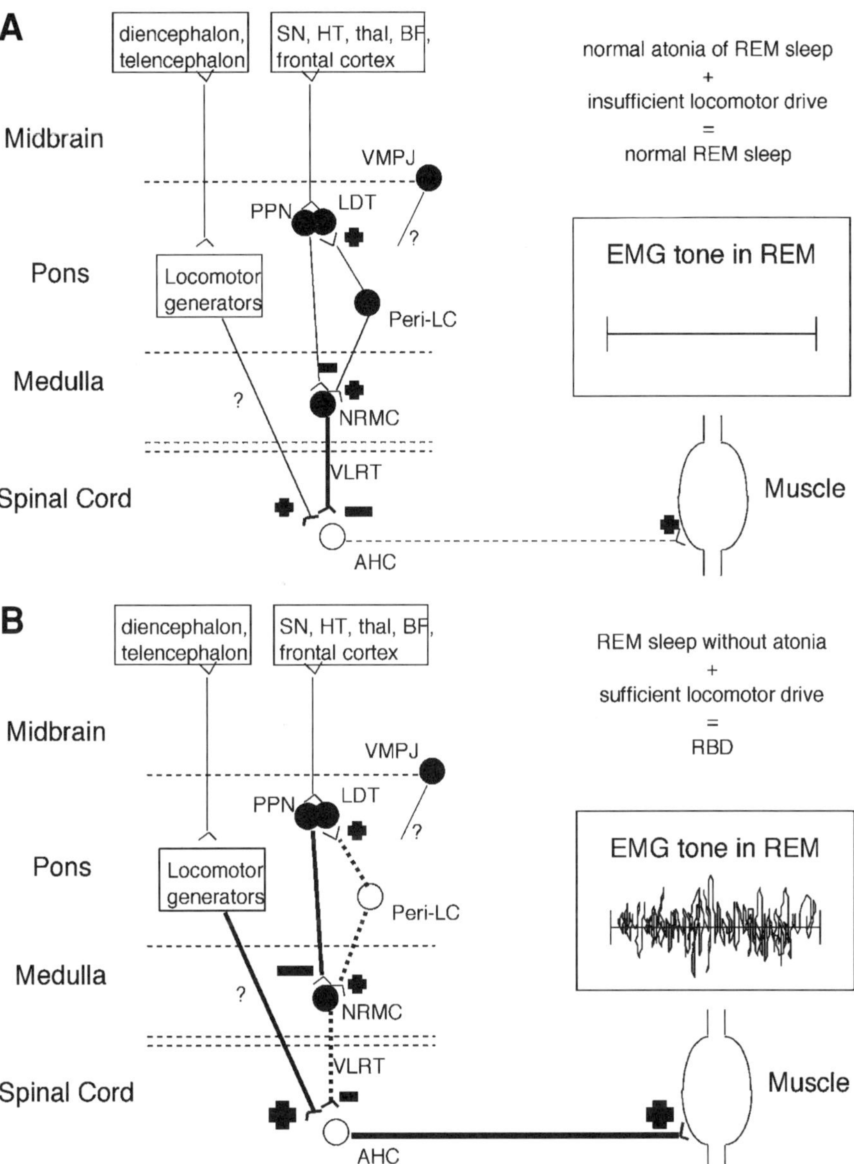

Fig. 2. Schematic of neuroanatomic connections underlying normal REM sleep (**A**) and RBD (**B**). See text for details.

reticular tract. Neurons in the peri-LC region are thought to inhibit the cholinergic pedunculopontine nucleus (PPN) and laterodorsal tegmental nucleus (LDTN) in the pons. The PPN is interconnected to the substantia nigra, hypothalamus, thalamus, basal forebrain, and frontal cortex. Locomotion involves pontine generators that have not been adequately characterized; the locomotor generator(s) likely receive input from supratentorial structures (particularly the forebrain and thalamus) and ultimately influence the spinal motorneurons. During REM sleep, phasic oculomotor and locomotor activity, such as rapid eye movements and muscle twitches, occurs, but more elaborate motoric activity is directly or indirectly suppressed *(5)*.

Several brainstem regions have been implicated in RBD pathophysiology, with most of the attention being directed toward the peri-LC region, PPN, and LDTN (Fig. 2B). In the cat model, lesions in the peri-LC region cause REM sleep without atonia, but the site of the lesion determines whether simple or complex behaviors are exhibited *(16)*. There is debate whether lesions in the PPN are sufficient to cause RBD *(14,17,18)*. Lesions in the ventral mesopontine junction (VMPJ) have recently been found to increase phasic REM sleep movements, suggesting this structure may be involved in RBD pathogenesis *(19)*. Mahowald and Schenck suggest that increased phasic locomotor drive and/or loss of REM sleep atonia underlies the clinical expression of RBD *(5)*. It should be noted, however, that some patients have PSG evidence of RSWA, yet have never exhibited dream enactment behavior. Thus, sufficient locomotor drive is likely necessary in the setting of RSWA to result in clinical RBD.

Using the activation–synthesis model of dream formation *(20)*, Mahowald and Schenck have theorized that alterations in the brainstem generators, activating locomotor, cognitive, affective, and other circuits, affect the synthesis of dreams in the forebrain, thus resulting in the altered dream content typical of human RBD *(5)*. These same brainstem alterations result in the simultaneous expression of complex motor behavior, thereby possibly explaining why the behaviors of RBD mirror dream content.

In the only human RBD case reported to date where detailed brainstem analyses were performed, a marked reduction in the number of neurons in the LC and marked increase in the number of neurons in the PPN and LDTN were found *(21)*. The authors proposed that the increased activity in cholinergic neurons and/or decreased disinhibition of the PPN and LDTN by the reduced monoaminergic activity of the LC led to the expression of RBD *(21)*.

The pathophysiologic underpinnings of human RBD are likely complex judging from the variable clinical response of RBD to agents affecting cholinergic, dopaminergic, and serotonergic networks. Any theory on pathophysiology must explain why clonazepam is most efficacious for RBD, yet elevated EMG tone during REM sleep still exists on PSG in those with excellent clinical response to the drug. Characterization of the pathophysiology of RBD is critical, as this knowledge may provide insights into the pathophysiology of certain neurodegenerative disorders (see Subheading 2).

1.7. Neuroimaging in RBD

Culebras and Moore reported on T2 signal changes on magnetic resonance imaging (MRI) in six patients with RBD and suggested vascular changes in the brainstem could disrupt REM sleep networks and result in RBD *(22)*. However, the vast majority of patients with RBD, in whom MRI has been done, have not corroborated this finding *(3,9,23)*.

Using dihydrotetrabenazine (DTBZ) positron emission tomography (PET), Albin et al. compared findings in elderly subjects with isolated RBD (i.e., not associated with another neurologic disorder) to those in similarly aged controls *(24)*. Striatal binding of DTBZ was reduced in the RBD subjects compared to controls, suggesting reduced dopaminergic substantia nigra neuron number. The authors concluded that this reduction is consistent with the hypothesis that RBD reflects an evolving degenerative parkinsonian disorder and suggested that RBD reflects either dysfunction of the PPN secondary to basal ganglia dysfunction or primary dysfunction of the PPN or other brainstem structures, which is temporally associated with basal ganglia dysfunction *(24)*.

Eisenher et al. used IPT-single photon emission computed tomography (SPECT), which reflects presynaptic dopaminergic transporter integrity, and IBZM-SPECT, which reflects postsynaptic dopaminergic D2 receptor integrity, to investigate dopaminergic parameters in patients with RBD, PD, and controls *(25)*. RBD cases had reduced striatal IPT uptake compared to controls, yet uptake was more similar (albeit symmetric) to PD cases. Furthermore, there was no significant difference in postsynaptic dopaminergic D2 receptors between RBD patients and controls. The reduction in dopaminergic transporters was thought to either be directly involved in RBD pathogenesis or that RBD is the initial manifestation of PD *(25)*.

2. RBD AND NEURODEGENERATIVE DISEASE

2.1. *Overview*

RBD has been described in dementing and parkinsonian disorders and has often been considered a nonspecific feature. However, the literature suggests that RBD may have a predilection for some neurodegenerative conditions and not others. In this section, we review data on those neurodegenerative disorders most commonly associated with RBD: PD, DLB, and MSA. We then review emerging data that suggests RBD may have particular pathophysiologic and clinical relevance in the synucleinopathies.

2.2. *RBD Associated with PD*

Schenck et al. characterized RBD as a clinical entity with key PSG findings in 1986 *(26,27)*. Several PD patients with clinically suspected, and PSG-confirmed RBD, have been reported *(8,9,11,26,28–33)*. Schenck et al. identified 38% of 29 patients with idiopathic RBD who subsequently developed a parkinsonian disorder, with a mean of 12.7 yr after the onset of RBD *(34)*. Others have also noted the tendency for RBD to precede parkinsonism *(9,31)*. Rye et al. reported a woman with juvenile PD whose clinical and PSG/Multiple Sleep Latency Test (MSLT) findings indicated the presence of both RBD and a narcolepsy-like illness *(32)*. Her monozygotic twin did not have evidence of any neurologic or sleep disorder. The authors suggest that the RBD and narcoleptic features were etiologically related to her PD, perhaps reflecting midbrain dopaminergic dysfunction *(32)*.

Comella et al. examined the occurrence of RBD and sleep-related injury (SRI) in consecutively evaluated patients with PD *(8)*. A structured questionnaire was used to determine the presence of RBD and SRI. Nine of 61 (15%) patients had responses suggesting RBD. SRI occurred more frequently in the group with RBD than those with no RBD, and 66% of the patients with SRI had features suggesting RBD. The authors concluded that SRI in PD patients likely reflects RBD and suggested treatment, such as clonazepam, to minimize future SRI risk *(8)*.

Sforza et al. reviewed the findings in 52 patients with RBD evaluated at their institution, of which 9 had PD *(31)*. Many findings were similar to those reported by Schenck et al. *(3)*.

Olson et al. analyzed the demographic, clinical, and laboratory features, and associated disorders in 93 consecutive patients with RBD *(9)*. Of the 25 with PD, 10 had subsequently developed dementia. RBD preceded the development of PD in 13 cases by a median of 3 yr. The frequency and severity of RBD waned with progression of PD in some of these cases *(9)*, which contrasts with the observation that no cases have been noted to spontaneously improve *(3)*.

Arnuf et al. investigated the relationship between hallucinations and sleep disorders by performing PSG and MSLT studies in 10 patients with PD and visual hallucinations (PD+VH) and 10 PD patients without hallucinations (PD-VH) *(33)*. All patients were on levodopa therapy, and none were considered to have dementia. PSGs revealed RBD in all PD+VH cases and 6 PD-VH cases. MSLT studies showed that approximately half in each group had excessive daytime somnolence (mean initial sleep latency <10 min; normal is 10 or more minutes). One or more sleep-onset REM periods occurred in eight of the PD+VH patients compared to two of the PD-VH patients (two or more sleep-onset REM periods and mean initial sleep latencies below 10 min are characteristic of patients with narcolepsy). The drowsiest patients had sleep-onset REM periods. Two patients reported hallucinations, and the hallucinations were immediately preceded by REM sleep. Delusions were also temporally associated with REM sleep. The authors conclude that visual hallucinations and delusions in patients with PD may reflect dream imagery, and suggest that psychosis reflects a narcolepsy-like REM sleep disorder *(33)*.

The findings of Arnulf et al. have several implications, many of which are acknowledged in their report *(33)*. From the treatment perspective, the principles of management in patients with narcolepsy may have applicability to patients with PD and DLB. First, daytime hypersomnolence may be intrinsic to Lewy body pathophysiology in some patients, and psychostimulants could minimize somnolence in such patients. There may be a general reluctance to use such agents in those who are already experiencing hallucinations and delusions, but if hallucinations and delusions represent features of REM sleep invading into wakefulness, REM sleep suppressants, such as selective serotonin re-uptake inhibitors and psychostimulants, may actually improve psychotic symptoms. Characterization of sleep–wake abnormalities in patients with PD and DLB may lead to treatments for challenging clinical problems.

2.3. RBD Associated with DLB

We originally appreciated the association of RBD and DLB in 1995 and have been actively studying patients with this association and reporting our findings since *(23,35–44)*. RBD is now regarded as a supportive feature for the diagnosis of DLB *(45)*. Importantly, most of the patients described in these reports began experiencing RBD years, sometimes decades, before their cognitive symptoms evolved.

We identified 37 patients with degenerative dementia +/– parkinsonism and RBD *(23)*. Neuropsychological testing demonstrated impaired visual perceptual–organizational skills, constructional praxis, and verbal fluency. There were no statistically significant differences in the frequency of clinical features or in neuropsychological performance between patients with or without parkinsonism. Thirty-four (92%) cases met criteria for clinically possible or probable DLB *(46)*. Three patients were autopsied: all had limbic with or without neocortical Lewy bodies. We concluded that the clinical and neuropsychometric features of the groups of patients with and without parkinsonism were similar, and hypothesized that the underlying pathology in these patients was DLB *(23)*.

We have subsequently compared the neuropsychometric profile of 31 patients with RBD/dementia to 31 with autopsy-proven Alzheimer's disease (AD), and have found a striking double dissociation with worse impairment on measures of attention, visual perceptual organization, and letter fluency for the RBD/dementia group, while the AD group showed significantly worse performance on confrontation naming and verbal memory *(41)*. We concluded that patients with RBD and degenerative dementia demonstrate a significantly different pattern of cognitive performance from AD. Most of the patients in this sample also met criteria for possible or probable DLB *(46)*, and the pattern of cognitive differences from AD is similar to reported comparisons between DLB and AD. The clinical and neuropsychometric data, therefore, provides evidence to suggest that the dementia associated with RBD may represent DLB *(41)*.

We recently analyzed the neuropsychometric performance on patients with dementia and RBD, who do not have parkinsonism or visual hallucinations, to see if they have a dementia that resembles probable DLB, which can be differentiated from the dementia of definite AD *(46a)*. Retrospective neurocognitive data was compared between patient groups of similar early dementia severity, including clinically probable DLB, dementia, and RBD without visual hallucinations or parkinsonism, and autopsy-confirmed AD. The neurocognitive profiles between probable DLB and dementia with RBD did not significantly differ. In contrast, when compared to AD, both groups demonstrated significantly worse visual perceptual organization and sequencing and significantly better confrontation naming and verbal memory. We conclude that patients with dementia and RBD, who do not have parkinsonism or visual hallucinations, have a dementia that is essentially neuropsychologically indistinguishable from that of probable DLB, and both groups differ significantly from AD *(46a)*. Therefore, in the absence of visual hallucinations or parkinsonism, the presentation of dementia and RBD may indicate underlying Lewy body disease.

Fluctuating cognition in DLB refers to recurrent alternating episodes of daytime confusion with periods of lucidity. The etiology of fluctuations is unclear, but one hypothesis involves disrupted mechanisms subserving sleep and arousal. An alternate hypothesis is that fluctuations may reflect disturbed sleep, associated with an underlying sleep disorder. We are testing the latter hypothesis, and data thus far suggest that sleep disorders, such as OSA and periodic limb movement disorder, may contribute, but do not entirely account for fluctuating cognition in DLB *(47)*.

Table 4
Clinical and Pathologic Diagnoses in 14 Patients with RBD

Case	Clinical diagnosis	Pathologic diagnosis	References
1	Normal	LBD (? brainstem)	*59*
2	Dementia	LBD (limbic) + AD	*21*, *60*, *23*-case 3, *44*-case 3
3	Dem with park	LBD (neocortical) + AD	*23*-case 1, *44*-case 1
4	DLB	LBD (neocortical) + AD	*23*-case 2, *44*-case 2
5	DLB	LBD	*48*, *49*
6	PD	LBD	*33*
7	PD	MSA	*44*-case 4
8	DLB	LBD (neocortical)	*44*-case 5
9	DLB	LBD (neocortical) + AGD	*44*-case 6
10	PD with dem	LBD (limbic) + AD	*44*-case 7
11	DLB	LBD (neocortical) + AD	*44*-case 8
12	Dem/park/MND	MND/LBD/NSP	*44*-case 9
13	Bins/AD	LBD/AD/Bins	*44*-case 10
14	DLB	LBD	*61*

Abbreviations: AD, Alzheimer's disease; AGD, agyrophilic grain disease; Bins, Binswanger's disease; Dem, dementia; DLB, dementia with Lewy bodies; LBD, Lewy body disease; MND, motor neuron disease; MSA, multiple system atrophy; NSP, nonspecific histopathology; park, parkinsonism; PD, Parkinson's disease.

Turner et al. described a case with a 17-yr history of RBD before typical DLB features evolved *(48)*. At autopsy, α-synuclein immunocytochemistry showed Lewy bodies in the substantia nigra, LC, and primarily limbic cortex (mild Alzheimer changes were also present) *(49)*. The authors suggested that the neuronal loss in the LC and substantia nigra may have disrupted cholinergic PPN functioning and led to RBD *(49)*.

2.4. RBD Associated with MSA

As in PD and DLB, numerous cases of RBD plus MSA have been described *(9,26,27,31,50–57)*, and one case, clinically suspected to have PD, had MSA identified at autopsy *(44)*. As noted above, RBD often precedes the onset of MSA features. The incidence and prevalence of RBD in MSA is not known, although Plazzi et al. reported historical features of RBD in 69% and PSG evidence of RBD in 90% of 39 consecutively examined patients *(50)*. Olson et al. *(9)* found that among 46 patients with RBD and a neurodegenerative disorder, 14 had MSA, of which 5 were female; this contrasted with 2 of the 32 patients with PD and/or dementia were female. These findings suggest that gender differences may exist in those with RBD and neurodegenerative disease.

Nocturnal stridor is a worrisome feature that sometimes evolves in MSA, and when present, sudden death can occur *(58)*. In patients with MSA, stridor, and RBD, clonazepam should be used with caution, if at all. Tracheostomy should be considered in all patients with MSA and stridor *(57)*.

2.5. Clinicopathologic Findings in Patients with RBD

To date, 14 autopsied patients with RBD have been reported (Table 4). The report of Uchiyama et al. involved a patient with a 20-yr history of RBD who had no cognitive or motor findings thoughout his clinical course *(59)*. At autopsy, Lewy bodies were identified, particularly in the brainstem. Schenck et al. reported a man with a 15-yr history of RBD before dementia evolved, and autopsy initially showed AD pathology *(21)*, but subsequently, ubiquitin immunocytochemistry revealed limbic Lewy bodies

(60). To date, we have identified nine other dementia cases, and all had Lewy body disease (LBD); coexisting AD pathology was present in five cases, argyrophilic grain pathology was present in one case, and Binswanger's pathology was present in one case *(44,61)*. Another patient with levodopa-responsive PD was found to have MSA at autopsy *(44,61)*. Turner et al. have provided detailed clinical and pathologic descriptions of their case with RBD and LBD *(48,49)*. The PD case reported by Arnulf et al. had LBD *(33)*. Therefore, all patients with RBD examined to date have had either Lewy body pathology or MSA at autopsy.

2.6. RBD and the Synucleinopathies: A Critical Association?

When associated with a neurodegenerative disorder, does RBD have a predilection for some disorders and not others? There are no published reports of RBD associated with pure AD (without co-existing Lewy bodies), MCI (which often reflects underlying AD), Pick's disease (Pick), frontotemporal dementia (FTD), progressive nonfluent aphasia (PNA), semantic dementia (SD), corticobasal degeneration (CBD), progressive subcortical gliosis, argyrophilic grain disease (AGD), or dementia lacking distinctive histopathology (DLDH). RBD has been reported in clinically suspected progressive supranuclear palsy (PSP) *(9,31)*, pure autonomic failure *(31)*, and amyotrophic lateral sclerosis *(31)*. REM sleep without atonia has been reported in single cases of CBD *(62)* and PSP *(63)*, but neither had clinical RBD features. As noted above, numerous cases of RBD have been reported in conjunction with MSA *(9,26,27,31,50–56)*, PD *(9,26,28–31,33,57)*, and DLB *(23,41,48,49,64)*. Furthermore, as shown above, all patients with RBD who have undergone autopsy have had either DLB or MSA. Therefore, there is considerable evidence indicating RBD occurs in association with PD, DLB (both forms of LBD), and MSA, and rarely if ever in other neurodegenerative disorders.

Recent immunocytochemical analyses have revealed that PD, DLB, and MSA share the similarity of α-synuclein positive intracellular inclusions *(65–68)*. Specifically, the oligodendroglial cytoplasmic filamentous inclusions in MSA and Lewy bodies and Lewy neurites in PD and DLB are comprised of the protein α-synuclein, and these disorders can be collectively considered as "synucleinopathies" *(67, 69–71)*. In contrast, the neurofibrillary tangles of AD, and the intracellular inclusions in Pick's disease, PSP, CBD, progressive subcortical gliosis, and AGD are made of the microtubule-associated protein tau in a hyperphosphorylated state, and these disorders can be characterized as "tauopathies" *(67,69–71)*.

A reasonable and testable hypothesis that stems from the published literature to date is the following: RBD occurs with disproportionally greater frequency, or is specific for, the synucleinopathies (e.g., MSA, PD, DLB) compared to those disorders that are nonsynucleinopathies (e.g., AD, Pick, PSP, CBD, progressive subcortical gliosis, AGD, and DLDH) *(44)*. Since the syndromes of MCI, FTD, PNA, and SD are typically manifestions of the nonsynucleinopathy disorders, one would also expect that RBD would be infrequent or absent in patients with these syndromes. We have performed three analyses to test this hypothesis.

We reviewed the clinical records of 398 consecutive patients evaluated at Mayo Clinic Rochester by a single neurologist (B.F.B.) for parkinsonism and/or cognitive impairment *(44)*. The frequency of suspected and PSG-confirmed RBD, among subjects with the synucleinopathies MSA, PD, or DLB, was compared to the frequency among subjects with the nonsynucleinopathies AD, FTD, CBD, PSP, MCI, primary progressive aphasia (PPA), and posterior cortical atrophy (PCA). The results indicate that patients with MSA, PD, or DLB were more likely to have probable and PSG-confirmed RBD compared to subjects with the nonsynucleinopathies (probable RBD 77/120 = 64% vs 7/278 = 3%, $p < 0.01$; PSG-confirmed RBD 47/120 = 39% vs 1/278 = <1%, $p < 0.01$) *(44)*.

We also reviewed the clinical records of 360 consecutive patients evaluated at Mayo Clinic Jacksonville for parkinsonism and/or cognitive impairment *(44)*. The frequency of probable RBD among patients with PD and DLB was compared to the frequency among patients with AD and MCI. Patients with PD and DLB were more likely to have probable RBD compared to those with AD and MCI (56 vs 2%, $p < 0.01$) *(44)*.

Finally, we reviewed the brain biopsy or postmortem autopsy diagnoses of 23 Mayo Clinic Rochester patients who had been clinically examined for possible RBD and a neurodegenerative disorder (this analysis includes 10 of the patients reported in the section under Subheading 2.5. *(44)*. Of the 23 autopsied patients who had been questioned about possible RBD, 10 were clinically diagnosed with RBD. The neuropathologic diagnoses in these 10 patients included LBD in 9 and MSA in 1. Of the other 13 cases, 12 did not have a history suggesting RBD, and the 1 case who did have normal EMG atonia during REM sleep on PSG, had autopsy findings of PSP *(44)*. Thus, the positive predictive values for RBD indicating a synucleinopathy exceeded 90% for each of these analyses.

In summary, the literature indicates that RBD is often associated with the synucleinopathies, but rarely if ever with the nonsynucleinopathies. Future clinicopathologic studies in patients with neurodegenerative disease, with and without RBD, will be necessary to test the hypothesis that in the setting of degenerative dementia and/or parkinsonism, the presence of RBD often reflects an underlying synucleinopathy *(44)*.

2.7. *Future Directions*

As noted above, more clinicopathologic studies are warranted to determine the predictive value of RBD for the synucleinopathies. The available data indicates that the onset of RBD often precedes (by decades in some cases) the onset of cognitive impairment or parkinsonism in MSA, PD, and DLB. Thus, if isolated RBD represents the earliest clinical manifestation of an evolving neurodegenerative disorder, the presence of RBD may be particularly relevant early in the course of a neurodegenerative disease when intervention may be most critical. The syndrome of MCI is considered by many to represent the earliest clinical manifestation of evolving AD *(72)*, and several treatment trials are currently in progress to potentially delay the progression of patients from MCI to AD. Perhaps RBD represents a similar early clinical manifestation of evolving LBD and MSA, and treatment of patients with isolated RBD could potentially delay or prevent the development of cognitive impairment or parkinsonism. Understanding the pathophysiologic substrate for RBD in animals and humans is critically important, as increased knowledge of what constitutes normal and abnormal REM sleep may ultimately lead to therapies for disabling neurodegenerative disorders.

ACKNOWLEDGMENTS

This work was supported by grants AG 16574, AG 06786, and AG 15866 from the National Institute on Aging.

REFERENCES

1. Schenck, C., Hurwitz, T., and Mahowald, M. (1993) REM sleep behaviour disorder: an update on a series of 96 patients and a review of the world literature. *J. Sleep Res.* **2,** 224–231.
2. Schenck, C.H., Milner, D.M., Hurwitz, T.D., Bundlie, S.R., and Mahowald, M.W. (1989) A polysomnographic and clinical report on sleep-related injury in 100 adult patients. *Am. J. Psychiatry* **146,** 1166–1173.
3. Schenck, C. and Mahowald, M. (1990) A polysomnographic, neurologic, psychiatric and clinical outcome report on 70 consecutive cases with REM sleep behavior disorder (RBD): sustained clonzepam efficacy in 89.5% of 57 treated patients. *Clev. Clin. J. Med.* **57(Suppl.),** 10–24.
4. Gross, P. (1992) REM sleep behavior disorder causing bilateral subdural hematomas [abstract]. *Sleep Res.* **21,** 204.
5. Mahowald, M. and Schenck, C. (2000) REM sleep behavior disorder, in *Principles and Practice of Sleep Medicine* (Kryger, M., Roth, T., and Dement, W., eds.), WB Saunders, Philadelphia, pp. 724–741.
6. Dyken, M., Lin-Dyken, D., Seaba, P., and Yamada, T. (1995) Violent sleep-related behavior leading to subdural hemorrhage. *Arch. Neurol.* **52,** 318–321.
7. Schenck, C.H. and Mahowald, M.W. (1996) REM sleep parasomnias. *Neurol. Clin.* **14,** 697–720.
8. Comella, C., Nardine, T., Diederich, N., and Stebbins, G. (1998) Sleep-related violence, injury, and REM sleep behavior disorder in Parkinson's disease. *Neurology* **51,** 526–529.
9. Olson, E., Boeve, B., and Silber, M. (2000) Rapid eye movement sleep behavior disorder: demographic, clinical, and laboratory findings in 93 cases. *Brain* **123,** 331–339.
10. International Classification of Sleep Disorders, Revised: Diagnostic and Coding Manual. (1997) American Sleep Disorders Association, Rochester, pp. 177–180.

11. Kunz, D. and Bes, F. (1999) Melatonin as a therapy in REM sleep behavior disorder patients: an open-labeled pilot study on the possible influence of melatonin on REM-sleep regulation. *Mov. Disord.* **14,** 507–511.
12. Boeve, B. (2001) Melatonin for treatment of REM sleep behavior disorder: response in 8 patients [abstract]. *Sleep* **24,** A374.
13. Ringman, J. and Simmons, J. (2000) Treatment of REM sleep behavior disorder with donepezil: a report of three cases. *Neurology* **55,** 870–871.
14. Rye, D. (1997) Contributions of the pedunculopontine region to normal and altered REM sleep. *Sleep* **20,** 757–788.
15. Bamford, C. (1993) Carbamazepine in REM sleep behavior disorder. *Sleep* **16,** 33–34.
16. Hendricks, J., Morrison, A., and Mann, G. (1982) Different behaviors during paradoxical sleep without atonia depend on pontine lesion site. *Brain Res.* **239,** 81–105.
17. Morrison, A. (1998) The pathophysiology of REM-sleep behavior disorder [letter]. *Sleep* **21,** 446.
18. Rye, D. (1998) The pathophysiology of REM-sleep behavior disorder [letter]. *Sleep* **21,** 446–449.
19. Siegel, J. (2001) REM Sleep Behavior Disorder, Associated Professional Sleep Societies, Chicago.
20. Hobson, J. and McCarley, R. (1977) The brain as a dream state generator: an activation-synthesis hypothesis of the dream process. *Am. J. Psychiatry* **124,** 1335–1348.
21. Schenck, C.H., Garcia-Rill, E., Skinner, R.D., Anderson, M.L., and Mahowald, M.W. (1996) A case of REM sleep behavior disorder with autopsy-confirmed Alzheimer's disease: postmortem brain stem histochemical analyses. *Biol. Psychiatry* **40,** 422–425.
22. Culebras, A. and Moore, J. (1989) Magnetic resonance findings in REM sleep behavior disorder. *Neurology* **39,** 1519–1523.
23. Boeve, B.F., Silber, M.H., Ferman, T.J., et al. (1998) REM sleep behavior disorder and degenerative dementia: an association likely reflecting Lewy body disease. *Neurology* **51,** 363–370.
24. Albin, R., Koeppe, R., Chervin, R., et al. (2000) Decreased striatal dopaminergic innervation in REM sleep behavior disorder. *Neurology* **55,** 1410–1412.
25. Eisensehr, I., Linke, R., Noachtar, S., Schwarz, J., Gildehaus, F., and Tatsch, K. (2000) Reduced striatal dopamine transporters in idiopathic rapid eye movement sleep behaviour disorder: comparison with Parkinson's disease and controls. *Brain* **123,** 1155–1160.
26. Schenck, C.H., Bundlie, S.R., Ettinger, M.G., and Mahowald, M.W. (1986) Chronic behavioral disorders of human REM sleep: a new category of parasomnia. *Sleep* **9,** 293–308.
27. Schenck, C.H., Bundlie, S.R., Patterson, A.L., and Mahowald, M.W. (1987) Rapid eye movement sleep behavior disorder. A treatable parasomnia affecting older adults. *JAMA* **257,** 1786–1789.
28. Silber, M. and Ahlskog, J. (1992) REM sleep behavior disorder in parkinsonian syndromes [abstract]. *Sleep Res.* **21,** 313.
29. Silber, M., Dexter, D., Ahlskog, J., Hauri, P., and Shepard, J. (1993) Abnormal REM sleep motor activity in untreated Parkinson's disease [abstract]. *Sleep Res.* **22,** 274.
30. Tan, A., Salgado, M., and Fahn, S. (1996) Rapid eye movement sleep behavior disorder preceding Parkinson's disease with therapeutic response to levodopa. *Mov. Disord.* **11,** 214–216.
31. Sforza, E., Krieger, J., and Petiau, C. (1997) REM sleep behavior disorder: clinical and physiopathological findings. *Sleep Med. Rev.* **1,** 57–69.
32. Rye, D., Johnston, L., Watts, R., and Bliwise, D. (1999) Juvenile Parkinson's disease with REM sleep behavior disorder, sleepiness, and daytime REM onset. *Neurology* **53,** 1868–1872.
33. Arnulf, I., Bonnet, A.M., Damier, P., et al. (2000) Hallucinations, REM sleep, and Parkinson's disease: a medical hypothesis. *Neurology* **55,** 281–288.
34. Schenck, C.H., Bundlie, S.R., and Mahowald, M.W. (1996) Delayed emergence of a parkinsonian disorder in 38% of 29 older men initially diagnosed with idiopathic rapid eye movement sleep behaviour disorder [published erratum appears in Neurology 1996 Jun;46(6):1787]. *Neurology* **46,** 388–393.
35. Ferman, T., Boeve, B., Silber, M., et al. (1997) Hallucinations and delusions associated with the REM sleep behavior disorder/dementia syndrome. *J. Neuropsychiatry Clin. Neurosci.* **9,** 692.
36. Boeve, B., Silber, M., Petersen, R., Kokmen, E., Parisi, J., and Olson, E. (1997) REM sleep behavior disorder and degenerative dementia with or without parkinsonism: a syndrome predictive of Lewy body disease? *Neurology* **48 (Suppl. 2),** 358–359.
37. Silber, M., Boeve, B., Petersen, R., Kokmen, E., Parisi, J., and Olson, E. (1998) REM sleep behavior disorder and dementia: a syndrome possibly predictive of Lewy body disease. *Sleep* **21,** 196.
38. Ferman, T.J., Boeve, B.F., Smith, G.E., et al. (1998) The REM sleep behavior disorder/dementia syndrome: neuropsychological differences when compared to Alzheimer's disease. *Neurology* **50(Suppl. 4),** A282.
39. Boeve, B.F., Silber, M.H., Ferman, T.J., et al. (1998) Further data supporting underlying Lewy body disease in the RBD/dementia syndrome. *Neurobiol. Aging* **19,** S205.
40. Ferman, T.J., Boeve, B.F., Smith, G.E., et al. (1998) RBD/dementia syndrome: a non-Alzheimer dementia. *Clin. Neuropsychol.* **12,** 257.
41. Ferman, T.J., Boeve, B.F., Smith, G.E., et al. (1999) REM sleep behavior disorder and dementia: cognitive differences when compared with AD. *Neurology* **52,** 951–957.
42. Boeve, B., Silber, M., Ferman, T., Lucas, J., and Parisi, J. (1999) Association of REM sleep behavior disorder and neurodegenerative disease [abstract]. *Sleep* **22(Suppl. 1),** S72.
43. Boeve, B., Silber, M., Ferman, T., Lucas, J., and Parisi, J. (2000) Association of REM sleep behavior disorder and neurodegenerative disease may reflect an underlying synucleinopathy [abstract]. *Mov. Disord.* **15,** 227–228.

44. Boeve, B., Silber, M., Ferman, T., Lucas, J., and Parisi, J. (2001) Association of REM sleep behavior disorder and neurodegenerative disease may reflect an underlying synucleinopathy. *Mov. Disord.* **16,** 622–630.
45. McKeith, I.G., Perry, E.K., and Perry, R.H. (1999) Report of the second dementia with Lewy body international workshop: diagnosis and treatment. Consortium on Dementia with Lewy Bodies. *Neurology* **53,** 902–905.
46. McKeith, I.G., Galasko, D., Kosaka, K., et al. (1996) Consensus guidelines for the clinical and pathologic diagnosis of dementia with Lewy bodies (DLB): report of the consortium on DLB international workshop. *Neurology* **47,** 1113–1124.
46a. Ferman, T.J., Boeve, B.F., Smith, G.E., et al. (2002) Dementia with Lewy bodies may present as dementia and REM sleep behavior disorder without parkinsonism or hallucinations. *J. Intl. Neuropsych. Soc.* **8,** 907–914.
47. Ferman, T., Boeve, B., Silber, M., Lin, S., and Fredrickson, P. (2001) Is fluctuating cognition in dementia with Lewy bodies attributable to an underlying sleep disorder? [abstract]. *Sleep* **24,** A374.
48. Turner, R.S., Chervin, R.D., Frey, K.A., Minoshima, S., and Kuhl, D.E. (1997) Probable diffuse Lewy body disease presenting as REM sleep behavior disorder. *Neurology* **49,** 523–527.
49. Turner, R., D'Amato, C., Chervin, R., and Blaivas, M. (2000) The pathology of REM sleep behavior disorder with comorbid Lewy body dementia. *Neurology* **55,** 1730–1732.
50. Plazzi, G., Corsini, R., Provini, F., et al. (1997) REM sleep behavior disorder in multiple system atrophy. *Neurology* **48,** 1094–1097.
51. Tachibana, N., Kimura, K., Kitajima, K., Shinde, A., Kimura, J., and Shibasaki, H. (1997) REM sleep motor dysfunction in multiple system atrophy: with special emphasis on sleep talk as its early clinical manifestation. *J. Neurol. Neurosurg. Psychiatry* **63,** 678–681.
52. Quera Salva, M. and Guilleminault, C. (1986) Olivopontocerebellar degeneration, abnormal sleep, and REM sleep without atonia. *Neurology* **36,** 576–577.
53. Tison, F., Wenning, G., Quinn, N., and Smith, S. (1995) REM sleep behavior disorder as the presenting symptom of multiple system atrophy. *J. Neurol. Neurosurg. Psychiatry* **58,** 379–380.
54. Wright, B., Rosen, J., Buysse, D., Reynolds, C., and Zubenko, G. (1990) Shy-Drager syndrome presenting as a REM behavioral disorder. *J. Geriatr. Psychiatry Neurol.* **3,** 110–113.
55. Manni, R., Morini, R., Martignoni, E., Pacchetti, C., Micieli, G., and Tartara, A. (1993) Nocturnal sleep in multisystem atrophy with autonomic failure: polygraphic findings in ten patients. *J. Neurol.* **240,** 247–250.
56. Coccagna, G., Martinelli, P., Zucconi, M., Cirignotta, F., and Ambrosetto, G. (1985) Sleep-related respiratory and haemodynamic changes in Shy-Drager syndrome: a case report. *J. Neurol.* **232,** 310–313.
57. Silber, M. and Levine, S. (2000) Stridor and death in multiple system atrophy. *Mov. Disord.* **15,** 699–704.
58. Isozaki, E., Naito, A., Horiguchi, S., Kawamura, R., Hayashida, T., and Tanabe, H. (1996) Early diagnosis and stage classification of vocal cord abductor paralysis in patients with multiple system atrophy. *J. Neurol. Neurosurg. Psychiatry* **60,** 399–402.
59. Uchiyama, M., Isse, K., Tanaka, K., et al. (1995) Incidental Lewy body disease in a patient with REM sleep behavior disorder. *Neurology* **45,** 709–712.
60. Schenck, C.H., Mahowald, M.W., Anderson, M.L., Silber, M.H., Boeve, B.F., and Parisi, J.E. (1997) Lewy body variant of Alzheimer's disease (AD) identified by postmortem ubiquitin staining in a previously reported case of AD associated with REM sleep behavior disorder [letter]. *Biol. Psychiatry* **42,** 527–528.
61. Boeve, B., Silber, M., Parisi, J., Dickson, D., Ferman, T., and Petersen, R. (2001) Neuropathologic findings in patients with REM sleep behavior disorder and a neurodegenerative disorder [abstract]. *Neurology* **56,** A299.
62. Kimura, K., Tachibana, N., Toshihiko, A., Kimura, J., and Shibasaki, H. (1997) Subclinical REM sleep behavior disorder in a patient with corticobasal degeneration. *Sleep* **20,** 891–894.
63. Pareja, J., Caminero, A., Masa, J., and Dobato, J. (1996) A first case of progressive supranuclear palsy and pre-clinical REM sleep behavior disorder presenting as inhibition of speech during wakefulness and somniloquy with phasic muscle twitching during REM sleep. *Neurologia* **11,** 304–306.
64. Negro, P. and Faber, R. (1996) Lewy body disease in a patient with REM sleep disorder [letter]. *Neurology* **46,** 1493–1494.
65. Spillantini, M., Crowther, R., Jakes, R., Cairns, N., Lantos, P., and Goedert, M. (1998) Filamentous alpha-synuclein inclusions link multiple system atrophy with Parkinson's disease and dementia with Lewy bodies. *Neurosci. Lett.* **251,** 205–208.
66. Baba, M., Nakajo, S., Tu, P., et al. (1998) Aggregation of alpha-synuclein in Lewy bodies of sporadic Parkinson's disease and dementia with Lewy bodies. *Am. J. Pathol.* **152,** 879–884.
67. Dickson, D.W. (1999) Tau and synuclein and their role in neuropathology. *Brain Pathol.* **9,** 657–661.
68. Dickson, D.W., Liu, W., Hardy, J., et al. (1999) Widespread alterations of alpha-synuclein in multiple system atrophy. *Am. J. Pathol.* **155,** 1241–1251.
69. Hardy, J. and Gwinn-Hardy, K. (1998) Genetic classification of primary neurodegenerative disease. *Science* **282,** 1075–1079.
70. Hardy, J. and Gwinn-Hardy, K. (1999) Neurodegenerative disease: a different view of diagnosis. *Mol. Med. Today* **5,** 514–517.
71. Hardy, J. (1999) Pathways to primary neurodegenerative disease. *Mayo Clin. Proc.* **74,** 835–837.
72. Petersen, R., Smith, G., Waring, S., Ivnik, R., Tangalos, E., and Kokmen, E. (1999) Mild cognitive impairment: clinical characterization and outcome. *Arch. Neurol.* **56,** 303–308.

30
Psychogenic Parkinsonism and Dystonia

Daniel S. Sa, MD and Anthony E. Lang, MD, FRCPC

1. INTRODUCTION

Psychogenic disturbances are a common differential diagnosis for almost every symptom known to medicine. Legal problems are frequently involved, either in the form of disability compensation or in other forms of compensation, for injuries sustained in accidents, work-related or not.

In neurology, and especially in movement disorders, these abnormalities pose a great dilemma, mainly due to the lack of widely available biological markers for the diseases being mimicked. Without these markers, it is always difficult to be certain about a diagnosis such as psychogenic movement disorder (PMD).

A great degree of diagnostic certainty is required in order that the patient is not denied potentially helpful treatment options. On the other hand, mistakenly diagnosing patients as having an organic disorder can be extremely hazardous. Indeed, patients with PMDs have been exposed to varied therapeutic trials with potential serious complications, including thalamotomies and possibly even cell transplantation procedures *(1,2)*.

The history of movement disorders is full of mistakes regarding the diagnosis of such syndromes. Dystonic syndromes were commonly regarded as psychogenic until the mid-20th century, and after it was established that dystonia had an organic basis, cases of psychogenic dystonia were frequently misdiagnosed as organic. Even with parkinsonian syndromes, which are not usually considered potentially psychogenic, there are important cases of misdiagnosis. The most striking example may have been one of the earliest patients undergoing adrenal cell transplantation for Parkinson's disease (PD); it is possible that one of the initial two cases reported to show marked benefit (thus generating tremendous enthusiasm about this new therapy) had a psychogenic syndrome *(2)*.

In this chapter, we begin with a review of some general aspects of PMDs followed by a more detailed discussion of the two most difficult to diagnose disorders: psychogenic dystonia and psychogenic parkinsonism. As mentioned, the former is relatively common, whereas the latter is one of the least common of the PMDs.

2. PREVALENCE

The data in the literature is limited, but psychogenic disorders seem to be relatively common; it is suggested that up to 25% of the population at some time or other would fulfill criteria for some psychogenic disorder *(3)*. In a hospital-based study, somatoform disorders were the main diagnoses at the time of discharge in 2.6% of 1801 patients *(4)*.

From: *Mental and Behavioral Dysfunction in Movement Disorders*
Edited by: M-A. Bédard et al. © Humana Press Inc., Totowa, NJ

Neurological complaints are not uncommon among these patients, accounting for 1–9% of all neurological diagnoses *(5–7)*. Among neurological complaints, movement disorders are not infrequently seen; in a group of 842 consecutive patients seen in a movement disorders clinic, 28 (3.3%) were ultimately diagnosed as having a PMD *(8)*. In this particular series, tremor was the most common manifestation, followed by dystonia, myoclonus, and parkinsonism in that order. A patient series published by Fahn and Williams, with 131 patients, had dystonia as the leading symptom *(9)*. However, referral bias may have contributed to this finding, since the study originated from a dystonia research clinic. It is also not infrequent in patients with PMDs to see a mixture of abnormal bizarre movement types, making an accurate classification impossible *(9)*.

In the Movement Disorders Clinic of The Toronto Western Hospital, of 33 patients with a diagnosis of PMD seen between July 2000 and June 2001, tremor was present in 13 patients (39.3%), dystonia in 10 patients (30.3%), myoclonus in 4 patients (12.1%), a gait disorder in 4 patients (12.1%), parkinsonism in 3 patients (9%), and tics in 1 patient (3%). Bizarre, unclassified movements accounted for 12% (4 patients), and 5 patients (15.1%) had a combination of different movement disorders. As in most series, women predominated, accounting for 69.6% (23) of the patients. Interestingly, in psychogenic parkinsonism, there is a small trend toward male preponderance (9:8 in a total of 17 patients) *(8,10,11)*.

A frequent confounding factor is the presence of concomitant organic and nonorganic symptoms. As in the case of pseudoseizures in epileptic patients, it is not uncommon to have both psychogenic and organic movement disorders in the same patient *(8,11–14)*. In fact, in the series of Factor and colleagues, 25% of the patients presented with a concomitant organic movement disorder along with the PMD *(8)*. However, we believe that this figure is too high. In our recent series, an underlying organic movement disorder was established in 3 out of 33 patients (9%). Therefore, one should exercise extreme caution when making the diagnosis; documenting a PMD does not exclude the possibility of a concomitant true organic disorder. On the other hand, where an underlying organic disorder is not evident, it is extremely rare for one to develop subsequently. Therefore, if the diagnosis of an isolated PMD can be made with confidence, the patient does not need to be followed and repeatedly investigated, searching for new evidence to support a diagnosis of a causative organic condition (e.g., multiple sclerosis) *(15)*. Underlying causative psychiatric disturbances are varied; most frequently, depression, anxiety, and personality disorders are reported *(1,7–9,16–18)*. Feinstein and colleagues, interviewing a sample of 42 patients with PMD seen in our unit, found a lifetime prevalence of anxiety disorders in 61.9% (26) of the patients and major depression in 42.9% (18 patients); a combination of both affected 28.6% of the patients (12). Other lifetime psychiatric diagnoses included adjustment disorder in 9.5% (4 patients), schizoaffective disorders in 2.4% (1 patient), bipolar disorder in 2.4% (1 patient) and alcohol or sedative abuse in 2.4% (1 patient) each *(18)*.

3. HISTORY AND PHYSICAL EXAMINATION

There are clues from the history and physical examination that should suggest the possibility of a psychogenic origin of the abnormal movement; most of these can be applied to all types of PMDs *(9,11, 14,16,19)*.

Because most organic movement disorders have a relatively slow onset and progression, an abrupt onset and very rapid progression to maximal severity are features suggestive of PMD. One should keep in mind that true organic diseases do occasionally begin abruptly and progress rapidly, including rapid-onset dystonia parkinsonism, Wilson's disease, and poststroke–lesional movement disorders. Paroxysmal movements (i.e., "attacks") are common in PMDs; however, organic causes of paroxysmal dyskinesias must be excluded. Spontaneous remissions, static course, relationship to minimal injury, and litigation are also suggestive of "psychogenicity" *(8,9,11,16,17,19–23)*.

Other evidence supportive of a diagnosis of a PMD include multiple somatic complaints and undiagnosed conditions, known psychiatric disorders, and clear secondary gain. Caution should be exercised, since a known hypocondriacal patient can eventually manifest a true organic disease.

Table 1
Comparative Clues in the Differentiation between Organic and PMDs

	Organic	Psychogenic
Typical patient	Variable	Young female (predominate) health care professional (occasional)
Onset	Insidious	Abrupt
Triggering factors	Not detectable	Trauma, psychological or physical
Course	Gradual	Static, erratic
Type of movement disorder	One dominant, definable	Multiple, difficult to classify
Suggestion/placebo	Minimal change	Can induce changes
Response to therapy	Reliable (but often variable)	Erratic[a]
Fluctuations/variations	Minimal	Frequent
Pending litigation	Unusual	Common
Additional complaints	Variable	Multiple, unrelated
Additional findings	Variable	Multiple, pseudoneurological common

[a]May get early profound improvement followed by subsequent loss of benefit typical of placebo responses.

On the examination, bizarre, mixed movement disorders should suggest this possibility. Inconsistencies such as variability, distractibility, entrainability (especially useful in the case of tremor), and movements that can be precipitated by suggestion and/or relieved by placebo should strongly suggest a PMD *(9,11,19–21,23)*. A selective disability, when the patient cannot perform simple tasks with a particular limb on examination, but seems to be unlimited in daily activities requiring the use of that limb, should also raise suspicion *(9,16)*. Organic task-specific movement disorders must be excluded in these circumstances.

Additional, atypical findings on the neurological examination, such as "give-way" weakness, sensory disturbances in a nonanatomical pattern, and extreme slowness of movements, typically with additional grimacing or sighing, are important clues. The classical "la belle indifference" may also be a helpful clue, although it is often not present and can be misleading in some patients with organic disorders. Obviously, the most definitive evidence is surreptitious observation of a symptom-free period in patients with otherwise continuous movements (i.e., not paroxysmal) *(24)*.

Table 1 provides some comparative clues in the differentiation between organic or PMD. Caution should be exercised, because all the characteristics seen in psychogenic disorders can be shared by organic diseases and vice-versa *(25)*.

4. DYSTONIA

In the case of dystonic syndromes, it is far more common to misdiagnose an organic disease as psychogenic than the other way around *(26)*. In fact, in his original description in 1908, Schwalbe considered dystonia to be a psychogenic disorder *(22)*. Reasons for this misdiagnosis include the following characteristics of organic dystonic syndromes *(22,27)*:

1. The bizarre nature of most postures and movements, including paroxysmal movements in some patients.
2. Relief by sensory tricks (gestes antagoniste).
3. The fact that dystonic movements and postures can improve with relaxation, sedation, and hypnosis.
4. The occurrence of spontaneous remissions (especially but not exclusively in patients with cervical dystonia).
5. Fluctuation of symptoms, especially in dopa-responsive dystonia (DRD).
6. Task specificity of some dystonic syndromes, e.g., writer's cramp.
7. Frequent coexistence of psychological or psychiatric illnesses.

Psychological and psychiatric disturbances are not uncommon in patients with movement disorders. It is obvious that this, in part, simply reflects the negative impact movement disorders can have on a patient's life *(28–30)*. This is especially the case with dystonia where, in addition to physical disability, negative psychological impact comes from alterations in self-image due to the abnormal movements and postures, delays in diagnosis, and sometimes even misdiagnosis of organic dystonia as being psychologically based. It should also be remembered that basal ganglia dysfunction on its own can cause a vast array of neuropsychiatric dysfunctions, and finally, some forms of primary hereditary dystonia may be associated with behavioral or psychiatric disturbances (e.g., hereditary myoclonus dystonia). Here, the psychiatric diagnosis can be considered a co-morbidity rather than an etiologic factor or secondary to the movement disorder *(31)*.

Finally, the lack of biological markers, with the exception of some specific genetic mutations, including those causing DYT1 and DRD, also contributes to the misdiagnosis of dystonia. Therefore, it is clear that a diagnosis of psychogenic dystonia should be made with extreme caution, in order to avoid imposing additional stressors on patients afflicted with a true disabling organic condition.

Features suggestive of the possibility of psychogenic dystonia include the following *(9,16,22)*:

1. Inconsistency of movements over time—although dystonia can vary over time, during the course of an interview, it should behave in a more or less stereotyped pattern.
2. Incongruity with the movements and postures seen in patients with organic dystonia, including such factors as the use of sensory tricks and the occurrence of task specificity. This important criteria emphasizes the critical need for considerable experience with patients suffering from organic dystonia on the part of the physician making a diagnosis.
3. A rapid onset or progression, with fixed postures from the beginning—it is known that most dystonic syndromes begin with action-induced dystonia that might later evolve into fixed postures.
   Caution: peripheral trauma-induced dystonia, rapid-onset dystonia-parkinsonism.
4. Severe pain—dystonia can manifest pain, but is usually not a major component of the disability.
   Caution: patients with cervical dystonia can have severe pain even out of proportion to the evident dystonic posture.
5. Adults presenting with lower limb dystonia—this is usually a presentation of childhood, genetic dystonias; adults will more frequently present with cranial, cervical or upper limb involvement.
   Caution: adults with a variety of parkinsonian disorders or with other basal ganglia diseases may present with lower limb dystonia.
6. Paroxysms of movements. Caution: the organic paroxysmal dyskinesias.
7. Marked resistance to passive movements without concomitant contractures.

Obviously, some of the observations mentioned earlier in describing PMDs in general also apply here, e.g., additional pseudoneurologic deficits, distractibility, induction by suggestion, relief by placebo, selective disability, and observation of a symptom-free period. Other helpful observations might include observations such as a tan in a site supposedly inaccessible due to dystonia (e.g., one side of the neck in severe fixed laterocollis) and an adequately clean or shaved area under the arm or in other body creases in a severely affected immobile limb (examples seen in our patients).

Among the many pitfalls in the diagnosis of psychogenic dystonia, besides the ones already mentioned, is the occurrence of dystonia following peripheral trauma. Peripheral trauma-induced dystonia is not uncommonnly associated with evidence of a complex regional pain syndrome (CRPS).

CRPS, formerly known as reflex sympathetic dystrophy, is divided into type I, when the clinical syndrome is not limited to the distribution of a peripheral nerve, and type II, formerly causalgia, after damage to a particular nerve. Abnormal movements, especially dystonia, have been frequently described in patients with CRPS. Many of the features described above as typical of psychogenic dystonia are characteristic of the movement disorder found in these patients. Some authors feel strongly that these patients represent an unequivocal organic disorder and any evidence of underlying psychopathology is no different that that found in other patients suffering from chronic pain syndromes *(32)*. On the other hand, ourselves and others believe that psychological factors may play a very important role in the genesis of this disorder. In an interesting study, Verdugo and Ochoa studied 53 patients with CRPS and abnormal involuntary movements *(33)*. Dystonia and muscle spasms were frequent findings, accounting for some or all the abnormal movements in 74.2%. Surprisingly, no patients with CRPS type II (documented nerve damage) had abnormal movements. Other signs of a psychogenic component were present in all patients including "give-way" weakness, erratic fluctuations of symptoms, distractibility, placebo-induced relief, nonanatomic sensory disturbances, and response to psychotherapy. An important feature was the occurrence of a minimal precipitating event, usually work-related, in the majority of cases (81%). Only 5.2% of cases completely lacked an overt triggering event.

In studying patients with peripheral trauma-induced cervical dystonia, we have observed similar findings suggestive of a psychogenic component to the syndrome *(34)*. In a group of 13 patients developing dystonic-like muscle spasms with abnormal posturing of the neck and shoulder soon after local injury, common characteristics were identified, as follows:

1. Precipitants were always trivial, usually work-related, and frequently involving the neck and/or shoulder area.
2. No serious injury was diagnosed at the time of the original accident, despite early medical visits.
3. Abnormal movements developed quickly, with a fixed posture consisting of shoulder elevation and head tilt being present no later than 2 wk after the inciting event.
4. Pain was a prominent feature.
5. Litigation or compensation were involved in all patients.
6. Other pseudoneurological findings were frequent, including "give-way" weakness and nonanatomic sensory loss.
7. Psychological interview utilizing the Minnesota Multiphasic Personality Inventory was suggestive of conversion disorders.
8. Sodium amytal interview resulted in improvement of pain and posture in most patients.
9. General anesthesia ruled out hypertrophy in four out of five patients.
10. Other findings included distractibility, improvement with sham botulinum toxin injections, symmetrical neck tan, and observation of a symptom-free period.

Range of motion was affected in all our patients; this finding raises concerns over "established" long-standing disability related to traumatic injuries; one recent study implicated impaired range of motion as a prognostic factor in whiplash injuries *(35)*.

It is important to realize that early medical visits, injury anatomically related to the site of dystonia, and the development of an abnormal (dystonic) posture within 1 yr of the trauma are currently accepted criteria for the diagnosis of peripheral trauma-induced dystonia *(36)*. Another interesting feature of our group of patients was the fact that, despite the clinical impression of muscle hypertrophy, amytal interview and/or general anesthesia ruled this out in all but one tested patient. Muscle hypertrophy has been suggested as a typical finding of posttraumatic dystonia in other series, although no previous attempt has been made to define its true existence *(37–39)*.

5. PSYCHOGENIC PARKINSONISM

A PMD is usually not considered in the differential diagnosis of parkinsonism. Although certainly less common than tremor or dystonia, it should always be considered, since a diagnosis of true parkinsonism usually dictates some diagnostic tests and initiation of therapy that can be both expensive and deleterious to a nonparkinsonian patient. Like any other incorrect diagnosis, labeling a PMD as true parkinsonism can have major effects on a patient and his family's lifestyle, including changes in job, financial arrangements, and social relationships.

There are few reports of psychogenic parkinsonism in the literature. Probably the first one was published in 1988 describing a 64-yr-old man with an atypical gait, stuttering and a tremor that would persist with rest, posture, and action *(10)*.

Later, Lang and colleagues published a series of 14 patients with a diagnosis of psychogenic parkinsonism, including one patient with psychogenic parkinsonism superimposed on true PD *(11)*. This was followed by other reports that generally included psychogenic parkinsonism in the description of series of PMD patients *(8)*. It is interesting to note that, distinct from other PMDs, most series show a slight male preponderance for psychogenic parkinsonism *(8,10,11)*.

Contrary to typical PD, most of these patients present with a tremor manifested not only at rest, but with postural maintenance and action, (generally equal amplitude in all states). The tremor has other features of a psychogenic tremor, including entrainment to a new frequency when a slower repetitive movement is performed in the opposite limb. Concentration or distraction, such as performing "serial sevens," decreases the tremor, just as contralateral movements often decrease the apparent rigidity. This "rigidity" usually gives the "feel" of active resistance, without clear "coghwheeling." These features should prompt consideration of a psychogenic diagnosis, since it is widely recognized that mental tasks increase parkinsonian tremor, and contralateral movement increases tone in typical PD.

Bradykinesia in these patients is generally an excessive slowness of motion, without the classical fatigue or motor blocks on repetitive movements. Speech can also be atypical, including features such as stuttering and excessive hypophonia.

Early changes of gait and postural stability, with multiple, bizarre findings on examination, such as a violent backward displacement on the pull test, but little evidence of a tendency to fall, or a very elaborate gait, with forceful sliding of one foot at a time, are also supportive of this diagnosis.

Other features suggestive of psychogenic parkinsonism include absence of clear demonstrable effects of levodopa, including fluctuations and dyskinesias. However, some patients will have a placebo effect of levodopa, and we have even seen patients who complained of "wearing-off" close to the time that they were due to take the next dose.

6. ESTABLISHING A DIAGNOSIS

As already mentioned, a diagnosis of PMD should be carefully established. An incorrect diagnosis either way will certainly subject the patient to additional psychological stress, possible increased costs of ancillary tests, and lifestyle changes, and even more harmful, either the denial of potentially helpful treatments or the occurrence of treatment-associated side effects.

A clinical diagnosis, as can be inferred from the previous sections, is extremely difficult and filled with pitfalls. It should be established carefully, by a neurologist and preferably by a movement disorders specialist, since most of the useful clues rely on the recognition of atypical manifestations of an expected finding (e.g., excessive slowness in psychogenic parkinsonism). Therefore, the diagnosis is most accurately established only in the hands of an experienced clinician, used to the common clinical manifestations of organic movement disorders.

Admission to hospital in complex or difficult cases can prove beneficial for a variety of reasons. First, it provides the physician with an opportunity for continuous observation of the patient, including possible surreptitious observation by team members. If even that fails, video monitoring can also prove helpful. Second, it will allow for any necessary diagnostic procedure to exclude other causes for the symptoms, and especially to convince the patient that such diseases have been carefully excluded *(9,22)*. However, once the diagnosis is made with certainty, performing additional investigations can be counterproductive and can convey a degree of diagnostic uncertainty to the patient that may negatively impact on the initiation of appropriate therapy.

Ancillary tests are occasionally helpful, especially in the case of parkinsonism. In the appropriate clinical setting, a normal, carefully evaluated and quantified single-photon emission computerized tomography (SPECT) or positron emission tomography (PET) scan of the presynaptic nigrostriatal dopamine system (e.g., fluorodopa or scans evaluating the dopamine transporter) is strongly supportive of a psychogenic origin. However, some causes of organic parkinsonism, including DRD, can have normal findings on these imaging studies. In addition, we have seen a small number of patients with unequivocal organic parkinsonism (presumed PD) in whom the PET scan was reported as normal, obviously reducing the sensitivity of the test to suboptimal levels.

Electrophysiological studies may be of help in evaluating PMDs, especially myoclonus and tremor *(40)*. A variety of physiological abnormalities have been described in organic dystonic syndromes. The extent to which these contribute to dystonia or are secondary to the abnormal postures is not clear. In a recent review, Brown and Thompson *(40)* point out that two findings show promise. Diminished reciprocal inhibition at intermediate and long latencies, as well as the absence of broad-peak synchronization of co-contracting antagonist muscles could be useful in this differentiation. However, because these findings were never controlled for voluntary mimicking of the abnormal activity nor used in a setting differentiating organic from PMDs, to date these have not been clinically useful in the diagnosis of psychogenic dystonia.

Psychiatric consultation should be obtained for assistance with primary diagnosis and therapy. An established psychiatric diagnosis is of paramount importance both in the diagnosis and the treatment of patients with PMDs; a positive response to psychotherapy lends further support to the PMD diagnosis. However, it is important to reiterate that patients with organic movement disorders may have additional psychopathology. The diagnosis of a PMD is made by an experienced neurologist and should not be made or refuted by a psychiatrist, especially one inexperienced in the field of movement disorders.

Utilization of placebo or suggestion is a more controversial subject. Suggestion is a relatively benign approach: the reinforcement that there is no serious underlying degenerative disease, coupled sometimes with directed physiotherapy training and biofeedback techniques, can be extremely helpful.

The use of placebos can be hazardous. First, there are ethical and legal concerns about the use of nonactive drugs, negating the patient's autonomy. Second, it can endanger the physician–patient relationship, with the latter feeling deceived and, therefore, abandoning treatment *(41)*. There is also the potential for both severe psychogenic "reactions" upon the challenge and false-positive responses in suggestible patients with organic disease. Placebo-effects are widely recognized in a variety of diseases, including movement disorders *(42)*.

On the other hand, the use of a placebo enables a direct observation and can establish a diagnosis and even a therapeutic approach. One must remember that as soon as the diagnosis of a PMD can be established with a reasonable degree of certainty, it is possible to both withdraw and avoid therapies with potential harmful side effects. As previously mentioned, patients have been subjected to hazardous treatments, including neurosurgical procedures, due to incorrect diagnoses.

7. DIAGNOSTIC CRITERIA

In 1988, Fahn and Williams published a set of clinical criteria for the diagnosis of psychogenic dystonia, subdividing the levels of diagnostic accuracy into documented, clinically established, probable, and possible *(9)*. Currently, these criteria are widely used and accepted for all PMDs, not only dystonia.

Documented includes cases in which the movement is persistently relieved by psychotherapy, suggestion, or placebo; alternatively, the patient is surreptitiously witnessed to be free of symptoms. Clinically established includes movements inconsistent over time or incongruous with classical definitions of movement disorders; additional evidence of a psychogenic illness, such as pseudoneurological findings are required. Probable refers to patients who fulfill only one criteria for clinically definite. Possible is applied to patients with an obvious psychiatric disturbance who show a movement disorder consistent with an organic disorder.

8. TREATMENT

Treatment of psychogenic disturbances can be challenging. Unlike most other diseases, there is no clear physiologic basis nor an established prognosis to be discussed. After it has been established beyond reasonable doubt, the diagnosis should be discussed thoroughly with the patient, including treatment options and expected prognosis, despite the complete lack of comparative data in the literature as to the results of different treatment approaches.

Nevertheless, the lack of an underlying serious progressive neurological disease should be emphasized, as well as the physician's empathy for the problem. It should be clear to the patient that because there is no definite brain lesion, a complete recovery is possible. There should be no question in the patient's mind as to the seriousness of the physician's approach to his or her problem nor as to the certainty of the diagnosis.

The subsequent treatment approach has to be individualized, based on the patient's characteristics, degree of disability, and underlying psychiatric diagnosis. Again, it should be emphasized that, due to lack of prospective studies on different treatment approaches, therapeutic trials will inevitably follow a trial-and-error approach.

Physiotherapy can be attempted in patients with long-standing abnormalities, which might have even progressed to contractures or bizarre compensation mechanisms. Biofeedback techniques can be extremely helpful in some patients.

Obviously, the underlying psychiatric illness should be treated aggressively, with antidepressants or other appropriate drugs. Psychotherapy is generally helpful in learning to cope with the stressors that precipitated the problem in different more appropriate ways.

Placebo and suggestion may also be helpful, but usually improvement is short-lived, and this should not be used as the maintenance therapy. Furthermore, there are ethical issues involved in the use of placebo as discussed previously.

9. PROGNOSIS

Very little is known about the long-term prognosis of these patients, both with respect to the movement disorders and the psychiatric features. Despite the suggestion that settlement resolves the problem in patients involved in legal or compensation issues, or the natural intuitive thinking that abnormal movements of psychogenic origin will eventually settle, and the previous uncontrolled findings that 25% of the patients improve, it now seems that quite a high proportion of these patients will continue to have disability *(18,22)*.

Feinstein and colleagues have attempted to shed some light on this issue and interviewed 42 patients out of a group of 88 subjects with either documented or clinically established PMD *(18)*. In that group of patients, 10 had dystonia (23.8%) and none had pure parkinsonism. At the time of the study interview, on average, 3.2 yr after the initial assessment, all but four patients still had the abnormal movement (90.5%). Of these four patients, two had replaced the abnormal movement by a different somatoform disorder. Although there was no formal assessment at baseline, the psychiatric status showed a significant array of disorders; only two patients did not have a psychiatric diagnosis at follow-up (4.8%). Diagnosis at the time of interview included anxiety disorders in 16 patients (38.1%), major depression in 8 patients (19.1%) and a combination of the two in 5 patients (11.9%). A schizoaffective disorder was diagnosed in one patient (2.4%).

Twenty-three of our previously diagnosed PMD patients (most of these participating in the study of Feinstein described previously) agreed to a follow-up detailed neurological examination *(43)*. In this subset, all patients were still manifesting PMD at the time of follow-up, with a mean duration of symptoms of 8.6 +/– 8.5 yr (range 1.5–43). Activities of daily living such as eating, dressing, and hygiene were reported impaired in 19 of the examined patients (82.6%). Of the patients whose symptoms had improved or stabilized, 66.6% experienced this change within the first year of illness. This overall poor prognosis for recovery and substantial disability has been reported by other groups, for example, studying psychogenic tremor *(20)*.

Thus, in summary, PMDs seem to carry a poor prognosis, both for psychiatric and motor function. Patients who do fare better seem to be the ones who have symptoms improved and stabilized within the first year, suggesting that long-standing disease, when first assessed, carries a particularly poor prognosis. Other studies have suggested that additional features that may predict a good outcome in psychogenic neurological syndromes, include a clear emotional trigger or precipitant, lack of long-standing psychopathology, improvement while in the hospital, and early spontaneous improvement (the latter similar to our findings) *(44)*.

Given the profound disability and poor prognosis found in many patients with PMDs, there is a great need for well-designed prospective studies that include longitudinal follow-up and carefully controlled evaluation of various treatment approaches.

REFERENCES

1. Batshaw, M.L., Wachtel, R.C., Deckel, A.W., et al. (1985) Munchausen's syndrome simulating torsion dystonia. *N. Engl. J. Med.* **312,** 1437–1439.
2. Lang, A.E. (2001) Evaluation of the state of the art in surgery for Parkinson disease: should we use the same criteria as for drug trials? *Arch. Neurol.* **58,** 315–316.
3. Schepank, H., Hilpert, H., Honmann, H., et al. (1984) The Mannheim Cohort Project—prevalence of psychogenic diseaes in cities. *Z. Psychosom. Med. Psychoanal.* **30,** 43–61.
4. Snyder, S. and Strain, J.J. (1989) Somatoform disorders in the general hospital inpatient setting. *Gen. Hosp. Psychiatry* **11,** 288–293.
5. Franz, M., Schellberg, D., Reister, G., and Schepank, H. (1993) Incidence and follow-up characteristics of neurologically relevant psycogenic symptoms. *Nervenarzt* **64,** 369–376.
6. Marsden, C.D. (1986) Hysteria—a neurologist's view. *Psychol. Med.* **16,** 277–288.
7. Lempert, T., Dieterich, M., Huppert, D., and Brandt, T. (1990) Psychogenic disorders in neurology: frequency and clinical spectrum. *Acta Neurol. Scand.* **82,** 335–340.
8. Factor, S.A., Podshalny, G.D., and Molho, E.S. (1995) Psychogenic movement disorders: frequency, clinical profile and characteristics. *J. Neurol. Neurosurg. Psychiatry* **59,** 406–412.
9. Fahn, S. and Williams, P.J. (1988) Psychogenic dystonia. *Adv. Neurol.* **50,** 431–455.
10. Walters, A.S., Boudwin, J., Wright, D., and Jones, K. (1988) Three hysterical movement disorders. *Psychol. Reports* **62,** 979–985.
11. Lang, A.E., Koller, W.C., and Fahn, S. (1995) Psychogenic parkinsonism. *Arch. Neurol.* **52,** 802–810.
12. Kurlan, R., Deeley, C., and Comon, P.G. (1992) Psychogenic movement disorder (pseudo-tics) in a patient with Tourette's syndrome. *J. Neuropsychiatry Clin. Neurosci.* **4,** 347–348.
13. Kanner, A.M., Parra, J., Frey, M., Stebbins, G., Pierre-Louis, S., and Iriarte, J. (1999) Psychiatric and neurologic predictors of psychogenic pseudoseizure outcome. *Neurology* **53,** 933–938.
14. Ranawaya, R., Riley, D., and Lang, A.E. (1990) Psychogenic dyskinesias in patients with organic movement disorders. *Mov. Disord.* **5,** 127–133.
15. Crimlisk, H.L., Bhatia, K., Cope, H., David, A., Marsden, C.D., and Ron, M.A. (1998) Slater revisited: 6 year follow up study of patients with medically unexplained motor symptoms. *BMJ* **316,** 582–586.
16. Lang, A.E. (1995) Psychogenic dystonia: a review of 18 cases. *Can. J. Neurol. Sci.* **22,** 136–143.
17. Williams, D.T., Ford, B., and Fahn, S. (1995) Phenomenology and psychopathology related to psychogenic movement disorders. *Adv. Neurol.* **65,** 231–258.
18. Feinstein, A., Stergiopoulos, V., Fine, J., and Lang, A.E. (2001) Psychiatric outcome in patients with a psychogenic movement disorder: a prospective study. *Neuropsychiatry Neuropsychol. Behav. Neurol.* **14,** 169–176.
19. Monday, K. and Jankovic, J. (1993) Psychogenic myoclonus. *Neurology* **43,** 349–352.
20. Deuschl, G., Köster, B., Lücking, C.H., and Scheidt, C. (1998) Diagnostic and pathophysiological aspects of psychogenic tremors. *Mov. Disord.* **13,** 294–302.
21. Koller, W.C. and Findley, L.J. (1990) Psychogenic tremors. *Adv. Neurol.* **53,** 271–275.
22. Marsden, C.D. (1995) Psychogenic problems associated with dystonia. *Adv. Neurol.* **65,** 319–326.
23. Marjama, J., Troster, A.I., and Koller, W.C. (1995) Psychogenic movement disorders. *Neurol. Clin.* **13,** 283–297.
24. Kurlan, R., Brin, M.F., and Fahn, S. (1997) Movement disorder in reflex sympathetic dystrophy: a case proven to be psychogenic by surveillance video monitoring. *Mov. Disord.* **12,** 243–245.
25. Gould, R., Miller, B.L., Goldberg, M.A., and Benson, D.F. (1986) The validity of hysterical signs and symptoms. *J. Nerv. Ment. Dis.* **174,** 593–597.
26. Lesser, R.P. and Fahn, S. (1978) Dystonia: a disorder often misdiagnosed as a conversion reaction. *Am. J. Psychiatry* **153,** 349–352.
27. Marsden, C.D. and Harrison, M.J.G. (1974) Idiopathic torsion dystonia (dystonia musculorum deformans). A review of forty-two patients. *Brain* **97,** 793–810.
28. Diamond, E.L., Trobe, J.D., and Belar, C.D. (1984) Psychological aspects of essential blepharospasm. *J. Nerv. Ment. Dis.* **172,** 749–756.
29. Wenzel, T., Schnider, P., Griengl, H., Birner, P., Nepp, J., and Auff, E. (2000) Psychiatric disorders in patients with blepharospasm. *J. Psychosom. Res.* **48,** 589–591.
30. Broocks, A., Thiel, A., Angerstein, D., and Dressler, D. (1998) Higher prevalence of obsessive-compulsive symptoms in patients with blepharospasm than in patients with hemifacial spasm. *Am. J. Psychiatry* **155,** 555–557.

31. Saint-Cyr, J.A., Taylor, A.E., and Nicholson, K. (1995) Behavior and the basal ganglia. *Adv. Neurol.* **65,** 1–28.
32. Van Hilten, J.J., Van de Beek, W.J.T., Vein, A.A., Van Dijk, J.G., and Middelkoop, H.A.M. (2001) Clinical aspects of multifocal or generalized tonic dystonia in reflex sympathetic dystrophy. *Neurology* **56,** 1762–1765.
33. Verdugo, R.J. and Ochoa, J.L. (2000) Abnormal movements in complex regional pain syndrome: assessment of their nature. *Muscle Nerve* **23,** 198–205.
34. Sa, D.S., Mailis, A., and Lang, A.E. (2001) Posttraumatic Cervical Spasm. *Neurology* **56(Suppl. 3),** A123 (abstract).
35. Kasch, H., Bach, F.W., and Jensen, T.S. (2001) Handicap after acute whiplash injury: a 1-year prospective study of risk factors. *Neurology* **56,** 1637–1643.
36. Jankovic, J. (1994) Post-traumatic movement disorders: central and peripheral mechanisms. *Neurology* **44,** 2006–2014.
37. Truong, D.D., Dubinsky, R., Hermanowicz, N., Olson, W.L., Silverman, B., and Koller, W.C. (1991) Posttraumatic torticollis. *Arch. Neurol.* **48,** 221–223.
38. Tarsy, D. (1998) Comparison of acute- and delayed-onset posttraumatic cervical dystonia. *Mov. Disord.* **13,** 481–485.
39. Goldman, S. and Ahlskog, J.E. (1993) Posttraumatic cervical dystonia. *Mayo Clin. Proc.* **68,** 443–448.
40. Brown, P. and Thompson, P.D. (2001) Electrophysiological aids to the diagnosis of psychogenic jerks, spasms, and tremor. *Mov. Disord.* **16,** 595–599.
41. Markus, A.C. (2000) The ethics of placebo prescribing. *Mt. Sinai J. Med.* **67,** 140–143.
42. Goetz, C.G., Leurgans, S., Raman, R., and Stebbins, G.T. (2000) Objective changes in motor function during placebo treatment in PD. *Neurology* **54,** 710–714.
43. Fine, J., Stergiopoulos, V., Nieves, A., Feinstein, A., and Lang, A.E. (2000) Long-term follow-up of psychogenic movement disorders. *Neurology* **54(Suppl. 3),** A50–A51.
44. Couprie, W., Wijdicks, E.F.M., Rooijmans, H.G.M., and vanGijn, J. (1995) Outcome in conversion disorder: a follow up study. *J. Neurol. Neurosurg. Psychiatry* **58,** 750–752.

31

Clinical Management of Psychosis and Mood Disorders in Huntington's Disease

Mark Guttman, MD, FRCPC, **Meneske Alpay,** MD,
Sylvain Chouinard, MD, **Peter Como,** PhD,
Anthony Feinstein, MPhil, PhD, MRCPsych, FRCPC,
Ira Leroi, MD, FRCPC, **and Adam Rosenblatt,** MD

1. THE CLINICAL MANAGEMENT OF PSYCHOSIS

1.1. *Introduction*

Patients with Huntington's disease (HD) experience psychotic symptoms more frequently than the general population. The clinical picture includes a broad spectrum of disorders including poorly systematized paranoia, isolated delusional states, and psychotic states. The challenge to the clinician is to be able to recognize and treat psychotic symptoms in HD patients, who have been diagnosed with this disorder, and also to consider these symptoms as the earliest manifestation of HD in patients, who are at risk. This chapter reviews the literature and clinical experience relating to HD and psychosis and offers a treatment management strategy based on the clinical experience of a multidisciplinary group that was assembled to discuss these issues.

1.1.2. *Epidemiology*

Some patients with HD present with psychotic symptoms resembling various types of schizophrenia *(1)*. A retrospective study of 110 patients with HD in 30 families found a lifetime prevalence of schizophrenia in 9% of HD patients *(1)*. In another study of 30 patients with HD, schizophrenia and atypical psychosis was seen in 5 patients *(2)*. In a review of 11 studies, Mendez noted that the prevalence of psychotic symptoms in HD ranged from 3.4–12% *(3)*. Other studies revealed that psychotic symptoms may be found in up to 30% of HD patients *(4)*. The prevalence of schizophrenia-like symptoms in HD patients is much higher than the expected 1% prevalence of schizophrenia in the general population. There is a familial aggregation of schizophrenia-like syndromes in HD families *(5)*. There has been no clear association between the presence of psychotic symptoms and the severity of motor manifestations or the number of CAG repeats *(6)*. Psychosis is more common among early-onset cases than among those whose disease begins in midlife or old age *(7,8)*. An early age of onset seem to be an increased risk for psychosis *(9)*.

1.1.3. *Pathophysiology*

The underlying neuropathology leading to psychosis in HD is not well understood, but there are several hypotheses. The psychosis may be due to dysfunction in the basal ganglia itself with the known

From: *Mental and Behavioral Dysfunction in Movement Disorders*
Edited by: M-A. Bédard et al. © Humana Press Inc., Totowa, NJ

pathological changes that occur in the caudate nucleus or to the altered pathways linking the basal ganglia to the limbic-associated cortex. It is possible that the psychosis may be due to cortical disease directly. Psychosis in HD has been correlated with medial caudate pathology and reduced anterior hemispheric metabolism *(10,11)*. Neurotransmitter alterations in these brain regions may also contribute to the occurrence of psychosis in HD. Dopamine has been implicated in the pathogenesis of psychosis. Dopamine, however, is relatively preserved in HD, whereas other neurochemical systems are affected. It has been postulated that the disproportionate preservation of dopamine may facilitate the occurrence of psychosis in HD *(7)*.

1.2. The Assessment of Psychosis in HD

1.2.1. Clinical Features

It may be difficult to diagnose schizophrenia vs a psychotic disorder due to HD in patients who have HD or are at risk for HD. It is possible that there may be an overrepresentation of schizophrenia in HD patients *(12)*. Psychosis can be the first manifestation in some cases and is part of the clinical spectrum *(13)*. It is also possible that there are other genetic factors that might predispose HD patients to psychosis *(6,9)*.

In patients with HD, the most common psychotic presentation is poorly systematized paranoia that is commonly seen with aggression, irritability, and poor impulse control. Patients tend to underreport paranoia and need to be asked specifically about increased suspiciousness and distrustfulness during their clinical evaluation. Family members may not be aware of the paranoia or minimize it. Overvalued ideas such as preoccupation with marital infidelity are seen and may border on psychotic states. Isolated well-defined delusional states and schizophrenia-like psychotic states are less common and, as just mentioned, may present diagnostic dilemmas. When a patient is at risk for HD and presents with psychosis, it is difficult to make a diagnosis in the absence of other symptoms of HD such as chorea. Symptoms such as apathy and flat affect are present both in HD as well as in schizophrenia and are not helpful in the differential diagnosis. In patients with HD, typical psychotic symptoms are more commonly persecutory delusions, and these usually do not interfere with day-to-day functioning. Patients with HD tend to lack premorbid conditions, such as schizotypal personality. Patients with HD typically do not report hallucinations as part of their psychosis. Auditory and visual hallucinations tend to point toward a diagnosis of schizophrenia rather than a psychotic disorder due to HD. Psychotic symptoms in HD patients have a more benign course and respond well to neuroleptic treatment compared to patients with schizophrenia. Another differentiating feature may be the age of presentation of the psychosis. HD patients may present much later in life with psychosis after having many years being successfully employed and becoming ill in their 40s or 50s. This would be an unusual presentation of schizophrenia. On the other hand, if a patient presents with a typical onset of first psychosis in the late teenage years or 20s with auditory hallucinations and other features of schizophrenia in a person at risk for HD who does not have any motor manifestations, one should consider the diagnosis of schizophrenia in isolation. Direct DNA testing will not be helpful in this situation, because a positive test will not predict if the psychosis is related to HD or other disorders.

1.2.2. Differential Diagnosis

Differential diagnosis of psychotic disorder due to HD includes psychotic depression, severe obsessive–compulsive disorder (OCD), drug-induced psychotic states (cocaine-induced paranoia), mania with psychotic features, and delirium. Acute-onset of confusion, agitation, and waxing and waning of the mental status are features of delirium. As in any other neurodegenerative disorder, patients with HD are susceptible to toxic or metabolic encephalopathy. In these cases physicians should look for a medical cause, such as an infection. Aspiration pneumonia in patients with swallowing difficulties and urinary tract infections in patients with incontinence are common causes of acute delirium in patients with HD. Other medical problems that should be eliminated include, electrolyte imbalance and drug-

Table 1
Neuroleptics for Use in HD

Name	Starting dose (mg/d)	Maximal dose (mg/d)
Quetiapine	12.5 mg	400 mg, rarely up to 600 mg
Olanzapine	2.5 mg	20 mg, rarely to 40 mg
Risperidone	0.5 mg	6 mg
Clozapine	6.25 mg	300 mg, rarely to 600 mg
Haloperidol equivalent (for typical neuroleptics)	0.5 mg	10 mg

induced encephalopathy, including medications and illicit drugs. In patients with gait problems and frequent falls, subdural hematoma should be considered, and neuroimaging studies need to be obtained if there is a change in their condition.

1.3. *Treatment*

The major treatment for all psychotic disorders in HD patients involves antipsychotic medication. They are also commonly used for irritability and agitation and are covered in the companion chapter. It is important to interview patients who are experiencing agitation and irritability in detail to identify if these individuals have undiagnosed generalized paranoia. In these patients, the behavioral disturbance may respond well to antipsychotic treatment rather than other agents.

Typical neuroleptic agents are used in HD to treat the psychotic symptoms as well as chorea. Side effects of the typical neuroleptics are very common, including lethargy, extrapyramidal side effects (EPS), and tardive dyskinesia (TD) *(14)*. Swallowing is another problem that may worsen with the initiation of typical neuroleptic treatment and must be closely followed. In those cases the neuroleptic dose may need to be decreased, or if the patient is on a typical neuroleptic, a change to an atypical neuroleptic may be more appropriate. Hypokinesia with typical antipsychotic agents may be a significant side effect especially as the HD advances in severity. A study showed that patients with HD who were on typical antipsychotic agents had more hypokinesia and lower scores of functional status compared to patients who were not on antipsychotics *(15)*. Typical antipsychotics were also reported to induce and worsen dystonia in patients with HD *(16)*. This emphasizes the potential problem with prescribing neuroleptic agents in HD. Caution is recommended to use these agents only when clinically necessary and to use the smallest dose possible. Typically, HD patients respond to much smaller doses compared to other patients with schizophrenia or other psychiatric disorders. The availability of depot forms of typical neuroleptics may be an advantage in noncompliant HD patients. Newer atypical agents such as clozapine, quetiapine, olanzapine, risperidone, and ziprasidone are better choices for patients with HD due to their side effect profile. See Table 1 for doses of these agents.

Atypical antipsychotics cause less EPS such as dystonia, TD, and parkinsonian symptoms *(17)*. Clozapine has a superior EPS profile as compared to other neuroleptics, but has the major disadvantage of blood monitoring for bone marrow suppression. Clozapine may be useful in treatment-resistant cases *(18)*. It was also shown to decrease choreiform movements *(19,20)*. The need to check weekly blood counts, due to the possibility of agranulocytosis, makes it difficult to use in patients with chorea and severe behavioral disturbances. Quetiapine also has a lower incidence of producing EPS symptoms and does not have the bone marrow suppression problems associated with clozapine. It is also useful for irritability, agitation, and insomnia. Olanzapine is also another reasonable choice of atypical neuroleptic, with a benign EPS profile, and has been used in HD to help with psychosis, irritability, insomnia, and obsessional thinking *(21)*. Quetiapine and olanzapine are considered the first-line choices

Table 2
Consensus Statement For the Treatment of Psychosis in HD

Treating the HD patients with neuroleptics remains an area of ongoing debate, and there is insufficient clinical evidence to promote an evidence-based treatment algorithm. Based on clinical experience:

1. We prefer the use atypical agents due to lower side effects of EPS, swallowing problems, and sedation.
2. The general principal of initiation with low dose treatment with cautious and slow dose escalation is important in this patient population.
3. Caution is also recommended in rendering a diagnosis of symptomatic HD based on isolated symptoms of psychosis without motor manifestations of this disorder. Since schizophrenia is more common than HD, it is possible to have co-existing problems. Ongoing prospective clinical studies of subjects at risk for HD have been designed to give more information on the initial presenting features of symptomatic HD. This will give important information on the prevalence and nature of psychiatric symptoms, which may predate the motor manifestations of this disorder. The current clinical consensus, however, is that symptomatic HD is not considered manifest unless there are motor manifestations apparent on the motor evaluation.

for the treatment of psychosis in HD patients. Risperidone may act like a typical neuroleptic, especially if it is used in higher doses. There is currently not enough data with ziprasidone to speculate on the usefulness in HD patients.

When treating patients with neuropleptic agents, physicians need to consider other side effects, such as neuroleptic malignant syndrome (NMS). The symptoms of NMS include acute mental status changes, lead-pipe rigidity, autonomic dysfunction, and increased creatine-phosphokinase (CPK). Patients may also experience neuroleptic-induced catatonia with mutism, waxy flexibility, psychomotor retardation or agitation, and autonomic instability. Patients treated with neuroleptics may also get TD, but the exact incidence in the HD population is unknown and may be difficult to diagnose.

1.4. Conclusions

Psychosis is more common in HD than in the general population. The type of psychotic symptoms, their frequency, and relationship to other variables have not been well studied. It is possible that there are genetic factors that might predispose to psychosis. Psychosis may be the first manifestation of HD in some cases. There are numerous methodological problems with the current literature in this area. This includes small study numbers, variability of diagnostic criteria, definition of psychosis, referral bias, and lack of prospective controlled studies. The consensus statement is in Table 2.

2. THE CLINICAL MANAGEMENT OF MOOD DISORDERS

2.1. Introduction

HD is associated with many neuropsychiatric sequellae, among which mood disorders feature prominently. This observation may be traced back to George Huntington's (1872) first description of the disease that bears his name, for in it he noted a tendency to insanity and suicide. Moreover, there remains a debate whether or not psychiatric changes represent the onset of disease manifestations in advance of the characteristic motor changes. This chapter reviews the literature pertaining to two major disturbances in mood and affect, namely depression and mania, and provide recommendations as to treatment. In common with many other neuropsychiatric disorders, there is a dearth of methodologically robust treatment trials to guide the clinician in their choice of the appropriate antidepressant or mood stabilizer. As such, the emphasis is on anecdotal clinical experience complemented by results from open label trials. This approach is applied to anxiety disorders, where a similar situation pertaining to a limited literature exists. These limitations should not, however, deter the clinician when it comes to treatment. Mood disorders are associated with significant morbidity and mortality, a situation that may be accentuated in patients with compromised neurological status. Thus, failure to recognize a concomitant mood disorder or provide adequate treatment to the HD patient, and his or her family, does a considerable disservice.

Anxiety symptoms and more defined anxiety syndromes are commonly seen in HD. As with depression, anxiety has been reported as a relatively frequent prodrome to the motor symptoms of HD *(22)*. Untreated anxiety has significant implications: (*i*) it can worsen the expression of the motor symptoms of HD; (*ii*) it can increase the risk of alcohol and other substance abuse; and (*iii*) it can have an adverse affect on quality of life. Hence, the recognition and management of anxiety in HD is crucial.

2.1.2. Epidemiology

2.1.2.1. Depression

Folstein and colleagues noted that 42% of all HD patients in Maryland ($n = 88$) had either a major depression or dysthymic disorder *(8)*. This figure overlaps with that of Shiwach (1994), who reported that the lifetime prevalence of major depression in 110 HD patients was 39% *(23)*. The relatively small sample sizes, for epidemiological purposes, are offset by the confluence of findings suggesting that a significant minority of HD patients, almost one in two, will suffer a clinically significant depressive illness during the course of their lifetime. The Huntington figures are, however, similar to that for other disabling, degenerative neurological disorders such as Parkinson's disease (PD) *(24)*, multiple sclerosis *(25)*, and Alzheimer's disease *(26)*.

2.1.2.2. Bipolar Affective Disorder

The prevalence of bipolar affective disorder has not been well researched. However, Folstein and colleagues *(8)* noted hypomanic or manic episodes in 10% of 88 patients, whereas Mendez examined seven studies of HD patients and, using a variable definition of mania, estimated the rate as 4.8% *(3)*.

2.1.2.3. Suicide

The suicide rate in HD is four to six times higher than in the general population and accounted for over 2% of deaths in a large sample of HD patients *(27)*.

2.1.2.4. Anxiety

Detailed epidemiological studies of the prevalence and incidence of anxiety in HD are lacking. However, clinical experience suggests that anxiety syndromes, such as social phobia and generalized anxiety disorders, are particularly prevalent. Panic attacks and more generalized "anxiety attacks" also occur. In addition, the frequent losses of all kinds experienced by those afflicted with the HD often lead to adjustment disorders with anxiety. Obsessions and compulsions in HD have been reported in the literature *(28)* and are commonly seen clinically. The phenomenology and management of the latter are dealt with later in this chapter. In general, the etiology of anxiety in HD is multifactorial. It ranges from increased worrying due to the very real psychosocial stress, to actual neurotransmitter changes resulting from the pathophysiology of HD.

As is the case with primary psychiatric disorders, anxiety in HD often exists as either a complication of, or a continuum with mood disorders. In particular, clinical experience suggests that untreated depression often underlies social phobia. At times it may be difficult to distinguish an anxiety symptom or syndrome from other behavioral changes seen in HD. For example, perseveration due to frontal lobe damage in HD may mimic the restlessness of an anxiety disorder.

2.1.3. Neuropathological Basis for Mood Disorder in HD

A number of key frontal-subcortical neural circuits are known to regulate mood and behavior *(29)*. The pathophysiology of HD disrupts the integrity of these pathways, leading to neuropsychiatric sequellae. Functional neuroimaging (positron emission tomography [PET]) has shown that HD patients with depression have lower metabolic activity in the orbitofrontal and inferior prefrontal cortex compared

Table 3
Consensus Statement on Mood Disorders in HD

1. Depression is a frequent concomitant of HD occurring three to four times more commonly than in the general population.
2. Depression may predate the onset of neurological symptoms, however, this is not sufficient to render the diagnosis of symptomatic HD (*see* Table 1).
3. Clinicians should also be alerted to the high suicide rate in HD.
4. Functional brain imaging points toward abnormalities in frontal brain circuits that underpin depressive disorders.
5. Mania, while not studied as often, also occurs more frequently than chance dictates.

to euthymic HD controls *(30)*. The importance of frontal system pathology in the pathogenesis of depression has also been noted in other neuropsychiatric disorders, namely PD *(31)*. Furthermore, these PET findings concur with data from patients with primary depression *(32)*. Interruption in the neural circuits probably translates into mood disturbance via a dysregulation in pivotal neurotransmitter such as serotonin, dopamine, and glutamate, among others.

There is evidence to suggest that depression in HD may be linked to early neuronal loss in the medial caudate, an area richly connected to limbic structures subserving mood and affect. Indeed, the part of the neostriatum damaged earliest in HD, the dorsal medial caudate, may provide a clue as to why mood disorder may be the first symptom of HD.

2.1.4. Temporal Association Between Mood and Neurologic Symptoms

There is an on-going debate as to whether a mood disorder preceding the onset of neurological symptoms should be considered part of the prodromal phase to HD. This question transcends mere academic interest and has important implications for treatment, because there are data showing that secondary depression (i.e., depression due to HD, in Diagnostic and Statistical Manual of Mental Disorders, fourth edition [DSM-IV] parlance) may respond to lower doses on antidepressant medication than primary depression (i.e., depression coexistent with HD) *(33)*.

Shiwach and colleagues reported that one-third of their depressed sample of HD patients presented with mood change on average 4.3 yr [range 1–8 yr] before the onset of motor symptoms *(23)*. Mindham and colleagues compared psychopathology prior to onset of confirmed disease in HD and Alzheimer patients and noted that the former were twice as likely to have a mood disorder, suggesting a more integral association between HD and depression as opposed to mood change as a nonspecific prodrome *(34)*. Table 3 identifies the consensus statement concerning these issues in mood disorder and anxiety.

2.2. The Assessment of Mood Disorder and Anxiety in HD

Mood disorders may be assessed by clinical interview or via rating scales that are either interview-driven or self-reporting. Before listing to some of the more useful diagnostic procedures, some clarification is needed with respect to the phenomenology of mood change associated with HD.

2.2.1. Phenomenology of Mood Change

2.2.1.1. The Typical ("Classic") Presentation

With respect to current psychiatric taxonomy, depressed or manic HD patients will, in most cases, be given the diagnosis of mood disorder due to a general medical condition, the latter referring to HD. Five criteria must be satisfied before this diagnosis is made, namely: (*i*) a prominent and persistent disturbance in mood predominates in the clinical picture and is characterized by one or both of the following: depressed mood or markedly diminished interest or pleasure in all, or almost all activities, and/or elevated, expansive, or irritable mood; (*ii*) there is evidence from the history, physical examination, or laboratory findings that the disturbance is the direct physiological consequence of the general medical condition; (*iii*) the disturbance is not better accounted for by another mental disorder (i.e., an adjustment disorder in response to the stress of having the general medical condition); (*iv*) the disturbance does not occur exclusively during a delirium; and (*v*) the disturbance causes clinically significant distress or impairment in social, occupational, or other important areas of functioning.

Significantly, the DSM-IV goes on to specify four subtypes to the above. The first, entitled "depressive features" requires the presence of depressed mood, but not the full criteria for major depression. With a major depression-like episode, the syndrome of low mood with ancillary features such as anhedonia, sleep, and appetite disturbance, poor concentration, fatigue, and suicidal ideation are required. The two remaining subtypes are called, "manic features," where the predominant mood is elevated, euphoric, or irritable, and "mixed features," where both mania and depression are present, but neither predominates.

The data from the HD literature is compatible with the first three subtypes. In addition, patients may present with clinical features that do not fit neatly into the DSM model. The situation is further complicated by the fact that not all researchers follow DSM terminology. Watt and Seller found both major depression (26%) and lesser degrees of depression (28%) *(35)*, the latter described as brief depressive reactions, neurotic depression, and adjustment disorder with depressed mood, in a sample of 65 patients with HD. Although major depression was considered an integral part of the HD pathology, the lesser degrees of depression were thought to be reactive in nature. Similarly, Leroi also noted both major depression (28.6%) and other lesser types of depression (brief recurrent depressive disorder, dysthymia) in a sample of 21 HD patients. Caine and Shoulson earlier noted both types of depression in a cohort of 30 HD patients *(2)*.

2.2.1.2. Atypical or Subsydromal Presentations of Mood Disorder

Subthreshold presentations of change in mood and affect may also occur. Here, the predominant features may be disturbances such as irritability or aggression, as opposed to sadness or elated mood. Lauterbach described cases in which guilty ruminations, low self-esteem, worthlessness, and neurovegetative changes (altered sleep and appetite) may feature more prominently than feelings of sadness or depression *(36)*. Hopelessness is a frequently encountered symptom. Analogous situations have been reported in other neuropsychiatric disorders. Thus, symptoms such as irritability and frustration have been found to occur more frequently than sadness in patients with multiple sclerosis *(37, 38)*. It may not always be clear whether these stem directly from the disease process or whether they are primarily driven by situational difficulties, i.e., a reaction to living with an incurable progressive degenerative disease, which is an observation as germane to HD as it is to other neurological diseases.

2.2.1.3. Conditions that Mimic Mood Disorders in HD

Diagnostic dilemmas may be frequently encountered in HD, because certain behavioral syndromes may phenotypically resemble mood disorders. Although these behavioral changes are regarded as distinct from mood change, this demarcation may be somewhat artificial given that the neural circuits underpinning mood and behavior overlap. A corollary is that core symptoms of HD, such as sleep and appetite disturbance, fatigue and apathy are also integral to patients with depression. Nevertheless, despite this overlap, a clinical distinction is important because treatments may differ.

Some common examples of these dilemmas are apathy masquerading as depression, the "frontal lobe" personality change of disinhibition, and facetiousness resembling mania, as may the hypersexuality or paraphilias encountered in HD patients *(35)*. Similarly, agitated delirium may also be mistaken for mania. A useful pointer that may guide the clinician when it comes to uncertainty with respect to a diagnosis of mania, is to remember that "classic" mania comprises a constellation of three essential elements, i.e., an elevated or irritable mood, a grandiose (or paranoid) thought content, and physical overactivity, which manifests typically as racing thoughts, pressured speech, less need for sleep, etc. This triad is frequently lacking in patients whose presentation is primarily one of frontal disinhibition.

2.2.2. *Rating Scales to Assess Mood*

The heterogeneity in presentation of depression in HD (major depression, dysthymia, subsyndromal depression, vegetative symptoms common to depression and HD) may create difficulties when it comes to use of rating scales in assessing mood. While self-report rating scales cannot generate a clinical diagnosis, they are nevertheless useful in monitoring response to medication, and as such, are invariably part of the methodology of treatment trials.

2.2.2.1. Depression Scales

There are several well-known scales to assess depression. These scales are typically administered by either a trained mental health profession or are self-rated by the subject. Although the use of rating scales can be helpful in diagnosing mood disorders or assessing response to a therapeutic intervention, one should not rely solely on rating scales in the clinical assessment of mood disorders in HD patients.

The Hamilton Rating Scale for Depression (HAM-D) is among the most widely used scale *(39)*. It requires administration by an experienced mental health clinician as it depends on interviewing skills and the ability to evaluate symptoms. The HAM-D is most often used in treatment studies to assess response to a clinical intervention for depression. This scale also remains the standard by which other scales are often validated against. The HAM-D tends to emphasize the somatic symptoms of depression and, therefore, may be less useful in the assessment of depression in patients with neurological disorders.

An alternative to the HAM-D for patients with neurological disease is the Montgomery-Asberg Depression Rating Scale (MADRS) *(40)*. The MADRS is also a widely used scale that was specifically designed to be sensitive to changes over time. This scale does not include somatic or psychomotor symptoms and, therefore, may have an advantage over HAM-D in neurological disorders with prominent motor features such as HD.

The Bech-Rafaelsen Melancholia Rating Scale (BRMS) *(41)* was developed based on the HAM-D and consists of 11 items, each rated on a five-point scale. The BRMS scale has the advantage of specific severity anchor points to guide raters in their clinical assessment. Finally, the Behavioral section of the Unified Huntington's Disease Rating Scale (UHDRS) *(42)* includes assessment of mood and suicidality, however, there are no published psychometric studies of its reliability or validity. The UHDRS Behavioral section primarily assesses frequency and severity of specific behavioral symptoms.

In addition, there are several self-rated depression scales. Scores on these scales typically require clinical confirmation, as subjects may either under- or overendorse symptoms. Among the most widely used self-rated depression scale is the Beck Depression Inventory (BDI) *(43)*. The BDI consists of 21 items, each rated on a three-point severity level. The BDI tends to have a greater focus on cognitive symptoms of depression (i.e., pessimism, diminished self-esteem) and is generally felt to be sensitive to response to therapy. The Hospital Anxiety and Depression Scale *(44)* was developed specifically to capture core symptoms of mood disturbance in medically ill patient populations. It excludes potential contaminating symptoms such as sleep, appetite, and cognitive difficulties.

Another common self-rated depression scale is the Zung Self-Rating Depression Scale (SDS) *(45)*. The SDS contains 20 items rated according to their frequency of occurrence, such that symptoms that are not severe or bothersome, but occur frequently, receive a higher rating. The sensitivity of the SDS has not been clearly established, and it is less suitable for drug trials, however, it may be an efficient screening tool. The Cornell Scale for Depression in Dementia *(46)* has been validated in patient populations with cognitive impairment, communication difficulties, and dementia and relies on both caregiver input and clinician assessment. This scale may be useful in HD given the well-known cognitive impairment associated with HD.

2.2.2.2. Mania Rating Scales

Fewer scales are available to rate mania, most likely due to the fluctuating nature of this condition. In addition, patients experiencing a hypomanic episode are less likely to endorse symptoms. Therefore, the available mania rating scales require administration by a trained mental health professional. The Manic State Rating Scale (MSRS) is an observer-rated scale and consists of 26 items rated from 0–5 on the basis of both frequency and intensity *(47)*. The focus is on behaviors that would be typically observed in an inpatient setting, which may be less common in HD population. The MSRS is best suited for use by trained psychiatric nurses. There are no anchor points for determining severity, and this scale can take a long time to administer.

The Bech-Rafaelsen Mania Scale *(48)* consists of 11 items rated on a five-point scale, with severity ratings that have well-described anchor points. This scale is recommended to be used in conjunction with HAM-D.

Finally, the Young Mania Rating Scale (Y-MRS) *(49)* is completed based on a clinical psychiatric interview and consists of 11 items. Four of the items (irritability, speech rate/amount, content of thought, disruptive–aggressive behavior) are given extra weight in scoring. The Y-MRS has clearly described anchor points. There is a reported high correlation between Y-MRS and length of hospitalization.

2.2.2.3. Anxiety Scales

As with all other psychiatric syndromes in HD, assessment of anxiety requires a thorough medical and psychiatric work-up. Reversible causes of anxiety, including environmental and medical causes, must be sought and removed. Common environmental precipitants of anxiety include toileting, social situations, and changes in daily routine. Another example of an environmental trigger is the fear of choking at meal times. Medical precipitants of anxiety include thyroid disease and infection, as well as substances, such as caffeine and nicotine, use or withdrawal. Recognition and management of an underlying mood disorder or adjustment disorder due to loss and grief must also be undertaken.

Rating instruments have been developed to quantify the amount of normal anxiety and to measure the severity of pathological anxiety states, such as obsessional behavioral, panic disorder, and phobic behaviors. Normal anxiety can be a symptom associated with a variety of medical conditions. In HD, anxiety is a common symptom associated with a variety of factors, such as course of the illness, disease progression and disability, and the risk status of any offspring.

Anxiety scales can be professionally administered or self-rated. Among the most widely used professionally administered anxiety rating scale is the Hamilton Rating Scale for Anxiety (HAM-A) *(50)*. The HAM-A was developed to rate anxiety for patients with anxiety syndromes and not for measuring generalized anxiety in other psychiatric and medical illness. Therefore, anxiety states specifically associated with medical conditions, such as HD, should not be assessed by the HAM-A. Moreover, the HAM-A resembles the HAM-D in its bias toward somatic symptoms and, therefore, is less suitable for patients with neurological disease.

An alternative to the HAM-A is the Anxiety Disorders Interview Scale-Revised (ADIS-R) *(51)*. The ADIS-R is administered as part of a semistructured interview and is based on DSM-IV criteria for anxiety disorders. An advantage of the ADIS-R is that it provides rich information about symptoms of anxiety disorders such as panic, generalized anxiety, and phobic avoidance. It also documents the disability incurred by the patient due to anxiety. This scale also includes the HAM-D and the HAM-A.

A modification of the Schedule for Affective Disorders and Schizophrenia–Lifetime Anxiety (SADS-LA) *(52)* was designed for use in epidemiological studies with a focus on the lifetime occurrence of anxiety symptoms and disorders. Thus, it may be less useful for assessing acute anxiety disorders in HD, but may be useful in establishing premorbid anxiety disorders in at-risk individuals considering presymptomatic gene testing.

Self-rated anxiety scales include the State-Trait Anxiety Inventory (STAI) *(53)*, the Fear Questionnaire *(54)*, and the UCLA 4-D Anxiety Scale *(55)*. The STAI differentiates between state anxiety, which may be experienced in specific situations (e.g., undergoing presymptomatic gene testing), and trait anxiety, which describes the anxiety experienced by the individual when there are no identifiable stressors. The Fear Questionnaire is used primarily for assessing specific phobias that tend to be relatively less common in HD. Finally, the UCLA 4-D Anxiety Scale is a more recently developed

Table 4
Consensus Statement on Assessment of Mood Disorders in HD

1. The DSM-IV offers a useful approach to the taxonomy of mood change associated with HD.
2. There are clinical presentations, such as subsyndromal depression, that will not be captured by the DSM-IV criteria, and clinicians should be alerted to their presence.
3. Rating scales that are useful in HD should include both interview-based and self-reported measures.

instrument designed to be more comprehensive than other anxiety scales by including measures of emotional, physiological, cognitive, and behavioral dimensions of anxiety. Please see Table 4 for the consensus statement.

2.3. *Treatment of Mood Disorders in HD*

Treatment of HD may be divided into two synergistic modalities, the pharmacologic (Table 5) and the psychosocial. In general, there is a paucity of literature pertaining to both, and as such, we have to often extrapolate from evidence obtained from primary psychiatric disorders or other neuropsychiatric conditions. Before outlining specific treatment recommendations, however, some basic principles need expounding: (*i*) HD patients may have an increased sensitivity to the side effects of medication, namely dehydration and/or delirium with lithium carbonate and agitation with the selective serotonin re-uptake inhibitors (SSRIs). In addition, central nervous system toxicity may be aggravated when the neurologic patient is depressed or already sedated by other drugs used, for example, to treat chorea *(56)*. (*ii*) Metabolism of drugs may be altered in HD for a number of reasons, such as low serum albumin, impaired renal clearance, and general physical debilitation. (*iii*) Psychotropic medication may further compromise an already impaired neurological status, i.e., the anticholinergic effects of tricyclic antidepressant (TCA) medication may aggravate cognitive impairment, whereas orthostatic hypotension, another side effect of TCAs, may further impair gait and balance. (*iv*) Dosage regimes should be conservative, i.e., start low and go slow. (*v*) Patients should have a physical examination and work-up prior to treatment, as some medical problems may affect the mental state and mislead the clinician. Examples are hypothyroidism mistaken for depression and hyperactive delirium caused by a pneumonia or urinary tract infection misdiagnosed as mania. (*vi*) Adequate attention should be directed at symptoms of HD that may be aggravating mood difficulties, i.e. insomnia leading to fatigue and demoralization, movement difficulties promoting irritability and frustration, and anorexia and weight loss exacerbating low self-esteem and fatigue.

2.3.1. *Pharmacologic Management*

There are no randomized controlled trials of treatment for either depression or mania in HD. Two published sets of guidelines *(57,58)* are based on anecdotal evidence and clinical expertise.

2.3.1.1. Depression

2.3.1.1.1. SSRIs

SSRIs are the first choice when it comes to treating depression (major depression and dysthymia). While there are no treatment trials with these drugs reported in the HD literature, there are data from other neuropsychiatric disorders, such as Alzheimer's disease *(59)* and multiple sclerosis *(60)*, that sertraline is effective. Anecdotal reports suggest the other SSRI drugs, such as fluoxetine *(61)*, are just as effective in patients with secondary depression. The SSRIs are generally well-tolerated. Problems may, however, occasionally occur with gastrointestinal side effects, in particular nausea and diarrhea, and vigilance is called for in HD patients with anorexia and weight loss. Treatment may increase agitation in some patients because of akathisia-like effects, but in others, the SSRIs may have a calming effect by ameliorating irritability *(62)*. Rarely, the SSRI drugs may induce apathy *(63)*. Theoretically,

Table 5
Consensus Statement on the Pharmacological Management of Mood Disorders and Anxiety

1. There is broad agreement that SSRI drugs are the treatment of choice in patients with depression and subsyndromal depression. Although empirical data are still awaited, clinical experience reveals this class of antidepressant is generally well-tolerated. Possible agitation with worsening in chorea may occur, albeit rarely. Maintenance treatment should be continued for at least 1 yr in a first episode of depression. Recurrent depressive episodes will require treatment of longer duration.
2. Sodium valproate and carbamazepine are recommended as first-choice mood-stabilizing drugs in mania associated with HD.
3. Should psychosis occur with mania, olanzapine or quetiapine are recommended as drugs of choice.
4. ECT is also a useful alternative in psychotic manic and/or depressed patients. Although generally well-tolerated, delirium is a possible side effect of treatment.
5. Acute anxiety may be treated with benzodiazepines and chronic anxiety with SSRIs.

all the SSRI's may improve motor symptoms probably by inhibiting dopamine release in the basal ganglia secondary to serotonin (5-HT_2) receptor stimulation *(64)*.

There are a choice of five SSRIs commercially available, fluoxetine, paroxetine, citalopram, fluvoxamine, and sertraline. It is recommended that initial dosing should be conservative, i.e., half the usual therapeutic dosage. In the case of fluoxetine, paroxetine, and citalopram, this means a starting dose of 10 mg/d, which may later be increased to 20 mg/d (the typical therapeutic dose for most patients with primary depression), depending on clinical response. Occasionally, clinical need may dictate higher doses, i.e., 40+ mg, but these instances are rare, and as always, the clinician should be alert to adverse reactions. With the remaining two SSRI drugs, the same principles apply, i.e., starting at half strength (25 mg) and increasing in increments of 25 mg until a therapeutic response is obtained, the latter usually obtained in a daily dose range of 50–150 mg/d. Nausea may prove problematic with higher doses, particularly with fluvoxamine.

2.3.1.1.2. Serotonin and Noradrenaline Re-Uptake Inhibitors

Venlafaxine can be tried if a patient does not respond to an SSRI, but gastrointestinal side effects may prove problematic. It may have some added benefit in patients whose depression is characterized by severe melancholia (i.e., prominent vegetative features). The benefits and risks to this class of drugs are similar to that of the SSRIs.

2.3.1.1.3. Serotonin Antagonism and Re-Uptake Inhibitors

Examples of this class of antidepressant are nefazadone and trazadone. Once again, these drugs should be considered only after a failed trial of an SSRI. They may prove helpful in depressed patients with prominent sleep disturbance.

2.3.1.1.4. Noradrenaline and Dopamine Re-Uptake Inhibitors

Given the dopaminergic effects of buproprion, choreiform movements may be exacerbated. However, on the plus side, the stimulant effects of the drug may reduce apathy and psychomotor retardation when present.

2.3.1.1.5. TCAs

These antidepressants have been around a long time, and imipramine was first synthesized in 1958 *(65)*. It is their longevity, as much as their utility, that explains their prominence in the HD literature published to date. Although these drugs are no less effective than the SSRI's in treating depression, their more troublesome side effects, particularly within the anticholinergic spectrum, have demoted them from their first choice slot, occupied until the late 1980s. A series of early case reports and one open trial in HD patients demonstrated their effectiveness in treating depression *(2,14,66–68)*, but sample sizes were small, and dosages plus length of treatment were not always stipulated. If tricyclic medication is to be used, we recommend desipramine and nortriptyline as drugs of choice, given their lesser propensity for anticholinergic side effects. Amoxapine, a metabolite of the antipsychotic loxapine, has some dopamine antagonistic properties in addition to being an antidepresaant and, thus, may be potentially useful in suppressing chorea while elevating mood at the same time. A single case report noted beneficial effects on mood *(69)*.

2.3.1.1.6. Monoamine Oxidase Inhibitors

Phenelzine, the most widely prescribed monoamine oxidase inhibitor (MAOI), may be tried if the HD patient has not responded to one of the antidepressants mentioned above. Unlike the newer treatments, there is some evidence to suggest it may prove effective *(69)*. However, there are a number of problems with taking MAOIs, foremost of which are the dietary restrictions. In patients already compromised cognitively, the added burden of having to watch what they eat in order to avoid a dietary-induced hypertensive crisis may prove impractical. Furthermore, drug interactions may also precipitate a hypertensive crisis. Conversely, orthostatic hypotension may lead to falls. For all these reasons, the recommendation is that MAOIs, despite their reported efficacy, should be used only if other antidepressants have failed and then, only under close supervision.

2.3.1.1.7. Other Antidepressants

There are a number of other antidepressant drugs available, but data on their effectiveness in HD is again lacking. Mirtazepine has the advantage of increasing appetite and may thus prove useful in depression associated with anorexia and weight loss. It is also sedating, suggesting a possible use in the agitated depressed patient. Psychostimulants are by themselves generally ineffective in treating depression, but may on occasion prove useful as an adjunct to an antidepressant drug. They may also help with fatigue and apathy. Although there are no data from HD patients, modafinil may reduce fatigue associated with MS *(70)* and augment antidepressant treatment *(71)*.

In general, antidepressants vary in their ability to sedate or activate patients. Thus, care should be taken in avoiding potentially stimulating drugs in the agitated patient, while conversely, more sedating agents such as mirtazepine would be ill-advised in patients with marked apathy.

2.3.1.1.8. Electroconvulsive Therapy

There are limited data from three published studies suggesting that electroconvulsive therapy (ECT) is effective in treating depression associated with HD. Folstein and Folstein in a single case study *(72)* and Folstein in a retrospective series of two patients *(67)* found treatment to be effective and without side effects. Ranen noted that five of six patients (five major depression and one bipolar affective disorder) improved with ECT, but delirium and deterioration in movements were reported in two patients *(73)*. Evans reported a single case of psychotic depression refractory to medication, but responsive to ECT *(74)*. There was no associated cognitive worsening and choreiform movements were only slightly exacerbated. On the basis of this limited data, ECT can be tried in HD, but only after failed treatment with an antidepressant medication. Ranen reported that psychotic depression responded particularly well, thus replicating a finding from the primary depression literature *(73)*.

2.3.1.2. Subsyndromal Depression

The question is whether to treat HD patients who present with symptoms, such as irritability and frustration, but who do not meet the criteria for depressive disorder, be it a major depression or dysthymia? Data from mood disorder researchers suggest that this constellation of symptoms may be regarded as subsyndromal depression and will adversely impinge on psychosocial outcome *(75)*. It has been shown that subsyndromal depression is more likely to be detected and treated in the mental health domain than in a general medical setting *(76)*. Given that depression and chronic medical conditions have unique and additive effects on patient functioning *(77)* and mortality *(78)*, the importance of detecting and treating subsyndromal depression needs emphasising. Treatment studies with SSRI and TCAs have shown that this can be done most effectively in conditions such as traumatic brain injury *(79)* and nicotine withdrawal *(80)*. Our clinical experience dictates a similar approach to patients with HD.

2.3.1.3. Depression and Psychosis

Should a HD patient develop a depression with either mood congruent of mood incongruent delusions (according to DSM-IV terminology), treatment requires the addition of an antipsychotic agent to the antidepressant medication. There is a wide choice of antipsychotic drugs available. The newer generation of drugs such as olanzapine, risperidone, and seroquel are to be preferred over the older preparations (chlorpromazine, haloperidol, and perphenazine among others) given their significantly lower incidence of EPS. A drawback to the newer drugs is that none are currently available in injectable form. However, the recent development of a rapidly dissolving form of olanzapine (dissolves orally within a few seconds) confers obvious advantages when it comes to treating the noncomplaint patient, whose psychosis has led to impaired insight. As with the antidepressant drugs, starting at a small dose of olanzapine (i.e., 2.5 mg/d) is recommended, with increments of 2.5 mg until clinical effect is obtained. Anecdotal experience suggests this usually occurs with 5–10 mg/d, although occasionally 10+ mg/d is required. Splitting the dose in a twice a day regime may prove helpful in reducing daytime agitation. ECT is also an effective treatment and should be considered if medication has failed.

2.3.1.4. Mania

The mainstay of treatment is a mood stabilizing agent. Concern has been expressed about the use of lithium carbonate because of poor response and possible toxicity that may arise should the patient become dehydrated, which is not an infrequent situation in HD patients *(58)*. However, there is, as yet, not enough evidence suggesting the hazards of lithium outweigh the benefits. As such, careful monitoring plus adopting a more cautious dosing schedule, as followed in geriatric patients, may prove helpful. The latter involves using smaller doses of lithium (450–600 mg/d), and waiting at least 7 d (as opposed to 5 d in younger patients) in achieving a steady state blood level of 0.4–0.8 mmol/L.

Alternatives to lithium carbonate include carbamazepine and valproic acid, although treatment trials in HD have not been carried out. Valproic acid may help with irritability, but the clinician has to watch out for increased gait impairment and falls due to valproic acid-induced ataxia.

Should mania occur with psychosis, antipsychotic medication will be required, and the choice of drug, as outlined in section 2.3.1.3 on psychotic depression, is equally applicable here. ECT may also prove effective.

2.3.1.5. Anxiety Disorder

For episodic anxiety, such as that triggered by short-term environmental changes, consider the use of short-acting benzodiazepines as necessary. These include lorazepam, oxazepam, and temazepam. Benzodiazepines should be used with caution, as they may worsen gait and cognition and may even lead to delirium. For anxiety caused by medical procedures or dental visits, consider using chloral hydrate as needed. However, due to the sensitivity of HD sufferers to medications of all types, the use of benzodiazepines should not become regular.

For chronic anxiety, consider using SSRIs as first-line agents. Within the SSRI class, activating agents, such as fluoxetine, should be avoided, as they may worsen anxiety. Because these agents do not provide immediate relief of anxiety symptoms, short-term benzodiazepines can be used as adjunctive agents. Other antidepressants, which may be beneficial for chronic anxiety, include venlafaxine, nefazodone, and mirtazepine.

2.3.2. Psychosocial Treatment

Similar to pharmacological treatment, there are no controlled studies that have investigated the efficacy of psychosocial treatment in HD. Nevertheless, a host of treatment modalities may prove useful, either as an adjunct to medication or as a stand alone approach. Supportive psychotherapy, grief counseling, and support groups for patients have potential utility, but may be limited by the presence of cognitive dysfunction and other markers of disease severity. Thus, traditional insight-oriented psychotherapy may be less useful in a cognitively compromised individual. In addition, varying degrees of motor disability might inadvertently increase mood disturbance among patients attending group counseling sessions, who might infer their future course by observing the severity of HD among their fellow patients. However, rehabilitation offering vocational assessment, retraining, and placement, social work interventions addressing financial and housing issues and respite care, and the input of occupational therapists, both on an outpatient basis and in the home, to assist with compensatory rehabilitation strategies, all have their place in the treatment of HD patients and their families. Psychosocial intervention might best be targeted towards caregivers, who are at an increased risk for caregiver burden related to psychological dysfunction. Clinicians may not always adequately assess the degree of caregiver burden. For HD clinics with multidisciplinary teams, referral to the psychologist, social worker, or psychiatrist for more detailed assessment and treatment for the caregiver should be considered. Group counseling for caregivers have great potential for a positive benefit given the mutual problems and needs among these individuals who care for HD patients.

To our knowledge, there have been no specific studies of the management of anxiety in HD. Hence, guidelines should follow standard clinical practice for the management of primary anxiety and anxiety disorders. There are two main approaches to management: (*i*) modifying environmental precipitants; and (*ii*) pharmacological management.

Management through the modification of environmental issues involve: (*i*) identifying environmental triggers of anxiety and making appropriate changes; (*ii*) considering the use of alternative therapies, such as music therapy, recreation therapy, and relaxation training; (*iii*) cognitive behavioral therapy, which may have a role in early HD; (*iv*) encouraging physical activity; and (*v*) creating a regular and structured daily routine, and if changes to the daily routine are required, give adequate warnings and undertake appropriate preparations.

2.4. Mood and Anxiety Disorders Associated with Presymptomatic DNA Testing

A direct gene test in presymptomatic at-risk individuals has been available since 1993. Despite the relative ease by which gene testing can now be completed, there has not been a dramatic increase in the number of at-risk individuals seeking presymptomatic gene testing. Nonetheless, as the availability of agents that may delay the onset or slow disease progression become available in the coming years, the number of individuals who pursue gene testing will undoubtedly increase. The treatment of mood dysfunction associated with presymptomatic gene testing will likely become an additional activity for the HD clinician.

A fairly substantial literature exists regarding the psychological consequences of gene testing in HD. There is consensus among published studies that psychological dysfunction is the potential consequence of both gene positive and gene negative results. More striking is the finding by Decruyenaere et al. *(81)* that 15% of participants in their predictive DNA program had at least mild depression or elevated scores for general anxiety during the pretest period. These authors concluded that individuals who are close to the perceived age of onset of HD and who have pessimistic risk perception (along with clinical features of depression and/or anxiety) are at increased risk for posttest psychological distress. Long-term follow-up of individuals with a positive gene test demonstrate that they appear to have greater psychological distress *(82)*. Codori et al. found that individuals with greater mood disturbance and poor adjustment had tested positive, were married, had no children, and were closer to their estimated age of disease onset *(83)*.

Among the individuals who receive a gene positive result, depression and anxiety are the commonest reported psychiatric symptoms typically occurring 2 to 3 mo following the test result *(84–86)*, but are reported to occur within 10 d following the test result *(87)*. These individuals are considered to be at a high risk for psychological dysfunction. However, there is no reported increased rate of catastrophic events, such as psychiatric hospitalization, increased suicide rate, or increased suicide attempts. However, evidence of anxiety and depression observed during the pretesting phase have been reported to persist up to 1 yr following testing *(88)*.

Among individuals with a gene negative result, psychological problems are reported to occur anywhere from 2–12 mo following the result being made known. Approximately 10% of individuals with gene negative results require on-going psychological treatment *(85)*. Common reasons for psychological dysfunction in the gene negative group include survivor guilt, results contradicting expected outcome, and regret over past decisions (e.g., sterilization). However, psychological test scores on depression and anxiety inventories competed during the pretesting phase are reported to normalize after 1 yr posttest results *(88)*.

Despite compelling evidence of increased mood and anxiety symptoms among individuals who pursue predictive testing, regardless of the test result, there are no reported treatment studies of this population. Several factors must be considered regarding the treatment of mood disorders in this population. These include, but are not limited to evidence of pretest mood disorder, level of psychosocial support, and proximity to disease onset. Without published studies of treatment in this population, treatment efforts should focus on "target" symptoms. Individuals with clinical evidence of an adjustment disorder (either with depressed mood, with anxiety, or with mixed anxiety and depressed mood) should receive short-term psychiatric intervention (e.g., 6–12 mo) following the test result, which may include both psychopharmacological and psychotherapeutic intervention. The choice of pharmacological agent is similar to that described earlier for patients with manifest HD. In general, serotonergic agents tend to be well-tolerated with good efficacy. Reevaluation of the need for pharmacological intervention in these individuals should be done on a regular basis, given the results of long-term follow-up studies, which suggest a general resolution of psychiatric dysfunction over time, regardless of the result.

2.5. Conclusions

Mood disorders are common in patients with HD, contributing significantly to the morbidity and mortality associated with the disease. We have provided recommendations as to how these disorders can be recognized and treated. We are cognisant of the fact that in the majority of the mood disorders described, empirical data recommending choice of drug and optimal dosage scheduling are lacking. Although further research is clearly needed to elucidate best clinical practice, there is in place a body of evidence, drawn from anecdote, clinical trials, and other neuropsychiatric disorders, that can provide working therapeutic guidelines. Close attention to the principles outlined in this chapter, coupled with a knowledge of each drugs' potential benefits and drawbacks, increases the likelihood of a patient responding favorably to treatment and remaining compliant with that treatment.

ACKNOWLEDGMENTS

This work was supported by the Huntington Society of Canada and the Huntington Disease Society of America.

REFERENCES

1. Shiwach, R.S. and Norbury, C.G. (1994) A controlled psychiatric study of individual at risk for HD. *Br. J. Psychiatry* **165,** 500–505.
2. Caine, E.D. and Shoulson, I. (1994) Psychiatric symptoms in HD. *Am. J. Psychiatry* **140,** 728–733.
3. Mendez, M.F. (1994) HD: update and review of neuropsychiatric aspects. *Int. J. Psychiatry Med.* **24,** 189–208.
4. Bolt, J.M.W. (1970) Huntington's chorea in the west of Scotland. *Br. J. Psychiatry* **116,** 259–270.
5. Tsuang, D., Almqvist, E.W., Lipe, H., et al. (2000) Familial aggregation of psychotic symptoms in Huntington's disease. *Am. J. Psychiatry* **157,** 1955–1959.
6. Weigell-Weber, M., Schmid, W., and Spiegel, R. (1996) Psychiatric symptoms and CAG expansion in Huntington's disease. *Am. J. Med. Genet.* **67,** 53–57.
7. Cummings, J.L. (1995) Behavioral and psychiatric symptoms associated with Huntington's disease. *Neurology* **65,** 179–186.
8. Folstein, S.E., Chase, G.A., Wahl, W.E., et al. (1987) HD in Maryland: clinical aspect of racial variation. *Am. J. Hum. Genet.* **41,** 168–179.
9. Lovestone, S., Hodgson, S., Sham, P., Differ, A.M., and Levy, R. (1996) Familial psychiatric presentation of Huntington's disease. *J. Med. Genet.* **33,** 128–131.
10. Vonsattel, J.P., Myers, R.H., Stevens, T.J., et al. (1985) Neuropathological classification of HD. *J. Neuropathol. Exp. Neurol.* **44,** 559–577.

11. Kuwert, T., Lange, H.W., Langen, K.J., et al. (1989) Cerebral glucose consumption measured by PET in patient with and without psychiatric symptoms of HD. *Psychiatry Res.* **29,** 361–362.
12. De Marchi, N. and Mennella, R. (2000) Huntington's disease and its association with psychopathology. *Harv. Rev. Psychiatry* **7,** 278–289.
13. Folstein, S. (1989) *Huntington's Disease: a Disorder of Families,* John Hopkins University Press, Baltimore.
14. Shoulson, I. (1981) HD: functional capacities in patients treated with neuroleptic and antidepressant drugs. *Neurology* **31,** 1333–1335.
15. van Vugt, J.P., van Hilten, B.J., and Roos, R.A. (1996) Hypokinesia in Huntington's disease. *Mov. Disord.* **11,** 384–388.
16. Schott, K., Ried, S., and Dichgans, J. (1989) Antipsychotically induced dystonia in Huntington's disease: a case report. *Eur. Neurol.* **29**, 39–40.
17. Kapur, S. and Seeman, P. (2001) Does fast dissociation from the dopamine d(2) receptor explain the action of atypical antipsychotics? A new hypothesis. *Am. J. Psychiatry* **158,** 360–369.
18. Sajatovic, M., Verbanac, P., Ramirez, L.F., et al. (1991) Clozapine treatment of psychiatric symptoms resistant to neuroleptic treatment in patients with Huntington's chorea. *Neurology* **41,** 156.
19. van Vugt, J.P., Siesling, S., Vergeer, M., van der Velde, E.A., and Roos, R.A. (1997) Clozapine versus placebo in Huntington's disease: a double blind randomised comparative study. *J. Neurol. Neurosurg. Psychiatry* **63,** 35–39.
20. Bonuccelli, U., Ceravolo, R., Maremmani, C., Nuti, A., Rossi, G., and Muratorio, A. (1994) Clozapine in Huntington's chorea. *Neurology* **44,** 821–823.
21. Squitieri, F., Cannella, M., Porcellini, A., et al. (2001) Short-term effects of olanzapine in Huntington's disease. *Neuropsychiatry Neuropsychol. Behav. Neurol.* **14,** 69–72.
22. Dewhurst, K., Oliver, J.E., and McKnight, A.L. (1970) Socio-psychiatric consequences of Huntington's disease. *Br. J. Psychl.* **116,** 255–258.
23. Shiwach, R. (1994) Psychopathology in Huntington's disease in patients. *Acta Psychiatr. Scand.* **90,** 241–246.
24. Starkstein, S.E. and Robinson, R.G. (1989) Depression and Parkinson's disease, in *Aging and Clinical Practice: Depression and Co-existing Disease* (Robinson, R.G. and Rabins, P.V., eds.), Igaku-Shoi, New York, pp. 213–248.
25. Sadovnik, A.D., Remick, R.A., Allen, J., et al. (1996) Depression and multiple sclerosis. *Neurology* **46,** 628–632.
26. Loreck, D.J. and Folstein, M.F. (1993) Depression in Alzheimer's disease, in *Depression and Neurologic Disease* (Starkstein, S.E. and Robinson, G., eds.), John Hopkins Press, Baltimore, pp. 50–62.
27. Schoenfield, M., Meyers, R.H., Cupples, R.A., et al. (1984) Increased rate of suicide among patients with Huntington's disease. *J. Neurol. Neurosurg. Psychiatry* **47,** 1283–1287.
28. Cummings, J.L. and Cunningham, K. (1992) Obsessive-compulsive disorder in Huntington's disease. *Biol. Psychiatry* **31,** 263–270.
29. Alexander, G.E. and Crutcher, M.D. (1990) Functional architecture of basal ganglia circuits: neural substrates of parallel processing. *Trends Neurosci.* **13,** 266–271.
30. Mayberg, H.S., Starkstein, S.E., Peyser, C.E., et al. (1992) Paralimbic frontal lobe hypometabolism in depression associated with Huntington's disease. *Neurology* **42,** 1791–1797.
31. Mayberg, H.S., Starkstein, S.E., Sadzot, B., et al. (1990) Selective hypometabolism in the inferior frontal lobe in depressed patients with Parkinson's disease. *Ann. Neurol.* **28,** 57–64.
32. Baxter, L.R., Schwartz, J.M., Phelps, M.E., et al. (1989) Reduction of prefrontal cortex metabolism common to three types of depression. *Arch. Gen. Psychiatry* **46,** 243–250.
33. Lakshmanan, M., Mion, L.C., and Frengley, J.D. (1986) Effective low dose tricyclic antidepressant treatment for depressed geriatric rehabilitation patients. A double-blind study. *J. Am. Geriatr. Soc.* **34,** 421–426.
34. Mindham, R.H.S., Steele, C., Folstein, M.F., and Lucas, J. (1985) A comparison of the frequency of major affective disorder in Huntington's disease and Alzheimer's disease. *J. Neurol. Neurosurg. Psychiatry* **48,** 1172–1174.
35. Watt, D.C. and Seller, A. (1993) A clinico-genetic study of psychiatric disorder in Huntington's chorea. *Psychol. Med,* **23(Suppl.),** 1–46.
36. Lauterbach, E.C. (ed.) (2000) *Psychiatric Management in Neurologic Disease,* American Psychiatric Press, Washington, DC.
37. Minden. S.L., Orav, J., and Reich, P. (1987) Depression in multiple sclerosis. *Gen. Hosp. Psychiatry* **9,** 426–434.
38. Feinstein, A. and Feinstein, K.J. (2001) Depression associated with multiple sclerosis: looking beyond diagnosis to symptom expression. *J. Affect. Disord.* **66,** 193–198.
39. Hamilton, M. (1960) A rating scale for depression. *J. Neurol. Neurosurg. Psychiatry* **23,** 56–62.
40. Montgomery, S.A. and Asberg, M. (1979) A new depression scale designed to be sensitive to change. *Br. J. Psychiatry* **134,** 383–389.
41. Bech, P. and Rafaelsen, O.J. (1980) The use of rating scales exemplified by a comparison of the Hamilton and the Bech-Rafaelsen Scale. *Acta Psychiatr. Scand.* **285(Suppl. 128),** 128–131.
42. Huntington Study Group. (1996) The unified Huntington's disease rating scale: reliability and consistency. *Mov. Disord.* **1,** 136–142.
43. Beck, A.T., Ward, C.H., Mendelson, M., Mock, J., and Erbaugh, J. (1961) An inventory for measuring depression. *Arch. Gen. Psychiatry* **4,** 53–63.
44. Zigmond, A.S. and Snaith, R.P. (1983) The Hospital Anxiety and Depression Scale. *Acta Psychiatr. Scand.* **67,** 361–370.
45. Zung, W.W.K. (1965) A self-rating depression scale. *Arch. Gen. Psychiatry* **12,** 63–70.
46. Alexopolous, G.S., Abrams, R.C., Young, R.C., et al. (1988) Cornell scale for depression in dementia. *Biol. Psychiatry* **23,** 271–284.

47. Beigel, A., Murphy, D., and Bunney, W. (1971) The manic state rating scale: scale construction, reliability, and validity. *Arch. Gen. Psychiatry* **25,** 256–271.
48. Bech, P., Rafaelsen, O.J., Kramp, P., and Bolwig, T.G. (1978) The mania rating scale: construction and inter-observer agreement. *Neuropharmacology* **17,** 430–431.
49. Young, R.C., Briggs, V.T., Ziegler, V.E., et al. (1978) A rating scale for mania: reliability, validity, and sensitivity. *Br. J. Psychiatry* **133,** 429–436.
50. Hamilton, M. (1959) The assessment of anxiety states by rating. *Br. J. Med. Psychol.* **32,** 50–60.
51. DiNardo, P.A., O'Brien, G.T., Barlow, D.H., et al. (1982) *The Anxiety Disorders Interview Schedule,* Center for Stress and Anxiety Disorders, Albany, NY.
52. Manuzza, S., Fyer, A., Klein, D., and Endicott, J. (1986) Schedule for affective disorders and schizophrenia—lifetime version modified for the study of anxiety disorders (SADS-LA): rationale and conceptual development. *J. Psychiatr. Res.* **20,** 317–337.
53. Spielberger, C.D. (1983) *Manual for the State-Trait Anxiety Inventory,* Consulting Psychologist Press, Palo Alto.
54. Marks, I.M. and Matthews, A.M. (1979) Brief standard self-rating for phobic patients. *Behav. Res. Ther.* **17,** 263–279.
55. Bystritsky, A, Linn, L.S., and Wane, J.E. (1990) Development of a multidimensional scale of anxiety. *J. Anx. Disord.* **4,** 99–115.
56. Fogel, B.S. (1996) Drug therapy in neuropsychiatry, in *Neuropsychiatry* (Fogel, B.S., Schiffer, R.B., and Rao, S.M., eds.), Williams & Wilkins, Baltimore.
57. Peyser, C.E. and Folstein, S.E. (1993) Depression in Huntington's disease, in *Depression in Neurologic Disease* (Starkstein, S.E. and Robinson, R.G., ed.), Johns Hopkins University Press, Baltimore, pp. 117–139.
58. Ranen, N.G., Peyser, C.E., and Folstein, S.E. (1993) *A Physician's Guide to the Management of Huntington's Disease: Pharmacologic and Non-pharmacologic Interventions,* Huntington's Disease Society of America, New York, NY.
59. Lyketsos, C.G., Sheppard, J.M., Steele, C.D., et al. (2000) Randomized, placebo controlled, double blind clinical trial of sertraline in the treatment of depression complicating Alzheimer's disease: initial results from the depression in Alzheimer's disease study. *Am. J. Psychol.* **157,** 1686–1689.
60. Scott, T.F., Nussbaum, P., McConnell, H., et al. (1995) Measurement of treatment response to sertraline in depressed multiple sclerosis patients using the Carrol scale. *Neurol. Res.* **1,** 421–422.
61. Flax, J.W., Gray, J., and Herbert, J. (1991) Effects of fluoxetine on patients with multiple sclerosis. *Am. J. Psychol.* **14,** 45,1603.
62. Ranen, N.G., Lipsey, J.R., Treisman, G., et al. (1996) Sertraline in the treatment of severe aggressiveness in Huntington's disease. *J, Neuropsychiatry Clin. Neurosci,* **8,** 338–340.
63. Hoehn-Saric, R., Lipsey, J.R., and McLeod, D.R. (1990) Apathy and indifference in patients in patients on fluoxetine and fluvoxamine. *J. Clin. Psychopharmacol.* **10,** 343–345.
64. Kapur, S. and Remington, G. (1996) Serotonin-dopamine interaction and its relevance to schizophrenia. *Am. J. Psychol.* **153,** 466–476.
65. Kuhn, R. (1958) The treatment of depressive states with G22355 (imipramine hydrochloride). *Am. J. Psychol.* **115,** 459–464.
66. Folstein, S.E., Folstein, M.F., and McHugh, P.R. (1979) Psychiatric syndromes in Huntington's disease, in *Huntington's Disease* (Chase, T.N., et al., eds.), *Adv. Neurol.* Raven Press, New York, pp. 281–289.
67. Folstein, S.E., Abbott, M.H., Chase, G.A., Jensen, B.A., and Folstein, M.F. (1983) The association of affective disorder with Huntington's disease in a case series and in families. *Psychol. Med.* **13,** 537–542.
68. Moldawsky, R.J. (1984) Effect of amoxapine on speech in a patient with Huntington's disease. *Am. J. Psychiatr.* **141,** 150.
69. Ford, M.F. (1986) Treatment of depression in Huntington's disease with monoamine oxidase inhibitors. *Br. J. Psychiatry* **14,** 654–656.
70. Rammohan, K.W., Rosenberg, J.H., Pollack, C.P., Lynn, J., Blumenfeld, A., and Nagaraja, H.N. (2000) Provigil (modafenil): efficacy and safety for the treatment of fatigue in patients with multiple sclerosis. Presented at the 52nd Annual Meeting of the American Academy of Neurology, San Diego, CA.
71. Menza, M.A., Kaufman, K.R., and Castellanos, A. (2000) Modafenil augmentation of antidepressant treatment in depression. *J. Clin. Psychiatry* **61,** 378–381.
72. Folstein, S. and Folstein, M. (1981) Diagnosis and treatment of Huntington's disease. *Comp. Ther.* **7,** 60–66.
73. Ranen, N.G., Peyser, C.E., and Folstein, S.E. (1994) ECT as a treatment for depression in Huntington's disease. *J. Neuropsychol.* **6,** 154–158.
74. Evans, D.L., Pedersen, C., and Tancer, M.E. (1987) ECT in the treatment of organic psychosis in Huntington's disease. *Convuls. Ther.* **3,** 145–150.
75. Judd, L., Paulus, M.P., Wells, K.B., et al. (1996) Socio-economic burden of sub-syndromal depressive symptoms and major depression in a sample of the general population. *Am. J. Psychol.* **15,** 1411–1417.
76. Sherbourne, C.D., Wells, K.B., and Hays, R.D. (1994) Subthreshold depression and depressive disorder: clinical characteristics of general medical and mental health specialty outpatients. *Am. J. Psychol.* **151,** 1777–1784.
77. Wells, K.B., Stewart, A., Hays, R.D., et al. (1989) The functioning and well being of depressed patients. Results from the Medical Outcome Study. *JAMA* **262,** 914–978.
78. Wells, K.B. (1995) The role of depression in hypertension-related mortality. *Psychosom. Med.* **57,** 436–438.
79. Silver, J.M. and Yudowsky, S.C. (1997) Aggressive disorders, in *Neuropsychiatry of Traumatic Brain Injury* (Silver, J.M., Yudowsky, S.C., and Hales, R.E., eds.), American Psychiatric Press, Washington, DC, pp. 313–353.

80. Prochazka, A.V., Weaver, M.J., Keller, R.T., et al. (1998) A randomized trial of nortriptyline for smoking cessation. *Arch. Int. Med.* **158,** 2035–2039.
81. Decruyenaere, M., Evers-Kiebooms, G., Boogaerts, A., et al. (1999) Psychological functioning before testing for Huntington's disease: the role of the parental disease, risk, perception, and subjective proximity of the disease. *J. Med. Genet.* **36,** 897–905.
82. Taylor, C.A. and Myers, R.H. (1997) Long-term impact of Huntington's disease linkage testing. *Am. J. Med. Genet.* **70,** 365–370.
83. Codori, A.M., Slavney, P.R., Young, C., Miglioretti, D.L., and Brand, J. (1997) Predictors of psychological adjustment to genetic testing for Huntington's disease. *Health Psychol.* **16,** 36–50.
84. Almquist, E.W., Bloch, M., Brinkman, R., Craufurd, D., and Hayden, M.R. (1999) A worldwide assessment of the frequency of suicide, suicide attempts, or psychiatric hospitalization after predictive testing for Huntington's disease. *Am. J. Hum. Genet.* **64,** 1293–1304.
85. Hayden, M.R., Bloch, M., and Wiggins, S. (1995) Psychological effects of predictive testing for Huntington's disease, in *Behavior Neurology of Movement Disorders.* (Weiner, W.J. and Lang, A.E., eds.), Raven Press, New York, pp. 201–210.
86. Mandich, P., Jacopini, G., DiMaria, E., et al. (1998) Predictive testing in Huntington's disease: ten years experience in two Italian centers. *Ital. J. Neurol. Sci.* **19,** 68–74.
87. Lawson, K., Wiggins, S., Green, T., Adam, S., Bloch, M., and Hayden, M.R. (1996) Adverse psychological events occurring in the first year after predictive testing for Huntington's disease: the Canadian collaborative predictive testing. *J. Med. Genet.* **33,** 862–862.
88. Decruyenaere, M., Evers-Kiebooms, G., Boogaerts, A., et al. (1996) Prediction of psychological functioning one year after the predictive test for Huntington's disease and impact of the test result on reproductive decision making. *J. Med. Genet.* **33,** 737–743.

32

Clinical Management of Aggression and Frontal Symptoms in Huntington's Disease

Adam Rosenblatt, MD, Karen Anderson, MD, Alex D. Goumeniouk, MD, FRCPc, Paul Lespérance, MD, MSc, Martha A. Nance, MD, Jane S. Paulsen PhD, Allen Rubin, MD, Jean A. Saint-Cyr, PhD, Russ Sethna, MD, and Mark Guttman, MD, FRCPc

1. INTRODUCTION

Patients with Huntington's disease (HD) and other brain conditions suffer from three categories of psychiatric symptoms. There are those problematic experiences and behaviors that can be seen as aspects of well-known psychiatric syndromes found in the general population, such as mania. There are those symptoms that have such a wide variety of causes or are a secondary aspect of so many different kinds of disease that they can properly be called nonspecific, such as insomnia. Finally, there are those symptoms, predominantly found in persons whose brains have been injured through trauma or disease, which appear to belong to psychiatric syndromes recognized by experienced clinicians, but not well described in terms of essential features, etiology, or therapeutics. An example of this kind of symptom would be apathy, arising out of the frontal syndrome of HD. The task at hand is to try to identify and group together this last category of symptoms, particularly with respect to aggression and the "frontal lobe" syndrome of HD, so as to pave the way for reliable diagnosis and rational therapeutics *(1)*.

2. AGGRESSION

2.1. *Scope of the Problem*

Difficulties with rage and aggression are one of the most problematic neuropsychiatric sequelae of Huntington's disease. These behaviors are a burden for caregivers and frequently result in placement of patients in a nursing home or chronic hospital setting. There is very little literature on the phenomenology and management of aggression in patients with HD, although there is much on the management of aggression in other dementing conditions, which may also be useful in understanding the phenomenon and devising treatment strategies.

2.2. *Description of Aggression in HD*

Aggressiveness in HD falls on a continuum of severity. At one end of this spectrum lie the assertiveness, willfulness, and effective defending of the self, which are a normal part of human experience. In the middle of the continuum there is a loosening of self-control and self-regulation, and the introduction

From: *Mental and Behavioral Dysfunction in Movement Disorders*
Edited by: M-A. Bédard et al. © Humana Press Inc., Totowa, NJ

of ego eccentricity, indifference to the consequences of actions, and a heightened level of reactivity so that assertive responses take on an autonomous quality, representing a shift of emotional state or a change in personality. At the far end of the spectrum lies overt aggression and violence, acted out in violation of social norms, which can carry the risk of harm to property or to other persons.

The most common form of aggression in HD might be described as "impulsive aggression." The aggressive behavior escalates quickly and is not controlled by the usual social inhibitions. The implication is that such episodes are, in fact, in response to a stimulus. However, this may not be immediately apparent because, to an outside observer, the provocation appears trivial. Persons with HD may experience a disproportionately angry reaction to disappointment, frustration, or perceived disregard in interpersonal situations. These outbursts are not usually effective in achieving the individual's goals and may be highly maladaptive. The episodes tend to be of relatively low frequency but high intensity, making them dangerous, difficult to predict, and difficult to assess for response to treatment.

2.3. *Biological Underpinning*

There are a number of biological models of aggression, including an important role for adrenergic receptors in the limbic forebrain and cerebral cortex *(2)*, and the observation that patients who exhibit aggressive outbursts have higher levels of five-3-methoxy-4-hydroxyphenylglcol (MHPG), a norepinepherine metabolite *(3)*. Low levels of serotonin (5-HT) activity, as well as dopamine dysfunction in the mesolimbic and mesocortical regions of the brain, have also been implicated in aggressive disorders *(4,5)*. In the typology of frontal lobe disorders postulated by Mega and Cummings, disinhibition and irritability are associated in particular with disorders of the lateral orbital prefrontal cortex *(6)*. Some of these hypotheses might have implications for treatment if proven true, but it is a complex challenge for the clinician to devise a regimen, taking into account these underlying factors and their relationship to the patient's environment.

2.4. *Predisposing Factors for Aggression in HD*

A number of factors can be identified which probably predispose persons with HD to aggressive behavior. HD patients suffer from a number of specific psychiatric syndromes that may result in aggression, including depression and mania, psychotic disorders, anxiety disorders, obsessive–compulsive disorders (OCD), and delirium. Commonly, the interplay of cognitive dysfunction, particularly the failure of frontal executive functions, and what might be called "frontal" personality changes, contribute to the process by which annoyance escalates to aggression. If obsessions or inflexibility are present, a person with HD has great difficulty adapting to a provocative situation. Failure of self-observation, which can occur to varying degrees of severity, results in a loss of self-regulation. A sense of being overstimulated or overwhelmed by multiple tasks can lead to a collapse of adaptive reserve. Rarely, misperception or misinterpretation of events may provoke aggressive behavior. These topics will be covered in much more depth in Subheading 3. Changes brought about by the physical manifestations of the disease, such as changes in institutional or home environments, interaction with strange healthcare personnel, difficulties with authority figures, and the supervision of children, may cause HD patients to experience high levels of stress, and the difficulty in satisfying basic needs (e.g., hunger, sex, hygiene, and insomnia) may result in frustration and contribute to aggressive outbursts. Many episodes are provoked by communications problems, in situations where the person with HD has dysarthria and has difficulty being understood, or is slow to answer due to a lack of initiation and slow mental processing. Finally, psychological factors having to do with a loss of autonomy and control, brought about by such issues as loss of a driver's license, inability to work, and marital difficulties, may result in decreasing frustration thresholds and breakthrough aggression.

2.5. *Differential Diagnosis of Aggression in HD*

Aggression in HD describes a symptom, rather than a syndrome, and is a nonspecific term. Therefore, a thorough differential diagnosis is of primary importance with respect to the evaluation and clinical management of aggression. The diagnostic impression will need to be reached after a longitudinal evaluation, tasking into account the patient's mental status prior to, during, and after the period of aggression, his or her preexisting personality, medical condition, and the environmental factors that may have come into play and serve to predispose, precipitate, or perpetuate the symptoms. Specific psychiatric diagnoses, such as depression or OCD, should be made where possible, because of the implications for prognosis and treatment strategy. This is especially true in the case of delerium.

Delerium should always be suspected in patients with HD who experience an acute change in mental state, particularly if accompanied by a fluctuating level of alertness, disorganization of thought, and visual and other sensory perceptual abnormalities (hallucinations and illusions). Persons with HD have many reasons to become delirious, including head injuries and subdural hematoma from falls, seizures, metabolic disorders, substance abuse, infections, malnutrition, or the side effects of medications. In the person with advanced HD, attention must be paid to basic biological drives and systemic factors, which contribute to the patient's agitation. These include pain, bladder and bowel discomfort and hunger. A large number of nursing home patients with HD have serum glucose in the hypoglycemic range, suggesting that the caloric demands of these patients exceed both attempts at augmented feeding and the body's capacity for gluconeogenesis.

2.6. *Assessment of Aggression in HD*

In assessing and rating aggression in HD, it can be difficult to account for the subjective impressions of the rater. Nevertheless, a number of potentially useful rating scales have been developed, although not specifically for HD, such as the Overt Aggression Scale *(7)*, the Neuro-Psychiatric Inventory *(8)*, and the RAGE Scale *(9)*, The Overt Aggression Scale was developed to attempt to evaluate the efficacy of different psychopharmacological interventions on four primary groups of aggressive behaviors: verbal aggression, physical aggression against the self, physical aggression against objects, and physical aggression against other people. In addition to identifying the type of aggressive behavior, the rater also lists the therapeutic intervention used.

Silver and Yudofsky and coworkers suggest that the Overt Aggression Scale be used to establish baseline criteria with respect to the aggressive behaviors so that subsequent documentation and pharmacological response or lack of response can be evaluated more efficaciously *(7)*. The Overt Aggression Scale has been used in HD research *(10)*. The HD irritability scale *(10)* may be the only instrument developed specifically to measure irritability in HD, but does not address the issue of overt aggression.

2.7. *Management of Aggression in HD*

The management of aggression in HD can be divided into short-(acute) and long-term (prophylactic) strategies, each of which may be divided into pharmacological and nonpharmacological interventions. The development of a strategy for managing aggression should begin with a period of observation, identification of precipitating and ameliorating factors, a review of relevant history, such as previous episodes of substance abuse, domestic disputes, or habitual fighting, and an assessment of personality vulnerabilities, which could lead to aggression. Nonpharmacological interventions could include reducing environmental stress, regularization of the affected person's schedule to avoid unpleasant surprises, and education and counseling of caregivers. Family members should be educated about the personality changes that may accompany HD, producing such symptoms as apathy, irritability, and perseveration, and should be encouraged to prioritize, so that limits can be set when necessary, but unnecessary confrontations can be avoided. For example, a stereotypical behavior occurs in some individuals with HD consisting of a perseverative, impatient, and irresolvable demand, which finally results in a temper outburst. Companions who attempt to reason, persuade, or intervene in the midst of one of these escalations often discover they contribute to further escalation. In contrast, when the companion can fall back to a momentary vacating from the argument or an expression of acquiescence, the episode may wane more quickly, again allowing rational discourse to emerge, and allowing the patient to assert wishes and values without the overtones of aggressiveness.

Acute pharmacological management of aggression in HD primarily relies on benzodiazepine agents and antipsychotic drugs. It is thought that the newer antipsychotic drugs such as risperidone, olanzapine, quetiapine, and ziprasidone may decrease the risk of disabling or dangerous side effects, such as acute dystonia, tardive dyskinesia, or neuroleptic malignant syndrome, in an already neurologically compromised individual. However, they are expensive and are generally not available in as great a range of doses or delivery systems, such as injectable and liquid forms, as the older agents. For this reason, a conventional neuroleptic, like haloperidol or fluphenazine, may at times be more practical. The sedative effects of these agents are of primary importance to the acute management of the aggression, whatever the cause, such as psychosis, mania, delirium, depression, or organic personality change. Benzodiazepines with relatively short half-lives, such as lorazepam, are most helpful in the acute management of aggression either in conjunction with neuroleptics or by themselves. However, benzodiazepines can also worsen motoric deficits and may result in increased postural instability in these patients.

There is very little published data on the efficacy of pharmacologic agents for aggression in HD, but agents with putative anti-aggressive properties include neuroleptics, benzodiazepines, antidepressants, lithium, anticonvulsants, adrenergic antagonists, psychostimulants, anti-androgens, opiate antagonists, and miscellaneous agents. Each class is dealt with in turn. Controlled trials are lacking, and there is no more than a relative consensus among experienced HD clinicians as to which classes are preferable. Obviously, when a specific psychiatric diagnosis or syndrome, such as major depression or command hallucinations, can be identified as the cause of the aggressive behavior, a standard therapy should be attempted if one exists. In cases where such a specific diagnosis cannot be made, a commonsensical strategy is proposed, which would still select the type of medication to begin with on the basis of the most salient features of the presentation. Patients who appear hallucinated, delusional, or suspicious would be given a neuroleptic. Patients who present with obsessions and compulsions would be given a serotonergic agent. Those with depressive symptoms would be given an antidepressant, and those who appear disinhibited, euphoric, or irritable would begin with an anticonvulsant.

2.8. Classes of Medications Used

2.8.1. Neuroleptics

These medications are mildly sedating and can be given primarily in the evening, building from low doses. The use of neuroleptics is linked to their effect on dopamine receptors. There are no controlled studies of antipsychotic treatment in HD. However, clinical experience suggests that the newer (atypical) agents, olanzepine, risperidone, quetiapine, and ziprasidone, are useful and generally better tolerated than the older neuroleptics. Clozapine is used uncommonly because of cumbersome monitoring procedures that particularly limit the most impaired patients. Clozapine also carries a stronger burden of anticholinergic adverse side effects, particularly in the nonambulatory or elderly patient. The older neuroleptics, such as haloperidol, are sometimes used for suppression of chorea, are less expensive, and come in a wider range of delivery systems, but new intramuscular formulations of several atypical agents are potential additions to the pharmacopoeia.

2.8.2. Benzodiazepines

This class of medication is often relied on as a first-line intervention in acute management. The effects of benzodiazepines on impulse control are primarily through their sedative and anxiolytic effects, resulting in a dampening of environmental influences on an individual's behavior. The use of oral and intramuscular lorazepam in a clinical practice starting at 0.5 mg twice daily and titrating upwards to maximum of 8 mg/d in divided doses is a popular strategy. There is a theoretical possibility of disinhibition, but this is rarely seen in clinical practice.

Clonazepam appears to be, in the setting of HD, a useful adjunctive medicine for prophylaxis of aggression. This is thought to be related to its anticonvulsant and antimanic properties. In clinical practice, dosing should start at 0.25 mg twice daily to a maximum of 6 mg/d. Longer acting benzodiazepines (e.g., diazepam) are not recommended due to their more profound effects of daytime sedation, and cognitive disruption, and the increased difficulty with postural instability.

The use of short-term benzodiazepines such as triazolam and alprazolam are not recommended because of difficulties with rebound anxiety and disinhibition.

2.8.3. *Antidepressants*

Antidepressants, even in HD patients who do not have an obvious depressive syndrome, may reduce aggressive behavior. The selective serotonin re-uptake inhibitors (SSRIs), including fluoxetine, sertraline, paroxetine, fluvoxamine, and citalopram, are thought to be particularly helpful. They seem to mitigate the frontal syndrome of HD, which produces irritability, apathy, perseveration, and disinhibition (see Subheading 3.), which may, in turn, lead to episodes of aggression and violence. There have been few systematic studies, but sertraline has been shown to reduce irritability and aggressiveness in HD patients *(11)*.

2.8.4. *Lithium*

Lithium was able to decrease aggression in a group of prison inmates with probable antisocial personality disorders *(12)*. It is postulated that lithium exerts its effects by 5-HT neurotransmitters augmentation and dampening catecholamine function. It may be useful in the long-term management of aggression in HD, but there are no controlled studies with lithium. Clinical dosing should start at 150 mg/d gradually increasing to an initial maintenance dose reflecting serum levels at the low end of the therapeutic range.

2.8.5. *Anticonvulsants*

These medications have been widely used in neuropsychiatry for aggressive conditions and for mood instability and cyclical mood disorders. Most commonly used are carbamazepine and valproic acid. These drugs probably represent the treatment of choice for the prophylaxis of HD-related aggression. Newer anticonvulsants including gabapentin, lamotrigine, and topiramate may also have a role, but experience in this regard is less well developed. Carbamazepine, in the clinical setting, possesses the most striking evidence of beneficial effects, and this is reflected in studies in individuals with a variety of other conditions, including borderline personality disorders *(13)*, organic brain disorders *(14)*, schizophrenia *(15)*, developmental disabilities *(16,17)*, and dementia *(18)*. Dosing of carbamazepine should start at 100 mg/d, preferably of a controlled-release preparation, titrating to the lower limits of the therapeutic range (by serum levels). Anticonvulsants likely exert their effects by enhancing 5-HT activity in the brain. Valproic acid is also frequently used based on studies in individuals with organic brain syndromes and mental retardation (MR) *(19,20)*.

2.8.6. *Adrenergic Antagonists*

There is no data on the use of β-blockers in Huntington's disease, but β-blockers such as propranolol and pindolol have been demonstrated to have anti-aggressive properties at higher doses in a variety of other neuropsychiatric condition. These medicines are postulated to work through both adrenergic and serotonergic mechanisms. Their efficacy in HD in unknown.

2.8.7. *Psychostimulants and Opiate Antagonists*

The use of psychostimulants in adults with attention deficit disorder (ADD) related aggression has been reported *(21)*. Opiate antagonists have been useful in self-injurious behaviors *(22)*.

2.8.8. *Anti-Androgens*

In aggressive males, an additional option is the use of anti-androgenic hormonal therapies, such as medroxyprogesterone. Such treatments can be used particularly when the aggression has sexual selectivity or sexualized content, but can also be applied to aggressiveness separate from these qualities. Sexual aggression is seen more commonly in men. Sexual acting out in persons with HD could be the result of hypofrontal phenomena, which result in interpersonal boundary dissolution and disinhibited behaviors. It appears that the fewer the social supports, the more at risk individuals are for sexually disinhibited behaviors. These behaviors can also be a result of psychotic symptoms such as delusional love or obsessive ruminative ideas regarding infidelity or impropriety in a spouse.

2.8.9. Miscellaneous

There have been anecdotal reports on the use of clonidine, guaifenesin, buspirone, and amantadine, to control aggressive behavior.

2.9. Summary

In summation, aggression in Huntington's disease is a multifactorial symptom, which requires a sophisticated approach. Detailed, longitudinal observations should be made, and precipitants and triggers should be identified. Coping strategies, management of the environment, and education and support of caregivers should be employed. Specific psychiatric diagnoses should be made where possible and treated accordingly. Pharmacologic management of aggression can be divided into acute strategies, mostly involving neuroleptics and benzodiazepines, and prophylactic treatment. The initial class of drug for long-term intervention can be selected on the basis of the most salient psychiatric symptoms associated with the aggression or, all things being equal, an anticonvulsant like carbamazepine or valproic acid is probably the first-line treatment of choice. Many aggressive behaviors in persons with HD appear to arise out of the frontal syndrome associated with the disease in which irritability, disinhibition, and a rigid style may interact with the individual's environment to produce aggressive outbursts. This frontal syndrome is dealt with much more fully in the next section.

3. FRONTAL LOBE DISORDERS IN HD

3.1. Introduction

Of all the behavioral and psychiatric aspects of HD, the ones that we have termed "frontal lobe disorders" are perhaps the most difficult to define, characterize, and treat and yet may be the most common psychiatric manifestations of the disease. They are so common, in fact, that they are often regarded as a personality change, rather than a set of discrete symptoms. Individuals with this syndrome may become apathetic, irritable, disinhibited, impulsive, obsessional, and perseverative. Given that the neuropathology of HD is characterized by selective death of the medium spiny neurons in the caudate nucleus, with a dorsomedial to ventrolateral and caudal-rostral progression of degeneration *(23)*, "frontal lobe" disorder, in this context, is really a pseudo-anatomical term for a syndrome also involving the basal ganglia and other parts of the brain. We refer to the symptoms by this name, not because the responsible structures have been definitively localized, but because of the syndrome's resemblance to that seen in a host of other conditions involving frontal-subcortical structures and usually accompanied by subcortical dementia, a term introduced by McHugh and Folstein in 1979 *(24)*. Such conditions could include Parkinson's disease, frontotemporal dementia, traumatic brain injury, cerebrovascular accident (CVA), human immunodeficiency virus (HIV) infection, and even, in some cases, Alzheimer's disease. Although it is difficult to define the borders of the frontal syndrome, the argument to be advanced in this chapter is that it is a useful clinical entity, worthy of continued research, and that there is an emerging pharmacopoeia for HD patients with frontal syndromes, sometimes involving drugs with dopaminergic effects.

There are at least five recognized discrete parallel circuits uniting regions of the frontal lobe (motor, frontal eye, dorsolateral, orbitofrontal, and anterior cingulate areas) with the striatum, globus pallidus, and thalamus in functional systems. The cognitive functions of planning, initiating, and completing activities, decision making, judgment, abstract thinking, set-shifting, keeping content "on-line" for the needed period of time, suppression of inappropriate content, and timing are recognized as "executive" or frontal lobe functions *(25)*. Three principal frontal lobe behavioral symptom complexes have been described: (*i*) a dorsolateral prefrontal circuit with functions involving fluency, motor programming, set-shifting, learning, memory retrieval, and problem solving; (*ii*) an orbitofrontal syndrome, with prominent disinhibition and irritability; and (*iii*) a medial frontal-anterior cingulate syndrome with apathy and diminished initiative *(6)*. We have included discussions of apathy, irritability, unawareness, and perseveration, or obsessive–compulsive symptoms as separate topics. We have not attempted an extensive separate treatment of the cognitive dysfunction that often coexists and certainly contributes to these behavioral problems. This topic is covered in detail in other chapters.

3.2. Apathy

3.2.1. Definition

Among the earliest to apply the term apathy in HD were McHugh and Folstein *(26)*, who described the dementia of HD as being characterized by "a prominent psychic apathy and inertia that worsens to an akinetic mute state." Caine et al. *(27)*, working from neuropsychometric studies, described in HD-affected individuals a "failure to initiate activities spontaneously," and hypothesized that this was related to both a "difficulty in organizing and planning and … a failure to recall information at a desired time," again suggesting that apathy has its basis in the loss of certain cognitive abilities. Burns et al. *(10)* defined apathy as a loss of emotion, characterized either by an internal feeling of disinterest or an external behavioral state of inaction. Marin has also emphasized that apathy may have an underlying cognitive, motor, sensory, or affective basis in different patients or patient groups. The differential diagnosis of apathy includes abulia, akinesia, depression, dementia, delirium, despair, and demoralization *(28,29)*. Rubin *(30)* pointed out the many ways that "lack of response" in an HD patient may be interpreted or described by different health practitioners, including depression and indifference (psychiatrist), bradykinesia and initiation defect (neurologist), abulia and inattention (neuropsychologist), resistance or lack of motivation (nurse or nursing assistant), processing or organization failure (physical, occupational, or speech therapist), or failure to comprehend (family).

3.2.2. Measurement

Burns et al. *(10)* attempted to quantify apathy in HD by means of a five-question caregiver survey, which asked about (*i*) loss of interest in activities; (*ii*) to what extent the affected individual "lies around"; (*iii*) to what extent the individual is less active than premorbidly; (*iv*) to what extent the individual keeps busy; and (*v*) whether the affected person seemed withdrawn. This scale has been subsequently expanded into a 15-item questionnaire, which has seen extensive use in the HD Center at Johns Hopkins. In the early 1990s, Marin et al. devised an Apathy Evaluation Scale, which has been validated in a series of patients with conditions other than HD (traumatic brain injury, stroke, and other dementias) *(31,32)*. This scale has subsequently been used by investigators to assess apathy in patients with Alzheimer's disease, HIV, lewy body disease (LBD), and myotonic dystrophy *(33–35)*. Although apathy in HIV was found to correlate with depression, in patients with LBD and other dementias, apathy did not always co-segregate with depression, aggression, or irritability. The Apathy Evaluation Scale, although not designed specifically for HD, has been applied more widely than the scale devised by Burns et al.

3.2.3. Apathy in HD

In HD, apathy can exist separately from depression *(36)*. Apathy also fails to co-segregate with irritability and aggression *(10)*. The same authors found that individuals with HD had a higher frequency of apathy (defined as being present if the score was >3 on a five-point scale on at least 3 out of 5 survey questions) than a group of Alzheimer's patients matched for Mini-Mental Status Exam Score, suggesting that apathy is not solely due to dementia. Apathy is thought to be very common in HD patients in clinical practice and is a significant source of distress to caregivers, although, by definition, not to the patients themselves.

3.2.4. Treatment

Apathy is usually far more distressing to caregivers, friends, and family members, than to the patient actually experiencing apathy. The question arises as to whether treatment is even necessary. Future studies of the treatment of apathy should attempt to demonstrate whether there are improvements in other measures of the quality of life. Sometimes the only necessary intervention is to educate caregivers, to explain that apathy is a common and even expected manifestation of HD, and that it is to be distinguished from depression. Expectations of the patient may need to be revised. In problematic cases, such as when the patient fails to eat or practice personal hygiene, more intervention may be required.

Anecdotal reports have been published of the successful treatment of apathy with amantadine, amphetamines, bromocriptine, bupropion, methylphenidate, selegiline, and hydroquinidine *(32,37)*. In a recent review, catecholaminergic agents were suggested as appropriate therapeutic agents, based on the current neuroanatomic and neurochemical understanding of apathy *(38)*. The use of stimulants such as methylphenidate, dextroamphetamine, or pemoline is appropriate in severe cases, but might carry a risk of increasing irritability or aggression. A relatively nonsedating SSRI, such as fluoxetine, sertraline, or citaprolam may also be considered, particularly if there is coexisting or underlying depression. Several authors have pointed out the importance of considering a reduction in medications that might blunt emotion or slow cognitive processing, such as the neuroleptics *(30,39)*. Nonpharmacologic approaches to increasing activity in patients with apathy include avoiding open-ended questions or tasks, providing cueing for patients for both simple questions and more complex acts, and maintaining a simple and regular daily schedule. Positive reinforcement for desired behaviors or actions can be helpful. Increased environmental stimulation, such as involvement in a sheltered workshop or day program may benefit some patients.

3.3. Irritability

3.3.1. Definition

Irritability is a ubiquitous human experience, found in both normal and pathological situations. As stated by Galbraith, although irritability is a common complaint in "general practitioners' surgeries, and the outpatient clinics of psychiatrists, neurologists, and neurosurgeons", studies specifically aimed at it are surprisingly scant *(40)*. In fact, Snaith and Taylor introduced a clinical working definition for irritability only in 1985. They define irritability as a "feeling state characterized by reduced control of the temper which usually results in irascible, verbal, or behavioral outbursts, or can be present without observed manifestations" *(41)*. For Burns and colleagues, aggression "is akin to irritability" but implies verbal or physical assaults. It is important to note that irritability may not be recognized by a patient, but only by the caregiver *(10)*. This is particularly often the case in HD patients.

3.3.2. Measurement

Although clinicians agree that it is important to distinguish irritability from other more classic mood states (sadness, elation) or behaviors (withdrawal, aggression), and it seems easily done in a clinical setting, the only published scale that partially addresses irritability was a scale meant to accompany the Yudofsky Overt Agression Scale *(7,10)* so as to elicit informants' evaluation of apathy and irritability. Inter-rater and test–retest reliability (1.00 and 0.81 for irritability) and validity of the scale are quite good, and administration takes only a few minutes. Both the resulting HD apathy and HD irritability scales have seen years of use as research instruments at the HD Center at Johns Hopkins and could be used to obtain objective measures of treatment response.

3.3.3. Irritability in HD

In an early multicenter study of 102 patients with HD, Dewhurst and others *(42)*, described irritability in half of their cohort of patients hospitalized for mental and behavioral manifestations associated with HD. Irritability appears to be very common in HD, and therapies to reduce this symptom may benefit a large proportion of HD patients. In the study of Burns et al. *(10)*, irritability, aggression, and apathy were independent of each other. This suggests that targeting irritability to reduce overt aggression in HD patients may not work (and vice-versa). Likewise, a study by Mayberg et al. *(43)* found that depression and irritability were not correlated in HD patients, suggesting that treatment of co-morbid depression may not reduce irritability in a direct way. Available treatment reports and studies of irritability in HD or neurologically impaired patients rarely address this point. Most recent papers have targeted irritability as both a mood or aggression by-product. Fortunately, there are many pharmacological agents whose secondary, if not primary, effects, may help to reduce irritability.

3.3.4. Treatment of Irritability

The first principle of treatment of irritability in HD is to identify and treat any underlying co-morbid conditions or environmental factors. Appropriate therapy for depression or bipolar disorder, or support for normal reactions to the losses and frustrations of HD, may result in a secondary reduction in irritability.

There have been few systematic studies of treatment for irritability in HD. In the published literature, sertraline successfully reduced irritability and aggressiveness in two HD patients *(11)*. Buspirone (up to 20 mg twice daily), a partial 5-HT1A agonist, was successful in treating outbursts of agitation and aggression in one juvenile-onset HD patient and in two aggressive patients with adult-onset HD *(44)*. Studies of the treatment of irritability in brain injury, Alzheimer's disease, and other psychiatric conditions supports consideration of various treatment regimens such as SSRIs, trazodone, and buspirone in the treatment of disturbed behaviors and irritability *(45)*.

Haloperidol and fluphenazine have proved useful in treating chorea, hallucinations, and delusions as well as irritability in HD *(46)*. Clozapine, risperidone, trazodone, propranolol (up to 600 mg/d), and pindolol have all shown benefits in the treatment of aggression and irritability in patients with Alzheimer's disease, other dementias, and other neurologic conditions *(47–53)*. In HD, both propranolol and pindolol have shown some efficacy on aggression *(54)*.

The anticonvulsant valproate has shown to improve irritability in borderline personality disorder and in one HD patient *(55,56)*. Although they have not been studied in HD, case reports have documented a reduction in aggression or irritable behavior in patients with other neurological conditions following the use of carbamazepine, gabapentin, and lamotrigine.

When treating irritability in a particular patient, a number of other factors such as anxiety, depressive states, and aggressive behavior should all be taken into consideration. For reasons of ease of use, applicability to other symptoms, such as anxiety and depression, and favorable side effect profile, an SSRI antidepressant would appear to be a good first agent. In some cases, improvement may be much more rapid than when SSRIs are used to treat classical instances of depression.

Anticonvulsants, sometimes used as "mood stabilizers" (valproate, carbamazepine, and to a lesser extent, lamotrigine, gabapentin, or topiramate), the newer better tolerated neuroleptics, and longer-acting benzodiazepines, such as clonazepam, would be appropriate second-line choices, depending on the specifics of the particular patient, including co-morbid conditions and the need to avoid certain side effects.

3.4. Unawareness

3.4.1 Definition, Measurement, and Unawareness in HD

One of the most frequent behavioral complaints about HD from family members is that the affected individual "refuses to accept" or "denies" the disease and its consequences. Evidence suggests that the apparent "denial" represents a neurologically based unawareness or anosognosia *(57–59)* and is to be distinguished from the more familiar type of psychological denial, which may also be present in persons with HD. In one recent study *(57)*, an eight-item self-rating scale was administered to 19 individuals with HD and 15 consecutive patients referred for neuropsychological assessment with non-HD diagnoses. HD patients showed higher anosognosia than the comparison patients did. In addition, performances on the Wisconsin Card Sorting Test and the visual–spatial subtests of the Wechsler

Adult Intelligence Scale-revised (WAIS-R) were significantly associated with levels of anosognosia for the HD patients. These findings suggest that unawareness in HD is likely to reflect dysfunction in the frontoparietal lobes and their connections and not merely an unwillingness to face the diagnosis of HD.

3.4.2. Treatment

Pharmacotherapy is not known to play a role in the management of unawareness. Helping caregivers to understand that the problem may have a neurological basis can help to reduce conflict. Some patients will describe and allow treatment of specific symptoms, such as chorea, depression, and dysphagia, without ever acknowledging the diagnosis of HD. Some HD patients have what appears to be unawareness or denial of their diagnosis, combined with either withdrawn, reclusive behavior, or aggressive, irritable, or even violent behavior. Patients in these two subgroups may be very difficult to manage, the first because they do not seek medical care, and the second because they actively or aggressively resist treatment. In some cases, the physician can work with the family to maintain safety in the home and to ensure the availability of emergency services. Involvement of community social services and consideration of the legal and public safety implications of such a patient in the community is also important.

3.5. Obsessions, Compulsions, and Perseveration

3.5.1. Definition

Obsessions are recurrent and persistent thoughts, impulses, or images that are experienced as intrusive and cause anxiety or distress. Compulsions, which often occur in response to an obsession, are repetitive behaviors such as handwashing, or mental acts, such as counting, that a person feels obligated to perform. To meet Diagnostic and Statistical Manual of Mental Disorders, fourth edition (DSM-IV) criteria for OCD *(60)*, the obsessions and compulsions must cause distress, be time-consuming, and interfere with normal daily functioning. The person experiencing them must regard them as excessive and unreasonable at some point in the illness. Since HD patients may experience obsessions and compulsions without meeting full criteria for OCD, due, for example, to lack of insight as to why the obsessions and compulsions are problematic, we will use the term "O/Cs" to denote obsessive and compulsive symptoms themselves. Persons with HD may also manifest behaviors, which seem phenomenologically, to lie along an O/C spectrum, but are different from true obsessions and compulsions. This would include the inflexibility, or "stickiness" often observed by family members, and the tendency to perseverate on topics of concern with a single-minded intensity that can interfere with other essential tasks, which is extremely distressing to caregivers.

Baxter and others proposed the idea that different pathways in the corticostriatal system might modulate different subtypes of symptoms in primary OCD. This is the "striatal topography" model of OCD *(61)*, which could explain the heterogeneity seen in that condition. Rauch and others, using symptom provocation paradigms with OCD patients, have proposed that the paralimbic system (posterior medial orbitofrontal cortex, cingulate, anterior temporal parahippocampal, and insular cortices) mediates affective states in OCD *(62)*. A ventral cognitive circuit (projections from the anterior and lateral orbitofrontal cortex via the ventral caudate nucleus, which possibly modulates context-related operations and response inhibition) is thought to mediate obsessional symptoms *(63)*, based on work by Alexander and others delineating frontal-striatal circuitry *(64)*. Cummings *(65)* has also suggested that cognitive deficits in HD result from involvement of the head of the caudate, which receives lateral prefrontal striatal projections, while personality changes reflect involvement of the ventromedial caudate region, which receive projections from the orbitofrontal cortex. The striatal location of the primary pathology in HD makes O/Cs a not-unexpected feature of the disease.

3.5.2. Measurement

The most widely used scale for measurement of O/Cs is the Yale–Brown Obsessive Compulsive Scale (Y-BOCS) *(66,67)*. The Y-BOCS has been studied for validity and reliability. It has been used in one study of O/Cs in HD, which is described in Subheading 3.5.3. *(68)*. Other studies of O/Cs in HD have relied on either the physician's assessment during an interview or the questions on the behavioral section of the Unified Huntington's Disease Rating Scale *(69)*. There is no instrument in widespread use that specifically addresses inflexibility and perseveration in HD.

3.5.3. Obsessions and Compulsions in HD

A recent review of 960 patients who were followed at 43 HD centers found that 22.3% had O/Cs at their first visit to a Huntington's Center *(70)* when simply asked during general evaluation whether or not they had O/Cs. The lifetime prevalence for primary OCD is 2 to 3% *(71)*. Thus, O/Cs may have a higher than normal prevalence in HD. Supporting this thought, Anderson and others *(68)* found that up to 50% of a group of 27 HD patients reported O/Cs when administered the Y-BOCS, suggesting that these symptoms may be among the most common behavioral features of HD. In this study, presence of O/Cs did not correlate with motor symptoms, duration of disease, or impairment in function, but more executive dysfunction was evident in the O/Cs group on neuropsychological tests. It is important to recognize that not all HD patients with O/Cs meet criteria for OCD. However, unrecognized symptoms may still cause major disability in HD and impose additional burdens on caregivers. Improper characterization of O/Cs as psychosis or other behaviors may lead to inappropriate treatment. Investigations of O/Cs in HD patients could lead to a better understanding of the neural basis of these symptoms.

In addition to HD, several other neurological disorders involving the striatum are known to produce O/Cs with high frequency. Tourette's disorder (TD) patients have a high prevalence of O/Cs. In a study of 134 TD patients, 23% met full OCD criteria, and 46% met criteria for subthreshold OCD *(72)*. Up to one-third of patients with Fahr's disease meet criteria for OCD *(73)*. Sydenham's chorea is also associated with OCD-like behavior *(74)*, as is carbon monoxide poisoning, which can cause globus pallidus damage *(75)*. Acquired OCD is also seen in patients with nonspecific basal ganglia lesions *(76)*.

Several case reports describe the features of O/Cs in HD. Cummings and Cunningham *(77)* described two patients with HD who had OCD. Both were belligerent when prevented from acting on their compulsions. Onset of symptoms began in mid-life, in contrast to primary OCD, which generally begins in the early twenties. Scicutella *(78)* also reports on a patient with onset of OCD and mild choreiform movements at age 70, who was subsequently diagnosed with HD. Dewhurst and others *(42)* listed "obsessional features" among a list of prodromal personality changes seen in HD patients. A case reported by Tonkonogy and Barreira *(79)* involved a clinical history and neuroimaging compatible with HD in a patient who had washing compulsion. De Marchi and others *(80)* reported a family with HD and a 34% lifetime prevalence of OCD. In their discussion of why O/Cs are rarely reported in HD, they suggest that it may be an embarrassing symptom for patients, who do not volunteer information about it *(81)*. Cummings and Cunningham *(77)* suggest several reasons why O/Cs are seldom reported in HD. These include lack of specific questioning, assignment of the symptoms to other categories of behavior (e.g. perseveration, psychosis), or the possibility that only a small number of HD patients develop O/Cs.

Examples of the types of O/Cs seen in HD include sexual images, aggressive obsessions (usually directed at others), compulsive consumption of cigarettes or beverages, frequently caffeinated, and "just so" or symmetry obsessions (which often produced compulsions to rearrange things to suit the obsessive feelings). At times, the O/Cs may border on delusional beliefs, as may occur when a physical complaint is the focus of the obsession. There does not appear to be any stage of HD at which these symptoms are more likely to appear, but O/Cs, like other psychiatric manifestations of HD, may, in some cases, predate the emergence of an obvious movement disorder.

3.5.4. Treatment

To date, there has been no systematized study of treatment for O/Cs or OCD in HD. Cummings and Cunningham *(77)* in their case reports note that haloperidol, which was given to one HD patient with OCD for choreiform movements early on in the illness, had no effect on the O/Cs. Scicutella notes that, due to lack of insight into his symptoms, the patient with late onset OCD and HD she described refused medication *(78)*. In their case series of patients with basal ganglia lesions (infarcts, calcifications, ischemia), which were associated with OCD or O/Cs, Chacko et al. *(76)* generally found that standard treatment with SSRIs or clomipramine resulted in improvement of these symptoms. One patient in the series failed to achieve lasting remission with various medication therapies, but showed a good response to electroconvulsive therapy (ECT).

The mainstays of pharmacotherapy for idiopathic OCD are serotonergic agents, including SSRI's and clomipramine. It seems reasonable to begin with one of these drugs when treating O/C's in HD. At least anecdotally, they also seem to be helpful with perseveration and inflexibility. SSRIs are safer and better tolerated than clomipramine. Some clinicians believe clomipramine to be slightly more efficacious, but not so much so that it makes sense to bypass the far less toxic SSRI's. As in idiopathic OCD, higher doses of medication may be required than when these drugs are used in the treatment of depression, but given the vulnerability of these patients, the titration should be slow. Monoamine oxidase inhibitors are thought to have some efficacy in idiopathic OCD. The dietary restrictions, side effect profile, and potential for lethality in overdose make them something of a last resort in HD. Potentially augmenting agents for partial responders include, in no particular order of preference, buspirone, lithium, benzodiazepines, and pindolol. While probably not effective for true obsessions and compulsions, the dopaminergic agent amantadine, in doses of 100–300 mg/d has been useful in the treatment of perseveration, behavioral rigidity, and stimulus bound behavior in patients with HD.

Cognitive behavioral therapy, which has been very useful in primary OCD, is probably of limited use to HD patients with O/Cs, since they often lack insight into the symptoms and may be too cognitively impaired to participate. However, family interventions, including psychoeducation and the establishment of reward-based environments, may be very beneficial.

3.6. Summary

There does appear to be a readily recognizable, if not precisely delineated, syndrome of problematic experiences and behaviors in persons with HD, which is similar to behavioral syndromes found in other diseases involving the frontal-subcortical circuitry. Characteristic symptoms include apathy, irritability, unawareness, obsessions and compulsions, perseveration, and behavioral inflexibility. Pharmacotherapy is, at this time, largely based on clinical experience and analogy with other conditions. We have tried to lay out some of the likeliest agents, but when controlled data, or even a professional consensus is lacking, it makes sense to start with the medications that are the safest and easiest to use. Avenues for future research include exploring the correlations between the cognitive dysfunction of HD and the frontal syndrome of HD, comparison of behavior, pathology, and neuroimaging data between frontal symptom patients with HD and those with other conditions, and controlled clinical trials for treatment of some of the most problematic frontal symptoms.

4. CONCLUSIONS

HD is a complex disease, with motor, cognitive, emotional, and behavior manifestations, all of which influence each other, interact with the patient's environment, and change over the longitudinal course of the illness. Persons with HD often have problems that defy the conventional diagnostic criteria, despite our best efforts to describe appropriate syndromes. At the same time, HD patients can be particularly vulnerable to the motor, cognitive, and metabolic consequences of drug therapy. When journeying into such "uncharted waters," the clinician would be advised to observe the following guidelines: Conduct a very thorough history and exam, including obtaining information from outside informants and making longitudinal observations of the patient. Make specific diagnoses where possible, since a well-known syndrome, such as major depression, has coherent therapeutics already associated with it. Always at least consider nonpharmacologic interventions before initiating drug therapy. All things being equal, start with the pharmacologic agent that offers the greatest ease of use and least noxious side effects. Finally, the clinician should persevere, while maintaining a hopeful attitude. The most successful treatments for symptoms of HD are to be found at this time in the psychiatric realm. Treatment of aggression or a frontal lobe syndrome in someone suffering from HD is not easy, but when successful, can make the difference between chronic institutionalization and what remains of a happy productive life.

ACKNOWLEDGMENTS

This work is supported by the Huntington Society of Canada and the Huntington Disease Society of America.

REFERENCES

1. Rosenblatt, A. and Leroi, I. (2000) The neuropsychiatry of Huntington's disease and basal ganglia disorders. *Psychosomatics* **41,** 24–30.
2. Comings, D.E., Johnson, J.P., Gonzalez, N.S., et al. (2000) Association between the adrenergic alpha 2A receptor gene (ADRA2A) and measures of irritability, hostility, impulsivity and memory in normal subjects. *Psychiatr. Genet.* **10,** 39–42.
3. Brown, G.L., Goodwin, F.K., Ballenger, J.C., Goyer, P.F., and Major, L.F. (1979) Aggression in humans correlates with cerebrospinal fluid amine metabolites. *Psychiatry Res.* **1,** 131–139.
4. Kavoussi, R., Armstead, P., and Coccaro, E. (1997) The neurobiology of impulsive aggression. *Psychiatr. Clin. N. Am.* **20,** 395–403.
5. Oquendo, M.A. and Mann, J.J. (2000) The biology of impulsivity and suicidality. *Psychiatr. Clin. N. Am.* **23,** 11–25.
6. Mega, M.S. and Cummings, J.L. (1994) Frontal-subcortical circuits and neuropsychiatric disorders. *J. Neuropsychiatry Clin. Neurosci.* **6,** 358–370.
7. Yudosky, S.C., Silver, J.M., Jackson, W., et al. (1986) The Overt Aggression Scale for the objective rating of verbal and physical aggression. *Am. J. Psychiatry* **143,** 35–39.
8. Cummings, J., Mega, M., Gray, K., et al. (1994) The neuropsychiatric inventory: comprehensive assessment of psychopathology in dementia. *Neurology* **44,** 2308–2314.
9. Patel, V. and Hope, R.A. (1992) A rating scale for aggressive behaviour in the elderly—the RAGE. *Psychol. Med.* **22,** 211–221.
10. Burns, A., Folstein, S., Brandt, J., and Folstein, M. (1990) Clinical assessment of irritability, aggression, and apathy in Huntington and Alzheimer disease. *J. Nerv. Ment. Dis.* **178,** 20–26.
11. Ranen, N.G., Lipsey, J.R., Treisman, G., and Ross, C.A. (1996) Sertraline in the treatment of severe aggressiveness in Huntington's disease. *J. Neuropsychiatry Clin. Neurosci.* **8,** 338–340.
12. Sheard, M.H., Marini, J.L., Bridges, C.I., and Wagner, E. (1976) The effect of lithium on impulsive aggressive behavior in man. *Am. J. Psychiatry* **133,** 1409–1413.
13. Cowdry, R.W. and Gardner, D.L. (1988) Pharmacotherapy of borderline personality disorder. Alprazolam, carbamazepine, trifluoperazine, and tranylcypromine. *Arch. Gen. Psychiatry* **45,** 111–119.
14. Mattes, J.A. (1988) Carbamazepine vs. propranolol for rage outbursts. *Psychopharmacol. Bull.* **24,** 179–182.
15. Hakola, H.P. and Laulumaa, V.A. (1982) Carbamazepine in treatment of violent schizophrenics. *Lancet* **1,** 1358.
16. Folks, D.G., King, L.D., Dowdy, S.B., et al. (1982) Carbamazepine treatment of selected affectively disordered inpatients. *Am. J. Psychiatry* **139,** 115–117
17. Yatham, L.N. and McHale, P.A. (1988) Carbamazepine in the treatment of aggression: a case report and a review of the literature. *Acta Psychiatr. Scand.* **78,** 188–190.
18. Gleason, R.P. and Schneider, L.S. (1990) Carbamazepine treatment of agitation in Alzheimer's outpatients refractory to neuroleptics. *J. Clin. Psychiatry* **51,** 115–118.
19. Giakas, W.J., Seibyl, J.P., and Mazure, C.M. (1990) Valproate in the treatment of temper outbursts. *J. Clin. Psychiatry* **51,** 525.
20. Mattes, J.A. (1992) Valproic acid for nonaffective aggression in the mentally retarded. *J. Nerv. Ment. Dis.* **180,** 601–602.
21. Wender, P.H., Reimherr, F.W., and Wood, D.R. (1985) Stimulant therapy of 'adult hyperactivity'. *Arch. Gen. Psychiatry* **42,** 840.
22. Konicki, P.E. and Schulz, S.C. (1989) Rationale for clinical trials of opiate antagonists in treating patients with personality disorders and self-injurious behavior. *Psychopharmacol. Bull.* **25,** 556–563.
23. Vonsattel, J.P., Myers, R.H., Stevens, T.J., Ferrante, R.J., Bird, E.D., and Richardson, E.P. (1985) Neuropathological classification of Huntington's disease. *J. Neuropathol. Exp. Neurol.* **44,** 559–577.
24. McHugh, P.R. and Folstein, M.F. (1979) Psychopathology of dementia: implication for neuropathology, in *Congenital and Acquired Cognitive Disorders* (Katzman, R. ed.), Raven Press, New York, pp. 17–30.
25. Alexander, M.P. and Stuss, D.T. (2000) Disorders of frontal lobe functioning. *Semin. Neurol.* **20,** 427–437.
26. McHugh, P.R. and Folstein, M.F. (1975) Psychiatric syndromes of Huntington's chorea: a clinical and phenomenological study, in *Psychiatric Aspects of Neurologic Disease* (Benson, D.F. and Blumer, D., eds.), Grune & Stratton, New York.

27. Caine, E.D., Hunt, R.D., Weingartner, H., and Ebert, M.H. (1978) Huntington's dementia: Clinical and neuropsychological features. *Arch. Gen. Psychiatr.* **35,** 377–384.
28. Marin, R.S. (1996) Apathy: concept, syndrome, neural mechanisms, and treatment. *Semin. Clin. Neuropsychol.* **1,** 304–314.
29. Marin, R.S. (1990) Differential diagnosis and classification of apathy. *Am. J. Psychol.* **147,** 22–30
30. Rubin, A.J. Lecture given to Huntington Society of Canada, October 24, 1992.
31. Marin, R.S., Biedrzycki, R.C., and Firinciogullari, S. (1991) Reliability and validity of the Apathy Evaluation Scale. *Psychol. Res.* **38,** 143–162.
32. Marin, R.S., Fogel, B.S., Hawkins, J., Duffy, J., and Krupp, B. (1995) Apathy: a treatable syndrome. *J. Neuropsychiatry Clin. Neurosci.* **7,** 23–30.
33. Rabkin, J.G., Ferrando, S.J., van Gorp, W., Rieppi, R., McElhiney, M., and Sewell, M. (2001) Relationships among apathy, depression, and cognitive impairment in HIV/AIDS. *J. Neuropsychiatry Clin. Neurosci.* **12,** 451–457.
34. Aarsland, D., Litvan, I., and Larsen, O.P. (2001) Neuropsychiatric symptoms of patients with PST and Parkinson's disease. *J. Neuropsychiatry Clin. Neurosci.* **13,** 42–49.
35. Starkstein, S.E., Petracca, G., Chemerinski, E., and Kremer, J. (2001) Syndromic validity of apathy in Alzheimer's disease. *Am. J. Psychiatry* **158,** 872–877.
36. Levy, M.L., Cummings, J.L., Fairbanks, L.A., et al. (1988) Apathy is not depression. *J. Neuropsychiatry Clin. Neurosci.* **10,** 314–319.
37. Di Costanzo, A., Mottola, A., Toriello, A., Di Iorio, G., Tedeschi, G., and Bonavita, V. (2000) Does abnormal neuronal excitability exist in myotonic dystrophy? II. Effects of the antiarrhythmic drug hydroquinidine on apathy and hypersomnia. *Neurol. Sci.* **21,** 81–86.
38. McAllister, T.W. (2000) Apathy. *Semin. Clin. Neuropsychiatry* **5,** 275–282.
39. Shoulson, I. (1990) Huntington's disease: cognitive and psychiatric features. *Neuropsychiatry Neuropsychol. Behav. Neurol.* **3,** 15–22.
40. Galbraith, S. (1985) Irritability. *BMJ* **291,** 1668–1669.
41. Snaith, R.P. and Taylor, C.M. (1985) Irritability: definition, assessment and associated factors. *Br. J. Psychiatry* **147,** 127–136.
42. Dewhurst, K., Oliver, J., Trick, K., et al. (1969) Neuro-psychiatric aspects of Huntington's disease. *Confin. Neurol.* **31,** 258–268.
43. Mayberg, H.S, Starkstein, S.E., Peyser, C.E., Brandt, J., Dannals, R.F., and Folstein, S.E. (1992) Paralimbic frontal lobe hypometabolism in depression associated with Huntington's disease. *Neurology* **2,** 91–1797.
44. Findling, R.L. (1993) Treatment of aggression in juvenile-onset Huntington's disease with buspirone. *Psychosomatics* **34,** 460–461.
45. Byrne, A.P., Martin, W., and Hnatko, G. (1994) Beneficial effects of buspirone therapy in Huntington's disease. *Am. J. Psychiatry* **151,** 1097.
46. Purdon, S.E., Mohr, E., Ilivitsky, V., and Jones, B.D.W. (1994) Huntington's disease: pathogenesis, diagnosis and treatment. *Psychiatr. Neurosci.* **19,** 359–367.
47. Fava, M. (1997) Psychopharmacologic treatment of pathological aggression. *Psychiatr. Clin. N. Am.* **20,** 427–451.
48. Kant, R., Smith-Seemiller, S.L., and Zeiler, D. (1998) Treatment of aggression and irritability after head injury. *Brain Inj.* **12,** 661–666.
49. Lebert, F., Pasquier, F., and Petit, H. (1994) Behavioral effects of trazodone in Alzheimer's disease. *J. Clin. Psychiatry* **55,** 536–538.
50. Michals, M.L., Crismon, M.L., Roberts, S., and Childs, A. (1993) Clozapine response and adverse effects in nine brain-injured patients. *J. Clin. Psychopharmacol.* **13,** 198–203.
51. Lerner, D.M., Schuetz, L., Holland, S., Rubinow, D.R., and Rosenstein, D.L. (2000) Low-dose risperidone for the irritable medically ill patient. *Psychosomatics* **41,** 69–71.
52. Schneider, L.S. and Sobin, P.B. (1992) Non-neuroleptic treatment of behavioral symptoms and agitation in Alzheimer's disease and other dementias. *Psychopharmacol. Bull.* **28,** 71–79.
53. Greendyke, R.M. and Kanter, D.R. (1986) Therapeutic effects of pindolol on behavioral disturbances associated with organic brain disease: a double-blind study. *J. Clin. Psychiatry* **47,** 423–426.
54. Stewart, J.T., Mounts, M.L., and Clark, J.L. Jr. (1987) Aggressive behavior in Huntington's disease: treatment with propranolol. *J. Clin. Psychiatry* **48,** 106–108.
55. Kavoussi, R.J. and Coccaro, E.F. (1998) Divalproex sodium for impulsive aggressive behavior in patients with personality disorder. *J. Clin. Psychiatry* **59,** 676–680.
56. Grove, V.E., Quintanilla, J., and DeVaney, G.T. (2000) Improvement of Huntington's disease with olanzapine and valproate. *N. Engl. J. Med.* **343,** 973–974.
57. Deckel, A.W. and Morrison, D. (1996) Evidence of a neurologically based "denial of illness" in patients with Huntington's disease. *Arch. Clin. Neuropsychol.* **11,** 295–302.
58. Frankenburg, F.R. (1989) A variation of Capgras syndrome with anosognosia in Huntington's disease: a case report. *Hillside J. Clin. Psychiatry* **11,** 121–126.
59. Snowden, J.S., Craufurd, D., Griffiths, H.L., and Neary, D. (1998) Awareness of involuntary movements in Huntington's disease. *Arch. Neurol.* **55,** 801–805.
60. American Psychiatric Association (1994) *Diagnostic and Statistical Manual of Mental Disorders, Fourth Edition,* American Psychiatric Press, Washington, DC.

61. Baxter, L.R., Schwartz, J.M., Guze, B.H., et al. (1990) Neuro-imaging in obsessive-compulsive disorder: seeking the mediating neuroanatomy, in *Obsessive Compulsive Disorder: Theory and Management,* ed. 2 (Jenike, M.A., Baer, L., and Minichiello, W.E, eds.), Mosby, Chicago, pp. 167–188.
62. Rauch, S.L., Jenike, M.A., Alpert, N.M., et al. (1994) Regional cerebral blood flow measured during symptoms provocation in obsessive-compulsive disorder using 0-15 labeled CO2 and positron emission tomography. *Arch. Gen. Psychiatry* **51,** 62–70.
63. Rauch, S.L., Whalen, P.J., Dougherty, D., et al (1998) Neurobiologic models of obsessive-compulsive disorder, in *Obsessive Compulsive Disorders: Practical Management,* 3rd ed (Jenike, M.A., Baer, L., and Minichiello, W.E., eds.), Mosby, Chicago, pp. 222–253.
64. Alexander, G.E., Crutcher, M.D., and DeLong, M.R. (1990) Basal ganglia-thalamocortical circuits: parallel substrates for motor, oculomotor, "prefrontal" and "limbic" functions. *Prog. Brain Res.* **85,** 119–146.
65. Cummings, J.L. (1993) Frontal subcortical circuits and human behavior. *Arch. Neurol.* **50,** 873–880.
66. Goodman, W.K., Price, L.H., Rasmussen, S.A., et al. (1989a) The Yale-Brown Obsessive Compulsive Scale: I. Development, use, and reliability. *Arch. Gen. Psychiatry* **46,** 1006–1011.
67. Goodman W.K., Price L.H., Rasmussen S.A., et al. (1989b) The Yale-Brown Obsessive Compulsive Scale. II. Validity. *Arch. Gen. Psychiatry* **46,** 1012–1016.
68. Anderson, K., Louis, E., Stern, Y., and Marder, K., (2001) Cognitive correlates of obsessive and compulsive symptoms in Huntington's disease. *Am. J. Psychiatry* **158,** 799–801.
69. Huntington Study Group (1996) Unified Huntington's disease rating scale: reliability and consistency. *Mov. Disord.* **11,** 136–142.
70. Marder, K., Zhao, H., Myers, R.H., et al (2000) Rate of functional decline in Huntington's disease. *Neurology* **54,** 452–458.
71. Karno, M., Goldin, J.M., Sorenson, S.B., and Burnom, A. (1988) The epidemiology of obsessive compulsive disorder in five U.S. communities. *Arch. Gen. Psychiatry* **45,** 1094–1099.
72. Leckman, J.F., Walker, D.E., Goodman, W.K., et al. (1994) Just right perceptions associated with compulsive behavior in Tourette's syndrome. *Am. J. Psychiatry* **151,** 675–680.
73. López-Villegas, D., Kulisevsky, J., Deus, J., et al. (1996) Neuropsychological alterations in patients with computed tomography detected basal ganglia calcification. *Arch. Neurol.* **53,** 251–256.
74. Swedo, S.E., Rapoport, J.L., Cheslow, D.L., et al. (1989) High prevalence of obsessive-compulsive symptoms in patients with Sydenham's chorea. *Am. J. Psychiatry* **146,** 246–249.
75. Laplane, D., Levasseur, M., Pillon, B., et al. (1989) Obsessive-compulsive and other behavioral changes with bilateral basal ganglia lesions. *Brain* **112,** 699–725.
76. Chacko, R.C., Corbin, M.A., and Harper, R.G. (2000) Acquired obsessive-compulsive disorder associated with basal ganglia lesions. *J. Neuropsychiatry Clin. Neurosci.* **12,** 269–272.
77. Cummings, J.L. and Cunningham, K. (1992) Obsessive-compulsive disorder in Huntington's Disease. *Biol. Psychiatry* **31,** 263–270.
78. Scicutella, A. (2000) Late life obsessive compulsive disorder and Huntington's disease. *J. Neuropsychiatry Clin. Neurosci.* **12,** 288–289.
79. Tonkonogy, J. and Barreira, P. (1989) Obsessive-compulsive disorder and caudate frontal lesion. *Neuropsychiatry Neuropsychol. Behav. Neurol.* **2,** 203–209.
80. De Marchi, N., Morris, M., Mennella, R., La Pia, S., and Nestadt, G. (1998) Association of obsessive-compulsive disorder and pathological gambling with Huntington's disease in an Italian pedigree: possible association with Huntington's disease mutation. *Acta Psychiatr. Scand.* **97,** 62–65.
81. De Marchi, N. and Mennella, R. (2000) Huntington's disease and its association with psychopathology. *Harv. Rev. Psychiatry* **7,** 278–289.

33
Heterogeneous Psychopathology of Tourette Syndrome

Mary M. Robertson, MBChB, MD, DPM, MRCPCH, FRCPsych

1. INTRODUCTION

Tourette syndrome (TS) is a complex inherited childhood-onset movement disorder. TS is, however, also a heterogeneous disorder. Several types of psychopathology are associated with TS. The psychopathologies are too, for the most part, heterogeneous. Controversy has always reigned as far as the links between the various psychopathologies associated with TS. Suggestions as to the etiologies of the various associated psychopathologies are given. Thereafter, a brief overview of the psychopathologies is given. Finally, the rationale is given for the decision, and three psychopathologies are described in detail, namely obsessive–compulsive disorder (OCD), depression, and autistic spectrum disorder (ASD). It is suggested that the psychopathology of TS may well be described and divided as follows: (*i*) obsessive–compulsive behaviors (OCB) (integral and genetically related); (*ii*) attention deficit hyperactivity disorder (ADHD) (common, and genetically related in some cases only); (*iii*) depression (common and multifactorial in etiology); (*iv*) anxiety (secondary to having TS); (*v*) other psychopathologies that may be related to co-morbidity rather than to TS *per se* (e.g., personality disorder); (*vi*) psychopathology as a result of referral bias; (*vii*) psychopathology secondary to medication; and (*viii*) other disorders, which require further investigation (e.g., ASDs, rage, and bipolar affective disorder [BAD]). These disorders and their relationships to TS are highlighted, as are suggestions for future research.

2. TS

TS is a common *(1,2)*, complex, childhood-onset movement disorder consisting of both multiple motor tics and one or more vocal tics, which must have been present for more than 1-yr duration *(3,4)*. The etiology has included both a genetic susceptibility and environmental factors. TS itself is a heterogeneous disorder with at least three types being described. They include "pure TS" (with only motor and vocal tics), "full blown TS" (with coprophenomena, echophenomena, and paliphenomena), and "TS plus" (with all the co-morbid disorders and psychopathologies) *(5)*.

The psychopathology of TS has always been controversial. Originally, psychological factors were seen as etiological in TS and, in fact, psychoanalytical speculation dominated the early literature. Thus, in 1921 Ferenci *(6)*, for example, expressed the opinion that "many tics may turn out to be stereotyped equivalents of onanism." The ideas were perpetuated by Mahler and colleagues in the 1940s

From: *Mental and Behavioral Dysfunction in Movement Disorders*
Edited by: M-A. Bédard et al. © Humana Press Inc., Totowa, NJ

Table 1
Suggested Relationships Between Psychopathology and TS

1. Generally accepted as an integral part of TS and genetically linked to TS
   - OCB/OCD
2. Common in TS and genetically linked in some cases
   - ADHD
3. Multifactorial depression
4. Secondary to having TS (e.g., anxiety)
5. Adult psychopathology as a result of the childhood co-morbid psychopathology (ADHD, ODD, CD) rather than the TS *per se*
   - Personality disorder
6. As a result of referral bias
   - CD
   - ODD
   - Personality disorder
7. Impulsivity plus rage, but not fulfilling criteria for ADHD
   - More research needed
8. Secondary to medication
   - Dysphoria
   - Anxiety (e.g., separation anxiety)
   - Cognitive impairment
9. Unknown as yet
   - Autism
   - AS
   - BAD
10. Rare and probably the association is by chance
   - Schizophrenia

who, although acknowledging that the symptoms of TS were probably mediated via striopallidal connections, also suggested that they occurred in highly narcisstic individuals with disturbed psychosexual development and parent–child relationships (for review see ref. *7*). This type of view continued, with Fenichel *(8)* suggesting that tics were involuntary motor equivalents of emotional activity, and Heuscher *(9)* seeing tics as a defense against becoming psychotic. OCBs were recognized as being an integral part of TS from the earliest writings of Gilles de la Tourette, Guinon, and Grasset *(10)*, and were to play a major role in the evolution of the psychopathological history of TS. The organic basis of TS was then recognized, with genetics *(11)* and possibly some infections *(12–14)* being invoked in the etiopathogenesis.

The domain of psychopathology associated with TS, however, has remained controversial. Shapiro and colleagues *(15,16)* always asserted that there was no specific psychopathology associated with TS. At the other end of the spectrum, Comings *(17–21)*, not only suggested that TS was associated with a wide variety of psychopathologies, but that these conditions were specifically and genetically related to TS, forming part of the "TS spectrum." The pendulum swung from this notion, with the Yale group *(22–24)* consistently demonstrating that that there was no genetic relationship between TS and, for example, ADHD, anxiety, depression, phobias, and panic disorder. OCB then reentered the TS stage, and, at last, there was some consensus of opinion; not only was OCB seen as integral to TS, but also that some types of OCB and TS were genetically related *(25–27)*.

The relationships between the various psychopathologies and TS are varied and intricate, but it is suggested that they include the disorders shown in Table 1. Of importance to highlight, however, is that not only is TS heterogeneous, but also almost all the psychopathologies associated with TS are themselves heterogeneous. In addition, it is important to state at the outset that the prognosis of TS is influenced by a variety of factors including psychopathology. The quality of life (QoL) of patients with TS has recently been studied and is also associated with some of the psychopathologies.

A recent study embraced 3500 TS individuals in clinics from 22 countries, and at all ages, about 12% of TS had no associated co-morbidity. In other words, the vast majority did have other psychopathological problems. The most commonly reported co-morbidity was ADHD (60%), with OCB being next common (32%), and OCD coming next (27%) *(28)*.

In this chapter, an introductory overview of the psychopathologies associated with TS is documented. Thereafter, three conditions or psychopathologies are examined in detail, namely, OCD, depression, and ASD. This is justified as: (*i*) one is undeniably and undisputedly related to TS and may even be a phenotype of the putative TS gene(s), i.e., OCD; and (ii) depression, although common, and which the author recognizes as important, is suggested to be multifactorial in etiology and not genetically related to TS; and finally (*iii*) the investigation of ASD in the setting of TS is, as yet, in its relative infancy despite a couple of rigorous studies.

The types of psychopathologies described in individuals with TS, which are briefly discussed, include ADHD, conduct disorder (CD) and oppositional disorder, anxiety disorders, and personality disorder. A few other types of psychopathology are also found in people with TS, but are somewhat rare or as yet not studied, such as psychosis or schizophrenia, and as thus, are not mentioned in any depth. They have been briefly discussed in Robertson *(7)*. Of importance is that in a recently published study embracing 3500 clinic patients from 22 countries, the vast majority (around 88%) had co-morbid psychopathology and associated behaviors *(28)*.

The relationships between TS and the psychopathologies associated with the disorder are summarized in Table 1. This chapter forms the basis of the rationale by which the author came to making the suggestions in the Table 1.

3. OCD

3.1. Definition and Clinical Features

OCD is characterized by persistent obsessions (recurrent intrusive senseless thoughts, which are ego-dystonic, unwelcome, and persistent) or compulsions (repetitive and purposeful behaviors, which are performed according to certain rules or in a stereotyped fashion); they are a significant source of distress to the individual, or they result in dysfunction *(3,29,30)*.

It is important at the outset to state that OCD itself is an heterogeneous disorder. However, exactly what constitutes the main subtype(s) has been somewhat controversial. For instance, early on, Hodgson and Rachmann *(31)* employed the Maudsley Obsessive Compulsive Inventory (MOCI) and described four OC factors: checking, cleaning, slowness, and doubting. Others, such as Khanna et al. *(32)*, later described a cluster analysis on more than 400 OCD patients and reported five subgroups: checking, washing, the past, death, and sex. Even later, it was suggested that there are essentially three main types of OCD: (*i*) familial type related to tic disorders; (*ii*) familial type unrelated to tic disorders; and (*iii*) nonfamilial type *(33)*. More recently, Summerfeldt et al. *(34)* investigated several models of symptoms in OCD by employing factor analysis. They documented that the models did not adequately fit the data when symptoms were examined individually and suggested that the dimensional structure should be examined at the most basic level, which is at the individual symptom level. Thus, even if there is some consensus as to what constitutes OCD, there are difficulties in subtyping the disorder. Thus, the relationship between the TS and OCD (although one of the most understood relationships) remains under investigation.

OCD, like TS, has a childhood-onset, with early descriptions mentioning young children of only 5 and 11 yr of age with OCD *(35–38)*.

3.2. Prevalence

Prevalence studies suggest that OCD is actually quite common. Early reports suggested a prevalence rate in the adult general population of 0.05%, but newer research suggests lifetime prevalence rates of between 1.9–3.2% *(39)* and from between 0.25% *(40)* to 1–4% of children and adolescents *(41)*; of interest is that these figures are about twice as much as for schizophrenia or panic disorder *(38)*. Of note is that from one-third to one-half of adult cases have their onset by the age of 15 *(38)*. In the first epidemiologic study of OCD in adolescents, Flament et al. *(38)* reported that the prevalence estimates range from 0.35% for current prevalence and 0.40% for lifetime prevalence. Of importance is that 15 out of 20 (75%) of the OCD group had one or more other lifetime diagnosis, whereas 10 out of 20 (50%) had at least one other current diagnosis. Associated disorders most frequently encountered included major depression (n = 5), overanxious disorder (n = 4), bulimia (n = 3), and dysthymia (n = 1). In this group, it is interesting that no case had TS or tics *(38)*. For a recent comprehensive review of OCD in children and adolescents, the reader is referred to Shafran *(41)*.

3.3. OCD and TS: the Evidence

It is becoming increasingly evident and persuasive that there is a clear and strong association between TS and OCD, both in TS patients and in their family members, with evidence for the association being obtained from historical writings, phenomenological, family–genetic, epidemiological, neurochemical, and neuroanatomical investigations *(5,42,43)*.

At the outset, it is important to note that the obsessive–compulsive symptoms (OCS) and OCBs encountered in TS may well be describing the same phenomenon, but, importantly, they are clinically and statistically significantly different from the symptoms encountered in primary OCD. Having said that, however, it may be simplistic to divide the groups into simply TS and OCD, as recent research suggests that there may well be more subgroups of each disorder.

Historical evidence for the association between TS and OCD goes back to the earliest patient described with TS. Thus, one of the first to acknowledge that obsessions and compulsions were an integral part of TS was Georges Gilles de la Tourette himself *(44,45)*, when he redescribed the case of the French noblewoman, the Marquise de Dampierre, described originally by Itard *(46)*, and who was the first person documented with TS in the medical literature. Other early historical writings describing OCS/OCB in people with TS, include those of Guinon *(47)*, Grasset *(48)*, Meige and Feindel *(49)*, Kinnear-Wilson *(50)*, Ascher *(51)*, and Bockner *(52)*. One of the famous, if not the most famous person in the literature with TS, is Samuel Johnson the prominent 18th-century literary figure *(53,54)* who, apart from his motor and vocal tics, had severe OCS/OCB/OCD.

Phenomenological evidence for the association between TS and OCD is strong and can now be viewed from several perspectives. Twelve studies conducted between 1969 and 1985, reported TS patients with OCS/OCB, traits or illnesses, varying from single-case reports to significant percentages of of TS populations, ranging from 11% to as high as 80% (for review see ref. *7*). In a similar but later review of 12 studies between 1978 and 1995 (excluding both the studies already mentioned, as well as excluding those of Shapiro), the range of OC symptoms found in TS cohorts ranged from 13–69% *(55)*. Substantial studies in the late 1980s not already mentioned also indicated that OCS/OCB were common in TS occurring in 47% *(56)* and 49% *(57)* of TS patients. As already stated, OCB and OCD occurred in 32 and 27%, respectively, of the 3500 clinic TS cases described by Freeman et al. *(28)*. Clearly, all these figures are way in excess of the 1.9%-3.2% for OCD in the general population *(39)*. Even though the OCS/OCB symptoms in TS are different from those in OCD (see Subheading 3.4.), the high rates in individuals with TS are remarkable.

3.4. OCD and TS: Relationships and Phenomenology

At least three studies have suggested that OCS/OCB in TS change with age or duration of TS. Montgomery et al. *(58)* and Nee et al. *(59)* both suggested that OCS/OCB increased with frequency with the duration of TS. Frankel et al. *(60)* suggested that younger TS patients exhibited OCS/OCB related to impulse control, while older patients were more concerned with checking and arranging *(5)*.

Robertson et al. *(61)* reported that coprolalia and echophenomena were significantly related to OCS/OCB. Robertson et al. *(62)* reported that the self-injurious behaviors (SIB) encountered in people with TS were significantly related to obsessionality. The only study to control for depression showed that TS patients are disproportionately obsessional, which is not accounted for by depression *(63)*.

At least four controlled studies have now also indicated that OCB/OCS in patients with TS is higher than in normal control individuals, or than assessment schedule scores documented for the general population *(20,63,64)*.

Despite the phenomenological similarities being important between the OCS/OCB encountered in TS and OCD, at least 10 investigations have now demonstrated significant phenomenologic differences between pure or primary OCD and the OCS/OCB encountered in TS *(65–74)*. In essence, the obsessions encountered in TS have to do with sexual, violent, religious, aggressive, and symmetrical themes; the compulsions are to do with checking, ordering, counting, repeating, forced touching, symmetry ("evening up"), getting things "just right," and self-damage or SIB. In contrast, the obsessions seen in pure or primary OCD are to do predominantly with contamination, dirt, germs, being neat and clean, fear of something going wrong or bad happening, and the fear of becoming ill; compulsions in pure OCD are consequently mainly to do with cleaning and washing. In OCD, the compulsions, in addition, are preceded by cognitions, autonomic anxiety, and and have fewer prior sensory phenomena.

Importantly, at a clinical level, the OCS/OCB in TS appear to be ego-syntonic, rather than the ego-dystonic symptoms, which characterize the stand-alone OCD. However, this summary may well be an oversimplification.

Swerdlow et al. *(75)* compared adults with OCD ($n = 103$) and TS ($n = 50$), plus TS children ($n = 11$), using structured interviews such as the Yale–Brown Obsessive Compulsive Scale (YBOCS), Children's YBOCS (C-YBOCS), and both the adult and children's Yale Global Tic Severity Scale (YGTSS). Children were also interviewed using the Diagnostic Interview Schedule for Children-Revised. The patients were categorized into five groups, namely OCD alone, OCD?Tic, OCD+Tic, TS+OCD, and TS alone. Both quantitative and qualitative differences, as well as differences of functional impact, were found between the groups. Thus, substantially higher YBOCS scores were associated with OCD alone or OCD+Tic group compared with the TS+OCD group. Of note is that the TS+OCD subjects had lower YBOCS scores compared with all other OCD groups and higher YGTSS scores (which correlated significantly with YBOCS scores). Thus, of importance, was the fact that for TS subjects, the presence of even mild OCD was associated with functional impairment. In addition, YGTSS impairment scores were substantially higher in TS+OCD when compared to TS alone subjects. Other differences were observed and one of the most obvious was in the content of severe aggressive and violent obsessions, which were most common in the OCD+Tic subjects (compared with only 4% in the TS alone group). The authors suggested that overall, their data may present a challenge to the notion of a continuous spectrum of OCD and TS *(75)*.

Other investigations have also highlighted the special phenomenology of the OCS/OCB seen in TS. Leckman et al. *(76)* have described the "just right" phenomenon in TS. For example, an individual would have to arrange, rearrange, and even rearrange things further, in a particular order and in certain positions or patterns, until they looked "just right" to the individual; the subtle differences in this rearranging would probably not be discernable to most other people watching. In the clinic, the author has encountered this phenomenon many times, but in most cases, it is not distressing to the patient, and the patients have said that no previous clinicians had noticed the behaviors. In another study in TS subjects with OCS/OCB, the most common obsessions concerned the fear that one might harm oneself or others, intrusive nonsense sounds, words or music, and thoughts that something terrible such as fire, death, or illness might happen; common compulsions included checking, excessive washing and toothbrushing, rituals of cleaning household or inanimate objects, counting and hoarding or collecting rituals *(77)*, (for review see ref. *5*).

In one study *(67)*, the TS group reported that their compulsions arose *de novo* or spontaneously, while the pure OCD group reported that their compulsions were frequently preceded by stimuli, such as guilt or worry. In another study *(71)*, those probands who shared a similar symptom profile to TS subjects, all had a positive family history of OCD; all other OCD probands were isolated cases *(5)*.

Guarda et al. *(78)* described five patients (four females and one male; ages 18–35 yr) with eating disorders (three with anorexia nervosa and two with bulimia nervosa) who also had OCS/OCB and TS. Following the identification of four similar cases in the literature obtained by MEDLINE and PSYCHLIT, the authors suggest this putatively marks a subset of eating disorders with a link to TS and OC sympatomatology. The authors stated that OCS/OCB were common in both TS and eating disorders.

Evidence from family and genetic studies has increased substantially ever since the early descriptions. There is general agreement now that at least some forms of OCS/OCB are genetically related to TS and may well be a phenotype of the putative TS gene(s). An argument for a clear association between TS and OCB/OCD came from family studies which demonstrated that relatives of TS individuals had OCB/OCD *(20,25,26,79–81)*. In contrast, one study found no increase of OCB/OCD in family members of TS probands *(77)*. It is also worth noting in this context, that in the TS twin study of Jenkins and Ashby *(82)*, both twins were described as "obsessional." Later complex and statistical studies confirmed that TS and OCS/OCB/OCD were indeed genetically related *(27,83)*.

Finally, it was suggested some time ago *(42)*, that there may be some neurochemical and neuroanatomical features that could be argued to be similar in TS and OCD, in that frontal and basal ganglia abnormalities had been described in both disorders. Thus, despite the differences in neurochemical pathways, with dopamine being primarily involved in TS and serotonin being involved in OCD, it was suggested that there may be common neurophysiological disturbances. The striatum and limbic system receive extensive projections, and disturbances in these parts of the brain could be responsible for dopamine-mediated tics and vocalizations and serotonin-mediated obsessions and compulsions in these patients *(42)*. Later, however, Swerdlow et al. *(75)* noted that neuroimaging studies, although not unanimous in their conclusions, suggested opposite patterns of brain metabolism within corticostriatal-pallidothalamic (CSPT) circuitry in OCD vs TS, with hyperfunction and hypermetabolism in OCD, vs hypometabolism and hypofunction in TS *(75)*.

In the recent epidemiological study of Kadesjo and Gillberg *(1)*, there were two parts. In the first (investigating true prevalence, which was 1.1% of children), no mention was made of either OCB/OCD. However, in their second study, during which all children who were registered with TS in the catchment area ($n = 58$), co-morbidity was examined. Of these, 22 (38%) were diagnosed as having OCD *(1)*.

A recent study *(84)*, the first to investigate QoL in patients with TS, used the Medical Outcomes Short Form (SF-36) and the Quality of Life Assessment Schedule (QoLAS) and other measures, such as the Leyton Obsessional Inventory, to investigate 90 patients with TS. The authors reported that patients with TS showed significantly worse QoL than a general population sample. They had better QoL than patients with intractable epilepsy as measured by the QoLAS, although the SF-36 showed significant differences on the subscales Role Limitation due to physical problems and Social Functioning only. Factors influencing QoL domains included employment status, tic severity, and OCB. Nineteen patients (21%) had high scores on the Leyton Obsessional Inventory. Patients with OCB had lower scores on the Vitality subscale of the SF-36 only ($p = 0.04$). No significant difference in TS severity was found.

Some years ago, Cummings and Frankel *(85)* commented on at least five similarities between TS and OCD including: (*i*) age at onset; (*ii*) lifelong course (although this has been latterly challenged [86]); (*iii*) waxing and waning of symptoms; (*iv*) involuntary, intrusive, ego-alien behaviors and experiences; and (*v*) worsening with depression and anxiety. Others have, however, highlighted differences between the two disorders including that: (*i*) OCD is more common than TS; (*ii*) TS is three to four times more common in males, whereas in pure OCD sex patterns are balanced; (*iii*) TS is typically diagnosed at about the age of 7 yr, compared with the age of 20 in OCD; and (*iv*) the neuroimaging differences *(75)*.

It would be worth mentioning that coprolalia (inappropriate and involuntary use of obscenities) occurs in about 10–30% of TS cases, but in few children or mild cases *(3,5)*. It is, however, almost considered pathognomonic when it does occur. In this context, it is interesting to note that Pitman and Jenike *(87)* documented coprolalia in a patient with OCD. This provides further evidence that TS and OCD are related.

An interesting paper illustrates another aspect of TS and OCD research. The relationship between OCD and performance on a test sensitive to frontal lobe function (The Wisconsin Card Sorting Test [WCST]) was investigated in 100 patients with TS between the ages of 6 and 18 yr. Performance on the WCST was correlated with ratings of OC characteristics, but not with other TS symptoms. The relationship was maintained even when the full scale intelligence quotient (IQ) and the total number of TS symptoms were controlled. The author also asserted that the effect could not be attributed to medication. The author speculated that different symptoms associated with TS may have different neuroanatomic substrates *(88)*.

In an elegant documentation, 54 children, who had been included in a study of OCD (in which TS was an exclusionary criterion), were evaluated 2–7 yr later with a structured interview to assess the presence of tics or TS. The children's first degree relatives (FDRs) (n = 171) were also investigated. At baseline, 57% (n = 31), and at follow-up, 59% (n = 32), had lifetime histories of tics; eight (all males) met diagnostic criteria for TS. One of the most relevant and most interesting facts was that patients with TS differed from other male patients only in having an earlier age at onset of OCD. Of the FDRs, 1.8% (n = 3) had TS, whereas 14% (n = 24) had a tic disorder *(89)*.

From the evidence to date, it would appear that OCS/OCBs are an integral part of TS, and in this context, it is interesting to note that in 1903 Pierre Janet *(37)*, in his treatise Les Obsessions et la Psychasthenie, described three clinical stages of psychasthenic illness: the first was the "psychasthenic state," the second "forced agitations," which included motor tics, whereas the third was obsessions and compulsions *(7,90)*.

It is important to briefly mention the treatment of the two disorders. Very simply, the treatment of the motor and vocal tics of TS for some time has been the dopamine antagonists (e.g., haloperidol, pimozide, sulpiride, and tiapride). The pharmacological treatment of OCD, on the other hand, has been with large doses of antidepressants, which primarily affect serotonin (i.e., above doses given for depression). These include the "older" tricyclic antidepressant, chlomipramine and the "newer" selective serotonin reuptake inhibitors (SSRIs), such as citalopram, fluoxetine, fluvoxamine, paroxetine, and sertraline. In patients with both disorders (i.e., TS and OCD), the concomitant use of both higher doses of antidepressants, as well as neuroleptics, has been stressed. For a full exposition of the treatment of all aspects of OCD and TS, the reader is referred to a thorough earlier review *(5)*.

3.5. Conclusion

In summary and conclusion, and in the author's opinion, it does appear that there are specific OCS/OCB in the majority of TS patients, but that they are significantly different to the obsessions and compulsions seen in pure and/or primary OCD. In addition, the OCS/OCB in TS seem clinically less egodystonic than those encountered in pure or primary OCD. Finally, there seems to be a genetic relationship between some types of OCS/OCB/OCD and TS. In addition, there are differences in management strategies in the two disorders. It may transpire with more time however, that the groups of disorders involved are not as simply divided into TS and OCD; there may well be further subgroups. The precise genetic mechanisms may well shed light on these discussions, as may more sophisticated neuroimaging studies using not only different ligands, but also more definite and different clinical subgroups of each separate disorder.

4. DEPRESSION

4.1. Prevalence of Depression

Depression is a common disorder with a lifetime risk of 7.5–10%, with rates even higher in women *(91)*. It is also common in children, with prevalence estimates varying between 1.8 and 8.9% *(92)*. It may be a mild disorder, but if severe, the lifetime suicide risk is about 15% *(93)*.

4.2. Clinical Spectrum of Depression

It is vital to acknowledge that depression is a spectrum disorder, with a variety of types of depression being described, including "endogenous" major depressive disorder (MDD), dysthymia, residual depression, masked depression, subthreshold depression, double depression, unipolar and/or bipolar depression, and neurotic and/or psychotic depression *(94–97)*. Winokur, moreover, suggests that MDD is not a disease, but a syndrome, which is clinically homogeneous, but etiologically heterogeneous *(97)*.

4.3. Etiology of Depression

The etiology of depression is often multifactorial, with a variety of contributory factors including genetic predisposition *(98)*, as well as psychosocial variables including serious adverse or negative life events *(99,100)*, adverse childhood circumstances (e.g., parental loss, stress, or abuse in childhood), and adverse current social circumstances *(93,101)*.

4.4. Depression and TS

Studies of depression in the setting of TS, to the best of the author's knowledge, have only been documented from the North American continent and Europe, especially from the United Kingdom. Although depression has been frequently studied in TS, the relationship between the two disorders remains unclear. The importance of depression in TS individuals has not been sufficiently highlighted, even though it has important treatment and probably prognostic implications.

Uncontrolled studies from North America have found depression to be prominent in TS. Thus, Stefl *(102)*, in a mailed questionaire survey, reported that one third of more than 400 TS respondents had prominent "mood swings." Ferrari et al. *(103)* reported "depression" in TS children, which was reported by their parents. Grossman et al. *(104)* also reported depressive symptoms in TS subjects using the self-report questionnaire, the Minnesota Multiphasic Personality Inventory (MMPI). Erenberg et al. *(105)* reported "severe mood swings" in 52% of their TS patients. Wand et al. *(106)* examined 446 TS patients who completed a 52-item self-report survey about tics and a variety of associated features. In the age group 6–17 yr, 27% had experienced mood swings often, whereas 41% had experienced them sometimes; only 32% had never experienced them. In the age group 18+, 23% had experienced mood swings often, 41% had experienced them sometimes, and 36% had never experienced them. Rosenberg et al. *(107)*, using the Child Behavior Checklist, documented that one-third of nearly 200 TS children had depressive symptomatology.

Several controlled investigations from North America have also found TS individuals to be more depressed than control subjects *(66,108)*. Wodrich et al. *(109)* reported that TS children were more depressed than controls, although this study relied on parents completing a questionaire (Personality Inventory for Children) about their children; the children did not personally complete the questionaire.

In an elegant study, Pauls et al. *(110)* interviewed three groups of subjects: (*i*) 338 biological FDRs of 85 TS probands; (*ii*) 92 biological FDRs of 27 unaffected control probands; and (*iii*) 21 nonbiological FDRs of 6 adopted TS probands. The relatives of the unaffected probands and adopted TS probands (i.e., groups *ii* and *iii*) served as a control sample of the whole data set. The authors examined rates of MDD, which were significantly higher for TS probands than controls. MDD was also significantly increased among relatives of TS probands. When this association was examined further, however, the rates of MDD in relatives of TS+MDD probands was higher than control subjects, but the rates of MDD in relatives of TS-MDD probands was no higher than controls. This is compatible with MDD being genetic in its own right, but not with the suggestion that TS and MDD are genetically related.

Spencer et al. *(111)* examined 32 TS children, 39 children with chronic tics, and 38 normal control children, who were matched for age and gender. Results showed that 9 (29%) of TS subjects, and 13 (33%) of tic children had severe major depression, which was significantly greater than the one (3%)

in a normal child ($X^2 = 12.4$; $p = 0.002$); there were no significant differences found with regards to dysthymia. In summary, from these studies, it seems that there is little doubt that depression is increased in TS individuals.

Another elegant controlled study examined depression in children with TS. Carter et al. *(112)* examined 16 children with TS only, 33 children with TS plus ADHD, and 23 children who had no psychiatric diagnoses, who served as the control group. All children completed the Kovacs Child Depression Inventory (CDI). Mean CDI scores for the groups were as follows: TS plus ADHD (10.97), GTS alone (8.19), and normal controls (4.43); the TS children scored significantly higher than the normal control children.

The other main studies of affective disorder in patients with TS have come from the author's clinic, the National Hospital for Neurology and Neurosurgery in London. The authors' group has investigated adult TS subjects, both in clinical and community settings. The TS subjects all fulfilled the appropriate Diagnostic and Statistical Manual of Mental Disorders (DSM) and World Health Organization (WHO) criteria, and depression was assessed using a variety of standardized self-report scales.

Robertson et al. *(61)* investigated consecutively referred TS patients to the clinic, and 54 adult TS patients were studied employing standardized psychiatric rating scales including the Beck Depression Inventory (BDI), the Mood Adjective Checklist (MACL), and the Crown Crisp Experiental Index (CCEI), formerly known as the Middlesex Hospital Questionaire, both the latter having depression subscales; on all three measures, the TS patients' scores were substantially higher than normative data. BDI and CCEI depression subscales were significantly higher in females, older people, and those exhibiting echophenomena. People with coprolalia had higher scores on the CCEI depression subscale, while the MACL depression scores did not relate to any demographic or TS variable. Depression was not related to medication; using the MACL (the only scale employed to differentiate between depression and fatigue), patients currently taking medication scored higher on the MACL fatigue subscale, but not on the MACL depression subscale. All 90 patients (adult and children) had full mental state examinations undertaken, and 15 out of 90 (17%) were judged clinically to have depressive symptoms severe enough to constitute a depressive illness. Of interest and note is that 43 out of 90 probands (48%) had a positive family history of psychiatric illness, of which the most common disorder was depression (the family history was by history, and not direct examination and, therefore, likely to be an underestimate).

In a controlled study, Robertson et al. *(63)* examined 22 TS adults (aged between 18 and 65), and compared them to 19 patients with MDD and 21 normal controls using the BDI. The mean BDI scores for the normal controls was 2.71, for the TS patients was 12.09, and for the MDD patients was 25.32. Analysis of variance showed a significant difference in BDI scores between the three groups. Post-hoc *t*-tests showed that both the TS and depressed patients scored significantly higher than the controls; the depressed subjects also scored significantly higher than the TS subjects.

In a further controlled study *(64)*, 39 consecutive TS patients in the clinic were compared to 34 control subjects (matched for age and gender), using the BDI, as part of a larger investigation into personality disorders in TS. The mean score of the Yale Global Tic Severity Scale in TS subjects was 26.2 (range 11–55), which is indicative of moderate severity. The mean BDI score for the TS cases was 12.3, while that of the control subjects was 0.7 ($t = 6.6$; $p < 0.001$; 95% confidence interval [CI], 8.1–15.1), indicating that TS subjects were significantly more depressed.

In the recent study of QoL in patients with TS in the author's clinic, which was already mentioned *(84)*, depression scores on the BDI significantly influenced the QoL domains. Nineteen patients (21%) had high scores on the BDI (>19) indicating the presence of depression. Patients with depression had significantly lower scores on all subscales of the SF-36 except for physical functioning, indicating worse QoL, in comparison to patients without depression. Patients with depression had significantly higher TS severity scores on the YGTSS than patients without depression ($p = 0.01$).

Few studies have examined mild TS cases for depression or psychopathology. In a group of mild TS cases (relatives of a TS proband in a family study), the authors examined a multiply affected British pedigree spanning six generations and consisting of 122 members *(80)*. The authors personally interviewed 85 individuals and obtained information on 25 via family members. Fifty individuals were diagnosed as "cases"; 48 were mild, one was moderate (proband), and one was severe (had attracted a previous diagnosis of schizophrenia). The adults completed the CCEI, and scores of the TS cases on the depression subscale were no different from the scores of family members who were non-TS cases *(80)*.

The limitations of self-report scales, such as the BDI, MACL, and CCEI, are acknowledged. The BDI in particular, however, has been shown to be a reliable *(113)* and valid measure of depression, with high correlations of scores, with the clinician-rated Hamilton Depression Rating Scale for Depression (e.g., *114,115*). It is suggested, therefore, that the depressive symptomatology scores reported in our studies are probably suggestive of a significant amount of depression in TS patients. Whether or not the TS patients would fulfill DSM research criteria for MDD in our clinic has not been established in a formal study, but in clinical practice many of our patients are diagnosed as having MDD and require treatment with antidepressant medications.

It is of interest that in the large multicenter study by Freeman et al. *(28)*, as high as 20% of the 3500 patients had co-morbid mood disorders.

4.5. Etiology of Depression in TS

In the author's opinion, there is no doubt that depression is common in TS patients, and this has been demonstrated in both controlled and uncontrolled settings. In the author's opinion, the depression in TS is highly likely to be multifactorial in origin, as is the depression in non-TS populations (e.g., *97,116,117*).

TS can be a very distressing condition, particularly if the symptoms are moderate to severe. This depression in TS clinic patients and probands could, therefore, be explained, at least in part, by the fact that sufferers have a chronic, socially disabling, and stigmatizing disease *(118)*. The depression in clinic TS patients may also be due to the side effects of neuroleptics, which have been reported with, for example, haloperidol *(119)*, pimozide *(120)*, fluphenazine *(121)*, tiapride *(122)* and sulpiride *(123)*. It has been clearly demonstrated that children who have been bullied at school may also become depressed *(124,125)*; some of our TS children in the clinic have been bullied, teased, and given perjorative nicknames, such as "Noddy" and "Nudge, nudge wink, wink," and thus, the depression may result from that. The high levels of depression may reflect the fact that clinic attenders (including TS patients) often have more than one problem and/or disorder and thus, are subject to ascertainment bias *(126)* in specialist centers. Next, ADHD is common in TS and has been shown to have a high co-morbidity with depression *(127)*, and thus, many of our TS patients could be depressed because of the co-morbidity with ADHD. Similarly, OCB is common in TS, although there are phenomenological differences between symptoms in TS and OCD, (as demonstrated above). Depressive symptoms occur in 20–30% of patients with OCD *(93)*; the depression therefore, could be partly explained by the OCB/OCD co-morbidity. It has been shown that family members of TS probands may also have a history of depression *(58,61)*, although it is not suggested that this has genetic and/or etiological implications. Finally, it has also been shown that depression is common, with a lifetime prevalence of 7.5–10% in adults *(91)* and 1.8–8.9% in children *(92)*; TS may also be more common than was previously recognized *(1,2)*. Thus, the two disorders could coexist by chance in some instances.

It has been demonstrated clearly that both depressive symptoms and depressive disorder are common in TS. It is suggested, in conclusion, that depression in the setting of TS is highly likely to be multifactorial (as is the case in primary depressive illness) and that the debate, as to whether or not TS and depression are genetically related or not, should be finally put to rest. Studies to be explored further may include the assessment of depression in nonclinic TS patients (such as mild relatives of patients in the clinic), as well as studies further examining the precise phenomenology of the depression in the context of TS. As in the case of OCB/OCD, the depressive symptoms in TS and those in MDD may be phenomenologically different. Once this is done, the treatment of the depression in TS may become clearer, and the prognosis of the individual may hopefully alter for the better.

4.6. Conclusion: Depression and TS

In summary and conclusion, depressive illness and depressive symptomatology are common in TS, but it is suggested that they are multifactorial in etiology. The depression can also be severe, and thus, recognition, appropriate antidepressant treatment, and psychosocial strategies are important in managing the patient.

5. BAD

5.1. Etiology of Bipolar Disorder

The etiology of BAD is also multifactorial, with both a genetic predisposition *(117)* and psychosocial factors, such as stressful life events and social rhythm disruption, being important in the episodes of depression and mania *(128)*.

5.2. Bipolar Disorder and TS

Several recent studies have suggested a relationship between TS and BAD. Burd and Kerbeshian *(129)* reported the case of a TS patient who also had BAD, in whom the frequency and intensity of motor and vocal tics were correlated positively with the presence of manic symptoms and inversely with depressive symptoms. The same authors *(130)* then documented three boys under the age of 14 yr who had both TS and BAD and in whose early life had also had ADHD. A subsequent epidemiological study, demonstrated a trend toward an association between TS and BAD. Kerbeshian et al. *(131)* studied 205 TS patients in the North Dakota TS Surveillance Project, and 15 patients (7%) had co-morbid BAD. The estimated risk of developing BAD in individuals with TS was more than four times higher than that expected by chance, but which failed to reach statistical significance; males with TS were at a greater risk for BAD than females. Spencer et al. *(111)*, in the study mentioned earlier, found BAD to occur in 4 (13%) of 32 TS children and 11 (28%) of 39 tic children, compared to only one (3%) normal child; this was statistically significant ($X^2 = 10.0$; $p = 0.006$). Berthier et al. *(132)* examined 30 adult TS patients with co-morbid TS and BAD, who were selected from a consecutive series of 90 TS patients. They thus reported that BAD was found to occur commonly in one-third of TS patients; the full spectrum of BAD was found, including bipolar 1 disorder, bipolar 11 disorder, schizoaffective bipolar disorder, and cyclothymic disorder. BAD mainly occurred in TS patients with mild tic symptomatology and was associated with a wide variety of other psychopathologies *(132)*. In this context, Comings and Comings *(108)* already proposed that a gene leading to the expression of TS may aditionally represent a locus for BAD. In conclusion, it does seem that BAD may well be over-represented in TS individuals.

With regard to TS and BAD, the reasons for the coexistence are unclear. Kerbeshian and Burd *(131)* have suggested that TS and BAD appear to share a number of neurophysiological features, including abnormalities in noradrenergic, dopaminergic, and serotonergic neurotransmission, and both have been shown to be responsive to a variety of medications including neuroleptics, clonidine, and lithium.

5.3. Conclusion Bipolar Disorder and TS

In summary and conclusion, it does seem that BAD may be related to TS in some individuals. However, numbers in the studies are small, and thus, more investigations are suggested.

6. ADHD

6.1. Prevalence of ADHD

ADHD is probably one of the most common psychiatric disorders affecting children, with prevalence estimates ranging from 1 to 2% (using the International Classification of Diseases [ICD] criteria) to 5–10% (DSM criteria) *(133)*.

6.2. *Etiology of ADHD*

The etiology of ADHD is not fully understood. As ADHD begins in early childhood, parents are often the first to note symptoms of clumsiness, excessive activity, low frustration tolerance, and "accident proneness" *(134)*.

6.3. *Phenomenology and Genetics of ADHD*

For a careful review of stand-alone hyperkinetic disorder (which includes ADHD), influences on pathogenesis, the history, prevalence, diagnosis, co-morbidity, differential diagnosis, work-up, and treatment guidelines, readers are referred to Swanson et al. *(133)* and Taylor et al. *(135)*, for an insight into phenomenology and genetics, Nadder et al. *(136)*, and for an historical note Palmer and Finger *(137)*.

Swanson et al. *(133)* point out that the behaviors of inattention, hyperactivity, and impulsivity in children are in fact recognized as a disorder when the behaviors are severe and developmentally inappropriate and impair function both at home and at school. Swanson and colleagues describe the history of the disorder noting that a century ago, Still in 1902, in *The Lancet* described "some physical conditions in children," attributing the symptoms to "defects of moral control" *(133)*. The expert authors also make the point that diagnosis of ADHD (and hyperkinetic disorder [HKD]) are essentially based on history, and they do not recommend either biological or psychological tests for routine clinical use. The ratio of boys to girls with ADHD is between 3:1 and 9:1, but this figure may decrease with age. They suggest that part of this difference between the sexes may be due to referral bias, related to disruptive behaviors, as boys have more hyperactive and/or impulsive symptoms and more conduct and oppositional symptoms than girls. The authors then go on to discuss the differences between the DSM and ICD (more rigorous) criteria, but suggest that there are sensible recommendations about making the diagnosis, including taking a good history from those people who know the children best, namely their parents and teachers *(133)*.

6.4. *ADHD and TS*

As early as 1973, it was generally accepted that a substantial proportion of children who have TS first manifest various behavioral disturbances often called minimal brain dysfunction (MBD), HKD, hyperactivity, or attention deficit disorder (ADD) *(138,139)*. Although diagnostic criteria have changed over time, in this section, for the sake of convenience, all these types of symptoms, unless otherwise specified, will be referred to as ADHD. For a detailed history of ADHD through the DSM variants, the reader is referred to Towbin and Riddle *(134)*.

It has been pointed out that of all the co-morbid conditions, ADHD is probably the most commonly encountered in TS, as evidenced by a vast literature on the subject *(28,134,140)*. Although early studies found ADHD in as few as 13% of TS patients *(141)*, it is now evident that ADHD occurs in a substantial proportion of TS patients, ranging from 21–90% *(142)* and 24–75% *(143)* of clinic populations and as high as 44–66% of school based studies *(143)*, clearly way in excess of the 1–10% *(133)* in the general population. Of importance as stated earlier, in the large study of Freeman et al. *(28)*, ADHD was the most common co-morbid disorder, occurring in 60% of the 3500 TS individuals.

Five epidemiological studies have, however, also examined ADHD in TS and, in the author's opinion are some of the strongest arguments for the possible integral relationship between TS and ADHD in some cases. Thus, Caine et al. *(57)* in an early epidemiological study in Monroe County, New York, investigated a population of more than 142,000, finding 41 individuals with TS, including 11 (27%) with symptoms of ADHD. Apter et al. *(144)* examined in excess of 28,000 recruits into the Israeli Defence Force during 1 yr and reported the rate of ADHD in people with TS to be 8.3%, which is much more than the population point prevalence of 3.9% at the time. The author's group conducted a postal survey in New Zealand, with a population of around 3.35 million, and documented 40 TS cases of whom 10 (25%) had symptoms of ADHD *(145)*. Mason et al. *(146)* undertook a school epidemiological pilot study examining TS and tics in West Essex, UK. Of the 30 out of 167 (18%) tic possibles, there was no increase in ADHD in tic possibles compared to the other children, as rated by the short Connors scale; there was also no increase in hyperactivity as assessed by both the General Health and Behavior Questionaire, and the Strength and Difficulty Questionaire of Goodman. Four out of five (80%) of the identified TS individuals (definite and probable) were, however, reported as hyperactive by their teachers, parents, or both; one satisfied DSM-IV criteria for ADHD *(146)*. Kadesjo and Gillberg *(1)* investigated a population of 435 children and reported that the prevalence of TS was five (1.1%); of these, one (20%) had a diagnosis of ADHD. In the second part of the study, during which all children who were registered with TS in the catchment area (n = 58), co-morbidity was examined. Of these, 37 (64%) were diagnosed as having ADHD *(1)*.

Symptoms of ADHD and poor impulse control frequently precede the emergence of the actual tics *(147,148)*. In fact, for the DSM-IV *(30)* diagnosis to be made, symptoms of ADHD must be present in two or more settings before the age of 7; the TS tic symptoms, however, often begin later (see previous reviews in refs. *5,7,120*).

Only one investigation to date has examined the phenomenology of "pure" ADHD and compared it to that of ADHD+TS *(149)*. It was reported that in TS, there were increased rates of both OCD and ADHD. In contrast to the co-morbidity with OCD, it was found that the other co-morbidities (such as disruptive behaviors, mood disorder, and anxiety disorders) were indistinguishable in between children with TS+ADHD and children with ADHD alone. This may suggest that some psychopathology (e.g., mood and anxiety) could be secondary to the co-morbidity with ADHD, rather than the TS *per se*. In addition, it was shown that children with TS+ADHD had lower psychosocial functioning than children with pure ADHD *(149)*. A more recent paper *(150)* compared 128 male children and adolescents with 110 controls at baseline and at 4 yr later. When compared to controls, AHDH youngsters had more tic disorders initially. Of interest is that tic disorders and ADHD had independent courses, with ADHD showing markedly less remission *(5,50)*.

Of interest is that in the elegant study referred to earlier *(112)*, TS-ADHD and TS+ADHD children were compared on a variety of structured interviews including the Child Behavior Checklist (CBCL). Children with TS+ADHD showed more externalizing and internalizing behavior problems and poorer social adaptation than children with TS only or normal controls. In addition, with the ADHD diagnosis, obsessional symptom severity and family functioning were significantly associated with social and emotional adjustment.

Several investigations (e.g., *151–153*) in non-TS youngsters have all demonstrated that childhood ADHD was predictive of antisocial personality disorder in adults. As so many TS children have ADHD symptoms, this may well account for the apparent increase in at least some of the adulthood psychopathologies (e.g., personality disorder) in TS (see below).

The precise relationship between ADHD and TS is complex and has long been debated. There appear to be four possibilities as to the nature of the relationship. There have (*i*) been suggestions that the two disorders are genetically related (e.g., *154,155*), although this has been disputed *(22,156,157)*. The data from another study, however, (*ii*) suggested that there may be two types of individuals with TS and ADHD; one in whom ADHD is independent of TS, and others in whom ADHD is secondary to TS *(158)*. (*iii*) A third possibility is that "pure" ADHD and TS+ADHD are different phenomenologically, but the exact relationship is unclear. (*iv*) A fourth possibility as to the cause of the apparent relationship has been put forward by Towbin and Riddle *(134)*, who suggested that TS individuals may have reduced capacities for concentration, attention, and impulse control, but at a level subthreshold for a DSM diagnosis of ADHD; the frequency of co-morbidity, therefore, depends on where the cut-off point for ADHD is set *(134)*. Possibilities *ii*, *iii*, and *iv* may well be related in some way, and more research needs to be undertaken.

Finally, it seems that ADHD may also be an heterogeneous disorder. It has been highlighted that ADHD has many co-morbid disorders other than TS. These include major depression, bipolar disorder, and generalized anxiety disorder *(127)*. Thus, the presence of ADHD in an individual with TS may also partly account for the presence of other psychopathologies.

6.5. Conclusions

In the author's opinion, ADHD or similar symptoms, are common in people with TS, and it appears that they may occur in even milder TS cases who are identified in epidemiological studies. It is unlikely, therefore, to be wholly due to referral bias. Whether or not the symptoms are sufficient, however, to warrant an actual ADHD diagnosis is as yet unknown, and whether or not the symptoms in TS+ADHD are identical to those seen in pure and/or primary ADHD has to be investigated further *(5)*.

7. CD AND OPPOSITIONAL DEFIANT DISORDER

7.1. Clinical Definitions

Oppositional Defiant Disorder (ODD) and CD are often suggested to be common in children with TS, but the area has in fact not been widely studied. The essential feature of ODD is a recurrent pattern of negativistic, defiant, disobedient, and hostile behavior, which persists for at least 6 mo and is characterized by the frequent occurrence of certain behaviors such as losing temper, being angry, resentful, and being spiteful and vindictive *(30)*. The essential feature of CD is a repetitive and persistent pattern of behavior in which the basic rights of others or major-age appropriate societal norms or rules are violated. There are four main groupings of these behaviors: (*i*) aggressive conduct that causes or threatens physical harm to persons or animals; (*ii*) nonaggressive conduct, which results in property loss or damage; (*iii*) deceitfulness or theft; and finally (*iv*) serious violations of rules *(30)*.

7.2. OD and CD and TS

An early controlled study suggested that ODD and CD were more common in TS subjects than in control individuals *(19)*. In the Freeman et al. *(28)* investigation, 15% of 3500 TS individuals had co-morbid ODD/CD, although 37% of patients had a history of anger control problems, and 26% currently had these problems.

In the epidemiological study of Kadesjo and Gillberg *(1)*, there were two parts. In the first part, no mention was made of either ODD or CD. However, in their second study, during which all children who were registered with TS in the catchment area ($n = 58$), of whom 21 (36%) were diagnosed as having CD.

7.3. Rage and Explosive Outbursts

Recently, explosive outbursts (also referred to as "rage" or "anger attacks") have also been described in a substantial proportion (possibly as high as one-third) of patients with TS *(159–162)*. These explosive outbursts are of unknown etiology, sudden onset, have no clear predisposing or precipitating immediate factors. If there are such factors, the attacks or outbursts are out of proportion to them. Often, the child with these attacks is apologetic and remorseful afterwards. In recent studies, these attacks in people with TS have been demonstrated to be associated with ADHD, OCD, and expressed emotion *(160,163)*. In a study of 105 children with TS aged 7–17 yr, the rage attacks were highly and specifically associated with, in particular, ODD, and it has been suggested that this episodic rage may be associated with disturbed serotonergic function *(163)*.

7.4. Conclusions

Thus, it does seem that in recent studies, where the disorders are being looked for and diagnostic criteria used, a substantial number of TS children are demonstrated to have ODD or CD. Clearly this has management and prognostic implications. More research into the area is required.

8. ANXIETY DISORDERS

8.1. Anxiety and TS

Anxiety is also common in TS patients and has been examined frequently, although by and large, not in great depth. Anxiety has been found in substantial proportions of several TS cohorts *(61,105, 164–166)*. In controlled investigations, more TS individuals have been shown to have increased anxiety when compared to control populations *(19,63,64,66)*. For a fuller exposition of the above studies, the reader is referred to a previous review by the author *(5)*. Thibert et al. *(167)* examined responses to a mailed questionaire and showed that the TS patients with high OCS/OCB, scored higher on social anxiety than did the general population. On the other hand, Robertson and Gourdie *(80)* demonstrated that, in a group of mild TS cases (relatives of a TS proband in the community), the scores of the TS cases on the three anxiety subscales of the CCEI were no different from the scores of non-TS cases.

Carter et al. *(168)* investigated the frequency of TS, tics, and other behavioral disorders among children at risk for TS, and assessed the association of family functioning with the children's diagnostic status. Young children who were not showing any tic behaviors, but who had an FDR with TS were recruited and evaluated with standardized instruments. Increased rates of tic disorders, OCS/OCB, and anxiety symptoms were reported. Family functioning, independent of parental psychopathology, was associated with anxiety disorders.

In the careful genetic study already described in the depression section, Pauls et al. *(24)* interviewed 338 biological FDRs of 85 TS probands, 92 biological FDRs of 27 unaffected control probands, and 21 nonbiological FDRs of 6 adopted TS probands. The relatives of the unaffected probands and adopted TS probands served as a control sample of the whole data set. The rates of generalized anxiety disorder (GAD) were nonsignificantly higher in the TS probands than controls. However, the rates of GAD were not significantly different between relatives of TS probands and controls, suggesting that GAD and TS are not genetically related.

It is of interest to note that in the large study by Freeman et al. *(28)*, as high as 18% of the 3500 patients had co-morbid anxiety disorders.

8.2. Conclusions

In summary and conclusion, in the author's opinion, it seems that anxiety is common in clinic TS patients, but its exact relationship to TS is as yet unclear. It may well be secondary to having moderate or severe TS *(5)*. The results of Carter et al. *(168)*, on the other hand, suggested that anxiety symptoms were observed in children who were at risk of developing TS. Thus, it seems that, although the majority of studies have concentrated on TS clinic patients, and there is no doubt that they have increased anxiety (this may in turn be associated with the onus of having TS or due to TS medications), future studies may well examine the phenomenology of anxiety in even more detail and, thus, give more clues to the relationship between TS and the subgroups of the anxiety disorders.

9. PERSONALITY DISORDER

There has been only one investigation of personality disorder in TS, but, as it has important clinical implications, the results will be discussed briefly. Robertson et al. *(64)* examined 39 adult TS patients of moderate severity of whom 79% were male, with 34 age- and sex-matched controls. TS patients and controls were examined using the Structured Clinical Interview for DSM-III-R Personality Disorders II (SCID-II), to systematically determine personality axis II personality disorders. Subjects also completed a self-rated scale for personality disorders (SCTPD). Results showed that, using the SCID-II, 64% of TS patients had one or more DSM-III-R personality disorders, compared with only 16% of control subjects which was highly statistically significant. The cause of this increase in personality disorder may well be the result of the long-term outcome of childhood ADHD, referral bias, or because of other childhood psychopathology (see below). Thus, it does appear that at least some clinic TS populations have personality disorders that have both treatment and prognosis implications *(64)*.

10. PERVASIVE DEVELOPMENTAL DISORDERS AND ASD

10.1. Clinical Definitions and Spectrum

The two main disorders included in this spectrum are autism and Asperger's syndrome. The notion of the ASD seems, however, also to be heterogeneous and controversial. The conditions are characterized by severe and pervasive impairment in several areas of development: reciprocal social interaction skills, communication skills, and the presence of stereotyped behavior, interests, and activities. Associated features of autism include mental retardation (IQ 35–50) in about 75%, as well as a variety of behavioral symptoms, including hyperactivity, short attention span, impulsivity, aggression, SIB, and temper tantrums. The onset by definition is under 3 yr old, males are more affected than females (5:1), and epidemiological studies suggest rates of 2–5 cases per 10,000. There is an increased risk of autistic disorder in siblings *(30)*. Asperger's syndrome (AS) is also included on the spectrum of pervasive developmental disorders (PDD). Unlike autism, however, there is no general delay in language and no clinically significant delay in cognitive development *(30)*.

10.2. Conditions Similar to Autism

Conditions with similarities to autism include elective mutism, attachment disorder, developmental receptive language disorder, HKD with stereotypies, disintegrative disorder, mental handicap and/or retardation, Rett's syndrome, and Landau-Kleffner syndrome *(169)*.

10.3. ASD and TS

Over the last 20 yr, there have been an increasing number of reports and series, including over 90 patients displaying features of both PDD and TS. The cases were almost all subjects with an established diagnosis of PDD, who then went on to display additional symptoms of TS. This sequence of events is in keeping with the diagnostic requirement for autistic disorder for onset before the age of 3 yr, whereas symptoms of TS begin at around 5–7 yr (for reviews see refs. *5,170*).

Only a few dedicated studies examining TS and ASD have, however, have been conducted in the area. In a pilot study, the investigators observed 37 children (pupils) at a special school for children and adolescents with autism for the presence of motor and vocal tics. Subsequent family interviews confirmed the diagnosis of co-morbid TS in three children, giving a minimum prevalence rate of 8.1% (3 out of 37 children). Family history data also suggested that the TS was inherited with positive family history of generally accepted TS spectrum. It was suggested that the rate of TS in autism may exceed that expected by chance, but the sample size was felt too small for the conclusion. The presence of TS was not associated with superior intellectual, language, or social development *(171)*. In the more recent large-scale definitive study, 447 pupils from 9 schools for youngsters with autism were investigated in a six-stage procedure involving both observational and family history methods *(172)*. Results showed that definite TS was diagnosed in 19 children, giving a prevalence rate of 4.0%; 10 more children were diagnosed as having probable TS (2.2%). Several other youngsters (34%) showed tics on observation (but not both motor and vocal tics), and thus, the observed rate of 6.48% of TS in autism may be an underestimate. Of importance is that family histories for tics or OCB were positive in 25 out of 32 youngsters (78%). TS was not related to the severity of the autism in the youngsters *(172)*. It is important to note that in both studies, the diagnoses of TS were made using standardized assessment schedules, but the autism and ASD were clinical diagnoses only.

In the recent epidemiological study of Kadesjo and Gillberg *(1)*, five children (four boys) with TS were identified. One of the four boys received a clinical diagnosis of Asperger's disorder and moreover met diagnostic criteria. One boy had a diagnosis of deficits in attention, motor control, and perception (DAMP). In their second part of the study, during which all children who were registered with

TS in the catchment area ($n = 58$), of whom, three (5%) were diagnosed as having Asperger's disorder and 10 (17%) had PDD not otherwise specified *(1)*.

Sverd *(173)* recently reported that in a group of 388 inpatients (aged 10–18 yr), eight of the boys met criteria for PDD, and five of these (62%) met criteria for TS, and two (25%) met criteria for chronic multiple tic (CMT) disorder. In a second group of 146 outpatients (aged 6–18 yr), 20 (13%) were diagnosed at having PDD. Five patients already attending the outpatient clinic were added to the sample. Of these 25 patients, six (24%) were diagnosed as having TS before referral, and an additional 12 children were subsequently diagnosed as having TS. In other words, 18 (72%) of outpatients with PDD showed evidence of a tic disorder *(173)*.

10.4. Conclusions

In summary and conclusion, it does seem as evidenced by at least 90 case reports, two dedicated studies by the author's group, and the epidemiological study of Kadesjo and Gillberg *(1)*, as well as that of Sverd *(173)*, that autism (or at least ASD and PDD) and TS occur together more commonly than would be expected by chance. At present, however, no further definitive conclusions can be made. Further studies are suggested to explore the occurrence from a different perspective (e,g., investigating autism or AS) in a TS clinic or grouping and assessing both conditions fully.

11. THE IMPACT OF CHILDHOOD PSYCHOPATHOLOGY ON ADOLESCENT AND ADULT FUNCTIONING AND PSYCHOPATHOLOGY

11.1. Introduction

The role of childhood behavior and psychopathology on outcome in later life has always been acknowledged and has received much attention in the literature, more so recently. A brief review of relevant literature in chronological order will be made.

11.2. Evidence from the Literature

In a classic paper, Robins *(174)* suggested that: (*i*) adult antisocial behavior requires childhood antisocial behavior; (*ii*) most antisocial children do not become antisocial adults; (*iii*) the variety of antisocial behavior in childhood is a better predictor of adult antisocial behavior than is any particular behaviour; (*iv*) adult antisocial behavior is better predicted by childhood behavior than by family background or social class; and (*v*) social class makes little contribution to the predication of serious adult antisocial behavior.

As part of a longitudinal study from childhood, Zoccolillo et al. *(175)* investigated the effect of childhood CD on adult social functioning in a variety of modalities, including work, interpersonal relationships, and criminality. The findings were based on 254 subjects: 171 who had been in care (those who had spent much of their childhhod in cottage children's homes) and 83 in the quasirandom comparison group, from economically deprived inner city areas, who had not been in care. Results showed that most subjects with conduct disorder (three or more DSM symptoms) had pervasive (but not necessarily severe) social difficulties compared to peers without conduct disorder. Of the 35 males with conduct disorder in childhood, 14 (40%) were rated as having an antisocial personality disorder as an adult, compared to only 9 out of 42 (4%) of those without conduct disorder. Similarly, for females, of the 26 with childhood CD, 9 (35%) showed adult antisocial personality disorder, compared with none in without childhood CD. To summarize, less than half of this group met DSM-III adult criteria for antisocial personality disorder, and just over half were given a diagnosis of personality disorder on interviewer clinical ratings.

It is important to note that many children with TS are very impulsive and have impaired attention, as well as, in some, a formal diagnosis of ADHD. In this context it is worth noting that Tremblay et al. *(176)* undertook a large longitudinal study of boys and showed that the impulsivity dimension was the best predictor of the early onset of stable highly delinquent behavior. Other studies have also documented that attentional difficulties in middle childhood were associated with risks of academic failure or difficulties, juvenile offending, and substance misuse in adulthood *(177)*. Others have demonstrated that childhood conduct problems as well as hyperactivity–impulsivity independently, as well as jointly, predict a greater likelihood of having an arrest record for males, but not females *(178)*.

Even more recently, several authors have addressed the issue. Stevenson and Goodman *(179)* examined the records of 828 criminals who had been assessed at the age of 3 yr and reported that the risk of having any adult conviction and criminality was related to activity level, management difficulties, and temper tantrums. Hofstra et al. *(180)* found that deviant scores of a self-report measure (Youth Self Report) completed between the ages of 10 and 19 yr, predicted deviant scores on another self-report measure (Young Adult Self Report) 10 yr later, and more deviant early scores also predicted adult DSM-IV diagnoses. Finally, Fombonne et al. *(181,182)* studied 149 subjects who were assessed between 1970 and 1983, 20 yr later. The two groups consisted of youngsters who had MDD+CD and MDD-CD. Results showed that adolescent depression carried an elevated risk of adult depression, but in the light of this chapter, almost more importantly, early CD resulted in higher rates of adult drug misuse and dependence, alcoholism, suicidal behaviors, adult personality disorders, criminal offences, and more pervasive social dysfunction in adulthood.

11.3. Conclusion

The author wishes to suggest that as many youngsters with TS indeed often have depression, OCS/OCB/OCD, impulsivity, poor attention, formal diagnoses of ADHD, as well as ODD and CD, and it may be these psychopathologies–co-morbidities that are the reason for referral to specialist clinics in the majority of cases. In addition, it is suggested that it is the co-morbidities that predict some of the adult psychopathologies and maladaptive social functioning, rather than the TS *per se*.

12. OVERALL CONCLUSIONS

TS is in itself heterogeneous, and currently, genetic studies are underway (e.g., Tourette Syndrome Association International Consortium for Genetics) hoping to identify more precisely the phenotype of not only TS, but also of the psychopathological disorders associated with TS. Structured assessment schedules are used for all diagnoses and are, thus, rigorous in their descriptions. However, it is acknowledged that other environmental factors, such as perinatal difficulties and/or certain infections, have recently been invoked as etiopathological, and whether or not the "genetic TS" will be of the same phenotype as "environmentally driven TS" has, as yet, to be discovered. How the heterogeneous psychopathology will be explained is even harder to debate. The author's current suggestions as to the psychopathology accompanying TS are shown in Table 1. It is suggested that future research examining the psychopathologies with more structured and rigorous methods, linking them to genetic, neuroimaging, neuroimmunological, and neuropsychological studies will be fruitful.

ACKNOWLEDGMENTS

The author wishes to thank the Tourette Syndrome Associations of the UK, USA, and Canada for their continuing encouragement. The author also wishes to thank John Ludgate for his support and patience.

REFERENCES

1. Kadesjo, B. and Gillberg, C. (2000) Tourette's disorder: epidemiology and comorbidity in primary school children. *J. Am. Acad. Child Adolesc. Psychiatry* **39,** 548–555.
2. Kurlan, R., McDermott, M.P., Deeley, C., et al. (2001) Prevalence of tics in school children and association with placement in special education. *Neurology* **57,** 1383–1388.
3. American Psychiatric Association. (2000) *Diagnostic and Statistical Manual of Mental disorders (fourth ed.-text revision) (DSM-IV-TR),* American Psychiatric Association, Washington DC.

4. World Health Organization. (1992) *International Classification of Diseases and Health Related Problems, tenth revision,* World Health Organization, Geneva.
5. Robertson, M.M. (2000) Invited Review. Tourette syndrome, associated conditions and the complexities of treatment. *Brain* **123,** 425–462.
6. Ferenczi, S. (1921) Psycho-analytic observations on tic. *Int. J. Psychoanalysis* **2,** 1–30.
7. Robertson, M.M. (1989) The Gilles de la Tourette syndrome: the current status. *Br. J. Psychiatry* **154,** 147–169.
8. Fenichel, O. (1945) *The Psychoanalytic Theory of Neurosis*, Norton and Company, New York.
9. Heuscher, J.E. (1953) Intermediate states of consciousness inpatients with generalised tics. *J. Nerv. Ment. Dis.* **117,** 29–38.
10. Robertson, M.M. and Reinstein, D.Z. (1991) Convulsive tic disorder. Georges Gilles de la Tourette, Guinon and Grasset on the phenomenology and psychopathology of Gilles de la Tourette syndrome. *Behav. Neurol.* **4,** 29–56.
11. Tourette Syndrome Association International Consortium for Genetics. (1999) A complete genome scan in sib pairs affected by Gilles de la Tourette syndrome. *Am. J. Hum. Genet.* **65,** 1428–1436.
12. Swedo, S.E., Leonard, L.H., Garvey, M., Mittleman, B.B., Allen, A.J., and Perlmutter, S. (1998) Pediatric autoimmune neuropsychiatric disorders associated with streptococcal infections: clinical description of the first 50 cases. *Am. J. Psychiatry* **155,** 264–271.
13. Muller, N., Riedel, M., Straube, A., Gunther, W., and Wilske, B. (2000) increased anti-streptoccal antibodies in patients with Tourette's syndrome. *Psychiatr. Res.* **94,** 43–49.
14. Cardono, F. and Orefici, G. (2001) Group A streptococcal infections and tic disorders in an Italian pediatric population. *J. Pediatr.* **138,** 71–75.
15. Shapiro, A.K., Shapiro, E.S., and Sweet, R.D. (1978) *Gilles de la Tourette Syndrome*, Raven Press, New York.
16. Shapiro, A.K. and Shapiro, E.S. (1982) Tourette syndrome: history and present status, in *The Gilles de la Tourette Syndrome. Advances in Neurology, 35* (Friedhoff, A.J. and Chase, T.N., eds.), Raven Press, New York, pp. 17–23.
17. Comings, D.E. (1990) *Tourette Syndrome and Human Behaviour*, Hope Press, Duarte, California.
18. Comings, D.E. (1995) Tourette syndrome: a behavioural spectrum disorder. *Adv. Neurol.* **65,** 293–303.
19. Comings, D.E. and Comings, B.G. (1987a) A controlled study of Tourette syndrome, I-VII. *Am. J. Hum. Genet.* **41,** 701–866.
20. Comings, D.E. and Comings, B.G. (1987b) Hereditary agoraphobia and obsessive-compulsive behaviour in relatives of patients with Gilles de la Tourette syndrome. *Br. J. Psychiatry* **151,** 195–199.
21. Comings, D.E., Wu, S., Chiu, C., Ring, R.H., Gade, R., Ahn, C., et al. (1996) Polygenic inheritance of Tourette syndrome, stuttering, attention deficit hyperactivity, conduct, and oppositional defiant disorder: the additive and subtractive effect of the three dopaminergic genes—DRD2, DâH, and DAT1. *Am. J. Med. Genet.* **67,** 264–288.
22. Pauls, D.L., Hurst, C.R., Kruger, S.D., Leckman, J.F., Kidd, K.K., and Cohen, D.J. (1986a) Gilles de la Tourette's syndrome and attention deficit disorder with hyperactivity. *Arch. Gen. Psychiatry* **43,** 1177–1179.
23. Pauls, D.L., Cohen, D.J., Kidd, K.K., et al. (1988) The Gilles de la Tourette syndrome [letter]. *Am. J. Hum. Genet.* **43,** 206–209.
24. Pauls, D.L., Leckman, J.F., and Cohen, D.J. (1994) Evidence against a genetic relationship between Tourette's syndrome and anxiety, depression, panic and phobic disorders. *Br. J. Psychiatry* **164,** 215–221.
25. Pauls, D.L., Leckman, J.F., Towbin, K.E., et al. (1986b) A possible genetic relationship exists between Tourette syndrome and obsessive-compulsive disorder. *Psychopharmacol. Bull.* **22,** 730–733.
26. Pauls, D.L., Towbin, K.E., Leckman, J.F., et al. (1986c) Gilles de la Tourette syndrome and obsessive-compulsive disorder: evidence supporting a genetic relationship. *Arch. Gen. Psychiatry* **43,** 1180–1182.
27. Eapen, V., Pauls, D.L., and Robertson, M.M. (1993) Evidence for autosomal dominant transmission in Gilles de la Tourette syndrome—United Kingdom cohort. *Br. J. Psychiatry* **162,** 593–596.
28. Freeman, R.D., Fast, D.K., Burd, L., Kerbashian, J., Robertson, M.M., and Sandor, P. (2000) An international perspective on Tourette syndrome: selected findings from 22 countries. *Dev. Med. Child Neurol.* **42,** 436–447.
29. American Psychiatric Association. (1987) Diagnostic and Statistical Manual of Mental Disorders (Third ed., Revised) (DSM-lll-R), American Psychiatric Association, Washington, DC.
30. American Psychiatric Association. (1994) Diagnostic and Statistical Manual of Mental disorders (Fourth ed.) (DSM-IV), American Psychiatric Association, Washington, DC.
31. Hodgson, R.J. and Rachmann, S. (1997) Obsessional-compulsive complaints. *Behav. Res. Ther.* **15,** 389–395.
32. Khanna, S., Kaliaperumal, V.G., and Channabasavanna, S.M. (1990) Clusters of obsessive-compulsive phenomena in obsessive compulsive disorder. *Br. J. Psychiatry* **156,** 51–54.
33. Pauls, D.L., Alsobrook, J.P. II, Goodman, W., Rasmussen, S., and Leckman, J.F. (1995) A family study of obsessive-compulsive disorder. *Am. J. Psychiatry* **152,** 76–84.
34. Summerfeldt, L.J., Richter, M.A., Antony, M.M., and Swinson, R.P. (1999) Symptom structure in obsessive-compulsive disorder: a confirmatory factor-analytic study. *Behav. Res. Ther.* **37,** 297–311.
35. Freud, S. (1955) Obsessions and phobias, in *Collected Papers 1* (Strachey, J., ed.), Hogarth Press, London, pp. 128–137.
36. Freud, S. (1958) The predisposition to obsessional neurosis, in *The Standard Edition of the Collected Works on Sigmund Freud,* vol. 12 (Strachey, J., ed.), Hogarth Press, London, pp. 311–326.
37. Janet, P. (1903) *Les Obsessions et la Psychasthenie,* vol 1, Arno 1976, New York.
38. Flament, M.E., Whitaker, A., Rapoport, J.L., Davies, M., et al. (1988) Obsessive compulsive disorder in adolescence: an epidemiological study. *J. Am. Acad. Child Adolesc. Psychiatry* **27,** 764–771.

39. Dinan, T.G. (1995) Obsessive compulsive disorder: the paradigm shift. *J. Ser. Res.* **1(Suppl. 1),** 19–25.
40. Heyman, I., Fombonne, E., Simmons, H., Ford, T., Meltzer, H., and Goodman, R. (2001) Prevalence of obsessive-compulsive disorder in the British nationwide survey. *Br. J. Psychiatry* **179,** 324–329.
41. Shafran, R. (2001) Obsessive compulsive disorder in children and adolescents. *Child Psychol. Psychiatr. Rev.* **6,** 50–58.
42. Robertson, M.M. and Yakeley, J. (1993) Obsessive-compulsive and self injurious behaviour, in *Handbook of Tourette's Syndrome and Related Tic and Behavioural Disorders* (Kurlan, R., ed.), Marcel Dekker, New York, pp. 45–87.
43. Robertson, M.M. (1995) The relationship between Gilles de la Tourette syndrome and obsessive compulsive disorder. *J. Ser. Res.* **11(Suppl.),** 49–62.
44. Gilles de la Tourette, G. (1885) Etude sur une affection nerveuse caracterisee par de l'incoordination motrice accompagnee d'echolalie et de copralalie. *Arch. Neurol.* **9,** 19-42, 158–200.
45. Gilles de La Tourette, G. (1899) La Maladie des tics convulsifs. *La Sem. Med.* **19,** 153–156.
46. Itard, J.M.G. (1825) Memoire sur quelques fonctions involontaires des appareils de la locomotion de la prehension etde la voix. *Arch. Gen. Med.* **8,** 385–407.
47. Guinon, G. (1886) Sur la maladie des tics convulsifs. *Rev. Med.* **6,** 50–80.
48. Grasset, J. (1890) Lecons sur un cas de maladie des tics et un cas de tremblement singulier de la tete et des membres gauches. *Arch. Neurol.* **20,** 27–45, 187–211.
49. Meige, H. and Feindel, E. (1907) *Tics and their Treatment* (Wilson, S.A.K., Trans. and ed.), William Wood and Co., New York.
50. Wilson, S.A.K. (1927) The tics and allied conditions. *J. Neurol. Psychopathol.* **8,** 93–109.
51. Ascher, E. (1949) Psychodyanmic considerations in Gilles de la Tourette's disease (maladie de tics). A report of five cases and discussion of the literature. *Am. J. Psychiatry* **105,** 267–276.
52. Bockner, S. (1959) Gilles de la Tourette's disease. *J. Ment. Sci.* **105,** 1078–1081.
53. McHenry, L.C. Jr. (1967) Samuel Johnson's tics and gesticulations. *J. Hist. Med.* **22,** 152–168.
54. Murray, T.J. (1979) Dr. Samuel Johnson's movement disorders. *BMJ* **1,** 1610–1614.
55. King, R.A., Leckman, J.F., Scahill, L., and Cohen, D.J. (1999) Obsessive-compulsive disorder, anxiety, and depression, in *Tourette's Syndrome. Tics, Obsessions, Compuslions* (Leckman, J.F. and Cohen, D.J., eds.), John Wiley & Sons, New York, pp. 43–62.
56. van der Wetering, B.J.M., Cohen, A.P., Minderaa, R.B., Roos, R.A.C., and van Woerkom, T.C.A.M. (1988) Het syndroom van Gilles de la Tourette—klinsche bevindingen. *Nederlands Tijdschrifte voor Geneeskinde* **132,** 21–25.
57. Caine, E.D., McBride, M.C., Chiverton, P., Bamford, K.A., Rediess, S., and Shiao, J. (1988) Tourette syndrome in Monroe County school children. *Neurology* **38,** 472–475.
58. Montgomery, M.A., Clayton, P.J., and Friedhoff, A.J. (1982) Psychiatric illness in Tourette syndrome patients and first-degree relatives, in *Gilles de la Tourette Syndrome. Adv. Neurology,* vol. 35 (Friedhoff, A.J. and Chase, T.N., eds.), Raven Press, New York, pp. 335–359.
59. Nee, L.E., Polinsky, R.J., and Ebert, M.H. (1982) Tourette syndrome: clinical and family studies, in *Gilles de la Tourette syndrome* (Friedhoff, A.J. and Chase, T.N., eds.), Reven Press, New York, pp. 291–295.
60. Frankel, M., Cummings, J.L., Robertson, M.M., Trimble, M.R., Hill, M.A., and Benson, D.F. (1986) Obsessions and compulsions in Gilles de la Tourette's syndrome. *Neurology* **36,** 378–382.
61. Robertson, M.M., Trimble, M.R., and Lees, A.J. (1988) The psychopathology of the Gilles de la Tourette syndrome: a phenomenological analysis. *Br. J. Psychiatry* **152,** 383–390.
62. Robertson, M.M., Trimble, M.R., and Lees, A.J. (1989) Self-injurious behaviour and the Gilles de la Tourette syndrome. A clinical study and review of the literature. *Psychol. Med.* **19,** 611–625.
63. Robertson, M.M., Channon, S., Baker, J., and Flynn, D. (1993) The psychopathology of Gilles de la Tourette syndrome: a controlled study. *Br. J. Psychiatry* **162,** 114–117.
64. Robertson, M.M., Banerjee, S., Fox-Hiley, P.J., and Tannock, C. (1997) Personality disorder and psychopathology in Tourette's syndrome: a controlled study. *Br. J. Psychiatry* **171,** 283–286.
65. Frankel, M., Cummings, J.L., Robertson, M.M., Trimble, M.R., Hill, M.A., and Benson, D.F. (1986) Obsessions and compulsions in Gilles de la Tourette's syndrome. *Neurology* **36,** 378–382.
66. Pitman, R.K., Green, R.C., Jenike, M.A., and Mesulam, M.M. (1987) Clinical comparison of Tourette's disorder and obsessive-compulsive disorder. *Am. J. Psychiatry* **144,** 1166–1171.
67. George, M.S., Trimble, M.R., Ring, H.A., Sallee, F.R., and Robertson, M.M. (1993) Obsessions in obsessive compulsive disorder with and without Gilles de la Tourette's syndrome. *Am. J. Psychiatry* **150,** 93–96.
68. Holzer, J.C., Goodman, W.K., McDougle, C.J., et al. (1994) Obsessive-compulsive disorder with and without a chronic tic disorder. A comparison of symptoms in 70 patients. *Br. J. Psychiatry* **164,** 469–473.
69. Leckman, J.F., Grice, D.E., Barr, L.D., et al. (1994-5) Tic-related vs. non-tic-related obsessive compulsive disorder. *Anxiety* **1,** 208–215.
70. Muller, N., Putz, A., Kathmann, N. et al. (1997) Characteristics of obsessive compulsive symptoms in Tourette's syndrome, Obsessive compulsive disorder and Parkinson's disease. *Psychiatr. Res.* **70,** 105–114.
71. Eapen, V., Robertson, M.M., Alsobrook, J.P., and Pauls, D.L. (1997) Obsessive compulsive symptoms in Gilles de la Tourette syndrome and obsessive compulsive disorder: differences by diagnosis and family history. *Am. J. Med. Genet.* **74,** 432–438.
72. Miguel, E.C., Baer, L., Coffey, B.J., et al. (1997) Phenomenological differences appearing with repetitive behaviours in obsessive-compulsive disorder and Gilles de la Tourette's syndrome. *Br. J. Psychiatry* **170,** 140–145.

73. Zohar, A.H., Pauls, D.L., Ratzoni, G., et al. (1997) Obsessive-compulsive disorder with and without tics in an epidemiological sample of adolescents. *Am. J. Psychiatry* **154,** 274–276.
74. Petter, T., Richter, M.A., and Sandor, P. (1998) Clinical features distinguishing patients with Tourette's syndrome and obsessive compulsive disorder from patients with obsessive compulsive disorder without tics. *J. Clin. Psychiatry* **59,** 456–459.
75. Swerdlow, N.R., Zinner, S., and Farber, R.H. (1999) Symptoms in obsessive-compulsive disorder and Tourette syndrome: a spectrum? *CNS Spectrums* **4,** 21–23.
76. Leckman, J.F., Walker, D.E., Goodman, W.K., Pauls, D.L., and Cohen, D.J. (1994) "Just right" perceptions associated with compulsive behavior in Tourette's syndrome. *Am. J. Psychiatry* **151,** 675–680.
77. Hebebrand, J., Klug, B., Fimmers, R., et al. (1997) Rates for tic disorders and obsessive compulsive symptomatology in families of children and adolescents with Gilles de la Tourette syndrome. *J. Psychiatr. Res.* **31,** 519–530.
78. Guarda, A.S., Treasure, J., and Robertson, M.M. (1999) Eating disorders and Tourette syndrome: a case series of comorbidity and associated obsessive-compulsive symptomatology. *CNS Spectrums* 4 **92,** 77–86.
79. Kurlan, R., Behr, J., Medved, L., et al. (1986) Familial Tourette's syndrome: report of a large pedigree and potential for linkage analysis. *Neurology* **36,** 772–776.
80. Robertson, M.M. and Gourdie, A. (1990) Familial Tourette's syndrome in a large British pedigree. Associated psychopathology, severity, and potential for linkage analysis. *Br. J. Psychiatry* **156,** 515–521.
81. Walkup, J.T., LaBuda, M.C., Singer, H.S., Brown, J., Riddle, M.A., and Hurko, O. (1996) Family study and segregation analysis of Tourette syndrome: evidence for a mixed model of inheritance. *Am. J. Hum. Gen.* **59,** 684–693.
82. Jenkins, R.L. and Ashby, H.B. (1983) Gilles de la Tourette syndrome in identical twins. *Arch. Neurol.* **40,** 249–251.
83. Pauls, D.L. and Leckman, J.F. (1986) The inheritance of Gilles de la Tourette syndrome and associated behaviours. *N. Engl. J. Med.* **315,** 993–997.
84. Elstner, K., Selai, C.E., Trimble, M.R., and Robertson, M.M. (2001) Quality of Life (QOL) of patients with Gilles de la Tourette's syndrome. *Acta Psych. Scand.* **103,** 52–59.
85. Cummings, J.L. and Frankel, M. (1985) Gilles de la Tourette syndrome and the neurological basis of obsessions and compulsions. *Biol. Psychiatry* **20,** 1117–1126.
86. Leckman, J.F., Zhang, H., Vitale, A., et al. (1998) Course of tic severity in Tourette syndrome: the first two decades. *Pediatrics* **102,** 14–19.
87. Pitman, R.K. and Jenike, M.A. (1988) Coprolalia in obsessive-compulsive disorder: a missing link. *J. Nerv. Ment. Dis.* **176,** 311–313.
88. Bornstein, R.A. (1991) Neuropsychological correlates of obsessive characteristics in Tourette syndrome. *J. Neuropsychiatry* **3,** 157–162.
89. Leonard, H.L., Lenin, M.C., Swedo, S.E., Rettew, D.C., Gershon, E.S., and Rapoport, J.L. (1992) Tics and Tourette's disorder: a 2 to 7 year follow-up of 54 obsessive-compulsive children. *Am. J. Psychiatry* **149,** 1244–1251.
90. Pitman, R.K. (1987) Pierre Janet on obsessive-compulsive disorder (1903); review and commentary. *Arch. Gen. Psychiatry* **44,** 226–232.
91. Kessler, R.C., Zhao, S., Blazer, D.G., and Swartz, M. (1997) Prevalence, correlates and course of minor depression and major depression in the National Comorbidity Survey. *J. Affect. Disord.* **45,** 19–31.
92. Angold, A. and Costello, E.J. (1995) The epidemiology of depression in children and adolescents, in *The Depressed Child and Adolescent; Developmental and Clinical Perspectives* (Goodyer, I.M., ed.), Cambridge University Press, Cambridge UK, pp. 127–147.
93. Katona, C. and Robertson, M.M. (1998) *Psychiatry at a Glance* (revised ed.), Blackwell Science, Oxford.
94. Akiskal, H.S., Judd, L.L., Gillin, C., and Lemni, H. (1997) Subthreshold depressions: clinical and polysomnographic validation of dysthymic, residual and masked forms. *J. Affect. Disord.* **45,** 53–63.
95. Angst, J. and Merikangas, K. (1997) The depressive spectrum: diagnostic classification and course. *J. Affect. Disord.* **45,** 31–40.
96. Keller, M.B., Hirshfield, R.M.A., and Hanks, D. (1997) Double depression: a distinctive subtype of unipolar depression. *J. Affect. Disord.* **45,** 65–73.
97. Winokur, G. (1997) All roads lead to depression: clinically homogeneous, etiologically heterogeneous. *J. Affect. Disord.* **45,** 97–108.
98. Kovacs, M. (1997) A controlled family history study of childhood-onset depressive disorder. *Arch. Gen. Psychiatry* **54,** 613–623.
99. Brown, G.W. and Harris, T. (1978) *The Social Origins of Depression*, Tavistock Press, London, UK.
100. Paykel, E., Myers, J.K., and Dienelt, M.N. (1969) Life events and depression; a controlled study. *Arch. Gen. Psychiatry* **32,** 327–333.
101. Katona, C. (1999) From the periphery to the core: a Cook's tour of affective disorders. *Curr. Opin. Psychiatry* **12,** 67–68.
102. Stefl, M.E. (1984) Mental health needs associated with Tourette syndrome. *Am. J. Public Health* **74,** 1310–1313.
103. Ferrari, M., Matthews, W.S., and Barabas, G. (1984) Children with Tourette syndrome: results of psychological tests given prior to drug treatment. *J. Dev. Behav. Pediatr.* **5,** 116–119.
104. Grossman, H.Y., Mostofsky, D.I., and Harrison, R.H. (1986) Psychological aspects of Gilles de la Tourette syndrome. *J. Clin. Psychol.* **42,** 228–235.
105. Erenberg, G., Cruse, R.P., and Rothner, A.D. (1987) The natural history of Tourette syndrome: a follow-up study. *Ann. Neurol.* **22,** 383–385.
106. Wand, R.R., Matazow, G.S., Shady, G.A., Furer, P., and Staley, D. (1993) Tourette syndrome: associated symptoms and most disabling features. *Neurosci. Biobehav. Rev.* **17,** 271–275.

107. Rosenberg, L.A., Brown, J., and Singer, H.S. (1995) Behavioral problems and severity of tics. *J. Clin. Psychology* **51,** 760–767.
108. Comings, D.E. and Comings, B.G. (1987c) A controlled study of Tourette syndrome, V; depression and mania. *Am. J. Hum. Genet.* **41,** 804–821.
109. Wodrich, D.L., Benjamin, E., and Lachar, D. (1997) Tourette's syndrome and psychopathology in a child psychiatry setting. *J. Am. Acad. Child Adolesc. Psychiatry* **36,** 1618–1624.
110. Pauls, D.L., Leckman, J.F., and Cohen, D.J. (1994) Evidence against a genetic relationship between Tourette's syndrome and anxiey, depression, panic and phobic disorders. *Br. J. Psychiatry* **164,** 215–221.
111. Spencer, T., Biederman, J., Harding, M., Wilens, T., and Faraone, S. (1995) The relationship between tic disorders and Tourette's syndrome revisited. *J. Am. Acad. Child Adolesc. Psychiatry* **34,** 1133–1139.
112. Carter, A.S., O'Donnell, D.A., Schultz, R.T., Scahill, L., Leckman, J.F., and Pauls, D.L. (2000) Social and emotional adjustment in children affected with Gilles de la Tourette's syndrome: associations with ADHD and family functioning. *J. Child Psychol. Psychiatry* **41,** 215–223.
113. Hamilton, M. (1969) Standardised assessment and recording of depressive symptoms. *Psychiatr. Neurol. Neurochir.* **72,** 201–205.
114. Schwab, J.J., Bialow, M.R., and Holzer, C.E. (1967) A comparison of two rating scales for depression. *J. Clin. Psychology* **23,** 94–99.
115. Williams, J.G., Baslow, D.H., and Agras, W.S. (1972) Behavioural measurement of severe depression. *Arch. Gen. Psychiatry* **27,** 330–333.
116. Zimmerman, M., Coryell, W., and Pfohl, B. (1986) Validity of familial subtypes of primary unipolar depression: clinical, demographic and psychosocial correlations. *Arch. Gen. Psychiatry* **43,** 1090–1096.
117. Strober, M. (1995) Family-genetic aspects of juvenile affective disorders, in *The Depressed Child and Adolescent; Developmental and Clinical Perspectives* (Goodyer, I.M., ed.), Cambridge University Press, New York, pp. 149–170.
118. Robertson, M.M. (1994) Annotation: Gilles de la Tourette syndrome—an update. *J. Child Psychol. Psychiatry* **35,** 597–611.
119. Caine, E.D. and Polinsky, R.J. (1979) Haloperidol-induced dysphoria in patients with Tourette syndrome. *Am. J. Psychiatry* **136,** 1216–1217.
120. Regeur, L., Pakkenberg, B., Fog, R., and Pakkenberg, H. (1986) Clinical features and long-term treatment with pimozide in 65 patients with Gilles de la Tourette's syndrome. *J. Neurol. Neurosurg. Psychiatry* **49,** 791–795.
121. Bruun, R.D. (1984) Gilles de la Tourette's syndrome: an overview of clinical experience. *J. Am. Acad. Child Adolesc. Psychiatry* **23,** 126–133.
122. Chouza, C., Romero, S., Lorenzo, J., et al. (1982) [Clinical trial of tiapride in patients with dyskinesia (author's transl).] *Sem. Hop.* **58,** 725–733.
123. Robertson, M.M., Schnieden, V., and Lees, A.J. (1990) Management of Gilles de la Tourette syndrome using sulpiride. *Clin. Neuropharmacol.* **13,** 229–235.
124. Salmon, G., James, A., and Smith, D.M. (1998) Bullying in schools: self-reported anxiety, depression and self-esteem in secondary school children. *BMJ* 924–925.
125. Bond, L., Carlin, J.B., Thomas, L., Kerryn, R., and Patton, G. (2001) Does bullying cause emotional problems? A prospective study of young teenagers. *BMJ* **7311,** 480–484.
126. Berkson, J. (1946) Limitations of the application of fourfold table analysis to hospital data. *Biometrics* **2,** 47–51.
127. Millberger, S., Biederman, J., Faraone, S.V., Murphy, J., and Tsuang, M.T. (1995) Attention deficit disorder and comorbid disorders: issues of overlapping symptoms. *Am. J. Psychiatry* **152,** 1793–1799.
128. Malkoff-Schwartz, S., Frank, E., Anderson, B., et al. (1998) Stressful life events and social rhythm disruption in the onset of manic and depressive bipolar episodes; a preliminary investigation. *Arch. Gen. Psychiatry* **55,** 702–707.
129. Burd, L. and Kerbeshian, J. (1984) Gilles de la Tourette's syndrome and bipolar disorder. *Arch. Neurol.* **41,** 1236.
130. Kerbeshian, J. and Burd, L. (1989) Tourette disorder and bipolar symptomatology in childhood and adolescence. *Can. J. Psychiatry* **34,** 230–233.
131. Kerbeshian, J.B., Burd, L., and Klug, M. (1995) Comorbid Tourette's disorder and bipolar disorder: an etiologic perspective. *Am. J. Psychiatry* **152,** 1646.
132. Berthier, M.L., Kulisevsky, J., and Campos, V.M. (1998) Bipolar disorder in adult patients with Tourette's syndrome: a clinical study. *Biol. Psychiatry* **43,** 364–370.
133. Swanson, J.M., Sergeant, J.A., Taylor, E., Sonuga-Barke, E.J.S., Jensen, P.S., and Cantwell, D.P. (1998) Attention-deficit hyperactivity disorder and hyperkinetic disorder. *Lancet* **351,** 429–433.
134. Towbin, K.E. and Riddle, M.A. (1993) Attention deficit hyperactivity disorder, in *Handbook of Tourette's Syndrome and Related Tic and Behavioral Disorders* (Kurlan, R., ed.), Marcel Dekker, New York.
135. Taylor, E., Sergeant, J., Doepfner, M., et al. (1998) Clinical guidelines for hyperkinetic disorder. *Eur. Child Adolesc. Psychiatry* **7,** 184–2000.
136. Nadder, T.S., Silberg, J., Rutter, M., Maes, H.H., and Eaves, L.J. (2001) Comparison of multiple measures of ADHD symptomatology: a multivariate genetic analysis. *J. Child Psychol. Psychiatry* **42,** 475–486.
137. Palmer, E.D. and Finger, S. (2001) An early description of ADHD (inattentive subtype): Dr. Alexander Crichton and "mental restlessness" (1798). *Child Psychol. Psychiatr. Rev.* **6,** 66–73.
138. Shapiro, A.K., Shapiro, E., and Wayne, H.L. (1973a) The symptomatology and diagnosis of Gilles de la Tourette's syndrome. *J. Am. Acad. Child Psychiatry* **12,** 702–723.

139. Shapiro, A.K., Shapiro, E., Wayne, H.L., Clarkin, J., and Bruun, R.D. (1973b) Tourette's syndrome; summary of data on 34 patients. *Psychosom. Med.* **35,** 419–435.
140. Freeman, R.D. (1997) Attention deficit hyperactivity disorder in the presence of Tourette syndrome. *Neurol. Clin.* **15,** 411–420.
141. Lieh Mak, F., Chung, S.Y., Lee, P., et al. (1982) Tourette syndrome in the Chinese: a follow-up of 15 cases, in *Gilles de la Tourette Syndrome, Adv. Neurol. 35* (Friedhoff, A.J. and Chase, T.N., ed.), Raven Press, New York.
142. Robertson, M.M. and Eapen, V. (1992) Current controversies in the use of stimulant medication in GTS. *Clin. Neuropharmacol.* **15,** 408–425.
143. Walkup, J.T., Khan, S., Schuerholz, L., Paik, Y.-S., Leckman, J.F., and Schultz, R.T. (1999) Phenomenology and natural history of tic-related ADHD and learning disabilities, in *Tourette's Syndrome: Tics, Obsessions, Compulsions. Developmental Psychopathology and Clinical Care* (Leckman, J.F. and Cohen, D.J., eds.), John Wiley & Sons, New York.
144. Apter, A., Pauls, D.L., Bleich, A., Zohar, A.H., Kron, S., and Ratzoni, G. (1993) An epidemiological study of Gilles de la Tourette's syndrome in Israel. *Arch. Gen. Psychiatry* **50,** 734–738.
145. Robertson, M.M., Verrill, M., Mercer, M., James, B., and Pauls, D.L. (1994) The Gilles de la Tourette syndrome in New Zealand: a postal survey. *Br. J. Psychiatry* **164,** 263–266.
146. Mason, A., Banerjee, S., Eapen, V., Zietlin, H., and Robertson, M.M. (1998) The prevalence of Tourette syndrome in a mainstream school population. *Dev. Med. Child Neurology* **40,** 292–296.
147. Jagger, J., Prusoff, B.A., Cohen, D.J., Kidd, K.K., Carbonari, C.M., and John, K. (1982) The epidemiology of Tourette's syndrome: a pilot study. *Schizophr. Bull.* **8,** 267–278.
148. Singer, H.S., Schuerholz, L.J., and Denckla, M.B. (1995) Learning difficulties in children with Tourette syndrome. *J. Child Neurol.* **10(Suppl. 1),** S58–S61.
149. Spencer, T., Biederman, J., Harding, M., et al. (1998) Disentangling the overlap between Tourette's disorder and ADHD. *J. Child Psychol. Psychiatry* **39,** 1037–1044.
150. Spencer, T., Biederman, J., Coffey, B., Geller, D., Wilens, T., and Faraone, S. (1999) The 4-year course of tic disorders in boys with attention-deficit/hyperactivity disorder. *Arch. Gen. Psychiatry* **56,** 842–847.
151. Weiss, G., Hechtman, L., Milroy, T., and Perlman, T. (1985) Psychiatric status of hyperactives as adults: a controlled prospective 15-year follow-up of 63 hyperactive children. *J. Am. Acad. Child Psychiatry* **24,** 211–220.
152. Mannuzza, S., Klein, R.G., Bessler, A., Malloy, P., and LaPadula, M. (1993) Adult outcome of hyperactive boys: educational achievement, occupational rank, and psychiatric status. *Arch. Gen. Psychiatry* **50,** 565–576.
153. Mannuzza, S., Klein, R.G., Bessler, A., Malloy, P., and LaPadula, M. (1998) Adult psychiatric status of hyperactive boys grown up. *Am. J. Psychiatry* **155,** 493–498.
154. Comings, D.E. and Comings, B.G. (1984) Tourette's syndrome and attention deficit disorder with hyperactivity: are they genetically related? *J. Am. Acad. Child Adolesc. Psychiatry* **23,** 138–146.
155. Knell, E.R. and Comings, D.E. (1993) Tourette's syndrome and attention-deficit hyperactivity disorder: evidence for a genetic relationship. *J. Clin. Psychiatry* **54,** 331–337.
156. Pauls, et al. 1988.
157. Eapen, V. and Robertson, M.M. (1996) Gilles de la Tourette syndrome and attention deficit disorder—no evidence for a genetic relationship. *J. Neuropsychiatry Neuropsychol. Behav. Neurol.* **9,** 192–196.
158. Pauls, D.L., Leckman, J.F., and Cohen, D.J. (1993) Familial relationship between Gilles de la Tourette syndrome, attention deficit hyperactivity disorder, learning disabilities, speech disorders and stuttering. *J. Am. Acad. Child Adolesc. Psychiatry* **32,** 1044–1050.
159. Bruun, R. and Budman, C. (1998) Paroxetine as a treatment for anger attacks in patients with Tourette syndrome. *J. Clin. Psychiatry* **59,** 581–588.
160. Budman, C., Park, K., Olson, M., and Bruun, R. (1998) Rage attacks in children and adolescents with Tourette syndrome. A pilot study. *J. Clin. Psychiatry* **59,** 576–580.
161. Budman, C., Bruun, R., Park, K., Lesser, M., and Olson, M. (2000) Explosive outbursts in children with Tourette's disorder. *J. Am. Acad. Child Adolesc. Psychiatry* **39,** 1270–1276.
162. Coffey, B., Biederman, J., Smoller, J., Geller, D., Schwartz, S., and Kim, G. (2000) Anxiety disorders and tic severity in juveniles with Tourette's disorder. *J. Am. Acad. Child Adolesc. Psychiatry* **39,** 526–568.
163. Budman, C., Feirmen, L., Bruun, R., Shi, Q., Lesser, M., and Olson, M. (2001) Clinical correlates of rage in Tourette syndrome. Abstract no. 6: International Symposium on Tourette Syndrome and other Neurodevelopmental Disorders, May 31–June 2, 2001, Toronto Canada.
164. Corbett, M.A., Mathews, A.M., Connell, P.H., and Shapiro, D.A. (1969) Tics and Gilles de la Tourette's syndrome: a follow-up and critical review. *Br. J. Psychiatry* **115,** 1229–1241.
165. Coffey, B., Frazier, J., and Chen, S. (1992) Comorbidity, Tourette syndrome, and anxiety disorders. *Adv. Neurol.* **58,** 95–104.
166. Chee, K.Y. and Sachdev, P. (1994) The clinical features of Tourette's disorder: an Australian study using a structured interview schedule. *Austr. N. Z. J. Psychiatry* **28,** 313–318.
167. Thibert, A.L., Day, H.I., and Sandor, P. (1995) Self-concept and self-consciousness in adults with Tourette syndrome. *Can. J. Psychiatry* **40,** 35–39.
168. Carter, A.S., Pauls, D.L., Leckman, J.F., and Cohen, D.J. (1994) A prospective longitudinal study of Gilles de la Tourette's syndrome. *J. Am. Acad. Child Adolesc. Psychiatry* **33,** 377–385.
169. Baron-Cohen, S. and Bolton, P. (1995) *Autism: The Facts*, Oxford University Press, Oxford, UK.

170. Stern, J.S. and Robertson, M.M. (1997) Tics associated with autistic and pervasive developmental disorders. *Neurol. Clin.* **15,** 345–355.
171. Baron-Cohen, S., Mortimore, C., Moriarty, J., Izaguirre, J., and Robertson, M. (1999a) The prevalence of Gilles de la Tourette's syndrome in children and adolescents with autism. *J. Child Psychol. Psychiatry* **40,** 213–218.
172. Baron-Cohen, S., Scahill, V.L., Izaguirre, J., Hornsey, H., and Robertson, M.M. (1999b) The prevalence of Gilles de la Tourette syndrome in children and adolescents with autism: a large scale study. *Psychol. Med.* **29,** 1151–1159.
173. Sverd, J. (2001) Comorbid pervasive developmental disorder and Tourette's disorder: frequency of cases presenting to a state children's psychiatric hospital. Abstract no. 7: International Symposium on Tourette Syndrome and other Neurodevelopmental Disorders, May 31–June 2, 2001, Toronto Canada.
174. Robins, L.N. (1978) Sturdy childhood predictors of adult antisocial behaviour: replications from longitudinal studies. *Psychol. Med.* **8,** 611–622.
175. Zoccolillo, M., Pickles, A., Quinton, D., and Rutter, M. (1992) The outcome of childhood conduct disorder: implications for defining adult personality disorder and conduct disorder. *Psychol. Med.* **22,** 971–986.
176. Tremblay, R.E., Pihl, R.O., Vitaro, F., and Dobkin, P.L. (1994) Predicting early onset of male antisocial behavior from preschool behaviour. *Arch. Gen. Psychiatry* **51,** 732–739.
177. Fergusson, D.M., Lynskey, M.T., and Horwood, L.J. (1997) Attentional difficulties in middle childhood and psychosocial outcomes in young adulthood. *J. Child Psychol. Psychiatry* **38,** 633–644.
178. Babinski, L.M., Hartsough, C.S., and Lambert, N.M. (1999) Childhood conduct problems, hyperactivity-impulsivity, and inattention as predicators of adult criminal activity. *J. Child Psychol. Psychiatry* **40,** 347–355.
179. Stevenson, J. and Goodman, R. (2001) Association between behaviour at age 3 years and adult criminality. *Br. J. Psychiatry* **179,** 197–202.
180. Hofstra, M.B., van der Ende, J., and Verhulst, F.C. (2001) Adolsecents' self-reported problems as predictors of psychopathology in adulthood: 10-year follow-up study. *Br. J. Psychiatry* **179,** 203–209.
181. Fombonne, E., Wostear, G., Cooper, R., Harrington, R., and Rutter, M. (2001a) The Maudsley long-term follow-up of child and adolescent depression. 1. Psychiatric outcomes in adulthood. *Br. J. Psychiatry* **179,** 210–217.
182. Fombonne, E., Wostear, G., Cooper, R., Harrington, R., and Rutter, M. (2001b) The Maudsley long-term follow-up of child and adolescent depression. 2. Suicidality, criminality and social dysfunction in adulthood. *Br. J. Psychiatry* **179,** 218–223.

34
In Search of the Pathophysiology of Tourette Syndrome

James F. Leckman, MD

1. INTRODUCTION

Despite the overt nature of tics and several decades of scientific scrutiny, ignorance concerning the pathophysiology of Tourette syndrome (TS) and other tic disorders remains profound. Notions of cause have ranged from an "irritation of the motor neural systems by toxic substances, of a self-poisoning bacteriological origin" to "hereditary degeneration" to "a constitutional inferiority of the subcortical structures …[that] renders the individual defenseless against overwhelming emotional and dynamic forces" *(1)*. Predictably, each of these etiological explanations has prompted new treatments and ways of relating to families. This chapter reviews the various risk factors that have been implicated in the development of TS before critically reviewing three current theories of TS pathogenesis.

2. RISK FACTORS

During the course of the past decade, TS and related conditions have emerged as model disorders for researchers interested in the interaction of genetic, neurobiological, and environmental (epigenetic) factors that shape clinical outcomes from health to chronic disability over the life span *(2)*.

2.1. Genetic Factors

Twin and family studies provide evidence that genetic factors are involved in the vertical transmission within families of a vulnerability to TS and related disorders *(3)*. The concordance rate for TS among monozygotic twin pairs is greater than 50%, whereas the concordance of dizygotic twin pairs is about 10% *(4,5)*. If co-twins with chronic motor tic disorder are included, these concordance figures increase to 77% for monozygotic and 30% for dizygotic twin pairs. Differences in the concordance of monozygotic and dizygotic twin pairs indicate that genetic factors play an important role in the etiology of TS and related conditions. These figures also suggest that nongenetic factors are critical in determining the nature and severity of the clinical syndrome.

At present, the nature of the vulnerability genes that predispose individuals to develop TS are unknown. The pattern of vertical transmission among family members is suggestive of major gene effects, and segregation analyses are consistent with models of autosomal transmission *(3,6)*. These findings have prompted the identification of large multigenerational families for genetic linkage studies. Historically, efforts to identify susceptibility genes within these high-density families using traditional linkage strategies have met with limited success *(7)*. More recently, investigators studying a large French Canadian family have reported evidence for linkage on chromosome 11 (11q23) *(8)*.

Recently, nonparametric approaches using families, in which two or more siblings are affected with TS, have been undertaken *(9)*. This sib-pair approach is suited for diseases with an unclear mode of

From: *Mental and Behavioral Dysfunction in Movement Disorders*
Edited by: M-A. Bédard et al. © Humana Press Inc., Totowa, NJ

inheritance and has been used successfully in studies of other complex disorders, such as diabetes mellitus and essential hypertension. In this study, two areas are suggestive of linkage to TS, one on chromosome 4q and another on chromosome 8p.

Identity-by-descent (IBD) approaches have also been utilized in population isolates in South Africa and Costa Rica. The South African study implicated regions near the centromere of chromosome 2, as well as on 6p, 8q, 11q, 14q, 20q, and 21q *(10)*. Of interest, the 11q marker in the French Canadian family that was associated with the highest logarithm of the odds (LOD) score was the same marker for which significant linkage disequilibrium with TS was recently detected in the Afrikaner population of South Africa.

It is also noteworthy that none of the chromosomal regions (3 [3p21.3], 8 [8q21.4], 9 [9pter], and 18 [18q22.3]), in which cytogenetic abnormalities have been found to co-segregate with TS, showed any convincing evidence for linkage in the high density families, the sib-pair study, or the IBD studies.

Finally, a number of candidate genes have been evaluated in TS, including various dopamine receptors (DRD1, DRD2, DRD4, and DRD5), the dopamine transporter, various noradrenergic genes (ADRA2a, ADRA2C, and DBH), and a smaller number of serotoninergic genes (5-HTT). To date, none of the reported associations have been replicated, and it appears unlikely that genetic variation at these loci is a major source of vulnerability to TS, although major single gene effects may be present in specific kindreds.

Future progress is anticipated, and clarity about the nature and normal expression of even a few of the TS susceptibility genes is likely to provide a major step forward in understanding the pathogenesis of this condition.

2.2. Epigenetic Risk Factors

A number of epigenetic factors have also been implicated in the pathogenesis of TS, and these include pre- and perinatal adverse events, sex-specific hormonal factors, psychosocial stressors, and immune-based mechanisms *(2)*.

2.2.1. Pre- and Perinatal Events

Interest on the potential role of adverse perinatal events in the pathogenesis of TS dates from the report of Pasamanick and Kawi who found that mothers of children with tics were 1.5 times more likely to have experienced a complication during pregnancy than the mothers of children without tics *(11)*. Other investigations have reported that among monozygotic twins discordant for TS, the index twins with TS uniformly had lower birth weights than their unaffected co-twins *(5,12)*. Severity of maternal life stress during pregnancy, severe nausea, and/or vomiting during the first trimester have also emerged as potential risk factors in the development of tic disorders *(13)*. In 1997, Whitaker and coworkers reported that premature and low birth weight children are at increased risk of developing tic disorders and attention deficit hyperactivity disorder (ADHD) *(14)*. This appears to be especially true of children who had ischemic parenchymal brain lesions. More recently, Burd and colleagues *(15)* presented the results of a case control study in which low Apgar scores at 5 min and more prenatal visits were associated with a higher risk of TS. Finally, there is limited evidence that smoking and alcohol use, as well as forceps delivery, can predispose individuals with a vulnerability to TS to develop comorbid obsessive–compulsive disorder (OCD) *(16)*.

2.2.2. Sex-Specific Risk Factors

Males are more frequently affected than females with TS *(17)*. Although this could be due to genetic mechanisms, frequent male-to-male transmissions within families appear to rule out the presence of an X-linked vulnerability gene. This observation has led us to hypothesize that androgenic steroids act at key developmental periods to influence the natural history of TS and related disorders *(18)*. These developmental periods include the prenatal period when the brain is being formed, adrenarche when adrenal androgens first appear at age 5–7 yr and puberty. Androgenic steroids may be responsible for these effects, or they may act indirectly through estrogens formed in key brain regions by the aromatization of testosterone.

The importance of gender differences in expression of associated phenotypes is also clear given the observation that women are more likely than men to develop obsessive–compulsive symptoms without concomitant tics *(19)* and that boys are much more likely than girls to display disruptive behaviors *(20)*. Surges in testosterone and other androgenic steroids during critical periods in fetal development are known to be involved in the production of long-term functional augmentation of subsequent hormonal challenges (as in adrenarche and during puberty) and in the formation of structural central nervous system (CNS) dimorphisms *(21)*. In recent years, several sexually dimorphic brain regions have been described, including portions of the amygdala (and related limbic areas) and the hypothalamus (including the medial preoptic area that mediates the body's response to thermal stress) *(22)*. These regions contain high levels of androgen and estrogen receptors and are known to influence activity in the basal ganglia both directly and indirectly *(23)*. Indeed, a proportion of TS patients appear to be uniquely sensitive to thermal stress, such that when their core body temperature increases and they begin to sweat, their tics increase *(24)*. It is also of note that some of the neurochemical and neuropeptidergic systems implicated in TS and related disorders, such as dopamine, serotonin, and the opioids, are involved with these regions and appear to be regulated by sex-specific factors.

2.2.3. *Psychosocial Stress*

Tic disorders have long been identified as "stress-sensitive" conditions *(17,25,26)*. Typically, symptom exacerbations follow in the wake of stressful life events. As noted by Shapiro and colleagues *(17)*, these events need not be adverse in character. Clinical experience suggests that, in some unfortunate instances, a vicious cycle is initiated in which tic symptoms are misunderstood by the family and teachers. This can lead, in turn, to active attempts to suppress the symptoms by punishment and humiliation. These efforts can lead to more stress and a further exacerbation of symptoms. Unchecked, this vicious cycle can lead to the most severe manifestations of TS and dysthymia, as well as maladaptive characterological traits. Although psychological factors are insufficient to cause TS, the intimate association of the content and timing of tic behaviors and dynamically important events in the lives of children make it difficult to overlook their contribution to the intramorbid course of these disorders *(27,28)*.

2.2.4. *Immune-Based Mechanisms*

Recent attention has focused on the possible role of poststreptococcal autoimmune phenomena in the development of TS. Speculation concerning the postinfectious (or at least the post-rheumatic fever [RF]) etiology for tic disorder symptoms dates from the late 1800s *(1)*. It is well established that group A β-hemolytic streptococci (GABHS) can trigger immune-mediated disease in genetically predisposed individuals. Acute RF is a delayed sequela of GABHS, occurring approx 3 wk following an inadequately treated upper respiratory tract infection. RF is characterized with inflammatory lesions involving the joints, heart, and/or CNS. Sydenham's chorea (SC) and TS share common anatomic areas, the basal ganglia of the brain and the related cortical and thalamic sites. Furthermore, some SC patients display motor and vocal tics, obsessive–compulsive, and ADHD symptoms, suggesting the possibility that, at least in some instances, these disorders share a common etiology. As in SC, antineural antibodies have been reported to be elevated in the sera of some patients with TS *(29–31)*. It has been proposed that pediatric autoimmune neuropsychiatric disorder associated with streptococcal infection (PANDAS) represents a distinct clinical entity and includes SC and some cases of TS and OCD. Further suggestive evidence comes from Swedo and colleagues, who reported that, in children who met PANDAS criteria, GABHS infection was likely to have preceded neuropsychiatric symptom onset for 44% of the children, whereas pharyngitis (no culture obtained) preceded onset for another 28% of the children *(32)*.

Although the etiological significance of the antineuronal antibodies and the association with prior GABHS infections remains a topic of considerable debate *(33)*, preliminary data from animal model systems provide limited support for the molecular mimicry hypothesis *(34,35)*, and therapeutic in-

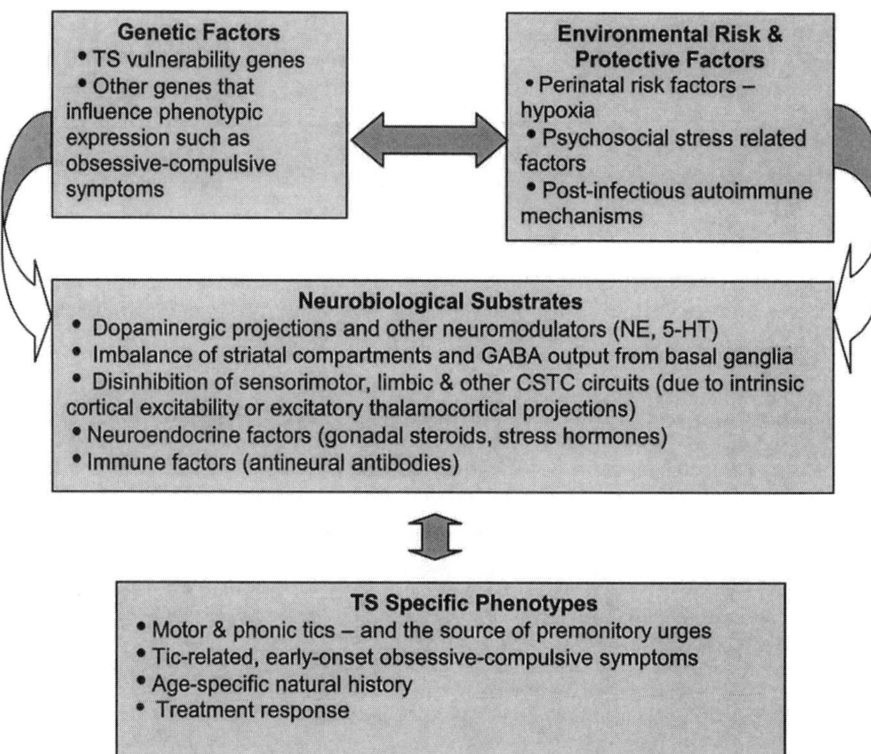

Fig. 1. Working model of TS pathogenesis. Unique features of this model include the role of the TS-specific genes (G_{TS}) and their putative interrelationship with the environmental factors that are active early in CNS development (RP_{PN}). A crucial question remains: do the TS vulnerability genes in any way set the stage for any of the perinatal risk factors or are they separate and independent mechanisms? Heuristically, it may be useful to consider that specific vulnerability TS genes are themselves involved in the development or remodeling of the CSTC circuits.

terventions based on this putative mechanism also show promise *(36)*. Further, if specific immunological alterations are associated with onset or acute clinical exacerbations, then the nature of these alterations should provide insight as to the genetic, neuroanatomic, and immunological mechanisms involved. This knowledge may provide a basis for the rational design of therapeutic and preventative interventions.

3. MODELS OF PATHOGENESIS

Figure 1 presents a general model of TS pathogenesis that emphasizes the likely role of gene–environment interactions taking place over the course of CNS development.

3.1. Dopaminergic Theories

Involvement of dopaminergic systems in the basal ganglia have long been suspected to be of etiologic importance in TS. Inputs from ascending dopamine pathways originating in the substania nigra, pars compacta, play a crucial role in coordinating the output from the striatum *(37)*. Explicit "dopamine" hypotheses for TS posit either an excess of dopamine or an increased sensitivity of D2 dopamine receptors. These hypotheses are consistent with multiple lines of empirical evidence. First, data implicating central dopaminergic mechanisms include the results of double-blind clinical trials in which haloperidol, pimozide, tiapride, and other neuroleptics, which preferentially block dopaminergic D2 receptors, have been found to be effective in the temporary suppression of tics for a majority of patients *(2)*. Second, tic suppression has also been reported following administration of agents such as tetrabenazine, which reduce dopamine synthesis *(17)*. Third, increased tics have been reported following withdrawal of neuroleptics or following exposure to agents that increase central dopaminergic activity, such as levadopa (L-dopa) and CNS stimulants, including cocaine *(38)*. Fourth, preliminary positron emission tomography (PET) studies of brain dopamine D2 receptors provide some evidence that the density and/or binding of D2 receptors in the striatum are associated with current levels of tic severity *(39,40)*. Finally, postmortem brain and ligand-based neuroimaging studies have reported alterations in the number or affinity of presynaptic dopamine carrier sites in the striatum *(41,42)* or the presynaptic processing of dopamine *(43)*. However, a recent assessment of the number of striatal vesicular monoamine transporter type-2 sites found no differences between TS patients and controls *(44)*.

Recently, another line of evidence has emerged that may clarify some aspects of the role of dopaminergic neurotransmission in the pathophysiology and natural history of TS. Clinical studies have documented that motor and phonic tics occur in bouts over the course of a day and wax and wane in severity over the course of weeks to months. There appears to be a "self-similarity" of these temporal patterns across different time scales, and the frequency distribution of inter-tic interval durations follow the inverse power law of temporal scaling *(45)*; observations are consistent with a fractal, nonlinear dynamical system. In addition, first return maps, in which the duration of one inter-tic interval is plotted against the duration of the next inter-tic interval, demonstrate both "burst-like" behavior and short-term periodicity, proving that successive tic intervals are not random events *(45)*. This pattern resembles the temporal patterning of the firing of dopaminergic neurons in the substania nigra *(46)*. A deeper understanding of the multiplicative processes that govern these timing patterns may clarify why tics occur in bouts and why tics wax and wane over the course of months.

In sum, while the evidence that dopaminergic pathways are intimately involved in the pathobiology of TS is compelling, the exact nature of the abnormality remains to be elucidated. It is also possible that, while the timing and expression of tics may be mediated by dopaminergic activity, the ultimate causes of TS may lie elsewhere.

3.2. The Formation of Habits and a Possible Imbalance in Striatal Compartments

Alterations in the function of the basal ganglia have long been thought to be key in understanding the pathophysiology of TS and related disorders *(47)*. The motor, sensorimotor, association, and inhibitory neural circuits that course through the basal ganglia are commonly referred to by their successive processing components and are, therefore, called "corticostriatothalamocortical" (CSTC) circuits. CSTC circuits are composed of multiple, partially overlapping, but largely "parallel" circuits that direct information from the cerebral cortex to the subcortex and then back again to specific cortical regions *(48–50)*.

Recently, Graybiel and colleagues have reviewed evidence that the basal ganglia contribute to habit and stimulus-response learning in animal model systems (see ref. *51* and Chapter 4 of this book). If habits are coordinated ensembles of thought and action, then conceptually, tics or stereotypies may be best seen as those prewired bits of behavior that are available to be assembled into habits *(2)*. Like habits, tic action sequences often arise from a heightened and selective sensitivity to environmental cues from within the body or from the outside world. These perceptual cues include faint premonitory feelings or urges that are relieved with the performance of tics and a need to perform tics or compulsions until they are felt to be "just right" *(52)*. Although the neural mechanisms that produce tics have yet to be precisely described, preliminary evidence suggests that they involve the same structures that underlie habit formation.

Ensemble recordings, in which the activity of multiple medium spiny neurons are recorded simultaneously, have begun to clarify the role of the striatum and related brain circuits in the learning and production of habitual or "automatic" behavioral responses such as tics. For example, Jog, Graybiel, and colleagues have recorded from ensembles of electrodes in the sensorimotor areas of rat striatum

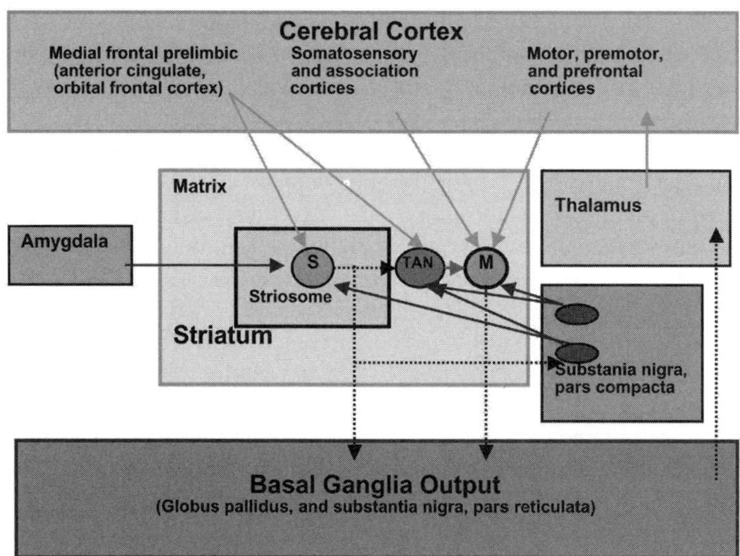

Fig. 2. Cortical-subcortical circuits implicated in tics and stereotypies. Schematic diagram illustrating the organization of the striatum and cortical-subcortical circuits *(37)*. Animal models indicate that the MSP neurons of the striatum exist within two closely intertwined compartments, striosomes (S) and the matrix (M). These two compartments differ with respect to their cortical inputs with the striosomal MSP neurons receiving limbic and prelimbic inputs and the MSP neurons in the matrix receiving from ipsilateral primary motor and sensory motor cortices and contralateral primary motor cortices. An imbalance in the functional activity of the MSP neurons within these two compartments has been implicated in stereotypies *(54)*. Similarly, changes in the responsiveness of tonically active neurons (TANs) located at the boundary between striosomes and matrisomes could selectively alter behaviors keyed to specific environmental perturbations. Dopaminergic projection neurons from the pars compacta of the substania nigra appear to tune this system to respond selectively to certain internal somatosensory or external perceptual cues.

during cued learning tasks, and their results demonstrated large-scale changes in recruitment and firing patterns of these neurons *(53)*. Of special interest was the tendency for the number of units firing at the start and end of goal-directed activity to increase asymptotically during successive stages of learning. Tonically active interneurons that are positioned at the interface of the two-striatal compartments (striosomes and matrix) also appear to play a key role in learning and production of habits *(37)*.

In addition, recent animal studies have also indicated that the balance of activity of medium spiny neurons located in the striosomes vs the matrix of the striatum may crucially determine an individual's vulnerability to dopamine-mediated stereotypies *(54)* (see Fig. 2). These stereotypies include a range of repetitive tic-like head and paw movements, as well as repetitive sniffing.

Advances in neuroimaging and neurophysiological techniques have made it possible to examine these circuits in living subjects. In TS, there is preliminary evidence that voluntary tic suppression involves activation of regions of the prefrontal cortex and caudate nucleus and bilateral deactivation of the putamen and globus pallidus *(55)*. If confirmed, these findings are consistent with the well-known finding that chemical or electrical stimulation of inputs into the putamen can provoke motor and vocal responses that resemble tics. They also suggest that prefrontal cortex-basal ganglia circuits participate in shaping of the inhibitory influence of the output neurons in the internal segment of the globus pallidus and the pars reticulata of the substania nigra.

Most functional magnetic resonance imaging (fMRI) studies to date have employed a block design in which the activation–deactivation signal reflects a presumed continuous mental state. More recently, event-related fMRI techniques have been developed that will greatly enhance the temporal resolution of these studies. Work in progress suggests that it should be possible to monitor individual tics as they occur in the magnet. These studies should permit investigators to begin to define the temporal sequence of activity within different portions of these cortical-subcortical loops. In this regard, it will be intriguing to study the involvement of the supplementary motor area as electrical stimulation of the supplementary motor area elicits a variety of bodily sensations, which include premonitory sensations or "urges" to perform a movement or a sense of anticipation that a movement is about to occur *(56)*.

In sum, efforts to clarify the role of the basal ganglia in the learning and production of habits show promise of elucidating the neural systems that underlie tics and compulsions. The importance of perceptual cues in this model is tantalizingly similar to what is known about the premonitory urges that precede tics. Animal models may result that may accelerate basic research on this complex multiplicative system. However, in vivo neuroimaging and neurophysiological studies also emphasize that a full understanding of these processes will depend on a deeper understanding of the roles of the cortex and thalamocortical projections.

3.3. *Intrinsic Cortical Hyperexcitability*

Two recent studies using transcranial magnetic stimulation (TMS) have documented defective paired-pulse inhibition and reduced motor thresholds in TS and early-onset tic-related OCD and suggest possible primary motor cortex abnormalities in these disorders *(57,58)*. That defective intracortical inhibition is found in both early-onset OCD and TS is consistent with the view that the similar and frequently overlapping symptoms and heritability of these two illnesses may reflect common pathophysiology in CSTC circuits *(19,59)*. Pharmacologic studies have shown that intracortical inhibition measured by TMS procedures depends, to a large degree, on a balance between inhibitory γ-amino butyric acid (GABA)ergic and excitatory glutaminergic mechanisms, so that the observed reduced intracortical inhibition could result from activity in thalamocortical inputs producing relatively less GABAergic inhibition or relatively more glutamate-mediated excitation of the cortical output neurons.

The results of neurosurgical treatments *(60,61)* and in vivo neuroimaging studies *(62)* are also highly suggestive that cortical activity *per se* and/or thalamic inputs to the cortex are key to understanding the pathophysiology of TS. For example, Vandewalle and colleagues recently reported that high frequency stimulation of the thalamus resulted in symptomatic improvement in a TS patient *(61)*. In addition, a recent MRI volumetric study found that TS subjects have larger volumes in dorsal prefrontal and parieto-occipital regions *(62)*. Age-specific and sex-specific differences in cortical morphometry were also detected in this large study. The dorsal prefrontal findings may be particularly germane to the neural mechanisms involved in voluntary tic suppression, while the parieto-occipital findings may contribute to a deeper understanding of the visuomotor deficits frequently encountered in TS patients *(63)*.

In sum, defective intracortical inhibition in TS is also consistent with long-standing proposals and recent neuroimaging and neuropsychological data that TS and related disorders involve basal ganglia dysfunction. Because a specific basal ganglia pathogenesis for TS remains to be established, however, other explanations of the TMS findings, including a primary cortical abnormality, remain possible. These data also suggest that medications modulating the GABA/glutamate balance might have therapeutic effects in TS.

4. SPECULATIONS: TOWARD AN INTEGRATED DEVELOPMENTAL THEORY

If tics, like stereotypies, vary according to the balance of activity of medium spiny neurons in the striosome and matrix compartments of the striatum (Fig. 2), then it should be possible to examine the clinical impact of genetic and/or developmental insults that affect the relative number and sensitivity of medium spiny neurons in the two striatal compartments. For example, perinatal ischemic and hypoxic insults involving parenchymal lesions increase the risk of tic disorders eightfold *(14)*. Do they also increase an animal's susceptibility to develop stereotypies in response to psychomotor stimulants? If so, is there evidence of a differential injury to medium spiny neurons in the matrix?

Further, this model may provide a meaningful integration of knowledge about tics drawn from a number of perspectives, including the stress responsiveness of tics (limbic activation), the presence of premonitory sensory urges (as sensory motor and primary motor cortical inputs converge on the fewer medium spiny neurons in the matrix), the reduction of tics when an individual is engaged in acts that require selective attention and guided motor action (heightened activity within the matrix compartment), and the need to "even-up" sensory and motor stimuli in a bilaterally symmetrical fashion (convergence of information from both ipsi- and contralateral primary motor neurons on medium spiny neurons within the matrix). The timing of tics and the course of tic disorders may be reflected in the collective burst firing of dopaminergic neurons *(45)*.

From a developmental perspective, it is clear that many of the GABAergic interneurons of the cerebral cortex migrate tangentially from the same embryonic regions in the ganglionic eminence that also give rise to the GABAergic medium spiny projection (MSP) neurons of the striatum *(64)*. Could adverse events occurring at a specific point in development account for both the striatal imbalance and the intracortical deficits inhibition seen in some patients with TS?

Finally, it is tempting to speculate that in SC and in postinfectious forms of TS, the functional activity of the medium spiny neurons of the matrix is differentially impaired as a result of the autoimmune response. Indeed, one plausible hypothesis is that the antineural antibodies found in a subset of TS patients may modulate synaptic transmission and alter the balance between the striosomal and matrisomal compartments of the striatum.

5. FUTURE PROSPECTS

Current conceptualizations of TS have been shaped by advances in systems neuroscience and the emerging understanding of the role of the basal ganglia in implicit learning and habit formation. Although the evidence that the same mechanisms are involved in both habit formation and tics is circumstantial, recent progress in neuroanatomy, systems neuroscience, and functional in vivo neuroimaging has set the stage for major advances in our understanding of TS. Continued success in these areas will lead to the targeting of specific brain circuits for more intensive study. Diagnostic, treatment, and prognostic advances can also be anticipated, e.g., which circuits are involved and to what degree? How does that degree of involvement affect the patient's symptomatic course and outcome? Will it be possible to track treatment response using neuroimaging techniques? Will specific circuit-based therapies using deep brain stimulation emerge to treat refractory cases?

The identification of susceptibility genes in TS will doubtless point in new therapeutic directions for treatment, as will the characterization of the putative autoimmune mechanisms active in the PANDAS subgroup of patients. Given this potential, TS can be considered a model disorder to study the dynamic interplay of genetic vulnerabilities, epigenetic events, and neurobiological systems active during early brain development. It is likely that the research paradigms utilized in these studies, and many of the empirical findings resulting from them, will be relevant to other disorders of childhood onset and to our understanding of normal development.

ACKNOWLEDGMENTS

This work was funded by grants from the National Institutes of Health MH-493515, MH-30929, and RR-06022, as well as contributions from members of the National Tourette Syndrome Association in the United States.

REFERENCES

1. Kushner, H.I. (1999) *A Cursing Brain? The Histories of Tourette Syndrome*, Harvard University Press, Cambridge, MA.
2. Leckman, J.F. and Riddle, M.A. (2000) Tourette's syndrome: when habit-forming systems form habits of their own? *Neuron* **28,** 349–354.

3. Pauls, D.L. and Leckman, J.F. (1986) The inheritance of Gilles de la Tourette syndrome and associated behaviors: evidence for autosomal dominant transmission. *N. Engl. J. Med.* **315,** 993–997.
4. Price, R.A., Kidd, K.K., Cohen, D.J., Pauls, D.L., and Leckman, J.F. (1985) A twin study of Tourette's syndrome. *Arch. Gen. Psychiatry* **42,** 815–820.
5. Hyde, T., Aaronson, B., Randolph, C., Rickler, K., and Weinberger, D. (1992) Relationship of birth weight to the phenotypic expression of Gilles de la Tourette's syndrome in monozygotic twins. *Neurology* **42,** 652–658.
6. Walkup, J.T., LaBuda, M.C., Singer, H.S., Brown, J., Riddle, M.A., and Hurko, O. (1996) Family study and segregation analysis of Tourette syndrome: evidence for a mixed model of inheritance. *Am. J. Hum. Genet.* **59,** 684–693.
7. Barr, C.L. and Sandor, P. (1998) Current status of genetic studies of Gilles de la Tourette syndrome. *Can. J. Psychiatry* **43,** 351–357.
8. Merette, C., Brassard, A., Potvin, A., et al. (2000) Significant linkage for Tourette syndrome in a large French Canadian family. *Am. J. Hum. Genet.* **67,** 1008–1013.
9. The Tourette Syndrome Association International Consortium for Genetics. (1999) A complete genome screen in sibpairs affected with Gilles de la Tourette syndrome. *Arch. Gen. Psychiatry* **65,** 1428–1436.
10. Simonic, I., Gericke, G.S., Ott, J., and Weber, J.L. (1998) Identification of genetic markers associated with Gilles de la Tourette syndrome in an Afrikaner population. *Am. J. Hum. Genet.* **63,** 839–846.
11. Pasamanick, B. and Kawi, A. (1956) A study of the association of prenatal and paranatal factors in the development of tics in children. *Pediatrics* **48,** 596–601.
12. Leckman, J.F., Price, R.A., Walkup, J.T., Ort, S., Pauls, D.L., and Cohen, D.J. (1987) Birthweights of monozygotic twins discordant for Tourette's syndrome. *Arch. Gen. Psychiatry* **44,** 100.
13. Leckman, J.F., Hardin, M.T., Dolansky, E.S., et al. (1990) Perinatal factors in the expression of Tourette's syndrome. *J. Am. Acad. Child Adolesc. Psychiatry* **29,** 220–226.
14. Whitaker, A.H., Van Rossem, R., Feldman, J.F., et al. (1997) Psychiatric outcomes in low-birth-weight children at age 6 years: relation to neonatal cranial ultrasound abnormalities. *Arch. Gen. Psychiatry* **54,** 847–856.
15. Burd, L., Severud, R., Klug, M.G., and Kerbeshian, J. (1999) Prenatal and perinatal risk factors for Tourette disorder. *J. Perinatol. Med.* **27,** 295–302.
16. Santangelo, S.L., Pauls, D.L., Goldstein, J., Faraone, S.V., Tsuang, M.T., and Leckman, J.F. (1994) Tourette's syndrome: what are the influences of gender and comorbid obsessive-compulsive disorder? *J. Am. Acad. Child Adolesc. Psychiatry* **33,** 795–804.
17. Shapiro, A.K., Shapiro, E.S., Young, J.G., and Feinberg, T.E. (eds.) (1988) *Gilles de la Tourette Syndrome, 2nd ed.,* Raven, New York.
18. Peterson, B.S., Leckman, J.F., Scahill, L., et al. (1992) Hypothesis: Steroid hormones and sexual dimorphisms modulate symptom expression in Tourette's syndrome. *Psychoneuroendocrinology* **17,** 553–563.
19. Pauls, D.L., Raymond, C.L., Stevenson, J., and Leckman, J.F. (1991) A family study of Gilles de la Tourette syndrome. *Am. J. Hum. Genet.* **48,** 154–163.
20. Comings, D.E. and Comings, B.G. (1987) A controlled study of Tourette syndrome. I. Attention-deficit disorder, learning disorders, and school problems, II. Conduct. *Am. J. Hum. Genet.* **41,** 701–760.
21. Sikich, L. and Todd, R.D. (1988) Are neurodevelopmental effects of gonadal hormones related to sex differences in psychiatric illness. *Psychiatr. Dev.* **6,** 277–310.
22. Boulant, J.A. (1981) Hypothalamic mechanisms in thermoregulation. *Fed. Proc.* **40,** 2843–2850.
23. Fehrbach, S.E., Morell, J.I., and Pfaff, D.W. (1985) Identification of medial preoptic neurons that concentrate estradiol and project to the midbrain in the rat. *J. Comp. Neurol.* **247,** 364–382.
24. Scahill, L., Lombroso, P.J., Mack, G., et al. (2001) Thermal sensitivity in Tourette syndrome. *Percept. Mot. Skills* **92,** 419–432.
25. Silva, R.R., Munoz, D.M., Barickman, J., and Friedhoff, A.J. (1995) Environmental factors and related fluctuation of symptoms in children with Tourette's disorder. *J. Child Psychol. Psychiatry* **36,** 305–312.
26. Jagger, J., Prusoff, B.A., Cohen, D.J., Kidd, K.K., Carbonari, C.M., and John, K. (1982) The epidemiology of Tourette's syndrome: a pilot study. *Schizophr. Bull.* **8,** 267–277.
27. Carter, A.S., Pauls, D.L., Leckman, J.F., and Cohen, D.J. (1994) A prospective longitudinal study of Gilles de la Tourette syndrome. *J. Am. Acad. Child Adolesc. Psychiatry* **33,** 377–385.
28. Carter, A.S., O'Donnell, D.A., Schultz, R.T., Scahill, L., Leckman, J.F., and Pauls, D.L. (2000) Social and emotional adjustment in children affected with Gilles de la Tourette's syndrome: associations with ADHD and family functioning. *J. Child Psychol. Psychiatry* **1,** 215–223.
29. Husby, G., van de Rijn, I., Zabriskie, J.B., Abdin, Z.H., and Williams, R.C. (1976) Antibodies reacting with cytoplasm of subthalamic and caudate nuclei neurons in chorea and acute rheumatic fever. *J. Exp. Med.* **144,** 1094–1110.
30. Singer, H.S., Giuliano, J.D., Hansen, B.H., et al. (1998) Antibodies against human putamen in children with Tourette syndrome. *Neurology* **50,** 1618–1624.
31. Morshed, S.A., Parveen, S., Leckman, J.F., et al. (2001) Antibodies against striatal, nuclear, cytoskeletal and streptococcal epitopes in children and adults with Tourette's syndrome, Sydenham's chorea, and autoimmune disorders. *Biol. Psychiatry* **50,** 566–577.
32. Swedo, S.E., Leonard, H.L., Garvey, M., Mittleman, B., Allen, A.J., and Perlmutter, S. (1998) Pediatric autoimmune neuropsychiatric disorders associated with streptococcal infections: clinical description of the first 50 cases. *Am. J. Psychiatry* **155,** 264–271.
33. Kurlan, R. (1998) Tourette's syndrome and 'PANDAS': will the relation bear out? Pediatric autoimmune neuropsychiatric disorders associated with streptococcal infection. *Neurology* **50,** 1530–1534.

34. Hallett, J.J., Harling-Berg, C.J., Knopf, P.M., Stopa, E.G., and Kiessling, L.S. (2000) Anti-striatal antibodies in Tourette syndrome cause neuronal dysfunction. *J. Neuroimmunol.* **111,** 195–202.
35. Taylor, J.R., Morshed, S.A., Parveen, S., Leckman, J.F., and Lombroso, P.J. (2002) An animal model of Tourette's syndrome. *Am. J. Psychiatry* **159,** 657–660.
36. Perlmutter, S.J., Leitman, S.F., Garvey, M.A., et al. (1999) Therapeutic plasma exchange and intravenous immunoglobulin for obsessive-compulsive disorder and tic disorders in childhood. *Lancet* **354,** 1153–1158.
37. Aosaki, T., Graybiel, A.M., and Kimura, M. (1994) Effect of the nigrostriatal dopamine system on acquired neural responses in the striatum of behaving monkeys. *Science* **265,** 412–415.
38. Anderson, G.M., Leckman, J.F., and Cohen, D.J. (1998) Neurochemical and neuropeptide systems, in *Tourette's Syndrome Tics, Obsessions, Compulsions—Developmental Psychopathology and Clinical Care* (Leckman, J.F. and Cohen, D.J., eds.), John Wiley & Sons, New York, pp. 261–281.
39. Wolf, S.S., Jones, D.W., Knable, M.B., et al. (1996) Tourette syndrome: prediction of phenotypic variation in monozygotic twins by caudate nucleus D2 receptor binding. *Science* **273,** 1225–1227.
40. Wong, D.F., Singer, H.S., Brandt, J., et al. (1997) D2-like dopamine receptor density in Tourette syndrome measured by PET. *J. Nucl. Med.* **38,** 1243–1247.
41. Singer, H.S., Hahn, I.-H., and Moran, T.H. (1991) Abnormal dopamine uptake sites in postmortem striatum from patients with Tourette's syndrome. *Ann. Neurol.* **30,** 558–562.
42. Malison, R.T., McDougle, C.J., van Dyck, C.H., et al. (1995) [I^{123}]β-CIT SPECT imaging demonstrates increased striatal dopamine transporter binding in Tourette's syndrome. *Am. J. Psychiatry* **152,** 1359–1361.
43. Ernst, M., Zametkin, A.J., Jons, P.H., Matochik, J.A., Pascualvaca, D., and Cohen R.M. (1999) High presynaptic dopaminergic activity in children with Tourette's disorder. *J. Am. Acad. Child Adolesc. Psychiatry* **38,** 86–94.
44. Meyer, P., Bohnen, N.I., Minoshima, S., et al. (1999) Striatal presynaptic monoaminergic vesicles are not increased in Tourette's syndrome. *Neurology* **53,** 371–374.
45. Peterson, B.S. and Leckman, J.F. (1998) The temporal dynamics of tics in Gilles de la Tourette syndrome. *Biol. Psychiatry* **44,** 1337–1348.
46. King, R., Barchas, J.D., and Huberman, B.A. (1984) Chaotic behavior in dopamine neurodynamics. *Proc. Natl. Acad. Sci. USA* **81,** 1244–1247.
47. Albin, R.L., Young, A.B., and Penney, J.B. (1989) The functional anatomy of basal ganglia disorders. *Trends Neurosci.* **12,** 366–375.
48. Alexander, G.E., DeLong, M.R., and Strick, P.L. (1986) Parallel organization of functionally segregated circuits linking basal ganglia and cortex. *Ann. Rev. Neurosci.* **9,** 357–381.
49. Parent, A. and Hazrati, L.-N. (1995) Functional anatomy of the basal ganglia: I. The cortico-basal ganglia-thalamo-cortical loop. *Brain Res. Rev.* **20,** 91–127.
50. Parent, A. and Hazrati, L.-N. (1995) Functional anatomy of the basal ganglia: II. The place of the subthalamic nucleus and the external pallidum in basal ganglia circuitry. *Brain Res. Rev.* **20,** 128–154.
51. Graybiel, A.M. (1998) The basal ganglia and chunking of action repertoires. *Neurobiol. Learn. Mem.* **70,** 119–136.
52. Leckman, J.F., Walker, D.E., and Cohen, D.J. (1993) Premonitory urges in Tourette's syndrome. *Am. J. Psychiatry* **150,** 98–102.
53. Jog, M.S., Kubota, Y., Connolly, C.I., Hillegaart, V., and Graybiel, A.M. (1999) Building neural representations of habits. *Science* **286,** 1745–1749.
54. Canales, J.J. and Graybiel, A.M. (2000) A measure of striatal function predicts motor stereotypy. *Nat. Neurosci.* **3,** 377–383.
55. Peterson, B.S., Skudlarski, P., Anderson, A.W., et al. (1998) A functional magnetic resonance imaging study of tic suppression in Tourette syndrome. *Arch. Gen. Psychiatry* **55,** 326–333.
56. Fried, I., Katz, A., McCarthy, G., et al. (1991) Functional organization of human supplementary motor cortex studied by electrical stimulation. *J. Neurosci.* **11,** 3656–3666.
57. Ziemann, U., Paulus, W., and Rothenberger, A. (1997) Decreased motor inhibition in Tourette's disorder: evidence from transcranial magnetic stimulation. *Am. J. Psychiatry* **154,** 1277–1284.
58. Greenberg, B.D., Ziemann, U., Cora-Locatelli, G., et al. (2000) Altered cortical excitability in obsessive-compulsive disorder. *Neurology* **54,** 142–147.
59. Nestadt, G., Samuels, J., Riddle, M., et al. (2000) A family study of obsessive-compulsive disorder. *Arch. Gen. Psychiatry* **57,** 358–363.
60. Rauch, S.L., Baer, L., Cosgrove, G.R., and Jenike, M.A. (1995) Neurosurgical treatment of Tourette's syndrome: a critical review. *Compr. Psychiatry* **36,** 141–156.
61. Vandewalle, V., van der Linden, C., Groenewegen, H.J., and Caemaert, J. (1999) Stereotactic treatment of Gilles de la Tourette syndrome by high frequency stimulation of thalamus. *Lancet* **353,** 724.
62. Peterson, B.S., Staib, L., Scahill, L., et al. (2001) Regional and ventricular volumes in Tourette syndrome. *Arch. Gen. Psychiatry* **58,** 427–442.
63. Schultz, R.T., Carter, A.S., Gladstone, M., et al. (1998) Visual-motor integration, visuoperceptual and fine motor functioning in children with Tourette's syndrome. *Neuropsychology* **12,** 134–145.
64. Anderson, S.A., Marin, O., Horn, C., Jennings, K., and Rubenstein, J.L. (2001) Distinct cortical migrations from the medial and lateral ganglionic eminences. *Development* **128,** 353–363.

35

Obsessive–Compulsive Disorder as a Frontostriatal-Thalamic Dysfunction

Tiffany R. Farchione, MD, **Shauna N. MacMillan,** BS, **and David R. Rosenberg,** MD

1. INTRODUCTION

Our understanding of the neurobiologic underpinnings of anxiety disorders including obsessive–compulsive disorder (OCD), has lagged far behind treatment development for these conditions. However, a multidisciplinary approach incorporating and translating advances in developmental neuroscience into treatment development is critical "to finally overcome the pervasive Cartesianism that continues to incubate stigma and ignorance about mental illness" *(1)*. This is especially true for a heterogeneous condition like OCD. OCD is by far the most investigated anxiety disorder in terms of both clinical treatment trials and examining the neurobiologic substrate.

1.1. Clinical Characterization and Assessment

OCD is a chronically disabling neuropsychiatric illness characterized by recurrent intrusive thoughts and repetitive ritualistic behavior *(2)*. The most commonly reported obsessions in children and adolescents are fears of contamination (35%), followed closely by thoughts of harming oneself or loved ones (30%). Frequent compulsions include washing and cleaning (75%), checking (40%), and straightening (35%) *(3)*.

In recent years, there has been increased recognition that OCD is not an illness merely of pedantic interest, but far more common than initially believed. Its lifetime prevalence is approx 2 to 3% *(4–6)*. Particularly relevant to healthcare professionals working with children and adolescents, at least 80% of all cases have their onset in childhood and adolescence *(7)*. Boys tend to have an earlier onset than girls, with a peak in puberty and in early adulthood *(8)*.

Co-morbid tic disorders are particularly common in childhood OCD, particularly in boys *(8)*. In a study by Swedo and collegues *(9)* examining co-morbidity in a group of 70 children with OCD, 30% of patients had a co-morbid tic disorder, whereas 26% had major depressive disorder (MDD), and 24% had some form of developmental disorder.

Recently, a potentially new subtype of OCD has been described. This subtype includes OCD and tic disorders associated with Group A β-hemolytic streptococcal infections (GABHS) and is referred to as pediatric autoimmune neuropsychiatric disorders associated with GABHS (PANDAS) *(10,11)*. This "immunologic" subtype of OCD is distinguished from "classic" OCD, in that the onset and emergence of symptoms in PANDAS is described as being sudden and abrupt, as opposed to the more insidious course characteristic of "classic" OCD. Although antibiotic treatment has not proved to be effective

From: *Mental and Behavioral Dysfunction in Movement Disorders*
Edited by: M-A. Bédard et al. © Humana Press Inc., Totowa, NJ

in treating PANDAS, plasmapheresis and intravenous immunoglobulin have been shown to be effective in some cases where standard treatments (e.g., selective serotonin [5-HT] re-uptake inhibitors [SSRIs] and cognitive behavioral therapy [CBT]) have proved to be ineffective *(12,13)*. Of note, these therapies do not alleviate symptoms in patients with non-PANDAS OCD *(13)*, underscoring the importance of characterizing the individual subtypes of OCD. Given that there may be multiple distinct subtypes of OCD, one must consider that treatment-refractory cases of OCD may actually be a separate biological subtype that has yet to be defined.

2. DEVELOPMENTAL NEUROBIOLOGY

For a comprehensive review of the developmental neurobiology of OCD, the reader is referred to the recent report by Fitzgerald and collegues *(14)*. We present an overview here.

Neurobiological studies using various techniques in several laboratories have provided converging lines of evidence supporting ventral prefrontal cortical-striatal-thalamic dysfunction as a basis for OCD *(15–18)*. Our neurology and neurosurgery colleagues, together with lesion studies in animals, have provided indirect support for ventral prefrontal-striatal-thalamic lesions being involved in the pathogenesis of OCD *(19–23)*. Neurosurgical lesions in these regions have, in fact, been reported to lead to improvement in some treatment-refractory OCD patients *(24,25)*. Functional neuroimaging studies in adult OCD patients have fairly consistently reported alterations in ventral prefrontal-striatal-thalamic circuits correlated with severity of illness and response to treatment intervention *(26–28)*. Recent investigation in children suggests a new clinical neurodevelopmental model for pediatric OCD, with differential brain mechanisms in OCD depending on the age of symptom onset *(29,30)*. Advances in technology, particularly brain imaging techniques (e.g., magnetic resonance imaging [MRI] and positron emission tomography [PET]) are making brain mechanisms involved in anxiety disorders, such as OCD, accessible as never before.

2.1. Volumetric Alterations in Childhood Onset OCD

2.1.1. Corpus Striatum

Using computerized tomography (CT), Behar and collegues *(31)* reported increased ventricular brain ratios (VBRs) in adolescent patients with OCD as compared to healthy comparison subjects. Although increased VBRs suggested reduced striatal (caudate and putamen) volumes in OCD patients, the authors did not present data on these regions of interest. A subsequent quantitative CT study conducted by Luxenberg and collegues *(32)* did, however, find bilaterally reduced caudate volumes in adolescent males with OCD as compared to healthy comparison subjects. Rosenberg and collegues *(33)* also demonstrated bilateral reductions in striatal volume in 19 nondepressed, treatment-naïve pediatric OCD patients, 7–17 yr vs 19 age- and sex-matched controls. Reduced striatal volumes were highly correlated with increased OCD symptom severity but not illness duration. This suggests that reduced striatal volume may represent an early developmental biomarker in pediatric OCD, rather than a degenerative effect of illness and/or medication intervention. Since central nervous system (CNS) active medications have been shown to lead to changes in caudate volume *(34,35)*, this underscores potential advantages in studying pediatric patients near illness onset before treatment intervention and long-term illness duration.

In contrast to the aforementioned findings in the striatum, Giedd and collegues *(36,37)* report strikingly different findings in the PANDAS subtype of OCD. Instead of reductions in striatal volumes, they observed a significant increase in basal ganglia volumes in PANDAS patients as compared to controls. Remarkably, effective treatment with plasmapheresis resulting in OCD symptom resolution was associated with a concomitant decrease in basal ganglia volume *(38)*. Relapse of the symptoms was associated with subsequent increase in basal ganglia volume. Chronic recurrent GABHS infections were recently observed to be associated with increased basal ganglia volumes in OCD patients, with increased basal ganglia volumes being correlated with increased antibody titers of antistreptolysin O and antideoxyribonuclease B *(39)*. These results underscore the importance of precise neurobiologic characterization of the somatic substrate underlying OCD. At some point, many different subtypes of OCD may be identified, and it is likely that treatment interventions will need to be individually tailored accordingly, rather than streamlined *(40)*.

2.1.2. Prefrontal Cortex

An initial volumetric MRI study report by Rosenberg and collegues *(33)* failed to identify alterations in prefrontal cortical volume in pediatric OCD patients as compared to age- and sex-matched controls. However, this investigation measured total prefrontal cortical volume so that alterations in specific subdivisions (e.g., ventral prefrontal cortex) may not have been detected. Subsequent investigation *(41, 42)* of the corpus callosum, which connects regions of the cerebral hemispheres to specific brain regions *(43)*, demonstrated alterations in the genu region of the corpus callosum in OCD patients compared to controls. This region connects ventral prefrontal cortex. Alterations in the genu region of the corpus callosum were associated with increased OCD symptom severity but not duration of illness. A striking age-related increase in corpus callosal area was observed in healthy pediatric controls. This age-related increase in corpus callosal area was absent in OCD patients. Interestingly, adults with OCD have not been found to have alterations in corpus callosal area as compared to healthy controls *(44,45)*. OCD clearly does not "go away" during adulthood. Thus, these data suggest that certain neurodevelopmental windows of aberrant maturation may "open and close" across the age span and may have potential implications for treatment intervention.

Rosenberg and Keshevan *(29)* examined specific subdivisions of the prefrontal cortex and observed localized increased anterior cingulate volumes in OCD patients as compared to controls (Fig. 1A). Case-control pairs did not differ in dorsolateral prefrontal cortical or posterior cingulate volumes. Consistent with the differential developmental maturation observed between OCD patients and controls in the corpus callosum, a similar developmental divergence was observed in maturation of anterior cingulate volumes in OCD patients and controls (Fig. 1B).

2.1.3. Thalamus

The thalamus serves as the final subcortical input to prefrontal cortex and promotes cortical output when released from basal ganglia inhibition *(16)*. The findings of increased anterior cingulate volume, which was correlated with reduced striatal volumes in pediatric OCD patients, led Gilbert and collegues *(46)* to conduct a volumetric MRI study of the thalamus in 21 nondepressed psychotropic-medication-naïve pediatric OCD patients, 8–17 yr of age, and 21 case-matched healthy pediatric controls (Fig. 2). Thalamic volumes were significantly increased in pediatric OCD patients as compared to controls. Moreover, a differential maturation of thalamic volume was observed between OCD patients and controls (Fig. 2). This may, in part, explain, why Jenike and collegues *(47)* found no significant differences in thalamic volume between adult OCD patients and controls. It should also be noted that most of these patients had been ill for a considerable period and were being treated with SSRI medication.

In fact, Gilbert and collegues *(46)* observed a significant decrease in thalamic volume in OCD patients after 12 wk of treatment with the SSRI, paroxetine, to levels comparable to those observed in controls. Decrease in thalamic volume in OCD patients was positively correlated with decrease in OCD symptom severity (Fig. 3). What is particularly intriguing about these findings is that the larger the thalamic volume pretreatment, the more likely was a child with OCD to respond to medication, whereas the smaller the pretreatment volume, the less likely was a child with OCD to respond to paroxetine. Thus, even though different patients may have the same cluster of signs and symptoms, the underlying neurobiology and treatment response may differ among patients with differential neuroanatomic alterations.

More recent investigation of the medial and lateral subcomponents of the thalamus demonstrated that reductions in thalamic volume associated with paroxetine treatment appeared to be localized to medial, not lateral, thalamus *(48)*. Medial thalamic regions, particularly the dorsomedial nucleus of the thalamus have been especially implicated in the pathogenesis of OCD *(15)*.

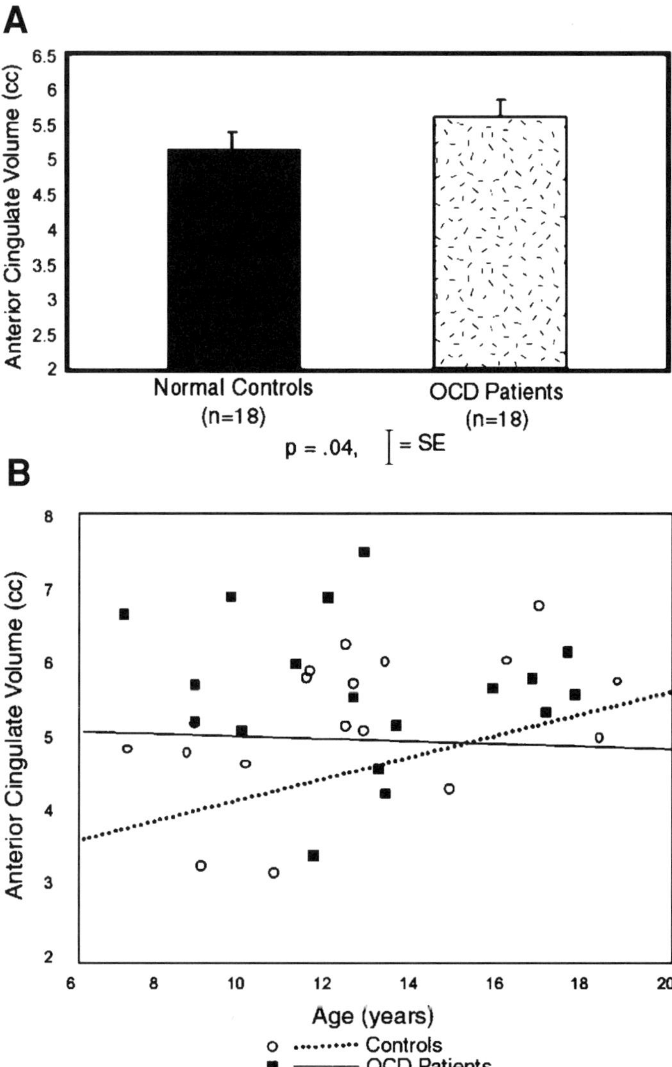

Fig. 1. (**A**) Anterior cingulate volume by group. (Adapted with permission from ref. *29*.) (**B**) Anterior cingulate volume as a function of age for pediatric OCD patients and normal controls. Note the trend for a significant correlation between age and anterior cingulate volume in controls but not in OCD patients. (Reprinted by permission of Elsevier Science from "Toward a neurodevelopmental model of obsessive-compulsive disorder," by D.R. Rosenberg & M.S. Keshavan, *Biological Psychiatry* **43,** 623–640, Copyright ©1998 by the Society of Biological Psychiatry.)

These results obviously require replication before definitive conclusions can be drawn, but provide the basis for testable hypotheses that might ultimately be incorporated into treatment development trials. Thalamic volume did not change significantly in pediatric OCD patients treated with cognitive behavioral therapy *(49)*, suggesting that this may represent a specific effect of SSRI treatment rather than a general treatment effect and/or spontaneous resolution of symptoms.

Recent investigation with a new more sophisticated MRI technique, proton magnetic resonance spectroscopy (^{1}H-MRS) has further delineated the role of the thalamus in pediatric OCD. ^{1}H-MRS has been found to be more sensitive than conventional structural neuroimaging techniques in identifying alterations in specific brain regions in neuropsychiatric disorders such as OCD (50). This technique has identified

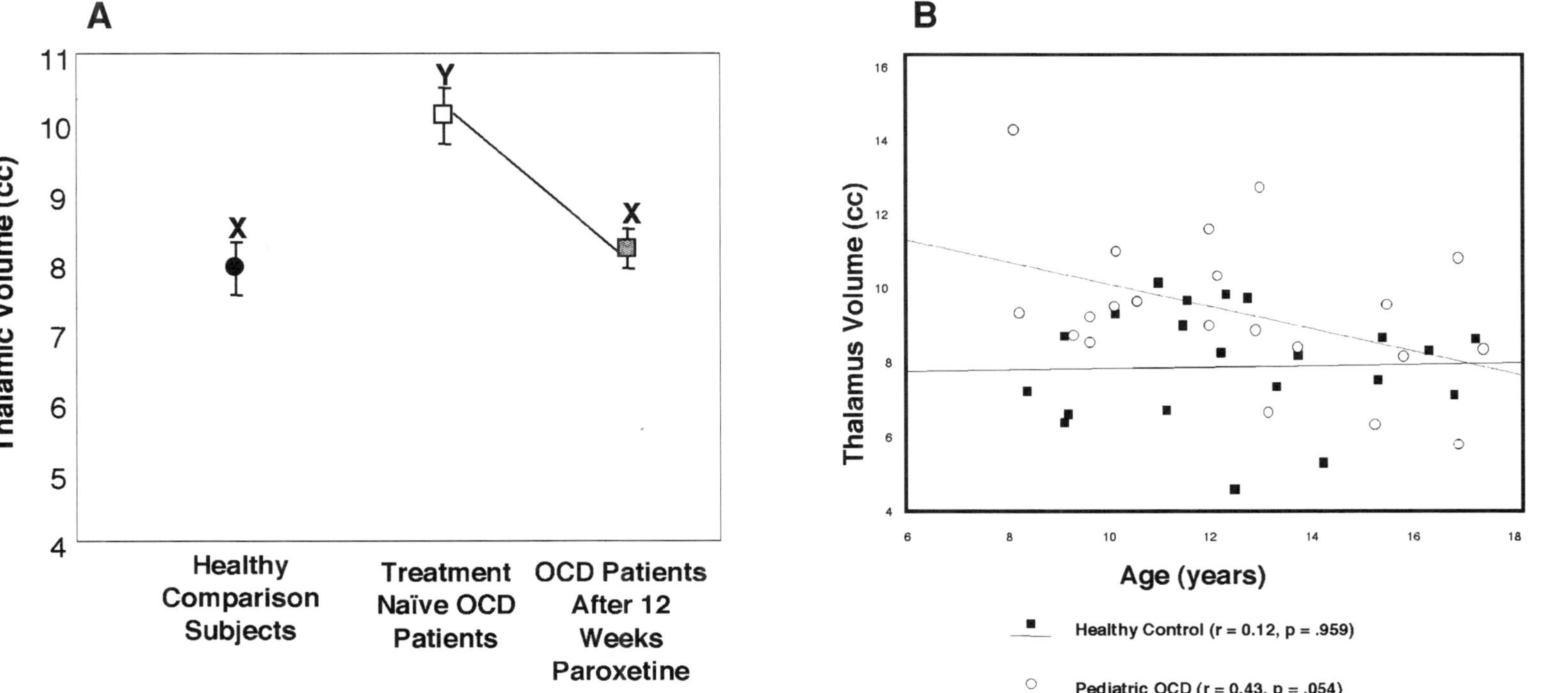

Fig. 2. (**A**) Thalamic volume by diagnostic and treatment condition. Groups not sharing the same letter are significantly difference at $p < 0.05$. OCD, obsessive–compulsive disorder. (**B**) Thalamic volume vs age in pediatric OCD patients vs healthy comparison subjects. [(**A**) Adapted with permission from ref. *46*. (**B**) Reprinted by permission of Elsevier Science from "Genetic and imaging strategies in obsessive-compulsive disorder: Potential implications for treatment development," by D.R. Rosenberg & G. Hanna, *Biological Psychiatry* **48,** 1210–1222, Copyright ©2000 by the Society of Biological Psychiatry.]

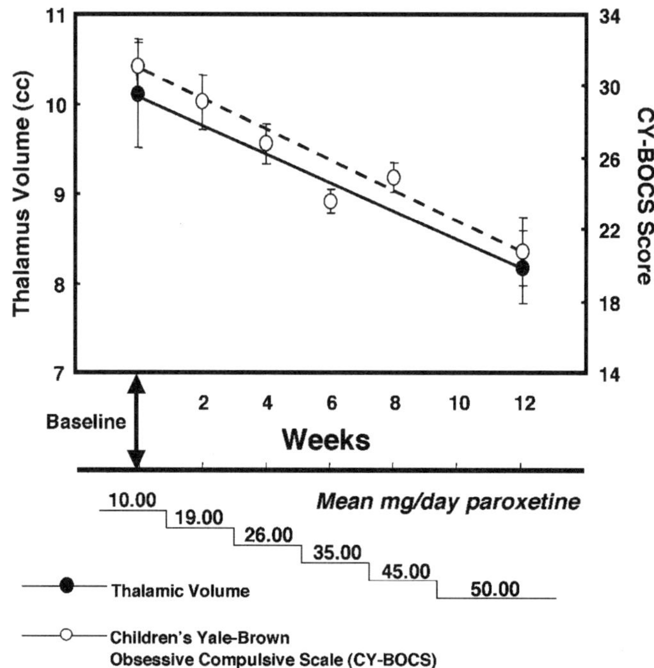

Fig. 3. Decrease in thalamic volume associated with reduction in Obsessive–Compulsive Score of the Children's Yale–Brown Obsessive–Compulsive Scales. (Reprinted by permission of the American Medical Association from "Decrease in thalamic volumes of pediatric patients with obsessive-compulsive disorder who are taxing paroxetine," by A.R. Gilbert, G.J. Moore, M.S. Keshavan, et al., *Archives of General Psychiatry* **57,** 449–456, Copyright ©2000, American Medical Association.)

localized functional neurochemical marker abnormalities in medial, rather than lateral, thalamus *(51,52)*. Preliminary ^{1}H-MRS investigation suggests that paroxetine treatment in pediatric OCD patients may result in an increase in N-acetyl-aspartate (NAA) concentrations in medial thalamus *(52)*. NAA is a reliable indicator of neuronal viability *(53)*, which suggests that effective paroxetine treatment may have a neurotrophic effect in certain brain regions. This is an active area of investigation in our laboratory.

3. NEUROCHEMISTRY

Pharmacologic studies still provide the most compelling evidence for a serotonergic role in OCD *(54)*. To date, the only medications that have been proven effective in adults and children with OCD are the 5-HT re-uptake inhibitors.

Platelet and cerebrospinal fluid (CSF) studies of serotonin have reported alterations in pediatric and adult OCD patients compared to controls *(55–58)*, although contrary reports exist *(59–62)*. Pharmacologic challenge studies, particularly with the mixed 5-HT agonist–antagonist, meta-chlorphenylpiperazide (mCPP), have demonstrated in some *(63–67)*, but not all, studies *(68,69)* that its administration results in exacerbation of OCD symptoms. However, these studies provide only a very peripheral window into brain chemistry. New advances in PET and MRS provide unprecedented opportunities for measuring brain chemistry before and after treatment intervention.

PET allows for the measurement of 5-HT synthesis and receptor function. Because of its putative ionizing radiation risks, it is often not feasible for study in pediatric populations, particularly in controls and for repeated measurement. Nonetheless, advances in technology coupled with the advent of three-dimensional PET, which substantially reduces radiation exposure, may make this technique more feasible.

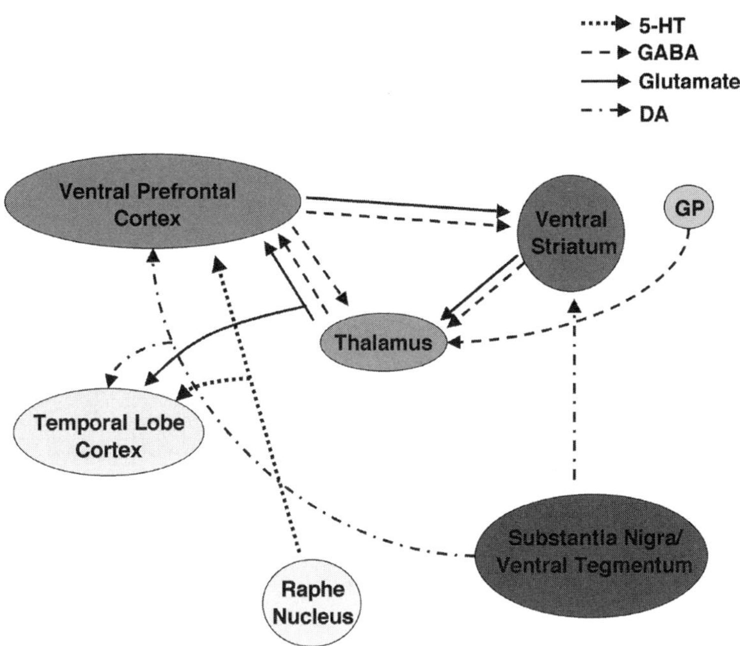

Fig. 4. Schematic diagram showing selected aspects of corticostriatal connections in the neurodevelopment of OCD. Neurotransmitters: DA, dopamine; 5-HT, serotonin. Brain regions: GP, globus pallidus. (Adapted with permission from ref. *29*.)

3.1. Glutamate

While MRS does not allow for direct measurement of 5-HT, it does permit the direct, in vivo and noninvasive measurement of neurochemical compounds, such as glutamate, that may be especially relevant to the pathophysiology of OCD. Corticostriatal glutamate has been shown to inhibit 5-HT release *(70–74)*, whereas medial prefrontal glutamate transmission is modulated by 5-HT *(75)*.

The developmental dysmaturation in ventral prefrontal-striatal-thalamic circuitry in pediatric OCD patients with increased thalamic and ventral prefrontal cortical volumes, coupled with reduced striatal volumes, led to the hypothesis of a "neural network dysplasia of OCD" *(29)*, which might result from abnormalities in glutamatergic modulation of serotonergic neurotransmission (Fig. 4). Glutamatergic involvement in OCD was suggested by several reports in the literature. The caudate nucleus, a region hypothesized to represent the primary locus of abnormality in OCD *(76)* receives an especially dense glutamatergic innervation from ventral prefrontal cortex *(70)*, which is a region also implicated in the pathogenesis of OCD *(26)*. Most of the axonal terminals in the caudate nucleus are, in fact, glutamatergic afferents *(77,78)*. Striking reductions in caudate glutamatergic concentrations are observed after frontal cortical ablation *(79,80)*. 5-HT neurons also influence glutamatergic concentrations *(75)*.

Rosenberg and collegues *(81)* conducted a ^{1}H-MRS study, which permits measurement of glutamatergic concentrations, and found that caudate glutamatergic concentrations were significantly elevated in pediatric OCD patients compared to healthy controls (Figs. 5 and 6). After 12 wk of monodrug therapy with paroxetine, caudate glutamatergic concentrations in pediatric OCD patients decreased to levels not significantly different from those observed in controls. Decrease in caudate glutamatergic concentrations was also robustly correlated with reduction in OCD symptom severity (Fig. 7). Glutamatergic alterations were not observed in the occipital cortex. This is consistent with basic neuroscience studies conducted by El Manasari and collegues *(82)*, which demonstrated that sustained administration of SSRIs

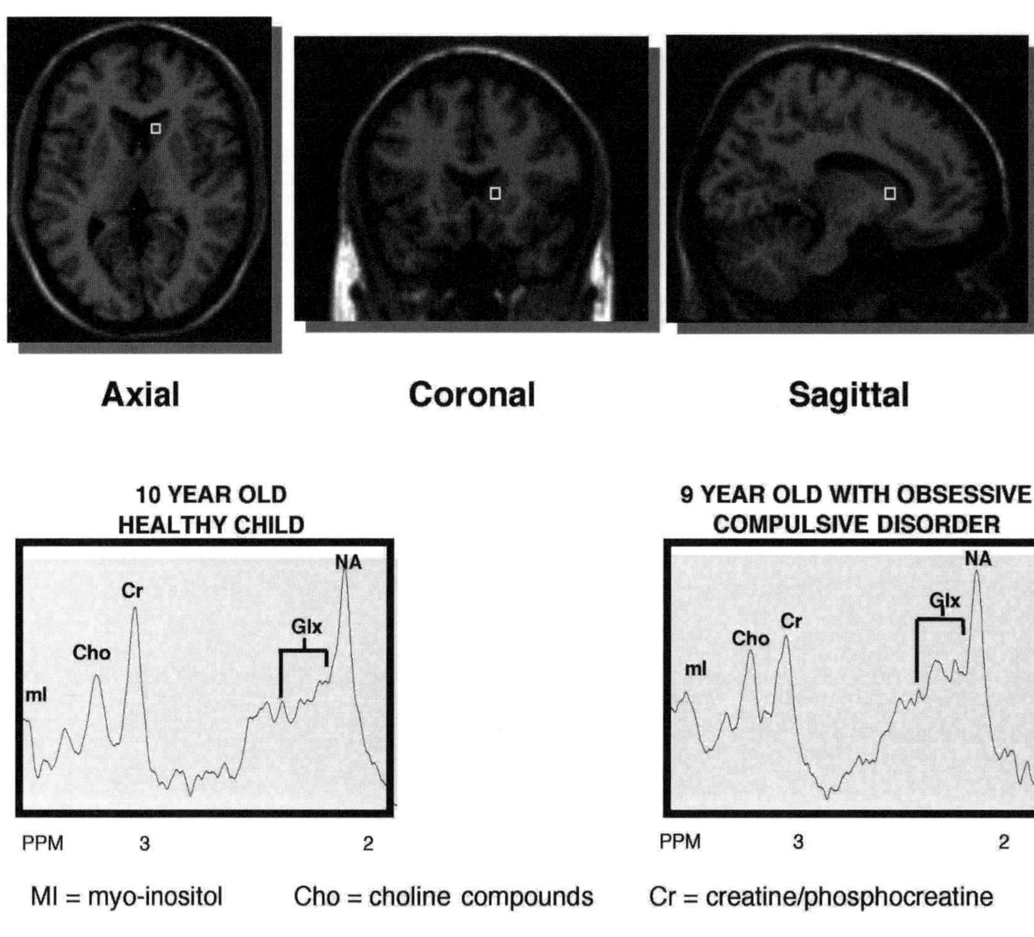

Fig. 5. (Top panel) Illustration of voxel placement in left caudate nucleus. (Bottom panel) ^{1}H-MRS of a 0.7-mL vol of interest centered in the left caudate in a 10-yr-old healthy control and a 9-yr-old treatment-naïve patient with OCD as shown on the T1-weighted MR images. (Reprinted by permission of Cambridge University Press from "Brain anatomy and chemistry may predict treatment response in paediatric obsessive-compulsive disorder," by D.R. Rosenberg, S.N. MacMillan, and G.J. Moore, *International Journal of Neuropsychopharmacology* **4,** 179–190, Copyright ©2001, CINP.)

increased 5-HT release from ventral prefrontal cortex. Because axonal terminals in the caudate nucleus are primarily glutamatergic, SSRI treatment could reduce glutamatergic efferents from the frontal cortex, which would result in reduced caudate glutamate *(81)*.

Perhaps even more intriguing, there is some preliminary evidence to suggest that, in children, these neurochemical changes persist in patients whose illness remains in remission even after discontinuation of pharmacotherapy *(83)*. It should be noted that studies in adults *(84)* suggest relapse rates as high as 90% when treatment is discontinued. Further study is warranted in pediatric OCD patients to determine the role of glutamate as a neurobiologic marker of treatment response (or lack thereof) and predicting longer term remission of symptoms.

Neurobiologic studies may ultimately prove helpful in identifying moderator (present at baseline) and mediator (changing with treatment) variables that might potentially identify surrogate biologic

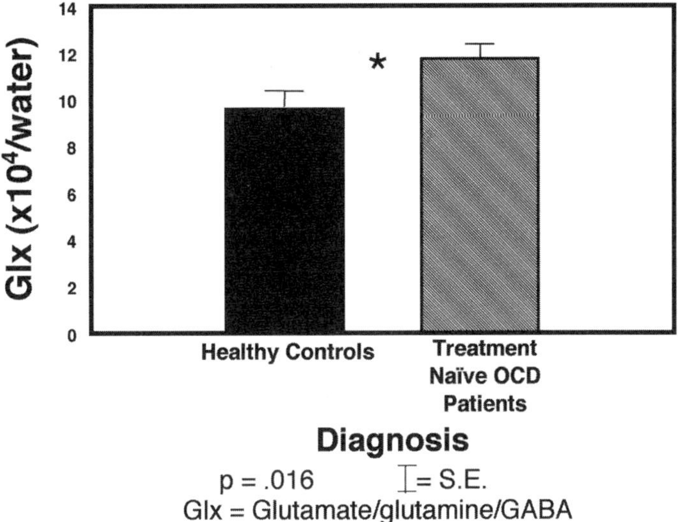

Fig. 6. Left caudate glutamatergic concentrations in treatment-naïve pediatric OCD patients and age- and sex-matched healthy comparison subjects. (Adapted with permission from ref. *81*.)

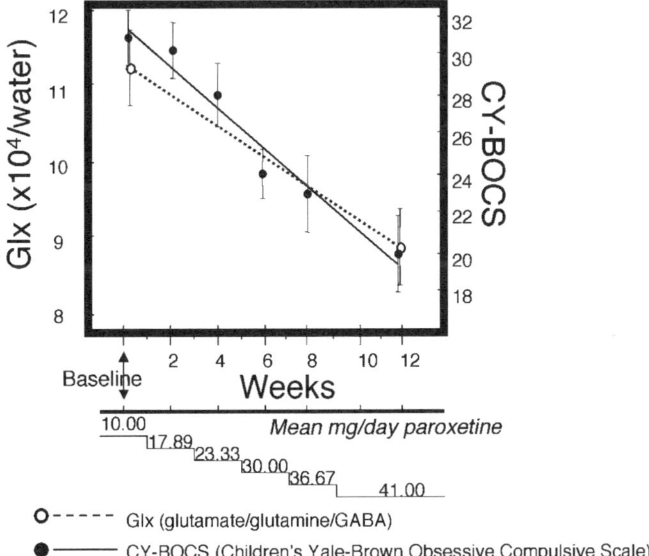

Fig. 7. Decrease in left caudate glutamatergic concentrations associated with reduction in Obsessive–Compulsive Score of the Children's Yale–Brown Obsessive–Compulsive Scales. (Reprinted by permission of Elsevier Science from "Genetic and imaging strategies in obsessive-compulsive disorder: Potential implications for treatment development," by D.R. Rosenberg & G. Hanna, *Biological Psychiatry* **48,** 1210–1222, Copyright ©2000 by the Society of Biological Psychiatry.)

markers predictive of treatment response (or lack, thereof). Differential patterns of brain anatomy, chemistry, and function may predict better response to a particular treatment (e.g., CBT vs pharmacotherapy vs combination therapy) *(85)*. We are not yet at such a stage, but exciting times clearly lie ahead in our efforts to integrate advances in developmental neuroscience into enhanced neurodiagnostic assessment and better treatments for the condition.

REFERENCES

1. Hyman, S.E. (2000) The millenium of mind, brain, and behavior. *Arch. Gen. Psychiatry* **57**, 88–89.
2. American Psychiatric Association. (1994) *DSM-IV: Diagnostic and Statistical Manual of Mental Disorders,* 4th ed., American Psychiatric Press, Washington, DC.
3. Castellanos, D. and Hunter, T. (1999) Anxiety disorders in children and adolescents. *South. Med. J.* **92,** 946–954.
4. Hanna, G.L. (1995) Demographic and clinical features of obsessive-compulsive disorder in children and adolescents. *J. Am. Acad. Child Adolesc. Psychiatry* **34,** 19–27.
5. Valleni-Basile, L.A., Garrison, C.Z., Jackson, K.L., et al. (1994) Frequency of obsessive-compulsive disorder in a community sample of young adolescents. *J. Am. Acad. Child Adolesc. Psychiatry* **33,** 782–791.
6. Flament, M.F., Whitaker, A., and Rapoport, J.L. (1988) Obsessive compulsive disorder in adolescence: an epidemiological study. *J. Am. Acad. Child Adolesc. Psychia*try **27,** 764–771.
7. Pauls, D.L., Alsobrook, J.P., Phil, M., et al. (1995) A family study of obsessive-compulsive disorder. *Am. J. Psychiatry* **152,** 76–84.
8. Zohar, A.H. (1999) The epidemiology of obsessive-compulsive disorder in children and adolescents. *Child Adolesc. Psychiatr. Clin. N. Am.* **8,** 445–460.
9. Swedo, S.E., Rapoport, J.L., Leonard, H., et al. (1989) Obsessive-compulsive disorder in children and adolescents. *Arch. Gen. Psychiatry* **46,** 335–341.
10. Swedo, S.E., Leonard, H.L., Garvey, M., et al. (1998) Pediatric autoimmune neuropsychiatric disorders associated with streptococcal infections: clinical description of the first 50 cases. *Am. J. Psychiatry* **155**, 264–271.
11. Allen, A.J., Leonard, H.L., and Swedo, S.E (1995) Case study: a new infection-triggered, autoimmune subtype of pediatric OCD and tourette's syndrome. *J. Am. Acad. Child Adolesc. Psychiatry* **34,** 307–311.
12. Perlmutter, S.J., Leitman, S.F., Garvey, M.A., et al. (1999) Therapeutic plasma exchange and intravenous immunoglobulin for obsessive-compulsive disorder and tic disorders in childhood. *Lancet* **354**, 1153–1158.
13. Nicolson, R., Swedo, S.E., Lenane, M., et al. (2000) An open trial of plasma exchange in childhood-onset obsessive-compulsive disorder without poststreptococcal exacerbations. *J. Am. Acad. Child Adolesc. Psychiatry* **39,** 1313–1315.
14. Fitzgerald, K.D., MacMaster, F.P., Paulson, L.D., and Rosenberg, D.R. (1999) Neurobiology of childhood obsessive-compulsive disorder. *Child Adolesc. Psychiatr. Clin. N. Am.* **8,** 533–75.
15. Modell, J.G., Mountz, J.M., Curtis, G.C., and Greden, J.F. (1989) Neurophysiologic dysfunction in basal ganglia/limbic striatal and thalamocortical circuits as a pathogenetic mechanism of obsessive-compulsive disorder. *J. Neuropsychiatry Clin. Neurosci.* **1,** 27–36.
16. Baxter, L.R., Saxena, S., Brody, A.L., et al. (1996) Brain mediation of obsessive-compulsive disorder symptoms: evidence from functional brain imaging studies in the human and nonhuman primate. *Semin. Clin. Neuropsychiatry* **1,** 32–47.
17. Insel, T.R. and Winslow, J.T. (1992) Neurobiology of obsessive compulsive disorder. *Psychiatr. Clin. N. Am.* **15,** 813–823.
18. Wise, S. and Rapoport, J.L. (1989) Obsessive-compulsive disorder: is it basal ganglia dysfunction?, in *Obsessive-Compulsive Disorder in Children and Adolescents* (Rapoport, J.L., ed.), American Psychiatric Press, Washington, DC, pp. 327–347.
19. Pitman, R.E., Green, R.C., Jenike, M.A., and Mesulam, M.M. (1987) Clinical comparison of Tourette's disorder and obsessive-compulsive disorder. *Am. J. Psychiatry* **144,** 1166–1171.
20. Swedo, S.E., Rapoport, J.L., and Cheslow, D.L. (1989) High prevalence of obsessive-compulsive symptoms in patients with Sydenham's Chorea. *Am. J. Psychiatry* **146,** 246–249.
21. von Economo, C. (ed.) (1931) Encephalitis Lethargica: Its Sequelae and Treatment. Oxford University Press, London.
22. Sasaki, K., Miyakawa, M., Sudo, T., and Yoshizaki, F. (1997) Evaluation of marble-burying behavior: induced alteration of monoamine metabolism in mouse brain. *Nippon Yakurigaku Zasshi* **110**, 205–213.
23. Bergmann, F., Chaimovitz, M., Pasternak, V., and Ramu, A. (1974) Compulsive gnawing in rats after implantation of drugs into the ventral thalamus. A contribution to the mechanism of morphine action. *Br. J. Pharmacol.* **51**, 197–205.
24. Jenike, M., Baer, L., and Ballantine, T. (1991) Cigulotomy for refractory obsessive-compulsive disorder: a long term follow-up of 33 patients. *Arch. Gen. Psychiatry* **48,** 548–555.
25. Chiocca, E.A. and Martuza, R.L. (1990) Neurosurgical therapy of obsessive compulsive disorder, in *Obsessive-Compulsive Disorders: Theory and Management* (Jenike, M.A., Baer, L., and Minichiello, W.E., ed.), Year Book Medical Publishing, Chicago, IL, pp. 283–294.
26. Baxter, L.R., Schwartz, J.M., Bergman, K.S., et al. (1992) Caudate glucose metabolic rate changes with both drug and behavior therapy for obsessive-compulsive disorder. *Arch. Gen. Psychiatry* **49,** 681–689.
27. Rauch, S.L., Jenike, M.A., Alpert, N.M., et al. (1994) Regional cerebral blood flow measured during symptom provocation in obsessive-compulsive disorder using oxygen 15-labeled carbon dioxide and positron emission tomography. *Arch. Gen. Psychiatry* **51,** 62–70.
28. Swedo, S.E., Pietrini, P., and Leonard, H.L. (1992) Cerebral glucose metabolism in childhood-onset obsessive-compulsive disorder: Revisualization during pharmacotherapy. *Arch. Gen. Psychiatry* **49,** 690–694.
29. Rosenberg, D.R. and Keshavan, M.S. (1998) Toward a neurodevelopmental model of obsessive compulsive disorder. *Biol. Psychiatry* **43**, 623–640.
30. Busatto, G.F., Buchpiguel, C.A., Zamignani, D.R., et al. (2001) Regional cerebral blood flow abnormalities in early-onset obsessive-compulsive disorder: an exploratory SPECT study. *J. Am. Acad. Child Adolesc. Psychia*try **40,** 347–354.

31. Behar, D., Rapoport, J.L., Berg, C.J., et al. (1984) Computerized tomography and neuropsychological test measures in adolescents with obsessive-compulsive disorder. *Am. J. Psychiatry* **141,** 363–369.
32. Luxenberg, J.S., Swedo, S.E., Flament, M.F., et al. (1988) Neuroanatomical abnormalities in obsessive-compulsive disorder determined with quantitative x-ray computed tomography. *Am J Psychiatry* **145**, 1089–1093.
33. Rosenberg, D.R., Keshavan, M.S., O'Hearn, K.M., et al. (1997) Fronto striatal measurement of treatment-naive pediatric obsessive compulsive disorder. *Arch. Gen. Psychiatry* **54,** 824–830.
34. Chakos, M.H., Lieberman, J.A., and Bilder, R.M. (1994) Increase in caudate nuclei volumes of first-episode schizophrenic patients taking antipsychotic drugs. *Am. J. Psychiatry* **151,** 1430–1436.
35. Keshavan, M.S., Bagwell, W.W., Haas, G.L., et al. (1994) Changes in caudate volume with neuroleptic treatment. *Lancet* **344,** 1434–1434.
36. Giedd, J.N., Rapoport, J.L., Kruesi, M.J.P., et al. (1995) Sydenham's chorea: magnetic-resonance-imaging of the basal ganglia. *Neurology* **45,** 2199–2202.
37. Giedd, J.N., Rapoport, J.L., Garvey, M.A., et al. (2000) MRI assessment of children with obsessive-compulsive disorder or tics associated with streptococcal infection. *Am. J. Psychiatry* **157**, 281–283.
38. Giedd, J.N., Rapoport, J.L., Leonard, H.L., et al. (1996) Case study: acute basal ganglia enlargement and obsessive-compulsive symptoms in an adolescent boy. *J. Am. Acad. Child Adolesc. Psychiatry* **35**, 913–915.
39. Peterson, B.S., Leckman, J.F., Tucker, D., et al. (2000) Preliminary findings of antistreptococcal antibody titers and basal ganglia volumes in tic, obsessive-compulsive, and attention deficit/hyperactivity disorders. *Arch. Gen. Psychiatry* **57,** 364–372.
40. Rosenberg, D.R. and Hanna, G.L. (2000) Genetic and imaging strategies in obsessive-compulsive disorder: potential implications for treatment development. *Biol. Psychiatry* **48,** 1210–1222.
41. Rosenberg, D.R., Keshavan, M.S., Dick, E.L., et al. (1997) Corpus callosal morphology in treatment niave pediatric obsessive compulsive disorder. *Prog. Neuropsychopharmacol. Biol. Psychiatry* **21,** 1269–1283.
42. MacMaster, F.P., Dick, E.L., Keshavan, M.S., and Rosenberg, D.R. (1999) Corpus callosal signal intensity in treatment naive pediatric obsessive compulsive disorder. *Prog. Neuropsychopharmacol. Biol. Psychiatry* **23**, 601–612.
43. Seltzer, B. and Pandya, D.N. (1986) The topography of commissural fibers., in *Two Hemispheres, One Brain. Functions of the Corpus Callosum* (Jasper, H.H., Lepore, F., and Ptito, M., eds.), Liss, New York, pp. 47–73.
44. Jenike, M.A., Rauch, S.L., Cummings, J.L., et al. (1996) Recent developments in neurobiology of obsessive-compulsive disorder. *J. Clin. Psychiatry* **57**, 492–503.
45. Breiter, H.C., Filipek, P.A., Kennedy, D.N., et al. (1994) Retrocallosal white matter abnormalities in patients with obsessive-compulsive disorder. *Arch. Gen. Psychiatry* **51,** 663–664.
46. Gilbert, A.R., Moore, G.J., Keshavan, M.S., et al. (2000) Decrease in thalamic volumes of pediatric obsessive compulsive disorder patients taking paroxetine. *Arch. Gen. Psychiatry* **57**, 449–456.
47. Jenike, M.A., Breiter, H.C., Baer, L., et al. (1996) Cerebral structural abnormalitites in obsessive-compulsive disorder: a quantitative morphometric magnetic resonance imaging atudy. *Arch. Gen. Psychiatry* **53,** 625–632.
48. Nolan, C.L., Moore, G.J., Daffu, G., et al. (2001) Localized reduction in medial thalamic volume with paroxetine treatment in pediatric obsessive compulsive disorder. *Biol. Psychiatry* **49(Suppl. 85),** 100S.
49. Rosenberg, D.R., Benazon, N.R., Gilbert, A.R., Sullivan, A., and Moore, G.J. (2000) Thalamic volume in pediatric obsessive compulsive disorder patients before and after cognitive behavioral therapy. *Biol. Psychiatry* **48,** 294–300.
50. Bartha, R., Stein, M.B., Williamson, P.C., et al. (1998) A short echo 1H spectroscopy and volumetric MRI study of the corpus striatum in patients with obsessive compulsive disorder and comparison subjects. *Am. J. Psychiatry* **155,** 1584–1591.
51. Fitzgerald, K.D., Moore, G.J., Paulson, L.D., et al. (2000) Proton spectroscopic imaging of the thalamus in treatment-naive pediatric obsessive compulsive disorder. *Biol. Psychol.* **47,** 174–182.
52. Rosenberg, D.R., Amponsah, A., Sullivan, A., et al. (2001) Increased medial thalamic choline in pediatric obsessive compulsive disorder as detected by quantitative in vivo spectroscopic imaging. *J. Child Neurol.* **16(9)**, 636–641.
53. Birken, D.L. and Oldendorf, W.H. (1989) N-acetyl-L-aspartic acid: a literature review of a compound prominent in 1H-NMR spectroscopic studies of brain. *Neurosci. Biobehav. Rev.* **13,** 23–31.
54. Grados, M., Scahill, L., and Riddle, M.A. (1999) Pharmacotherapy in children and adolescents with obsessive-compulsive disorder. *Child Adolesc. Psychiatr. Clin. N. Am.* **8**, 617–634.
55. Sallee, F.R., Hilal, R., Dougherty, D., et al. (1998) Platelet serotonin transporter in depressed children and adolescents: 3H-paroxetine platelet binding before and after sertraline. *J. Am. Acad. Child Adolesc. Psychiatry* **37**, 777–784.
56. Marazziti, D., Hollander, E., Lensi, P., et al. (1992) Peripheral markers of serotonin and dopamine function in obsessive compulsive disorder. *Psychiatry Res.* **42,** 41–51.
57. Insel, T.R., Mueller, E.A., Alterman, I., et al. (1985) Obsessive-compulsive disorder and serotonin: is there a connection? *Biol. Psychiatry* **11,** 1174–1188.
58. Thoren, P., Asberg, M., Cronholm, B., et al. (1980) Clomipramine treatment of obsessive compulsive disorder: I. A controlled clinical trial. *Arch. Gen. Psychiatry* **37,** 1281–1285.
59. Black, D.W., Kelly, M., Myers, C., and Noyes, R. Jr. (1990) Tritiated imipramine binding in obsessive-compulsive volunteers and psychiatrically normal controls. *Biol. Psychiatry.* **27,** 319–327.
60. Kim, S.W., Dysken, M.W., Pandey, G.N., and Davis, J.M. (1991) Platelet 3H-imipramine binding sites in obsessive–compulsive behavior. *Biol. Psychiatry* **30,** 467–474.
61. Vitiello, B., Shimon, H., Behar, D., et al. (1991) Platelet imipramine binding and serotonin uptake in obsessive-compulsive patients. *Acta Psychiatr. Scand.* **84,** 29–32.

62. Leckman, J.F., Goodman, W.K., Anderson, G.M., et al. (1995) Cerebrospinal fluid biogenic amines in obsessive sompulsive disorder, Tourette's syndrome, and healthy controls. *Neuropsychopharmacology* **12,** 73–86.
63. Hollander, E., Mullen, L., DeCaria, C.M., et al. (1991) Obsessive compulsive disorder, depression, and fluoxetine. *J. Clin. Psychiatry* **52,** 418–422.
64. Hollander, E., DeCarla, C.M., Nitescu, A., et al. (1995) Increased cerebral blood flow during m-CPP exacerbation of obsessive compulsive disorder. *J. Neuropsychiatry Clin. Neurosci* **7,** 485–490.
65. Pigott, T.A., Pato, M.T., L'Heureux, F., et al. (1991) A controlled comparison of adjuvant lithium carbonate or thyroid hormone in clomipramine-treated patients with obsessive compulsive disorder. *J. Clin. Psychopharmacol.* **11**, 242–248.
66. Grady, T.A., Pigott, T.A., L'Heureux, F., et al. (1993) Double-blind study of adjuvant buspirone for fluoxetine-treated patients with obsessive compulsive disorder. *Am. J. Psychiatry* **150**, 819–821.
67. Zohar, J. and Insel, T.R. (1987) Obsessive compulsive disorder: psychobiological approaches to diagnosis, treatment, and pathophysiology. *Biol. Psychiatry* **22,** 667–687.
68. Goodman, W.K., McDougle, C.J., Price, L.H., et al. (1995) m-Chlorophenylpiperazine in patients with obsessive-compulsive disorder: absence of symptom exacerbation. *Biol. Psychiatry* **38,** 138–149.
69. Ho Pian, K.L., Westenberg, H.G.M., den Boer, J.A., et al. (1998) Effects of meta-chlorophenylpiperazine on cerebral blood flow in obsessive-compulsive disorder and controls. *Biol. Psychiatry* **44,** 367–370.
70. Becquet, D., Faudon, M., and Hery, F. (1990) In vivo evidence for an inhibitory glutamatergic control of serotonin release in the cat caudate nucleus: involvement of GABA neurons. *Brain Res.* **519,** 82–88.
71. Fonnum, F., Storm-Mathisen, J., and Divac, I. (1981) Biochemical evidence for Glx as neurotransmitter in cortico-striatal and corticothalamic fibres in rat brain. *Neuroscience* **6,** 863–873.
72. Koller, K.J., Zeczek, R., and Coyle, J.T. (1984) N-acetyl-aspartyl-glutamate: regional levels in rat brain and the effects of brain lesions as determined by a new HPLC method. *J. Neurochem.* **43,** 1136–1142.
73. McLennan, H. and Curry, K. (1988) The actions of cyclopentane analogues of glutamic acid at binding sites for kainic and glutamic acids. *Exp. Brain Res.* **72,** 436–438.
74. Watkins, J.C. and Evans, R.H. (1981) Excitatory amino acids transmitters. *Annu. Rev. Pharmacol. Toxicol.* **21,** 165–204.
75. Edwards, E., Hampton, E., Ashby, C.R., et al. (1996) 5-HT3-like receptors in the rat medial prefrontal cortex: further pharmacological characterization. *Brain Res.* **733,** 21–30.
76. Rauch, S.L., Whalen, P.J., Dougherty, D.D., and Jenike, M.A. (1998) Neurobiological models of obsessive compulsive disorders, in *Obsessive Compulsive Disorders: Practical Management* (Jenike, M.A., Baer, L., and Minichiello, W.E., eds.), Mosby, Boston, pp. 222–253.
77. Parent, A., Cote, P.Y., and Lavoie, B. (1995) Chemical anatomy of primate basal ganglia. *Prog. Neurobiol.* **46,** 131–197.
78. Parent, A. and Hazrati, L.N. (1995) Functional anatomy of the basal ganglia. I. The cortico-basal ganglia-thalamo-cortical loop. *Brain Res.* **20,** 91–127.
79. Kim, J.S., Hassler, R., Haug, P., and Paik, K.S. (1977) Effect of frontal cortex ablation on striatal glutamic acid level in rat. *Brain Res.* **132,** 370–374.
80. Calabresi, P., Pisani, A., Mercuri, N.B., and Bernardi, G. (1996) The corticostriatal projection: from synaptic plasticity to dysfunction of the basal ganglia. *Trends Neurosci,* **19,** 279–280.
81. Rosenberg, D.R., MacMaster, F.P., Keshavan, M., et al. (2000) Decrease in caudate glutamatergic concentrations in pediatric obsessive compulsive disorder patients taking paroxetine. *J. Am. Acad. Child Adolesc. Psychiatry* **39,** 1096–1103.
82. El Mansari, M., Bouchard, C., and Blier, P. (1995) Alteration of serotonin release in the guinea pig orbito-frontal cortex by selective serotonin reuptake inhibitors: relevance to treatment of obsessive compulsive disorder. *Neuropsychopharmacology* **13,** 117–127.
83. Bolton, J., Moore, G.J., MacMillan, S., et al. (2001) Caudate glutamatergic changes with paroxetine persist after medication discontinuation in pediatric OCD. *J. Am. Acad. Child Adolesc. Psychiatry* **40,** 903–906.
84. Pato, M.T., Zohar-Kadouch, R., Zohar, J., and Murphy, D.L. (1988) Return of symptoms after discontinuation of clomipramine in patients with obsessive-compulsive disorder. *Am. J. Psychiatry* **145,** 1521–1525.
85. Saxena, A., Brody, A.L., Schwartz, J.M., and Baxter, L.R. (1998) Neuroimaging and frontal-subcortical circuitry in obsessive-compulsive disorder. *Br. J. Psychiatry* **173,** 26–37.

36

Dyskinesia in Patients with Schizophrenia Never Treated with Antipsychotics

Conceptual and Pathophysiological Implications

Christian Bocti, MD, **Deborah N. Black,** MD, MSc, **and John L. Waddington,** PhD, DSc

1. INTRODUCTION

Schizophrenia is a devastating mental disorder. Despite the fact that abnormal movements have been described in patients with schizophrenia for more than a century *(1,2)*, the significance and scope of this clinical reality is considerably under-represented in much of the medical literature. Because of the initial description of the extrapyramidal side effects of the first antipsychotic chlorpromazine by Steck in 1954 *(3)*, and of tardive dyskinesia by Schonecker in 1957 *(4)*, the focus of much research has been the presumed causal role of antipsychotics in the generation of abnormal movements in schizophrenia. Thus, although tardive dyskinesia has been the focus of a substantial number of studies, spontaneous dyskinesias in schizophrenia have received less consideration *(5,6)*.

2. HISTORICAL BACKGROUND: FROM KRAEPELIN AND BLEULER TO THE CONFLICT OF PARADIGMS

In 1873, Kahlbaum described the motor disorders of severe psychiatric illness and created the term catatonia *(7)*. Subsequently, Kraepelin *(1)* provided many clinical observations of abnormal movements among patients with schizophrenia, some of which appear to be indistinguishable from tardive dyskinesia: "the face is distorted by spasmodic grimacing," "wrinkling of the forehead, distortion of the mouth, irregular movements of the tongue and lips," "making faces," "rhythmic twitchings of the lips." Kraepelin was convinced that these abnormal movements were an integral part of what was then called dementia praecox, and described them as "reminding one of choreic movements." Furthermore, he conceived dementia praecox as a disease of the brain: "We arrive at the conclusion that, in dementia praecox, partial injury or destruction of neurons of the cortex must probably occur" *(1)*.

This conception of schizophrenia, however, did not prevail. During the following years, Bleuler introduced the term "schizophrenia" and along with it, a psychodynamic interpretation of abnormal movements of patients *(8)*. It is interesting to compare the phenomenological descriptions of movements by Bleuler and Kraepelin, which are very similar, and the interpretation of these movements, which are completely opposed *(9)*. Whereas Kraepelin understood them as "choreic movements" or "athetoid ataxia," Bleuler considered abnormal movements in schizophrenia as psychotic mannerisms, accessory symptoms to psychosis. This is the origin of the "conflict of paradigms" *(2)* concerning the nature of

From: *Mental and Behavioral Dysfunction in Movement Disorders*
Edited by: M-A. Bédard et al. © Humana Press Inc., Totowa, NJ

movement disorders in schizophrenia. Since the time of Kraepelin and Bleuler, diverging neurological and psychiatric traditions have produced diverging vocabularies for the description of either organic or psychogenic movement disorder, and this divergence has prevented the development of a common descriptive vocabulary for abnormal movements in schizophrenia.

Psychodynamic explanations of so-called mannerisms were to dominate, such that there was relatively little interest in studying such movements from a neurological perspective *(10)*. Though some authors considered antipsychotics to influence the course of disease-related motor disorders, soon after the introduction of antipsychotics and the description of their side effects of parkinsonism and tardive dyskinesia, the majority perspective was of an essentially, if not exclusively, causal role for antipsychotics in their genesis. Despite the difficulty of distinguishing dyskinesia from complex tics, mannerisms, and other motor phenomena using several different structured rating scales *(11)*, the conceptual distinction between presumed antipsychotic-induced tardive dyskinesia and psychogenic posturing, mannerisms, tics, and other unusual movements continued to dominate the psychiatric literature. This has remained the case until recently, when a series of publications began to challenge this notion.

3. CONTEMPORARY STUDIES OF SPONTANEOUS DYSKINESIA IN SCHIZOPHRENIA

Several recent studies have demonstrated a significant prevalence of spontaneous dyskinesia in patients with schizophrenia who were never exposed to antipsychotic drugs (Table 1). These drug-naïve patients come from four different groups: (*i*) patients from the preneuroleptic era; (*ii*) patients never treated with antipsychotics because of physician preferences; (*iii*) patients during their first psychotic episode; (*iv*) and patients from developing countries where use of these drugs is not ubiquitous. Most studies have used the Abnormal Involuntary Movement Scale (AIMS) *(12)* to assess involuntary movement disorder in a standardized fashion. Otherwise, there are substantial methodological differences among these studies, compounded by the difficulty of defining what constitutes an abnormal movement; accordingly, the reported prevalence varies greatly from one cohort to the other. Nevertheless, review of these reports enables one to extract converging evidence supporting the existence of at least a subgroup of patients with schizophrenia and movement disorders that cannot be attributed to antipsychotic medication exposure.

3.1. Spontaneous Dyskinesia in Patients from the Preneuroleptic Era

In one of the first contemporary studies of the subject, Owens and colleagues *(13)* examined 47 drug-naïve elderly schizophrenic inpatients with the AIMS and Rockland Scales in a blinded fashion relating to medication history. The patients were diagnosed according to standard criteria for schizophrenia (Feighner criteria and Present State Examination) and the possibility of undiagnosed neurological disorders was excluded by detailed history and complete neurological examination. Medication history was gathered from hospital records (average hospitalization 27 yr), and corroborated by nurses and patients when possible. The main result was the presence of abnormal involuntary movements in 51% of drug-naïve patients using a criterion of at least 3 (moderate severity) on one or more of the seven regions of the AIMS; furthermore, this challenging prevalence was only slightly, though significantly, exceeded by involuntary movements among antipsychotic-treated patients of the same cohort after adjustment for age *(14)*. The phenomenology, the distribution, and the severity of abnormal movements were indistinguishable from classic tardive dyskinesia, including orofacial involvement. This study provides strong evidence supporting the presence of abnormal movements in elderly patients with schizophrenia never treated with antipsychotics. Possible confounding factors were excluded, and the quality of the drug exposure history among these patients renders the conclusions robust.

In 1985, Rogers *(2)* published a conceptually critical study in which he described the motor disorders of severe psychiatric illness based on careful study of medical records and examination of 100 patients. The patients had been hospitalized since the preneuroleptic era, for an average of 40 yr. Nearly

Table 1
Prevalence of Spontaneous Dyskinesia in Patients with Schizophrenia but Never Exposed to Antipsychotic Drugs

Study (reference)	Patients	Mean age (yr) ± SD	n	Criteria	Prevalence (%)
Owens et al. *(13)*	Chronic inpatients	67 ± 12	47	AIMS,	
				2 on 1 item	53
				Schooler and Kane	51
Rogers *(2)*	Chronic inpatients	71	100	Clinical description	15–48
Chorfi and Moussaoui *(17)*	First episode	24	50	AIMS	0
Fenton et al. *(16)*	Chronic inpatients	28	100	Clinical description,	
				loosely defined	28
				narrowly defined	15
McCreadie et al. *(20)*	In/outpatients	45 ± 14	12	AIMS	0
Caligiuri and Lohr *(26)*	Chronically ill	37 ± 12	21	Quantitative battery	52
Chatterjee et al. *(22)*	First psychotic episode	26	89	Simpson-Dyskinesia Rating Scale,	
				1 on one item	1.1
Fenn et al. *(18)*	Acute inpatients	28 ± 5	22	AIMS,	
				Schooler and Kane	14
				2 on 1 item	37
McCreadie et al. *(21)*	Inpatients/outpatients	65	21	AIMS,	
				Schooler and Kane	38
Gervin et al. *(23)*	First psychotic episode	28 ± 10	49	AIMS,	
				Schooler and Kane,	10
				any dyskinesia	19
Puri et al. *(24)*	First episode	27 ± 8	27	AIMS,	
				2 on 1 item	7

SD, standard deviation.

all (92%) had a diagnosis of schizophrenia in their medical record. No attempt was made to apply modern diagnostic criteria for schizophrenia; however, clinical data did not suggest an alternative neurologic diagnosis. Motor disorders were defined broadly, in descriptive terms, with the conscious attempt to avoid the pitfall of the dualism of vocabulary, which pervades the neurological and psychiatric literature (e.g., mandibular tic vs grimacing mannerism). Motor behavior was considered under 10 categories, covering nearly all aspects of motor behavior: (*i*) posture; (*ii*) tone; (*iii*) purposive movement; (*iv*) overactivity; (*v*) abnormal movement of head, trunk and limbs; (*vi*) gait; (*vii*) abnormal eye movements; (*viii*) abnormal blinking; (*ix*) abnormal orofacial movements and posture; and (*x*) abnormal speech production. The retrospective review of disorders recorded before the introduction of antipsychotics in 1955 revealed that virtually every patient had a disturbance of motor function at admission, 71% having an abnormality in at least five of the defined categories. All patients were re-examined at the time of the study. Ninety-one percent had abnormalities in at least five categories of motor behavior. Interestingly, there was no significant difference in frequency or type of movements between patients currently on antipsychotic medication and those with no or minimal exposure to antipsychotics. Abnormal movements ranged from simple tic-like movements to complex postures and attitudes, with dyskinesia-like movements in between. Rogers argued that if both motor disorders and mental disorders are considered to be expressions of cerebral dysfunction, the separation between psychiatric and neurological diseases becomes superfluous. The very high prevalence of abnormalities in all aspects of motor control before any antipsychotic treatment argues in favor of including movement disorders as an integral part of severe psychiatric illness, with schizophrenia being the most prevalent clinical entity of this group. The systematic and very detailed phenomenological evaluation of motor behavior in this cohort of patients provides strong support for the existence of a pervasive disorder of motor control in schizophrenia; the scope of this conceptual approach goes beyond, but includes, the existence of spontaneous dyskinesia in schizophrenia.

As part of a larger study on tardive dyskinesia, Waddington and Youssef *(15)* described four elderly patients with schizophrenia who had never been exposed to antipsychotics and one who had received such treatment for only 2 mo. Orofacial dyskinesia, which is indistinguishable from tardive dyskinesia, was present in four of five patients. Severity scores (AIMS total) for their movements were indistinguishable from among age-matched counterparts who had received long-term exposure to antipsychotics.

A retrospective review of medical records of 94 chronically-ill patients from a private psychiatric hospital in Maryland, who met contemporary diagnostic criteria for schizophrenia, was undertaken by Fenton and colleagues *(16)*. From the time of first admission in the 1950s these patients did not receive antipsychotic medication. Patients with potentially confounding neurologic disorders were excluded. These investigators identified some form of movement disorder in 28%. Narrowly defined orofacial dyskinesia, indistinguishable from classic tardive dyskinesia, was present in 15% of patients. The particularly extensive medical records of this cohort of patients allowed the extraction of verbatim descriptions of abnormal movements, several of which were clearly compatible with contemporary definitions of tardive dyskinesia. While the retrospective nature of this study limits the precision of the results, although probably underestimating the prevalence, the unusually high quality of the medical records coupled with the stringency of the criteria used to define abnormal movements provide supporting evidence for the existence of spontaneous dyskinesia in a subgroup of patients with schizophrenia.

3.2. Spontaneous Dyskinesia in Patients from Developing Countries

Though an initial first-episode study in Morocco appeared negative *(17)*, Fenn and colleagues *(18)* subsequently examined 22 drug-naïve patients systematically and found choreoathetoid movements that met criteria for definite spontaneous dyskinesia in 14% of patients. These movements were qualitatively identical to tardive dyskinesia, as evaluated by clinicians experienced in assessment of movement disorders, but differed in distribution, being more prominent in the limbs with milder severity in the orofacial region. Of note, an additional 23% of patients presented moderate dyskinesia in only one body region, thus not meeting the stringent research criteria for tardive dyskinesia *(19)*. All patients met the Diagnostic and Statistical Manual of Mental Disorders, third edition (DSM-III) criteria for schizophrenia, and those with possible confounding factors were excluded. While a small initial study in Nigeria appeared negative *(20)*, a prevalence of spontaneous dyskinesia of 38% was reported by McCreadie and colleagues *(21)* in a larger study of drug-naïve elderly patients with schizophrenia in southeast India. This prevalence was comparable to that found in patients exposed to antipsychotics. Once again, spontaneous dyskinesia appeared indistinguishable from classic tardive dyskinesia by an experienced clinician blind to the medication history. The prevalence of similar movements among normal elderly controls of the same area (15%) was unusually high. These studies of drug-naïve patients provide prospective data supporting the existence of spontaneous dyskinesia in a significant proportion of schizophrenic patients.

3.3. Spontaneous Dyskinesia in First-Psychotic Episode Patients

The prevalence of spontaneous dyskinesia in patients with schizophrenia at the time of their first psychotic episode has been studied with objective clinical scales in four cohorts. In the first such study, Chatterjee and colleagues found only one of 89 patients with such movements *(22)*. However, in another study, Gervin and colleagues found spontaneous orofacial dyskinesia in 10% of 49 drug-naïve patients *(23)* using Schooler and Kane criteria *(19)*. Interestingly, this rate was lower (3%) among a group of similar patients who had been minimally medicated with antipsychotics before assessment;

this raises the possibility that antipsychotics may mask mild dyskinesia in young patients. The overall rate of spontaneous dyskinesia was 19% among all patients (drug-naïve and minimally treated) when mild forms of dyskinesia were included. In the third study of 27 patients, Puri and colleagues found 7% with spontaneous dyskinesia using a criterion of 2 on one or more AIMS items *(24)*; the rate of spontaneous dyskinesia was 11% if mild dyskinesia was included. Similarly, Lang and colleagues *(25)* reported that over one-third of never-medicated first-episode schizophrenic patients had extrapyramidal movement disorders. Thus, there is converging evidence from these prospective studies that a substantial minority of first-episode patients who meet clinical criteria for schizophrenia do exhibit spontaneous dyskinesia when evaluated with clinical scales.

In contrast, another group of investigators used innovative quantitative measurements to assess the presence of dyskinesia in antipsychotic-naïve patients with schizophrenia *(26)*, including accelerometry and spectral analysis of the frequency of movements, as validated for the study of tardive dyskinesia *(27)*. These authors found a significant instability of steady-state muscular force in 52% of patients, which was interpreted as subclinical spontaneous dyskinesia. This quantitative technique demonstrates a greater sensitivity compared to clinical assessment, and thus reveals subtle dysfunction of motor control in a relatively high proportion of first episode patients. These results have yet to be replicated.

In summary, spontaneous dyskinesia in young unmedicated patients with schizophrenia seems to be present to a previously unappreciated extent, though in a minority of patients, with this rate rising markedly with increasing chronicity of untreated illness.

4. CORRELATES OF SPONTANEOUS DYSKINESIA IN SCHIZOPHRENIA

There is a significant positive correlation between age and the reported prevalence of spontaneous dyskinesia *(18,23,28)*. Older age, which may be related to longer duration of untreated illness, appears to be a major risk factor for the appearance of spontaneous dyskinesia. This may account for the low prevalence of dyskinesia in studies of first-episode patients *(22–24)*. Other factors associated with spontaneous dyskinesia may include greater severity of negative symptoms, poorer prognosis, and cognitive dysfunction, such as reduced educational attainment *(16,21,23)*. Similar positive correlations between motor features and poor premorbid adjustment, longer duration of hospitalization, greater illness severity, and poor response to treatment were also found in a group of 187 psychotic inpatients, the majority of whom (77%) had schizophrenia or schizophrenia spectrum disorders *(29)*. Although 90% of this population were receiving antipsychotics, no correlations were found between motor symptoms and antipsychotic medications.

The association of spontaneous dyskinesia with cognitive impairment, negative symptoms, and disease severity appears similar to that reported previously for tardive dyskinesia *(30)*. This implies that such motor signs of schizophrenia may be a marker for greater cerebral dysfunction. In two recent studies, tardive dyskinesia was more strongly associated with impaired frontal lobe executive functions than with antipsychotic treatment *(31)*. A substantial body of evidence supports an association between impaired executive function and dyskinesia in schizophrenia *(30,32)*. It seems that the prevalence of spontaneous dyskinesia increases over the lifetime trajectory of schizophrenia in both treated and untreated patients and converges with increasing cognitive impairment in both groups with advancing age and chronicity of illness *(31)*. Thus, antipsychotic treatment may precipitate the appearance of abnormal movements in schizophrenic patients with an intrinsic vulnerability to them.

5. SPECIFICITY OF SPONTANEOUS DYSKINESIA TO SCHIZOPHRENIA

Spontaneous dyskinesia in the healthy elderly is infrequent, with a prevalence of 1.2–7.8% *(33–35)*; the prevalence and severity rise considerably in organic brain disease *(8,30,36)*. In the only systematic comparative study of which we are aware *(37)*, a higher prevalence of spontaneous dyskinesia was reported in schizophrenia (23%) relative to other diagnostic groups (7%), primarily affective and personality disorders.

6. SPONTANEOUS DYSKINESIA BEFORE ADULT ONSET OF SCHIZOPHRENIA AND IN SCHIZOPHRENIA SPECTRUM DISORDERS

The prevalence of spontaneous dyskinesia or dyskinetic-like movements has also been found to be elevated in two groups of individuals prior to the onset of schizophrenia. In a unique study, Walker and colleagues *(38)* reviewed childhood home movies of adult patients who were subsequently diagnosed with schizophrenia. More neuromotor abnormalities in the first 2 yr of life were found in preschizophrenic subjects compared to various control groups. Abnormalities included choreoathetoid movements and posturing of the upper limbs. Similarly, Jones and colleagues *(39)* in a birth cohort study found that infants and children who went on to develop schizophrenia in early adulthood showed an excess of grimacing and/or twitching movements. Other investigators have reported an increased prevalence of spontaneous dyskinesia in schizotypal personality disorder *(40,41)*, which is believed to represent a subclinical manifestation of the schizophrenia phenotype *(42)*.

7. PARKINSONISM IN DRUG-NAÏVE PATIENTS WITH SCHIZOPHRENIA

Although earlier authors noticed similarities between some clinical characteristics of schizophrenia and parkinsonism *(43)*, Caligiuri and colleagues *(44)* published the first contemporary report of parkinsonism in antipsychotic-naïve patients. They evaluated 24 newly diagnosed patients using clinical scales and a quantitative measurement battery. Clinical evaluation revealed a prevalence of 21% for rigidity and 12% for bradykinesia, while quantitative methods revealed a prevalence of 29% for rigidity and 37% for tremor; in contrast, the same quantitative methods revealed a 4% prevalence of rigidity, and no other abnormality, in a control group.

Two later studies looked at the prevalence of parkinsonism in first-episode patients using clinical scales. The first study *(22)* found a prevalence of 17% among 89 patients, mostly in the form of mild rigidity and akinesia; this was associated with less favorable response to therapy, and a higher risk of developing drug-induced parkinsonism. The second study *(24)* found a prevalence of only 4% for rigidity among 22 patients. Two other studies of drug-naïve patients with schizophrenia of various ages and disease chronicity *(18,21)* revealed parkinsonism in 18% and 24% of cases, respectively.

8. RELATIONSHIP OF SPONTANEOUS DYSKINESIA TO NEUROLOGICAL "SOFT SIGNS"

Neurological "soft signs" are subtle alterations in muscle tone, posture, and coordination, which imply nonlocalizing disorders of "complex learned patterns of motor adjustments" *(45)*. Disruptions of motor circuits linking the cerebellum, basal ganglia, and cerebral cortex are probably involved in their genesis *(46,47)*. Developmental (primitive) reflexes, such as snout, sucking, grasp, palmomental, and corneomandibular, reflect re-emergence of hard-wired motor patterns, normally suppressed during the course of brain maturation, in the presence of cerebral degeneration, aging, and brain disease; like soft signs, they do not have strict localizing value *(48)*. In a study of 152 individuals who were antipsychotic drug-free and at high risk of schizophrenia, neurological soft signs were not correlated with psychosis or with genetic liability to schizophrenia. Soft signs were, however, more frequent in subjects at high risk for schizophrenia than in normal controls, suggesting that soft signs in these high-risk individuals reflect a generalized subtle disorder of central nervous system development *(49)*.

Gupta and colleagues *(46)* examined soft signs in patients with schizophrenia, with or without exposure to antipsychotic medication. Twenty-three percent of antipsychotic-naïve patients had soft signs compared to 46% of antipsychotic-treated patients; developmental reflexes were present in 19 and 12%, respectively. In the antipsychotic-treated group, AIMS score was positively correlated with soft signs, while data for the antipsychotic-naïve group were not reported.

In a group of 66 antipsychotic-treated patients, Youssef and Waddington *(48)* reported that developmental reflexes were correlated with the presence of tardive dyskinesia, suggesting that both developmental reflexes and tardive dyskinesia in this population reflect an associated burden of cerebral dysfunction. Neurological soft signs, tardive dyskinesia, and cognitive impairment were also highly intercorrelated in a population of chronically ill, medicated patients *(50)*; soft signs were correlated with low IQ and asociality in unmedicated patients *(51)*. Although there was a trend for soft signs to be associated with the duration of antipsychotic medication, this may reflect earlier onset and more severe psychopathology in patients with soft signs *(50)*.

In a carefully designed study of 35 unmedicated first-episode patients with schizophrenia, Browne and colleagues *(52)* reported that one or more neurological soft signs were present in 34 (97%) patients, and two or more soft signs were present in 22 (63%). There were positive correlations between soft signs, mixed-handed dominance, severity of psychosis, fewer years of education, and poorer premorbid social adjustment compared to nonmixed-handed patients.

Rossi and colleagues found a higher incidence of soft signs in 58 treated patients relative to normal controls *(47)*. Cox and Ludwig *(53)* and Browne and colleagues *(52)* failed to find any relationship between antipsychotic medication and soft signs in schizophrenia.

9. PATHOPHYSIOLOGY OF MOVEMENT DISORDER INTEGRAL TO SCHIZOPHRENIA: ROLE OF THE BASAL GANGLIA IN CORTICAL-SUBCORTICAL NETWORKS

The studies cited above indicate that patients with schizophrenia can exhibit abnormal involuntary movements that are phenomenologically indistinguishable from tardive dyskinesia. A correlation exists between spontaneous dyskinesia and aging, disease chronicity, severity of negative symptoms, and indices of cognitive and neurological dysfunction, as has been reported for tardive dyskinesia. This constellation of abnormal involuntary movements, negative symptoms and cognitive dysfunction of the frontal–executive type is compatible with current concepts of frontal-subcortical network dysfunction *(54,55)*.

"Positive" motor phenomena of schizophrenia, including mannerisms, stereotypies, rituals, tics, dyskinesias, and verbigeration, and "negative" manifestations including mutism, postural perseveration, bradykinesia, rigidity, and parkinsonism, all share links to the basal ganglia and imply disturbance of frontosubcortical circuits *(11,56)*. Conversely, in clinical disorders known to affect the basal ganglia, psychotic and schizophreniform disorders are encountered in a significant minority of patients. For example, the misdiagnosis of Huntington's disease as schizophrenia has been reported several times *(57–59)*. In this neurodegenerative disease, the most striking atrophy is observed in the caudate and putamen. When psychiatric features antedate movement disorders by several years, the clinical picture may indeed be very similar to schizophrenia, emphasizing the role of basal ganglia dysfunction in psychosis.

Recent functional imaging data have provided further support for this association. Menon and colleagues *(60)* used a motor sequencing task to investigate activation of the caudate, putamen, globus pallidus, and thalamus in eight patients with schizophrenia and 12 controls. In patients, but not in controls, functional magnetic resonance imaging (fMRI) during the task showed bilateral hypoactivation in the posterior putamen-globus pallidus and secondary hypoactivation of the thalamus, which receives major input from the globus pallidus. In contrast, Manoach and colleagues demonstrated increased activation of basal ganglia and thalamus relative to controls on a cognitive (working memory) task *(61)*. The resolution of this fMRI study did not permit anatomical differentiation of basal ganglia structures. An innovative investigation by another group *(62)*, using a combination of proton magnetic resonance spectroscopy (^{1}H-MRS) and radioreceptor imaging, demonstrated a relationship between prefrontal cortex N-acetyl-aspartate, a marker of neuronal integrity, and striatal dopamine activity in schizophrenic patients. These results clearly point to a dysfunction of the basal ganglia and/or of associated neuronal networks in schizophrenia.

The data presented here enable us to speculate that functional or microstructural disconnection among neural networks involved in the integration of sensory signals and motor output may underlie the simple and complex abnormalities of motor behavior in schizophrenia. These data also suggest that the idea that antipsychotic drugs alone are the cause of tardive dyskinesia and parkinsonism in schizophrenia should be abandoned. This view should be replaced by a model in which antipsychotic drugs interact with the underlying neurodevelopmentally mediated disease process to accentuate motor phenomena *(11,31)*.

10. CONCLUSION

Schizophrenia is increasingly defined as a complex disorder having a neurodevelopmental basis. This conclusion is supported by a plethora of recent studies spanning neuropathology, neurobiology, functional and structural neuroimaging, neuropsychology, and genetics *(60,63–65)*.

One clinical counterpart of the reconceptualization of schizophrenia as a developmental disorder is the inclusion of a neuromotor component reflecting basal ganglia pathology. The motor disorders of schizophrenia thus join other markers of subtle but pervasive cerebral dysfunction, which are detectable well before the appearance of psychosis, including craniofacial dysmorphogenesis, poor social adjustment, mixed-handed dominance, reading and language difficulties, and poor visuomotor coordination *(65)*. In this perspective, antipsychotics promote dyskinesia by acting on disordered frontosubcortical circuits, but they are not the cause of dyskinesia. The paradigm shift, which places schizophrenia in the spectrum of developmental disorders, allows abnormalities of movement to be included as an integral feature of this disease.

REFERENCES

1. Kraepelin, E. (1919) *Dementia Praecox and Paraphrenia* (Trans. Barclay, R.M.), Livingstone, Edinburgh.
2. Rogers, D. (1985) The motor disorders of severe psychiatric illness: a conflict of paradigms. *Br. J. Psychiatry* **147,** 221–232.
3. Steck, H. (1954) Le syndrome extrapyramidal et diencéphalique au cours des traitements au largactil et au serpasil. *Ann. Med. Psychol.* **112,** 737–743.
4. Schonecker, V.M. (1957) Ein eigentümliches syndrom in oralen bereich bei megphen applikation. *Nervenarzt* **28,** 35–43.
5. Baldessarini, R.J. and Taresy, D. (1976) Mechanisms underlying tardive dyskinesia, in *The Basal Ganglia* (Yahr, M.D., ed.), Raven Press, New York, pp. 433–446.
6. Kane, J.M. (1999) Tardive dykinesia, in *Movement Disorders in Neurology and Neuropsychiatry* (Joseph, A.B. and Young, R.R., eds.), Blackwell Science, Oxford, pp. 31–35.
7. Kahlbaum, K.L. (1973) *Catatonia* (Trans. Levij, Y. and Priden, T.), Johns Hopkins University Press, Baltimore.
8. Waddington, J.L. and Crow, T.J. (1988) Abnormal involuntary movements and psychosis in the preneuroleptic era and in unmedicated patients: implications for the concept of tardive dyskinesia, in *Tardive Dyskinesia: Biological Mechanisms and Clinical Aspects* (Wolf, M. and Mosnaim, A.D., eds.), American Psychiatric Press, Washington, DC, pp. 51–66.
9. Casey, D.E. (1985) Spontaneous and tardive dyskinesias: clinical and laboratory studies. *J. Clin. Psychiatry* **46,** 42–47.
10. Flinn, D. and Bazzell, W. (1983) Psychiatric aspects of abnormal movement disorders. *Brain Res. Bull.* **11,** 153–161.
11. McKenna, P.J., Lund, C.E., Mortimer, A.M., and Biggins, C.A. (1991) Motor, volitional and behavioural disorders in schizophrenia 2: the "Conflict of Paradigms" hypothesis. *Br. J. Psychiatry* **158,** 328–336.
12. Guy, W., ed. (1976) *Abnormal Involuntary Movements Scale (AIMS). ECDEU Assessment Manual.* U.S. Department of Health, Education, and Welfare, Rockville, Maryland.
13. Owens, D.G., Johnstone, E.C., and Frith, C.D. (1982) Spontaneous involuntary disorders of movement: their prevalence, severity, and distribution in chronic schizophrenics with and without treatment with neuroleptics. *Arch. Gen. Psychiatry* **39,** 452–461.
14. Crow, T.J., Cross, A.I., Johnstone, E.C., Owen, F., Owens, D.G.C., and Waddington, J.L. (1982) Abnormal involuntary movements in schizophrenia: are they related to the disease process or its treatment? Are they associated with changes in dopamine receptors? *J. Clin. Psychopharmacol.* **2,** 336–340.
15. Waddington, J.L. and Youssef, H.A. (1990) The lifetime outcome and involuntary movements of schizophrenia never treated with neuroleptic drugs. *Br. J. Psychiatry* **156,** 106–108.
16. Fenton, W.S., Wyatt, R.J., and McGlashan, T.H. (1994) Risk factors for spontaneous dyskinesia in schizophrenia. *Arch. Gen. Psychiatry* **51,** 643–650.

17. Chorfi, M. and Moussaoui, D. (1989) Lack of dyskinesia in unmedicated schizophrenics [letter]. *Psychopharmacology* **97,** 423.
18. Fenn, D.S., Moussaoui, D., Hoffman, W.F., et al. (1996) Movements in never-medicated schizophrenics: a preliminary study. *Psychopharmacology* **123,** 206–210.
19. Schooler, N.R. and Kane, J.M. (1982) Research diagnoses for tardive dyskinesia. *Arch. Gen. Psychiatry* **39,** 486–487.
20. McCreadie, R.G. and Ohaeri, J.U. (1994) Movement disorder in never and minimally treated Nigerian schizophrenic patients. *Br. J. Psychiatry* **164,** 184–189.
21. McCreadie, R.G., Thara, R., Kamath, S., et al. (1996) Abnormal movements in never-medicated Indian patients with schizophrenia. *Br. J. Psychiatry* **168,** 221–226.
22. Chatterjee, A., Chakos, M., Koreen, A., et al. (1995) Prevalence and clinical correlates of extrapyramidal signs and spontaneous dyskinesia in never-medicated schizophrenic patients. *Am. J. Psychiatry* **152,** 1724–1729.
23. Gervin, M., Browne, S., Lane, A., et al. (1998) Spontaneous abnormal involuntary movements in first-episode schizophrenia and schizophreniform disorder: baseline rate in a group of patients from an Irish catchment area. *Am. J. Psychiatry* **155,** 1202–1206.
24. Puri, B.K., Barnes, T.R., Chapman, M.J., Hutton, S.B., and Joyce, E.M. (1999) Spontaneous dyskinesia in first episode schizophrenia. *J. Neurol. Neurosurg. Psychiatry* **66,** 76–78.
25. Lang, D.J., Kopala, L.C., Vandorpe, R.A., et al. (2001) An MRI study of basal ganglia volumes in first-episode schizophrenia patients treated with risperidone. *Am. J. Psychiatry* **158,** 625–631.
26. Caligiuri, M.P. and Lohr, J.B. (1994) A disturbance in the control of muscle force in neuroleptic-naive schizophrenic patients. *Biol. Psychiatry* **35,** 104–111.
27. Caligiuri, M.P., Lohr, J.B., Rotrosen, J., et al. (1997) Reliability of an instrumental assessment of tardive dyskinesia: results from VA Cooperative Study #394. *Psychopharmacology* **132,** 61–66.
28. Fenton, W.S. (2000) Prevalence of spontaneous dyskinesia in schizophrenia. *J. Clin. Psychiatry* **61(Suppl. 4),** 10–14.
29. Peralta, V. and Cuesta, M.J. (2001) Motor features in psychotic disorders. I. Factor structure and clinical correlates. *Schizophr. Res.* **47,** 107–116.
30. Waddington, J.L. (1995) Psychopathological and cognitive correlates of tardive dyskinesia in schizophrenia and other disorders treated with neuroleptic drugs, in *Advances In Neurology*, vol. 65 (Weiner, W.J. and Lang, A.E., eds.), Raven Press, New York, pp. 211–229.
31. Quinn, J., Meagher, D., Murphy, P., Kinsella, A., Mullaney, J., and Waddington, J.L. (2001) Vulnerability to involuntary movements over a lifetime trajectory of schizophrenia approaches 100%, in association with executive (frontal) dysfunction. *Schizophr. Res.* **49,** 79–87.
32. Brown, F.W. (1992) The neurobiology of late-life psychosis. *Crit. Rev. Neurobiol.* **7,** 275–289.
33. D'Alessandro, R., Benassi, G., Cristina, E., Gallasi, R., and Manzaroli, D. (1986) The prevalence of lingual-facial-buccal dyskinesia in the elderly. *Neurology* **36,** 1350–1351.
34. Kane, J.M., Weinhold, P., Kinon, B., Wegner, J., and Leader, M. (1982) Prevalence of abnormal involuntary movements ("spontaneous dyskinesias") in the normal elderly. *Psychopharmacology* **77,** 105–108.
35. Klawans, H.L. and Barr, A. (1982) Prevalence of spontaneous lingual-facial-buccal dyskinesias in the elderly. *Neurology* **32,** 558–559.
36. Waddington, J.L. (1989) Schizophrenia, affective psychoses and other disorders treated with neuroleptic drugs: the enigma of tardive dyskinesia, its neurobiological determinants and the "conflict of paradigms." *Int. Rev. Neurobiol.* **31,** 297–353.
37. Fenton, W.S., Blyler, C.R., Wyatt, R.J., and McGlashan, T.H. (1997) Prevalence of spontaneous dyskinesia in schizophrenic and non-schizophrenic psychiatric patients. *Br. J. Psychiatry* **171,** 265–268.
38. Walker, E.F., Savoie, T., and Davis, D. (1994) Neuromotor precursors of schizophrenia. *Schizophr. Bull.* **20,** 441–451.
39. Jones, P., Rodgers, B., Murray, R., and Marmot, M. (1994) Child developmental risk factors for adult schizophrenia in the British 1946 birth cohort. *Lancet* **344,** 1398–1402.
40. Cassady, S.L., Adami, H., Moran, M., Kunkel, R., and Thaker, G.K. (1998) Spontaneous dyskinesia in subjects with schizophrenia spectrum personality. *Am. J. Psychiatry* **155,** 70–75.
41. Walker, E., Lewis, N., Loewy, R., and Palyo, S. (1999) Motor dysfunction and risk for schizophrenia. *Dev. Psychopathol.* **11,** 509–523.
42. Kendler, K.S., McGuire, M., Gruenberg, A.M., O'Hare, A., Spellman, M., and Walsh, D. (1993) The Roscommon Family Study. III. Schizophrenia-related personality disorders in relatives. *Arch. Gen. Psychiatry* **50,** 781–788.
43. Mettler, F.A. (1955) Perceptual capacity, functions of the striatum and schizophrenia. *Psychiatr. Q.* **29,** 89–110.
44. Caligiuri, M.P., Lohr, J.B., and Jeste, D.V. (1993) Parkinsonism in neuroleptic-naive schizophrenic patients. *Am. J. Psychiatry* **150,** 1343–1348.
45. Kennard, M.A. (1960) Value of equivocal signs in neurologic diagnosis. *Neurology* **10,** 753–764.
46. Gupta, S., Andreasen, N.C., Arndt, S., et al. (1995) Neurological soft signs in neuroleptic-naive and neuroleptic-treated schizophrenic patients and in normal comparison subjects. *Am. J. Psychiatry* **152,** 191–196.
47. Rossi, A., DeCataldo, S., DeMichele, V., et al. (1990) Neurological soft signs in schizophrenia. *Br. J. Psychiatry* **157,** 735–739.
48. Youssef, H.A. and Waddington, J.L. (1988) Primitive (developmental) reflexes and diffuse cerebral dysfunction in schizophrenia and bipolar affective disorder: overrepresentation in patients with tardive dyskinesia. *Biol. Psychiatry* **23,** 791–796.
49. Lawrie, S.M., Byrne, M., Miller, P., et al. (2001) Neurodevelopmental indices and the development of psychotic symptoms in subjects at high risk of schizophrenia. *Br. J. Psychiatry* **178,** 524–530.

50. King, D.J., Wilson, A., Cooper, S.J., and Waddington, J.L. (1991) The clinical correlates of neurological soft signs in chronic schizophrenia. *Br. J. Psychiatry* **158,** 770–775.
51. Quitkin, F., Rifkin, A., and Klein, D.F. (1976) Neurological soft signs in schizophrenia and character disorders. *Arch. Gen. Psychiatry* **33,** 845–853.
52. Browne, S., Clarke, M., Gervin, M., et al. (2000) Determinants of neurological dysfunction in first episode schizophrenia. *Psychol. Med.* **30,** 1433–1441.
53. Cox, S.M. and Ludwig, A.M. (1979) Neurological soft signs and psychopathology, I: findings in schizophrenia. *J. Nerv. Ment. Dis.* **167,** 161–165.
54. Busatto, G.F. and Kerwin, R.W. (1997) Schizophrenia, psychosis and the basal ganglia. *Psychiatr. Clin. N. Am.* **20,** 897–910.
55. Frith, C.D. (1995) Schizophrenia: functional imaging and cognitive abnormalities. *Lancet* **346,** 615–620.
56. Krüger, S., Bräunig, P., Höffler, J., Shugar, G., Borner, I., and Langkrar, J. (2000) Prevalence of obsessive-compulsive disorder in schizophrenia and significance of motor symptoms. *J. Neuropsychiatry Clin. Neurosci.* **12,** 16–24.
57. Lovestone, S., Hodgson, S., Sham, P., Differ, A.M., and Levy, R. (1996) Familial psychiatric presentation of Huntington's disease. *J. Med. Genet.* **33,** 128–131.
58. Shiwach, R. (1994) Psychopathology in Huntington's disease patients. *Acta Psychiatr. Scand.* **90,** 241–246.
59. Tsuang, D., DiGiacomo, L., Lipe, H., and Bird, T.D. (1998) Familial aggregation of schizophrenia-like symptoms in Huntington's disease. *Am. J. Med. Genet.* **81,** 323–327.
60. Menon, V., Anagnoson, R.T., Glover, G.H., and Pfefferbaum, A. (2001) Functional magnetic resonance imaging evidence for disrupted basal ganglia function in schizophrenia. *Am. J. Psychiatry* **158,** 646–649.
61. Manoach, D.S., Gollub, R.L., Benson, E.S., et al. (2000) Schizophrenic subjects show aberrant fMRI activation of dorsolateral prefrontal cortex and basal ganglia during working memory performance. *Biol. Psychiatry* **48,** 99–109.
62. Bertolino, A., Knable, M.B., Saunders, R.C., et al. (1999) The relationship between dorsolateral prefrontal N-acetylaspartate measures and striatal dopamine activity in schizophrenia. *Biol. Psychiatry* **45,** 660–667.
63. Bullmore, E.T., Frangou, S., and Murray, R.M. (1997) The dysplastic net hypothesis: an integration of developmental and dysconnectivity theories of schizophrenia. *Schizophr. Res.* **28,** 143–156.
64. Paulsen, J.S., Heaton, R.K., Sadek, J.R., et al. (1995) The nature of learning and memory impairments in schizophrenia. *J. Int. Neuropsychol. Soc.* **1,** 88–99.
65. Waddington, J.L., Lane, A., Scully, P., et al. (1999) Early cerebro-craniofacial dysmorphogenesis in schizophrenia: a lifetime trajectory model from neurodevelopmental basis to 'neuroprogressive' process. *J. Psychiatr. Res.* **33,** 477–489.

VII
Quality of Life in Parkinson's Disease

37

Medical and Psychosocial Determinants of Quality of Life in Parkinson's Disease

Anette Schrag, MD, PhD **and Caroline Selai,** PhD

1. INTRODUCTION

In the last 20 yr, there has been an explosion of interest in the measurement of quality of life (QoL). Although this elusive concept proved difficult to operationally define and its measurement raises a number of complex technical and ethical issues, progress in the field has been rapid, and there are now more than 1000 QoL instruments available *(1)*. Well-validated measures of QoL now exist for many health conditions (e.g., cancer and cardiovascular disorders), but attention has only relatively recently turned to the assessment of QoL in neurological conditions *(2)*. As it has become clear that subjective patient-rated evaluation of well-being may differ considerably from the judgement by medical observers, the assessment of QoL is becoming increasingly important in the management of patients with Parkinson's disease (PD).

In this chapter, after reviewing a number of conceptual and methodological issues, we discuss the medical and psychosocial factors that have been found to be related to QoL of patients with PD.

2. MEASURING QoL IN PD

2.1. *Definition of QoL*

Although the definition of this somewhat elusive term is still discussed in the literature, there is general consensus on some fundamental points. First, QoL is a multidimensional construct comprising a variety of factors, including environmental, economic, spiritual, geographic, and political variables *(3)*. In the medical context, research has focused on the narrower concept of health-related quality of life (Hr-QoL), which comprises physical, psychological, and social well-being. While there is no absolute agreement about the subcomponents of each domain, most Hr-QoL scales include items such as physical fitness, main activity (work and social life), cognitive functioning, mood, and pain. Although not strictly identical, in the medical context the terms quality of life, health-related quality of life, and health status are used somewhat interchangeably.

Second, appraisal of Hr-QoL is highly subjective, and since research has shown that proxy ratings of Hr-QoL often do not correlate with patients' own answers, any appraisal of Hr-QoL should rely, where possible, on the perception of the individual patient.

2.2. *Types of Hr-QoL Measures*

There is no "gold standard" for measuring Hr-QoL, and the range of instruments available is remarkable in terms of both quantity and heterogeneity. The categories of Hr-QoL measures have been comprehensively reviewed elsewhere *(4)*. In brief, *generic* instruments cover a broad range of Hr-QoL domains

From: *Mental and Behavioral Dysfunction in Movement Disorders*
Edited by: M-A. Bédard et al. © Humana Press Inc., Totowa, NJ

in a single instrument. Their chief advantage is in facilitating comparisons between different disease groups. *Disease-specific* instruments are more specific, because they include only items relevant for a particular illness, but their main disadvantage is the lack of comparability of results with those from other disease groups. *Health profiles* provide separate scores for each of the dimensions of Hr-QoL, whereas a *health index*, which is a type of generic instrument, gives a single summary score, usually from 0 (death) to 1 (perfect health). A further category, developed within the economic tradition, is that of *utility* measures. These are preference-weighted measures, which are used for calculations of the allocation of healthcare resources in society. The choice of measure will depend on the goal of the study; a common recommendation is to include both disease-specific and generic measures in an investigation.

2.3. Measurement Issues

The psychometric testing of a measure is a labor-intensive exercise, and the evaluation of a measure's performance in a number of situations is an ongoing process. This testing has not uniformly been conducted with all instruments, particularly older instruments. In considering the psychometric properties of an instrument, the basic criteria are that the measure be valid, reliable, and sensitive. For a comprehensive review of the statistical procedures, see Streiner and Norman *(5)*. In brief, *validity* is how well the instrument measures what it purports to measure. There are various statistical procedures for testing different aspects of an instrument's validity. The terminology is somewhat confusing, but Streiner and Norman provide a useful guide to the various types (e.g., *face* validity, *construct* validity, *criterion* validity, *concurrent* validity, and *predictive* validity). *Reliability* assesses whether the same measurement can be obtained on other occasions and concerns the amount of error inherent in any measurement. Two basic reliability tests are the *internal consistency* of a test, measured by coefficient α, and *test–retest* reliability, where scores taken on two occasions are compared. There are problems in assessing the test–retest reliability of Hr-QoL measures, where genuine changes in the patient's well-being may have occurred before the follow-up assessment, making it difficult to distinguish measurement error from genuine change in health or Hr-QoL. *Sensitivity* is concerned with how sensitive the measure is in detecting clinically relevant changes in Hr-QoL. This is important for monitoring benefits of treatment.

2.4. QoL Measures Used in PD

Two approaches have been taken to the measurement of Hr-QoL in PD. Existing generic Hr-QoL measures such as the Sickness Impact Profile (SIP) *(6)*, the Nottingham Health Profile (NHP) *(7)*, the Medical Outcomes Short Form (SF-36) *(8)*, and EuroQoL (EQ-5D) *(9)*, have all been used, and to varying degrees been shown to be valid, in patients with PD. More recently, PD-specific Hr-QoL measures have been developed. Table 1 briefly describes the currently available PD-specific Hr-QoL measures. Out of these, only the Parkinson's Disease Questionnaire (PDQ-39) *(10)* and the Parkinson's Disease Quality of Life Questionnaire (PDQL) *(11)* have been validated by additional authors other than the developers. The differences between the contents and psychometric properties of these two scales have been reviewed elsewhere *(12)*.

Measurement of the impact of PD on Hr-QoL is important for assessing the outcome of treatment trials, planning provision of healthcare resources, and managing patients in clinical practice. We will discuss studies that have assessed HR-QoL of patients with PD.

2.5. Methodological Issues

In comparing studies, some methodological issues need to be borne in mind. For example, none of the available instruments is all-inclusive, so that issues important to individual patients may, therefore, be missed. Only limited comparisons can be made between studies using different types of instruments, studies with different sample sizes, and studies conducted in different settings (clinic-based or

Table 1
Disease-Specific Hr-QoL Measures Developed for PD

PD-specific measure	Number of items	Domains of Hr-QoL covered by scale	Reference
Parkinson' Disease Questionnaire 39-item version (PDQ-39)	39	Mobility, ADL, emotional well-being, stigma, social support, cognition, communications, bodily discomfort	Peto et al. *(10)*
Parkinson' Disease Questionnaire 8-item version (PDQ-8)	8	Mobility, ADL, emotional well-being, stigma, social support, cognition, communications, bodily discomfort	Peto et al. *(75)*
Parkinson' Disease Quality of Life Questionnaire (PDQL)	37	Parkinsonian symptoms, systemic symptoms, emotional functioning, social functioning	de Boer et al. *(11)*
Parkinson's Impact Scale (PIMS)	10	Self (positive), self (negative), family relationships, community relationships, work, leisure, travel, safety, financial security, sexuality; differentiates between on- and off-states	Calne et al. *(76)*
Parkinson's Disease Quality of Life Scale (PDQUALIF)	Not reported (abstract only)	Not reported	Welsh et al. *(64)*
Parkinson's Disease Symptom Inventory (PDSI)	51	Frequency and distress of symptoms, further analysis on scoring ongoing	Hogan et al. *(77)*

population-based samples). Thus, some complications of PD, which are not common in the overall population of patients with PD, may be very important to subgroups of patients. Studies investigating Hr-QoL in these subgroups would, therefore, yield different results than investigations in the overall population. For example, if hallucinations are a severe problem to some patients with PD, but uncommon, the presence of hallucinations would not influence the Hr-QoL score of the overall population, but may be reflected in an analysis of this subgroup. In addition, treatment trials for alleviation of a particular symptom, e.g., psychosis, will need to use a Hr-QoL instrument sensitive to this issue. Also, it should be kept in mind when comparing mean group scores, individual patients will differ from the overall population.

3. MEDICAL AND PSYCHOSOCIAL CONSEQUENCES OF PD

PD and its treatment can be associated with a wide range of symptoms, including the cardinal features of bradykinesia, rigidity, tremor, and postural instability, nonmotor symptoms, such as depression, insomnia, sexual, and autonomic dysfunction, and complications of the disease and its treatment, such as motor fluctuations, dyskinesias, hallucinations, and dementia. Physical symptoms mainly lead to impairment of Hr-QoL in the physical domain, but can also lead to increased dependence on others, a diminished sense of autonomy and self-image *(13)*, impairment of role functioning, emotional disturbances, fear of social stigma associated with physical symptoms, and withdrawal from social interactions *(10,14)*. Nonmotor symptoms such as depression, anxiety, and pain often lead to impaired emotional well-being, sexual dysfunction, and impairment of social functioning.

There is ample evidence that all areas of Hr-QoL can be affected by having PD, but the main areas of impairment lie in physical functioning, emotional reactions, social isolation, and energy. Other domains of impairment of Hr-QoL in PD identified include bodily discomfort and/or pain, self-image, cognitive function, communication, sleep, role function, and sexual function *(15–18)*.

Table 2 gives examples of features of PD and its treatment, domains of Hr-QoL, which can be affected, and demographic and psychosocial variables, which may influence Hr-QoL in patients with PD.

4. MEDICAL AND PSYCHOSOCIAL DETERMINANTS OF HR-QoL IN PD

The effect on Hr-QoL of having PD is likely to be dependent on a complex interaction of disease- and treatment-related demographic and psychosocial factors. Although no study can assess the relationship between all of these factors, a number of studies have provided information on factors relevant to the Hr-QoL of patients with PD. The results from a selection of studies are summarized in Table 3.

4.1. *Disease-Related*

In interpreting these studies, it should be remembered that a relationship between Hr-QoL and other factors is often complex, and, especially as most studies are cross-sectional, causality is difficult to establish.

4.1.1. Disease Severity

It is hardly surprising that Hr-QoL deteriorates with advancing disease and increasing disease severity as measured by the Hoehn and Yahr (HY) or Webster scales. However, this association differs according to the instruments used to assess Hr-QoL in patients with PD. Generally, the association between objective disease severity and Hr-QoL scores is stronger with disease-specific instruments, which enquire about physical problems related to PD, particularly in the areas of physical function, such as mobility, activities of daily living (ADL), and physical and social functioning *(16,18–21)*. Studies using generic instruments have also found associations between HY stage and all aspects of the generic Hr-QoL measures or their physical subscores, although the mental subscore of the SF-36 generally has, as might be expected, been shown to correlate less strongly with HY score and Webster scales *(22,23)*.

Table 2
Examples of Factors Relevant to HR-QoL in PD

Symptoms of PD and its treatment	Domains of HR-QoL that may be affected	Demographic variables	Psychosocial variables
Motor symptoms	Physical function, e.g., mobility, bodily discomfort	Age	Personal, e.g., coping strategies, personal attitudes, expectations, level of optimism
Speech impairment	Psychological, e.g., stigma, self-image	Gender	
Autonomic function	Social, e.g., family life, dependence on others, social interaction	Socioeconomic class	
Cognitive impairment	Role functioning, e.g., emotional, physical	Area of residence	
Affect, e.g., depression	ADL, e.g., self-care		
Sexual dysfunction	Emotional well-being, e.g., depression, isolation, fear of future		
Insomnia			
Motor fluctuations			
Dyskinesias			
Treatment-induced psychiatric complications			

Table 3
Main Findings of Selected Studies on Factors Associated with HrQoL in Patients with PD

Reference	Hr-Qol measure used	Study population	Main results
Kuopio et al. (2000) *(18)*	SF-36	Population-based	Depression was the most important factor associated with poor HrQoL. Association of disease severity with HrQoL exceeded that of depression only on the dimension of physical functioning. Women rated their HrQoL worse than men, but also had worse depression scores. The variance of HrQoL scores was predicted in a higher proportion of patients for the dimension of physical function than for other dimension.
Kuopio (2000) *(26)*	SF-36	Population-based	Depression was the most significant explanatory factor for all dimensions of HrQoL. Association of ADL with HrQoL scores only exceeded that of depression on tte dimensions measuring physical capacity. Freezing, night-time akinesia, and early morning akinesia were associated with worse HrQoL. Dystonia was associated with lower scores on the dimensions of mental health and health perceptions.
Karlsen et al. (1999) *(27)*	NHP	Population-based	Patients with PD had higher distress scores than elderly controls in all NHP dimensions. Lack of energy was reported by half of all patients with PD. The strongest predictor for total NHP scores were depression scores, self-reported insomnia, and a low degree of independence. Disease severity contributed to a lesser degree to prediction of Hr-QoL scores than depression, insomnia, and loss of independence.
Karlsen et al. (2000) *(25)*	NHP	Population-based	After 4 yr follow-up, there was a significant deterioration of total HrQoL scores and the subscores of physical mobility, emotional reactions, painand social isolation. No clinical or demographic factors predicted the decline of HrQoL scores. Change in HrQoL scores correlated with deterioration of disease severity. Depression, disability, and insomnia were the most important predictive factors for poor HrQoL scores at both points, but there was no correlation between change in depression and HrQoL scores.
Schrag et al. (2000) *(23)*	PDQ-39, SF-36, EQ-5D	Population-based	HrQoL scores were most strongly related to depression scores, disability, postural instability, and cognitive impairment. Patients with akinetic-rigid parkinsonism had worse HrQoL scores than those with tremor-dominant disease.

Schrag et al. (2000) *(17)*	PDQ-39,SF-36, EQ-5D	Population-based	Greatest impairment of Hr-QoL as compared to the general population was seen in the areas of physical and social functioning, physical role limitations, and general health perceptions.
Damiano et al. (2000) *(16)*	PDQ 39, SF-36	Clinic-based	Patients with dyskinesias reported significantly poorer PDQ-39 but not SF-36 scores than patients without dyskinesias. Patients with self-reported comorbidities reported worse physical function and general health scores on the SF-36.
Hobson et al. (1999) *(31)*	PDQL	Clinic-based	Poorer HrQoL was associated with increasing disease severity, more severe depressive symptomatology, and impaired cognitive functioning. Patients aged 75 or older had worse Hr-QoL scores in the dimensions of parkinsonian symptoms, systemic symptoms, and social functioning, but not emotional functioning.
Findley (1999) *(32)*	PDQ 39	Clinic-based	Hoehn and Yahr stage and medication together explained only 17% of the variability in Hr-QoL. Depression was the most significant predictor of variability in Hr-QoL, but patients' satisfaction with the explanation of the condition at diagnosis and current feelings of optimism also contributed to prediction of Hr-QoL scores.
Rubenstein et al. (1998) *(28)*	SF-36	Clinic-based	Poorer Hr-QoL scores were associated with disease stages in all dimensions. Patients with off-periods, dyskinesias, dystonia, and sleep disturbances had poorer Hr-QoL scores than those without.
Lyons et al. (1998) *(24)*	PDQ-39	Clinic-based	Postural instabilty, gait abnormalities, bradykinesia, and disease duration were the best predictors of Hr-QoL in PD. Tremor, rigidity, age, and units of PD medication were not strongly associated with Hr-QoL.

Abbreviations: SF-36, Medical Outcomes Short Form; NHP, Nottingham Health Profile; PDQ-39, Parkinson's Disease Questionnaire 39-item version; EQ-5D, EuroQoL.

4.1.2. Disease Duration

Most studies have not found a strong relationship between disease duration and Hr-QoL, although severity of disease and disability increase with longer disease duration *(23,24)*. An exception is a study from Finland *(18)*, in which the subscores of social functioning, physical functioning, and physical role limitations correlated significantly with longer disease duration, which the authors inter-preted as an increasing tendency toward unsociable behavior with advancing disease. This weak association between disease duration and Hr-QoL may indicate that through mediating factors, such as acceptance of illness, coping mechanisms, appropriate treatment, or change of environmental circumstances, longer disease duration has less impact on perceived health state. Another explanation may be that the relationship between longer disease duration and greater impairment of Hr-QoL may also be missed in cross-sectional samples due to the great variability in progression rates and poor recall of the time of onset. The only longitudinal study to date *(25)*, which assessed Hr-QoL after a follow-up of 4 yr, reported a significant increase in overall NHP scores, reflecting a decreased Hr-QoL and a deterioration in the dimensions of physical mobility, emotional reactions, pain, and social isolation, with a simultaneous increase in disease severity. This suggests that longer disease duration leads to worsening Hr-QoL, at least when there is an increase in disease severity. Studies adjusting for the effect of disease severity and disability using multivariate analyses, however, did not find any influence of disease duration on Hr-QoL scores once disease severity or disability were accounted for, indicating that disease duration itself does not seem an independent factor in patients' Hr-QoL *(23)*.

4.1.3. Age of Onset

An influence of age at onset on Hr-QoL scores has been reported only rarely. Kuopio *(26)* found that younger age at onset was associated with better Hr-QoL in the dimension of physical functioning but with worse scores on the dimension of mental functioning of the SF-36. They concluded that this may reflect a slower rate of progression in patients with younger age at onset of disease, on the one hand, and perhaps a more difficult adaptation to this chronic disease with a lower threshold for recognizing subtle mental difficulties than in older patients, on the other.

4.1.4. Disability

Stronger correlations with Hr-QoL scores than with measures of objective disease severity were seen with measures of disability such as the Schwab and England scale, the ADL section of the Unified Parkinson's Disease Rating Scale, or the North Western Disability Scale *(10,18,23,27,28)*. These scales measure the degree of independence or ability to perform tasks of daily life. However, they are completed by assessors rather than patients themselves and primarily assess physical functioning, and therefore stand in between measures of impairment and Hr-QoL. Kuopio *(26)*, found that, after depression, poor ADL score as measured on the Unified Parkinson's Disease Rating Scale ADL section, was the next powerful predictor to associate with six of the eight dimensions of the SF-36. It was better than the objective motor performance, as measured on the UDPRS motor part, at predicting low scores on all dimensions of the SF-36. Similarly, although disability is also associated with depression, most studies have found that disability makes an additional contribution to Hr-QoL scores even when depression is accounted for *(23,26,27,29)*. Thus, most studies show the importance of disability for Hr-QoL in patients with PD.

4.1.5. Motor Features

Among the cardinal features of PD, bradykinesia has shown the strongest correlation with Hr-QoL scores, whereas tremor scores appear less important. Peto et al. *(10)* described increasing Hr-QoL scores with increase in self-reported tremor and stiffness, but less than with slowness. Others found that tremor and rigidity scores did not correlate with Hr-QoL scores, whereas bradykinesia and gait were associated with worse Hr-QoL *(23,24)*. In one population-based study, patients with tremor-dominant disease also had better Hr-QoL than those with the akinetic subtype *(23)*, and another population-based study also found a tendency for patients with tremor-dominant disease to have better SF-36 Hr-QoL scores than those with the akinetic-rigid subtype, but this difference did not reach significance *(26)*.

4.1.6. *Laterality of Symptoms*

The laterality of symptoms does not appear to influence the Hr-QoL on any dimension *(23,26)*

4.1.7. *Falls and Postural Stability*

Postural instability with falls was one of the most important factors associated with Hr-QoL scores after depression and disability in a population-based study in London *(23)*. The occurrence of falls was also a common problem in this elderly community-based sample of patients with PD. A study by Lyons et al. similarly found that the postural instability and gait abnormalities score was the strongest predictor of Hr-QoL, accounting for 36% of the the total variance, even after disease duration had been adcounted for *(24)*. Although this association was not reported by other studies, few studies have investigated the association of falls with Hr-QoL, and it highlights the importance of addressing this common complication of PD in the community.

4.1.8. *Sleep Problems*

Insomnia is known to be associated with PD, but is assessed by only some Hr-QoL instruments. In studies using the NHP, which has a large section on sleep and energy, insomnia and fatigue have been found to make significant contributions to the Hr-QoL scores of patients with PD. Thus, the presence of sleep disturbances, as reported by patients, was found to be the second most predictive factor of poor Hr-QoL scores after depression scores, particularly of the dimensions of sleep, physical mobility, and social isolation *(27)*.

4.1.9. *Autonomic Dysfunction*

Symptoms of dysfunction of the autonomic nervous system in PD have not been found to be associated with Hr-QoL scores. Such symptoms include hypersalivation, constipation, sexual dysfunction, urinary disturbance, orthostatic hypotension, hyperhidrosis, and seborrhoea. With the exception of urinary incontinence, drooling and feeling unpleasantly hot or cold, which are covered by the disease-specific instruments, and sexual dysfunction, which is also included on many generic instruments, these symptoms are, however, scarcely covered by the available rating scales, and their impact on patients' well-being may, therefore, be missed. Furthermore, although these items might not be associated with group Hr-QoL scores, they may be significant for individual patients.

4.1.10. *Mental Disturbances*

4.1.10.1. Cognitive Function

Studies of Hr-QoL in dementia show that cognitive decline is associated with impairment of Hr-QoL *(30)*. However, most studies in PD excluded patients with severe cognitive impairment due to the difficulties in measuring Hr-QoL in people with dementia. In studies of Hr-QoL in patients with severe cognitive impairment, a proxy rating is often obtained. Caution is required in interpreting such data, because proxy scores may be biased. With this proviso, some studies have found a relationship between cognitive score and Hr-QoL *(15,18,23,31)*. In these studies, cognitive scores contributed to prediction of Hr-QoL scores even after accounting for depression scores, disease severity, and age, which are often correlated with cognitive scores *(18,23)*. Therefore, despite the limitations in assessing patients with severe cognitive decline, there appears to be an association between overall cognitive score and Hr-QoL in patients with PD.

4.1.10.2 Depression

Depression has been shown to be the factor most closely associated with poor Hr-QoL in patients with PD in the majority of studies, affecting all subscales to varying degrees *(15,18,23,26,27,31–33)*.

As this association was found irrespective of instruments used to assess depression, Hr-QoL, PD severity or disability, this appears to be a robust finding.

The relationship between depression and Hr-QoL is, however, complex, and the interpretation of these results is difficult. There is considerable overlap between the symptoms of depression and PD, particularly in rating scales that are weighted towards the physical symptoms of depression. Likewise, there is overlap between the questions assessing emotional well-being on Hr-QoL scales and depression scales. In addition, the direction of causality between Hr-QoL, depression, and disability is difficult to establish. Longitudinal follow-up data are, therefore, of particular interest. The only longitudinal study to date reported that depression and insomnia were the most important factors associated with poor Hr-QoL both at the initial assessment and 4 years later *(25)*. However, deterioration of Hr-QoL scores was not correlated with increasing depression scores, although this may reflect a lack of responsiveness of the depression scale. Further evidence for the importance of depression for Hr-QoL comes from another study *(34)*, published in abstract from, which reported that improvement of PDQ-39 scores after subthalamic nucleus stimulation was most strongly predicted by change in depression scores, particularly in the subscales of ADL, mobility, cognition, and emotional well-being. Although it is not possible to impute a causal relationship, the consistent association of poor Hr-QoL and depression, which frequently remains untreated *(35–38)*, therefore highlights the need to diagnose and treat depression in patients with PD.

4.2. Treatment-Related

4.2.1. Levodopa Dose

In the population-based study by Karlsen et al. *(27)*, higher levodopa doses, in addition to depression scores, sleep problems, and disability, predicted NHP scores, particularly in the subscores of vitality, physical mobility, and sleep. However, a multiple regression analysis did not show a significant contribution of levodopa score to overall Hr-QoL *(27)*. No other study found an independent contribution of levodopa dose to Hr-QoL scores.

4.2.2. Motor Fluctuations

Motor fluctuations and dyskinesias have been the focus of attempts to improve treatment for patients with PD using new pharmacological *(39,40)* and surgical *(41–44)* treatments. These complications of treatment are major challenges in the long-term treatment of PD, but little is known about their overall impact on patients' Hr-QoL.

In a population-based study in London *(23)*, no differences in Hr-QoL scores between patients with and without fluctuations was found. Similarly, the presence or absence of motor fluctuations did not contribute to Hr-QoL scores in another population-based study in Rogaland *(27)*. On the other hand, in a clinic-based study using the SF-36, the presence of off-periods was associated with worse scores on all subscales of the SF-36, except for those of mental health and vitality *(28)*. In a population-based study in Finland using the Sf 36, Kuopio *(26)* also found that freezing, nighttime akinesia, and early morning akinesia increased the disposition to lower Hr-QoL, whereas the more common wearing-off fluctuations did not. These findings are consistent with those of a different population-based study using the NHP, which reported that sleep problems were associated with poorer Hr-QoL *(15)*, possibly reflecting such nighttime mobility problems as nighttime and early morning akinesia.

These results indicate that, although overall occurrence of motor fluctuations is not a major determinant of Hr-QoL in patients with PD, these complications appear important in subgroups of patients with more severe motor fluctuations.

Indirect evidence for an association of Hr-QoL with motor fluctuations also comes from treatment trials, which found that improvement of Hr-QoL scores related to the improvement of severity of disease in the "off" state *(41,45)* or improvement of "off"-motor score and depression *(34)*.

4.2.3. Dyskinesias

Less evidence is available for the impact of treatment-induced dyskinesias on Hr-QoL. As with motor fluctuations, no overall association of presence of dyskinesias with Hr-QoL scores has been reported *(23,27)*. However, dystonia was associated with worse scores in the subdimenions of mental health and health perception of the SF-36 in a Finish population-based study *(26)*. Additionally, Damiano et al. *(16)* found, in a clinic-based study, that patients with dyskinesias had significantly poorer scores for four of the eight PDQ-39 subscales and the summary index, whereas there was no difference between patients with and without dyskinesias on SF-36 scale. In another clinic-based study *(28)*, dyskinesias were associated with worse SF-36 subscores in the dimensions of physical role limitations, bodily pain, social function, and emotional role limitations. Similarly, painful or disabling dyskinesias, as assessed on the Unified Parkinson's Disease Rating Scale, were associated with worse Hr-QoL in all dimensions apart from general health, mental health and emotional role limitations, and early morning dystonia was associated with worse scores on all subscales of the SF-36.

In the interpretation of these results, it should be noted that no adjustment for disease severity was made in these studies, and it is, therefore, possible that higher rates of dyskinesias and motor fluctuations reflected greater disease severity. Additionally, patients with these complications, as well as those with more severe disease, are likely to be over-represented in clinic-based samples. In contrast, the usually mild dyskinesias and motor fluctuations, which were mostly seen in population-based samples *(23,46)*, contributed little to overall Hr-QoL. Although further studies are required to assess the impact of fluctuations on patients with this complication, it appears that dyskinesias, as well as motor fluctuations, do not have a major impact on Hr-QoL in the overall population of patients with PD, but have an important influence on Hr-QoL in the subgroups of patients who have developed severe forms of these complications.

4.2.4. Psychiatric Complications of Treatment

Hallucinations or delusions have been shown to be associated with greater nursing home placement and higher mortality *(47–49)*. In one study, hallucinations were found to be associated with worse PDQ 39 scores, although this finding was not significant *(23)*. However, the impact of psychiatric side effects of medication, such as psychosis and hallucinations, on Hr-QoL requires further evaluation.

4.3. Factors Unrelated to PD

4.3.1. Comorbidity

Although co-morbidity is common in people of the age group of patients with PD and is likely to influence Hr-QoL, this has been assessed in few studies. Rubenstein et al. *(28)* failed to find an impact of co-morbidity on the Hr-QoL of patients with PD. In a study by Damiano et al. *(16)* however, patients with self-reported co-morbidities reported poorer Hr-QoL on some subscales of the SF-36.

4.3.2. Sociodemographic Factors

4.3.2.1. Gender

Most studies on Hr-QoL in PD have not found significant differences between men and women in their perceived Hr-QoL *(23,27)*. Exceptions are the studies by Peto et al. *(10)*, in which women rated their Hr-QoL worse than men on some dimensions of the PDQ-39, and by Kuopio et al., in which women considered their Hr-QoL, as measured on the SF-36, lower than men on most dimensions *(18)*. Women, who were also slightly older than men, were significantly more depressed than men in that study, which may partly explain these findings.

4.3.2.2. Age

Associations between increasing age and worse Hr-QoL have been found in most studies, mainly in the dimension of physical aspects of Hr-QoL, vitality, and occasionally, overall Hr-QoL scores

(15,18,23,32). However, age is also often correlated with higher depression scores, greater disease severity, and longer disease duration *(18,23)*. When these factors are accounted for in multiple regression analyses, age no longer contributes to Hr-QoL. In addition, as Hr-QoL is known to deteriorate with advancing age in the general population, it is difficult to distinguish between the effects of aging from the consequences of PD, and the results of studies are, therefore, difficult to interpret when no age-matched control group is used *(31)*.

4.3.2.3. Socioeconomic Group and Area of Residence

Lower socioeconomic group tended to be associated with lower Hr-QoL in patients with PD in London in the study by Schrag et al., but this difference did not reach significance *(23)*. Area of residence was assessed in the study by Kuopio et al. in Finland, in which rural patients with PD reported better Hr-QoL than urban patients in the dimension of emotional role limitations on the SF-36, but not in other dimensions *(18)*.

4.3.3. *Psychosocial Factors*

Even when accounting for multiple medical and demographic factors in a multivariate model to explain the variation of Hr-QoL scores, between 20 and 70% of the variance of Hr-QoL remains unexplained *(18,23,27)*. This supports the assumption that Hr-QoL also depends on factors other than those related to disease and its symptoms or demographic variables. This is to be expected as life satisfaction, and well-being in PD is also influenced by other psychosocial variables such as personal expectations, social interactions, and family worries *(50)*. Personal and social resources in coping with a chronic handicap may be crucial in determining patients' emotional reactions and perception of their own health and Hr-QoL *(51)*. Although such factors have not been assessed systematically in studies using Hr-QoL measures, evidence from studies using measures of general well-being, life satisfaction, and adjustment give important information on psychosocial factors that may contribute to patients' Hr-QoL.

4.3.4. *Personal Factors*

4.3.4.1. Perceived Control Over Symptoms

Patient-perceived control over symptoms and the related psychological concept of "mastery" have been shown to be significantly associated with patient and caregiver well-being, and less caregiver burden *(52–54)*.

4.3.4.2. Level of Optimism

Increased levels of optimism have been shown to be associated with decreased perceived severity even after controlling for negative affect *(55)*. Thus, more optimistic individuals reported less need for assistance with basic functional abilities than less optimistic individuals. In a similar vein, the Global Parkinson's Disease Steering Committee found in a large multinational study, which was published in abstract form, that level of optimism contributed to Hr-QoL scores even after depression, disease severity, and medication were accounted for *(32)*.

4.3.4.3. Coping Strategies and Personal Attitudes

It has been demonstrated that patients with PD employ a number of coping strategies including "distancing" *(56)*, sustaining a sense of continuity with their preparkinsonian self *(57)*, and various aspects of psychological adjustment *(58)*. In addition, different patterns of adaptation and personal attitudes *(54)* exist in patients with PD. It has been suggested that these differences in adaptation and coping strategies affect people's reaction to having PD and impaired well-being *(58)*.

4.3.5. *Social and Environmental Factors*

Social and environmental factors, such as the explanation and counseling given to patients at the time of diagnosis, access to clinics, neurological advice and therapy, instrumental support, financial situation, adaptation of patients' homes, support from a PD nurse, support in the community, housing, family support, and number of friends, have all been related to the well-being of patients with PD *(32,58,59)*, but the impact on these factors on Hr-QoL, as measured by the new Hr-QoL scales, has not been investigated in detail.

An important factor for patients Hr-QoL is also their caregivers' Hr-QoL. Patients' Hr-QoL directly depends on the strength of the spouse *(60,61)*, and, conversely, caregivers providing a lot of care experience worse health and have fewer contacts, outings, and holidays compared to noncaregiver spouses *(60)*.

These studies on psychosocial factors in patients with PD, which were mostly conducted before Hr-QoL measures were available, using measures of well-being and overall satisfaction, suggest that a number of nonpharmacological and nonsurgical interventions may be successful in improving patients' overall Hr-QoL. Counseling at the time of initial diagnosis and an opportunity to discuss current problems, fears of the future, and changes in self-image and role may also be beneficial *(50)*.

5. THE ROLE OF TREATMENT AND IMPACT ON HR-QOL

Although a detailed discussion of changes in Hr-QoL scores following treatment is beyond the scope of this chapter, a number of treatment trials with a variety of pharmacological and surgical interventions have shown that improvement of objective disease severity can be associated with improvement of overall Hr-QoL or individual domains of Hr-QoL measures *(41,42,45,62–68)*.

Hr-QoL measures may also pick up issues missed by other scales. Thus, adrenal medulla implantation led to improvement of sleep and rest, social isolation, and emotional well-being on the SF-36 after 1 yr, although this benefit was lost subsequently. The authors remarked that this would have remained unnoticed in the absence of an appropriate Hr-QoL evaluation *(69)*. Block et al. *(70)* reported that scores of emotional reactions and social situation on the NHP had improved after 5 yr of treatment with controlled-release carbidopa/levodopa, and Baron et al. reported that pallidotomy led to improvement of physical role, social function, and vitality subscales of SF-36 *(63)*. On the other hand, a deterioration of nonmotor aspects of functioning, which may not be reflected in clinical rating scales, may be captured by Hr-QoL assessments *(71)*. It is, therefore, increasingly advocated that Hr-QoL instruments are used as secondary or even primary treatment outcomes in clinical trials, reflecting patients' subjective evaluation of their own health *(72)*.

In addition to clinical trials of specific interventions, there is evidence for the benefit of adjustment of drug regimes. Larsen et al. *(73)* showed that among residents of nursing homes, definite improvement in function and better Hr-QoL was achieved with simple adjustments of drug treatment in 62% of patients in whom it was modified.

Nonpharmacological treatment may also improve HrQoL, as demonstrated in a study by Sitzia et al. *(74)* who found that a multidisciplinary inpatient rehabilitation treatment program for patients with PD resulted in measurable change in patients' Hr-QoL, particularly in the area of emotional reaction as measured on the NHP. However, data on nonpharmacological and nonsurgical treatment effects on Hr-QoL are scarce.

Finally, psychological counseling and the teaching of new coping strategies to patients and caregivers may help patients counteract negative effects of social and emotional stressors, which affect their overall well-being *(50)*, but systematic assessment of such effects has not yet been performed.

6. CONCLUSION

Despite the conceptual and methodological complexities, a number of psychometrically tested instruments to assess Hr-QoL in PD are now available. These tools have greatly improved our understanding of subjectively experienced difficulties associated with this disease. We have a clearer understanding of what aspects Hr-QoL are important to patients with PD and how the illness affects these.

Hr-QoL data can inform clinical and health-economic decisions. For example, recognizing the effect of depression on Hr-QoL in patients with PD should lead to greater efforts in diagnosing and treating this problem. It has become clear that it is not disease severity and presence of symptoms that primarily determines patients' Hr-QoL, but the disability associated with these symptoms and the emotional response to them. Some symptoms, which have received little attention, such as postural instability and falls, impaired cognition, and insomnia, have been found to be highly relevant to patients. These might be more important to Hr-QoL than those that have been the focus of many treatment trials, such as dyskinesia and motor fluctuations. These findings have implications for the setting of priorities in trials of new treatments and in the clinical management of patients. It should, however, be remembered that Hr-QoL is highly subjective, and caution is urged when group scores are applied to the individual or subgroups of patients.

Although there are fewer data on personal, social, and environmental factors, and their influence on Hr-QoL in PD, the information that is available suggests that the impact of the disease can be alleviated. There is some evidence that counseling at the time of diagnosis, psychological treatment, the acquisition of coping strategies, and the alleviation of caregiver burden may improve patients' Hr-QoL. Further research is also required to investigate whether modifications at the societal level, such as greater integration, day centers, better access to physiotherapy, speech therapy or occupational therapy, home assessment, and specialist care may improve Hr-QoL of patients with PD.

REFERENCES

1. Hedrick, S.C., Taeuber, R.C., and Erickson, P. (1996) On learning and understanding quality of life: a guide to information sources, in *Quality of Life and Pharmacoeconomics in Clinical Trials,* 2nd ed (Spilker, B., ed.), Lippincott-Raven Publishers, Philadelphia.
2. Swash, M. (ed.) (1998) *Outcomes in Neurological and Neurosurgical Disorders,* Cambridge University Press, Cambridge.
3. Spilker, B. and Revicki, D.A. (1996) Taxonomy of quality of life, in *Quality of Life and Pharmacoeconomics in Clinical Trials, 2nd ed.* (Spilker, B., ed.), Lippincott-Raven Publishers, Philadelphia.
4. Brooks, R.G. (1995) *Health Status Measurement: A Perspective on Change,* Macmillan Press Ltd., Philadelphia.
5. Streiner, D.L. and Norman, G.R. (1995) *Health Measurement Scales: A Practical Guide To Their Development and Use,* 2nd ed. Oxford Medical Publications, Oxford.
6. Bergner, M., Bobbitt, R.A., Carter, W.B., et al. (1981) The Sickness Impact Profile: development and final revision of a health status measure. *Med. Care* **19,** 787–805.
7. Hunt, S.M., McEwen, J., and McKenna, S.P. (1985) Measuring health stats: a new tool for clinicians and epidemiologists. *J. R. Coll. Gen. Pract.* **35,** 185–188.
8. Ware, J.E. and Sherbourne, C.D. (1992) The MOS 36-item short form health survey (SF 36). I. Conceptual framework and item selection. *Med. Care* **30,** 473–483.
9. EuroQoL Group. (1990) EuroQoL: a new facility for the measurement of health-related quality of life. *Health Policy* **16,** 199–208.
10. Peto, V., Jenkinson, C., Fitzpatrick, R., and Greenhall R. (1995) The development and validation of a short measure of functioning and well being for individuals with Parkinson's disease. *Qual. Life Res.* **4,** 241–248.
11. de Boer, A.G., Wijker, W., Speelman, J.D., and de Haes, J.C. (1996) Quality of life in patients with Parkinson's disease: development of a questionnaire. *J. Neurol. Neurosurg. Psychiatry* **61,** 70–74.
12. Damiano, A.M., Snyder, C., Strausser, B., and Willian, M.K. (1999) A review of health-related quality-of-life concepts and measures for Parkinson's disease. *Qual. Life Res.* **8,** 235–243.
13. Fitzsimmons, B. and Bunting, L.K. (1993) Parkinson's disease—quality of life issues. *Nurs. Clin. N. Am.* **28,** 807–818.
14. Jenkinson, C., Peto, V., Fitzpatrick, R., Greenhall, R., and Hyman, N. (1995) Self-reported functioning and well-being in patients with Parkinson's disease: comparison of the short-form health survey (SF-36) and the Parkinson's Disease Questionnaire (PDQ-39). *Age Ageing* **24,** 505–509.
15. Karlsen, K.H., Larsen, J.P., Tandberg, E., and Maland J.G. (1998) Quality of life measurements in patients with Parkinson's disease: a community-based study. *Eur J. Neurol.* **5,** 443–450.
16. Damiano, A.M., McGrath, M.M., Willian, M.K., et al. (2000) Evaluation of a measurement strategy for Parkinson's disease: assessing patient health-related quality of life. *Qual. Life Res.* **9,** 87–100.
17. Schrag, A., Jahanshahi, M., and Quinn. N. (2000) How does Parkinson's disease affect quality of life? A comparison with quality of life in the general population. *Mov. Disord.* **15,** 1112–1118.
18. Kuopio, A.M., Marttila, R.J., Helenius, H., Toivonen, M., and Rinne, U.K. (2000) The quality of life in Parkinson's disease. *Mov. Disord.* **15,** 216–223.
19. Fitzpatrick, R., Peto, V., Jenkinson, C., Greenhall, R., and Hyman, N. (1997) Health-related quality of life in Parkinson's disease: a study of outpatient clinic attenders. *Mov. Disord.* **12,** 916–922.

20. Martinez-Martin, P., Frades Payo, B., Fontan Tirado, C., Martinez Sarries, F.J., Guerrero, M.T., and del Ser Quijano, T. (1997) Assessing quality of life in Parkinson's disease using the PDQ-39. A pilot study. *Neurologia* **12,** 56–60.
21. Harrison, J.E., Preston, S., and Blunt, S.B. (2000) Measuring symptom change in patients with Parkinson's disease. *Age Ageing* **29,** 41–45.
22. Chrischilles, E.A., Rubenstein, L.M., Voelker, M.D., Wallace, R.B., and Rodnitzky, R.L. (1998) The health burdens of Parkinson's disease. *Mov Disord.* **13,** 406–413.
23. Schrag, A., Jahanshahi, M., and Quinn, N. (2000) What contributes to quality of life in patients with Parkinson's disease? *J. Neurol. Neurosurg. Psychiatry* **69,** 308–312.
24. Lyons, K.E., Pahwa, R., Troester, A.E., et al. (1998) A comparison of Parkinson's disease symptoms and self-reported functioning and well being. *Parkinsonism Rel. Disord.* **3,** 207–209.
25. Karlsen, K.H., Tandberg, E., Arsland, D., and Larsen, J.P. (2000) Health related quality of life in Parkinson's disease: a prospective longitudinal study. *J. Neurol. Neurosurg. Psychiatry* **69,** 584–589.
26. Kuopio, A.M. (2000) *Parkinson's Disease: Occurrence, Risk Factors and Quality of Life,* Doctoral dissertation, Turun Yliopisto, Turku.
27. Karlsen, K.H., Larsen, J.P., Tandberg, E., and Maeland, J.G. (1999) Influence of clinical and demographic variables on quality of life in patients with Parkinson's disease. *J. Neurol. Neurosurg. Psychiatry* **66,** 431–435.
28. Rubenstein, L.M., Voelker, M.D., Chrischilles, E.A., Glenn, D.C., Wallace, R.B., and Rodnitzky, R.L. (1998) The usefulness of the Functional Status Questionnaire and Medical Outcomes Study Short Form in Parkinson's disease research. *Qual. Life Res.* **7,** 279–290.
29. Cole, S.A., Woodard, J.L., Juncos, J.L., Kogos, J.L., Youngstrom, E.A., and Watts, R.L. (1996) Depression and disability in Parkinson's disease. *J. Neuropsychiatry Clin. Neurosci.* **8,** 20–25.
30. Selai, C.E., Trimble, M.R., Rossor, M., and Harvey, R. (2000) The Quality of Life Assessment Schedule (QOLAS)—a new method for assessing quality of life (QOL) in dementia, in *Assessing Quality of Life in Alzheimer's Disease* (Albert, S.M. and Logsdon, R.G., eds.), Springer Publishing Company, New York, pp. 31–48.
31. Hobson, P., Holden, A., and Meara, J. (1999) Measuring the impact of Parkinson's disease with the Parkinson's Disease Quality of Life questionnaire. *Age Ageing* **28,** 341–346.
32. Findley, L. (1999) Global Parkinson's Disease Steering Committee. Investigating factors which may influence quality of life in Parkinson's disease. *Parkinsonism Rel. Disord.* **5(Suppl.),** 146.
33. Caap-Ahlgren, M. and Dehlin O. (2001) Insomnia and depressive symptoms in patients with Parkinson's disease. Relationship to health-related quality of life. An interview study of patients living at home. *Arch. Gerontol. Geriatr.* **32,** 23–33.
34. Troster, A.I., Fields, J.A., Lyons, K., et al. (2001) Predictors and correlates of quality of life improvements after subthalamic deep brain stimulation in Parkinson's disease. *Neurology* **65(Suppl. 3),** A277.
35. Livingston, G., Watkin, V., Milne, B., Manela, M.V., and Katona C. (1997) The natural history of depression and the anxiety disorders in older people: the Islington community study. *J. Affect. Disord.* **46,** 255–262.
36. Miyoshi, K., Ueki, A., and Nagano, O. (1996) Management of psychiatric symptoms of Parkinson's disease. *Eur. Neurol.* **36(Suppl. 1),** 49–48.
37. Tandberg, E., Larsen, J.P., Aarsland, D., and Cummings, J.L. (1996) The occurrence of depression in Parkinson's disease. A community-based study. *Arch. Neurol.* **53,** 175–179.
38. Liu, C.Y., Wang, S.J., Fuh, J.L., Lin, C.H., Yang, Y.Y., and Liu, H.C. (1997) The correlation of depression with functional activity in Parkinson's disease. *J. Neurol.* **244,** 493–498.
39. Rascol, O., Brooks, D.J., Korczyn, A.D., De Deyn, P.P., Clarke, C.E., and Lang, A.E. (2000) A five-year study of the incidence of dyskinesia in patients with early Parkinson's disease who were treated with ropinirole or levodopa. 056 Study Group. *N. Engl. J. Med.* **342,** 1484–1491.
40. Parkinson Study Group. (1997) Safety and efficacy of pramipexole in early Parkinson disease. A randomized dose-ranging study. *JAMA* **278,** 125–130.
41. D'Antonio, L.L., Zimmerman, G.J., and Iacono, R.P. (2000) Changes in health related quality of life in patients with Parkinson's disease with and without posteroventral pallidotomy. *Acta Neurochir.* **142,** 759–767.
42. Scott, R., Gregory, R., Hines, N., et al. (1998) Neuropsychological, neurological and functional outcome following pallidotomy for Parkinson's disease. A consecutive series of eight simultaneous bilateral and twelve unilateral procedures. *Brain* **121,** 659–675.
43. Fine, J., Duff, J., Chen, R., Chir, B., Hutchison, W., Lozano, A.M., and Lang, A.E. (2000) Long-term follow-up of unilateral pallidotomy in advanced Parkinson's disease. *N. Engl. J. Med.* **342,** 1708–1714.
44. Limousin, P., Krack, P., Pollak, P., et al. (1998) Electrical stimulation of the subthalamic nucleus in advanced Parkinson's disease. *N. Engl. J. Med.* **339,** 1105–1111.
45. Pahwa, R., Lyons, K., McGuire, D., et al. (1997) Comparison of standard carbidopa-levodopa and sustained-release carbidopa-levodopa in Parkinson's disease: pharmacokinetic and quality-of-life measures. *Mov. Disord.* **12,** 677–681.
46. Larsen, J.P., Karlsen, K., and Tandberg, E. (2000) Clinical problems in non-fluctuating patients with Parkinson's disease: a community-based study. *Mov. Disord.* **15,** 826–829.
47. Goetz, C.G. and Stebbins, G.T. (1993) Risk factors for nursing home placement in advanced Parkinson's disease. *Neurology* **43,** 2227–2229.
48. Goetz, C.G. and Stebbins, G.T. (1995) Mortality and hallucinations in nursing home patients with advanced Parkinson's disease. *Neurology* **45,** 669–671.
49. Aarsland, D., Larsen, J.P., Tandberg, E., and Laake, K. (2000) Predictors of nursing home placement in Parkinson's disease: a population-based, prospective study. *J. Am. Geriatr. Soc.* **48,** 938–942.

50. Ellgring, H., Seiler, S., Perleth, B., Frings, W., Gasser, T., and Oertel, W. (1993) Psychosocial aspects of Parkinson's disease. *Neurology* **43(Suppl. 6),** S41–S44.
51. Gotham, A.M., Brown, R.G., and Marsden, C.D. (1986) Depression in Parkinson's disease: a quantitative and qualitative analysis. *J. Neurol. Neurosurg. Psychiatry* **49,** 381–389.
52. Wallhagen, M.I. and Brod, M. (1997) Perceived control and well-being in Parkinson's disease. *West J. Nurs. Res.* **19,** 11–25.
53. Koplas, P.A., Gans, H.B., Wisely, M.P., et al. (1999) Quality of life and Parkinson's disease. *J. Gerontol. A Biol. Sci. Med. Sci.* **54,** M197–M202.
54. Dakof, G.A. and Mendelsohn, G.A. (1989) Patterns of adaptation to Parkinson's disease. *Health Psychol.* **8,** 355–372.
55. Shifren, K. (1996) Individual differences in the perception of optimism and disease severity: a study among individuals with Parkinson's disease. *J. Behav. Med.* **19,** 241–271.
56. Frazier, L.D. (2000) Coping with disease-related stressors in Parkinson's disease. *Gerontologist* **40,** 53–63.
57. Habermann, B. (1999) Continuity challenges of Parkinson's disease in middle life. *J. Neurosci. Nurs.* **31,** 200–207.
58. MacCarthy, B. and Brown, R. (1989) Psychosocial factors in Parkinson's disease. *Br. J. Clin. Psychol.* **28,** 41–52.
59. Clarke, C.E., Zobkiw, R.M., and Gullaksen, E. (1995) Quality of life and care in Parkinson's disease. *Br. J. Clin. Pract.* **49,** 288–293.
60. O'Reilly, F., Finnan, F., Allwright, S., Smith, G.D., and Ben-Shlomo, Y. (1996) The effects of caring for a spouse with Parkinson's disease on social, psychological and physical well-being. *Br. J. Gen. Pract.* **46,** 507–512.
61. Carter, J.H., Stewart, B.J., Archbold, P.G., et al. (1998) Living with a person who has Parkinson's disease: the spouse's perspective by stage of disease. Parkinson's Study Group. *Mov. Disord.* **13,** 20–28.
62. Durif, F., Devaux, I., Pere, J.J., Delumeau, J.C., and Bourdeix, I. (2001) Efficacy and tolerability of entacapone as adjunctive therapy to levodopa in patients with Parkinson's disease and end-of-dose deterioration in daily medical practice: an open, multicenter study. *Eur. Neurol.* **45,** 111–118.
63. Baron, M.S., Vitek, J.L., Bakay, R.A., et al. (2000) Treatment of advanced Parkinson's disease by unilateral posterior GPi pallidotomy: 4-year results of a pilot study. *Mov. Disord.* **15,** 230–237.
64. Welsh, M.D., Dorflinger, E., Chernik, D., and Waters, C. (2000) Illness impact and adjustment to Parkinson's disease: before and after treatment with tolcapone. *Mov. Disord.* **15,** 497–502.
65. Straits-Troster, K., Fields, J.A., Wilkinson, S.B., et al. (2000). Health-related quality of life in Parkinson's disease after pallidotomy and deep brain stimulation. *Brain Cogn.* **42,** 399–416.
66. Hagell, P., Crabb, L., Pogarell, O., et al. (2000) Health-related quality of life following bilateral intrastriatal transplantation in Parkinson's disease. *Mov. Disord.* **15,** 224–229.
67. Grandas, F., Martinez-Martin, P., and Linazasoro, G. (1998) Quality of life in patients with Parkinson's disease who transfer from standard levodopa to Sinemet CR: the STAR Study. The STAR Multicenter Study Group. *J. Neurol.* **245(Suppl. 1),** S31–S33.
68. Martinez-Martin, P., Valldeoriola, F., Molinuevo, J.L., Nobbe, F.A., Rumia, J., and Tolosa, E. (2000) Pallidotomy and quality of life in patients with Parkinson's disease: an early study. *Mov. Disord.* **15,** 65–70.
69. Wilson, R.S., Goetz, C.G., and Stebbins, G.T. (1996) Neurological illness, in *Quality of Life and Pharmacoeconomics in Clinical Trials* (Spilker, B., ed.), Lippincott-Raven, Phildadelphia, pp. 903–908.
70. Block, G., Liss, C., Reines, S., Irr, J., and Nibbelink, D. (1997) Comparison of immediate-release and controlled release carbidopa/levodopa in Parkinson's disease. A multicenter 5-year study. The CR First Study Group. *Eur. Neurol.* **37,** 23–27.
71. McRae, C., O'Brien, C., and Freed, C. (1996) Qualtiy of life among persons receiving neural implant surgery for Parkinson's disease. *Mov. Disord.* **11,** 605–606.
72. Swash, M. (1997) Health outcome and quality-of-life measurements in amyotrophic lateral sclerosis. *J. Neurol.* **244 (Suppl. 2),** S26–S29.
73. Larsen, J.P. (1991) Parkinson's disease as community health problem: study in Norwegian nursing homes. The Norwegian Study Group of Parkinson's Disease in the Elderly. *BMJ* **303,** 741–743.
74. Sitzia, J., Haddrell, V., and Rice-Oxley, M. (1998) Evaluation of a nurse-led multidisciplinary neurological rehabilitation programme using the Nottingham Health Profile. *Clin. Rehabil.* **12,** 389–394.
75. Peto, V., Jenkinson, C., and Fitzpatrick, R. (1998) PDQ 39: a review of the development, validation and application of a Parkinson's disease quality of life questionnaire and its associated measures. *J. Neurol.* **245(Suppl. 1),** S10–S14.
76. Calne, S., Schulzer, M., Mak, E., et al. (1996) Validating a quality of life rating scale for idiopathic parkinsonism: Parkinson's Impact Scale. *Parkinsonism Rel. Disord.* **2,** 55–61.
77. Hogan, T., Grimaldi, R., Dingemanse, J., Martin, M., Lyons, K., and Koller, W. (1999) The Parkinson's disease symptom inventory (PDSI): a comprehensive and sensitive instrument to measure disease symptoms and treatment side-effects. *Parkinsonism Rel. Disord.* **5,** 93–98.

38
Sexuality and Parkinson's Disease

Gila Bronner, MPH, MSW, **Vladimir Royter,** MD,
Amos D. Korczyn, MD, MSc, **and Nir Giladi,** MD

1. SEXUALITY AND SEXUAL HEALTH

There is increasing public awareness that sexual dysfunction is a real problem affecting the health, wellness, and emotional well-being of innumerable women and men. Sexual function is an aspect of human behavior that encompasses relationship, physical and emotional intimacy, feelings, thoughts and interpersonal interaction. According to the World Health Organization (WHO) declaration *(1)*, fundamental rights exist for the individual, including the right to sexual health and the capacity to enjoy and control sexual and reproductive behavior. Individuals are entitled to be free of fear, shame, guilt, false beliefs, and organic disorders that might inhibit normal sexual response and impair sexual relationships and reproductive function. Because healthy sexual functioning is an integral part of normal life, it should be incorporated into health care plans along with other factors ensuring quality of life. Health professionals, being at the front line of health care services, should play a major role in advocating sexual health rights.

In this chapter, we review the effects of Parkinson's disease (PD) on the sexuality of patients and their sexual partners and evaluate possible treatment options. Initial results from our study evaluating sexual functioning of male and female patients in the Movement Disorder Unit are presented. We also describe our experience with implementation of sexual counseling service within the framework of the Movement Disorders Unit.

2. *The Effect of Chronic Disease on Sexual Function*

Sexual functioning is an important aspect in the quality of one's life *(2–4)*. Due to the effects of disease on sexual functioning, the quality of life of ill people and their spouses is at high risk for deterioration *(3,5–8)*. Four factors are involved in the deterioration of the sexual health of patients with chronic illness *(2,5,9)*: (*i*) sexual dysfunction caused directly by the illness itself; (*ii*) by treatment methods; (*iii*) by the general consequences of chronic illness (fatigue, weakness, concentration problems); and (*iv*) by psychological problems accompanying the illness (loss of control, loss of self-esteem, depression, body image problems, difficulties due to role changes). The active combat and the emotional crisis accompanying a chronic illness leaves patients with chronic and relentless fatigue and stress. They may fear resuming sexual activity and be nervous when they try to participate in any intimate activity.

Normal sexual function requires intact physiological function of the autonomic, sensory, and motor system, proper arterial blood supply to and venous returns from the genital organs, balanced hormonal

From: *Mental and Behavioral Dysfunction in Movement Disorders*
Edited by: M-A. Bédard et al. © Humana Press Inc., Totowa, NJ

profile, and a healthy emotional state. Age-related decline in most body systems may cause some sexual dysfunction in elderly people. The decline rate is increased when chronic illness is associated with the process of aging. Middle-aged men with subjective poor health had a sixfold increase in the likelihood of being sexually dysfunctional, and the increase was 40-fold in those over the age of 75 *(8)*. Sexual dysfunction has been reported in different diseases, e.g., multiple sclerosis *(10,11)*, arthritis *(12)*, diabetes mellitus *(13)*, cancer *(14)*, cardiovascular diseases *(3)*, and chronic renal failure *(5)*. Sexual dysfunction has been recognized as a complication of neurological disorders, although physicians and other health care providers treating patients with neurological diseases are often unaware of this association *(10)*. In addition, drugs may impair sexual function *(15,16)*. Several groups have reported on sexual dysfunctioning among people with PD *(6,10,12,17–22)*. However, PD as a chronic progressive neurological illness is a classical disorder in which the disease itself, the antiparkinsonian drugs, and the mental and psychological burdens are playing a role together.

2. 1. Aspect of PD Affecting Sexual Functioning

PD, a neurodegenerative disorder, is one of the most common neurological diseases affecting an estimated 1% of the population over 65 yr. In the general population, 20 new cases per 100,000 are diagnosed every year. The frequency is slightly higher for men *(23)*. Symptoms usually appear at the sixth decade of life, while many patients still work, and some even take care of young children. The pathophysiology of PD is characterized primarily by loss of dopaminergic neurons in the substantia nigra in the midbrain. The motor symptoms of PD include muscle rigidity, rest tremor, bradykinesia, postural reflexes abnormalities, and gait disturbances. In addition, autonomic dysfunction is common in PD patients. It includes abnormalities of bladder detrusor muscle and sphincter problems, gastrointestinal manifestations (drooling, difficulty swallowing, nausea, constipation), and orthostatic and postprandial hypotension *(24,25)*. Additionally, PD patients experience sensory disturbances (mainly pain), mood and cognitive disturbances, sleep difficulties, and eventually dementia *(26)*. The multisystemic nature of PD has a marked effect on the quality of life of patients and their families and on their sexual life *(27,28)*.

Motor symptoms such as bradykinesia, rigidity, and tremor contribute to sexual dysfunction, because they disturb normal sexual performance. Sixty-nine percent of male patients with PD had autonomic nervous system dysfunction, and 70% had sexual dysfunction *(18)*. About one-third of men and women felt that their motor disturbances were the main cause of their sexual problems *(6)*, and half of young patients with PD felt that their rigidity accounted for their sexual dysfunction *(21)*. Other motor disturbances can also influence sexual life of PD patients. Drooling, as well as sloppy dressing and walking, can make the PD patient unattractive, while masked face can be interpreted as lack of sexual interest *(6)*. Motor complications, including motor fluctuations and dyskinesias, often develop with chronic dopaminergic treatment. These complications can be disabling and contribute to low self-esteem, which will reflect on the overall performance of PD patients *(29)*. The excessive salivation and sweating can be very disturbing to sexual attractiveness. The bradykinesia and rigidity cause patients to be more passive *(6)*, thus imposing a more active role on the healthy partner. Role changes can also impede the normal sexual activity. Tremor and sleep disturbances cause many couples to separate their beds or bedrooms and, thus, decrease opportunities for intimate touch and sexual activity.

Depression, stress, and fatigue can damage sexuality profoundly, and masked depression and tension states frequently contribute to sexual dysfunctions *(30)*. When severely depressed, sex is the furthest thing from the mind. Even moderately depressed patients lose interest in pursuing sexual activity and are very difficult to seduce and arouse. Not surprisingly, there is a strong association between depression and sexual dysfunction in PD *(18)*. Depression was found in about 30% of advanced PD patients *(31)*. Unemployment and depression are some of the factors affecting sexuality in younger parkinsonian patients *(32)*. Increased age, severity, or duration of illness and depression were associated with reduced sexual function *(12)* and lower quality of sexual life *(28)*.

According to our clinical experience, spouses of parkinsonian patients, who serve as caregivers, feel rejected and insulted when their partners ignore them sexually. On the other hand, the patients may refrain from making sexual advances for the fear of rejection or failure.

2. 2. *Sexual Dysfunction in Women with PD*

Satisfactory sexual functioning is an important part of a women's personal health and well-being, with "satisfactory" being an individual's self-assessment in the context of her personal expectations and desires *(33)*. Female sexual dysfunction is a highly prevalent and significant age-related progressive problem *(34)*. The diagnostic categories of sexual problems delineated in the Diagnostic and Statistical Manual of Mental Disorders, fourth edition (DSM-IV) *(35)* include sexual desire disorders, sexual arousal disorders, orgasmic disorders, and sexual pain disorders (including dyspareunia and vaginismus). The recent National Health and Social Life Survey *(36)* found that 43% of 1749 American women aged 18–59 yr have sexual function complaints, which is more than in men. Women reported on low sexual desire (22%), arousal problems (14%), and dyspareunia (7%), with older women reporting less overall sexual dysfunction, although arousal insufficiency and vaginal dryness were more prevalent in older age (27 vs 18%).

The female sexual response is initiated by neurotransmitter-mediated vascular and nonvascular smooth muscle relaxation, resulting in increased pelvic blood flow, vaginal lubrication, and clitoral and labia engorgement. Impairments of the normal female sexual response bring about complaints associated with diminished sexual arousal, libido, vaginal lubrication, genital sensation, and ability to achieve orgasm *(34)*. Due to this complicated and comprehensive mechanism, women with neurological diseases are at high risk for development of sexual dysfunction. Yet, this area has attracted little interest and has been poorly studied.

Sexual problems were reported by 34–75% of parkinsonian women *(6,12,17,18,20,21)*. Decrease in intercourse frequency occurred in 43–82% of PD female patients, reduction in sexual drive occurred in about 70%, difficulty to get aroused in 67%, and about 35% of the women reported on vaginal dryness. Seventy-five percent stated that the frequency of orgasm was less since the parkinsonism started, and 38% were unable to reach orgasm *(6,18)*. They often reported changed orgasms, as the sexual tension no longer reached a definite peak, but rather a number of high points and then abrupt decline *(37)*. Other problems in arousal, such as vaginal tightness *(19)* and vaginismus were reported *(6)*. Welch, Hung, and Waters *(19)* compared women with PD with community controls, matched for age and marital status. They found that women with PD were less satisfied with the quality of their sexual experiences. There were significant differences between the two groups with respect to vaginal tightness, involuntary urination, anxiety, and depression. All changes in sexual function in women with PD were increased as the disease progressed and with duration of treatment.

A study carried out among patients in our Movement Disorder Unit suggests that 25% of women with PD stopped having sex since the onset of the disease. Half of the women who were still sexually active reported difficulties to get aroused during sexual activity, in comparison to 15% before the onset of PD. Whereas 37% of the women had difficulties reaching orgasm before the onset of PD, 74% reported on such difficulties since the onset of the disease. A significant decrease in the desire to have sex was found since the onset of PD ($p = 0.0019$, Fisher Exact Test). Seventy-four percent of the women reported that, before the onset of PD, they felt a frequent desire to have sex, and only 18.5% felt the same at present. A decrease in the frequency of sexual activity and in satisfaction with sexual life were reported by the women in our study. For about half the women, the frequency of sexual activity decreased from 2–7 times a week to less than twice a month. Although 78% of the women were very satisfied with their sexual life before the onset of PD, only 18% felt satisfied at present. Health was perceived by 89% women as an important factor disturbing their sexual life, 78% of them reported that physical parkinsonian symptoms increased during sexual activity, and 70% said that, due to their health state, they sometimes refrained from having sex. It is of interest that in spite of the marked decrease in satisfaction with sexual life, there was only a slight decrease in satisfaction with the quality of marriage life or couplehood. Seventy-eight percent (before PD onset) and 71% (at present) reported that they were very satisfied with the quality of their relationship.

2.3. *Sexual Dysfunction in Men with PD*

Recent studies indicate that sexual problems are experienced by many men of all ages. According to Laumann et al. *(36)*, sexual dysfunction is reported by 31% of men aged 18–59 yr. Five percent of men had low interest in sex and 21% reported premature ejaculation. The frequency of sexual dysfunction increased with age. Of 225 elderly men in a geriatric ambulatory care clinic surveyed by Mulligan et al. *(8)*, loss of libido was reported by 31% of those aged 65–75 yr and by 47% of those over 75 yr. Data from the Massachusetts Male Aging Study (MMAS) *(38)* indicates that 52% of the 1290 men aged 40–70 yr experienced minimal, moderate, or complete erectile dysfunction (ED). Complete ED, defined as the total inability to obtain or maintain erections during sexual stimulation, occurred in 10% of the subjects. Similar rates of ED were obtained by the National Health and Social Life Survey *(39)* in a nationally representative probability sample of respondents aged 18–59 yr. These studies indicate a strong association between aging and sexual dysfunction. Complete ED was tripled between the age of 40–70 yr (5–15%) *(38)*. The National Institutes of Health (NIH) Consensus Panel reported that ED may affect as many as 30 million men in the United States *(39)*.

The prevalence of sexual dysfunction is even higher when health factors intervene and outweigh the factor of aging *(3,5,8,40,41)*. In the MMAS, Feldman et al. *(38)* observed significant association between ED and chronic illness. Although complete impotence was found in 10% of the research population, the rate was 28% for diabetic men, 39% for cardiac patients, and 15% for hypertensive men. Atherosclerosis, hyperlipidemia, endocrine and neurological disorders, trauma and surgery, mental illness (depression, anxiety, stress), and drug or alcohol abuse are also major factors for ED *(3,5,29,38,42–45)*.

Complete impotence is significantly more prevalent in men taking certain medications, including hypoglycemic agents (26%), antihypertensive drugs (14%), vasodilators (36%), or cardiac drugs (28%).

Sexual function appears to be reduced in men with PD. Sexual dysfunction was reported by 65–80% *(6,18)*. Decreased sexual drive occurred in 44%, ED was experienced by 54%, whereas 50% were unable to have an ejaculation *(18)*. About 75% of men had trouble getting aroused and reaching orgasm. Delayed orgasm and ejaculatory delay are common in men with PD and cause a lot of frustration *(37)*.

Jacobs et al. *(32)* compared the personal opinion about sexual function and general health of 121 young patients with PD (mean age 45 yr) with 126 age- and sex-matched healthy controls. They found that more patients than controls indicated dissatisfaction with their current sexual life. Depressed and unemployed patients were more often dissatisfied with their sexual relationships. Men more often expressed dissatisfaction than women.

Brown et al. *(6)* conducted a study of PD patients and their partners. The highest scores indicating dissatisfaction from sexual life was reported by 59% of male patients and 58% female spouses, and sexual dysfunction was reported by 65% male patients and by 52% female spouses of parkinsonian patients.

A study carried out among patients in our Movement Disorder Unit suggests that 24% of men with PD stopped having sex since the onset of the disease. Although only 8% of the men who were still sexually active had ED during sexual activity before the onset of PD, 68% reported ED at present. (ED is of course a hallmark of multiple system atrophy, but the high frequency of ED found by us and others far exceeds the expected number of patients with undiagnosed multiple system atrophy.) Seventy-one percent of the men had difficulties reaching orgasm in comparison to 26% before the onset of PD. Significant decrease in sexual desire since the onset of PD was reported by men in our study ($p =$ 0.018, Fisher Exact Test). Forty-five percent of them reported that before the onset of PD, they always wanted to have sex, but no one felt the same at the time of the study. In our sample, there was no case of increase in sexual desire since the onset of PD. Men also reported on decrease in frequency of sexual activity and in satisfaction with their sexual life. Before the onset of PD, most men (84%) had sex two to seven times a week. Only 21% continued with this sexual frequency at present, and more than half of the men had sex less than twice a month. The decrease in their sexual desire was also reflected in the male sexual initiative behavior. Men with PD were initiating sex less and ignored sexual initiation by their spouses ($p = 0.083$, Fisher Exact Test). Whereas 87% of the men were very satisfied with their sexual life before the onset of PD, only 16% felt satisfied at present. Health was perceived by 71% of men as an important factor disturbing their sexual life, 58% of them reported that parkinsonian physical symptoms occurred during sexual activity, and 55% said that, due to their health state, they sometimes refrained from having sex. Despite the marked decrease in satisfaction with sexual life, many men (71%) reported that they were very satisfied with the quality of their married life or couplehood.

2. 4. *Hypersexuality and PD*

Reports about increased libido and hypersexuality in parkinsonian patients have attracted the attention of health care professionals due to its impact on patients and their families (almost all cases reported so far were males). Bearing in mind the role of hypothalamic dopamine on sexual function *(37)*, it was of interest to study how levodopa (L-dopa) treatment acts on the sexual function of parkinsonian patients. Revival of sexual interest and potency in conjunction with antiparkinsonian therapy is described in the literature *(23,46)*. Hyppä et al. *(46)* found increased libido in 10 (7 men and 3 women) of 41 patients treated with L-dopa. Uitti et al. *(47)* studied 13 cases of significant hypersexuality as reported by the family or the parkinsonian patient. Six patients clearly demonstrated sexual interest or behavior far in excess of their premorbid state. Hypersexuality, according to this study, occurs in a small number of patients treated with L-dopa and dopamine agonists. An attempt to characterize these patients who are prone to develop hypersexuality revealed no clear pattern, except for young age of PD onset (mean age 49.5 vs 61.8 yr in the general population) and male preponderance *(47)*.

In one study, about half of the patients reported an increase in sexual desire since acquiring parkinsonism *(37)*. These patients found it impossible to be sure it was the drugs affecting desire rather than the disease itself. Usually those months or years with undiagnosed symptoms were extremely stressful, possibly affecting sexual desire and certainly clouding recall as to its level during pretreatment period.

There are also single case reports. Two male patients with intact sexual function experienced increased sexual interest and activity with L-dopa treatment *(48)*. A PD patient's wife complained of aggressive demands for intercourse several times a day, which appeared a few days after administration of moclobemide *(49)*. In our recent study, 3 of 36 women reported an increase in their sexual drive since the onset of PD symptoms, but none of 50 men reported such changes.

Psychosexual disorders have also been reported in four men treated with apomorphine. An acute episode in each case had led them to the hospital in the context of a psychiatric emergency (after punishable sexual acts in two cases). In each case, this episode had been preceeded by an increase of self-administered apomorphine, whereas other antiparkinsonian drugs remained unchanged *(50)*. A case of zoophilia in a PD patient, which appears to have risen in a setting of increasing dopaminergic medication, was reported by Fernandez and Durso *(51)*. This behavior was successfully treated with clozapine. Sexual paraphilia can account for up to 3% of all neuropsychiatric complications of antiparkinsonian therapy *(52)*.

The exact mechanism of how these medications cause hypersexuality remains unknown, but prevalence is more common in men with early age of symptoms onset and has been reported to occur with all dopaminergic medications *(37,47,52)*. However, investigators seem to agree that the increase in sexual behavior is not explained merely by the physical and the mental improvement associated with the treatment of PD. Denervation supersensitivity offers a possible theoretical explanation for dopaminergic drugs increasing libido to premorbid levels or beyond *(37)*.

3. TREATMENT OF SEXUAL DYSFUNCTION

Treatment of sexual dysfunction is directed to healthy persons as well as to people who suffer from chronic diseases or disabilities. Today, many treatment options are available *(30,53,54)*. The behavioral therapy assumes that sexual dysfunction is a learned maladaptive behavior and prescribes specific exercises for the couple in order to experience and adapt new sexual habits. Pharmacologic treatment has two facets: (*i*) the elimination of drugs that compromise sexual function; and (*ii*) the introduction of drugs that enhance sexual function. Oral agents include antianxiety and antidepressant agents and hormonal agents. Men can benefit from sildenafil citrate, intracavernosal injections, intraurethral applications (alprostadil), and vaccum constriction devices, which are used to locally treat ED. Surgical therapies for ED include microvascular arterial bypass, venous ligation surgery, and penile implants.

The treatment of sexual dysfunction of parkinsonian patients and their partners demands a multidisciplinary approach. There are only few studies describing the outcomes of the treatment of sexual dysfunction of parkinsonian patients, and most of them deal with male problems, mainly ED. Neurogenic ED is due to imbalance between neurotransmitters favoring erection (notably nitrous oxide [NO]) and those favoring flaccidity (notably norepinephrine) *(29)*. Therefore, sildenafil, a NO-enhancing drug, is likely to be effective in PD. Neurogenic ED, in contrast to vasculogenic ED, enables also the use of lower dosage of intracavernosal injections of prostaglandin E1 (PGE1) to relax smooth muscle around the sinusoids to cause erection.

Zesiewicz et al. *(22)* investigated the effect of sildenafil citrate in an open label study on 10 men with PD and ED. They found significant improvement in sexual satisfaction, in the ability to achieve and maintain erections, and in the ability to reach orgasm. There was no significant change in the level of sexual desire. It is interesting to note that patients reported improved satisfaction with the same level of desire, possibly because they functioned better. Unified Parkinson's Disease Rating Scale (UPDRS) and Beck's Depressions Inventory (BDI) scores were not significantly changed. Side effects of sildenafil consisted of only one case of mild headache.

Other oral agents are still under investigation. As noted previously, apomorphine, a dopaminergic agonist acting on the central nervous system, was reported as inducing penile erections by subcutaneous injections in five patients with PD *(55)*. Apomorphine has shown efficacy in placebo-controlled fixed and dose escalation studies in the form of sublingual pill *(56)*. Further studies are needed to investigate the use of apomorphine for the benefit of PD patients with ED.

3.1. *Integration of Treatment Methods into Sex Life of the Parkinsonian Couple*

The implementation and integration of a chosen treatment method is one of the issues that are rarely addressed while treating sexual dysfunction. Patients having ED should undergo medical evaluation to uncover possible associated conditions that might induce ED and to exclude contraindications to sildenafil citrate use (concurrent nitrate administration or unstable heart disease). Men who suffer from ED are offered local PGE1 (as intracavernosal injection or intraurethral instillation of alprostadil) and oral sildenafil citrate. The use of PGE1 is effective in producing erection *(54)* independent of the arousal level of the men or their sexual partner. Therefore, it is very important to discuss the problem and the proposed treatment options with both partners. Such a discussion can help the couple integrate the injection or instillation into their existing sexual habits. For example, they can prepare the preloaded syringe and place it at the bedside, and the sexual partner can help with the injection *(29)*. In case alprostadil is used, a light massage over the penis is needed after it is applied, to facilitate spread of the medication. This can become part of a pleasuring foreplay.

When sildenafil is recommended, patients should be informed that the drug would enhance penile erection only in response to sexual arousal. The drug's maximal action begins about 30–60 min after it is taken, and its effect lasts approx 4 h *(57)*. Delayed absorption due to impaired gastrointestinal motility, as in some PD patients *(58)*, may delay its effect *(29)*. Informing patients about these possible changes and planning different timing for sexual activities in relation to sildenafil use will spare the couple from unnecessary sexual frustration and feelings of failure.

4. OUR CLINICAL EXPERIENCE

Our approach for treating sexual problems, when one partner is a PD patient, is based on a multidisciplinary team work and cooperation with other specialists (urologist, gynecologist, psychiatrist). We believe that despite their disabilities, patients with PD are still sexual beings with the ability to share love, bonding, intimacy, and sexual experiences. Our sexual counseling is comprised of the intercourse–outercourse approach, which offers patients and their partners a special training based on the concept of sexual flexibility. The intercourse–outercourse training enables a choice of two sexual options for those couples who cope with sexual dysfunctions. They can either have intercourse with or without medical treatment for their sexual dysfunction or enjoy a variety of pleasuring sexual activities without penetration (outercourse). Outercourse includes various methods of touching and pleasuring at all levels of sexual excitement. Through genital rubbing, oral stimulation of genitals, or manual stimulation, each partner can reach orgasm or stop at a lower level of pleasure and enjoyment.

In the Movement Disorders Unit, we offer inhouse sex therapy and counseling service to patients and their spouses in order to promote sexual health and contribute to improving our patients' quality of life.

We believe that physicians should directly question their patients about sexual concerns and problems. Despite the high frequencies of sexual concerns, it is still difficult for many patients to initiate discussions about sexuality *(59,60)*. These difficulties originate in shame to discuss sex and to admit the existence of a sexual problem, language difficulties, and low self-esteem with fear to look ridiculous. In addition, many patients have limited knowledge about the ability to help them, and often their spouses are not open to bring up the sexual difficulties either. In our study, half of the patients with PD reported that they have never or rarely discussed sexual issues with their partners before the onset of the disease. The frequency of sexual discussions was significantly decreased since then ($p = 0.0001$ for men and $p = 0.035$ for women, Fisher Exact Test). The combination of sexual life deterioration along the course of PD and the decrease in the couple's ability to discuss sexual issues emphasizes their increased need for assistance in coping with their sexuality. This is a role which must be attained by health care professionals, who should initiate a discussion on sexual issues with PD patients and their partners on a routine basis. Physicians can also use the guidelines for clinical approach to patients *(61)*.

Therefore, the service initiated short training sessions on an individual basis for physicians in the Movement Disorders Unit to increase the awareness to sexual disturbances and to assist them to improve their communication with their patients on sexual issues. They were presented with practical tools to bridge the communication gap that exists between an embarrassed patient and doctor. For example, after asking questions regarding various aspects of the disease, physicians were encouraged to ask: "How did your illness affect your intimate life?" or "Are you experiencing any problems in your sexual relations?" Another approach is to make the patient feel he/she is not the only person with sexual problems by asking: "Maybe you are unaware, but many men (women) with PD frequently find that it affects their sexual functioning. If you feel any changes, please tell me. Today we can treat sexual problems. " In case the patient complains of a sexual problem, he/she can be further evaluated and diagnosed by the physician or referred to the inhouse sex therapy clinic. The fact that patients can get sexual consultation at the same clinic where they have their routine medical follow-up made patients feel much more comfortable. Seventy-five percent of those who received sexual counseling in our unit said that they preferred the inhouse location of the sex clinic. Up to now, 36 PD patients (two women) received sex counseling of two sessions on average. Most of them were married, the average age was 61 yr (range 50–81), 53% of them came alone to the counseling session, 40% arrived with their spouse, and the rest (7%) were spouses who came for sex counseling without sharing this fact with the PD patient. Thirty-seven percent requested to continue with the sex therapy. Most patients complained on more than one sexual problem. The most frequent combinations of problems were ED with low sexual desire (21%) and ED with premature ejaculation (12%). Fifty-one percent of the men complained on ED, 31.5% on desire problems, and 7% on premature ejaculation. The desire problems consisted of low level of sexual desire in 14% of men and high level of sexual desire in comparison to their spouse in 17. 5% of them. The two women who came for consultation were both 50 yr old. One of them had difficulties to reach orgasm, and the other experienced a high sexual desire, which did not coordinate with her husband's libido.

The intercourse–outercourse intervention was used with 42% of our patients, 15% were referred to urologists for further evaluation, and one-quarter received special instruction of how to successfully use sildenafil for their ED by adopting the intercourse–outercourse principle. The acquired sexual flexibility enabled the PD couple to increase their sexual satisfaction, intimacy, and self-esteem, and decrease anxiety and marital tensions.

For example, Mr. B. is 60 yr old and has had PD for 11 yr. His wife is 56 yr old. They complained about his ED, which prevented them from having intercourse, and of the decrease of her sexual desire. In the last year, they had almost no sexual relations. Mr. B's physician offered him sildenafil, but he was afraid of getting addicted and losing his ability to function sexually without the drug. Evaluation of the couple revealed that he had good erections during foreplay, but he stopped the sexual activity because of loss of erection when he tried to move over to the missionary position. In order to help this couple regain confidence in their ability to enjoy sex and to pleasure one another, they were instructed to stop any effort of having intercourse and to shift to outercourse sexual activity. During the next few weeks, they practiced various types of body touching and pleasuring, shifting from nonsexual touch to more stimulating touch. They also had an opportunity to communicate frankly and to become more intimate. Mrs. B found oral sex to be a very effective way for her to reach orgasm, thus increasing her husband's self-esteem as an adequate sexual partner. The patient found that manual stimulation during outercourse enabled him reach orgasm without losing erection. The new definitions for successful sexual activity contributed to the couple's sexual satisfaction and gave them an opportunity for positive intimate experience. At this point, the use of sildenafil as an optional choice was successfully integrated. Sex intervention was concluded by giving the couple a choice of two options for sexual activity: having planned intercourse with the use of sildenafil to enhance the erection or having outercourse.

The short type of intervention (two-four sessions) used in our clinic was effective for many patients. It was found that 80% of the patients who were treated with the intercourse–outercourse approach were satisfied with the treatment, despite the fact that only half of them reported improvement in their sexual function. Maybe the increased experience of pleasuring touch and closeness explains the high rate of satisfaction. In addition, the use of sildenafil seems very effective. Ninety percent of those who received instruction for sildenafil use in combination with intercourse–outercourse training were satisfied with the treatment, and 64% of them actually experienced an improvement in their sexual functioning.

Our counseling service was dealing also with desire problems. About 17% of the 36 parkinsonian patients who requested sex counseling complained of desire problems. Usually, the long stressful period of undiagnosed symptoms was possibly affecting sexual desire. The medical treatment of PD caused improvement in patients feeling and helped the PD patient regain his previous level of sexual interest, whereas his spouse felt no change or even decrease in her sexual interest. The gap created caused a lot of distress and tension, thus deteriorating the couple's quality of life.

Hypersexuality was also an issue addressed in the staff education, because one hypersexual patient can cause a lot of disturbances to the routine nursing work in the neurological department. The counseling is aimed to defend nurses, hospitalized patients, and caregivers from any kind of sexual harassment created by uncontrolled sexual behavior. Many nurses, as well as family members, were ashamed to complain about such harassment, therefore the service initiated short training for the nursing staff to increase their awareness and decrease their embarrassment.

5. CONCLUSION

In our Movement Disorder Unit, inhouse sexual counseling and treatment is part of a comprehensive approach to the PD patient care. The physical and emotional changes in PD, as well as treatment of the disease, have a dramatic effect on sexual functioning of patients and their partners. PD patients experience sexual dysfunction on all levels of the sexual response: desire, arousal, orgasm, and satisfaction. Because sexual dysfunction is associated with low self-esteem, depression, and marital tension, it affects the quality of life of the patients and their families. Given the high prevalence of sexual dysfunction, physicians and other health care providers must include sexual health issues in the treatment process of their PD patients. Intervention can be done by providing information, recognizing sexual needs of PD patients and their partners, by letting them express their difficulties, and referring them to specialists.

REFERENCES

1. World Health Organization. (1987) Fertility awareness methods—report on a WHO workshop. World Health Organization, Regional Office for Europe Copenhagen, pp. 11–13.
2. Gregoire, A. (1999) ABC of sexual health: male sexual problems. *BMJ* **318,** 245–247.
3. Taylor, H.A. (1999) Sexual activity and the cardiovascular patient: guidelines. *Am. J. Cardiol.* **84,** 6N–10N.
4. Thirlaway, K., Fallowfield, L., and Cuzick, J. (1996) The sexual activity questionnaire: a measure of women's sexual functioning. *Qual. Life Res.* **3,** 81–90.
5. Uttley, L. (1996) Assessment and treatment of sexual dysfunction in chronic renal failure. *Dial. Transplant.* **25,** 19–35.
6. Brown, R.G. Jahanshahi, N., Quinn, N., and Marsden, C.D. (1990) Sexual function in patients with Parkinson's disease and their partners. *J. Neurol. Neurosurg. Psychiatry* **53,** 480–486.
7. Jensen, S.B. (1992) Sexuality and chronic illness: biospychosocial approach. *Semin. Neurol.* **12,** 135–140.
8. Mulligan, T., Retchin, S.M., Chinchilli, V.M., and Bettinger, C.B. (1988) The role of aging and chronic disease in sexual dysfunction. *J. Am. Geriatr. Soc.* **36,** 520–524.
9. Butcher, J. (1999) ABC of sexual health: female sexual problems I: loss of desire—what about the fun? *BMJ* **318,** 41–43.
10. Kalayjian, L.A. and Morrell, M.J. (2000) Female sexuality and neurological disease. *J. Sex Education Therapy* **25,** 89–95.
11. Hutler, B.M. and Lundberg, P.O. (1995) Sexual function in women with advanced multiple sclerosis. *J. Neurol. Neurosurg. Psychiatry* **59,** 83–86.
12. Lipe, H., Longstreth, W.T., Bird, T.D., and Linde, M. (1990) Sexual function in married men with Parkinson's disease compared to married men with arthritis. *Neurology* **40,** 1347–1349.
13. Romeo, J.H., Seftel, A.D., Madhun, Z.T., and Aron, D.C. (2000) Sexual function in men with diabetes type 2: association with glycemic control. *J. Urol.* **163,** 788–791.
14. Cull, A.M. (1992) The assessment of sexual function in cancer patients. *Eur. J. Cancer* **28A,** 1680–1686.
15. Broderick, G.A. and Foreman, M.M. (1994) Iatrogenic male sexual dysfunction: drug induced and operative, in *Sexual Dysfunction: a Neuro-Medical Approach* (Singer, C. and Weiner, W.J., eds.), Futura Publishing, Armonk, New York, pp. 299–331.
16. Oshry, A., Rabinowitz, R., and Korczyn, A.D. (1980) Serum dopamine beta hydroxylase (DBH) levels during tilting in patients with spinal cord injuries. *Clin. Exp. Pharmacol. Physiol.* **7,** 367–371.
17. Wermuth, L. and Stenager, E. (1995) Sexual problems in young patients with Parkinson's disease. *Acta Neurol. Scand.* **91,** 453–455.
18. Koller, W.C., Vetere-Overfield, B., Williamson, A., Busenbark, K., Nash, J., and Parrish, D. (1990) Sexual dysfunction in Parkinson's disease. *Clin. Neuropharmacol.* **13,** 461–463.
19. Welch, M., Hung, L., and Waters, C.H. (1997) Sexuality in women with Parkinson's disease. *Mov. Dis.* **12,** 923–927.
20. Longstreth, W.T. and Linde, M. (1984) Sickness impact profile in Parkinson's disease. *Neurology* **34,** 207–208.
21. Wermuth, L. and Stenager, E. (1992) Sexual aspects of Parkinson's disease. *Semin. Neurol.* **12,** 125–127.
22. Zesiewicz, T.A., Helal, M., and Hauser, M.D. (2000) Sildenafil citrate (Viagra) for the treatment of erectile dysfunction in men with Parkinson's disease. *Mov. Dis.* **15,** 305–308.
23. Duvoisin, R.C. and Yahr, M.D. (1972) Epidemiological approach to Parkinson's disease. *Lancet* **1,** 1400–1401.
24. Murata, Y., Haranda, T., Ishizaki, F., et al. (1997) Autonomic dysfunction in Parkinson's disease and vascular parkinsonism. *Acta Neurol. Scand.* **96,** 359–365.
25. Korczyn, A.D. (1987) Autonomic manifestations in Parkinson's disease, in *Handbook of Parkinson's Disease. Morbo di Parkinson e Malattie Extrapiramidali* (Nappi, G. and Caracenti, T. eds.), Edizioni Mediche Italiane, Pavia, pp. 205–210.
26. Korczyn, A.D. (1990) Cognitive dysfunction: the spectrum of parkinsonian syndromes, in *Mental Dysfunction in Parkinson's Disease II* (Wolters, E.C., Scheltens, P.H., and Berendse, H.W., eds.), Academic Pharmaceutical Productions, Utrecht, The Netherlands, pp. 209–214.

27. Damiano, A.M., Snyder, C., Strausser, B., and Willian, M.K. (1999) A review of health-related quality of life concepts and measures for Parkinson's disease. *Qual. Life Res.* **8,** 235–243.
28. Moore, O., Gurevitch, T., Korczyn, A.D., Anca, M., Shabtai, H., and Giladi, N. (2000) Quality of sexual life in Parkinson's disease. *Mov. Dis.* **15(Suppl. 2),** 170.
29. Basson, R. (2001) Sex and idiopathic Parkinson's disease. *Adv. Neurology* **86,** 295–300.
30. Kaplan, H.S. (1974) *The New Sex Therapy*, Brunner Mazel, New York, pp. 185–248.
31. Giladi, N., Treves, T.A., Paleacu, D., et al. (2000) Risk factors for dementia, depression and psychosis in long-standing Parkinson's disease. *J. Neural. Transm.* **107,** 59–71.
32. Jacobs, H., Vieregge, A., and Vieregge, P. (2000) Sexuality in young patients with Parkinson's disease: a population based comparison with healthy controls. *J. Neurol. Neurosurg. Psychiatry* **69,** 550–552.
33. Davis, S. (2000) Testosterone and sexual desire in women. *J. Sex Education Therapy* **25,** 25–32.
34. Berman, J.R., Adhikari, S.P., and Goldstein, I. (2000) Anatomy and physiology of female sexual function and dysfunction: classification, evaluation and treatment options. *Eur. Urol.* **38,** 20–29.
35. American Psychiatric Association. (1994) *Diagnostic and Statistical Manual of Mental Disorders, 4th ed.,* American Psychiatric Association, Washington, DC.
36. Lauman, E.O., Paik, A., and Rosen, R.C. (1999) Sexual dysfunction in the United States: prevalence and predictors. *JAMA* **281,** 537–544.
37. Basson, R. (1996) Sexuality and Parkinson's disease. *Parkinsonism Rel. Dis.* **2,** 177–185.
38. Feldman, H.A., Goldstein, I., Hatzichristou, D.G., et al (1994) Impotence and its medical and psychosocial correlates: results of the Massachusetts male aging study. *J. Urol.* **151,** 54–61.
39. National Institutes of Health Consensus Development Panel on Impotence. (1993) Impotence. *JAMA* **270,** 83–90.
40. Fogel, C.I. and Lauver, D. (1990) *Sexual Health Promotion*, W. B. Saunders, Philadelphia.
41. Mueller, J.E. (1999) Sexual activity as a trigger for cardiovascular events: what is the risk? *Am. J. Cardiol.* **84,** 2N–5N.
42. Greenstein, A., Chen, J., Miller, H., Matzkin, H., Villa, Y., and Braf, Z. (1997) Does severity of ischemic coronary disease correlate with erectile function? *Int. J. Impot.* **9,** 123–126.
43. Goldstein, I. (2000) The mutually reinforcing triad of depressive symptom cardiovascular disease and erectile dysfunction. *Am. J. Cardiol.* **86,** 41F–45F.
44. Phillips, R.L. and Slaughter, J.R. (2000) Depression and sexual desire. *Am. Fam. Physician* **62,** 782–786.
45. Jackson, G., Betteridge, J., Dean, J., et al. (1990) A systematic approach to erectile dysfunction in the cardiovascular patient: a consensus statement. *Int. J. Clin. Pract.* **53,** 445–451.
46. Hyppä, M., Rinne, U.K., and Sonninen, V. (1970) The activating effect of L-Dopa treatment on sexual functions and its experimental background. *Acta Neurol. Scand.* **46,** 223–224.
47. Uitti, R.J., Tanner, C.M., Rajut, A.H., Goetz, C.G., Klawan, H.L., and Thiessen, B. (1989) Hypersexuality in antiparkinsonian therapy. *Clin. Neuropharmacol.* **12,** 375–383.
48. Brown, E., Brown, G.M., Kofman, O., and Quarington, B. (1978) Sexual function and affect in parkinsonian men treated with L-Dopa. *Am. J. Psychiatry* **135,** 1552–1557.
49. Korpelainen, J.T., Hiltunen, P., and Myllyla, V.V. (1998) Moclobemide-induced hypersexuality in patients with stroke and Parkinson's disease. *Clin. Neuropharmacol.* **21,** 251–254.
50. Courty, E., Durif, F., Zenut, M., Courty, P., and Lavarenne, J. (1997) Psychiatric and sexual disorders induced by apomorphine in Parkinson's disease. *Clin. Neuropharmacol.* **20,** 140–147.
51. Fernandez, H.H. and Durso, R. (1998) Clozapine for dopaminergic-induced paraphilias in Parkinson's disease. *Mov. Disord.* **13,** 597–598.
52. Cummings, J.L. (1991) Behavioral complications of drug treatment of Parkinson's disease. *J. Am. Geriatr. Soc.* **39,** 708–716.
53. Kaplan, H.I. and Sadock, B.J. (1991) *Synopsis of Psychiatry*, Williams & Wilkins, Baltimore, pp. 438–465.
54. Lechtenberg, R. and Ohl, D.A. (1994) *Sexual Dysfunction—Neurologic, Urologic and Gynecologic Aspects,* Lea & Febiger, Philadelphia.
55. O'Sullivan, J.D. and Hughes, A.J. (1998) Apomorphine—induced penile erection in Parkinson's disease. *Mov. Disord.* **13,** 536–539.
56. Jardin, A., Wagner, G., Khoury, S., et al. (eds.) (2000) Recommendations of the 1st International Consultation on Erectile Dysfunction, Health Publication Ltd.
57. Pfizer. (1998) *Sildenafil Citrate Prescribing Information*, Pfizer Inc., New York.
58. Hardoff, R., Tamir, A., Sula, M., et al. (2001) Gastric emptying time and gastric motility in patients with Parkinson's disease. *Mov. Disord.,* in press.
59. Bronner, G. (1995) Helping health care professionals on issues of intimacy and sexuality among the aging. *Siecus Rep.* **25,** 4–7.
60. Bronner, G. (2001) Sexual health promotion—an inductive intervention model. *Harefuah* **140,** 72–76.
61. Lundberg, P.O., Ertekin, C., Ghezzi, A., Swash, M., and Vodusek, D. (2001) Neurosexology- guidelines for neurologists. *Eur. J. Neurol.* **8(Suppl. 3),** 2–24.

39

Daytime Sleepiness and Sleep Attacks in Idiopathic Parkinson's Disease

David B. Rye, MD, PhD, Joseph T. Daley, BS,
Amanda A. Freeman, BS, and Donald L. Bliwise, PhD

1. INTRODUCTION

The prevalence of disturbed sleep in idiopathic Parkinson's disease (PD) approaches 100% *(1)*. Sleep abnormalities include decrements in total sleep time, sleep spindling, stages 3 and 4 slow-wave sleep, and rapid eye-movement (REM)-sleep accompanied by sleep fragmentation and poor sleep efficiency *(2,3)*. As primary sleep disorders, which interfere similarly with sleep, are associated with pathological levels of excessive daytime sleepiness (EDS), EDS might be expected to be relatively commonplace in PD. Suprisingly, EDS in PD has received little prior attention. Only quite recently has subjective *(4,5)* and objective *(6–8)* documentation of EDS and intrusion of REM-sleep into daytime naps in PD rekindled interest and a decades-long debate as to whether dopamine (DA) participates in behavioral state control, and if it does, what its role(s) might be. Current heuristic models of behavioral state control have restricted themselves to prominent roles for acetylcholine and other monoamines (e.g., serotonin, norepinephrine, and histamine). Exclusion of DA from these models derives largely from an inability to reconcile acknowledged influences of exogenous DA upon behavioral state with reported invariability of endogeneous DA activity across unique behavioral states. Lacking a comprehensive conceptual framework that incorporates DA in a sleep–wake state or circadian rhythm modulation, clinical recognition of thalamocortical arousal impairments in PD has been met with surprise and no single parsimonious explanation. It has become increasingly clear, however, that wake (i.e., a thalamocortical-aroused state characterized by electroencephalography [EEG] desynchronization) is strongly influenced by DA *(9–11)*.

Parkinsonism provides a unique window in which to elucidate DA's modulation of behavioral state, as it is well studied and generally accepted as the prototypical hypodopaminergic condition reflecting a selective loss of mesostriatal DA neurons. Age, co-morbid conditions, medications, progression of DA neural loss, and extranigral neuropathological heterogeneity may independently contribute or interact to impair thalamocortical arousal in PD. It is, therefore, reasonable to expect that PD-associated decrements in waking arousal, REM-sleep expression, and an inability to initiate and maintain sleep might be a transient phenomena or even describe a continuum within an individual patient. This being said, significant insights into the pathophysiology of these impairments are beginning to emerge from studies of patients, animal models of PD, critical reappraisal of existing data, and the elucidation of novel anatomical and physiological features of mesostriatal pathways.

From: *Mental and Behavioral Dysfunction in Movement Disorders*
Edited by: M-A. Bédard et al. © Humana Press Inc., Totowa, NJ

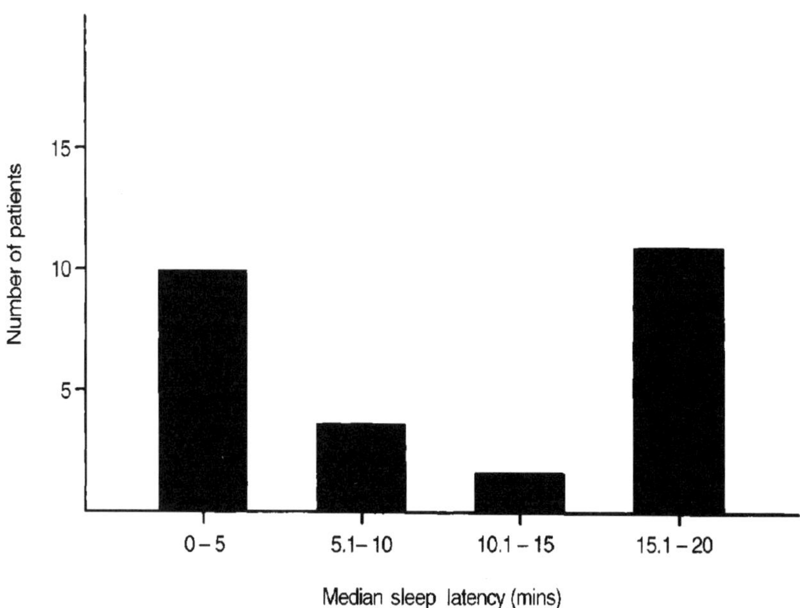

Fig. 1. Frequency histogram demonstrating median daytime sleep latencies in 27 PD patients. Note the biphasic distribution: 37% had a median latency ≤5 min (i.e., pathologic sleepiness), while 41% had a median latency >15 min.

2. EPIDEMIOLOGY AND CLUES TO THE PATHOPHYSIOLOGY OF SLEEPINESS IN PD

Questionnaire-based surveys of sleepiness in the general PD population are in disagreement. One community-based study of 245 PD patients reported a 15.5% prevalence of EDS that was more frequent than in elderly controls and more common with advanced disease and cognitive decline *(4)*. Another contends that fatigue related to the parkinsonian motor disability, but not EDS, is more common *(12)*. Prompted by reports of D2/D3 agonist-associated "sleep attacks" in PD, one recent assessment of 55 PD patients reported a 7% prevalence of EDS unrelated to the pharmacological profile of dopaminomimetics and more common with advanced disease *(5)*. Another prospective study identified EDS in 30.5% of 236 patients also unrelated to a specific dopaminomimetics and more common in patients with autonomic failure *(13)*. Objective measures are preferred, given the unreliability of subjective reports and the variability in terms that patients choose to describe sleepiness *(14)*. Given this void in knowledge, we recently reported a series of 27 adult idiopathic PD patients in whom polysomnography was performed followed by an evaluation of daytime sleepiness with a standardized physiological measure: the mean sleep latency test (MSLT) *(7)*.

Impairments in thalamocortical arousal state were common in this group of 27 patients and manifested as daytime sleepiness (Fig. 1) and intrusion of REM-sleep into daytime naps. Pathological sleepiness (i.e., sleep latency <5 min) was evident in 40 of 134 nap opportunities, with at least one such nap occurring in 14 of 27 patients. Intrusion of REM-sleep in daytime sleep, namely, sleep-onset REM-sleep (SOREMs), was evident in 13 of 134 nap opportunities and occurred in 6 of 27 patients. It is noteworthy that 15% of our study population (4 of 27) exhibited a narcolepsy-like phenotype (i.e., MSL <8 min and 2 SOREMS). These physiological tendencies bore little relationship to the primary motor manifestations of disease (e.g., disability scale, medication burden) or sleep architecture measures (e.g., total sleep time, stage %, etc.). In fact, contrary to what might have been expected based upon the demands of sleep homeostatic mechanisms, poor nocturnal sleep was associated with greater, rather than lesser, degrees of daytime alertness. The six patients exhibiting SOREMs were sleepier than the other 21 patients and differed in only one other important respect: longer disease duration (11.8 vs 6.1 yr). This confirms reports that subjective EDS is more common with advanced disease. The dissociation of arousal state from the motor manifestations of disease and homeostatic sleep drives (i.e., sleep propensity should be predicated upon the quality and quantity of prior sleep amounts) in PD has several implications. First, it argues that the integrity of DA pathways is essential to the maintenance of homeostatic sleep mechanisms. Second, it points to the pathophysiological basis of impaired thalamocortical arousal state residing outside of the sensorimotor subcircuit of nigrostriatal pathways traditionally thought to underlie parkinsonian motor disabilities. It is generally believed that a threshold of 60–90% of DA loss in the sensorimotor putamen needs to be exceeded before the emergence of waking clinical mainfestations *(15–17)*. Loss of DA is then believed to proceed in an orderly fashion through associative (i.e., caudate) and eventually limbic (i.e., nucleus accumbens) striatal subcircuits. Thus, it is the loss of DA in these latter circuits, which is characteristic of advanced disease, that is a potential factor in the expression of EDS and SOREM in PD.

Impaired maintenance of wakefulness in PD is supported by reported decrements in α-EEG power associated with wakefulness *(18)* and a recently described diffuse phenomenon coined "thalamocortical dysrhythmia" by Llinas *(19)*. At the level of single neurons in motor thalamic nuclei, this manifests as a decrement in neural activity and/or a shift to a burst firing mode similar to low-threshold spike driven low-frequency slow wave sleep-like synchronized oscillations *(20,21)*. These findings suggest a more generalized inhibition or disfacilitation of thalamocortical neurons secondary to mesostriatal DA loss, which are not satisfactorily accounted for by altered synaptic transmission solely in pallido- and nigrothalamic motor pathways. Widespread alterations in thalamocortical firing in PD might be more reflective of loss of nigrostriatal collateral innervation of the midline, prinicipal, and reticular thalamic nuclei that we have recently described *(22)*. When unaffected by disease, these novel DA pathways might otherwise serve to maintain normal states of thalamocortical excitability (see Subheading 6.2).

3. EFFECTS OF DISEASE

The parkinsonian condition itself appears to contribute to the expression of sleepiness and SOREMs. Five of the 27 PD patients that we examined were medication-free and afforded unambiguous controls for the potential confound of medications. Their mean and median MSLs did not differ significantly from the 22 medicated patients, although their disease duration was shorter and Hoehn-Yahr score lower. Pathological sleepiness was evident in 6 of 24 naps and in 2 of the 5 unmedicated patients. Only 1 of these 24 naps demonstrated a SOREM. This experience extends our earlier recognition of sleepiness and SOREMs expression in a single unmedicated 18-yr-old patient *(6)*.

4. EFFECTS OF MEDICATION

Differentiation of disease from medication-induced state-related phenomena can be obscured, in part, by dopaminomimetic treatments that have their own effects upon thalamocortical arousal state. Dopaminomimetics induce biphasic effects on sleep, such that low doses decrease wakefulness and increase sleep, including REM-sleep, whereas higher doses promote wakefulness at the expense of sleep (reviewed in refs. *2,23,24*). These dose-related behavioral effects exhibit complementary responses as assessed by EEG power spectral changes in the prefrontal cortex of experimental rats *(25)*. Systemic and local administration of low-doses of DA agonists are well known to suppress midbrain DA neural activity due to the presence of pharmacologically defined D2-like inhibitory autoreceptors *(26,27)*. The soporific effects of systemic administration of low-dose DA agonists are mimicked by bilateral local infusions into the ventral tegmental area (VTA) and are blocked in a dose-dependent fashion by local applications of D2-like receptor antagonists into the same loci *(28)*. Corresponding decrements in DA released from the terminal fields of mesocorticolimbic VTA neurons might, therefore, attend low-dose dopaminomimetic, particularly D2-like receptor agonist, use in PD. Whether this translates into sleepiness and SOREMs expression in PD is unsubstantiated, and if it does, the cellular and subcellular substrates responsible remain ill-defined. These phenomena may reflect decrements or loss of DA's effects upon neural excitability in any one of a number of nuclei targeted by surviving midbrain DA neurons. In addition to actions of systemic dopaminomimetics upon presynaptic autoreceptors, the additional potential actions at postsynaptic receptors rendered hypersensitive secondary to DA loss must also be considered.

The underlying diathesis to sleepiness and SOREMs expression in PD may be exaggerated by concomitant use of dopaminomimetics. A recent report of sleep attacks with pramipexole and ropinirole, which were dose-related in a small group of patients was initially interpreted as a novel idiosyncratic response specific to the newer nonergot-derived D2/D3 agonists *(29)*. The controversy generated by this report heightened awareness to sleepiness complaints in PD patients and has prompted a critical reappraisal of the underlying contributing factors, including the potential contribution of medications. Clinical experience and more comprehensive assessments agree that sleepiness has long been under-recognized in PD and that it is a phenomenon not restricted to a specific class of dopaminomimetics *(5,7,13,30–36)*. Although many clinicians have commented that sleepiness observed with dopaminomimetic use in PD is related to increasing dose, it remains unresolved how much this use contributes and if it is unique to PD. It cannot be overstated that sleepiness with SOREMs expression can express itself in drug-free patients and that sleepiness accompanies levodopa (L-dopa) exposure in drug naïve controls *(37)*.

Comparisons between our 22 patients receiving vs those not receiving medications indicated that mean and median MSL were unassociated with L-dopa/carbidopa, the D2-like agonist pergolide, amantadine, serotonin re-uptake inhibitors, or antipsychotic (e.g., clozapine, risperidone) use. The likelihood of SOREMs was greater in patients prescribed the monoamine oxidase B inhibitor selegiline; 3 of 4 patients using this medication exhibited SOREMs on MSLT vs 3 of 23 patients not using selegiline ($\chi^2 = 7.5, p < 0.01$). This most probably reflects REM-sleep rebound, given selegeline's metabolic conversion to methamphetamine and amphetamine *(38)*, which are well-established REM-sleep suppressants. Enhanced sleepiness in the four patients prescribed benzodiazepines (either temazepam or clonazepam) was also evident on both mean (5.8 [1.2] vs 11.9 [6.2], $t = 4.35$, $p < 0.005$) and median (5.5 [1.1] vs 12.1 [7.4], $t = 4.03$, $p < 0.0005$) MSL, but without any association with SOREMs.

5. DISTURBANCES OF THALAMOCORTICAL AROUSAL STATE IN ANIMAL MODELS OF PD

Differentiation of the neural substrates underlying disturbances of thalamocortical arousal in PD has been significantly advanced by investigations of animal models of disease. These models afford the ability to control for potentially confounding variables such as age, co-morbid conditions and medications, and, therefore, unambiguous associations of state-related phenomena to disease rather than other factors. Electrolytic lesions centered upon midbrain DA neurons decrease "behavioral arousal" *(39)*, with larger lesions of the ventral mesencephalon, including the substantia nigra (SN) producing a wake–sleep disruption remarkably similar to that seen in PD *(40)*. More selective destruction of nigrostriatal pathways with bilateral intrastriatal infusions of the DA toxin 6-hydroxydopamine (6-OHDA) in rats results in their spending more of their subjective day asleep *(41)*. Similarly, systemic delivery of the DA neurotoxin 1-methyl,4-phenyl-1,2,3,6-tetrahydropyridine (MPTP) in one nonhuman primate led to the expression of daytime sleepiness and SOREMs *(42)* (Fig. 2). These impairments in thalamocortical arousal were reversible with the DA precursor L-dopa, the DA re-uptake blocker bupropion, but not the D2 agonist pergolide *(42)* (Fig. 3). L-dopa and bupropion require presynaptic integrity to enhance synaptic availability of DA by promoting its synthesis or by blockade of the DA transporter, respectively. Thus, the abilities of these agents to reverse sleepiness and REM-sleep propensity in this parkinsonian nonhuman primate likely reflects actions upon surviving mesocorticolimbic DA circuits,

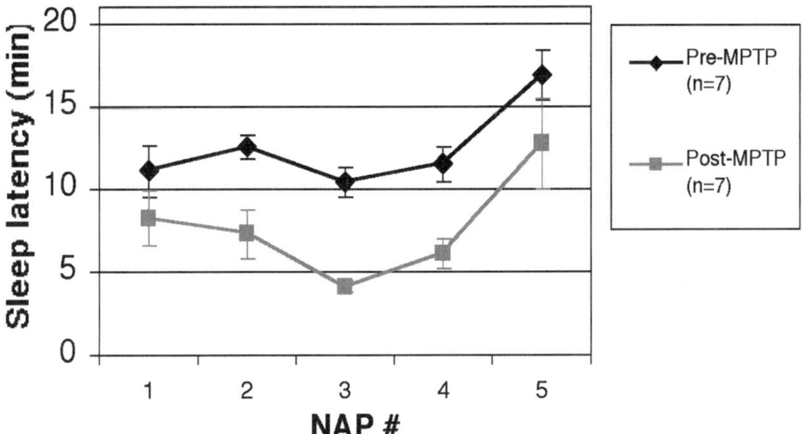

Fig. 2. Impaired daytime alertness was observed 2 to 3 mo following systemic treatment with the neurotoxin MPTP. Overall MSL dropped from 12.5 min at baseline to 7.7 min after MPTP treatment. Mean latency of the naps at midday (nap 3) was pathologic (<5 min). Of the 35 naps recorded following MPTP treatment, 14 had a latency of <5 min and 5 demonstrated REM-sleep. Data is presented as mean +/– standard error of the mean (SEM).

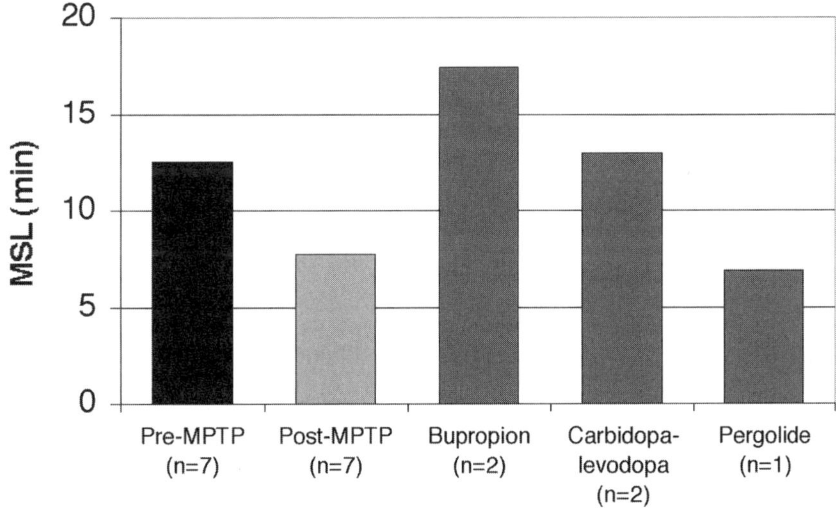

Fig. 3. The effects of dopaminomimetics on MPTP-induced daytime sleepiness were investigated. L-dopa/carbidopa (4.2/16.7 mg/kg by mouth [p.o.] three times daily [tid]) increased the MSL from the 7.7 min, observed with placebo, to pretreatment levels (13.0 min; (*n* = 2). In contrast, pergolide, a D2 agonist (0.004 mg/kg p.o. twice daily [bid]) failed to reverse the impairment, with a MSL of 6.9 min (*n* = 1). Daytime alertness was improved with bupropion (0.5–0.6 mg/kg intramuscularly [i.m.]), in fact, exceeding pretreatment levels (17.2 min; *n* = 2).

which are less vulnerable to MPTP. These disturbances in thalamocortical arousal persisted for approx 3 mo, at which time subsequent MSLT testing revealed a normal, if not heightened, level of daytime alertness and absence of SOREMs. It is tempting to speculate that this behavioral plasticity has its origin in compensatory sprouting within surviving DA axons known to occur with severe MPTP-induced loss of DA axons *(43)*.

6. PATHOPHYSIOLOGICAL BASIS OF DISTURBED THALAMOCORTICAL AROUSAL IN PD

The pathophysiological bases underlying the spectrum of PD-related changes in sleep–wake tendencies are likely complex. Consistent with the experience in obstructive sleep apneics *(44)*, much of the variation in sleepiness severity in PD is not explained by nocturnal arousals. Thus, individual patient differences in premorbid arousal traits are likely important determinants. These interact with unique disease-related brain pathologies that can be categorized into direct or indirect effects of the disease. Potential primary substrates include: (*i*) extranigral pathology in nuclei comprising the traditional ascending reticular activating system; (*ii*) degeneration of novel mesothalamic dopaminergic collaterals emanating from nigrostriatal axons; and (*iii*) degeneration of VTA dopaminergic neurons in mesocorticolimbic circuits that parallels disease progression. Alternatively, dysregulation of the pedunculopontine nucleus (PPN) tegmental region, an area known to promote thalamocortical arousal and REM-sleep, may occur secondary to its position as a principal brainstem target of pathological basal ganglia outflow.

6.1. *Extranigral Pathology: Involvement of Components of the Ascending Reticular Activating System*

Cortical EEG-defined and behavioral wakefulness are critically dependent upon a collection of neurochemically defined subcortical nuclei comprising the so-called ascending reticular activating system (ARAS) (namely, histamine, serotonin, norepinephrine, and acetylcholine cell groups). These nuclei share in common features such as: (*i*) axon pathways that collateralize extensively to many brain regions disparate in location and principal function; (*ii*) modulation of the responsiveness of target neurons to other stimuli, often in the context of behavioral state (e.g., wake vs sleep); and (*iii*) dense interconnectivity *(45)*. Cell loss in the ARAS commonly accompanies nigrostriatal DA neuron degeneration in PD, and individual components are variably involved *(46,47)* (reviewed in ref. *2*) and, therefore, might be expected to underlie specific disturbances of thalamocortical arousal in PD. Loss or dysfunction of histaminergic neurons of the hypothalamic tuberomamillary nucleus, for example, might contribute to decrements in waking arousal state in PD, since these neurons are selectively wake active and provide excitatory influences to the cortex and several wake-promoting nuclei *(48)*. Alternatively, loss of REM-sleep inhibitory serotonergic dorsal raphe and noradrenergic locus coeruleus influences might account for SOREM expression via disinhibition of the cholinergic PPN region. These are plausible clinicopathophysiological postulates, but lacking rigorous analysis of state-related clinical and physiological variables in concert with quantitative analysis of cell integrity in the ARAS, they remain purely conjectural.

6.2. *Loss of Novel Nigrostriatal Collateral Innervation of the Thalamus*

Individual mesencephalic DA neurons have the potential to modulate normal and pathologic behavior not only through traditional nigrostriatal pathways, but also by way of axon collaterals that innervate the thalamus *(22)*. As other monoamines generally facilitate thalamocortical transmission *(49)*, widespread reductions in thalamic DA innervation observed in animal models of parkinsonism might be a parsimonious explanation for the diffuse "thalamocortical dysrhythmia" *(19)*, impairments of wakefulness *(7)*, and loss of sleep spindles reflective of rhythmic bursting in the thalamic reticular nucleus (RTn). Although largely uninvestigated, DA's influences upon thalamic neurons are likely to be complex, given the differential thalamic distribution of DA receptor subtypes (D1–D5) and their unique effects on ion conductances and second messenger systems. Activation of D1-like receptors, for example, is positively coupled to adenylyl cyclase and depolarizes neurons, while D2-like receptors produce hyperpolarization via inhibition of 3',5'-cyclic adenosine monophosphate (cAMP) formation *(50)*. Thalamic relay and RTn cells fire in two distinct modes, tonic or burst, with the operative mode dictated by the state of low-threshold voltage-gated T-type Ca^{2+} channels. Thus, tonic firing, which is

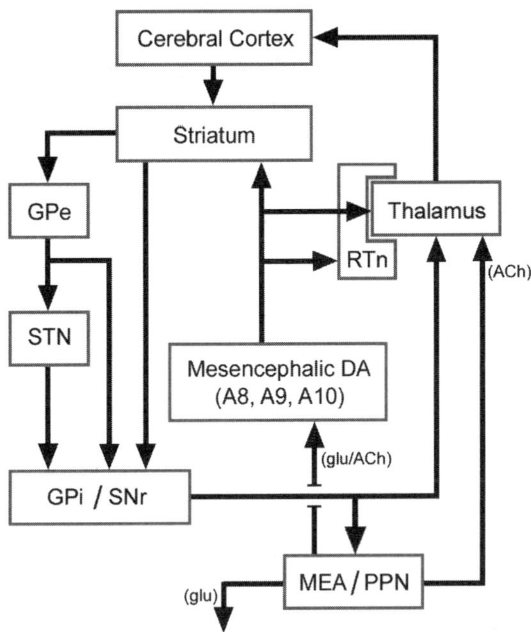

Fig. 4. Diagram of basal ganglia circuitry, including nigrostriatal collaterals innervating the thalamus. Dopaminergic projections from the retrorubral field (A8), SN pars compacta (A9), and VTA (A10) innervate functionally segregated striatal and thalamic regions. Basal ganglia influences on brainstem centers known to modulate thalamocortical arousal (midbrain extrapyramidal area [MEA]/PPN) are established via collaterals of basal ganglia output pathways to thalamus.

seen when the T channels are inactivated via membrane depolarization, and burst firing, when the T channels are activated from a hyperpolarized state, will very much depend upon the DA receptor subtype expressed by individual thalamic neurons. A preponderance of D1-like receptors in the ventral lateral nucleus pars oralis (VLo) *(51,52)*, suggests that here, DA mediates depolarization, thereby enhancing the likelihood of excitatory postsynaptic potentials (EPSP)-generated action potentials and sensorimotor processing during thalamocortical-aroused states. In contrast, D2-like receptors predominate in the limbic-related mediodorsal nucleus and midline nuclei *(51,53)*, suggesting that, here, DA promotes a shift to a burst firing mode similar to low-frequency slow-wave sleep-like synchronized oscillations reported in subprimates in vitro *(54)*. Critical to determining the role of DA in arousal state control will be its influences on the RTn, which, when in a bursting mode, inhibits large numbers of thalamocortical neurons via widespread and recurrent γ-amino butyric acid (GABA) innervation (Fig. 4). The latter is well known to promote synchronized and rhythmic occurrence of spindle-waves, the electrographic signature of wake–sleep transitions *(55)*. The presence of both D1 *(56)* and D4 *(57)* receptor subtypes in the RTn, with opposing physiological effects, renders this a challenging endeavor. To probe these considerations, preliminary experiments in a single hemiparkinsonian non-human primate demonstrate that DA has potent effects not only on the rate, but also on the pattern of thalamic neural firing (Fig. 5A–D). The altered firing patterns in the cerebellar recipient zone, i.e., the ventral posterior lateral nucleus pars oralis (VPLo), previously reported in PD, appear to be a more widespread phenomenon, as evidenced by markedly reduced RTn activity during wakefulness (1–4 Hz vs 15–30 Hz) (Fig. 5B). Focal applications of the D1 agonist SKF-82958 enhance firing of RTn and VPLo neurons (Fig. 5A,B) and have no effect upon the prinicipal thalamic sensory relay nucleus, the ventral posterior lateral pars caudalis (VPLc), which is devoid of DA innervation (Fig. 5C). Hyperpolarization of RTn neurons, secondary to DA loss, may account not only for their depressed activity, but also burst firing in response to a typical depolarizing effect of a D1 agonist (Fig. 5B).

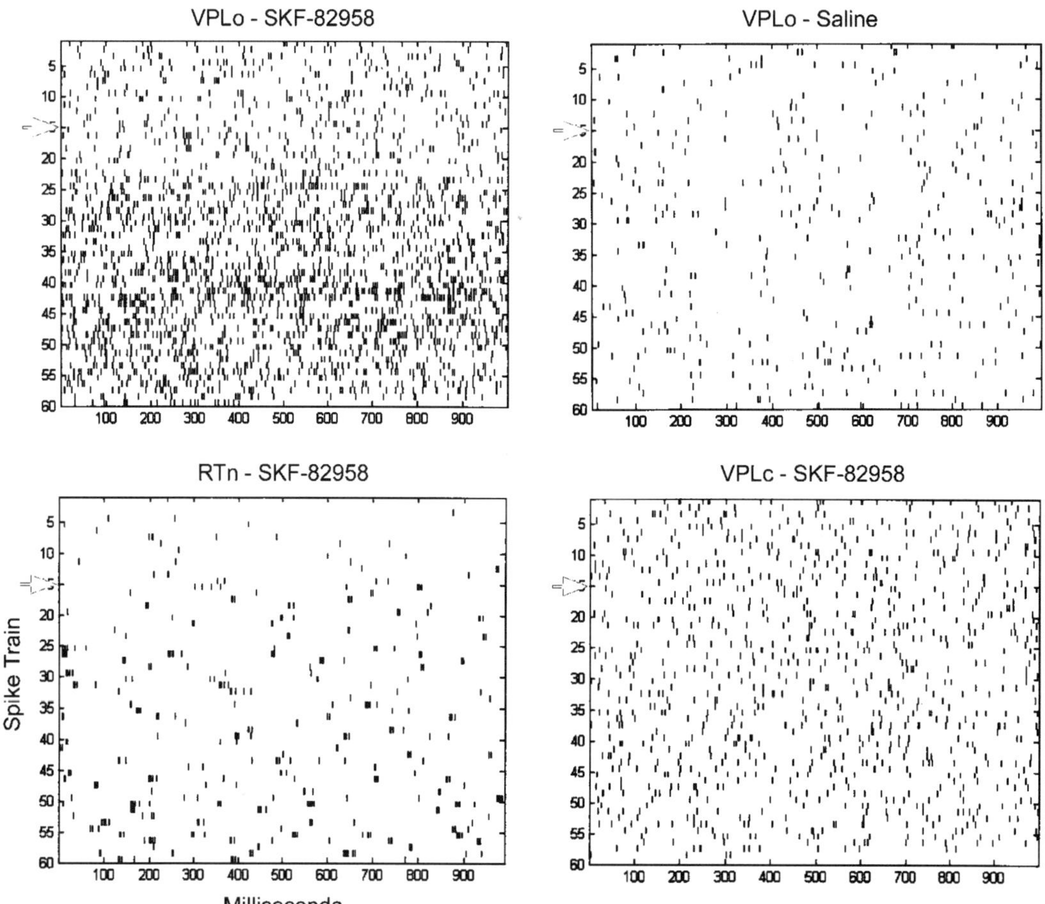

Fig. 5. Modulation of thalamic neuron responsivity in an awake parkinsonian nonhuman primate by local microinjection of a D1 agonist, SKF-82958. Each raster displays the firing rate for a single cell over a 1-min period; following 15 s of baseline activity, the drug was injected (indicated by arrow), and the activity of the cell was monitored for 45 s. In the cerebellar recipient area, VPLo, the firing rate increased in response to the D1 agonist. An injection within the RTn, considered to be the thalamic pacemaker, altered the firing pattern from tonic firing to burst firing as evidenced by enhanced clustering of the tick marks representative of individual action potentials. Similar to a control injection of saline, the VPLc, a sensory nucleus with no evidence of dopaminergic innervation, lacked firing rate and pattern changes in response to the drug.

Thalamic DA loss in idiopathic PD, therefore, appears likely to interfere with the normal relay of information to the cortex and, thereby, with behavioral consequences that potentially include thalamocortical arousal state disturbances. The consensus mode of thalamocortical excitability will depend upon which thalamic circuit predominates, recognizing that response modes of thalamocortical neurons to DA appear modality specific (e.g., differential modes in motor vs limbic vs state-related [midline nuclei and RTn]). In the disease-free state, modulation of thalamocortical arousal state by DA will depend upon the extent to which individual circuits function in parallel or independently, which DA receptors are expressed in these circuits, and the differential affinities of receptor subtypes to endogenous DA. In PD, the contribution of thalamic pathology to disturbances of thalamocortical arousal will be difficult to discern, given the dynamic compensatory responses to maintain synaptic DA transmission, such as increased synthesis, release and turnover of DA, axonal sprouting, and receptor up-regulation, particularly in the face of dopaminomimetic use. Disease progression from the ventral tier of the SN medially to the VTA is another modifying variable and commands that much more attention, given that sleepiness is more common with disease advancement, as noted above. The thalamic targets of the VTA, the midline paraventricular *(58)* and mediodorsal nuclei *(59)*, therefore, may be particularly relevant to the pathophysiology of disturbed thalamocortical arousal state in PD. While experimental and clinical experience supports a role for these thalamic nuclei in maintaining arousal *(60–62)*, the relevance of DA in these loci to arousal state control requires elucidation.

6.3. Degeneration of Mesocorticolimbic Neurons Paralleling Disease Progression

Degeneration of DA neurons, which is the hallmark of PD, occurs first in the ventral tier of the SN, which projects preferentially to sensorimotor circuits within the putamen. Cell loss then progresses through the dorsal tier, which projects upon ventral "limbic" striatal circuits, and eventually the contiguous VTA, whose cell bodies and diffuse projections comprise the mesocorticolimbic pathways *(63–65)*. These latter circuits are particularly intriguing when considering the phenomenon of EDS and SOREM expression in PD for several reasons. First, as noted above, it is fairly well established that the VTA is the locus through which D2-like receptor agonists evoke their soporific effects *(28)*. Second, sleepiness is more common with disease advancement as noted earlier. Thus, it is loss of DA in targets of VTA-DA neurons that potentially contributes to EDS and SOREM expression in PD. While the behavioral consequences of selective destruction of VTA-DA neurons in animals has not been investigated, several experimental observations support the contention that integrity of VTA-DA neurons is critical to the expression of arousal and suppression of REM-sleep. Enhancement of extracellular DA locally within the medial basal forebrain terminal fields of VTA-DA neurons, for example, has recently been shown to initiate and maintain alert waking *(66)*. Reduction of DA tone in these same circuits also exacerbates REM-sleep lack of control in narcolepsy *(67,68)*, a condition which, incidentally, shares many state-related disturbances with PD including sleepiness, SOREMs, periodic leg movements in sleep, and REM-sleep behavior disorder. As the VTA is more resistant to the neurodegenerative process and exhibits more pronounced compensatory responses, including sprouting *(43)*, surviving axons provide a potential substrate for treatment-based reversals of sleepiness and SOREM expression in PD. Enhancement of synaptic DA availability in mesocorticolimbic circuits, in fact, may underlie the success of the DA transport blocker bupropion (personal observations) and amphetamines in the treatment of PD *(69,70)*, thus providing beneficial alerting effects in truly "sleepy" patients.

6.4. Influences of Pathological Basal Ganglia Outflow Upon Brainstem Thalamocortical Arousal Sites

Functional anatomical models of the basal ganglia, which emphasize relationships with thalamocortical circuits, largely ignore one multisynaptic pathway through which DA-responsive striatal circuits might influence thalamocortical arousal state. This multisynaptic pathway links the striatum with the PPN region of the upper brainstem via the main output nuclei of the basal ganglia, the internal segment of the globus pallidus (GPi) and SN pars reticulata (SNr) (reviewed in ref. *71*). The PPN region contains both "wake-on" and "REM-on" cholinergic and glutamatergic neurons that are uniquely positioned to receive basal ganglia output and to reflect these influences, in turn, either back upon forebrain circuits, which modulate thalamocortical arousal, or to nuclei further down the neural axis. Heightened discharge of GABAergic GPi/SNr neurons secondary to nigrostriatal DA loss underlies many of the waking motor manifestations of parkinsonism *(72)*, yet the relevance to the physiological measures of thalamocortical arousal state remains ill-defined. Alleviation from parkinsonism, whether the treatment be medical, as noted upon the seminal introduction of L-dopa *(73)*, or surgical (e.g., pallidotomy; DeLong, Vitek and Rye, personal observations), is often described as an "awakening" by patients. This nearly immediate perception of improved daytime alertness could conceivably reflect restoration of excitability in wake-on and REM-on cholinergic neurons in the PPN region. Restoration of daytime alertness and REM-sleep, following lesions centered upon the sensorimotor GPi, has indeed been documented in two cases of idiopathic PD *(71,74)*. Disinhibition of the PPN region via

DA-mediated attenuation of GABAergic GPi output, however, selectively engages glutamatergic, rather than cholinergic, neurons in the PPN region *(71)*. The functional anatomy of this glutamatergic subpopulation is more centered upon sensorimotor subcircuits and, therefore, is better positioned to modulate motor activity in a state-dependent fashion *(71)*. Considerably more work is, therefore, warranted in order to establish which behavioral state-related functions these multisynaptic circuits subserve and the precise cellular and pharmacological substrates involved.

7. SUMMARY

Daytime somnolence experienced by idiopathic PD patients is very real, common, and potentially as severe as that manifested by narcoleptics. Clinical recognition is extremely challenging, as in our experience, PD patients and their caregivers infrequently volunteer complaints of excessive sleepiness, and, if they can be prompted to, the severity of sleepiness is typically underestimated. This is consistent with a growing realization that truly sleepy patients prefer the terms "fatigue" and "lack of energy" to describe their sleepiness *(14)* and may account for discrepancies in previous surveys of sleepiness in the general PD population. Proper treatment can dramatically enhance quality of life and prevent the significant morbidity and mortality that attends pathological sleepiness. We advocate a careful medication review, as dosage reduction or discontinuation of selegeline, benzodiazepines, and dopaminomimetics might be expected to reverse sleepiness. Benzodiazepine use, intended to improve daytime alertness by lengthening total sleep time and preventing nocturnal arousals, is particularly unwarranted, given the strong inverse correlation of parkinsonian sleepiness with the quantity or quality of prior night's sleep. If medication adjustments are ineffectual, the diagnostic "yield" for routine polysomnography and MSLT evaluation of PD patients is likely to be considerable. Treatment strategies that until now have focused primarily on minimizing waking motor disability may need to include agents specifically designed to promote daytime alertness. Identification of a narcolepsy-like phenotype or an MSL <5 min in the absence of SOREMS in PD would appear to justify prescribing wake-promoting agents such as bupropion, modafinil, or traditional psychostimulants.

ACKNOWLEDGMENT

This work was supported by United States Public Health Service grants NS-36977 and NS-40221 (D.B.R.), 2T32GM08169 (J.T.D.), MH-64312 (A.A.F.), NS-35345 and AG-10643 (D.L.B.), and the Restless Legs Syndrome Foundation.

REFERENCES

1. Lees, A., Blackburn, N., and Campbell, V. (1988) The nightime problems of Parkinson's disease. *Clin. Neuropharmacol.* **11,** 512–519.
2. Rye, D. and Bliwise, D. (1997) Movement disorders specific to sleep and the nocturnal manifestations of waking movement disorders, in *Movement Disorders: Neurologic Principles and Practice* (Watts, R. and Koller, W., eds.), McGraw-Hill, New York, pp. 687–713.
3. Greulich, W., Schafer, D., Georg, W.M., and Schlafke, M.E. (1998) Schlafverhalten bei patieten mit Morbus Parkinson. *Somnologie* **2,** 163–171.
4. Factor, S., McAlamey, T., and Sanchez-Ramos, J.R. (1990) Sleep disorders and sleep effect in Parkinson's disease. *Mov. Disord.* **5,** 280–285.
5. Pal, S., Bhattacharaya, K.F., Agapito, C., and Chaudhuri, K.R. (2001) A study of excessive daytime sleepines and its clinical significance in three groups of Parkinson's disease patients taking pramipexole, cabergoline and levodopa mono and combination therapy. *J. Neural. Transm.* **108,** 71–77.
6. Rye, D.B., Johnston, L.H., Watts, R.L., and Bliwise, D.L. (1999) Juvenile Parkinson's disease with REM behavior disorder, sleepiness and daytime REM-onsets. *Neurology* **53,** 1868–1870.
7. Rye, D.B., Bliwise, D.L., Dihenia, B., and Gurecki, P. (2000) FAST TRACK: daytime sleepiness in Parkinson's disease. *J. Sleep Res.* **9,** 63–69.
8. Arnulf, I., Bonnet, A.M., and Damier, P. (2000) Hallucinations, REM sleep, and Parkinson's disease: a medical hypothesis. *Neurology* **55,** 281–288.
9. Nishino, S., Mao, J., Sampath Kumaran, R., and Shelton, J. (1998) Increased dopaminergic transmission mediates the wake-promoting effects of CNS stimulants. *Sleep Res. Online* **1,** 49–61.

10. Kanabayashi, T., Honda, K., Kodama, T., Mignot, E., and Nishinol, S. (2000) Implication of dopaminergic mechanisms in the wake-promoting effects of amphetamine: a study of D- and L-derivatives in canine narcolepsy. *Neuroscience* **99,** 651–659.
11. Wisor, J.P., Nishino, S., Sora, I., Uhl, C.H., Mignot, E., and Edgar, D.M. (2001) Dopaminergic role in stimulant-induced wakefulness. *J. Neurosci.* **21,** 1787–1794.
12. van Hilten, J.J., Weggeman, M., van der Velde, E.A., Middelkoop, H.A., Kerkhof, G.A., and Roos, R.A. (1993) Sleep, excessive daytime sleepiness and fatigue in Parkinson's disease. *J. Neural. Transm.* **5,** 235–244.
13. Montastruc, J.-L., Brefel-Courbon, C., and Senard, J.M. (2001) Sleep attacks and antiparkinsonian drugs: a pilot prospective pharmacoepidemiologic study. *Clin. Neuropharmacol.* **24,** 181–183.
14. Chervin, R.D. and Aldrich, M.S. (1999) The Epworth Sleepiness Scale may not reflect objective measures of sleepiness or sleep apnea. *Neurology* **52,** 125–131.
15. Agid, Y. (1991) Parkison's disease: pathophysiology. *Lancet* **337,** 1321–1324.
16. Elsworth, J.D., Deutch, A.Y., Redmond, D.E. Jr., Taylor, J.R., Sladek, J.R. Jr., and Roth, R.H. (1989) Symptomatic and asymptomatic 1-methyl-4-phenyl-1,2,3,6-tetrahydropyridine-treated primates: biochemical changes in striatal regions. *Neuroscience* **33,** 323–331.
17. Marek, K. (1999) Dopaminergic dysfunction in parkinsonism: new lessions from neuroimaging. *Neurscientist* **5,** 333–339.
18. Myslobodsky, M., Mintz, M., Ben-Mayor, V., and Radwan, H. (1982) Unilateral dopamine deficit and lateral EEG asymmetry: sleep abnormalities in hemi-parkinson's patients. *Electroencephalogr. Clin. Neurophysiol.* **54,** 227–231.
19. Llinas, R.R., Ribary, U., Jeanmonod, D., Kronberg, E., and Mitra, P.P. (1999) Thalamocortical dysrhythmia: a neurological and neuropsychiatric syndrome characterized by magnetoencephalography. *Proc. Natl. Acad. Sci. USA* **96,** 15,222–15,227.
20. Vitek, J.L., Ashe, J., and Kaneoke, Y. (1994) Spontaneous neuronal activity in the motor thalamus: alteration in pattern and rate in parkinsonism. *Soc. Neurosci. Abstr.* **20,** 561.
21. Raeva, S., Vainberg, N., and Dubinin, V. (1999) Analysis of spontaneous activity patterns of human thalamic ventrolateral neurons and their modifications due to functional brain changes. *Neuroscience* **88,** 365–376.
22. Freeman, A., Ciliax, B., Bakay, R., et al. (2001) Nigrostriatal collaterals to thalamus degenerate in parkinsonian animal models. *Ann. Neurol.* **50,** 321–239.
23. Gillin, C., van Kammen, D.P., Post, R.M., Sitaram, N., Wyatt, R.J., and Bunney, W.E. (1981) What is the role of dopamine in the regulation of sleep-wake activity? in *Apomorphine and Other Dopaminomimetics* (Corsini, G. and Gessa, G., eds.), Raven Press, New York, pp. 157–164.
24. Gaillard, J.-M., Nicholson, A., and Pascoe, P. (1994) Neurotransmitter systems, in *Principles and Practice of Sleep Medicine* (Kreiger, M., Roth, T., and Dement, W., eds.), WB Saunders Company, London, pp. 338–348.
25. Sebban, C., Zhang, X.O., Tesolin-Decros, B., Millan, M.J., and Spedding, M. (1999) Changes in EEG spectral power in the prefrontal cortex of conscious rats elicited by drugs interacting with dopaminergic and noradrenergic transmission. *Br. J. Pharmacol.* **128,** 1045–1054.
26. Grace, A. and Bunney, B. (1980) Nigral dopamine neurons: intracellular recording and identification with L-dopa injection and histofluorescence. *Science* **210,** 654–656.
27. Steinfels, G.F., Heym, J., Strecker, R.E., and Jacobs, B.L. (1983) Behavioral correlates of dopaminergic unit activity in freely moving cats. *Brain Res.* **258,** 217–228.
28. Bagetta, G., De Sarro, G., Priolo, E., and Nistico, G. (1988) Ventral tegmental area: site through which dopamine D_2-receptor agonists evoke behavioral and electrocortical sleep in rats. *Br. J. Pharmacol.* **95,** 860–866.
29. Frucht, S., Rogers, J.D., Greene, P.E., Gordan, M.F., and Fahn, S. (1999) Falling asleep at the wheel: motor vehicle mishaps in persons taking pramipexole and ropinirole. *Neurology* **52,** 1908–1910.
30. Clarenbach, P. (2000) Parkinon's disease and sleep. *J. Neurol.* **247(Suppl. 4),** IV20–IV23.
31. Clarenbach, P., Greulich, W., and Meinck, H.M. (2000) Workshop I: Parkinson's disease and sleep—results of the group discussion. *J. Neurol.* **274(Suppl. 4),** IV34–IV35.
32. Ryan, M., Slevin, J., and Wells, A. (2000) Non-ergot dopamine agonist-induced sleep attacks. *Pharmacotherapy* **20,** 724–726.
33. Schafer, D. and Greulich, W. (2000) Effects of parkinsonian medication on sleep. *J. Neurol.* **247(Suppl. 4),** IV24–IV27.
34. Pirker, W. and Happe, S. (2000) Sleep attacks in Parkinson's disease. *Lancet* **356,** 597–598.
35. Schapira, A. (2000) Sleep attacks (sleep episodes) with pergolide. *Lancet* **355,** 1332–1333.
36. Ferreira, J.J., Galitzky, M., Montastruc, J.L., and Rascol, O. (2000) Sleep attacks and Parkinson's disease treatment. *Lancet* **355,** 1333–1334.
37. Andreau, N., Chale, J.J., Seward, J.M., Thalamas, C., Montastruc, J.L., and Rascol, O. (1999) L-dopa induced sedation: a double-blind cross-over controlled study versus triazolam and placebo in healthy volunteers. *Clin. Neuropharmacol.* **22,** 15–23.
38. Karoum, F., Chuang, L.W., and Eisler, T. (1982) Metabolism of (-) deprenyl to amphetamine and methamphetamine may be responsible for deprenyl's therapeutic benefit: a biochemical assessment. *Neurology* **32,** 503–509.
39. Jones, B.E., Bobillier, P., Pin, C., and Jouvet, M. (1973) The effect of lesions of catecholamine-containing neurons upon monoamine content of the brain and EEG and behavioral waking in the cat. *Brain Res.* **58,** 157–177.
40. Lai, Y.Y., Shalita, T., and Hajnik, T. (1999) Neurotoxic N-methyl-D-aspartate lesion of the ventral midbrain and mesopontine junction alters sleep-wake organization. *Neuroscience* **90,** 469–483.
41. Decker, M., Keating, G.L., Freeman, A.A., and Rye, D.B. (2000) Parkinsonian-like sleep-wake architecture in rats with bilateral striatal 6-OHDA lesions. *Soc. Neurosci. Abstr.* **26,** 1514.

42. Daley, J., Turner, R.S., Bliwise, D.L., and Rye, D.B. (1999) Nocturnal sleep and daytime alertness in the MPTP-treated primate. *Sleep* **22(Suppl.)**, S218–S219.
43. Song, D. and Haber, S. (2000) Striatal responses to partial dopaminergic lesion: evidence for compensatory sprouting. *J. Neurosci.* **20**, 5102–5114.
44. Aldrich, M., ed. (1999) *Sleep Medicine, Vol. 53,* Oxford University Press, New York.
45. Steriade, M. and McCarley, R. (1990) *Brainstem Control of Wakefulness and Sleep,* Plenum Press, New York.
46. Langston, J.W. and Forno, L.S. (1978) The hypothalamus in Parkinson disease. *Ann. Neurol.* **3,** 129–133.
47. Jellinger, K. (1991) Pathology of Parkinson's disease. Changes other than the nigrostriatal pathway. *Mol. Chem. Neuropathol.* **14,** 153–197.
48. Brown, R., Stevens, D., and Haas, H. (2001) The physiology of brain histamine. *Prog. Neurobiol.* **63,** 637–672.
49. Steriade, M. and McCarley, R.W. (1990) *Brainstem Control of Wakefulness and Sleep,* Plenum Press, New York.
50. Missale, C., Nash, S.R., and Robinson, S.W. (1998) Dopamine receptors: from structure to function. *Physiol. Rev.* **78,** 189–225.
51. Choi, W., Machida, C., and Ronnekleiv, O. (1995) Distribution of dopamine D1, D2, and D5 receptor mRNAs in the monkey brain: ribonuclease protection assay analysis. *Mol. Brain Res.* **31,** 86–94.
52. Fremeau, R.T. Jr., Duncan, G.E., and Fomaretto, M.G. (1991) Localization of D1 dopamine receptor mRNA in brain supports a role in cognitive, affective, and neuroendocrine aspects of dopaminergic neurotransmission. *Proc. Natl. Acad. Sci. USA* **88,** 3772–3776.
53. Gurevich, E.V. and Joyce, J.N. (1999) Distribution of dopamine D3 receptor expressing neurons in the human forebrain: comparison with D2 receptor expressing neurons. *Neuropsychopharmacology* **20,** 60–80.
54. Lavin, A. and Grace, A.A. (1998) Dopamine modulates the responsivity of mediodorsal thalamic cells recorded in vitro. *J. Neurosci.* **18,** 10,566–10,578.
55. Steriade, M., McCormick, D., and Sejnowski, T. (1993) Thalamocortical oscillations in the sleeping and aroused brain. *Science* **262,** 679–684.
56. Huang, Q., Zhou, D., Chase, K., Gusella, J.F., Aronin, V., and DiFiglia, M. (1992) Immunohistochemical localization of the D1 dopamine receptor in rat brain reveals its axonal transport, pre- and postsynaptic localization, and prevalence in the basal ganglia, limbic system, and thalamic reticular nucleus. *Proc. Natl. Acad. Sci. USA* **89,** 11,988–11,992.
57. Mrzljak, L., Bergson, C., Pappy, M., Huff, R., Levenson, R., and Goldman-Rakic, P.S. (1996) Localization of dopamine D4 receptors in GABAergic neurons of the primate brain. *Nature* **381,** 245–2489.
58. Takada, M., Campbell, K.J., Moriizumi, T., and Hatton, M. (1990) On the origin of the dopaminergic innervation of the paraventricular thalamic nucleus. *Neurosci. Lett.* **115,** 33–36.
59. Beckstead, R.M., Domesick, V.B., and Nauta, W.J.H. (1979) Efferent connections of the substantia nigra and ventral tegmental area in the rat. *Brain Res.* **175,** 191–217.
60. Bassetti, C., Mathis, J., Gugger, M., Lovblad, K.O., and Hess, C.W. (1996) Hypersomnia following paramedian thalamic stroke: a report of 12 patients. *Ann. Neurol.* **39,** 471–480.
61. Bouyer, J.J., Montaron, M.F., Buser, P., Durand, C., and Rugeul, A. (1992) Effects of mediodorsalis thalamic nucleus lesions on vigilance and attentive behavior in cats. *Behav. Brain Res.* **51,** 51–60.
62. Lugaresi, E., Tobler, I., Gambetti, P., and Montagna, P. (1998) The pathophysiology of fatal familial insomnia. *Brain Pathol.* **8,** 521–526.
63. Kish, S., Shannak, K., and Hornykiewicz, O. (1988) Uneven pattern of dopamine loss in the striatum of patients with idiopathic Parkinson's disease. *N. Engl. J. Med.* **318,** 876–880.
64. Gibb, W. and Lees, A. (1991) Anatomy, pigmentation, ventral and dorsal subpopulations of the substantia nigra, and differential cell death in Parkinson's disease. *J. Neurol. Neurosurg. Psychiatry* **54,** 388–396.
65. Lynd-Balta, E. and Haber, S. (1994) The organization of midbrain projections to the striatum in the primate: sensorimotor-related striatum versus ventral striatum. *Neuroscience* **59,** 625–640.
66. Berridge, C., O'Neil, J., and Wifler, K. (1999) Amphetamine acts within the medial basal forebrain to initiate and maintain alert waking. *Neuroscience* **93,** 885–896.
67. Honda, K., Riehl, J., Mignot, E., and Nishino, S. (1999) Dopamine D3 agonists into the substantia nigra aggravate cataplexy but do not modify sleep. *Neuroreport* **10,** 3717–3724.
68. Reid, M., Tafti, M., Nishino, S., Sampath Kumaran, R., Siegel, J.M., and Mignot, E. (1996) Local administration of dopaminergic drugs into the ventral tegmental area modulates cataplexy in the narcoleptic canine. *Brain Res.* **133,** 83–100.
69. Miller, E. and Nieburg, H. (1973) Amphetamines. Valuable adjunct in treatment of Parkinsonism. *NY State J. Med.* **73,** 2657–2661.
70. Parkes, J.D., Tarsy, D., and Marsden, C.D. (1975) Amphetamines in the treatment of Parkinson's disease. *J. Neurol. Neurosurg. Psychiatry* **38,** 232–237.
71. Rye, D. (1997) Contributions of the pedunculopontine region to normal and altered REM sleep. *Sleep* **20,** 757–788.
72. Wichmann, T. and DeLong, M.R. (1996) Functional and pathophysiological models of the basal ganglia. *Curr. Opin. Neurobiol.* **6,** 751–758.
73. Sacks, O.W., Kohl, M.S., Messeloff, C.R., and Schwartz, W.F. (1972) Effects of levodopa in Parkinsonian patients with dementia. *Neurology* **22,** 516–519.
74. Rye, D., Dempsay, J., Dihenia, B., DeLong, M., and Bliwise, D.L. (1997) REM-sleep dyscontrol in Parkinson's disease: case report of effects of elective pallidotomy. *Sleep Res.* **26,** 591.

40

Natural Evolution and Life Expectancy in Parkinson's Disease

Werner Poewe, MD

1. INTRODUCTION

A significant proportion of basic research in the field of Parkinson's disease (PD) is related to identify underlying mechanisms responsible for nigral cell loss in this disorder. The ultimate goal of such research is to identify agents that will modify or hold the progression of the disease. At present, no candidate has yet emerged for which clinical studies would have demonstrated sustained and marked effects on the progressive course of PD. At the same time, data concerning the natural history of PD are limited, and there is considerable uncertainty in a number of important areas, including possible duration of a preclinical phase, linear vs exponential rates of progression, different progression rates in subtypes of the disease, as well as risk factors and predictors for different rates of progression and mortality.

2. PROGRESSION OF MOTOR DISABILITY IN UNTREATED DISEASE

Two early studies have assessed the rates of progression of disability of patients with PD in the pre-levodopa (L-dopa) area. Hoehn and Yahr, in their 1967 paper, studied a subgroup of 183 patients using their newly developed Hoehn and Yahr scale *(1)*. Progression to stages IV and V had occurred in 16% of patients with disease duration of less than 5 yr, increasing to 37 and 42% after 10 and 15 yr, respectively. Median delays before reaching Hoehn and Yahr stages IV and V were 9 and 14 yr, respectively and even shorter in the series reported by Martilla and Rinne in 1977 *(2)*. However, there was large interindividual variability, and about a third of patients with durations of disease for 10 yr or longer were still in stages I and II. Similar percentages have also been reported in a more recent series by Hely and coworkers *(3)*.

More recent studies have assessed the rate of progression of Unified Parkinson's Disease Rating Scale (UPDRS) motor scores in a prospective fashion. Data from the seminal Deprenyl and Tocopherol Antioxidative Therapy of Parkinsonism (DATATOP) study comparing the impact of deprenyl and tocopherol vs placebo on the progression of PD have provided adequate data to estimate the annual rates of decline in untreated disease. Again, these were not uniform and differed from 3.5–8%/yr according to whether or not patients had reached the endpoint *(4)*.

Besides such interindividual variation, there is also evidence that progression of motor scores, when measured in treated patients during the off stage, is dynamic, with faster rates early vs later in the disease *(5–7)*. Nevertheless, available data on annual rates of motor UPDRS scores in untreated PD would predict severe disability within 10 yr of disease duration, which is rather in line with the early observations published by Hoehn and Yahr *(1)*.

From: *Mental and Behavioral Dysfunction in Movement Disorders*
Edited by: M-A. Bédard et al. © Humana Press Inc., Totowa, NJ

Table 1
Progression of Disability in IPD Latencies to Reach Successive Hoehn and Yahr Stages (Years)

Study (reference)	HY 1	HY 2	HY 3	HY 4	HY 5
Hoehn and Yahr *(1)*	3.0	6.0	7.0	9.0	14.0
Marttila and Rinne *(2)*	—	2.9	5.5	7.5	9.7
Hoehn *(15)*	—	9.0	12.0	12.0	18.0
Hely et al. *(3)*	—	—	4.0	7.0	6.0
Müller et al. *(14)*	—	3.0	5.5	14.0	15.0
Lücking et al. *(8)*	—	11.0	19.0	26.0	40

HY, Hoehn and Yahr stage.

3. IMPACT OF TREATMENT

When comparing disease progression in 282 patients receiving L-dopa therapy to cohorts of patients from the pre-L-dopa era, Hoehn and Yahr found that L-dopa-treated patients had latencies to reach successive Hoehn and Yahr stages that were prolonged by about 3–5 yr/stage compared to untreated patients. In addition, the percentages of patients who had become severely disabled or had died in successive 5-yr epochs of disease duration up to 15 yr was reduced by 30–50%/epoch compared to patients from the pre-L-dopa era. Several studies, but not all *(3)*, have found similar latencies to the different Hoehn and Yahr stages in PD patients receiving L-dopa plus additional dopaminergic and/or nondopaminergic drugs. The slowest rates of progression have been reported by Lücking et al. *(8)* in a cohort of young-onset PD patients with and without the Parkin-mutation, in which latencies to Hoehn and Yahr IV or V were 40 yr or longer. This is likely to reflect a different rate of progression in subtypes of PD, rather than impact of treatment alone (see Table 1).

Recent studies have focused on the impact of drug treatment on rates of progression of UPDRS score after temporary drug washout or rates of decline of surrogate markers of nigrostriatal dysfunction using 18-6-fluoro dopa positron emission tomography (FD-PET) or β-2 β-carbomethoxy-3β-(4-iodophenyl)tropane single-photon emission computed tomography (CIT-SPECT) (see below). Deprenyl treatment was found to delay the need for L-dopa by about 9 mo and also appeared to reduce the annual rate of decline of UPDRS motor scores by up to 50%. These findings, however, could also be explained by the drug's symptomatic effects and clearly do not seem to extend beyond 12 mo of treatment. Quite contrary to the findings of reduced progression of disability by L-dopa therapy, there has been renewed debate regarding a neurotoxic potential of L-dopa by virtue of its oxidative metabolism. A double-blind randomized prospective placebo-controlled trial designed to assess L-dopa's effects on natural disease (ELLDOPA) is currently underway. Results from another randomized double-blind prospective 12-mo trial have, however, failed to indicate any difference in the effects of deprenyl versus L-dopa on rates of progression of motor scores *(9)*.

Nevertheless, L-dopa therapy has introduced an additional source of progressive disability into the natural evolution of PD through its potential to induce abnormal involuntary movements as well as motor response oscillations. A larger number of retrospective series in the 1970s and 1980s have found rates of these motor complications generally above 50% after more than 5 yr of treatment *(10)*. More recent prospective double-blind trials with durations of 2–5 yr and L-dopa as an active treatment arm, suggest somewhat lower rates between less than 20 and up to 50% (see Table 2). In a recent community-based study, Schrag and coworkers assessed 124 PD patients, 87 of whom had received L-dopa preparations in order to define the prevalence of dyskinesias and motor fluctuations, as well as the factors determining their occurrence. Dyskinesias were present in 28% of patients, while 40% had developed motor fluctuations. Main predictors for the evolution of motor fluctuations and/or dyskinesias were duration of disease and treatment and L-dopa dose *(11)*.

Table 2
Incidence of Motor Complications in Recent Controlled Trials (% of Patients)

	Dyskinesias	Motor fluctutations
DA-agonists	4–10	23–25
LD	8–36	21–59
LD-CR preparations	10–34	22–57

References (author / drugs / study duration):
Rinne et al. *(16)* / CAB vs LD / 3.8 yr
Rascol et al. *(17)* / ROP vs LD / 5 yr
Oertel et al. *(18)* / PER vs LD / 3 yr
PSG *(19)* / PRA vs LD / 2 yr
Dupont et al. *(20)* / LD-CR vs LD / 5 yr
Koller et al. *(21)* / LD-CR vs LD / 5 yr

Abbreviations: DA, dopamine; LD, L-dopa; CAB, cabergoline; ROP, ropinirole; PER, pergolide; PRA, pramipexole; CR, carbidopa; PSG, Parkinson Study Group.

4. PROGRESSION OF SURROGATE MARKERS

Fearnley and Lees *(12)* have studied the subregional topography and progression rates of nigral cell loss in postmortem brain material at the UK PDS BRC and found a global rate of cell loss of 40%/decade. There was an exponential decline of the rate of attrition, which appeared much faster early in the disease compared to later stages, which is suggestive of a preclinical window of approx 5 yr. The latter was also suggested by sequential 18-FD-PET studies approx 18 mo apart, which found an approximate decline of putaminal Ki values for tracer uptake of 9%/annum. Assuming linear decline extrapolation of these results would again imply a preclinical phase of approx 5 to 6 yr.

Subsequent studies of rate of progression of nigrostriatal dysfunction as assessed by either sequential 18-FD-PET or β-CIT-SPECT have all found annual rates of decline in the order of 6–10%. In addition, there is evidence in these studies, that progression rates may be faster early in the disease compared to later. All patients studied so far have been under treatment, so that the impact of dopaminergic therapy on progression rates relative to untreated PD is unknown. A recent trial has assessed comparative rates of progression in patients receiving L-dopa vs dopamine agonist monotherapy with pramipexole using Beta-Cit-SPECT imaging as a surrogate marker. Results at 2, 3, and 4 yr of follow-up show a significantly greater decline in tracer binding in patients receiving L-dopa compared to those randomized to pramipexole *(12a)*. Interpretation of these results, however, is difficult owing to a lack of a placebo arm in this particular trial.

5. RISK FACTORS FOR RAPID PROGRESSION

A number of studies have assessed risk factors predicting faster progression of disability in idiopathic Parkinson's disease (IPD). They have consistently identified older age at onset and cognitive decline and dementia as being associated with rapid progression of motor disability.

Age, dementia, and hallucinosis have also been found to be the most relevant predictors for institutional care in PD. Hely and coworkers *(3)* in their 10-yr follow-up of a prospectively studied cohort of 146 patients found 23% having been admitted to nursing homes by 10 yr of diseases. Eighty-six percent of these patients had died by the time of the last follow-up, and mean survival in nursing home care was 34 mo.

Table 3
Mortality Ratios in Untreated vs Treated PD

Study (reference)	Mortality ratio	N
Hoehn and Yahr *(1)*	2.9	672
Nobrega et al. *(22)*	1.6	331
Marttila et al. *(23)*	1.8	349
Hoehn *(15)*	1.5	182
Shaw et al. *(24)*	1.5	178
Diamond et al. *(25)*	1.4–2.7	359
Ebmeier et al. *(26)*	2.3	267
PSG *(27)*	0.8	800
Hely et al. *(3)*	1.6	130

PSG, Parkinson Study Group.

Table 4
Causes of Death in PD

Cause of death	Percent
Pneumonia	9–45
Cardiovascular	10–26
Stroke	3–16
Cancer	2–20
"Parkinsonism"	5–38

Pooled data from Louis et al. *(28)*, Ben-Shlomo et al. *(29)*, and Hely et al. *(3)*.

6. MORTALITY

In their seminal paper, Hoehn and Yahr found an excess mortality in PD patients over the age-matched normal population of about threefold and concluded that "... the state of parkinsonism severely limits life expectancy" *(1)*. Most studies in the post-L-dopa era have found reduced excess mortality, but mortality ratios were still between 1.5 and 2.5 (see Table 3). The most notable exception is the 9-yr follow-up data of the DATATOP study cohort, which found a death rate of 2.1%/yr and a standard mortality ratio of 0.9, most likely reflecting the initial selection criteria excluding all significant co-morbidity. Cognitive decline and dementia, as well as older age at onset have been identified as predictors of decreased survival in several studies, including our own, and we and others have also found improved survival in patients presenting with tremor-dominant disease. In a series of 200 cases with pathologically confirmed Parkinson's disease, Jellinger and colleagues investigated the impact of clinical dementia and Alzheimer pathology on survival. Mean survival was around 10 yr in patients whose brains were free of Alzheimer-type pathology, but only half that long (4.9 yr) in patients with Alzheimer's disease (AD) pathology of Consortium to Establish a Registry for Alzheimer's Disease (CERAD) grade B or C *(13)*.

Pneumonia is the leading cause of death in PD, followed by cardiovascular events, stroke, and cancer in most surveys (see Table 4). In a recent population-based study of causes of death in PD, 245 patients were followed over a period of 4 yr. Causes of death among PD patients were identified from death certificates and compared to a population-based control group of 4491 individuals. Mortality was greater in male PD patients (41%) compared to females (28%) and age, and UPDRS scores and Hoehn and Yahr stage at baseline were greater in the PD patients who had died during follow-up compared to survivors. More PD patients (20%) died from pneumonia than controls (9%), while more controls (23%) had died from coronary heart disease compared to patients with PD (13%).

The relevance of aspiration pneumonia as a contributor to the increased mortality in PD is also suggested by a postmortem study showing a tight correlation between the onset of clinically relevant dysphagia and survival time across a group of 77 postmortem-confirmed cases of different degenerative parkinsonian disorders, including IPD, multiple system atrophy (MSA), progressive supranuclear palsy (PSP), corticobasal degeneration (CBD), and dementia with Lewy bodies (DLB) *(14)*.

REFERENCES

1. Hoehn, M.M. and Yahr, M.D. (1967) Parkinsonism: onset, progression, and mortality. *Neurology* **15,** 427–442.
2. Martilla, P.J. and Rinne, U.K. (1977) Disability and progression in Parkinson's disease. *Acta Neurol. Scand.* **56,** 159–169.
3. Hely, M.A., Morris, J.G., Traficante, R., et al. (1999) The sydney multicentre study of Parkinson's disease: progression and mortality at 10 years. *J. Neurol. Neurosurg. Psychiatry* **67,** 300–307.
4. Parkinson Study Group (1998) Mortality in DATATOP: a multicenter trial in early Parkinson's disease. *Ann. Neurol.* **43,** 318–325.
5. Bonnet, A.M., Loria, Y., Saint-Hilaire, M.H., Lhermitte, F., and Agid, Y. (1987) Does long-term aggravation of Parkinson's disease result from nondopaminergic lesions? *Neurology* **37,** 1539–1542.
6. Lee, C.S., Schulzer, M., Mak, E.K., et al. (1994) Clinical observations on the rate of progression of idiopathic parkinsonism. *Brain* **117,** 501–507.
7. Goetz, C.G., Tanner, C.M., and Shannon, K.M. (1987) Progression of Parkinson's disease without levodopa. *Neurology* **37,** 695–698.
8. Lücking, C.B., Durr, A., Bonifati, V., et al. (2000) Association between early-onset Parkinson's disease and mutations in the parkin gene. French Parkinson's Disease Genetics Study Group. *N. Engl. J. Med.* **342,** 1560–1567.
9. Olanow, C.W., Hauser, R.A., Gauger, L., et al. (1995) The effect of deprenyl and levodopa on the progression of Parkinson's disease. *Ann. Neurol.* **38,** 771–777.
10. Poewe, W.H., Lees, A.J., and Stern, G.M. (1986) Low-dose l-dopa therapy in Parkinson's disease: a 6-year follow-up study. *Neurology* **36,** 1528–1530.
11. Schrag, A. and Quinn, N. (2000) Dyskinesias and motor fluctuations in Parkinson's disease: a community-based study. *Brain* **123,** 2297–2305.
12. Fearnley, J.M. and Lees, A.J. (1991) Ageing and Parkinson's disease: substantia nigra regional selectivity. *Brain* **114,** 2283–2301.

12a. Marek, K., Seibyl, J., Shoulson, I., et al. (2002) Dopamine transporter brain imaging to assess the effects of pramipexole vs levodopa on Parkinson disease progression. *JAMA* **287,** 1653–1661.

13. Jellinger, K.A., Seppi, K., Wenning, G.K., and Poewe, W. Impact of coexistent Alzheimer pathology on the natural history of Parkinson's disease. *J. Neural. Transm.,* in press.
14. Müller, J., Wenning, G.K., Verny, M., et al. (2001) Progression of dysarthria and dysphagia in post-mortem confirmed parkinsonian disorders. *Arch. Neurol.* **58,** 259–264.
15. Hoehn, M.M. (1983) Parkinsonism treated with levodopa: progression and mortality. *J. Neurol. Transmiss.* **19,** 253–264.
16. Rinne, U.K., Bracco, F., Chouza, C., et al. (1998) Early treatment of Parkinson's disease with cabergoline delays in onset of motor complications. Results of a double-blind levodopa controlled trial. *Drugs* **55,** 23–30.
17. Rascol, O., Brooks, D.J., Korczyn, A.D., et al. (2000) A five-year study of the incidence of dyskinesia in patients with early Parkinson's disease who were treated with ropinirole or levdodopa. *N. Engl. J. Med.* **342,** 1484–1491.
18. Oertel, W.H. (2000) Pergolide versus L-Dopa (PELMOPET) [abstract]. *Mov. Disord.* **15(Suppl. 3),** 4.
19. Parkinson Study Group (2000) Pramipexole vs. Levodopa as initial treatment for Parkinson's disease. *JAMA* **284,** 1931–1938.
20. Dupont, E., Anderson, A., Boqs, J., et al. (1996) Sustained-release Madopar HBS compared with standard Madopar in the long-term treatment of de novo parkinsonian patients. *Acta Neurol. Scand.* **93,** 14–20.
21. Koller W.C., Hutton, J.T., Tolosa, E., Capildeo, R., and Carbidopa/Levodopa Study Group. (1999) Immediate-release and controlled-release carbidopa/levodopa in PD: a 5-year randomized multicenter study. *Neurology* **53,** 1012–1019.
22. Nobrega, F.T., Glattre, E., Kurland, L.T., and Okazaki, H. (1969) Comments on the epidemiology of parkinsonism including prevalence and incidence statistics for Rochester, Minnesota, 1935-1966, in *Progress in Neurogenetics* (Barbeau, A. and Brunette, J.R., eds.), Proceedings of the Second International Congress of Neurogenetics and Neuro-Ophthalmology. Amsterdam, Excerpta Medicina.
23. Martilla, R.J., Rinne, U.K., Surtola, T., et al. (1977) Mortality of patients with Parkinson's disease treated with levodopa. *J. Neurol.* **216,** 147–153.
24. Shaw, K.M., Lees A.J., and Stern G.M. (1980) The impact of treatment with levodopa on Parkinson's disease. *Q. J. Med.* **49,** 283–293.
25. Diamond, S.G., Markham, C.H., Hoehn, M.M., et al. (1987) Multi-center study of Parkinson mortality with early versus later dopa treatment. *Ann. Neurol.* **22,** 8–12.
26. Ebmeier, K.P., Calder, S.A., Crawford, J.R., et al. (1990) Parkinson's disease in Aberden: survival after 3.5 years. *Acta Neurol. Scand.* **81,** 294–299.
27. Parkinson Study Group. (1998) Mortality in DATATOP: a multicenter trial in early Parkinson's disease. *Ann. Neurol.* **43,** 318–325.
28. Louis, E.D., Marder, K., Cote, L., Tang, M., and Mayeux, R. (1997) Mortality from Parkinson's disease. *Arch. Neurol.* **54,** 260–264.
29. Ben-Shlomo, Y., Churchyard, A., Head, J., et al. (1998) Investigation by Parkinson's Disease Research Group of United Kingdom into excess mortality seen with combined levodopa and selegiline treatment in patient with early, mild Parkinson's disease: further results of randomised trial and confidential inquiry. *BMJ* **316,** 1191–1196.

INDEX

D

Q

T